.....
Cardiovascular Pathology

. . . . .

Cardiovascular Pathology

Malcolm D. Silver, M.B., B.S., M.D., Ph.D.
Professor Emeritus, Department of Laboratory Medicine
and Pathobiology
University of Toronto Faculty of Medicine
Toronto, Ontario, Canada

Avrum I. Gotlieb, M.D., C.M.
Professor and Chair, Department of Laboratory Medicine
and Pathobiology
University of Toronto Faculty of Medicine
Staff Pathologist, University Health Network
Toronto General Hospital
Toronto, Ontario, Canada

Frederick J. Schoen, M.D., Ph.D.
Professor, Department of Pathology, Harvard Medical
School
Director, Cardiac Pathology, and Vice-Chairman,
Department of Pathology
Brigham and Women's Hospital
Boston, Massachusetts

™ ℬ CHURCHILL LIVINGSTONE
A Harcourt Health Sciences Company
New York   Edinburgh   London   Philadelphia

CHURCHILL LIVINGSTONE
A Harcourt Health Sciences Company

The Curtis Center
Independence Square West
Philadelphia, Pennsylvania 19106

Library of Congress Cataloging-in-Publication Data

Cardiovascular pathology/[edited by] Malcolm D. Silver, Avrum I. Gotlieb, Frederick J. Schoen—3rd ed.

p.;   cm.

Includes bibliographical references and index.

ISBN 0–443–06535–7

1. Cardiovascular system—Diseases. I. Silver, Malcolm D. II. Gotlieb, Avrum I.   III. Schoen, Frederick J.

[DNLM: 1. Cardiovascular Diseases—pathology. WG 142 C264 2001]

RC669.9.C37 2001

616.1—dc21   2001025319

Acquisitions Editor Marc Strauss
Production Editor Mary Reinwald
Production Manager Carolyn Naylor
Illustration Specialist John S. Needles, Jr.
Book Designer Matt Andrews

CARDIOVASCULAR PATHOLOGY   ISBN 0–443–06535–7

Last digit is the print number: 9   8   7   6   5   4   3   2   1

Dedication

This book is dedicated to our wives and families; to colleagues who contributed; and to all those, past and present, whose intellectual curiosity allowed its contained knowledge to evolve.

Contributors

Giorgio Baroldi, M.D., Ph.D.
Professor Emeritus, Faculty of Medicine, University of Milan, Milan; Associate Professor, Institute of Clinical Physiology, National Research Council, Pisa and Milan, Italy
Myocardial Cell Death, Including Ischemic Heart Disease and Its Complications

Cristina Basso, M.D.
Contract Professor, Postgraduate School, Cardiology, and Consultant Cardiologist, Institute of Pathological Anatomy, University of Padua Medical School, Padua, Italy
Cardiovascular Causes of Sudden Death

Saroja Bharati, M.D.
Professor of Pathology, Rush-Presbyterian-St. Luke's Medical Center, Rush Medical College, Chicago; Clinical Professor of Pathology, Chicago Medical School, North Chicago; Visiting Professor of Pathology, University of Illinois at Chicago; Director, Maurice Lev Congenital Heart and Conduction System Center, The Heart Institute for Children; Hope Children's Hospital; Christ Hospital and Medical Center, Oak Lawn, Illinois
Pathology of the Conduction System

Allen P. Burke, M.D.
Adjunct Professor, Georgetown University School of Medicine; Associate Professor, Uniformed Services University of the Health Sciences, Washington, District of Columbia
Nonatherosclerotic Diseases of the Aorta and Miscellaneous Diseases of the Main Pulmonary Arteries and Large Veins • Tumors and Tumor-Like Conditions of the Heart

J. Butany, M.B., B.S., M.S.
Associate Professor, Department of Laboratory Medicine and Pathobiology (University of Toronto); Staff Pathologist, University Health Network (Toronto General Hospital), Toronto, Ontario, Canada
The Pericardium and Its Diseases

Domenico Corrado, M.D.
Contract Professor, Postgraduate School, Cardiology, and Consultant Cardiologist, Department of Cardiology, University of Padua Medical School, Padua, Italy
Cardiovascular Causes of Sudden Death

Giulia d'Amati, M.D., Ph.D.
Assistant Professor, Department of Experimental Medicine and Pathology, "La Sapienza" University; Staff Pathologist, "Polyclinic Umberto I" University Hospital, Rome, Italy
Cardiomyopathies

William D. Edwards, M.D.
Professor, Department of Pathology, Mayo Medical School and Mayo Graduate School of Medicine, Rochester, MN; Consultant in Anatomic Pathology, Mayo Clinic, Rochester, MN
Valvular Heart Disease: General Principles and Stenosis • Pathology of Cardiovascular Interventions, Including Endovascular Therapies, Revascularization, Vascular Replacement, Cardiac Assist/ Replacement, Arrhythmia Control, and Repaired Congenital Heart Disease

Pietro Gallo, M.D.
Professor, Cardiovascular Pathology, Department of Experimental Medicine and Pathology, "La Sapienza" University; Head, Division of Anatomical Pathology, "Polyclinic Umberto I" University Hospital, Rome, Italy
Cardiomyopathies

Feroze N. Ghadially, M.B., B.S. (Bom. and Lon.), M.D., Ph.D., D.Sc. (Can.)
Professor Emeritus, Department of Pathology, University of Saskatchewan College of Medicine, Saskatoon, Saskatchewan; Adjunct Professor, Department of Pathology and Laboratory Medicine, University of Ottawa, Ottawa, Ontario, Canada
Light Microscopy and Ultrastructure of the Blood Vessels and Heart

Avrum I. Gotlieb, M.D., C.M.
Professor of Laboratory Medicine and Pathobiology, University of Toronto Faculty of Medicine; Staff Pathologist, University Health Network (Toronto General Hospital), Toronto, Ontario, Canada
Atherosclerosis: Pathology and Pathogenesis • Diseases of Medium- and Small-Caliber Vessels Including Small Arteries, Arterioles, and Capillaries • Cardiovascular Effects of Systemic Diseases and Conditions

H. Alexander Heggtveit, M.D.
Professor Emeritus, Department of Pathology and Molecular Medicine, McMaster University Faculty of Health Sciences; Consultant Pathologist, Hamilton Health Sciences Corporation, Hamilton, Ontario, Canada
Cardiovascular Trauma

Reza Jahan, M.D.
Assistant Professor, Department of Radiological Sciences, School of Medicine, University of California, Los Angeles, Los Angeles, California
Interactions Between Heart and Brain

Wanda M. Lester, M.D.
Associate Professor, Department of Pathology and Medicine (Cardiology), University of Calgary; Pathologist, Calgary Laboratory Services, Calgary, Alberta, Canada
Age-Related Cardiovascular Changes • Cardiovascular Effects of Systemic Diseases and Conditions

William Lewis, M.D.
Professor, Department of Pathology, Emory University School of Medicine; Director, Cardiovascular Pathology, The Emory Clinic, Atlanta, Georgia
Adverse Effects of Drugs on the Cardiovascular System

Francesca V. O. Lobo, M.B., B.S.
Associate Professor, Department of Pathology and Molecular Medicine, McMaster University, Faculty of Health Sciences; Staff Pathologist, Hamilton Health Sciences Corporation, Hamilton, Ontario, Canada
Cardiovascular Trauma

Bruce M. McManus, M.D., Ph.D.
Professor and Head, Department of Pathology and Laboratory Medicine, University of British Columbia; Director, Cardiovascular Research Laboratory and Registry, and Co-Director, Vancouver Vascular Biology Research Center, St. Paul's Hospital-Providence Health Care, Vancouver, British Columbia, Canada
Myocarditis

Alan G. Rose, M.D., M.Med., M.B., Ch.B.
Professor of Pathology, University of Minnesota Medical School; Director of Cardiovascular Pathology and Autopsy Service, Department of Laboratory Medicine and Pathology, Fairview-University Medical Center, Minneapolis, Minnesota
Disease of Medium- and Small-Caliber Vessels Including Small Arteries, Arterioles, and Capillaries • Diseases of the Pulmonary Circulation

Barbara Sampson, M.D., Ph.D.
Office of the Chief Medical Examiner of the City of New York, New York, New York
Genetic Causes of Diseases Affecting the Heart and Great Vessels

Frederick J. Schoen, M.D., Ph.D.
Professor, Department of Pathology, Harvard Medical School; Director, Cardiac Pathology, and Vice Chairman, Department of Pathology, Brigham and Women's Hospital, Boston, Massachusetts
Valvular Heart Disease: General Principles and Stenosis • Pathology of Heart Valve Substitution With Mechanical and Tissue Prostheses • Pathology of Cardiovascular Interventions, Including Endovascular Therapies, Revascularization, Vascular Replacement, Cardiac Assist/Replacement, Arrhythmia Control, and Repaired Congenital Heart Disease • Pathology of Cardiac Transplantation

Christine Seidman, M.D.
Professor, Departments of Medicine and Genetics and Genetics, Harvard Medical School; Director, Cardiovascular Genetics Center, Brigham and Women's Hospital, Department of Medicine, Cardiovascular Division, Boston, Massachusetts
Genetic Causes of Diseases Affecting the Heart and Great Vessels

Malcolm D. Silver, M.B., B.S., M.D., Ph.D.
Professor Emeritus, Department of Laboratory Medicine and Pathobiology, Faculty of Medicine, University of Toronto, Toronto, Ontario, Canada
Examination of the Heart and of Cardiovascular Specimens in Surgical Pathology • Atherosclerosis: Pathology and Pathogenesis • Valvular Heart Disease: Conditions Causing Regurgitation • Adverse Effects of Drugs on the Cardiovascular System

Meredith M. Silver, M.B., B.S., M.Sc.
Professor Emerita, Department of Laboratory Medicine and Pathobiology, Faculty of Medicine, University of Toronto, Toronto, Ontario, Canada
Examination of the Heart and of Cardiovascular Specimens in Surgical Pathology; Valvular Heart Disease: Conditions Causing Regurgitation

Gaetano Thiene, M.D.
Full Professor, Department of Cardiovascular Pathology, and Director, Institute of Pathological Anatomy, University of Padua Medical School, Padua, Italy
Cardiovascular Causes of Sudden Death

John P. Veinot, M.D.
Associate Professor, Department of Pathology and Laboratory Medicine, University of Ottawa; Anatomic/Cardiovascular Pathologist, Ottawa Hospital and University of Ottawa Heart Institute, Ottawa, Ontario, Canada
Light Microscopy and Ultrastructure of the Blood Vessels and Heart

Harry V. Vinters, M.D.
Professor, Departments of Pathology and Laboratory Medicine and Neurology, and Chief, Section of Neuropathology, University of California, Los Angeles, UCLA School of Medicine; Member, Brain Research Institute, Mental Retardation Research Center, and Neuropsychiatric Institute, Los Angeles, California
Interactions Between Heart and Brain

Renu Virmani, M.D.
Clinical Professor of Research, Vanderbilt University, Nashville, Tennessee; Chairperson, Department of Cardiovascular Pathology, Armed Forces Institute of Pathology, Washington, District of Columbia
Nonatherosclerotic Diseases of the Aorta and Miscellaneous Diseases of the Main Pulmonary Arteries and Large Veins • Tumors and Tumor-Like Conditions of the Heart

Virginia M. Walley, M.D.
Chief, Department of Laboratory Medicine, Peterborough Regional Health Center, Peterborough, Ontario, Canada
Light Microscopy and Ultrastructure of the Blood Vessels and Heart

Gayle L. Winters, M.D.
Associate Professor, Department of Pathology, Harvard Medical School; Cardiovascular Pathologist and Director, Autopsy Division, Brigham and Women's Hospital, Boston, Massachusetts
Myocarditis • Pathology of Cardiac Transplantation

A. Woo, M.D.
Assistant Professor, Division of Cardiology, Department of Medicine, University of Toronto; Staff Cardiologist, Division of Cardiology, University Health Network (Toronto General Hospital), Toronto, Ontario, Canada
The Pericardium and Its Diseases

Preface

In this edition, I welcome as coeditors Avrum I. Gotlieb (Toronto) and Frederick J. Schoen (Boston).

The text has been revised and condensed to present a single volume. The book offers a comprehensive review of cardiovascular diseases in adults but includes discussion of congenital lesions that permit survival to adulthood and the effects of surgical procedures that allow those afflicted with congenital heart disease to reach an older age. New information and chapters have been added to deal with advances in clinical practice and, in particular, in therapeutic intervention. New pathology is defined. When possible, the molecular biology of disease is emphasized, and newly understood pathologic mechanisms are defined. Segments are included to help pathologists in daily practice in autopsy or surgical pathology suites. Many illustrations are in color. To forestall reviewers' criticisms, we have deliberately omitted the magnification of illustrations, because that supplied for a figure changed by photographic or other manipulation is always suspect. Small-, medium-, and high-power microscopic magnifications are obvious.

We welcome and thank new contributors and mourn those who have died since the last edition was published. We thank colleagues who referred cases to us, thereby helping to expand the knowledge of all of us. Discussion of cases with clinical colleagues continues to be invaluable in the practice of pathology. Thanks, too, to our students whose perspicacious questions provided another view and a challenge both to find answers and to seek the truth.

The editors would particularly like to thank Dr. Meredith M. Silver (Toronto) and Drs. Richard N. Mitchell and Gayle L. Winters (Boston) for their invaluable assistance. We appreciate the wonderful help given us by secretarial staff Diana Houghton, Sursattie Sarju (Toronto), and Claudia Davis (Boston).

MALCOLM D. SILVER

Contents

EXAMINATION AND STRUCTURE

Chapter 1

Examination of the Heart and of Cardiovascular Specimens in Surgical Pathology

Meredith M. Silver • Malcolm D. Silver

During the 50 years following the first successful "open heart" surgery, which closed a ductus arteriosus,[1] the operation has evolved into a day surgery procedure performed via a percutaneous intravascular approach to insert an umbrella stent.[2, 3] This technologic advance reflects a vast and accelerating change in the diagnosis and treatment of cardiovascular disease during the past several decades. Although the cardiac autopsy may have changed little during that period, the pathologist's role on the cardiac team has changed dramatically. Nowadays, the cardiovascular pathologist has an audience who are often fully aware of the altered cardiac anatomy and who well understand the heart's altered function preceding the patient's death. The pathologist must understand the functional changes in these cases, preferably before an autopsy is performed, so that accurate functional-morphologic correlations can be made. The excised heart, displayed grossly, recorded photographically, measured carefully, and studied histologically, remains the gold standard against which antemortem cardiologic findings are measured.[4–20] Exact sizes and relationships, measured to the nearest millimeter, are important to confirm, for example, a "critical" valve stenosis, a "restrictive" shunt, or the proximity of a potential site of surgery to anatomic markers of the conduction system. Of course, anatomic pathology is not perfect. For example, in reading necropsy reports in which the severity of coronary artery stenosis is recorded, cardiologists must be aware that the method pathologists use in estimating stenosis on histologic slides overestimates the degree of stenosis in comparison with the method employed by angiographers.[21] Furthermore, an echocardiographic recording is more accurate than physical measurement of a septal defect in a tiny fetal heart viewed at midgestation. Nevertheless, the principle remains: Clinical findings need validation by pathologic examination.

Using a sophisticated array of investigative tools that are constantly being refined or replaced, the clinician views images of the pumping heart. Echocardiography, axial cineangiography, computed tomographic (CT) radi-

ology, and magnetic resonance imaging (MRI) all provide two-dimensional views, in any number of planes, of cardiac anatomy. Reviews of current investigative techniques may be found in a textbook.[22] Recently, color flow Doppler and transesophageal echocardiography have become standard techniques. Also, three-dimensional echocardiography (static) reconstruction appears to be evolving into dynamic ("four-dimensional") cardiac imaging.[20, 23, 24] Other imaging techniques of particular interest to pathologists include the delineation of myocardial perfusion, metabolism, and tissue characteristics.[17, 25–28]

Understanding three-dimensional structure is the aim of all clinicians who study altered cardiac anatomy. A prosector displays the opened heart in three dimensions but can imitate, by slicing a perfusion-fixed heart in various planes, the two-dimensional studies done during life.[5, 6, 29–31] Thus, to help clinicians in current and future interpretations, a pathologist must, before examination, consider known or anticipated pathologic anatomy and plan the method of dissection for a particular heart that best displays lesion(s) and imitates clinical image(s). In this instance, one wonders whether three-dimensional echocardiography might be usefully applied to certain excised hearts before dissection, such as fetal hearts with complex malformations.[32]

A pathologist must keep abreast of technologic advances in diagnostic cardiology, interventional radiology, and cardiovascular surgery, to understand their diagnostic and therapeutic limitations and complications. After any invasive cardiac procedure, the pathologist who examines a heart at autopsy or an explanted heart in surgical pathology needs to know *what* was placed *where* in case of a local complication. Failures are not often published. By direct participation as a cardiac team member, the pathologist can learn, and perhaps record for the literature, such failures.

The various guidewires, catheters, balloons, electrodes, pacing wires, blades, stents, and devices threaded into the heart for diagnostic, monitoring, and therapeutic purposes are all more or less rigid foreign bodies that are often advanced through heart chambers and along vessels under fluoroscopic or ultrasonographic control. They can irritate, contuse, lacerate, rupture, or perforate a heart, its valves, or blood vessels. Furthermore, they may provoke vascular spasm, introduce infection, cause vessel wall dissection or hemorrhage, or induce thrombosis or thromboembolism. The body has its own way of dealing with plastics, metals, woven cloth, and tissue grafts. Also, these substances are variously subject to fatigue, wear, fracture, disintegration, or calcification. Hence, a pathologist must be prepared to relate any lesions discovered at autopsy to an interventional procedure or a prosthetic insert. Pathologic features related to interventional cardiology and cardiovascular surgery have been collated in a monograph[33] and are further discussed in Chapters 21 to 23.

Examining a heart after recent or remote cardiac surgery requires skill and patience as well as previous knowledge of cardiac incision sites, surgical procedures, and placement of cannulas, grafts, and prosthetic devices. If a patient dies soon after open heart surgery has been performed, a pathologist needs to know the details of the procedure, including anesthesia and perfusion techniques, the amount of time that the patient was on cardiopulmonary bypass, the amount of cross-clamp time, and the status of hemodynamic stability both during and after surgery. Such data not only help when gross examination is performed but also aid correlations with microscopic findings. Remote open heart surgery leaves dense pericardial adhesions that may make dissection difficult. Often, it is better to wash out heart chambers through atrial incisions and fix them before dissection. Sometimes, pressure perfusion–fixation of a heart and coronary arteries is indicated (Table 1-1). In cases of cardiac malformation, the lungs must be left attached, either inflated with fixative or sliced to allow good penetration. In cases of ischemic heart disease or coronary artery bypass surgery, postmortem coronary angiography is indicated (see Table 1-1).

GROSS EXAMINATION OF THE HEART

A pathologist must dissect the heart so that it best displays and records alterations of cardiac structure wrought by disease. Numerous special pathologic techniques are available to do this and the prosector must choose the best method for a particular heart (see Table 1-1). If a good understanding of clinical events and of functional alterations is attained, the gross findings can be confirmed and extended by well-chosen histologic, ultrastructural, and immunocytochemical studies, as well as by collecting samples that may be required for microbiologic, serologic, biochemical, or molecular and genetic studies. Even if there has been no forewarning of suspected heart disease, forethought on the part of the team (including the pathologist) may result, for example, in the preservation of cells for culture or provision of snap-frozen tissues that can be used for future diagnostic or research studies (see also Chapter 24). Ultimately, every member of the cardiac team studies cardiac cells and their adaptation, injury, or death. The pathologist is the team member best acquainted with cell morphology and best trained to interpret the cause and mechanism of disease at the cellular level. In the heart, more than in any other organ, cellular adaptations are attended by gross alterations in a highly predictable way because of their effect on its pumping function.

Clinical Anatomy of the Heart

A pathologist needs access to some of the several atlases available in cardiac anatomy and pathology.[51, 75, 81–86] In describing a heart, he or she can then use the same terminology employed by clinical colleagues; thus, clinical information can be readily understood.

Cardiologic investigative methods require interdisciplinary agreement on the correct use of anatomic terminology and acceptance of new tomographic nomenclature. The heart may be visualized not merely in silhouette, as in a standard chest radiograph, but in an infinite number of thin, two-dimensional (tomographic) slices in any chosen plane. These planes, and the direction of view used in each, are expressed in terms of the standard anatomic position; that is, the natural position of the heart within the chest of an erect subject viewed from the front.[51] Thus, the anteroposterior and lateral views show frontal (or coronal) and sagittal planes of the cardiac silhouette. Standard radiographic views, including right and left lateral oblique views, are used to visualize the relationship between cardiac segments. Transecting a perfusion-fixed heart in the same radiographic planes reveals those relationships to a prosector. Photographs are taken with the heart in its natural anatomic position.[51] The prosector is able to see, for example, the sigmoid shape of the interventricular septum and the normal overriding of the interventricular septum by the aortic valve.[50] In addition, tomographic imaging permits views of nonattitudinal planes that are also revealed by slicing the perfusion-fixed heart in the same planes[6, 29–31, 51] (see Chapter 10 for examples).

CT and MRI examinations permit views of the heart in horizontal (transverse of the body) slices, suited to viewing relationships between the heart and adjacent organs. They also reveal very clearly the internal anatomic features of the pair of segmented intertwined conduits that constitute the heart. Echocardiography is a most useful imaging technique; moreover, it appears capable of further development. MRI also holds great promise. Each major diagnostic mode has chosen standard views to obtain desired planes and nomenclature developed to relate those findings to natural cardiac anatomy. Pathologists must also relate the features of the *excised* heart to natural cardiac anatomy. McAlpine refers to this as the attitudinal position of the heart.[51] The names given its various surfaces were chosen because they were the best among the three pairs of standard anatomic directions of view (anterior/posterior, right/left, superior/inferior) of the heart in its normal position in situ. Thus, the undersurface, mainly with the right ventricle resting on the diaphragm, is now universally referred to as the inferior surface. In the past, pathologists wrongly called this the *posterior* surface; they were accustomed to view and photograph

TABLE 1-1 • **Special Autopsy Techniques and Their Indications**

Technique	Indication	References
Postmortem plain/contrast radiography	Calcification in coronary tree, valve cusps, and valve rings	34, 35
Postmortem coronary angiography	Localization and quantitation coronary artery stenosis/thrombosis	13, 21, 34–48
Pressure perfusion-fixation of the heart and coronary arteries	Measurement of chamber volumes, valve rings, and coronary arteries	9, 29, 42, 49–52
Coronary casts/selective perfusion	As above	18, 36–39, 45, 53
Standard measurements of ventricles and valve rings	Documentation of size and shape of chambers and valves	4, 10, 50, 54–56
Casts of heart chambers	Analysis of chamber size, shape, and volume	34, 36, 49, 56–59
Decalcification of coronary artery tree before gross sectioning	Microscopic quantification of coronary atherosclerosis	34, 36, 56, 59
Transverse ventricular slicing	Gross quantitation of focal lesions and sampling myocardium for histology	34, 60–64
Tomographic display of perfusion-fixed heart	Correlation with antemortem anatomic findings	29–31, 52
Special staining of ventricular slices or paraffin sections	Identification of recent myocardial infarcts	34, 63–68
Separate weights of right ventricle, septum, and left ventricle	Quantitation of right and left ventricular hypertrophy	58, 69–72
Examination of the conduction system	Histopathology of conduction system in case of fixed conduction defect	73–75
Special fixatives for preserving color and plasticity	Preliminary to photography, for teaching and preservation	76
Photography of the heart	Documentation of anatomic findings and teaching	51, 73, 75, 77
Dry preservation of the heart	Permanent specimen for teaching	59, 78–80

the heart as if illustrated on a Valentine card, with its apex pointing straight down.[77]

At autopsy, hearts are most commonly opened in the direction of blood flow. Then, microscopic sections may be chosen in the exact transverse or longitudinal orientation best suited to the histology of any hollow viscus. Therefore, it is likely that pathologists will continue to photograph excised hearts in nonattitudinal positions. Indeed, cardiac anatomy atlases for surgeons are composed entirely of photographs and diagrams of hearts viewed in the supine body from above right or left.[83, 86]

Historic Review

Cardiac dissection methods are best learned from personal communication and experience rather than from books or journal articles. Nevertheless, it is of interest to review methods on record with the idea of incorporating useful techniques into one's chosen method. In 1959, Lev and McMillan surveyed the literature to investigate incisions used by our predecessors for opening each heart chamber.[87] The authors reviewed included those found in the German literature dating mainly from the first half of the 20th century, but the reviewers researched as far back as 1815 to investigate authors who contributed to Marjolin's *Manuel d'Anatomie*. Special methods of studying the myocardium and the coronary arteries, of making coronary artery casts, and of performing angiography in one plane were included. After they completed their review, Lev and McMillan proposed inflow-outflow transvalvular incisions that preserved the conduction system and also allowed prompt gross diagnosis and selection of microscopic sections.

In another review of cardiac dissection methods, Chapman pointed out that the transvalvular slicing technique, which he attributed to Mallory and Wright, did not necessarily reveal subtle anomalies of spatial relationships within heart chambers and valves.[78] This is true if the prosector mechanically opens a heart by any method learned by rote: Anomalies go unnoticed if they are not carefully sought. We think the shape of the heart chambers is better preserved by lateral inflow incisions (along the acute and obtuse borders) than by the paraseptal incisions attributed to Virchow by Chapman.[78]

The method for opening a heart described later in this chapter is, for all intents, identical to that described by Lev and McMillan.[87] Historically, their method owes much to Oppenheimer, who in 1912 warned pathologists that the then newly introduced string galvanometer and polygraph, which were forerunners of electrocardiography, demanded that they open the heart by a method that would not destroy the conduction system.[88]

Dissection Method for an Adult Heart

The prosector should proceed systematically with a chosen technique but be flexible when necessary.[6, 61, 71, 73, 78, 87] The prosector must look, feel, and probe before cutting, and must open the heart in a manner that best displays lesions and causes the least amount of destruction of valves, vessels, or conduction system. The following method is conventional, easy, and logical in that it follows the direction of blood flow. The terms proximal and distal may be conveniently used (clinically, "upstream" and "downstream") to describe the position of lesions relative to fixed structures and to blood flow through the heart. In addition, such terminology allows the pathologist to correlate morphology with function as recorded by clinical investigations. The scheme is essentially the same whether performed on the heart of an infant examined in situ or on the excised heart of an older child or adult. Also, it is as easily applied to congenitally malformed as to anatomically normal hearts.

Heart Position

The heart lies in the anterior mediastinum. Anteriorly, it is overlaid on either side by the lungs and pleura and is related to the sternum, ribs, and intercostal muscles. Laterally, there are the hila of the lungs and the related hilar structures, the phrenic nerves, the pericardiophrenic vessels, and the lungs themselves; posteriorly, the heart is related to the lower esophagus, the descending aorta, and both the azygos and the hemiazygos veins.

Pericardium, Great Vessels

If there is no reason to suspect a major cardiac malformation (see later), the heart is best examined either after its removal from the chest or from the thoracic organ block and before fixation. If indicated and before proceeding, a pericardial fluid sample can be obtained by needling through an area of the pericardium that has been seared for sterilization. The anterior fibrous pericardium is then incised in situ and the pericardial contents are noted; 15 to 50 ml of clear, straw-colored fluid is a normal finding.[89] Adhesions may be present or the pericardial cavity may be distended with fluid or blood. If such distention occurs very rapidly, cardiac tamponade usually develops when 250 to 300 ml of fluid have collected. However, if the fluid accumulates slowly, a much greater volume (1 to 2 L) may be present without causing tamponade (see Chapter 12). The pericardium is a roughly conical, fibroserous sac with its base on the diaphragm. Its narrower superior end surrounds the great arteries at the base of the heart. The pericardium consists of two distinct layers: an outer one, the fibrous pericardium; and an inner one, which is invaginated by the heart to form the serous pericardium. The fibrous pericardium is attached to the central tendon of the diaphragm and the adjacent diaphragmatic muscle and to the sternum through the superior and inferior sternopericardial ligaments. The serous pericardium consists of a parietal layer that lines the fibrous pericardium and the epicardium, which is a visceral layer that covers the heart and is separated from the myocardium by a variable amount of epicardial fat containing vessels and nerves (see Chapters 2 and 12).

Before the heart is removed, the right atrium at its junction with the inferior vena cava may be needled, after its surface is seared, to obtain a sample of heart blood for microbiologic culture. However, the blood stream is rapidly colonized by microorganisms post mortem, so blood culture should be used selectively. Aerobic and anaerobic cultures may be appropriate, but there is little purpose in culturing blood post mortem if extensive microbiologic studies were done in the terminal part of a patient's life or if the interval between death and autopsy was long. The parietal and visceral pericardial serosal membranes are inspected in situ; their surface is normally smooth and shiny. Papilliform fibrous tags, which are of no significance, are often observed on the visceral pericardium covering the atrial appendages.[90] The vascular connections of the heart are defined in situ, including the ligamentum arteriosum that joins the origin of the left main pulmonary artery to the aortic arch, in case there is a patent ductus arteriosus. A persistent left superior vena cava, seen externally to join the left atrium, is sometimes found in an otherwise normal cardiovascular system; it drains into the coronary sinus, which, as a result, has a prominent and enlarged ostium in the right atrium. Azygos and hemiazygos veins are viewed in situ while they are still filled with blood. The main pulmonary artery is then opened, and its lumen and those of its right and left

branches are explored for thrombus, embolus, or other pathology. Similarly, the superior vena cava is opened into the innominate and right azygos veins to search for any solid contents. The vascular connections of the heart are cut one at a time while lifting the organ anteriorly and cranially, starting with the inferior vena cava as it passes through the diaphragm. Next, the pulmonary veins, usually two on each side, are transected at the roots of the lungs. The aorta and the pulmonary artery are then transected 2 cm distal to their valves. The latter transection is done by inserting the first and second fingers along the transverse sinus to display the pedicle formed by the two great arteries at the base of the heart. The pedicle is then transected transversely by cutting between the two fingers. Lastly, the superior vena cava is divided at least 2 cm proximal to its junction with the right atrium.

The relationship between the great vessels and the investing pericardium is best understood when their roots are viewed after the heart's removal (see Figs. 1-1; and 12-2). One investment of serous pericardium encloses the great arteries, and a second contains all the veins. Thus, the pericardium encloses the distal half of the superior vena cava, the greater part of the ascending aorta, and almost the entire pulmonary trunk. It is at the vascular roots that the parietal serous pericardium becomes continuous with the visceral pericardium, or epicardium, thereby investing the heart. One must remember that the pericardial space includes the proximal or distal 3 to 4 cm of these vessels.

The amount of epicardial fat should be gauged at this stage. Normally, it fills the atrioventricular (coronary) sul-

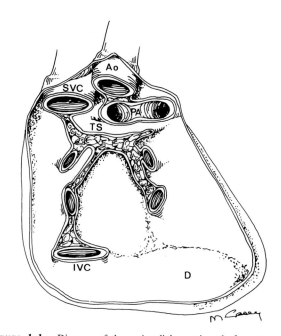

Figure 1-1 • Diagram of the pericardial sac viewed after removal of the heart by transecting the great vessels. Note the diaphragmatic surface (D), which is related to the inferior surface of the heart. The transverse sinus (TS) separates the two great arteries, the aorta (Ao) and the pulmonary artery (PA), from the two great veins—superior (SVC) and inferior vena cava (IVC)—which are enclosed in a common sheath with the four pulmonary veins.

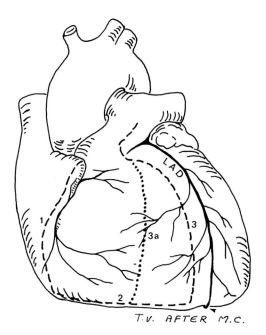

Figure 1-2 • Diagram of the anterior surface of the heart with dotted lines (1, 2, 3, 3a) indicating the incisions used to open the right heart chambers; incision 3a is an alternate path for incision 3. The left anterior descending coronary artery (LAD) indicates the anterior edge of the interventricular septum and usually rounds the acute border of the heart at the cardiac notch (arrowhead).

cus and extends along the anterior and posterior interventricular sulci toward the apex. When fat is increased, as in an obese person, it may blanket the epicardial surface of all chambers, especially along the course of coronary blood vessels; in extreme cases, more than half of the heart weight may be composed of fat.[91] Fat also extends anterior to the hilar lung vessels and spreads into the myocardium between the myofibers and along the intra-myocardial vessels, particularly in the right ventricle and interatrial septum.[92-96] This contrasts with the change seen in arrhythmogenic cardiomyopathy (see Chapters 10 and 11). Grossly, in a "fatty heart" (also called pathologic adiposity), only the outer half or two thirds of the myocardium is invaded by adipocytes.

External Features

The external surface of the heart is examined visually and by palpation. Myocardial lesions may be detected at this stage, and the sites of incisions to open chambers may be chosen accordingly. The location and relative size of the four heart chambers are assessed during the external examination, as are anomalies of the chamber shape, which may be a guide to the internal configuration. Any focal or diffuse disease that affects the epicardium is also apparent. Tendon-like white patches of epicardium (soldier's patches) are common, especially over the anterior surface of the right ventricle (see Chapter 12).

The coronary artery distribution should be noted (see Chapters 8 and 11), and the epicardial vessels should be palpated. A decision is made, based on clinical information and gross findings up to this point, about whether to perform postmortem coronary angiography before dissec-

tion of the coronary arteries, whether to examine the vessels in situ, or whether to excise the epicardial coronary tree for decalcification (see Table 1-1).

Opening the Heart Chambers

Having completed the external examination, the prosector holds the heart in one hand while using a knife—preferably a long, thin, pointed, and very sharp knife held in the other hand—to open the heart chambers. Scissors should not be used for this purpose because their blades crush tissue and leave jagged cut edges that are neither photogenic nor precisely radial. The incisions in the heart are made as illustrated in Figures 1-2 and 1-3. There are six incisions in all, three on each side. The knife is used correctly if its tip is stabbed through the organ at the distal end of a planned incision, and it is held with the cutting edge upward as the heart drops across the blade by its own weight and falls into the prosector's other hand. If the knife is sharp, very little retraction is needed to open a chamber. While doing so, the prosector frequently washes out or extracts postmortem clots found in cavities. The first incision in the right atrium is made 2 cm proximal and parallel to the atrioventricular groove. It passes from 1 cm anterior to the ostium of the inferior vena cava to the tip of the right atrial appendage (see Fig. 1-2, incision 1). This is also the incision surgeons use when repairing, for example, an atrial septal defect. This incision gives good exposure with no danger of damaging the sinoatrial node.[83] It is preferred to one that joins the superior and inferior venae cavae, because the latter incision destroys the valve of the inferior vena cava, makes it difficult to determine whether a Chiari net (see later) is present, and often destroys the sinoatrial node. This node may sometimes be visible, especially in infants or in nonfatty hearts of older subjects.[97] It usually lies to the right of the crest of the atrium.[86, 98] After viewing the interior of the right atrium and the tricuspid valve from that chamber, the prosector palpates the right ventricular

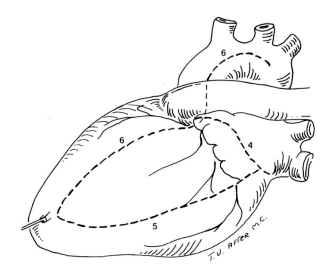

Figure 1-3 • Diagram of the left surface of the heart viewed in situ with the apex retracted toward the right. Incisions 4, 5, and 6 are indicated by dotted lines. Incision 6 passes between the (transected) pulmonary artery and the left atrial appendage.

inflow cavity and gauges the diameter of the valve; its ring normally admits the middle three fingers.

If the tricuspid valve or any valve examined subsequently should prove diseased, or if it is the site of a prosthetic heart valve, the prosector should leave the valve ring intact and recommence opening the heart by puncturing the right ventricle distal to the valve and then following the course of the incision usually made in that chamber. If vegetations are seen on the tricuspid valve or any other valvular or endocardial site, they should be sampled for microbiologic culture. To obtain better results, collect a sample of a vegetation by using instruments that have been flame sterilized at their ends and allowed to cool rather than swabbing with a sterile swab. If the tricuspid valve is normal, the second incision is made along the acute (right) border of the heart or up to 1 cm posterior to it (see Fig. 1-2, incision 2). This incision extends from the proximal end of the first incision to the right ventricular apex and transects the tricuspid ring and the posterior tricuspid leaflet. The inflow portion of the right ventricle, the tricuspid valve, and its tensor apparatus are thus exposed.

A third incision is made in the anterior right ventricle parallel to and 1 cm to the right of the interventricular septum from the right ventricular apex to the transected end of the main pulmonary artery. Care must be taken to keep the knife edge vertical to the heart wall (see Fig. 1-2, incision 3). Alternatively, the cut may be made from the midpoint of the second incision, keeping the knife anterior to the anterior papillary muscle (see Fig. 1-2, incision 3a). The triangular flap formed by incisions 2 and 3a is tethered to the septum by the moderator band, which joins the base of the anterior papillary muscle from the distal end of the septal band. The angle between the inflow and outflow tracts of the right ventricle is better appreciated by leaving the free wall attached to the anterior papillary muscle. The outflow tract (infundibulum), the pulmonary valve, and the proximal main pulmonary artery are examined at this stage.

The incision opening the left atrium must also open the left atrial appendage to enable the prosector to search for thrombus. A common technique is to join the superior or inferior pair of pulmonary veins and to extend the incision to the tip of the appendage, parallel to the atrioventricular groove. A disadvantage of this method is that the incision destroys the ostia of the pulmonary veins. A better method is to incise the atrium parallel to the atrioventricular groove, 1 cm proximal to it, and extend the incision to the tip of the atrial appendage. The mitral valve is examined from the left atrial cavity; its valve ring should admit two fingers.

Normally, the fifth incision is made through the mitral annulus and along the obtuse border of the heart to the left ventricular apex (see Fig. 1-3, incision 5). The best position for this cut is judged by palpating the two papillary muscles within the left ventricle through the mitral valve and guiding the knife between them. The inflow portion of the left ventricle and the mitral valve and its tensor apparatus are then examined.

The sixth and last incision opens the left ventricular outflow tract and is made from the apex to the aorta, parallel to and 1 cm to the left of the interventricular septum (see Fig. 1-3, incision 6). Anatomically, the incision passes between the pulmonary artery to the right and the left atrial appendage to the left (however, in this particular position, with the heart now held in the hand for the incision, the pulmonary artery seems to be located to the left of the incision and the left atrial appendage seems to be located to the right) and along the left side of the aorta dividing the left coronary cusp, usually very close to the left coronary artery ostium. Although the use of scissors has been advocated for this incision,[51] we prefer to use a knife in the unfixed heart; its blade converts the sinuous track into a straight cut exactly vertical to the aortic valve ring, through the middle of the left aortic cusp. Many pathologists dissect the pulmonary artery from the aortic root before making this incision to avoid damaging the pulmonary valve, but this is not really necesary. Occasionally, to protect the ostia of the coronary arteries and if the mitral valve is normal, the outflow tract may be opened more anteriorly through the center of the anterior mitral leaflet and the noncoronary cusp of the aortic valve. The left ventricular outflow cavity, the aortic valve, the sinuses of Valsalva, the coronary ostia, and the proximal aorta are examined.

Coronary Tree

The coronary arteries are now examined, Ideally, this examination is preceded by postmortem coronary angiography. If a patient had ischemic heart disease, or if the vessels are firm to palpation, or if the first section is gritty when cut, or if an angiogram or plain radiogram demonstrates severe coronary artery calcification, the entire epicardial arterial tree *must* be dissected from the heart and decalcified (see Table 1-1). Each artery should be placed in a separate container. Decalcification prevents artifactual damage that would be caused by cutting through a calcified arterial wall and crushing the lumen. Performing decalcification is the best way to prepare for serial blocking of the entire coronary tissue for histologic examination. This procedure is not difficult to perform because many sections may be included in a histologic block. If vessel decalcification is deemed necessary, it is best to remove the coronary tree before opening the heart (see Table 1-1). In the absence of any suspicion of coronary artery disease, especially if the patient is young and vessels are supple to palpation, they may be opened in situ, preferably by transverse cuts at 0.2 to 0.5 cm intervals. Alternatively, they may be opened longitudinally with iris scissors. We reserve the latter examination for the heart of fetuses and young children who do not have congenital heart disease.

Myocardium

A very useful incision, particularly if myocardial disease (e.g., ischemic damage, cardiomyopathy) is suspected, may be made either before opening the heart or before opening its left side. This incision transects the apices of both ventricles or the apex of the left ventricle at one third of the distance to the atrioventricular groove.[71] The apical mass remains hinged to the rest of the heart by means of the inferior epicardium and the outer inferior left ventricular myocardium. The incision permits inspection of the myocardium, examination of the tensor apparatus of the atrioventricular valves, and cap-ture of correctly oriented sections for microscopic study. Furthermore, it allows the prosector to judge the state of contraction of the ventricles by enabling him or her to view the degree of separation between the trabeculae carneae and the papillary muscles. Making a judgment about the degree of separation is basic for the prosector in estimating the degree of ventricular dilation or hypertrophy. This incision also permits excision of a transverse myocardial slice for gross stains that can help define the presence and extent of early ischemic damage.[63–67] When the prosector views the mitral valve apparatus through the ventricular cavity from the apical region after sectioning the apex, a ruptured papillary muscle or avulsed or ruptured chordae tendineae or a ruptured interventricular septum may be seen. This range of visibility allows the prosector to make a choice of the best site for the subsequent opening of the atrioventricular ring that will display but not disrupt such lesions. Furthermore, this short-axis view of the ventricular myocardium may lead the prosector to cut the ventricles entirely into transverse slices of 1 cm each, so that myocardial pathology can be mapped and quantitated accurately. Filleting incisions that are made parallel to the endocardium and that split the interventricular septum or ventricular free walls should not be used. They do not enable the prosector to estimate the size and position of a myocardial lesion accurately, nor do they permit correct orientation of histologic sections because they inevitably split deep myocardial lesions and fail to reveal small subendocardial ones.

Once it has been decided that an examination of the opened ventricular cavities is more or less desirable than one resulting from transverse incisions made across the ventricles, it may be necessary, after photographing the cavities, to incise endocardial or myocardial lesions. After their areas are measured, patches of opaque endocardium or mural thrombi are incised to facilitate study of the adjacent myocardium. Such incisions may transect the papillary muscles horizontally or split them vertically. In general, transversely oriented microscopic sections of the ventricles are preferable, except that the atrioventricular rings should be incised vertically (i.e., radially).

Although the method just described is used most often in practice, other techniques of dissecting may be better under certain circumstances (see Table 1-1). We reemphasize, for example, that myocardial injury is often best demonstrated and measured by means of transverse sections made at regular intervals across a myocardial injury. A prosector must choose the best dissection method, but in doing so, he or she must be practical. It could be argued that not all of the techniques defined in Table 1-1 may be available to a pathologist who practices at a smaller center. Nevertheless, many techniques can be established with ingenuity. We observe that for the best clinical pathologic correlations, it is better to forward an unopened heart for consultative study than one that has been sliced and diced.

Heart Weight

The opened heart, emptied of postmortem clot, is weighed; measurements of valve rings and ventricular wall thicknesses are made and the results are compared with accepted norms.[54, 71, 73, 75, 76, 99, 100] In individual cases, however, normality of heart weight may need to be judged by consideration of body size, weight, and gender. Hudson[73] gave the following useful guide to *fresh heart weight:*

Adult male heart weight: 0.45% of body weight, average 300 g, range 250 to 350 g.

Adult female heart weight: 0.40% of body weight, average 250 g, range 200 to 300 g.

An old study[101] that found that heart weight was related to body weight has been confirmed.[54, 102] Table 1-2 predicts a normal (*formalin-fixed*) heart weight from the body weight of adult men and women; it is based on a large study group.[54] Hutchins and Anaya noted that formalin fixation caused unpredictable changes in heart weight but on average induced a 5.4% increase.[99] Hort, however, found an average 6% decrease in the weights of normal hearts fixed in formalin for 1 month.[103] Heart weight is also related to body length[54, 100] but less so than to body weight.[54] Hangartner and associates discovered that body weight was superior to height as a predictor of total heart and isolated ventricular weights.[102] Although heart weight is said to increase with age,[100] this is more likely true in women than in men, and it decreases in the elderly of both genders[54] (see Chapter 3). Whether heart weight increases[100] or decreases[104] with increasing age in normal elderly subjects presumably depends on the definition of *normal* (see Chapter 3). Adult heart weight is reached between the ages of 17 and 20 years.[73] Heart weight in children is related to age and body size.[55, 105] Table 1-3 shows normal (*formalin-fixed*) *heart weights* predicted from body weights of male and female subjects up to 19 years of age.[55]

Although total heart weight has a wide normal range, it is the most practical and reproducible guide to myocardial hypertrophy when combined with a visual assessment of heart chamber musculature. It should be remembered that total heart weight reflects left rather than right ventricular hypertrophy. Visual assessment is particularly needed to judge the presence of right ventricular hypertrophy. Hypertrophied muscle produces brawny and prominent trabeculae carneae. More accurate measurements of hypertrophy in the individual ventricles, such as those obtained by dissecting the ventricles apart and weighing them separately, may be needed but are not readily applied at routine autopsy (see Table 1-1).

Wall Thickness

The thickness of ventricular walls is measured between vertically opposed surfaces at standard sites, such as those located midway between the base and the apex,[55] or at the thickest or thinnest (i.e., apical) parts of the ventricular free wall.[106] We measure at sites in each ventricle: 2 cm distal to the atrioventricular valves on acute and obtuse borders and 2 cm proximal to semilunar valves along incisions opening ventricular outflow tracts. Septal thickness is measured with calipers or a needle probe.[106] Septal thickness must not include trabeculated subendocardial muscle (trabeculae or columnae carneae), which makes up more than two thirds of the wall of the right ventricle but less than one third of the total width of the left. The normal thickness of compact muscle of the formalin-fixed right ventricle is 0.38 to 0.45 cm, and of the

TABLE 1-2 • **Predicted Normal Heart Weight (g) as a Function of Body Weight in 392 Women and 373 Men**

Body Weight		Women			Men		
kg	*lb*	L95	P	U95	L95	P	U95
30	66	133	196	287	162	213	282
32	71	137	201	295	167	220	291
34	75	141	206	302	172	227	300
36	79	144	211	310	177	234	309
38	84	148	216	317	182	240	317
40	88	151	221	324	187	247	325
42	93	154	226	331	191	253	334
44	97	157	230	337	196	259	341
46	101	160	234	344	200	265	349
48	106	163	239	350	205	270	357
50	110	166	243	356	209	276	364
52	115	169	247	362	213	281	371
54	119	171	251	368	217	287	379
56	123	174	255	374	221	292	386
58	128	177	259	379	225	297	392
60	132	179	262	385	229	302	399
62	137	182	266	390	233	307	406
64	141	184	270	395	237	312	412
66	146	187	273	401	240	317	419
68	150	189	277	406	244	322	425
70	154	191	280	411	248	327	431
72	159	194	284	416	251	331	437
74	163	196	287	420	255	336	444
76	168	198	290	425	258	341	450
78	172	200	293	430	261	345	455
80	176	202	297	435	265	349	461
82	181	205	300	439	268	354	467
84	185	207	303	444	271	358	473
86	190	209	306	448	275	362	478
88	194	211	309	453	278	367	484
90	198	213	312	457	281	371	489
92	203	215	315	461	284	375	495
94	207	217	318	465	287	379	500
96	212	219	320	470	290	383	506
98	216	221	323	474	293	387	511
100	220	222	326	478	296	391	516
102	225	224	329	482	299	395	521
104	229	226	331	486	302	399	526
106	234	228	334	490	305	403	531
108	238	230	337	494	308	406	536
110	243	232	339	497	311	410	541
112	247	233	342	501	314	414	546
114	251	235	345	505	316	418	551
116	256	237	347	509	319	421	556
118	260	239	350	513	322	425	561
120	265	240	352	516	325	429	566
122	269	242	355	520	327	432	570
124	273	244	357	523	330	436	575
126	278	245	360	527	333	439	580
128	282	247	362	531	335	443	584
130	287	249	364	534	338	446	589
132	291	250	367	537	341	450	593
134	295	252	369	541	343	453	598
136	300	253	371	544	346	456	602
138	304	255	374	548	348	460	607
140	309	257	376	551	351	463	611
142	313	258	378	554	353	466	616
144	317	260	381	558	356	470	620
146	322	261	383	561	358	473	624
148	326	263	385	564	361	476	629
150	331	264	387	567	363	479	633

Abbreviations: P, predicted normal heart weight; L95, lower 0.95% confidence limit; U95, upper 95% confidence limit.

From Kitzman DW, Scholz DG, Hagen PT, et al: Age-related changes in normal human hearts during the first 10 decades of life. Part II. Maturity: A quantitative anatomic study of 765 specimens from subjects 20 to 99 years old. Mayo Clin Proc 63:137, 1988.

**TABLE 1-3 • Predicted Normal Heart Weight (g) as a Function
of Body Weight in 100 Females and 100 Males Under 20 Years**

Body Weight		Females			Males		
kg	*lb*	**L95**	**P**	**U95**	**L95**	**P**	**U95**
3	7	13	19	29	11	16	24
4	9	16	24	37	14	21	31
5	11	19	29	44	18	26	38
6	13	22	33	51	21	30	45
7	15	25	38	58	24	35	51
8	18	28	42	64	27	39	58
9	20	30	46	71	30	44	64
10	22	33	50	77	33	48	71
12	26	38	58	89	39	57	83
14	31	43	66	101	45	65	96
16	35	48	74	113	50	74	108
18	40	53	81	124	56	82	120
20	44	58	88	135	61	90	132
22	49	62	95	146	67	98	143
24	53	67	102	156	72	106	155
26	57	71	109	166	78	111	167
28	62	76	116	177	83	122	178
30	66	80	122	187	89	130	190
32	71	84	129	197	94	137	201
34	75	88	135	207	99	145	212
36	79	93	142	216	104	153	223
38	84	97	148	226	110	160	235
40	88	101	154	236	115	168	246
42	93	105	160	245	120	175	257
44	97	109	166	254	125	183	268
46	101	113	172	264	130	190	279
48	106	117	179	273	135	198	289
50	110	121	184	282	140	205	300
55	121	130	199	304	153	224	327
60	132	140	214	326	165	242	354
65	143	149	228	348	178	260	380
70	154	158	242	370	190	278	406
75	165	167	256	391	202	295	432
80	176	176	269	412	214	313	458
85	187	185	283	432	226	331	484
90	198	194	296	453	238	348	509
95	209	202	309	473	250	365	535
100	220	211	322	493	262	383	560

Abbreviations: P, predicted normal heart weight; L95, lower 0.95% confidence limit; U95, upper 95% confidence limit.

From Scholz DG, Kitzman DW, Hagen PT, et al: Age-related changes in normal human hearts during the first 10 decades of life. Part I. Growth. A quantitative anatomic study of 100 specimens from subjects from birth to 19 years old. Mayo Clin Proc 63:126, 1988.

left, 1.23 to 1.50 cm.[50, 54, 71] The ventricular septum is 1.26 to 1.5 cm thick.[54, 71] Hutchins and Anaya found that by measuring wall thickness using postmortem radiographs, a normal right ventricle was 0.39 cm (range 0.2 to 0.7 cm) and a normal left ventricle was 1.5 cm thick (range 1.0 to 2.0 cm).[99] These investigators attributed, in part, the large variation to the different positions (systole-diastole) in which ventricles may be fixed in rigor. Measuring ventricular thickness is a poor method of assessing ventricular hypertrophy.[102] Measurements of the same heart at autopsy correlate only with echocardiographic measurements obtained during systole, probably because rigor imitates systolic contraction.[55] The consistency of heart muscle at autopsy reflects the stage of rigor or autolysis more than the stage of muscle tone during life. In fact, before the onset of rigor and after it has passed off, the heart quite lacks tone. Should it feel stiff, a prosector should consider whether an infiltrative process is present in the myocardium.

Valve Measurements

According to a large study, normal valve circumferences, which vary with age and gender, are as presented in Table 1-4.[54] In children, normal valve circumferences relate to age and to body weight and length.[55, 105] Unless

TABLE 1-4 • Normal Valve Circumferences

	Circumference (cm)	
Valve	*Women*	*Men*
Tricuspid	10–11.1	11.2–11.8
Pulmonary	5.7–7.4	6.1–7.5
Mitral	8.2–9.1	9.2–9.9
Aortic	5.7–7.9	6.0–8.5

From Kitzman DW, Scholz DG, Hagen PT, et al: Age-related changes in normal human hearts during the first 10 decades of life. Part II. Maturity: A quantitative anatomic study of 765 specimens from subjects 20 to 99 years old. Mayo Clin Proc 63:137, 1988.

it is either extremely small or large, the size of a heart valve ring does not help to determine whether the valve was stenosed or incompetent during life. In the past, pathologists tested valve competence by filling the great vessels with fluid, but this "water test" was abandoned as unnecessary during the early 20th century.[78] Direct viewing and palpation of each valve remain the best ways to judge antemortem function. In contrast to this subjective assessment, valvular regurgitation is now measured accurately in life by Doppler echocardiography technique.

Atrioventricular valve circumferences, measured at the level of their rings, are probably of no more value than those of ventricular wall thicknesses, since they also depend on the state of contraction of the heart when stiffened by rigor. Valve ring circumferences (particularly the circumference of the tricuspid ring) are not easily measured accurately, especially in the presence of rigor. It is more precise to use graduated cylinders and measure the valve ring diameter before opening it. However, the overlap between the range of valve measurements in health and acquired heart diseases is very great.[99] They are usually greater in men than women and tend to increase with age in both sexes (see Chapter 3 also).[54, 107] They increase in hearts manifesting congestive heart failure.[107]

Semilunar valve ring measurements are not affected by the state of ventricular contraction and correlate well with age and heart size, with the pulmonary valve "rather consistently exceeding the aortic valve by a factor of 1.1."[99] Semilunar valve ring circumferences also increase with age, and the circumference of the aortic valve is usually greater than that of the pulmonary valve after age 40.[54]

Photography

Color photography may be improved if a heart is fixed for a few hours or overnight in Jores or Klotz solution, because either of these solutions subdues highlights while retaining color and plasticity. Even if the heart is placed in any fixative for a few minutes, bright reflections are quenched. To subdue highlights on a fresh heart, filter screens should be used to polarize the illuminating light. Before the picture is taken, a polarizing filter on the camera should be rotated until highlights disappear. This method is quick, does not require drying of the specimen's surface, and enriches color; Ektachrome tungsten 50 film gives good color accuracy. An excellent guide for photographing medical specimens recommends the use of screens to diffuse highlights,[77] but these screens reduce both contrast and color saturation. We agree with Edwards' use of an unobtrusive matte black background rather than backlighting through translucent colored panels. We use black flocked paper, which is easily blotted dry.[77]

Storage

If a heart is to be stored as an anatomic specimen, it should be transferred to Kaiserling III solution. Formulas for all the fixative solutions mentioned are available.[76] An alternative to the wet museum specimen is dry preservation by plastination.[79, 80]

Summary

After the heart has been opened in the manner described, either general or local alterations of color and consistency may readily be defined in the myocardium, the endocardium, the epicardium, the heart valves, and the valvular tensor apparatus. Any lesions that are found may be displayed in a way that is conducive to good photography, gross demonstration, measurement, and description; eventually, correctly oriented microscopic sections can be prepared. Most importantly, the conduction system (see Chapter 20) and coronary vessels can be preserved, keeping them available for detailed study if needed.

Dissection Method for Fetal and Infant Hearts

Although this book is primarily devoted to examination of heart disease in adults, a method for examining fetal and infant hearts is included for the sake of completeness. Also, in this era of aggressive treatment, patients with congenital heart disease reach adult age increasingly often. Therefore, a method of examination that applies to both congenital and acquired heart disease is of value to a pathologist. A key point in these examinations is to keep the heart attached to the lungs (see discussion in Chapter 22 also).

Methods are available that have been designed specifically for the malformed perinatal heart[108, 109] and for normally formed but ischemically damaged infant hearts.[42] We prefer the transvalvular slicing method that is used in an adult heart (see earlier), but we modify incisions according to the kind of malformation. This modification requires the prosector to have full clinical information before autopsy. A perinatal cardiovascular pathologist is able to judge what to expect from the external features of a malformed heart. A less experienced prosector may first prefer to wash blood clots from chambers that show abnormal external morphology and then fix the heart in Klotz or Jores solution with a view to seeking help.

Initially, the position of the heart is noted in relation to the thoracic and abdominal viscera. The normal visceroatrial situs (situs solitus) refers to the inferior vena cava's attachment to a morphologic right atrium on the right side of the chest. Thus, the superior surface of the liver must be viewed to find the attachment of the inferior vena cava to the systemic atrium. Situs inversus is easily understood as the condition opposite to situs solitus. In situs ambiguus, as seen in defects of laterality typified by asplenia and polysplenia, it is not possible to identify separate right and left atria by morphologic criteria. Dissection of hearts from fetuses or infants with these conditions can be difficult even for experts.

Whether or not congenital heart disease is suspected, the heart of a fetus or neonate is best opened either in situ or en bloc with the lungs. The venous system can be examined adequately only in situ before blood loss is caused by dissection. The right side of the heart may be opened in situ and the left side after removal of the thoracic organ block from the chest, but the lungs must remain attached to the heart by the pulmonary vessels

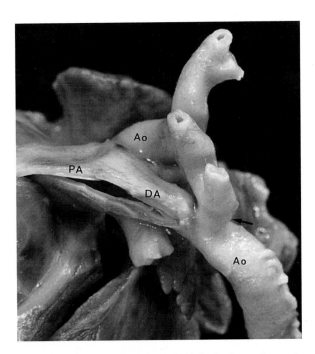

Figure 1-4 • The ductus arteriosus (DA) in the heart of a newborn infant joins the pulmonary artery to the isthmus (arrow) of the aorta (Ao). The main pulmonary artery (PA) has been opened lengthwise and the incision continued into the proximal part of the ductus so that the thick muscular wall of the ductus is visible on the cut edges. The left branch of the pulmonary artery is seen below the ductus, and part of the right branch is visible between the ductus and the aorta. The three great arteries to the head and arms ascend from the aortic arch proximal to the isthmus.

until dissection is complete. Again, it is especially important to look, feel, and probe before cutting, and to leave intact any site of stenosis.

Before opening the pericardium, the thymus is dissected from the anterior mediastinum. This must be done carefully to avoid damaging the innominate vein, which lies immediately deep to the junction of the thoracic and cervical lobes of the organ. Some blood is lost when the thymus is removed because the internal mammary vessels must be cut. At this stage, one looks for a persistent left superior vena cava that connects the innominate vein to the coronary sinus anterior to the left pulmonary veins. Its presence accentuates a fold of the pericardium (Marshall's fold), which marks this normally vestigial venous connection to the coronary sinus.[51] The pericardial sac is opened and its lining and the fluid contents are examined. The anterior parietal pericardium is dissected off the heart to the roots of the great vessels and the hilus of each lung. The azygos and hemiazygos veins are inspected by turning each lung anteriorly. The course and branches of the aorta are examined and the external surface of the ductus arteriosus is defined. In a newborn, the ductus appears to be a direct continuation of the main pulmonary artery and is hardly smaller than that artery in external diameter (Fig. 1-4).

Careful inspection of the heart's external surface usually reveals anomalies in the position of chambers and great vessels and prevents mistakes such as opening a ventricular outflow tract across a ventricular septal defect and into the wrong great vessel. In particular, the shape and position of the atrial appendages should be noted. The right one is a simple cone, whereas the left is hooked and has a narrow base; with its multiple lobes, it looks like a cock's comb. Morphology of the atrial appendage is a highly reliable guide to the atrium to which it attaches.[110] Juxtaposed atrial appendages lie together on one or other side of the great arteries. Left juxtaposition of the right appendage is far more common and almost always signals the presence of other severe malformations, such as abnormal atrioventricular connections.[86, 111] Right juxtaposition of the left appendage is less common and more likely associated with normal chamber connections.[86, 111] The position of the left anterior descending coronary artery normally marks the anterior edge of the interventricular septum. It is placed more to the left in a normal newborn than in an adult heart, because the right ventricle is as large as the left at birth. The great arteries, which are identified by their branches,[110] normally twist about each other, with the pulmonary artery being anterior proximally but posterior to the aorta at its bifurcation. Their relationship in a malformed heart depends on the ventricle they drain. We note that as with situs ambiguus, conotruncal malformations provide a semantic minefield.

Instruments used to open a tiny heart vary with the prosector. Many prosectors employ scissors rather than a knife. A scalpel, by cutting down onto a probe placed along the passage to be opened, can be used to prevent crushing. The first incision made in an infant heart as it lies in situ (see Fig. 1-2) starts just anterior to the ostium of the inferior vena cava. This incision spares the eustachian valve, which, in the fetus, directs blood from that vein through the foramen ovale and into the left atrium. The second incision is the same as that used in the adult heart, along the acute border to the right ventricular apex. The third incision, preferably done to spare the moderator band (see Fig. 1-2, incision 3a), is extended from the main pulmonary artery into the left pulmonary artery at the hilus of the left lung so that the proximal end of the ductus arteriosus can be inspected. The incision into the left atrium may be made from the tip of the left atrial appendage parallel to the atrioventricular groove and distal to the connections of the four pulmonary veins so that a congenital stenosis of these vessels, if patent, may be noted. Also, any membranous partition separating the proximal (posterior) from the distal (anterior) part of the atrium may be demonstrated (cor triatriatum sinister).

The left ventricular inflow tract is opened along the obtuse border of the heart as in an adult. The sixth incision, opening the left ventricular outflow, may be extended through the isthmus of the aorta after this area is inspected and probed for coarctation. In the newborn, a tubular narrowing of the isthmus to approximately two thirds the diameter of the ascending aorta is normal,[112] and there is a slight posterior fold or shelf of the aortic lining opposite the aortic end of the ductus arteriosus.

At this stage, a decision can be made whether to open the ductus arteriosus longitudinally or whether to fix it before transverse sectioning. Probing for patency is not

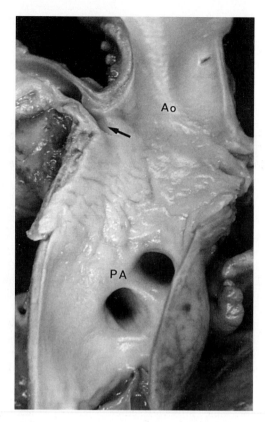

Figure 1-5 • The lining of the ductus arteriosus in a newborn infant, viewed after opening the ductus lengthwise in continuity with the main pulmonary artery (PA) and the descending thoracic aorta (Ao). The ostium of the right pulmonary artery is slightly proximal to that of the left, which is seen directly to the right of the PA. The arch of the aorta with the great branches to the head and arms is seen on the left of the narrow aortic isthmus (arrow). The corrugated lining of the ductus indicates contracted medial muscle in its wall (see Fig. 1-4).

advised, because this may dislodge thrombus and give a false impression of patency. A widely patent ductus is tortuous and soft-walled, but normal closure by medial muscular contraction shortens it, thickens its walls, and narrows its lumen. A widely patent ductus (as seen in the asphyxiated newborn) is very friable; it is wise to fix it before opening.[113] A normally closing ductus is narrower than the main pulmonary artery; it feels firm to palpation and has a corrugated lining (Fig. 1-5) because of the contraction of medial muscle squeezing intimal cushions into folds. The lumen becomes increasingly narrow and tortuous until anatomic closure is completed a few weeks after birth.[113]

After the newborn heart has been opened in situ following the course of the blood stream, any congenital anomalies are evident. If there are anomalies, the heart should be fixed en bloc with the lungs rather than dissected off for organ weighs; this may be done later on when the organs are fixed. Describing and classifying cardiac malformations is best done by direct description and simple box diagrams, or by using photocopied diagrams available for this purpose.[114] Recognition of the salient features that identify each chamber and great artery requires skill and practice.[109, 115] Anderson summarized the anatomic components that are most constant in

defining the morphology of an atrium (the shape of its appendage), a ventricle (its apical trabecular morphology), and a great vessel (its branching pattern).[110] Another good rule is that, except in cases of situs ambiguus, the atrioventricular valve morphology is concordant with that of the ventricle into which it opens.

The tinier a fetal heart, the harder it is to dissect. We follow the method described earlier if the heart comes from a fetus at approximately 17 weeks of gestation or older or if the heart weight is greater than 1 g, but we use a dissecting microscope if necessary. Smaller hearts may be totally embedded and examined histologically in step-serial sections. Echocardiographic examination of the excised heart is worth considering in such cases.[32]

If congenital malformations are found, it is best to leave sites of stenosis intact, at least initially, and to continue the dissection beyond them. The smaller the heart, the more delicate the tissue and the greater the need to probe with care and not produce false passages. The septum primum, which fills the fossa ovalis, is so delicate, translucent, and mobile in a perinatal heart that it is best visualized by squeezing the lungs, to distend the left atrium with blood, while viewing the fossa ovalis from the right atrium to determine whether the septum primum is valve-competent. An obliquely probe-patent but valve-competent foramen ovale is normal at this age; it is obligatory before birth. A foramen closed prenatally or a restrictive foramen is associated with congestive heart failure in some fetuses and is found in a substantial number of hearts with left heart hypoplasia.

Weights and Measurements

A normal newborn heart may be removed from the lungs for weighing, but most prosectors include the proximal great vessels and ductus arteriosus in this weight. Nevertheless, normal fetal and perinatal hearts, including these vessels, often weigh less than norms tabulated in the literature.[105, 116] Normal heart weight in infants and children is related to body weight and length as well as to age.[55, 105] Table 1-3 shows the normal range of heart weights predicted from body weight between birth and 19 years.[55] The circumference of the valve rings and the thickness of the ventricles may be measured as in an adult heart and compared with published norms.[4, 10, 55, 105] Tabulated normal heart valve circumferences are available from subjects ranging from 1 month to 12 years of age[105] and from birth to 19 years of age.[55] It is better to measure valve ring diameters before cutting them by using graduated metal cylinders rather than measuring valve ring circumferences after they are opened.[99]

INTERNAL CONFIGURATION OF THE HEART

Gross examination of the interior of the heart involves a basic understanding of normal anatomy [51, 75, 81, 84, 117–120] and embryology[81, 84–86, 116, 119, 121] as well as congenital heart anomalies.[82, 84, 122–124] In describing malformed hearts, however, we agree with Anderson that a pathologist should use simple terms that do not rely on concepts of development.[110] A prosector must note the individual features of each chamber and valve to decide on their normality and locate any lesions. By reducing the whole to its components, deviations from normal can be learned quickly, and acquired lesions and congenital malformations described; moreover, normal anatomic variations can be distinguished from true malformations (i.e., growth abnormalities that begin during embryonic development). Angelini proposed a useful rule of thumb for variations that have no functional significance in themselves but need recognition in, for example, diagnostic imaging procedures. If the variation affects less than 1% of a population, it may be arbitrarily classed as an anomaly, and if it affects more than 1%, it is called a normal variation.[125] Common examples of the latter are a double right coronary ostium and myocardial bridging over the middle segment of the left anterior descending coronary artery.[7, 125]

Malformations are often difficult to distinguish from deformations (i.e., disturbances of growth that occur after embryonic life). Deformations result from abnormal physical forces acting on growing tissues. In a fetal heart, abnormal blood flow resulting from a malformation is the most obvious cause of deformation. Deformations also supervene in the postnatal heart that is still growing or, at any age, in a heart undergoing hypertrophy.

Abnormal hemodynamic forces also disturb tissue organization at the cellular level during fetal life. Tissue disorganization at the microscopic level is correctly termed *dysplasia*. In the heart, the term is often used to describe cardiac valves scarred by abnormal blood flow secondary to a congenital malformation; such valves may well be disorganized at the microscopic level, but the more obvious diagnosis is that they are deformed by scar tissue. The term *dysplasia* is also correctly applied to the disarrayed cardiac muscle seen in hypertrophic cardiomyopathy and, arguably, to ventricular dysplasia or arrhythmogenic cardiomyopathy (see Chapter 10).

Right Atrium

The right atrium,[51, 81, 83, 85, 86, 126–129] the wall of which is approximately 0.2 cm thick, lies superior and posterior to the right ventricle and anterior to the left atrium. Its external relationships are to the anterior chest wall and to the medial aspect of the right lung.

This chamber receives systemic venous blood via the superior and inferior venae cavae, which respectively enter the proximal and distal extremities of its free wall posteriorly, close to the interatrial septum. The right atrium also receives the venous return from the heart itself via the coronary sinus. The smooth posterior atrial wall between the great veins (sinus venarum) is derived embryologically from the sinus venosus, whereas the remaining free anterior wall and appendage are trabeculated (pectinate muscles) and derived from the primitive atrium.

Trabeculae are oriented at right angles to the crista terminalis, a prominent muscle bundle that marks the junction of the two segments. Trabeculations of the right atrial appendage, also called the auricle, extend laterally just proximal to the atrioventricular junction, and they end just anterior to the orifice of the inferior vena cava.

On the acute border of the heart, a shallow pouch with trabeculated lining is called the subeustachian sinus of Keith, and just posterior to it is an even less obvious pouch, termed the fossa of His.[51, 86]

The right valve of the sinus venosus forms the crista terminalis, which is marked externally by a shallow groove, the sulcus terminalis, as well as by the valves of the inferior vena cava (eustachian) and coronary sinus (thebesian). These valves vary greatly in size and may be fenestrated or absent, but the eustachian valve is well developed in approximately 90% of normally formed hearts.[130] Thebesian valves are generally less well developed, covering the ostium in approximately 40% of subjects with normal heart weight.[131] A Chiari net, usually a lace-like veil of tissue, may span the atrial cavity from the region of the thebesian or the eustachian valve to insert into the crista terminalis.[127] The Chiari net represents a remnant of the right sinus venosus valve (Fig. 1-6). The left sinus venosus valve is usually absorbed into the right surface of the septum secundum, but remnants are often found as bands, or a net, of tissue bridging the posteroinferior margin of the fossa ovalis (Fig. 1-7).[128]

The fossa ovalis, which is the central landmark on the right side of the interatrial septum, can be as large as 3.5 cm in diameter and is usually well defined superiorly and anteriorly by the limbus of the fossa ovalis, formed by infolded atrial walls (Figs. 1-7 and 1-8).[132] Tiny vascular remnants, which may persist along its posteroinferior margin, may become thrombosed[133, 134] (see Fig. 1-8). Probing under the limbus anteriorly shows whether the foramen ovale is obliterated or valve-competent; the latter is a normal finding in as many as 31% of adult hearts (see Fig. 1-8).[129, 135] Possibly, a probe-patent foramen ovale is not totally innocuous in adult life because, as shown by contrast echocardiography, it is statistically

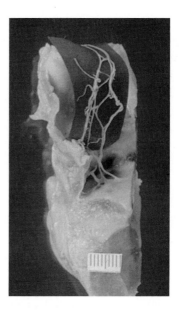

Figure 1-6 • Lace-like Chiari network excised from an adult heart with a block, including part of the tricuspid valve and the right atrium. It has its origin at the ostium of the coronary sinus and crosses the atrium to insert into the crista terminalis. Black paper covers the orifice of the inferior vena cava to emphasize the net. Scale indicates 1 cm.

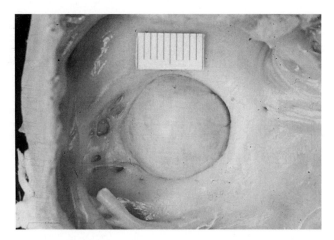

Figure 1-7 • Remnants of the left valve of the sinus venosus form bands across the posterior limbus of the fossa ovalis. A smooth-surfaced aneurysm of the septum primum projects into the right atrial cavity. Scale indicates 1 cm.

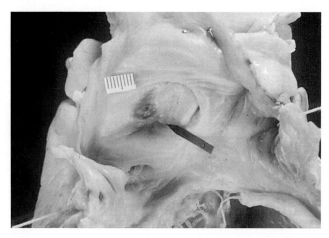

Figure 1-8 • Interatrial septal wall showing the fossa ovalis region. A venous remnant forms a nodule at the posterior limbus (pointer). The patient also had a valvular, probe-patent foramen ovale at the anterior edge of the fossa to the right of the pointer tip. Scale indicates 1 cm.

more common in young people who have suffered a stroke than in controls (see Chapter 15).[136]

Defects in the fossa ovalis are commonly called ostium secundum defects, because the fossa ovalis is the ostium secundum of embryonic life. The septum primum is membranous and hence transilluminable. Defects in this septum may be membranous fenestrations, or, at the foramen ovale, they may represent valvular incompetence. Other types of atrial septal defects are much less common than those occurring in the fossa ovalis. An ostium primum defect is closely related to the tricuspid valve ring and is usually part of an atrioventricular septal defect, which was formerly called an endocardial cushion defect, or persistent atrioventricular canal. Interatrial septal defects may also occur in the region of the coronary sinus or the superior vena cava.

An aneurysmal bulge of the septum primum may occur through the fossa ovalis into either atrium (although usually into the right atrium see Fig. 1-7).[137] The association in adults of aneurysms of the fossa ovalis with increased frequency of embolic stroke has been attributed to its significant association with mitral valve prolapse, dilated atria, intracardiac thrombi, and patent foramen ovale; the latter condition is present in 70% of such subjects.[138] An aneurysm of the fossa ovalis bulging to the left atrium is also seen during fetal life and is associated with fetal tachydysrhythmias and other causes of fetal heart failure.[139, 140]

Tiny holes (smaller than 0.05 cm diameter) that are apparent in the endocardium at variable sites in the right atrium are the entrance points of the thebesian veins. The most constant are a pair that drain the region of the sinoatrial node. Two larger holes, between 0.2 and 0.3 cm (foramina of Lannelongue), are often seen superior to the fossa ovalis and the opening of the coronary sinus. These holes also belong to the thebesian venous system.[135] This system intercommunicates extensively with the definitive cardiac venous sytem.[141]

The size of the coronary sinus opening is important. It may be larger than normal if it drains anomalous vessels (e.g., a persistent left superior vena cava via an oblique vein of Marshall, as seen in Fig. 1-9, or vessels from the

lung) or in the presence of severe right heart failure. Alternatively, the coronary sinus opening may be smaller than normal or even atretic if coronary sinus blood is passing from the heart through a persistent left superior vena cava to the innominate vein and, thence, via a right superior vena cava to the right atrium. The coronary sinus may be absent, as in those conditions in which a left superior vena cava connects directly to the left atrium. Such variations in the size of the coronary sinus may be isolated and unimportant but often accompany serious cardiac malformations.

By transillumination, part of the membranous interven-

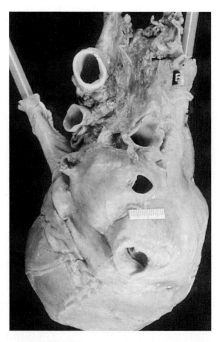

Figure 1-9 • Posteroinferior surface of the heart showing a superior vena cava (right cannula); an inferior vena cava orifice (lowermost orifice); a persistent left superior vena cava (left cannula), which joins the coronary sinus; four pulmonary vein orifices (above the inferior vena cava); and the transected aorta (top left). Scale indicates 2 cm.

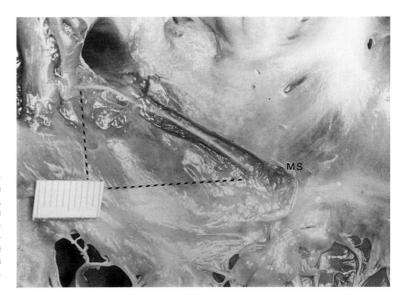

Figure 1-10 • The tendon of Todaro revealed by dissection through the endocardium of the right atrium. The atrioventricular node is found in the interatrial septum, within the triangle formed by the tendon of Todaro, the tricuspid annulus (horizontal dotted line), and a line joining this annulus to the mouth of the coronary sinus (vertical dotted line). The apex of this triangle is at the posterior edge of the membranous septum (MS), which can be confirmed by transilluminating this structure. Marker indicates 1 cm.

tricular septum is seen in the right atrium just proximal to the tricuspid annulus where it forms the base of the septal leaflet of the tricuspid valve. A defect in this area permits communication between the left ventricle and the right atrium, whereas a defect distal to the septal leaflet is a ventricular septal defect at its most common location. Usually, the anterior and septal leaflets of the tricuspid valve cross the membrane to meet at their commissure. Rarely, they insert at the edge of the membrane without forming a commissure. This does not produce valvular regurgitation. The right sinus of Valsalva of the aortic valve is also closely related to the right atrium and may cause a smooth protuberance of the right side of the anterosuperior atrial septum, the torus aorticus.[135, 142]

The tendon of Todaro is a ligament attached to the fibrous skeleton of the heart. It may represent the commissure of the eustachian and thebesian valves. This tendon probably functions during fetal life by strengthening the free edge of the eustachian valve and helping to direct venous return from the inferior vena cava across the foramen ovale.[143] The tendon of Todaro is sometimes seen in adult hearts, but it is more obvious in those of children. The tendon is a white cord deep to the right atrial endocardium, passing from the sinus septum, which separates the ostia of the inferior vena cava and the coronary sinus, toward the membranous septum.[135, 144] When this tendon is visible, it is a useful landmark for the atrioventricular node, which lies within the triangle (Koch's triangle) formed by Todaro's tendon, the tricuspid ring, and the coronary sinus orifice (Fig. 1-10). Todaro's tendon joins the right trigone of the central fibrous body and is seen microscopically in transverse section when the atrioventricular node is examined.

Tricuspid Valve

The tricuspid valve[51, 81, 83, 86, 145–148] (Fig. 1-11) is based on a ring (annulus) that points anteriorly, inferiorly, and to the left. Its normal annular circumference is 10 to 11.1 cm in women and 11.2 to 11.8 cm in men.[54] The three leaflets hang from the valve ring like a veil, and the

three commissures are almost as long as the posterior and septal leaflets. To define the leaflets, one must understand chordal attachments; the three leaflets are separated by commissures tethered by fan-shaped chordae tendineae.[148] Each leaflet has a distal rough zone and a proximal basal zone into which the chordae insert, as well as a clear zone free of chordal insertions that lies between the rough and the basal zones. The anterior leaflet is usually the longest (average 2.2 cm). It is semicircular or quadrangular and is 3.7 cm in average width at its base. Rarely, it has a distinct scallop in its medial side near the anteroseptal commissure. The septal leaflet is semioval and is 1.6 cm long by 3.6 cm wide on average. It shows a characteristic fold on its atrial surface in the angle where its base passes from the posterior ventricular free wall to the membranous area. The posterior leaflet, which averages 2.0 cm long by 3.6 cm wide at its base, has a variable number of scallops, usually two or three, produced by clefts or indentations in its free edge. These clefts are marked by small fan-shaped chordae that tether the leaflets. In all, 17 to 36 chordae are found, with an average number of 25.[148] There are five types of chordae: fan-shaped, rough-zone, basal, free-edge, and deep; of these, free-edge and deep chordae are unique to the tricuspid valve.[148] The chordae are of varying length (0.3 to 2.2 cm) and thickness (0.05 to 0. 15 cm). They arise from one large anterior papillary muscle. There is a relatively constant septal papillary muscle that is named for both Lancisius and Luschka[85]; it may be double or multiple and arises high on the septal band (see later), with several small posterior papillary muscles. Linear endocardial thickenings or "friction" lesions may be found between the chordae and the adjacent septal ventricular wall in hypertrophied hearts; sometimes, the two become tethered by scar tissue at these points.

Right Ventricle

The right ventricle[81, 83, 86, 118, 145, 146, 149–153] lies anterior to the other heart chambers. Its free wall forms an acute angle, which is the acute border, or margo acutus, of the

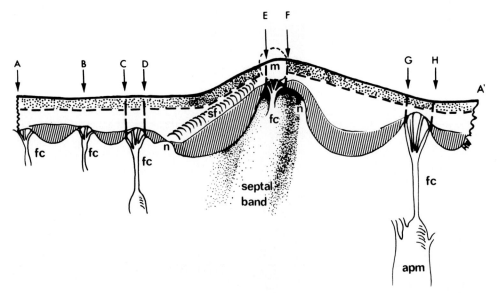

Figure 1-11 • Diagrammatic representation of the tricuspid valve opened through the acute margin of the right ventricle. Abbreviations: A-B, B-C, and H-A′, middle, posteroseptal commissural, and anteroposterior commissural scallops of posterior leaflet, defined by clefts at A or A′ and B; C-D, posteroseptal commissure; D-E, septal leaflet; E-F, anteroseptal commissure related to the membranous interventricular septum (dotted circle m); F-G, anterior leaflet; G-H, anteroposterior commissure. The commissures and clefts in the posterior leaflet are defined by fan-shaped chords (fc). Anterior and septal leaflets have notches (n) in their free margins. The anterior papillary muscle (apm), the most medial papillary muscle on the posterior wall (to the left of the diagram), a fold in the septal leaflet (sf), and the membranous interventricular septum (m) are auxiliary landmarks to the commissures. Cross-hatching indicates the rough zone of the leaflets; stippling indicates the basal zone. The intervening area is the clear zone. (From Silver MD, Lam JHC, Ranganathan N, Wigle ED: Morphology of the human tricuspid valve. Circulation 43:333, 1975.)

heart, between the anterior and the inferior, or diaphragmatic, external surfaces. Posteriorly and to the left, it is related to the left ventricle from which it is separated by the interventricular septum, which lies at a 45-degree angle to the median plane. The right ventricle is crescentic in transverse section, with its septal wall applied to the exterior of the convex septal surface of the conical left ventricle.

The anatomic right ventricle has an inflow portion, or sinus, and an outflow portion, the infundibulum or conus (Fig. 1-12). It has been suggested that the right ventricle is a tripartite structure with a confluent inlet and trabeculated apical and outflow segments.[81, 86] Blood flowing through the right ventricle changes direction in passing the free edge of the anterior tricuspid leaflet by 145 degrees in a child and 125 degrees in an adult.[85] The infundibulum is separated anatomically from the sinus by a muscular crest or arch, the crista supraventricularis. This crest, which separates tricuspid and pulmonary valves, merges medially where it meets the septum, with muscular ridges of variable prominence called the septal and parietal bands that course in those walls of the right ventricle. The site of insertion of the crest between these trabeculations may be smooth or marked by either a vertical ridge or a groove. The papillary muscle of the conus, Lancisi's muscle, arises from the septal wall just proximal to the crista; it is an important surgical landmark for the conduction system.[8, 50, 81, 83]

The junction of the sinus with the infundibulum is defined anteriorly by the upper edge of another smooth arch of muscle formed by the junction of the septal band,

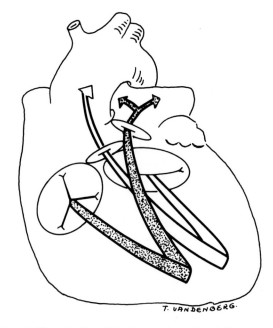

Figure 1-12 • Position of heart valve rings viewed diagrammatically from the front. The two atrioventricular valve rings point forward to the left and slightly downward. The aortic valve ring is fused to the tricuspid and mitral annuli, but the pulmonary valve ring is separated from it and lies at the higher level. Arrows indicate the direction of blood flow through the ventricles and the valve rings; the stippled arrow is in the right heart.

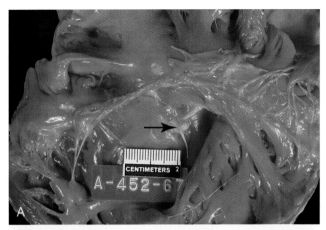

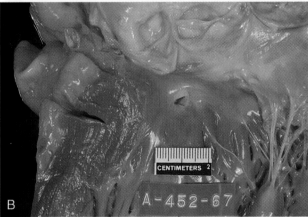

Figure 1-13 • Spontaneous closure of a small ventricular septal defect. Seen as a small septal aneurysm (arrow) in the right ventricular outflow tract (*A*) and from the left ventricle (*B*). Note the smooth-surfaced distal third of the septal wall in the outflow tract of the left ventricle. A 61-year-old male with 2:1 heart block who died of ventricular fibrillation. Scale indicates 2 cm.

the moderator band, and the anterior papillary muscle. The apex of the papillary muscle often points toward the commissure between the anterior and posterior tricuspid valve leaflets (see Fig. 1-11). The moderator band is not always as distinct in human hearts as in those of animals. The entire luminal surface of the right ventricle, with the exception of the septal and parietal bands and the posterior wall of the infundibulum above the crest (conus muscle), is coarsely trabeculated and, on section, the trabeculations form the inner two thirds or three fourths of the ventricular wall. Aberrant ventricular bands, usually muscular rather than fibrotic, are common in the distal part of the right ventricle and may be congenital or acquired.[154] The conus muscle separates the pulmonary valve ring from the aortic valve ring and is responsible for the higher position by approximately 1.5 cm of the former structure (see Fig. 1-16). Within this muscle is a variable fibrous attachment between the rings of the two semilunar valves; this is the conus ligament.

Ventricular septal defects or the sites of their patch repair may be seen proximal to, or, rarely, distal to the crest. If there are defects between the inflow portions of the ventricles, they will open among the trabeculations on

the interventricular septum.[152] Such defects may be multiple, small, and tortuous. Small ones often close spontaneously, being obliterated either by adherent tricuspid leaflet tissue or by endocardial proliferation about their edges; sometimes, small aneurysms result (Fig. 1-13).

Pulmonary Valve

The pulmonary valve[51, 81, 83, 86, 135, 142, 146, 155, 156] lies between the infundibulum and the pulmonary artery and is attached to the pulmonary annulus, which points posteriorly, superiorly, and to the left. Its ring circumference is 5.7 to 7.4 cm in women and 6.0 to 7.5 cm in men.[54] The pulmonary infundibulum winds across the anterior aspect of the aortic root, with the annulus approximately 1.5 cm higher than the aortic annulus (Figs. 1-12 and 1-14). The three cusps are named the anterior, the right (closest to the right coronary aortic cusp), and the left (closest to the left coronary aortic cusp). Figure 1-14 shows these relationships and that of the commissures between the right and the left cusps of each semilunar valve. The three pulmonary cusps have a U-type insertion, with the commissures inserting on the most distal part of the cylindrical fibrous pulmonary annulus; at midpoint, each is 1.5 to 2.0 cm tall. Rarely, there is a fourth pulmonary cusp, which is usually small and of no functional significance (Fig. 1-15); even more rarely, the pulmonary valve is bicuspid.[155] The pulmonary cusps demarcate shallow sinus pockets and are structurally similar to the aortic cusps, although they are more filmy and, like the aortic cusps, are often fenestrated in the lunulae (i.e., the part of the

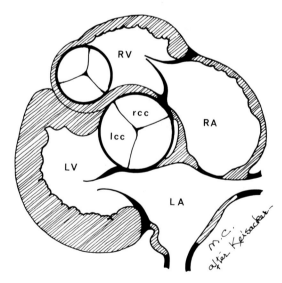

Figure 1-14 • Diagram of the heart valve rings seen from above. The pulmonary infundibulum of the right ventricle (RV) winds across the front of the aortic root, bringing the pulmonary annulus to a higher level (see Fig. 1-12); the conus muscle separates these two valve rings, whereas the tricuspid and mitral valve rings are in fibrous continuity (black areas) with the aortic annulus. The right atrium (RA) lies anterior to the left atrium (LA); the black area in the interatrial septum indicates the fibrous part of the septum primum within the fossa ovalis. The aortic and pulmonary cusps are named according to their relationship to the coronary ostia: right aortic coronary cusp (rcc), left aortic coronary cusp (lcc), noncoronary or posterior aortic cusp, right pulmonary cusp, left pulmonary cusp, and anterior pulmonary cusp. LV, left ventricle.

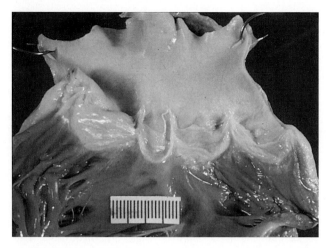

Figure 1-15 • Quadricuspid pulmonary valve is an incidental finding in a 63-year-old male who died of metastatic lung cancer. Scale indicates 2 cm.

valve between the line of closure and the free edge). Fibrocartilaginous nodules, named for both Morgagni and Arantius, are located centrally on the free edge of each cusp. They are larger than similar nodules on the aortic valve, but the linea alba, or line of closure, is barely visible (see Chapter 3).

Left Atrium

The left atrium,[51, 81, 83, 86, 129, 157] with a wall 0.3 cm in average thickness, lies posterior to both ventricles and to the right atrium and immediately anterior to the lower esophagus. The left side of the interatrial septum has the septum primum attached to the septum secundum by fibrous bands that radiate forward and upward on either side of the free edge of the septum primum; the latter forms a crescentic ridge, the valve of the foramen ovale if the septum is open (see Fig. 1-8). The remainder of the luminal surface of the left atrium is smooth, being derived from the absorbed primitive single pulmonary vein.

It shows the ostia of the four pulmonary veins and the base of the left atrial appendage. The latter structure has a narrow opening and divides into several lobules. It is lined by fine pectinate muscles like those in the right atrial appendage, but unlike the right atrium, the free wall of the left atrium lacks pectinate muscles. There may be tiny ostia of thebesian veins in the left atrium as there are in the right; the largest, the ostia of Lannelongue, are central in the wall. The endocardial lining of the left atrium is thicker and more opaque than that of the right atrium, in keeping with the higher pressure within the left side of the heart. A patch of thickened, rough endocardium on the posterior atrial wall just proximal to the mitral ring is a consequence of mitral regurgitation. Endocardial pockets may develop here, opening toward the regurgitant stream of blood.

Mitral Valve

The mitral valve[51, 81, 86, 147, 158–163] (Fig. 1-16) is based on a fibrous tissue ring that points anteriorly, inferiorly, and to the left (see Figs. 1-12 and 1-14). The valve's normal annular circumference is between 8.2 and 9.1 cm in women and 9.2 and 9.9 cm in men.[54] The two leaflets are joined by commissures almost as long as the posterior leaflet, so that the valvular tissue forms a continuous veil suspended from the ring. As with the tricuspid valve, the extent of each leaflet is defined by observing its chordal attachments. The commissures are tethered by fan-shaped chordae (see Fig. 1-16). The lateral spread of attachment of branches from these commissural chordae determines the lateral extent of the commissural areas; the branches of the posteromedial commissural chorda are larger and thicker and have a wider spread than do those of the anterolateral commissural chorda. In many, but not all hearts, the apices of the left ventricular papillary muscles point toward the commissures.

The anterior, or aortic, mitral leaflet has a variable degree of fibrous continuity with the aortic valve proximal to its noncoronary and left coronary cusps[164] (see Fig. 1-18). It is long (average 3 cm) and triangular, or

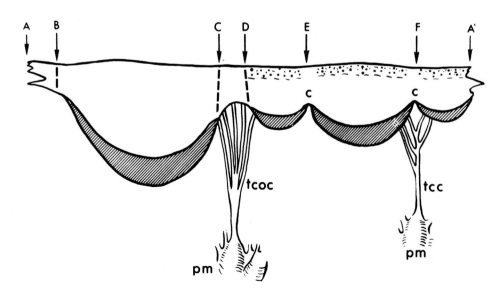

Figure 1-16 • Diagram of a mitral valve with typical commissural and cleft chordae tendineae attached. A-B, anterolateral commissure; B-C, anterior leaflet; C-D, posteromedial commissure; D-A', posterior leaflet; D-E, posteromedial commissural scallop; E-F, middle scallop; F-A', anterolateral commissural scallop; c, cleft; pm, papillary muscle; tcoc, typical commissural chorda; tcc, typical cleft chorda. Dotted area shows the basal zone; cross-hatching shows the rough zone. Intervening areas on the leaflets are the clear zones. (From Rangarathan N, Lam JHC, Wigle ED, Silver MD: Morphology of human mitral valve. II. The valve leaflets. Circulation 41:459, 1970.

almost square, having an average width of 3.3 cm at its base. A ridge on its atrial aspect, 0.8 to 1.0 cm from the free edge, defines the line of closure. The rough zone of chordal attachment on the ventricular surface lies between the line of closure and the free edge. The remaining valve tissue is a smooth membrane, clear on transillumination and devoid of chordal attachments. The leaflet hangs like a veil into the left ventricular cavity, dividing it into inflow and outflow portions; its ventricular surface forms part of the aortic vestibule.

The posterior mitral leaflet attaches to the parietal part of the mitral annulus; it is also called the mural leaflet. It is divided into scallops, usually three, by clefts defined by small fan-shaped cleft chordae. The leaflet has an average width of 4.8 cm, and the longest scallop, usually the middle one, has an average length of 1.3 cm. Unlike the anterior leaflet, the posterior leaflet has a basal zone of chordal attachment that is separated from the rough zone near the free edge by a narrow clear zone. The line of closure, located on the atrial surface of the leaflet, lies approximately 0.2 cm from the free edge.

In addition to the commissural and cleft chordae already described, there are basal chordae that originate directly from the trabeculae carneae and insert on the basal zone of the posterior leaflet. There are also rough zone chordae, with the two thickest and largest inserting into the anterior leaflet at the 4 and 8 o'clock positions; these are called strut chordae. Rough zone chordae tether the tips of each papillary muscle to the anterior mitral leaflet at its free margin, near its line of closure and between. The advantage of this chordal nomenclature[159, 160, 162] over the old terminology, which recognized first-, second-, and third-order chordae,[135, 146, 163] is not only in providing anatomic definition of the valve leaflets but also in allowing a better correlation of function with structure. Abnormal insertion of chordae into prolapsed mitral valves is documented.[165, 166] The chordae of the mitral valve vary in number, length, and thickness.[159] Except for the basal type, they arise from the two papillary muscles of the left ventricle; these are named the anterior, or anterolateral, and the posterior, or posteromedial muscles. They are of approximately equal size and are often double throughout or bifid at their tips, the posterior muscle showing subdivision into two or more columns more often than the anterior muscle.[161, 163] The papillary muscles have broad bases in the apical trabecular muscle, and their tips give attachment to chordae that tether the adjacent halves of each mitral leaflet; those chordae from the anterior papillary muscle attach to the anterior halves of each leaflet. "False" chordae, which do not insert into valve leaflets, are frequently seen, particularly passing between the posterior papillary muscle and the smooth part of the septum.[167, 168] They are also termed ventricular aberrant bands and are usually fibrotic rather than muscular; their attachment sites help distinguish congenital from acquired bands.[154]

Left Ventricle

The left ventricle[51, 81, 83, 86, 145, 150] forms part of the anterior surface and most of the left lateral surface of the heart. It is a symmetrical cone in cross section; one sixth is interventricular septum and five sixths is free wall. The inflow portion has finer and more numerous trabeculations than the right ventricle. They make up less than the inner one fourth of the wall; the outer three fourths is composed of compact muscle. The outflow portion has a smooth septal wall formed by the upper third of the interventricular septum anteriorly and to the right, and by the ventricular surface of the anterior mitral leaflet posteriorly and to the left (see Fig. 1-13B). Blood flowing through the left ventricle changes direction by nearly 180 degrees in passing the free edge of the anterior mitral leaflet (see Fig. 1-12). The inflow or sinus portion of the left ventricle contains two papillary muscles, described earlier; in a contracted heart, they abut on each other and on the interventricular septum to virtually obliterate the ventricular cavity. As in the right ventricle, "friction" lesions can develop between the chordae and the endocardium (see Fig. 3-2). In this ventricle, they are most often found on the endocardium related to the posterior mitral leaflet; in some instances, attachments form between the chordae and the endocardium. The smooth muscular interventricular septum bulges somewhat into the left ventricular outflow tract and may become more prominent with increasing age, producing a sigmoid septum (see Chapter 3).[104, 150, 169] This muscular septal bulge must be distinguished from that caused by idiopathic hypertrophic cardiomyopathy (see Chapter 10). The triangular membranous septum lies proximal to and between the noncoronary and right coronary cusps of the aortic valve and can be transilluminated. A ventricular septal defect may occur in the membranous septum but commonly involves the muscular septum immediately proximal and anterior to this region. Small muscular ventricular septal defects often heal spontaneously and may be marked by gray-white endocardial dimples or small septal aneurysms (Fig. 1-13A and B). An unusually large membranous septum may be seen in persons with Down syndrome. If the aortic valve is incompetent, endocardial thickenings, which often resemble pockets opening toward regurgitant blood jet streams, may be apparent proximal to the aortic valve, either on the septal wall (Fig. 1-17) or on the ventricular surface of the anterior mitral leaflet. If there is a history of recent cardiac ischemia, heart slices may be incubated in nitro-blue tetrazolium or 2,3,5 triphenyl tetraxolium chloride[170] to demonstrate lesions (see Table 1-1).

Aortic Valve

The aortic valve,[51, 83, 86, 107, 123, 142, 146, 156, 171–174] lies between the left ventricular outflow tract and the aorta. Its normal annular circumference is 5.7 to 7.9 cm in women and 6.0 to 8.5 cm in men.[54] The valve ring points posteriorly, superiorly, and to the right (see Fig. 1-12). It is a fibrous cylinder that gives a U-shaped attachment to the valve cusps with the commissures of related cusps attached distally on the annulus. The valve may have one cusp; bicuspid aortic valves are relatively common and may lead to calcific aortic stenosis (see Chapter 13); four or five cusps have been seen occasionally.[171] Even when there are three cusps, they may be unequal in size, either

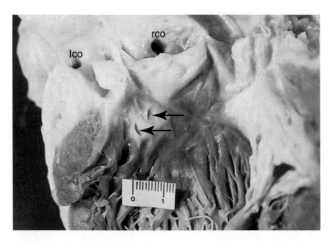

Figure 1-17 • Endocardial "jet lesions" (arrows) forming pockets of endocardial scarring on the muscular septum of the left ventricle in a patient with healed aortic rheumatic disease and aortic valve regurgitation. Left (lco) and right (rco) coronary artery ostia are defined. (Courtesy of E.M. Davies, MD, London, Ontario, Canada.)

in width or length. In some instances, this leads to calcific aortic stenosis.[172] The aortic and mitral valve rings are fused (intervalvular fibrosa) over the length of attachment of the anterior mitral leaflet, the latter of which has a variable degree of fibrous continuity with the adjacent halves of the noncoronary and left coronary aortic cusps (Fig. 1-18).[164] The noncoronary cusp is posterior in position, and the right and left coronary cusps are anterior (see Fig. 1-18).

The three semilunar cusps have well-marked nodules at the center of their free edge. A white ridge, the linea alba, that marks the line of closure is seen on their ventricular aspect just proximal to the free edge. The cusps, which are 1.5 to 2.2 cm tall at their midpoints, are filmy and commonly fenestrated, particularly close to their commissures and between the linea alba and the free edge (i.e., in the lunulae) (see Fig. 3-4). The nodules (of Arantius or Morgagni) at the center of the free edge of each cusp are somewhat triangular and fill the three-cornered defect that would occur in their absence when cusps are in the closed position. Lambl's excrescences are common on the nodules and along the line of closure (see Ch. 19).

The sinus (of Valsalva) of each aortic cusp is the pocket enclosed by the cusp attachment proximally and a ridge encircling the aortic lining at the level of the commissures. The sinus portion of the aorta or bulb of the aorta is 1.5 times wider than the proximal tubular ascending aorta, but this is better appreciated in angiograms taken during life than in the opened heart at necropsy. As mentioned previously (see Right Atrium), the right coronary aortic sinus is closely related to the right atrial septal wall (see Fig. 1-14).[142, 175] Mechanisms of valve closure are discussed in Chapter 13.

The coronary ostia may be quite variable in number, position, and size. The mean diameter of the right vessel is 0.32 cm, and of the left, 0.40 cm. They are usually single, centrally located within the wall of the sinus of Valsalva, and approximately equal in size.[38, 176] If unequal, the left is more often larger, but the right is more commonly double, with one ostium, usually a conal artery, for its first branch.

Normal variations of coronary ostia are distinguished from anomalies (e.g., both the left anterior descending artery and the circumflex coronary artery arising from the same coronary sinus.)[125] Nevertheless, a solitary coronary ostium, an acute angulation, or an intussusception of ostia may be associated with sudden death[177-179] (see Chapter 11).

Coronary Blood Vessels

The coronary arteries[38, 51, 73, 81, 83, 86, 125, 178, 180, 181] form a ring, or crown, as they course in the atrioventricular or coronary groove, giving off branches to the atria and the ventricles (Fig. 1-19). The right half of the ring is formed by the right coronary artery, which usually reaches the crux of the heart and then turns abruptly toward the heart's apex to become the posterior descending coronary artery. It usually gives origin to a penetrating artery that supplies the atrioventricular node at a U-bend along its course.[73, 125] Again, the sinoatrial node is supplied by the right coronary artery more frequently than by the left.[182] The left half of the ring is formed by the circumflex branch of the left coronary artery, which leaves the parent vessel at a right angle, where it becomes the (left) anterior descending coronary artery. The latter descends into the epicardium anterior to the interventricular septum, supplying branches to the anterior part of both ventricles and to the anterior septum. At the acute border of the heart, at the notch between the apices of the two ventricles, it usually continues onto the heart's inferior surface for a short distance.

Coronary veins follow the course of the arteries. They are more superficial in the epicardial fat and eventually join the coronary sinus, which passes from left to right in the posterior atrioventricular sulcus to open into the posterior wall of the right atrium just anterior to the inferior vena cava. Some small (accessory) coronary veins drain the free wall of the right ventricle and open directly into the anterior wall of the right atrium. The smallest veins

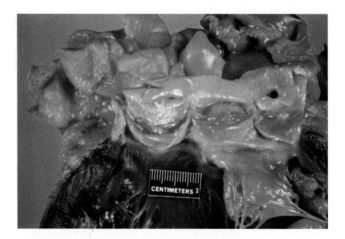

Figure 1-18 • Outflow tract of the left ventricle, the aortic valve, and the proximal ascending aorta. The right coronary cusp is on the left side of the photograph, the posterior or noncoronary cusp is in the middle, and the left coronary cusp is on the right. Note that the anterior mitral valve leaflet has fibrous continuity with the noncoronary right half of the left coronary cusp.

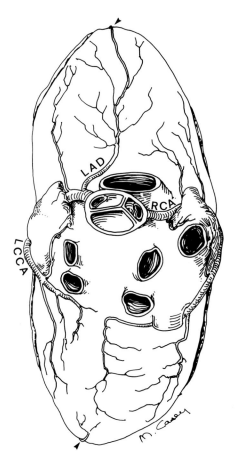

Figure 1-19 • Drawing of the coronary circulation as viewed when the ventricles are bivalved. The right (RCA) and left circumflex coronary arteries (LCCA) form a ring in the atrioventricular edge of the interventricular septum, round the apex of the heart at the cardiac notch (arrowhead), and ascend along the posterior edge (see also Fig. 1-2). Abbreviation: LAD, left anterior descending (artery).

are those of the thebesian, or luminal, system that form within the myocardium and drain directly into each of the heart chambers.[135, 141] They are remnants of sinusoidal intramyocardial blood vessels present in the embryonic heart, at the stage of the spongy myocardium.

The coronary blood vessels are also discussed in Chapter 8. A cardiac lymphatic system has been well described.[183, 184]

Cardiac Skeleton

To understand relationships between the heart chambers and the valves, one must study the fibrous cardiac skeleton.[81, 83, 85, 86, 135, 144, 154] Few have reconstructed the cardiac skeleton from serial sections or demonstrated it by dissection, but it is seen in many histologic sections; for example, in the valve rings and the atrioventricular node. It supports all valve cusps and leaflets, has the atrioventricular conduction system passing through it, and provides attachment for the cardiac muscle fibers. When viewed from above (see Fig. 1-14), the conal muscle is seen to separate the pulmonary valve ring from the aortic valve ring. The rings are joined, however, by a conal ligament that is variably developed in human hearts.

Microscopically, one may see fibrocartilage, or pseudo-cartilage, in the right fibrous trigone, where it is penetrated by the bundle of His, especially in the newborn. The right trigone region may become ossified in man as is common in some animals. This central fibrous body is continuous with the membranous septum and forms part of the interatrial septum, the atrioventricular septum, and the right wall of the aorta. It may truly be called the core of the heart. The valve rings in the right side of the heart are thinner than those in the left, and both atrioventricular rings are thinner laterally than in their medial regions, where they fuse together with the aortic valve ring and the membranous septum. Calcification occurs in aortic tissue, particularly in mitral annular fibrous tissue (see Chapter 3). A plain radiogram of the postmortem heart wall helps to define its extent.

Cardiac Innervation

The nerve supply to the heart is autonomic, including both a sympathetic and a parasympathetic supply via both efferent and afferent fibers.[74, 81, 84, 185-187] It is conveyed to the cardiac plexus in branches from the vagus and phrenic nerves and also from the cervical and thoracic cardiac nerves. The cardiac plexus is a group of nerve ganglia located between the arch of the aorta and the bifurcation of the trachea. The largest ganglion, that of Wrisberg, lies below the arch of the aorta. Nerve ganglia are seen frequently in microscopic sections of the subendocardial muscle of the right atrium, particularly in the interatrial septum and in the epicardium near the roots of the great vessels. Both sympathetic and parasympathetic nerves supply the sinoatrial and atrioventricular nodes. Newer immunohistochemical and enzyme histochemical techniques can distinquish nerve subpopulations and cellular electrophysiology of the conducting system.[188, 189] A report by Marron and colleagues discussed the innervation of atrioventricular and semilunar valves.[190]

Histology of the Heart

This topic is fully discussed in Chapter 2.

The correct choice of histologic blocks for microscopic section depends on the presence of lesions found by gross examination. If a heart is not needed as an anatomic specimen and no lesions are observed, we believe transverse sections across the midregions of the anterior and posterior papillary muscles, including the adjacent left ventricular wall, suffice. These sections are most likely to demonstrate acute myocardial damage. If cardiac lesions are observed, we institute a wider examination, collecting six or seven histologic blocks and adding to them sections from lesions. These blocks include one from each valve ring with the ventricular myocardium and the adjoining atrial myocardium, or great vessel. These atrioventricular blocks include the coronary vessels in the atrioventricular grooves. They are best taken from the edges of incisions used to open the heart and should be precisely vertical to the valve rings. In addition, routine transverse blocks of left ventricular myocardium should be collected at the level where papillary muscles take origin (i.e., between the apical and middle thirds of the ventricular wall) and should include the papillary muscle. In an adult, a block should be taken from the septum at the same level. A right ventricular myocardial block cut transversely across the midpart of the anterior papillary muscle and adjacent free wall may be useful. All of the nonatrioventrcular blocks are taken conveniently from a single transverse ventricular slice. In cases of myocarditis and cardiomyopathy, additional sections should be taken from the atria, for example, transversely across the atrial appendages. We have mentioned previously the case for embedding the whole coronary artery system.

On occasion, whole-mount sections of a transverse ventricular block or a block placed radial to an atrioventricular ring and extending to the apex of the ventricle may be of value for morphometry of lesions or for teaching purposes. In newborn and fetal hearts, transverse ventricular slices fit on normal microslides or on 2-inch-square, whole-mount slides suitable for 35-mm projection.

Examination of standard heart blocks, as described earlier, enables a pathologist to acquire an understanding of the normal variations in histology. Occasionally, the conduction system is examined histologically (see Chapter 20 for details). In our opinion, this procedure does not often yield results unless the documented conducting system abnormality was permanent rather than transitory.

Stains that are used in microscopy of the heart are hematoxylin and eosin, a connective tissue stain; a combination of Masson's trichrome and Verhoeff's elastic stain is most useful. The ideal stain for heart valves is the Movat pentachrome[191] because it differentiates between muscle, collagen, elastin, and ground substance. Quantitative results should be used in reporting histologic findings. They can be presented as a grade of change or by direct morphometric measurement.

EXAMINATION OF CARDIOVASCULAR SPECIMENS IN SURGICAL PATHOLOGY

The nature of surgical pathology specimens taken from cardiovascular cases has also changed markedly in recent years as a result of more aggressive treatment; also, because of the greater use of plastic and reconstructive procedures to improve postoperative function, surgeons may conserve valvular tissue and papillary muscles rather than totally excising them. Moreover, many prosthetic devices have been introduced while endomyocardial biopsy and heart transplantation have become accepted modes of diagnosis and therapy, respectively. The processing of these specimens in surgical pathology is considered under a series of headings, and then the handling of particular specimens is discussed.

Practical Considerations

General

When handling specimens, a pathologist always practices universal safety precautions.[192] Appropriate protective clothing and items should be worn. No tissue, even fixed material, should ever be handled with bare hands. It must be kept in mind that noxious agents are present in the laboratory. They must be treated with respect and appropriate precautions. Pathologists are not immune to illness. Formaldehyde solution soon irritates nasal mucosa, making its presence known, but long exposure can lead to debilitating corneal ulceration, respiratory problems, dermatitis, or other pathology. Other agents are flammable and still others toxic. Potential untoward actions must be recognized and prevented. Knowledge of safety regulations is essential, and the location of safety features in the laboratory should be known by all. It is especially important to be cognizant of the procedures to be followed by individuals and staff if a toxic spill occurs or a fire starts. The significance of various hospital alarms must be understood, and expected responses to them must be known. Escape routes must be memorized.

A pathologist must know when to consult colleagues in the field, when to participate in quality assurance exercises, and how to ensure correct data collection for departmental and hospital statistics and potential research endeavors. Keeping current with the literature and continuing education are important activities. Pathologists teach, regardless of the type of hospital where they practice, so it is vital that they understand effective pedagogic methods and the best ways of presenting data.

Receipt/Accession of Specimens

Specimens, irrespective of their nature, are received with a consultation request bearing details about the patient as well as brief clinical data. All this information is vital and is incorporated into the final pathology report. Surgeons should know that they will not receive a final pathology report or that it will be delayed unless this information is provided. The pathologist must ensure that specimen containers are correctly labeled and must not accept tissue from more than one anatomic site in a container. Errors at this stage are best dealt with by returning both the consultation request and the containers to the operating room for correction. The tissue is usually in a fixative solution and is given a laboratory accession number; correct identification must be maintained at all subsequent stages of the process. However, in some cases, before collection is made, and in many others, before dissection and blocking for histology are performed, the pathologist must consider the need for any other action. For example, should an individual specimen be collected fresh or should it be placed in a special fixative? Is it appropriate to photograph a specimen for a subsequent teaching session or presentation at rounds? Edwards[77] provides guidance for this type of activity. Good-quality 35-mm color photographs can supply black and white negatives for prints, but some pathologists prefer separate color and black and white photographs if the latter are to be published. A radiographic examination can determine the degree of calcification in the cusps and leaflets of natural or prosthetic heart valves and help identify the latter. Also, radiography can locate stents or other prostheses in vessels or coronary arteries of excised hearts. Microbiologic examinations or use of electron microscopy may be indicated, and frozen tissue is required for some examinations.

Gross Examination

Economically responsible practice is good practice. Therefore, consideration must be given as to whether to perform histologic sections on all specimens. For medicolegal purposes, pathologists must practice according to the norms established in their communities. In other words, if all cardiovascular pathologists in a city or region submit every specimen for histology, it would be prudent to do so. On the other hand, city-wide or regional groups may decide, after consideration, that it is appropriate to omit some histologic examinations. If they establish guidelines for the examinations to be performed, it is appropriate to use them. For example, some groups do not perform routine histologic examinations of heart valves, varicose veins, thrombus removed from the lumen of an aneurysm, and so forth. Nevertheless, as a consultant, the pathologist must make case-by-case decisions. For our part, if we are fully satisfied, for example, that no vascular wall adheres to an excised luminal thrombus taken from an abdominal aneurysm, we settle for a gross description. However, if the thrombus has vessel wall attached to it, we do a histologic examination, because added information could help establish the type of aneurysm that contained the thrombus. Again, we do not often examine excised natural heart valves histologically. Nevertheless, if there is any unusual abnormality or deposit in or on the tissue, we always section it. In such a case, use of a strong magnifying glass in examination is essential. If gross examination alone is performed, this point should be noted in a rider added to the report. The rider should indicate that the specimen has been subjected to gross examination only, with no histologic sections made. The surgeon or physician should be advised that the specimen will be saved for a month. If the clinician believes there is reason to examine the specimen histologically, he or she should, within the month, contact the pathologist who signed the report. If the preceding statements seem heretical, a practitioner's conscience may be salved by taking histologic sections and blocking, but not sectioning, them. In our view, specialist societies should take a lead in defining acceptable practice in this area.

Cleanliness at the workbench when making gross descriptions is essential, to prevent contamination of the area and to prevent the spread of contamination from one case to another. Copious use of water and handling each specimen on a new paper towel help to maintain a clean working environment. No more than one specimen container should be open at a time.

In examination, the description must be exact and detailed. The pathologist may be aided, in part, by points defined by Bailey & Love[193] and used clinically to describe an ulcer. Thus, the description must include information about the source of the specimen, the number and size of fragments included in the container with its/their measurements and (if appropriate) weight, and its/their shape, surface, edge, color, consistency, and relationships. Even though photographs are better, diagrams may aid

the description and localize the sites of subsequent histologic sampling.

Histologic sampling must be representative. In some instances, all of a specimen, especially if it is small, is embedded, with that fact noted in the report. Very small specimens may be wrapped in tissue paper and stained grossly with 10% eosin to help identification when the paper is unwrapped. Tissue blocks must be no thicker than 3 mm and should not overfill the cassette in which they are placed. Histopathology technicians cannot be expected to deliver good sections if the material supplied to them is less than ideal. Tissue should always be decalcified if the cutting knife grates in passage; rapid decalcification does not delay processing. Only rarely, when calcification is very extensive (e.g., calcification that affects the posterior mitral annulus), need processing be prolonged and done before sections are cut. Metal staples should be removed from blocks. Also, if blocks must include suture, cloth, or other unusual material, the histopathology laboratory should be advised of their presence. Processing may be completed overnight or by more rapid methods.

Of the routine stains available, we use hematoxylin and eosin (H&E). We find a combined Verhoeff elastic–Masson trichrome stain and Movat stain the most useful ancillary ones. The former helps to define layers in vessel walls or other cardiovascular tissues, permitting orientation, whereas the latter is invaluable in demonstrating proteoglycans. It is unwise to rely solely on one or the other of these to the exclusion of H&E. For example, *medionecrosis* may be suspected because of the condensation of elastic lamellae in connective tissue stains, but only H&E allows true definition. In examining cardiovascular lesions, a pathologist employs the full barrage of other histochemical, immunohistochemical, and molecular diagnostic techniques available and may employ morphometry or other techniques in examination.

For some specimens, protocol examinations and "canned" diagnoses may be appropriate. Protocol examinations help to teach residents, to ensure consistency, and to allow technicians to deal with some specimens, whereas canned diagnoses speed report preparation. Again, time can be saved by predetermining the type of special stains that are required for certain gross findings and by ordering stains when blocks are submitted.

Reporting

Whether the pathologist supplies both gross and microscopic descriptions with diagnosis in a report or, as we prefer, a gross description with a diagnosis, depends on local practice. In either instance, an explanatory comment relating clinical and pathologic findings is often pertinent.

When the pathologist dictates reports, it is appropriate to establish both the patient's name and surgical accession number. Use of short sentences is best, with avoidance of traditional yet nonsensical duplications, such as, "yellow *in color*" or "*measures* 2x4x5 cm." A typed report, whether on screen or on paper, should always be read, both to correct typographic errors and to shorten it. If a report is unnecessarily long, the pathologist's or the secretary's time is wasted in preparing it, and time is wasted in reading it. Only rarely can a report not be shortened, even if it is dictated by an experienced pathologist. Ultimately, the pathologist is responsible for the report. If the report is not prepared carefully, the pathologist may be embarrassed in court or on another occasion if typographic errors or other inconsistencies are drawn to his or her attention.

Handling Particular Specimens

In discussing the handling of particular groups of cardiovascular specimens, no mention is made in this chapter of the various devices used to treat or ameliorate cardiovascular disease, or of native or donor hearts from patients who have received a transplant, or of endomyocardial biopsies. That information is presented in Chapters 21 to 23.

Vascular Structures

Because all organs have blood vessels, there may be some desire on the part of a renal pathologist to see kidney vessels, and on the part of a neuropathologist to examine temporal artery biopsies. Interestingly, few seem delighted to examine amputation specimens from patients with peripheral vascular disease, even though these specimens often provide fascinating histopathology. At individual centers, a satisfactory modus vivendi must be decided upon by colleagues. Our arrangements produce healthy interaction with frequent consultation. We embed all of a temporal artery biopsy, process it rapidly, and make sections at several levels through the block, reporting on H&E sections. These and endomyocardial biopsies are the only ones in which rapid processing is employed, so that reporting can be done the same day. Luminal contents may be received separately or included with vascular tissue. If received separately, the thrombus/clot is weighed, and, if it is included with vascular tissue, a record is made of whether the material is mural and whether it stenoses the lumen or occludes it. Formaldehyde fixation changes the color of clots and thrombi. Information is needed about intimal lesions and those that are located in the vessel wall and its adventitia. For example, measuring the aortic wall thickness, which is normally 2 to 3 mm, may indicate whether all is present or whether the specimen is from a dissecting aneurysm. We embed all of an endarterectomy, irrespective of its length or source, as well as the full length of arteries recovered from amputation specimens removed for peripheral vascular disease. The reason is that vascular pathology may change along a specimen's length. Many transverse sections can be included in a single cassette. Incidentally, because of religious beliefs, some patients seek to bury amputated limbs after examination. A means of satisfying their requests must be available. As indicated earlier, connective tissue stains are de rigueur, to help define wall components and aid interpretation. When histologic examination of luminal contents is performed, it must always be kept in mind that there is a possibilty of an embolism of one type or another. Signs of infection and atheromatous or tumorous embolisms must be investigated.

Native Heart Valves

Mitral and aortic valve components are received most frequently. Their leaflets and cusps are usually orientated easily by defining the chordae tendineae of atrioventricular valves or the semilunar lines of closure, and the corpus Arantius of the semilunar valves. Correct anatomic location of the anterior and posterior mitral leaflets and those of the tricuspid valve is often possible, especially if they are intact, by defining strut chordae attached to the anterior mitral leaflet and the scallops of the posterior leaflet, but such localization is virtually impossible with the semilunar valve cusps. Intact valves also allow description of commissural areas, and their correct anatomic location is important. In our view, the term *commissural fusion* is a misnomer, indicating, as it does, *fusion of adjacent sides of leaflets/cusps at a commissural area.* Nevertheless, we use the term in this sense. In some cases, luminal diameter may be determined by graded cones. The appearance of the free margin and both the flow and nonflow surfaces of leaflets/cusps must be described. Thickening of the free margin of a semilunar cusp may indicate valvular regurgitation, whereas examination of the inflow surface of an atrioventricular leaflet may allow comment as to whether it bulged toward the left atrium. Radiographic examination allows quantification of calcification.

When atrioventricular valves that are not attached to papillary muscles are evaluated, a magnifying glass should be used for careful examination of the ends of the chordae tendineae. Most of those cut by a surgeon's knife have clean, square-cut or angled ends. Depending upon the timing of the event before the examination, ruptured chordae tendineae, which are most commonly located on mitral valves, are usually shortened and have an elongated, whisker-like appearance or a frayed end, whereas others have a tiny knob of thrombus or connective tissue expanding the free end, and still others may recurve to reattach to the nonflowing surface of the leaflet. A chorda that is avulsed from a papillary muscle presents its full length with a tiny lump of tissue attached to it. If rupture or avulsion is suspected, that chorda should be separated from the specimen, embedded individually, and sectioned at multiple levels through the block. This demonstrates pathologic changes needed to confirm suspicion; the examination increases the yield of ruptured chordae. Movat stain indicates that most ruptures are associated with myxomatous changes in the valve and the chordae. If papillary muscle tissue is attached to leaflets, it must always be examined histologically to determine whether it is ruptured, infarcted, or atrophic. If it is ruptured, attached chordae may be twisted about the long axis of the muscle. We always section such tissue in its long axis. With increasing age, the apices of left ventricular papillary muscles fibrose, with tiny foci of calcification in the scar (see Chapter 3).

Of the semilunar valves, the aortic valve is received most frequently. An examiner must determine the number of cusps present and the pathologic changes that they display. See Chapters 13 and 14 for more details. Any vegetation attached to a valve must be sectioned and assumed to be infected until proved otherwise. If no previous microbiologic studies have been done, part of a vegetation should be sent for examination from the surgical pathology suite. A native valve may appear normal on external examination yet be excised because there is functional regurgitation or because changes beyond the valve caused dysfunction.

Myocardium

Tissue that is received ranges in size from an endomyocardial biopsy (see Chapter 23) to large blocks from left ventricular aneurysms. Tissue recovered from a left ventricular outflow tract myotomy must always be cut transversely to the endocardial surface. This may increase the probability of diagnosing hypertrophic cardiomyopathy. A connective tissue stain is required if the endocardium is thickened or the ventricular wall is markedly thinned. This stain determines, in the first instance, the nature of the thickening, and in the latter instance, layers in the ventricular wall. Contraction band change is a common histologic artifact at the edges of tissue cut from living myocardium (see Chapter 8). Myocarditis is discussed in Chapter 9.

Pericardium

Pericardial tissue is usually dealt with easily but may be heavily calcified. In trying to determine the cause of pericarditis, it is better to see H&E sections before ordering special stains that may define pathogenesis. A flamboyant proliferation of mesothelial cells may make differential diagnosis from malignant cells perplexing (see Chapter 12).

Endocardium

It is unusual to receive endocardium except as part of an endomyocardial biopsy (EMB). Connective tissue stains are vital in its examination.

Endomyocardial Biopsy

The endomyocardial biopsy (EMB) is an important adjunct to clinical practice and research endeavors. Biopsies are usually obtained from the septal wall of a ventricle, and although they may be collected from the left ventricle during other diagnostic procedures, they much more frequently have their origin from the right ventricle, with a bioptome introduced through the right internal jugular vein either during a concomitant cardiac catheterization or as an outpatient procedure.

EMBs are used for diagnostic purposes in cases of congenital and acquired heart diseases and in pediatric and adult practices. They are particularly employed in diagnosing myocarditis (see Chapter 9), cardiomyopathies (see Chapter 11), and storage diseases (see Chapter 16). EMBs are also used to monitor drug therapy (see Chapter 17 and especially cardiac rejection (see Chapter 23). Nevertheless, EMBs have other uses. Tissue fragments can be studied with use of any of the ancillary techniques mentioned earlier and applied to other tissue specimens.

In Chapter 23, which discusses cardiac transplantation, Winters and Schoen provide exact details regarding the limitations of EMB, the size of biopsies, methods of processing them, common findings and artifacts encountered, interpretation of diffuse and focal diseases, and complications of the biopsy procedure. They emphasize that fewer than three fragments, or those consisting predominantly of blood clot and endothelial cells or fat, should be regarded as unsatisfactory for diagnosis if not prohibiting descriptive findings. The latter, in either a satisfactory EMB, or one that is unsatisfactory but includes some myocardium, should present a systematic evaluation. For example, myocardial architecture should be considered before details are provided about myocardial cell size, cellular contents and components, interstitium, blood vessels, nerves, and endocardium. In general, the finding of hypertrophied myocardial cells implies that a process has been active for a long time, whereas normal-sized fibers may indicate a process of rapid onset. Even without a definitive diagnosis, a full description of findings may help a clinician. Again, a definitive diagnosis may not be possible because of nonspecific findings, especially in cases of congestive cardiomyopathy, but the pathologist describing them may comment that although they are not specific, they are compatible with a particular diagnosis.

In dealing with biopsies from cases of suspected cardiomyopathy, we employ a barrage of histologic stains, including a connective tissue stain and others for iron, amyloid, and glycogen. Electron microscopy is employed if a distinct diagnosis cannot be made by light microscopy or if the latter findings require further study. We urge the use of electron microscopy in all cases of restrictive cardiomyopathy, because, in the past, the diagnosis of amyloid was sometimes missed because light microscopy stains were not diagnostic. There may be sufficient biopsy fragments to embed for electron microscopic examination immediately after they are collected, but if taken in a universal fixative, fragments may be recovered and satisfactorily processed for electron microscopy from a paraffin block. Alternatively, unstained/destained histologic slides may be used.

Tumor and Tumor-like Conditions

A pathologist may be asked to examine a frozen section. Cardiac and vascular tumors are not common and usually present no difficulty in diagnosis. Resection margins are as important as they are in the excision of any other tumor. Because tumor-like conditions in small blood vessels sometimes give trouble in diagnosis, consultation with the local soft tissue expert at a cancer hospital may be appropriate.

Limbs Excised for Peripheral Vascular Disease

A report must include a description of the type of amputation, appropriate measurements of leg and foot, details of previous surgical sites, and current areas of necrosis or gangrene. If possible, it is appropriate to indicate the race of the patient from whom the specimen was removed. We collect specimens from the proximal resection margin and the site of any area of necrosis. Stains for microorganism are important. We excise the vascular system intact, noting any anastomoses or other surgical procedures. We serially section vessels and embed them totally. In reporting, we note the source of the specimen and give general diagnoses (e.g., atherosclerosis of peripheral arteries with locally severe stenosis); we provide specific diagnoses if particular vessels are occluded or thrombosed. Examination of an appropriate number of both large and small vessels is important if atheromatous emboli are to be recognized frequently.

REFERENCES

1. Gross RE, Hubbard JP: Surgical ligation of a patent ductus arteriosus: Report of first successful case. JAMA 112:729, 1939
2. Rashkind WJ, Cuaso CC: Transcatheter closure of patent ductus arteriosus. Successful use in a 3.5 kilogram infant. Pediatr Cardiol 1:3, 1979
3. Mullins CE: Pediatric and congenital therapeutic cardiac catheterization. Circulation 77:1153, 1989
4. Rowlatt UF, Rimaidi MJA, Lev J: The quantitative anatomy of the normal child's heart. Pediatr Clin North Am 10:499, 1963
5. Tajik AJ, Seward JB, Hagler DJ, et al: Two-dimensional real-time ultrasonic imaging of the heart and great vessels. Technique, image orientation, structure, identification and validation. Mayo Clin Proc 53:271, 1978
6. Edwards WD, Tajik AJ, Seward JB: Standardized nomenclature and anatomic basis for regional tomographic analysis of the heart. Mayo Clin Proc 56:479, 1981
7. Isner JM, Donaldson RF: Coronary angiographic and morphologic correlation. Cardiol Clin 2:571, 1984
8. Tamiya T, Yamashiro T, Matsumoto T, et al: A histological study of surgical landmarks for the specialized atrioventricular conduction system, with particular reference to the papillary muscle. Ann Thorac Surg 40:599, 1985
9. Thomas AC, Davies MJ, Dilly S, et al: Potential errors in the estimation of coronary arterial stenosis from clinical arteriography with reference to the shape of the coronary arterial lumen. Br Heart J 55:129, 1986
10. Alvarez L, Ardnega A, Saucedo R, Contreras JA: The quantitative anatomy of the normal human heart in fetal and perinatal life. Int J Cardiol 17:57, 1987
11. Rosenberg MC, Klein LW, Agarwal JB, et al: Quantification of absolute luminal diameter by computer-analyzed digital subtraction angiography: An assessment in human coronary arteries. Circulation 77:484, 1988
12. Sharif DS, Huhta JC, Marantz P, et al: Two-dimensional echocardiographic determination of ventricular septal defect size: Correlation with autopsy. Am Heart J 117:1333, 1989
13. Johnson DE, Alderman EL, Schroeder JS, et al: Transplant coronary artery disease: Histopathologic correlations with angiographic morphology. J Am Coll Cardiol 17:449, 1991
14. Siegel RJ, Ariani M, Fishbein MC, et al: Histopathologic validation of angioscopy and intravascular ultrasound. Circulation 84:109, 1991
15. Coy KM, Park JC, Fishbein MC, et al: In vitro validation of three-dimensional intravascular ultrasound for the evaluation of arterial injury after balloon angioplasty. J Am Coll Cardiol 20:692, 1992
16. Oberhoffer R, Cook AC, Lang D, et al: Correlation between echocardiographic and morphological investigations of lesions of the tricuspid valve diagnosed during fetal life. Br Heart J 68:580, 1992
17. Delbeke D, Lorenz CH, Votaw JR, et al: Estimation of left ventricular mass and infarct size from nitrogen-13-ammonia PET images based on pathological examination of explanted human hearts. J Nucl Med 34:826, 1993
18. Haese J, Slager CJ, Keane D, et al: Quantification of intracoronary volume by videodensitometry: Validation study using fluid filling of coronary casts. Cathet Cardiovasc Diagn 33:89, 1994
19. Matar FA, Mintz GS, Douek P, et al: Coronary artery lumen volume measurement using three-dimensional intravascular ultrasound: Validation of a new technique. Cathet Cardiovasc Diagn 33:214, 1994
20. Vogel M, Ho SY, Lincoln C, et al: Three-dimensional echocardiography can simulate intraoperative visualization of congenitally malformed hearts. Ann Thorac Surg 60:1282, 1995
21. Mann JM, Davies MJ: Assessment of the severity of coronary artery disease at postmortem examination. Are the measurements clinically valid? Br Heart J 74:528, 1995
22. Braunwald E (ed): Heart Disease A Textbook of Cardiovascular Medicine. 5th ed. WB Saunders Co, Philadelphia, 1997
23. Belohlavek M, Foley DA, Gerber TC, et al: Three-dimensional ultrasound imaging of the atrial septum: Normal and pathologic anatomy. J Am Coll Cardiol 22:1273, 1993
24. Wang X-F, Li Z-A, Cheng TO, et al: Four-dimensional echocardiography: Methods and clinical application. Am Heart J 132:672, 1996
25. Skorton DJ, Brundage BH, Schelbert HR, Wolf GL: Relative merits of imaging techniques. In: Braunwald E (ed): Heart Disease. A Textbook in Cardiovascular Medicine. 5th ed. WB Saunders, Philadelphia, 1997, p 349
26. Hoff SJ, Stewart JR, Frist W, et al: Noninvasive detection of acute rejection in a new experimental model of heart transplantation. Ann Thorac Surg 56:1074, 1993
27. van der Wall EE, Vliegen HW, de Roos A, Bruschke AV: Magnetic resonance imaging in coronary artery disease. Circulation 92:2723, 1995
28. Taylor AM, Pennell DJ: Recent advances in cardiac magnetic resonance imaging. Curr Opin Cardiol 11:635, 1996
29. Thomas AC, Davies MJ: The demonstration of cardiac pathology using perfusion-fixation. Histopathology 9:5, 1985
30. Ackerman DM, Edwards WD: Anatomic basis for tomographic analysis of the pediatric heart at autopsy. Perspect Pediatr Pathol 12:44, 1988
31. Waller BF, Taliercio CP, Slack JD, et al: Tomographic views of normal and abnormal hearts: The anatomic basis for various cardiac imaging techniques. Part I. Clin Cardiol 13: 804, 1990
32. Vogel M, Ho SY, Anderson RH: Comparison of three dimensional echocardiographic findings with anatomical specimens of various congenitally malformed hearts. Br Heart J 73:566, 1995
33. Schoen FJ: Interventional and Surgical Cardiovascular Pathology: Clinical Correlations and Basic Principles. Philadelphia, WB Saunders, 1989
34. Lichtig C, Glagov S, Feldman S, Wissler RW: Myocardial ischemia and coronary artery atherosclerosis. A comprehensive approach to postmortem studies. Med Clin North Am 57:79, 1973
35. Russell GA, Berry PJ: Post mortem radiology in children with congenital heart disease. J Clin Pathol 41:830, 1988
36. Robbins SL, Fish SJ: A new angiographic technic providing a simultaneous permanent cast of the coronary arterial lumen. Am J Clin Pathol 42:156, 1964
37. Robbins SL, Solomon M, Bennett A: Demonstration of intercoronary anastomoses in human hearts with a low viscosity perfusion mass. Circulation 33:733, 1966
38. Baroldi G, Scomazzani G: Coronary Circulation in the Normal and Pathologic Heart. Washington, D.C., Armed Forces Institute of Pathology, 1967
39. Rodriquez FL, Robbins SL: Post mortem angiographic studies on the coronary arterial circulation. Intercoronary arterial anastomoses in adult human hearts. Am Heart J 70:348, 1965
40. Suberman CO, Suberman RI, Dalldorf FG, Gabriele OF: Radiographic visualization of coronary arteries in postmortem hearts. A simple technique. Am J Clin Pathol 53:254, 1970
41. Hutchins GM, Bulkley BH, Ridolfi RL, et al: Correlation of coronary arteriograms and left ventriculograms with postmortem studies. Circulation 56: 32, 1977
42. Donnelly WH, Hawkins H: Optimal examination of the normally formed perinatal heart. Hum Pathol 18:55, 1987
43. Cliff WJ, Heathcote CB, Moss NS, Reichenbach DD: The coronary arteries in cases of cardiac and noncardiac sudden death. Am J Pathol 132:319, 1988
44. Katsuragawa M, Fujiwara H, Miyamae M, Sasayama S: Histologic studies in percutaneous transluminal coronary angioplasty for chronic total occlusion: Comparison of tapering and abrupt types of occlusion and short and long occluded segments. J Am Coll Cardiol 21:604, 1993
45. Grande NR, Taveira D, Silva AC, et al: Anatomical basis for the separation of four cardiac zones in the walls of human heart ventricles. Surg Radiol Anat 16:355, 1994

46. Kunamoto M, Nakashima Y, Sueishi K: Intimal neovascularization in human coronary atherosclerosis: Its origin and pathophysiological significance. Hum Pathol 26:450, 1995

47. Reig J, Jornet A, Petit M: Direct connection between the coronary arteries in the human heart. Intercoronary arterial continuity. Angiology 46:235, 1995

48. Farb A, Tang AL, Burke AP, et al: Sudden coronary death. Frequency of active coronary lesions, inactive coronary lesions, and myocardial infarction. Circulation 92:1701, 1995

49. Glagov S, Eckner FAO, Lev M: Controlled pressure fixation apparatus for hearts. Arch Pathol 76:640, 1963

50. Eckner FAO, Brown BW, Davidson DL, Glagov S: Dimensions of normal hearts after standard fixation by controlled pressure coronary perfusion. Arch Pathol 88:497, 1969

51. McAlpine WA: Heart and Coronary Arteries. New York, Springer-Verlag, 1975

52. Edwards WD. Anatomic basis for tomographic analysis of the heart at autopsy. Clin Cardiol 2:485, 1984

53. Piek JJ, Becker AE: Postmortem quantification of collateral vessels in the human heart. A new approach. Am J Cardiovasc Pathol 2:301, 1989

54. Kitzman DW, Scholz DG, Hagen PT, et al: Age-related changes in normal human hearts during the first 10 decades of life. Part II. Maturity: A quantitative anatomic study of 765 specimens from subjects 20 to 99 years old. Mayo Clin Proc 63:137, 1988

55. Scholz DG, Kitzman DW, Hagen PT, et al: Age-related changes in normal human hearts during the first 10 decades of life. Part I (growth): A quantitative anatomic study of 200 specimens from subjects from birth to 19 years old. Mayo Clin Proc 63:126, 1988

56. Wissler RW, Lichtig C, Hughes R, et al: New methods for determination of postmortem left ventricular volumes: Clinico-pathologic correlations. Am Heart J 89:625, 1975

57. Lange PE, Onnasch D, Farr FL, et al: Analysis of left and right ventricular size and shape, as determined from human casts. Description of the method and its validation. Eur J Cardiol 8:431, 1978

58. Rahlf G: Chronic cor pulmonale. Weight and intraventricular volume of the right ventricle in chronic pulmonary diseases. Virchows Arch [A] 378:273, 1978

59. Kilner PJ, Ho SY, Anderson RH: Cardiovascular cavities cast in silicone rubber as an adjunct to postmortem examination of the heart. Int J Cardiol 22:99, 1988

60. Achor RWP, Futch WD, Burchell HB, Edwards JE: The fate of patients surviving acute myocardial infarction. Arch Intern Med 98:162, 1956

61. Layman TE, Edwards JE: A method for dissection of the heart and major pulmonary vessels. Arch Pathol 82:314, 1966

62. Hackel DB, Ratcliff NB Jr: A technic to estimate the quantity of infarcted myocardium post mortem. Am J Clin Pathol 61:247, 1974

63. Lie JT, Titus JL: Pathology of the myocardium and the conduction system in sudden coronary death. Circulation 52(suppl 6):III41, 1975

64. Boor PJ, Reynolds ES: Myocardial infarct size: Clinicopathologic agreement and discordance. Hum Pathol 8:685, 1977

65. Brody GL, Belding A, Belding M, Felman SA: The identification and delineation of myocardial infarcts. Arch Pathol 84:312, 1967

66. Harnaryan C, Bennett MA, Pentecost BL, Brewer DB: Quantitative study of infarcted myocardium in cardiogenic shock. Br Heart J 18:320, 1970

67. Derias NW, Adams CWM: Nitro blue tetrazolium test: Early gross detection of human myocardial infarcts. Br J Exp Pathol 59:254, 1978

68. Bardales RH, Hailey LS, Xie SS, et al: In situ apoptosis assay for the detection of early acute myocardial infarction. Am J Pathol 149:821, 1996

69. Fulton RM, Hutchinson EC, Jones AM: Ventricular weight in cardiac hypertrophy. Br Heart J 14:413, 1952

70. McPhie J: Left ventricular hypertrophy with special reference to preponderance of one or other chamber. Aust Ann Med 6:328, 1957

71. Reiner L: Gross examination of the heart. In: Gould SE (ed): Pathology of the Heart and Blood Vessels. 3rd ed. Springfield, IL, Charles C. Thomas, 1968, p 1111

72. Dadgar SK, Tyaki SO: Importance of heart weight, weights of cardiac ventricles and left ventricle plus septum/right ventricle ratio in assessing cardiac hypertrophy. Jpn Heart J 20:63, 1979

73. Hudson R: Structure and function of the heart. In: Cardiovascular Pathology. Vol. 1. London, Edward Arnold, 1965

74. Canale ED, Campbell GR, Smolich JJ, Campbell JH: Part 7: Cardiac muscle. In: Oksche A, Voilrath L (series eds): Handbook of Microscopic Anatomy. Vol. 2. Springer Verlag, Berlin, 1986

75. Davies MJ: Colour Atlas of Cardiovascular Pathology. Oxford, Harvey Miller Publishers and Oxford University Press, 1986

76. Ludwig J, Lie JT: Current Methods of Autopsy Practice. 2nd ed. Philadelphia, WB Saunders, 1979

77. Edwards WD: Photography of medical specimens: Experiences from teaching cardiovascular pathology. Mayo Clin Proc 63:42, 1988

78. Chapman CB: On the study of the heart. A comment on autopsy techniques. Arch Intern Med 113:318, 1964

79. Hagens GV, Tiedemann K, Kritz W: The current potential of plastination. Anat Embryol 175:411, 1987

80. Öostrom K: Plastination of the heart. J Int Soc Plastination 1:12, 1987

81. Anderson RH, Becker AE: Cardiac Anatomy. An Integrated Text and Colour Atlas. London, Churchill Livingstone, 1980

82. Becker AE, Anderson RH: Cardiac Pathology. An Integrated Text and Color Atlas. New York, Raven Press, 1982

83. Bharati S, Lev M, Kirklin JW: Cardiac Surgery and the Conduction System. New York, Churchill Livingstone, 1983

84. Netter FH: The Heart. The CIBA Collection of Medical Illustrations. Vol. 6. New York, CIBA Publications, 1969

85. Walmsley R, Watson H: Clinical Anatomy of the Heart. Edinburgh, Churchill Livingstone, 1978

86. Wilcox BR, Anderson RH: Surgical Anatomy of the Heart. Edinburgh, Churchill Livingstone, 1985

87. Lev M, McMillan JB: A semiquantative histopathologic method for the study of the entire heart for clinical and electrographical correlations. Am Heart J 58:140, 1959

88. Oppenheimer BS: A routine method of opening the heart with conservation of the bundle of His and the sinoauricular node. JAMA 59:937, 1912

89. Holt JO: The normal pericardium. Am J Cardiol 26:455, 1970

90. Rodriquez FL, Robbins SL. Papilliform fibrous tags on atrial appendages. Arch Pathol 74:537, 1962

91. Shirani J, Berezowski K, Roberts WC: Quantitative measurement of normal and excessive (cor adiposum) subepicardial adipose tissue, its clinical significance, and its effect on electrocardiographic QRS voltage. Am J Cardiol 76:414, 1995

92. Reiner L, Mazzoleni A, Rodriquez FL, Fruendenthal RR: The weight of the human heart. 1. "Normal" cases. Arch Pathol 68:58, 1959

93. Page DL: Lipomatous hypertrophy of the cardiac interatrial septum: Its development and probable clinical significance. Hum Pathol 1:151, 1970

94. Crocker DW: Lipomatous infiltrates of the heart. Arch Pathol Lab Med 102:69, 1978

95. Shirani J, Roberts WC: Clinical, electrocardiographic and morphologic features of massive fatty deposits ("lipomatous hypertrophy") in the atrial septum. J Am Coll Cardiol 22: 226, 1993

96. Burke AP, Litovsky S, Virmani R: Lipomatous hypertrophy of the atrial septum presenting as a right atrial mass. Am J Surg Pathol 20:678, 1996

97. Chiu I-S, Hung C-R, How S-W, Chen M-R: Is the sinus node visible grossly? A histological study of normal hearts. Int J Cardiol 22:83, 1989

98. Anderson KR, Has Y, Anderson RH: Location and vascular supply in sinus node in human heart. Br Heart J 41:28, 1979

99. Hutchins GM, Anaya OA: Measurements of cardiac size, chamber volumes and valve orifices at autopsy. Johns Hopkins Med J 133: 96, 1973

100. Zeek PM: Heart weight. 1. The weight of the normal human heart. Arch Pathol Lab Med 34:820, 1942

101. Smith HL: The relation of the weight of the heart to the weight of the body and of the weight of the heart to age. Am Heart J 4:79, 1928

102. Hangartner JR, Marley NJ, Whitehead A, et al: The assessment of cardiac hypertrophy at autopsy. Histopathology 9:1295, 1985

103. Hort W: Quantitative morphology and structural dynamics. Methods Achiev Exp Pathol 5:3, 1971

104. Kitzman DW, Edwards WD: Age-related changes in the anatomy of the normal human heart. J Gerontol 45: M33-M39, 1990

105. Schulz DM, Giordano DA: Hearts of infants and children. Arch Pathol 74:464, 1962

106. Lev M, Simkins CS: Architecture of the human ventricular myocardium. Technic for study using a modification of the Mall-MacCullum Method. Lab Invest 5:396, 1956

107. Westaby S, Karp RB, Blackstone EH, Bishop SP: Adult human valve dimensions and their surgical significance. Am J Cardiol 53: 552, 1984

108. Lev M, Rowlatt UF, Rimoldi HJA: Pathologic methods for study of congenitally malformed heart. Arch Pathol 73:493, 1961

109. Devine WA, Debich DE, Anderson RH: Dissection of congenitally malformed heart, with comments on the value of sequential segmental analysis. Pediatr Pathol 11:235, 1991

110. Anderson RH: How should we optimally describe complex congenitally malformed hearts? Ann Thorac Surg 62:710, 1996

111. Anjos RT, Ho SY, Anderson RH: Surgical implications of juxtaposition of the atrial appendages. A review of forty-nine autopsied hearts. J Thorac Cardiovasc Surg 99:897, 1990

112. Rosenberg HS: Coarctation of the aorta. Morphology and pathogenetic considerations. In: Perspectives in Pediatric Pathology. Vol. 1. Chicago, Year Book Medical Publishers, 1973, p 339

113. Silver MM, Freedom RM, Silver MD, Olley PM: Morphology of the human newborn ductus arteriosus: Reappraisal of its structure and closure with special emphasis on prostaglandin E1 therapy. Hum Pathol 12:1123, 1981

114. Mullins CE, Mayer DC: Congenital Heart Disease; A Diagrammatic Atlas. New York, Alan R. Liss, 1989

115. Shinebourne EA, Macartney FJ, Anderson RH: Sequential chamber localization—logical approach to diagnosis in congenital heart disease. Br Heart J 38:327, 1976

116. Schulz DM, Giordano DA, Schulz DH: Organ weights of fetuses and infants. Arch Pathol 74:244, 1962

117. Van Mierop LHS: Anatomy of the heart. Ciba Found Symp 18:67, 1966

118. Van Mierop LHS: Anatomy and embryology of the right ventricle. In: Edwards JE (ed): The Heart. Baltimore, Williams & Wilkins, 1974

119. Van Mierop LHS, Kutsche LM: Embryology of the heart. In: Hurst JW (ed): The Heart. 6th ed. New York, McGraw-Hill, 1986, p 3

120. Walmsley R, Watson H: The clinical anatomy of the heart. In: Watson H (ed): Paediatric Cardiology. St. Louis, CV Mosby, 1968

121. Los JA: Embryology. In: Watson H (ed). Pediatric Cardiology. St. Louis, CV Mosby, 1968, p 1

122. Becker AE, Anderson RH: Cardiac Pathology. In: Berry CL (ed): Paediatric Pathology. New York, Springer-Verlag, 1981, p 15

123. Edwards JE: Congenital malformations of the heart and great vessels. In: Gould SE (ed): Pathology of the Heart and Blood Vessels. 3rd ed. Springfield, IL, Charles C. Thomas, 1968, p 262

124. Edwards JE: Survey of operative congenital heart disease. Am J Pathol 82:408, 1976

125. Angelini P: Normal and anomalous coronary arteries: Definitions and classifications. Am Heart J 117:418, 1989

126. Hickie JB: Anatomy of the right atrium. Br Heart J 18:320, 1956

127. Powell EDU, Mullaney JM: The Chiari network and the valve of the inferior vena cava. Br Heart J 22:579, 1960

128. Drury RAB: Persistent venous valves. J Pathol 61:449, 1978

129. Sweeney LJ, Rosenquist GC: The normal anatomy of the atrial septum in the human heart. Am Heart J 98:194, 1979

130. Remmell-Dow DR, Bharati S, Davis JT, et al: Hypoplasia of the eustachian valve and abnormal orientation of the limbus of the foramen ovale in hypoplastic left heart syndrome. Am Heart J 130: 148, 1995

131. Silver MA, Rowley NE: The functional anatomy of the human coronary sinus. Am Heart J 115:1080, 1988

132. Wang K, Ho SY, Gibson DG, Anderson RH: Architecture of atrial muscle in humans. Br Heart J 73:559, 1995

133. Rose AG: Venous malformations of the heart. Arch Pathol Lab Med 103:18, 1979

134. Harrity PJ, Tazelaar HD, Edwards WD, et al: Intracardiac varices of the right atrium: A case report and review of the literature. Int J Cardiol 48:177, 1995

135. Walmsley T: Part III: The heart. In: Quain's Elements of Anatomy. Vol. IV. London, Longmans, Green, 1929

136. Lechat PH, Mas JL, Lascault G, et al: Prevalence of patent foramen ovale in patients with stroke. N Engl J Med 318:1148, 1988

137. Silver MD, Dorsey JS: Aneurysms of the septum primum in adults. Arch Pathol Lab Med 102:62, 1978

138. Shirani J, Zafari AM, Roberts WC: Morphologic features of fossa ovalis membrane aneurysm in the adult and its clinical significance. J Am Coll Cardiol 26:466, 1995

139. Stewart PA, Wladimiroff JW: Fetal atrial arrhythmias associated with redundancy/aneurysm of the foramen ovale. J Clin Ultrasound 16:643, 1988

140. Silver MM, Zielenska, M, Perrin D, MacDonald JK: Association of prenatal closure of the foramen ovale and fetal parvovirus infection in hydrops fetalis. Cardiovasc Pathol 4:103, 1995

141. von Ludinghausen M, Ohmachi N, Besch S, Mettenleiter A: Atrial veins of the human heart. Clin Anat 8:169, 1995

142. Reid K: The anatomy of the sinus of Valsalva. Thorax 25:79, 1970

143. Voboril ZB: Todaro's tendon in the heart. 1. Todaro's tendon in the normal human heart. Folia Morphol 15:187, 1967

144. Zimmerman J: A new look at cardiac anatomy. J Albert Einstein Med Ctr 7:77, 1959

145. Allwood SP, Anderson RH: Developmental anatomy of the membranous part of the ventricular septum in the human. Br Heart J 41:275, 1979

146. Gross, L, Kugel MA: Topographic anatomy and histology of the valves in the human heart. Am J Pathol 7:445, 1931

147. Rosenquist GC, Sweeney LJ: Normal variation in tricuspid valve attachments to the membranous ventricular septum: A clue to the etiology of left ventricle-to-right atrium communication. Am Heart J 89:186, 1975

148. Silver MD, Lam JHC, Ranganathan N, Wigle ED: Morphology of the human tricuspid valve. Circulation 43:333, 1971

149. Anderson RH, Becker AE, Van Mierop LHS: What should we call the "crista?" Br Heart J 39:856, 1977

150. Goor DA, Edwards JE: The spectrum of transposition of the great arteries. With special reference to the developmental anatomy of the conus. Circulation 48:406, 1973

151. Van Praagh R, Van Praagh S, Nebesar RA, et al: Tetralogy of Fallot: Under-development of the pulmonary infundibulum and its sequelae. Am J Cardiol 26:25, 1970

152. Wenink AC, Oppenheimer-Dekker A, Moulaert AJ: Muscular ventricular septal defects: a reappraisal of the anatomy. Am J Cardiol 43:259, 1979

153. Dean JW, Ho SY, Rowland E, et al: Clinical anatomy of the atrioventricular junctions. J Am Coll Cardiol 24:1725, 1994

154. Keren A, Billingham ME, Popp RL: Ventricular aberrant bands and hypertrophic trabeculations. Am J Cardiovasc Pathol 1:369, 1988

155. Hurwitz LE, Roberts WC: Quadricuspid pulmonary valve. Am J Cardiol 31:623, 1973

156. Maron BJ, Hutchins GM: The development of the semilunar valves in the human heart. Am J Pathol 74:331, 1974

157. Nathan H, Eliakim M: The junction between the left atrium and the pulmonary veins. Circulation 34:412, 1966

158. Brock RC: The surgical and pathological anatomy of the mitral valve. Br Heart J 14:489, 1952

159. Lam JHC, Ranganathan N, Wigle ED, Silver MD: Morphology of the human mitral valve. 1. Chordae tendineae: A new classification. Circulation 41:449, 1970

160. Ranganathan N, Lam JHC, Wigle ED, Silver MD: Morphology of human mitral valve. II. The valve leaflets. Circulation 41:459, 1970

161. Perloff JK, Roberts WC: The mitral apparatus: Functional anatomy of mitral regurgitation. Circulation 46:227, 1972

162. Ranaganathan N, Silver MD, Wigle ED: Recent advances in the knowledge of the anatomy of the mitral valve. In: Kalmanson D (ed): The Mitral Valve. Acton, MA, Publishing Sciences Group, 1976, p 1

163. Rusted IE, Scheifley CH, Edwards JE: Studies of the mitral valve. 1. Anatomic features of the normal mitral valve and associated structures. Circulation 6:825, 1952

164. Rosenquist GC, Clark EB, Sweeney LJ, McAllister HA: The normal spectrum of mitral and aortic valve discontinuity. Circulation 54:298, 1976

165. Bel Kahn JVD, Duran DR, Becker AE: Isolated mitral valve prolapse: Chordal attachment as an anatomic basis in older patients. J Am Coll Cardiol 5:1335, 1985

166. Virmani R, Atkinson JB, Byrd BF, et al: Abnormal chordal insertion: A cause of mitral valve prolapse. Am Heart J 113:851, 1987

167. Gerlis LM, Wright HM, Wilson N, et al: Left ventricular bands: A normal anatomical feature. Br Heart J 52:641, 1984

168. Luetmer PH, Edwards WD, Seward JB, Tajik AJ: Incidence and distribution of left ventricular false tendons: An autopsy study of 483 normal human hearts. J Am Coll Cardiol 8:179, 1986

169. Toth, AB, Engel JA, McManus AM, McManus BM: Sigmoidity of the ventricular septum revisited: progression in early adulthood, predominance in men, and independence from cardiac mass. Am J Cardiovasc Pathol 2:211, 1988

170. Adegboyega PA, Adesokan A, Haque AK, Bloor PJ: Sensitivity and specificity of triphenyl tetrazolium chloride in the gross diagnosis of acute myocardial infarcts. Arch Pathol Lab Med 121: 1063, 1997

171. Roberts WC: The congenitally bicuspid aortic valve. Am J Cardiol 26:72, 1970

172. Vollebergh FEMG, Becker AE. Minor congenital variations of cusp size in tricuspid aortic valves. Possible link with isolated aortic stenosis. Br Heart J 39:1006, 1977

173. Silver MA, Roberts WC: Detailed anatomy of the normally functioning aortic valve in hearts of normal and increased weight. Am J Cardiol 55:454, 1985

174. Sutton JP III, Ho SY, Anderson RH: The forgotten interleaflet triangles: A review of the surgical anatomy of the aortic valve. Ann Thorac Surg 59:419, 1995

175. Edwards JE, Birtchell HB: The pathological anatomy of deficiencies between the aortic root and the heart, including aortic sinus aneurysms. Thorax 12:125, 1957

176. Bergmann SR, Fox KAA, Geltman EM, Sobel BE: Positron emission tomography of the heart. Prog Cardiovasc Dis 28:165, 1985

177. Virmani R, Chun PKC, Goldstein RE, et al: Acute takeoffs of the coronary arteries along the aortic wall and congenital coronary ostial valve-like ridges: Association with sudden death. J Am Coll Cardiol 3:766, 1984

178. Shirani J, Roberts WC: Solitary coronary ostium in the aorta in the absence of other major congenital cardiovascular anomalies. J Am Coll Cardiol 21:137, 1993

179. Taylor AJ, Byers JP, Cheitlin MD, Virmani R: Anomalous right or left coronary artery from the contralateral coronary sinus: "High-risk" abnormalities in the initial coronary artery course and heterogeneous clinical outcomes. Am heart J 133:428, 1997

180. Hutchinson MCE: A study of the atrial arteries in man. J Anat 125:39, 1978

181. Vlodaver Z, Neufeld HD, Edwards JE: Coronary Arterial Variations in the Normal Heart and in Congenital Heart Disease. Orlando, FL, Academic Press, 1975

182. DiDo LJ, Lopes AC, Caetano AC, Prates JC: Variations of the origin of the artery of the sinoatrial node in normal human hearts. Surg Radiol Anat 17:19, 1995

183. Bradham RR, Parker EF, Barrington BA Jr, et al: The cardiac lymphatics. Ann Surg 171:899, 1970

184. Johnson RA, Blake TM: Lymphatic system of the heart. Circulation 33:137, 1966

185. James TN: Cardiac innervation: anatomic and pharmacologic relationships. Bull NY Acad Med 43:1041, 1967

186. Crick SJ, Wharton J, Sheppard MN, et al: Innervation of the human cardiac conduction system. A quantitative immunohistochemical and histochemical study. Circulation 89:1697, 1994

187. Chow LT, Chow SS, Anderson RH, Gosling JA: The innervation of the human myocardium at birth. J Anat 187:107, 1995

188. Imaizumi S, Mazgalev T, Dreifus LS, et al: Morphological and electrophysiological correlates of atrioventricular nodal response to increased vagal activity. Circulation 82:951, 1990

189. McGuire MA, de Bakker JM, Vermeulen JT, et al: Atrioventricular junctional tissue. Discrepancy between histological and electrophysiological characteristics. Circulation 94:571, 1996

190. Marron K, Yacoub MH, Polak JM, et al: Innervation of human atrioventricular and arterial valves. Circulation 94:368, 1996

191. Russell HK: A modification of Movat's pentachrome stain. Arch Pathol 94:187, 1972

192. Centers for Disease Control and Prevention: Guidelines for prevention of transmission of human immunodeficiency virus and hepatitis B virus to health care and public safety workers. MMWR 38:1, 1989

193. Mann CV, Russell RCG (eds): Bailey & Love's Short Practice of Surgery. 21st ed. New York, Chapman and Hall Medical, 1992, pp 152–153

Chapter 2

Light Microscopy and Ultrastructure of the Blood Vessels and Heart

....

John P. Veinot • Feroze N. Ghadially • Virginia M. Walley

All but unicellular and the simplest multicellular animals need a circulatory system, a series of pumps and tubes, to transport nutrients and oxygen to the tissues and to remove waste products. The functions of such a system are listed in Table 2-1. In humans, the pump function of the circulation is provided by the heart. Collection and distribution are performed by the arteries, arterioles, veins, and venules. Small capillary vessels serve gas and nutrient exchange. The circulatory system must also be capable of buffering the pulsatile blood flow to ensure steady capillary flow, to regulate blood pressure and volume, to maintain circulatory continuity while allowing gas and nutrient exchange, and to control hemostasis. Temperature regulation and an immunologic/inflammatory role are also important.

The heart consists of pumps in series with a set of valves to ensure unidirectional flow. The right-sided pumps receive deoxygenated, waste-rich blood from the systemic venous circulation. The right atrium serves as a primer pump for pushing the blood through the tricuspid valve to the right ventricle. The right ventricle then pumps the blood through the pulmonary valve to the pulmonary arteries of the lungs for oxygenation. Oxygenation occurs at the capillary level. The oxygenated blood returns to the heart via the pulmonary veins, entering the left atrium, which is the primer pump for pushing blood through the mitral valve to the left ventricle. The left ventricle receives the oxygenated blood and distributes it to the body's systemic arterial circulation, where oxygen and nutrients are extracted and waste products are removed from tissues. Initially, the flow from the left ventricle is directed through the aorta. From there, blood flows into arteries and then arterioles en route to the capillary beds where the exchanges occur. The arterioles, as discussed later, form the main resistance in the system; they are responsible for the control of blood flow into the capillary bed and help in blood pressure regulation. The pressure in the pulmonary artery circulation is a fraction of the systemic pressure, so as to protect the delicate pulmonary capillary network from fluid seepage and subsequent pulmonary edema. However, both ventricles pump the same amount of blood, albeit at different pressures. The systemic venous system is distensible and therefore functions as a reservoir for blood.

This chapter deals with the important light and ultrastructural characteristics of the blood vessels and the heart. Pathologic states are not discussed (see Chapters 4 to 8, 22, and 23).

BLOOD VESSELS

Organization

Arteries and veins of varied size share many similarities of architecture and functional organization; their differences are dictated by the vessel size, the peculiarities of individual function, the blood pressure carried, and the nature of the pulse wave experienced. Veins are more numerous and generally have larger caliber and thinner walls with less muscle and elasticity than their arterial counterparts, because they carry more volume at lower pressure.

Each vessel usually has an intima with luminal endothelial cells and subendothelial fibroelastic connective tissue, a media formed of smooth muscle cells and connective tissue, and an adventitia formed of connective tissue that may blend with supporting soft tissues.[1] These layers vary in thickness and structural complexity from vessel to vessel. The American Heart Association Committee on Vascular Lesions defines the border between the intima and the media as being marked by the internal elastic lamina.[2] The existence or prominence of the internal elastic lamina (between intima and media) and the external elastic lamina (between media and adventitia) varies considerably as well.

Many arteries gradually taper in caliber, and a sharp point of distinction (e.g., from large elastic to muscular) cannot be made. Those in the transitional regions (e.g., popliteal, iliac, carotid, axillary) may be called arteries of "mixed type." Some arteries, either elastic or mixed, give off muscular branches at sharp angles (e.g., the visceral branches of the abdominal aorta), and their transitional regions are quite short. These may be referred to as arteries of "hybrid type"; they may have an inner muscular media and an outer elastic media. Veins, as a group, show even greater variability. In a single vein, or among veins of similar caliber, there may be considerable morphologic diversity.

In the evaluation of vessels by routine techniques, histologic artifacts may be encountered. Smooth muscle contraction bands are exceedingly common at autopsy and in surgically removed material. Vascular "telescoping" with apparent onion-skin or multilayered intima may be seen in arteries. Telescoping results when a small portion of the vessel is traumatically pushed or contracts into the lumen of an adjacent segment, most often in the context of biopsy.

TABLE 2-1 • **Properties of the Circulatory System**

Distribution of blood to and from viscera and the body periphery
Capillary exchange of oxygen, wastes, nutrients, and cells
Some immunologic/immune functions
Regulation of blood pressure
Hemostasis
Some endocrine functions
Regulation of body temperature

Light Microscopy

Aorta and Other Elastic Arteries

General Features

These arteries are in continuity with the heart and include the pulmonary artery along with the aorta and its largest branches: the brachiocephalic, common carotid, subclavian (with vertebral and internal mammary/thoracic branches), and common iliac arteries. These vessels are also referred to as conducting arteries. Their organization, with a large elastic tissue component, functions to absorb the pulse wave during cardiac systole. The vessels tend not to contract but rather recoil during diastole. They are often more than 1.0 cm in diameter and have relatively thin walls in relation to their large overall diameters. Distally, elastic arteries ramify as muscular arteries.

Intima

The intimal thickness may be up to 100 μm in the aorta. On the luminal surface, polygonal endothelial cells are arranged over a subendothelial layer composed of collagen, elastic fibers, scattered fibroblasts, and, in the deep layers, a few longitudinally oriented smooth muscle cells and macrophages. Macrophages play a role as scavengers and are involved in phagocytosis or storage of lipid.[2] In the deep intima, some elastic fibers join the innermost medial elastic fiber network. An internal elastic lamina is not well delineated because of the prominence of elastic in the media, but it can be arbitrarily defined as the innermost of the medial elastic lamellae. The intimal thickness of the aorta and other arteries varies with age (see Chapter 3) and with pathologic conditions.

Media

The media may be up to 500 nm thick and is formed of numerous and distinct concentric elastic lamellas, up to 2.5 nm thick and spaced 6 to 18 nm apart, that anastomose to form a network (Fig. 2-1). The interspaces contain amorphous ground substance, a fine elastic network, and spirally arranged smooth muscle cells with surrounding collagen. There are fewer smooth muscle cells per square unit of area than in muscular arteries. As pressures drop after birth, the histology of the pulmonary artery trunk becomes less uniform, tending to have wider spaced elastic lamellas of more irregular width and smooth muscle cells that may be irregularly orientated (see Fig. 2-1); the intrapulmonary elastic arteries have a more uniform appearance. Near the heart, the media of the pulmonary artery and aorta may contain a few cardiac myocytes. Usually, there is no clearly discernible external elastic lamina, but, again, it is arbitrarily defined as the outermost of the elastic lamellas.

The aorta by dry weight is composed of 20% smooth muscle proteins and 60% collagen and elastic lamellae, with more elastic in the thoracic portion and more collagen in the abdominal aorta. The relation between the

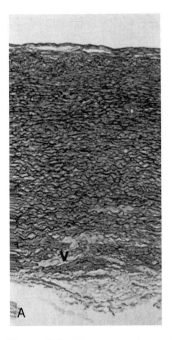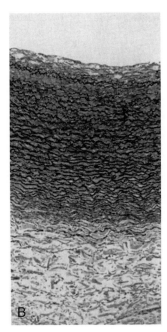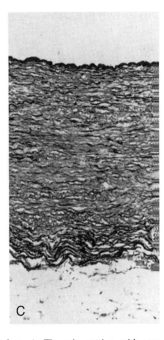

Figure 2-1 • Light photomicrographs. *A* and *B*, The aorta of a human infant. *A*, Thoracic portion with vasa vasorum (V). Note thicker media with more and thinner elastic lamellar units than in the abdominal aorta *(B)*. *C*, Pulmonary artery of a human adult. Note the less regular elastic and smooth muscle in its media (all Movat stain).

medial lamellar units (each unit comprising an elastic lamella and the cells and other material in its adjacent interlamellar zone) and the medial thickness, or aortic diameter, is linear.[3] The elastic and other elements in the media take on an artifactually wrinkled appearance in the usual histologic sections, whereas at physiologic pressures they are straight, more tightly and regularly spaced, and circumferential. Differences in medial thickness between the thoracic and the abdominal aorta relate to the larger numbers of lamellar units in the former structure, even though they are thinner than those in the abdominal aorta. Minor degrees of elastic fragmentation, medial fibrosis, medionecrosis, and accumulation of glycosaminoglycans (cystic medial necrosis) are normal findings and show an increase with patient age.[4]

Adventitia

The adventitia is a thin layer containing collagen, elastic fibers, and macrophages. It restrains the vessel from excessive extension and recoil.[1] Lymphatics run in this layer, as do vasa vasorum. The vasa form a thin-walled vascular network with arterial and venous components that penetrates the adventitia episodically and arborizes as a capillary network to nourish the deeper layers of the media. The vasa take origin from branches of the vessel served or from neighboring arteries. In the ascending aorta, vasa vasorum originate from the coronary arteries, in the arch from the great vessels of the neck, and in the thoracic aorta from the intercostal arteries.[5] Similar vessels with diameters of 0.1 cm or more serve those arteries and veins. Removal of the vasa vasorum experimentally leads to medial necrosis and decreased distensibility of the aorta. Intimal thickening may also occur if the vasa network is not functional, highlighting its role in transport functions. If the transarterial transport of macromolecules, such as fibrinogen and low-density lipoproteins (LDL), is impeded, these substances may accumulate in the vessel wall.[6] Vasa vasorum increase in number and density and become mesh-like in areas of arterial lesions, such as atherosclerotic plaques.[7]

Unmyelinated nerve fibers from sympathetic ganglia may penetrate the adventitia and end in the media. Myelinated sensory fibers may also be identified in the adventitia. Several other cell types seen occasionally in the adventitia of blood vessels, and at times also in other layers, particularly in pathologic states, include macrophages, plasma cells, mast cells, eosinophils, lymphocytes (occasionally in perivascular aggregates), and, rarely, neutrophils.

Internal Thoracic Artery

The internal thoracic or mammary arteries are unusual in that they have a small-caliber but elastic architecture. Along their length, the morphology is variable, with transitions between elastic, musculoelastic, and muscular types, depending on the number of elastic lamellae. The intima of these arteries is thickest in the muscular areas where there are discontinuities in the innermost elastic lamina.[8]

Muscular Arteries

General Features

These muscular, thick-walled branches of elastic arteries include most of the grossly visible and named arteries (Figs. 2-2 and 2-3). They are also referred to as distributing arteries. The vessels are capable of active contraction and to some extent may control blood flow to individual organs or body sites. They vary from 1.0 cm to as little as 0.05 cm in diameter and have relatively thick walls compared with their overall diameters. Distally, they blend with arterioles.

Intima

Intimal endothelial cells tend to be elongated and aligned with the long axis of the vessel. In smaller vessels their basal lamina may rest on the internal elastic lamina, whereas in larger ones it is separated from the latter by a subendothelial layer of elastic and collagen with occasional fibroblasts. In some larger muscular arteries (e.g., coronary, splenic, renal), there may be some longitudinally arranged smooth muscle in this layer. This

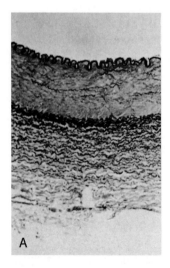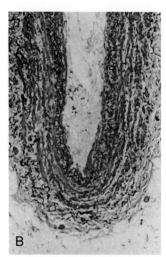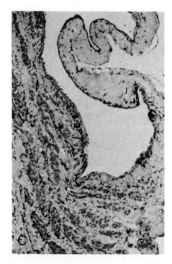

Figure 2-2 • Light photomicrographs. *A,* Medium-sized muscular femoral artery of human infant; *B,* medium-sized tibial vein of human adult; *C,* venous valve of human adult (all Movat stain).

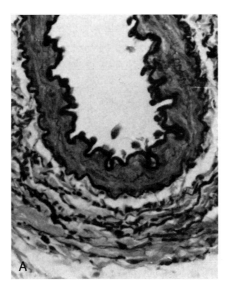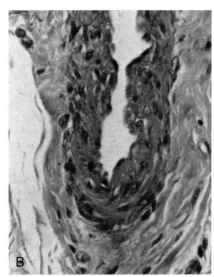

Figure 2-3 • Light photomicrographs. *A,* Small muscular artery of human infant; *B,* small vein of human infant (both Movat stain).

muscle may also be present in the carotid, axillary, iliac, and popliteal arteries. In penile, uterine, and palmar arteries, smooth muscle cells may be disproportionately represented, producing a very thick intima.

The prominent internal elastic lamina is an important feature in identifying these vessels. It is a thick, fenestrated layer of interwoven elastic fibers, which by light microscopy have a crenelated appearance due to artifactual contraction. This layer may appear to be absent at branch points and forks in the vessels; such areas are termed medial raphes and may mimic sites of old injury.[2] Intimal fibrosis is a common aging change and may be marked in some vessels, such as those in the myometrium and thyroid.[9] Medial fibrosis also occurs with aging; histologically, the internal elastic lamina may appear fragmented, reduplicated, or multilayered; and there may be calcification of the lamina.

Media

The chief component of the media is the spirally arranged smooth muscle, from three to four cell layers thick in the smallest-caliber vessels to 40 layers in the largest. Large amounts of ground substance or proteoglycans may be present. For their caliber, intracranial arteries have a disproportionately thin media. Pulmonary artery branches have thinner muscular walls than their systemic arterial counterparts. In umbilical, axillary, and popliteal arteries, which are subjected to repeated flexion, there is an inner, longitudinally arranged layer in addition to the spirally arranged one. Only relatively small amounts of collagen and a few elastic fibers are present in the media of muscular arteries, although in some larger-caliber ones (e.g., renal, popliteal) there may be prominent circularly oriented elastic lamellae between smooth muscle cells. Concentration of these and adventitial elastic fibers may form a definite external elastic lamina; this is more easily distinguished in larger-caliber arteries. With aging there may be medial fibrosis.

Adventitia

In muscular arteries, the adventitia is often as thick as the media. Longitudinally or helically arranged collagen and elastic fibers constitute much of the adventitia. Occasional smooth muscle cells may be present in coronary and splenic arteries. Unmyelinated nerve fibers may be seen. The adventitia blends with supporting soft tissues, and its limit may be difficult to define. Although the vasa vasorum network is not morphologically prominent in normal arteries, it has important transport and nutritional properties similar to those of elastic arteries. In diseased arteries, the vasa vasorum may be very prominent.[7, 10] With aging, pericytes of the vasa vasorum may migrate through the vascular wall, producing areas of intimal thickening.[11–13]

Arterioles

Arterioles are the smallest arterial vessel, with a diameter of less than 100 μm. Their intima includes the endothelium and a subendothelial connective tissue layer. The media is of variable thickness and may be prominent or reduced to a few layers of smooth muscle cells. The muscular layer is an important component of the precapillary sphincter mechanism, a variable resistance function further discussed in the next section. The adventitia is thin and composed of collagenous fibers and cellular elements, including macrophages, mast cells, plasma cells, fibroblasts, and unmyelinated nerve fibers. Hyalinization of arteriolar walls is a common accompaniment of aging. Plasma proteins and lipids accumulate in the media, giving it an eosinophilic, glassy appearance. Intimal fibrosis and fragmentation of the elastic lamina are normal aging changes.

Capillaries

Capillaries are the blood vessels with the smallest diameters, but they have a great surface area, hundreds of times larger than that of the aorta. Capillaries function in tissue/blood exchange and, therefore, are vital to the body's metabolic and homeostatic mechanisms. In general, the more metabolically active an organ is, the richer is its capillary bed. The transition between an arteriole and a capillary occurs when the muscularis layer of the arteriole disappears. The transition from a capillary to a venule is poorly defined.

Capillaries have no media or elastic lamellae. Their basic structure consists of an endothelial cell layer, a basal lamina, and supporting cells termed pericytes. Capillaries vary in size from 5 to 40 μm; the larger ones are termed sinusoids. There are three types of capillaries: continuous, fenestrated/perforated, and sinusoidal.

Continuous capillaries, without fenestrations, are the most common type and are found in muscular and nervous tissues. The basement lamina of their endothelial cells encloses the pericytes. Plasmalemmal vesicles (for transport) and zona occludens (to present a variable permeability) are present. The thin adventitia contains collagen, fibroblasts, mast cells, macrophages, and ground substance.

Fenestrated capillaries are characterized by the presence of fenestrae, or pores, 60 to 90 nm in diameter. Some pores have sieve-like diaphragms. Micropinocytotic vesicles for transport are also present; they further allow rapid exchange of substances between blood and tissues. This type of capillary is found in metabolically active organs, including the kidney and endocrine organs.

Sinusoidal capillaries are large-diameter, tortuous vessels 30 to 40 μm in diameter. They have no continuous lining and therefore have large, open spaces between cells where the capillary contents communicate directly with the tissues. Phagocytic cells are usually seen. This type of capillary is commonly found in the liver, spleen, and bone marrow.

Pericytes are mesenchymal cells commonly found at the arteriolar and capillary levels of the circulation. These cells have long cytoplasmic processes that encircle the endothelial cells. Because they possess filaments, they may provide the endothelial cells with a means of contracting. Pericytes are also capable of differentiating into other cells, including smooth muscle cells and fibroblasts. Pericytes may function in the production of cell membrane and in transport, because they often contain many plasmalemmal vesicles.[14] They also may inhibit the proliferation of endothelial cells, perhaps through alterations in their common extracellular matrix.[15, 16]

The precapillary sphincter consists of active smooth muscle in the arteriole just proximal to the capillary bed. The flow through a capillary bed depends on precapillary sphincter activity, neural and hormonal stimuli, and the state of arteriovenous anastomoses. These anastomoses allow arteriolar blood to empty directly into venules, bypassing capillary beds. Capillary tissue barriers exist in the brain (the blood-brain barrier) and in other tissues, including eye, thymus, nerve, and testes.

Venules

The transition from capillary to venule is gradual with the accumulation of a medial layer. The venule intima has an endothelial layer and a thin layer of collagen in the subendothelial space. Small venules may participate in interchange of metabolites between the blood and tissues. Pericytes, as defined in the previous section, are present at this diameter of vessel. The venular endothelial intercellular junctions are loosely organized, giving rise to very permeable endothelium. The endothelium of larger venules is not as porous, and both gap and occluding-type junctions are present. The media starts as a single layer of smooth muscle cells, and in venules of about 200 μm in diameter a continuous circular media is present. The myocytes are separated by collagenous and elastic fibers. The adventitia, the thickest layer, is composed of collagen, elastic fibers, and fibroblasts.

Veins

This group of vessels serves to drain the venules throughout the body. They are often named and accompany their arterial counterparts, compared with which they have thinner walls and larger caliber (see Figs. 2-2 and 2-3). The veins vary in diameter from 0.1 to 1.0 cm and carry large volumes of blood at low pressure. Many, even large-sized veins, contain valves. Valves (see Fig. 2-2) are particularly obvious in the veins of the lower limbs but are common in others such as subclavian and jugular veins.[17] The valves are formed most often of paired infoldings of intima, the subendothelial layer of which, on the side facing the current of blood, contains a fine elastic fiber network. These veins empty into large veins more centrally.

In the intima, polygonal endothelial cells rest on an inconspicuous subendothelial layer. Smooth muscle cells, longitudinally or circularly deployed, may be seen in this layer in veins of the extremities. There may be some fine elastic fibers present, but they do not form a well-defined internal elastic lamina. The media is thin compared with that of similar-sized arteries, but it is well developed in lower limb veins. Similarly, the veins of the gravid uterus, the umbilical vein, and some mesenteric veins have a prominent muscular media. Other veins, such as the cerebral and meningeal vessels, the dural sinuses, and the retinal, bony, and penile veins, are virtually devoid of a muscular media. The adventitia forms the bulk of the wall in veins of this caliber. It comprises thick, longitudinally arranged collagen with interspersed coarse elastic fibers and a few smooth muscle cells in small fascicles. Unmyelinated nerve fibers are seen.

With age, phlebosclerosis is commonly noted and is not thought to represent a disease state. The most common associated finding is intimal thickening, eccentric or less commonly concentric, rarely with calcification. Both the adventitia and the media develop increased amounts of collagen. Elastic fibers in vein walls become atrophic and less distinct.[18]

Large Veins

Large veins, usually greater than 1.0 cm in diameter, include the pulmonary veins, the portal vein, and the venae cavae and their main branches. They drain medium-sized veins and empty into the atria of the heart.

A simple endothelial layer makes up the intima. In some larger trunks, large amounts of connective tissue may thicken it to up to 65 μm. In many of these vessels (e.g., venae cavae), the media is very poorly developed and is composed of a few smooth muscle cells or is absent. In the pulmonary veins, circularly arranged smooth muscle may be prominent.

The adventitia is the thickest layer and has three zones. The first is an inner one formed of dense fibroelastic connective tissue, often with large collagen bundles arranged in an open spiral. The middle zone is formed of longitudinally disposed smooth muscle cells. Coarse collagen and thick elastic fibers form the outer zone. Cardiac muscle cells may extend from the heart for short distances into the venae cavae and pulmonary veins. Vasa vasorum and lymphatics are prominent in this layer, and in some large veins they may penetrate and extend as far as the intima.

Intrapulmonary Vessels

Adult Circulation

The pulmonary blood vessels in the adult have many characteristics in common with the systemic vessels; however, because they exist in a system with relatively high flow and low pressure, there are important differences. Although it is responsible for the same blood flow as the systemic vessels, the resistance in the pulmonary vasculature is about one-sixth that in the systemic circulation, with the result that pulmonary vascular walls seem thin and the vessels dilated.[19]

The arterial side of the pulmonary circulation consists of the arteries and arterioles that lead to the capillaries in alveolar walls. On the venous side, after the capillary bed, are venules and then veins, which reenter the heart at the left atrium. In addition, the bronchial arteries, small branches directly off the thoracic aorta, are present in the adventitia of bronchi and bronchioles. Bronchial veins, which drain to the left atrium, and azygous and hemiazygous veins provide accessory drainage of the bronchial tree.

In general, pulmonary arteries and veins have a similar structure, and any differences are very much less pronounced compared with the corresponding vessels in the systemic periphery. The location of vessels in the lung is the best indicator of their identity. The arteries and arterioles follow the bronchial tree, whereas pulmonary veins are located at the periphery of the lung lobules in the interlobular septa.[20]

The elastic arteries are those with an external diameter greater than 1000 μm. These vessels follow bronchi to the level of subsegmental bronchi. Muscular arteries extend from the subsegmental bronchi to the respiratory bronchi level; they have both an internal and external elastic lamina and an external diameter of 100 to 1000 μm. Arterioles are those vessels smaller than 100 μm that extend from the respiratory bronchi to the alveoli; they have only a single elastic lamina and often no muscularis layer.[19]

The arteries have more pronounced smooth muscle and more elasticity than pulmonary veins. An internal elastic lamina is present. As the vessels decrease in size and branch, their intimal thickness and the number of elastic fibers decrease. The lumens of the arteries are large in comparison with their wall thicknesses. Elastic fibers are detected in the very small arteries, even up to 0.5 to 1.0 mm in diameter. In larger muscular arteries, the adventitia may be quite prominent, up to two to three times the medial thickness. The media has circularly oriented smooth muscle with some collagen fibers. This medial layer is bound on either side by elastic laminas. The transition from artery to arteriole level is not a sharp distinction. The media becomes gradually discontinuous, and the vessels become nonmuscular. At this level, there is no adventitia and no media.

The capillaries of the alveolar spaces are fenestrated, in contrast to those of the bronchial tree, which are continuous. The capillaries make up a part of the alveolar wall and are responsible for gas exchange. They are metabolically active, for instance providing angiotensin conversion. At rest, the capillary bed is partially closed. With exercise, the capillary bed opens, with vascular redistribution and recruitment, thereby allowing increased flow with no pressure change.

The pulmonary veins have longitudinally oriented intimal elastic fibers and contain moderate amounts of elastic fibers in the muscularis layer. There is usually an indistinct external elastic lamina and no internal elastic lamina. The adventitia of pulmonary veins may be the thickest layer, and near the left atrium it may contain cardiac myocytes, as an extension of left atrial tissues. Pulmonary veins have no valves. In general, vein walls are thinner and have a more haphazard histologic arrangement than that of the arteries. The media-adventitia boundary is indistinct, and this layer contains elastic fibers, smooth muscle, and collagen.

With age, elastic arteries develop intimal thickening and the amount of medial collagen increases. The pulmonary trunk dilates, and a few shallow atheromas may occur. The muscular arteries show an increased thickness of the muscularis layer, and there may be eccentric intimal fibrous thickening. The capillaries develop some age-related thickening. The veins show patchy or circumferential hyalinization.[19]

Lymphatics are also present in the lung parenchyma. They are located primarily in the interlobular septa, around the tracheobronchial tree, and in the pleura. They differ morphologically from veins in that they possess valves and do not contain blood. Their function is to drain excess fluid from the pulmonary interstitium. The system has been divided into deep components, which follow the tracheobronchial tree, and superficial components, which are based in the visceral pleura. Lymphatic vessels do not extend beyond the level of the alveolar ducts.

Fetal Circulation

In the fetal state, the ductus arteriosus allows free communication between pulmonary and systemic circulations. In the fetus, the media of elastic and muscular arteries is pronounced, but this layer begins to widen and thin shortly after birth.[19, 20] As the lung expands, regression allows a low-pressure, low-resistance milieu to develop. The muscular arteries are one of the main determinants of pulmonary vascular resistance, because the media is responsive to oxygen level and other vasoactive mediators.

Ultrastructure

Endothelium

General Features

The endothelium, which lines the inner or adluminal surface of the heart and blood vessels, is composed of a

TABLE 2-2 • **Properties of Endothelial Cells**

Regulation of blood flow via dilatation and constriction of vessels
Modulation of selective permeability and substance transfer
Gas, nutrient, and waste exchange
Lipid metabolism
Extracellular matrix production and modulation
Growth factor secretion and regulation; smooth muscle cell regulation
Some immunologic functions
Some regulation of inflammatory reactions
Variable coagulant and thrombotic functions
    Prothrombotic
    Antithrombotic/anticoagulant

single layer of flat endothelial cells. The endothelium has many purposes, including structural, hemostatic, and immune functions (Table 2-2).[1] (Aspects of endothelial cell function are presented in Table 4-2.) Endothelial cells also produce endothelin, a vasoconstrictor, and nitric oxide, a vasodilator.[21] The cells are polygonal or elongated in the direction of blood flow. They are about 25 to 50 μm long and 10 to 15 μm wide. In addition to an unremarkable nucleus and a small nucleolus, these cells contain sparse cisterns of rough endoplasmic reticulum, ribosomes and polyribosomes lying free in the cytoplasmic matrix, a few mitochondria, a small Golgi complex, and, at times, some smooth endoplasmic reticulum. Lysosomes and residual bodies (lipofuscin granules) are more frequently seen in arterial than in venous endothelium. Multivesicular bodies, a variety of lysosome, are also at times seen in vascular endothelial cells. A few glycogen particles (monoparticulate form) and, rarely, lipid droplets are present in the cytoplasm. The endothelium produces fibronectin and basement membrane material.[2]

Endocytotic Structures

Endocytosis of fluids is carried out by structures called pinocytotic vacuoles and micropinocytotic vesicles (Figs. 2-4 through 2-7). Slender cell processes seen on the surface of endothelial cells are processes or folds of the cell membrane called lamellipodia; they impound fluid from the blood and transport it into the cell in a single-membrane–bound vacuole called a pinocytotic vacuole.

Much smaller than vacuoles, 60 to 70 nm in diameter, are the micropinocytotic vesicles or caveolas. These appear as flask-shaped invaginations of the adluminal and abluminal cell membrane and as rounded vesicles lying free in the cell cytoplasm. The microvesicles arise from the latter by a process of "pinching off." It is thought that most of these vesicles are involved in the transport of fluid to and from blood and tissues, by shuttling of vesicles from one cell front to another or fusion of vesicles to form transendothelial channels. Clefts between the endothelial cells may also aid in intercellular transport.[22] Membrane receptors, specifically for LDL, are also present.[2]

Filaments and Microtubules

A few intermediate filaments, 8 to 10 nm in diameter, termed vimentin filaments, are frequently seen in endothelial cells as part of the cytoskeleton. They may be numerous and appear as fascicles or as whorls filling the cell cytoplasm (see Fig. 2-5). Such an excess of intermediate filaments in various cell types has been regarded as a regressive change associated with aging and disease processes.[23]

As in most cells, some randomly oriented thin filaments, actin filaments about 5 nm thick, are present just deep to the plasma membrane; however, in routine preparation, even at moderately high magnifications, they are not prominent.[24] The filaments are readily demonstrated in immunohistochemical preparations of whole endothelial cells lining blood vessels or endothelial cells in culture. Actin filaments are a part of the cytoskeleton, and a few may be discerned in the cell cytoplasm also.[25] More readily visualized are fibrils formed by parallel aggregation of these filaments, particularly when they also bear focal densities along their course. Such actin fibrils are infrequently encountered in endothelial cells. Tropomyosin and viniculin are also present.[2, 24]

Weibel-Palade Bodies

Weibel-Palade bodies—long, cylindrical, rod-shaped, microtubulated bodies bound by a single membrane and containing 6 to 26 microtubules per set in a matrix—are

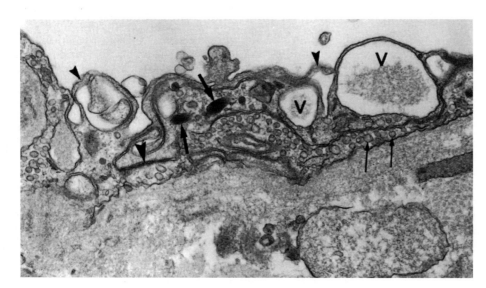

Figure 2-4 • Electron micrograph of a human femoral vein. Endothelial cells showing cell processes (small arrowheads), pinocytotic vacuoles (V), micropinocytotic vesicles (thin arrows), and Weibel-Palade bodies (thick arrows). Note also the tight junction (large arrowhead).

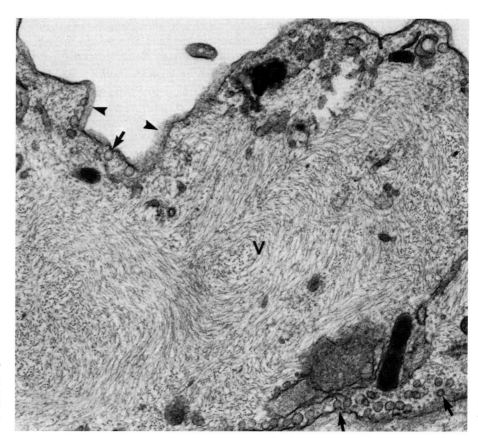

Figure 2-5 • Electron micrograph of a human femoral vein. The cytoplasm of the endothelial cell is packed with whorls of vimentin filaments (V). Note also the surface coat (arrowheads) and micropinocytotic vesicles (arrows).

present in endothelial cells (see Figs. 2-6 and 2-7).[26] As a rule, they appear randomly scattered in the cytoplasm of endothelial cells of arteries, veins, capillaries, and endocardium but not lymphatics. At times, they are seen clustered in the neighborhood of the Golgi complex, from which they are known to develop.[27] Weibel-Palade bodies are rarely cut along their entire length, which therefore is difficult to ascertain, but its maximum is probably 3.2

μm. The diameter of these bodies ranges from 0.1 to 0.5 μm (about 0.15 μm in humans), and that of the microtubules in their substance from 12 to 27 nm (about 20 nm in humans). The matrix varies from moderately to highly electron-dense, so that the microtubules in their substance are often difficult to demonstrate. A central filament has been observed within the microtubules.[26] Not every electron microscopic section through an endothelial cell

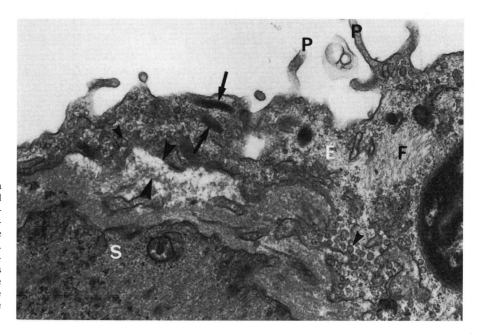

Figure 2-6 • Electron micrograph of a human femoral vein. Endothelial cell showing cell processes (P), micropinocytotic vesicles (small arrowheads), Weibel-Palade bodies (arrows), and intermediate filaments (i.e., vimentin filaments) (F). Thickening of the lamina densa is evident adjacent to the smooth muscle cells (S) and endothelial cell (E). In one zone (between large arrowheads), both the lamina lucida and the lamina densa are thickened.

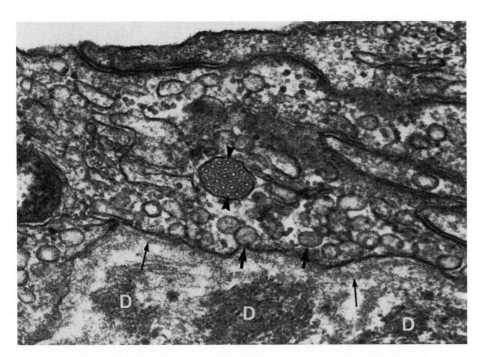

Figure 2-7 • Electron micrograph of a muscular artery from human leg. Endothelial cell showing numerous micropinocytotic vesicles (thick arrows) and a cross-cut Weibel-Palade body containing several microtubules (arrowheads) in its interior. Note also the basal lamina (thin arrows) and the obliquely cut electron-dense fibrils (D).

reveals Weibel-Palade bodies, and usually no more than one or two are seen in endothelial cells in normal tissues. However, at times the bodies are numerous, particularly in blood vessels in some benign vasoformative tumors.

The current view about the function of these organelles is that they may be involved in blood coagulation. Immunoelectron microscopic studies show that the bodies contain factor VIII–related antigen and von Willebrand factor, known to affect platelet binding to arterial subendothelium in vivo and to interact with fibronectin and fibrinogen in mediating platelet binding to solid substrata in vitro.[2, 28]

Cell Membrane, Surface Coat, and Basal Lamina

Like all cells, endothelial cells are bounded by a trilaminar cell membrane. The specialization of the polysaccharide-rich cell coat, the glycocalyx, at the cell surface forms the surface coat, while that at the base forms the basal lamina.

The adluminal surface of endothelial cells bears a slender, fuzzy surface coat about 5 nm thick. The surface coat covers cell processes and extends into pinocytotic vacuoles and micropinocytotic vesicles. As in other epithelia, the basal lamina of endothelial cells is composed of a lamina lucida and a lamina densa (see Fig. 2-6). Usually, the basal lamina forms a continuous layer, but it can also be attenuated, interrupted, thickened, or reduplicated. In arterioles and capillaries, at various sites, thickening and reduplication of the basal lamina are associated with disease processes such as diabetes, rheumatoid arthritis, and perhaps aging, but information on such matters in large vessels is lacking. Both surface coat and basal lamina are produced by, and firmly attached to, the cell membrane. They are considered part of the cell itself and not of the extracellular matrix or milieu.

Cell Junctions

Only two types of junctions occur between endothelial cells of human blood vessels—tight junctions (occluding junctions) and gap junctions (communicating junctions). Freeze-cleaved preparations are needed to confidently and accurately evaluate these structures. When tissue preservation and processing are adequate and the plane of sectioning is favorable (i.e., normal to the cell membranes), the tight junction is seen as a zone of punctate and/or linear fusion of the outer leaflets of the apposed cell membranes of adjacent cells, whereas the gap junction appears as a structure in which the intercellular gap is narrowed to about 20 nm. A polygonal lattice is at times discernible in the gap of gap junctions.[29]

Studies on freeze-cleaved tissues show that tight junctions have a meshwork of ridges and matching grooves.[30] Gap junctions have a lattice-like area with particles and matching pits. At the center of each particle that penetrates the cell membrane, a pore or channel is present. Small molecules of molecular weight up to about 1200 can pass through these channels. The passage of fluorescent dyes, amino acids, sugars, cyclic adenosine monophosphate, and other nucleotides has been demonstrated. Thus, the gap junction is a permeable structure that facilitates diffusion of ions and small molecules from cell to cell through low-resistance pathways.

To a greater or lesser extent, all intercellular junctions, including tight and gap junctions, provide some mechanical coupling. In addition, the gap junction provides electrical coupling. The basic function of a tight junction is to provide an effective, watertight seal that occludes the lumen of a viscus (e.g., gut, acinus, duct) from the intercellular spaces; but this is not always so, and in several sites, including blood vessels, the situation is more complex. The available morphologic evidence indicates that in arteries and veins the junctions are quite tight. However, in most capillaries (i.e., except capillaries of the blood-brain barrier), the junctions are readily permeated or circumvented by tracers. Therefore, one of the factors contributing to the permeability of capillaries is the structure and deployment of the tight junction. (See Chapter 4 for further discussion of endothelial cell function.)

Smooth Muscle

General Features

Except for their smaller size, vascular smooth muscle cells (Fig. 2-8) are similar to those found elsewhere. These cells occur in all vessels except capillaries and pericytic venules. The relaxed smooth muscle has an oval or elongated nucleus, but in the contracted state the nucleus is folded and has a concertina-like appearance (Fig. 2-9). Most of the cell cytoplasm is occupied by myofilaments, but in favorable sections one can see, usually but not invariably, in the juxtanuclear or perinuclear position, rough endoplasmic reticulum, polyribosomes lying free in the cytoplasm, Golgi complex, mitochondria, and an occasional lysosome or lipofuscin granule (residual body). The lipofuscin granule is easily identified as a single-membrane–bound body containing electron-dense material (particles, granules, and masses) and an electron-lucent or medium-density lipid (triglyceride) droplet or droplets (see Fig. 3-13).

The monoparticulate glycogen in these cells appears as rows or aggregates of electron-dense particles in the cytoplasm between myofilaments and/or as aggregates in the juxtanuclear cytoplasm. An occasional lipid droplet is present in normal cells, but in aging and in atherosclerosis, large numbers of lipid droplets accumulate, transforming them into foam cells. Because the smooth muscle cell is the only one present in the media of most vessels, this is the cell that synthesizes and secretes the precursors of

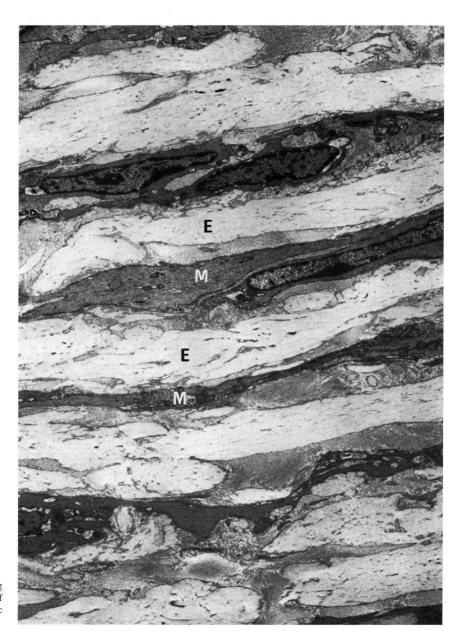

Figure 2-8 • Electron micrograph of a pig aorta. Seen here are the alternate layers of smooth muscle cells (M) and elastic lamellae (E) that make up the media.

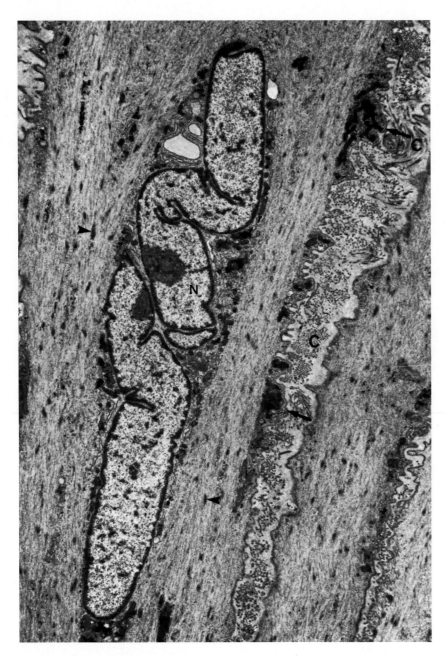

Figure 2-9 • Electron micrograph of a muscular artery of a human leg. Seen here are smooth muscle cells set in a collagenous matrix (C). Note the characteristic folded nucleus (N) and perinuclear collection of organelles. In the contracted muscle cell, some organelles are also seen in pockets (arrows) under the crenated cell membrane. The cell cytoplasm is packed with thin filaments bearing focal densities (arrowheads) along their course.

matrical collagen fibers, elastic fibers, and proteoglycans, thereby assuming the function of fibroblasts elsewhere.

In atherosclerosis, there is an increase of rough endoplasmic reticulum in these cells, which come to resemble myofibroblasts or are thought to have transformed into myofibroblasts.[31, 32] Myofibroblasts occur in many sites and situations but are best known for their occurrence in granulation tissue. Like smooth muscle cells, myofibroblasts contain tracts of actin filaments that permit them to contract like smooth muscle cells; they also have both a well-developed rough endoplasmic reticulum and Golgi complex (as in fibroblasts) that permit them to synthesize precursors of matrix components as do fibroblasts. This transformation may play a key role during vascular remodeling.[2]

Endocytotic Structures

Although a few short, at times bifurcating, cell processes are seen on the surfaces of smooth muscle cells, they do not appear to be engaged in pinocytotic activity. However, numerous micropinocytotic vesicles are of common occurrence. Their function seems to be the transport of fluid in and out of the cell.

Filaments

The most prominent or characteristic feature of the smooth muscle cell is a cytoplasm packed with bundles of parallel filaments called thin filaments (see Fig. 2-9) or actin filaments, also containing tropomyosin, with focal densities containing α-actinin (similar to Z lines of striated muscle) along their course. Such densities are also seen deep to the cell membrane, where they are called subplasmalemmal densities. They serve as anchoring sites for filaments.

Thick myosin filaments are difficult to find or confidently identify as such in routine electron micrographs of smooth muscle. For this reason, it was thought at one time that myosin was not present in vertebrate smooth muscle. However, it is now accepted that the difficulty of demonstrating myosin filaments is a result either of preparative procedures or of the occurrence of myosin in a depolymerized state, forming filaments only during contraction. The general view now is that, as in skeletal muscle, contraction occurs by a sliding filament mechanism.

Intermediate filaments, desmin and vimentin, occur in vascular smooth muscle cells but again are difficult to identify confidently in routine electron micrographs. Finally, because of random sectioning and the thinness of the actin filaments, they too are only occasionally adequately resolved, even at moderately high magnification. However, their presence is easily sensed by the "gray areas," devoid of common organelles, in the cell and the telltale focal densities.

Cell Membrane and External Lamina

Smooth muscle cells are bounded by a trilaminar cell membrane. Each cell is surrounded by a lamina that is morphologically similar to the basal lamina seen at the base of epithelial cells. This is usually called the basal lamina; however, because the membrane covers the entire cell surface, a more apt term is external lamina. In human material, the lamina densa is often quite thick and, unless the plane of sectioning is favorable, the lamina lucida is not visualized.

Cell Junctions

Freeze-fracture studies demonstrate only gap or communicating junctions between vascular smooth muscle cells. They are more frequent in arterioles and small arteries than in large vessels. Therefore, the gap junctions between vascular smooth muscle cells are not only instrumental in conducting impulses but also provide mechanical coupling between these cells. Obviously, such electrical and mechanical coupling is essential if cell contraction is to be coordinated.

Matrix Elements

General Features

Where exactly a cell ends and the extracellular compartment begins was a subject of controversy in the past, but it is now widely accepted that this boundary is the cell membrane with its coat. The extracellular matrix of connective tissues and the vessel wall have two main components: (1) the fibrous component, consisting of collagen and elastic fibers, sometimes referred to as the fibrous matrix or fibrillary matrix (Fig. 2-10; see Figs. 2-8 and 2-9), and (2) the ground substance or "interfibrillary matrix," which contains mainly proteoglycans, solutes, and water (Figs. 2-11 and 2-12). The predominant form of proteoglycans in arteries is chondroitin sulphate, and in veins, dermatan sulphate. The concentration of glycosaminoglycans is higher in arteries than in veins. The static mechanical properties of the vessel wall, largely the media, are dependent on the physical characteristics of matrix components. For example, the stretching and recoil of the walls of conducting vessels with each heartbeat is facilitated by elastic fibers and lamellae, whereas the tensile strength that prevents overstretching and possible rupture is mediated by collagen fibrils and fibers.

Collagen

In this discussion, the nomenclature used defines a filament as "a solitary thread-like structure," a fibril as "a thread-like structure composed of an aggregate of filaments," and a fiber as "a thread-like or rope-like structure composed of an aggregate of fibrils." Native collagen fibrils are readily identified in electron micrographs by their banded or cross-striated appearance. They exhibit, on both low-angle x-ray diffraction and electron microscopy, a marked axial periodicity. In suitably stained preparations, each period is seen to consist of a light and a dark band, sometimes referred to as the major bands; some fine, dark cross-striations (minor bands) can also be discerned within each period. The length of each period (i.e., one dark band and one light band) depends on the state of hydration of the collagen fibril. It has long been recognized that the structural units of collagen are synthesized intracellularly, but polymerization to form collagen fibrils occurs extracellularly. The first step is the synthesis of polypeptide α chains by the polyribosomes of the rough endoplasmic reticulum to form procollagen. This is transported to the Golgi complex, where it is modified, packaged in secretory vacuoles, and discharged into the matrix like any merocrine secretion. In the matrix, the procollagen is converted into tropocollagen by the action of procollagen peptidase, which removes most of the nonhelical terminal extension on the ends of the rod-like procollagen molecule. Once the tropocollagen molecules are formed, they aggregate in a quarter-staggered arrangement to form native fibrils of characteristic periodicity, when conditions are physiologic.

It is apparent that cells that synthesize collagen must have a fair amount of rough endoplasmic reticulum and a Golgi complex. Fibroblasts, cells characterized by an abundance of these organelles, produce collagen found in many connective tissue matrices, including that of the adventitia of blood vessels. In the media, this function is performed by smooth muscle cells. Type III collagen is the principal collagen found in blood vessels. Type I collagen also occurs, particularly in vessels of older persons.[33] Type IV collagen, produced by endothelial cells, occurs in the basal lamina and external lamina.

It is not possible to say which type of collagen is present by simply looking at electron micrographs; however, fibrils composed of type III collagen tend to be somewhat more slender than those composed of type I collagen, which is found principally in skin, bone, and tendon. Differentiation is possible with the use of immunohistochemistry techniques. Most collagen fibrils seen in the vascular wall are quite thin, but occasionally much thicker fibrils, called giant collagen fibrils, are encoun-

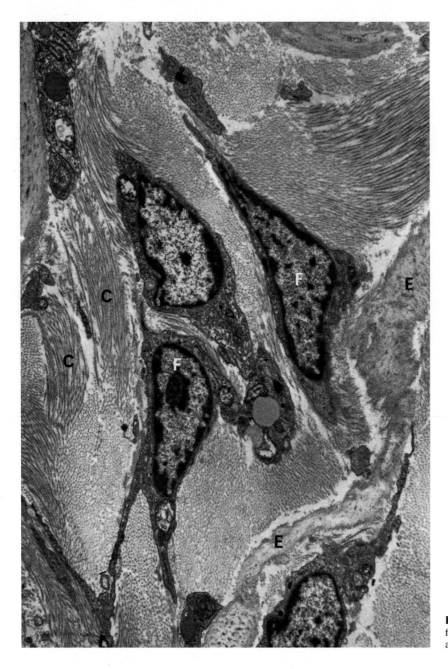

Figure 2-10 • Electron micrograph of a human femoral vein. Fibroblasts (F), collagen fibers (C), and elastic fibers (E) are found in the adventitia.

tered. It is now known that, with age, collagen fibrils become more crystalline through cross-linking and that the fibrils thicken. It seems that an age-associated thickening of collagen occurs in blood vessels also and may be engendered by pathologic states.

Collagen fibrils and fibers are flexible, so they are of little value in resisting a compressive load. Nevertheless, they offer great resistance to a pulling force, and their function in blood vessels is to resist tensile forces that might otherwise overstretch and tear the vessel wall.

Elastic

Both thread-like elastic fibers and sheet-like elastic lamellas occur in the walls of blood vessels (see Fig. 2-10). Elastic fibers occur principally in the adventitia, whereas elastic lamellas occur in the media. Elastic lamellae may

appear as solitary structures, internal elastic lamina, external elastic lamina, or lamellas regularly alternating with sheets of muscle cells (see Fig. 2-8). The lamellae are extensively fenestrated and interconnected by branches so that they form a three-dimensional meshwork. The number and distribution of lamellae and fibers vary with the type of vessel.

Ultrastructural studies show that elastic fibers and lamellas have two distinct morphologic components, and it is now established that they represent two discrete proteins.[34] In mature elastic fibers, about 90% of the elastic fiber consists of the well-known protein elastin. In routine electron microscopic preparations, this component has an amorphous appearance, with electron density ranging from lucent to moderately electron-dense. The other component of the elastic fiber is an electron-dense filament

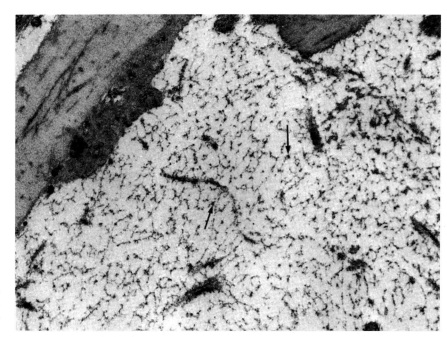

Figure 2-11 • Electron micrograph of a human carotid artery. Proteoglycan particles (arrows) and associated filaments are forming a loose network in the interfibrillary matrix.

about 11 nm in diameter. Filaments and aggregates of such filaments (i.e., fibrils) occur on the surface and within the amorphous elastin of elastic fibers and are also found lying free in the extracellular matrix. During elastogenesis, the electron-dense filaments and fibrils are laid down first, and later the elastin is laid down within the fibrils, which serve as a scaffolding or template for its deposition. In the aorta, the elastic laminae are preceded by sheet-like aggregates of electron-dense filaments. However, not all electron-dense fibrils are pre-elastic fibrils, and some persist as such throughout life.

The elasticity of elastic fibers converts the highly pulsatile cardiac output in arterial vessels into a more continuous flow. In popular usage, elasticity means the ability to be stretched easily by a small force and to spontaneously recover normal bulk and shape when the force is removed, rather like a rubber band. Elastic fibers can be stretched to about 150% of their original length before they break.

MYOCARDIUM

Organization

The arrangement of myocardial fibers has been studied for hundreds of years. It is clear from careful anatomic studies using dissecting microscopic, histologic, and scanning electron microscopic observations that the myocardium of the two ventricles is interrelated.[35-37] Some studies divided the myocardium into distinct muscles, the superficial and deep sinospiral and bulbospiral muscles and the scroll muscle.[38] More recent studies differ slightly, describing three layers or groups of fibers: the superficial subepicardial, the middle, and the subendocardial (or deep). Although investigators may disagree about the arrangement of muscle fibers, there is much agree-

ment concerning their distribution and function. The layers are extensively shared by both ventricles, with the exception of the left ventricular middle layer, which is mainly left-sided. The superficial layer travels from the base of the ventricles to the apex of the heart in an oblique right-to-left or left-to-right direction. At the apex, these fibers invaginate and become the deep (or subendocardial) layer of the left and right ventricles. The deep layer forms the subendocardium and the papillary muscles of the left ventricle. On the right side, the subendocardium also receives a major contribution of fibers from an invagination of the middle layer, which runs deeply at the anterior interventricular sulcus. The middle-layer fibers run transversely and form a cylinder, open at both ends, from the base to the apex. The subendocardial fibers anchor to the atrioventricular and arterial rings of the fibrous skeleton and to the chordae tendineae. The change of direction of the fibers is gradual with no distinct cleavage planes present.[35]

Contraction of the ventricles begins in the subendocardium, pulling the apex of the heart toward the base. The middle muscle layer contraction constricts the ventricle. The contraction of the superficial layer squeezes or wrings the ventricle, providing the final contribution to ventricular systole.[36] Muscle fiber distribution also probably plays a role in the determination of stress and strain on the ventricular wall.[39]

The atrial muscles are circumferential or transverse and longitudinal. The circumferential muscles cross and interconnect the atria. In the right atrium, the crista terminalis, with its pectinate muscle branches, forms the most prominent muscle structure. On the left atrial side, the circumferential muscles are most prominent. The atrial muscles are distinct from those of the ventricles.[40] Contraction of the atrial muscles during atrial systole draws the ventricles to the heart base, most markedly on the right side.

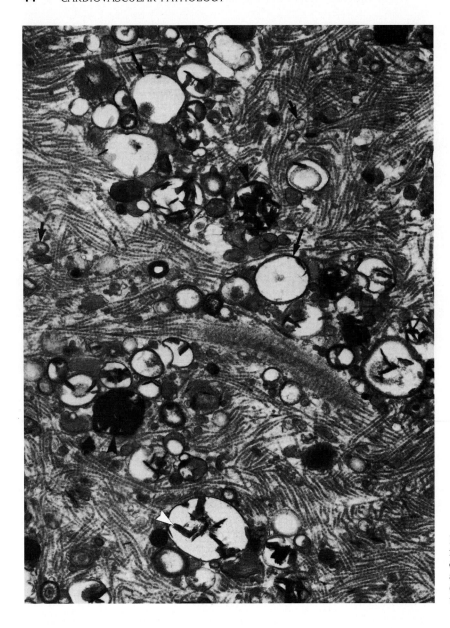

Figure 2-12 • Electron micrograph of a human femoral artery. In this higher-power view, matrical cell debris appears as vesicles (short arrows) and vacuoles (long arrows). Crystalline deposits (arrowheads) of calcium salts are seen in several vacuoles.

The myocardium is formed of muscle cells and a connective tissue interstitium. Myocytes make up about one third of the cells in the myocardium (Fig. 2-13). The interstitium is formed mainly of fibroblasts with smaller numbers of other cells, including adipocytes and a few leukocytes. The interstitium also has a rich capillary network originating from the epicardial coronary arteries. Although some authors recognize the presence of myocardial sinusoids, coexisting with the thebesian veins, this is controversial.[41] Lymphatics have also been noted in mammalian hearts, although their significance is incompletely understood.[42, 43]

Light Microscopy

The contractile proteins in the myofibers, the myofilaments, are arranged into groups that cause the cytoplasm to appear repetitively banded. Distinct bands, termed in-

tercalated disks, are a unique finding in cardiac muscle. As discussed later, these bands provide important structural support. The myocytes often have a step-like arrangement, because of the staggered location of their intercalated discs. Myocardial contraction bands (see Chapter 8) are an almost universal finding in endomyocardial biopsy specimens where they are artifactual. Unlike skeletal muscle, in cardiac muscle one or two nuclei are situated centrally in the cytoplasm. Lipofuscin, a golden-brown pigment, is often found in a perinuclear position.

Although cardiac muscle cells are seen bound end-to-end, there is also considerable branching that forms a complex network of interconnected cells. This prominent degree of cellular connection is not surprising when one considers that the function of the heart is not organized contractile strength but rather highly efficient repetitive contraction. The high degree of intercellular intertwining also means that myocytes are not organized into distinct

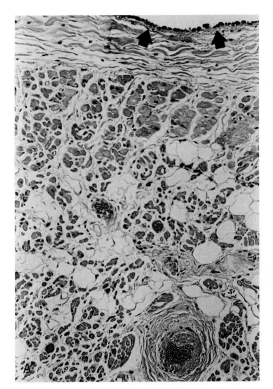
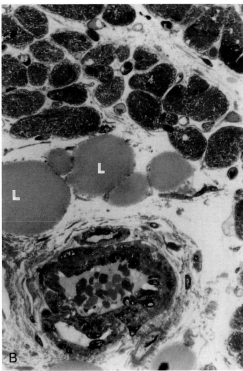

Figure 2-13 • Light micrograph of the atrial myocardium. *A,* The overlying thin pericardium is covered by a single layer of cuboidal mesothelial cells. Note that the myocardial interstitium contains small vessels and adipose tissue. This is also evident in *B,* in which lipid in adipocytes (L) was not extracted by the routine light microscopic processing, as occurred in *A. (A,* hematoxylin-phloxine saffron; *B,* methylene blue, electron microscopic "thick" section.)

fibers covered by a connective sheath, as is the case in other muscles.

There are no great differences between atrial and ventricular myocytes at the light microscopic level. Atrial fibers tend to be a smaller size than ventricular cardiomyocytes. The specialized cells of the conduction system, which are noted in the subendocardium, do possess a unique appearance; however, these are the topic of Chapter 20 and are not further discussed here.

Ultrastructure

Cell Membrane

The sarcolemma is composed of the trilaminar plasma membrane and the external lamina of the cardiomyocyte. The external lamina extends into the T-tubule system, as outlined later.

Nucleus

The nucleus of the myocyte is usually oval with its long axis oriented in the direction of the long axis of the cell. There is evenly distributed fine chromatin, often with central condensation. A single nucleolus is present. Nuclear pores for continuity of the nucleoplasm and the cytoplasm are present. The nucleus often has a close relationship to microtubules and cytoskeleton filaments. Because the cytoskeleton is connected to Z lines, the nucleus of the cell shows conformational changes depending on the state of contraction or relaxation of the

cell.[44] A cell may have more than one nucleus, as is found in 2 to 10% of myocytes in the adult myocardium. The number of nuclei is greater in children, and an association with hypertrophy has also been noted.[45] Polyploidy of the nucleus (diploidy to tetraploidy) is also quite common in normal hearts and in hearts with hypertrophy and overload.[46, 47] These changes are reflected by nuclear hyperchromasia and irregularity of nuclear shape.

Sarcoplasmic Reticulum

The sarcoplasmic reticulum (Fig. 2-14) is a complex network of specialized smooth endoplasmic reticulum that is important in transmitting the neural impulse to contract and in the storage of calcium ions to allow contraction. These longitudinal tubules form a membrane-bound system of tubules and cisterns that surround the myocytes. The sarcoplasmic reticulum is not as well developed in cardiac muscle as in skeletal muscle.

At the Z line, a T tubule (see Fig. 2-14), formed by an invagination of the sarcolemma, extends into the myocytes and makes contact with the sarcoplasmic reticulum. The T tubules spread a received electrical impulse through the myofiber, whereas the sarcoplasmic reticulum releases calcium for excitation (contraction) coupling. This overall configuration of the sarcoplasmic reticulum is similar to that of skeletal muscle, except it has a less well developed organization and the T tubules are larger in the heart.[48]

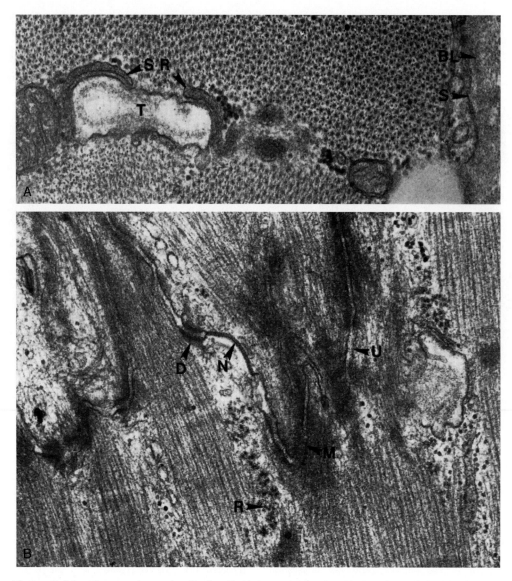

Figure 2-14 • Electron micrographs showing T tubules, sarcoplasmic reticulum, intercellular junctions, and cytoskeletal filaments. *A,* Cross-section of muscle cell showing sarcolemma (S), basement membrane (BL), thick and thin myofilaments, and T tubule (T), which form a triad with two closely apposed elements of sarcoplasmic reticulum (SR). *B,* Part of intercalated disk showing nexus (N), undifferentiated region (U), desmosome (D), and myofibrillar insertion sites (M) with dark material resembling that in Z-bands. Also note T tubule and free ribosomes (R) (*A,* ×49,000; *B,* ×45,000). (*A* and *B* courtesy of Victor J. Ferrans, MD, PhD.)

Cell Junctions

The intercalated disc (see Fig. 2-14), which occurs in place of a Z line in the region where two myocytes meet, is the most prominent junctional complex of cardiac muscle. These discs connect myocytes and organize them into myofibers[49]; they have structural, mechanical, and physiologic functions. The disks are composed of a fascia adherens that is responsible for end-to-end cell anchoring of actin filaments to one another. Between the myofibers, the macula adherens (or desmosome) binds the cells and is responsible for anchoring the intermediate-filament cytoskeleton proteins, vimentin and desmin.

Gap junctions, forming longitudinal communications between the cells, are responsible for the ionic continuity of the cells and, therefore, are important in contraction.

These structures, which have been studied extensively by freeze-fracture technique, were described previously. In the myocardium, the junctions may be associated with clusters of mitochondria, reflecting their role in calcium transport and production of energy in the cell.[49, 50] A typical myocyte is connected to an average of 9 to 11 other myocytes.[50] Age-related changes in gap junctions occur. Fetal cells possess gap junctions over their entire surface, whereas by age 6 years, the junctions are predominantly at cell ends and around intercalated discs.[51] In disease states, such as healing infarcts, the number, size, and spatial pattern of the gap junctions change and may contribute to arrhythmogenesis. Connexin, the major protein of the gap junction, is of multiple subtypes, with variation between different types of myocytes.[50]

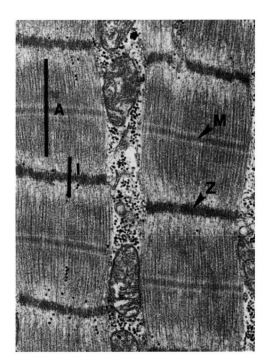

Figure 2-15 • Electron micrograph showing the structure of the sarcomeres. Note the A-, I-, M-, and Z-bands. Darkly stained granules are present between myofilaments. (Courtesy of Victor J. Ferrans, MD, PhD.)

Contractile Elements

Two types of myofilaments—thick and thin, or myosin and actin—are arranged in a highly ordered fashion to form contractile elements called myofibrils. Numerous myofibrils occur in the cytoplasmic matrix (sarcoplasm) of the muscle fiber. Under polarized light, the myofibrils and myofibers display alternating bright anisotropic bands, called A-bands, and dark isotropic bands, or I-bands. Other features shown in suitable preparations by light microscopy, but more clearly demonstrable by electron microscopy (Figs. 2-15 and 8-1), include (1) a dark line, the Z line (or Zwischenscheibe), which transverses the middle of the I-band; (2) a pale zone, the H-band (or Hensen's stripe), which bisects the A-band; and (3) a narrow, dark line, the M line (or Mittelscheibe), which transverses the center of the H-band. The portion of a myofibril between two consecutive Z lines is called a sarcomere. This is the contractile unit of striated muscle. At the Z line, the thin actin filaments from two neighboring sarcomeres are believed to be attached laterally to one another. In cross section, the Z line shows a lattice pattern. The relative lengths of the I- and A-bands depend on the state of contraction or relaxation of the myofibril. The A-band remains constant in length, but the I-band is longest when the muscle is stretched, medium-sized when it is relaxed, and shortest when it is contracted. The thin actin filaments in the I-band extend into the A-band, which contains the thick myosin filaments. Cross-sections through the A-bands of vertebrate skeletal and cardiac muscle show that the thick filaments form a hexagonal array or lattice.

During contraction, thin filaments slide over thick fila-ments and extend deeper into the A-band. This draws the two Z lines closer together and reduces the length of the sarcomere with resultant shortening of the fiber. In relaxed muscle, the thin filaments extending into the A-band from opposite ends do not meet at the M line but leave a gap that determines the width of the H-band. The H-band is the region of the A-band from which thin filaments are absent at any given moment. This explains why the H-band is wide in stretched muscle, of a medium size in relaxed muscle, and very narrow or entirely absent when the muscle is contracted.

The widely accepted view is that in vertebrate (including human) striated muscle, each thick myosin filament is surrounded by six thin actin filaments occupying the trigonal position (i.e., equidistant from and shared by three thick myosin filaments), with the ratio of thin to thick filaments being 2:1. However, this perfect pattern often is not demonstrable; frequently, there seem to be too few or too many thin filaments around the thick filaments, and thin filaments are not as regularly or equidistantly spaced between thick filaments.

Actin filaments are formed of two protofilaments wound around each other in a double helix arrangement. Tropomyosin filaments run in thin chains over the surface of the actin filaments. Troponin has three components: troponin T, which binds to tropomyosin; troponin C, which binds calcium; and troponin I, which inhibits the actin-myosin interaction.[52] Myosin is composed of two light and two heavy chains. Myosin possesses an adenosine triphosphatase (ATPase) site and has the ability to bind actin filaments. Titin, the third most abundant protein in the myocardium after myosin and actin, extends from the Z line to the area adjacent to the M line. Titin centers the A-band, is responsible for the structural continuity of the sarcomere, and forms the template for actin and myosin organization. Titin is responsible for the elastic recoil of the sarcomere and therefore influences compliance.[53]

Contraction of cardiac muscle involves neuromuscular communication, the sarcoplasmic reticulum, and interaction between actin and myosin filaments. Neural activity causes depolarization of the T-tubule system, which releases calcium from the sarcoplasmic reticulum to the myofilament areas. The calcium binds to troponin and changes its configuration, forcing the tropomyosin deeper into the actin filaments. This exposes a site with which myosin may bind. As this occurs, ATP is split, energy is released, and the myosin head bends and pulls the actin filaments past the myosin. This sliding-filament method of contraction ceases when new ATP is replenished and the filaments detach.[52, 54, 55]

Other Cytoplasmic Elements

The cytoplasm contains a cytoskeletal network of microtubules and intermediate filaments, chiefly vimentin and desmin. It also contains numerous organelles, especially mitochondria. This abundance probably reflects the oxidative metabolism and high energy requirements of the heart. The sarcoplasm contains glycogen and lipid, which are also sources of energy through fatty acid oxidation. Golgi apparatus and secondary lysosomes, or residual

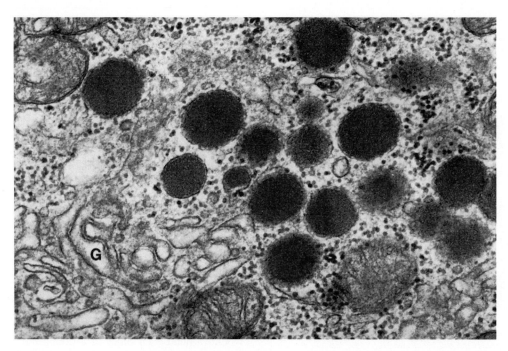

Figure 2-16 • Electron micrograph showing Golgi complex (G) and numerous darkly stained specific atrial granules found in the perinuclear region of an atrial myocyte. (Courtesy of Victor J. Ferrans, MD, PhD.)

bodies, commonly occur in the perinuclear region. These lysosomes give rise to lipofuscin, the "wear and tear pigment" commonly noted in the perinuclear region. This pigment increases with age and may be quite prominent.[46] It is not of homogenous composition and is best thought of as representing undigested residues from lysosomal actions. Polyglycosan may also accumulate, causing basophilic degeneration of the myocardium. This is found to a variable degree in all hearts of patients older than 60 years.[46, 56]

Atrial Granules

Atrial myocardium is similar to ventricular myocardium with a few exceptions. The myocytes are usually smaller, and the sarcoplasmic reticulum–T-tubule system is poorly developed. Perhaps the most important difference is that the atria of the heart have an important endocrine function and are known to possess secretory granules (Fig. 2-16). These granules play an important role in blood pressure regulation. They contain a polypeptide hormone, atrial natriuretic factor (ANF), which induces a diuresis when the atria are distended. The actions of ANF include (1) promotion of sodium and water excretion, (2) an increase in glomerular filtration rate, (3) renin secretion and aldosterone secretion inhibition, and (4) a decrease in systemic blood pressure.[57] The largest site of concentration is the atrial appendages, but secretory granules are also detected in the main body of the atria and in parts of the pulmonary circulation and the conduction system. Ultrastructurally, the granules are centered in a perinuclear location, adjacent to the secretory Golgi apparatus. The granule contents affect blood pressure by antagonizing vasoconstrictive substances, decreas-

ing vasopressin (antidiuretic hormone) secretion, and affecting aldosterone and renin secretion at the juxtaglomerular apparatus.[57] Studies have shown that the amount and distribution of ANF are altered in diseased hearts.[57–59] The number of granules in the atria decreases and the plasma ANF level increases in congestive heart failure.[57, 59]

INTERSTITIUM

The interstitium is composed of an extracellular matrix of fibrous proteins, both structural (collagen and elastin) and adhesive (fibronectin), as well as proteoglycans and cellular components. Although by volume the myocytes constitute about 75% of the wall of each cardiac chamber, they account for only about one third of the cells. The right atrium is notable for the relative prominence of fibrous tissue in its interstitium.

Extracellular Components

Collagen and Other Fibers

The heart has a well-developed interstitium of supportive connective tissue, chiefly collagen fibers with a much smaller component of elastic fibers. The interstitial collagen is part of the collagenous network of the heart, along with the collagen of the valves and the chordae.[60] The right ventricle has a higher amount of collagen than the left ventricle does.[61] Collagen is important in maintaining the geometry of the heart, to keep proper cell-to-cell alignment, to prevent overdistention and deformation during filling, and to prevent slippage of the myocytes from each other.[62]

The structure of collagen fibers was discussed previously. The two major collagen types in the myocardial interstitium are types I and III. Three important structural components can be discerned: small struts interconnecting the myocytes, small struts connecting the myocytes with the capillaries, and a complex series of sheaths encircling small groups of myocytes.[60, 63] The collagen fibers attach to the cell membrane adjacent to the Z lines, with linkage to integrins through vinculin, talin, and α-actinin.[62] Collagen deposition and degradation are influenced by mediators such as α_1-angiotensin, transforming growth factor-β, and matrix metalloproteinases—collagenase, gelatinase, and stromeolysin.[62] The collagen content of the myocardium generally increases with age.[46]

The other fiber types in the interstitium include elastic and fibronectin. Fibronectin forms a bridge from the myocyte to the extracellular matrix and is important in cell migration and healing. Laminin is an important component of the cell coat of myocytes and fibroblasts. Laminin binds collagen and is important in cellular adhesion, migration, growth, and differentiation.[62]

Proteoglycan Particles

Proteoglycans, once called mucoproteins or protein-polysaccharides, are an important constituent of the interfibrillary matrix. Their morphology is variable, but in many tissues they appear as round, oval, triangular, or stellate electron-dense, non–membrane-bound particles associated with filaments about 5 nm thick. Such a demonstration of proteoglycan particles is often difficult because a substantial loss of carbohydrates, and hence proteoglycans, occurs during routine fixation. Proteoglycans are complexes of covalently bound glycosaminoglycans inserted at regular intervals along a protein core.

Matrical Lipidic Debris, Spherical Microparticles, and Matrix Vesicles

In 1965, osmiophilic granular and membranous material (i.e., vesicles, myelinoid membranes, and figures) was reported in the matrix of human and rabbit articular cartilage.[64] This was called "matrical lipidic debris," and it was postulated that it derived from extruded cell processes of chondrocytes and also from in situ necrosis of chondrocytes. Since then, such cellular debris found in the basal lamina and matrix in various tissues and organs (e.g., kidney, heart, placenta, nerves, menisci, blood vessels, tumors) has been referred to as spherical microparticles or matrix vesicles. In most sites, such debris has a strong tendency to calcify, so these structures have also at times been called calcifying vesicles.

In the heart, spherical microparticles are looked upon as debris cast off by cells, particularly injured cells in pathologic states. Alternatively, the shedding of small numbers of spherical microparticles may be a normal biologic phenomenon involved in remodeling of cell surfaces and junctions whereby obsolescent areas of membrane are cast off by budding.[65] The occurrence of much larger numbers of spherical microparticles in diseased hearts probably represents an exaggeration of this phenomenon.

Cellular Components

The cellular elements of the interstitium include adipocytes, fibroblasts, histiocytes, veil cells, myofibroblasts, smooth muscle cells, undifferentiated mesenchymal cells, and mononuclear inflammatory cells including mast cells and lymphocytes.[66, 67]

Mature adipose tissue is found in all layers of the myocardium, especially the epicardium, in and on both atria and ventricles, and is concentrated around the heart base and along the courses of epicardial coronary arteries. Small sheaths of adipose tissue may extend into the myocardium from the epicardium around penetrating intramural coronary arteries. The right ventricle particularly may have a large proportion of its wall thickness constituted by such adipose tissue. Adipose tissue may account for 4 to 52% of the heart weight; its amount increases with patient age. Many studies also found a relationship between the amount of adipose tissue and patient gender, body weight, and, in some cases, drug therapy (e.g., corticosteroid treatment).[46, 68–71] Epicardial lymphocytes are normal and often have an association with the coronary arterial adventitia.[72] Age-related amyloid (see Chapter 3) may deposit in either an intravascular or an interstitial location.[73] Ganglia are commonly noted in the epicardial adipose tissue and sometimes in the superficial myocardium. They are concentrated near the sinoatrial and atrioventricular nodes, the left atrial surface, the appendage-atrium junction, and around the base of the great arteries.[74]

Fibroblasts are elongated, often bearing long polar cell processes. They are characterized by the absence of an external lamina, an abundance of rough endoplasmic reticulum, and a prominent Golgi complex. The latter two structures are needed to produce precursors of the matrix components and are best developed in metabolically active fibroblasts; the scant cytoplasm of quiescent or resting fibroblasts contains few organelles. Scattered actin filaments may be noted, but these are more marked in myofibroblasts.

The histiocytes of the interstitium are phagocytic and, therefore, are characterized by their irregular cell membrane and prominent cytoplasmic lysosome contents. Mast cells are found in a perivascular location, in the endocardium, and in small numbers in myocardial interstitium. Their importance or function is unknown.

Myofibroblasts resemble fibroblasts with some characteristics of smooth muscle cells, including tracts of actin filaments with focal densities along their course. The veil cells have thin, elongated cytoplasmic processes that wrap around myocytes and are thought to play a role similar to that of pericytes.

ENDOCARDIUM

The endocardial layer lines the atria, the atrial appendages, and the ventricles. The endocardium's structure in those sites is similar, but the endocardium is thicker in the left-sided chambers, and it is thicker in the atria compared with the ventricles. Outflow tract endocardium is noticeably thicker than that of the inflow tracts. There are three recognized layers: an endothelial layer, a subendothelial layer, and an elastic layer. These layers are sometimes ill defined, and there is some variation even within the same chamber.

The endothelial layer consists of a single layer of flat, parallel endothelial cells. These are similar to endothelial cells described elsewhere, with an irregular cell membrane, Weibel-Palade bodies, pinocytotic vesicles, and a cell membrane. Complex lateral interdigitations are common in this site.[75] Occasionally, the cytoplasm of the atrial endothelial cells contains microtubules and microfilaments, structures usually not found in ventricular endothelial cells.[75] Pinocytotic vesicles suggest that these cells may be active in transport of materials. The subendothelial layer contains delicate collagen fibrils, loosely dispersed and multidirectional, often with fibroblasts. This layer is also more prominent in the atrial endocardium.[75] The elastic layer, the thickest, contains prominent elastic fibers that increase in size from the endothelial layer to the area adjacent to the myocardium. Collagen fibers and groups of smooth muscle cells are also noted. The smooth muscle may be prominent, especially in the left atrium and in the left ventricular septal region.

Between the endocardium and myocardium is another layer, the subendocardium, which binds the true endocardium to the myocardium. This contains thick elastic and collagen fibers and a prominent number of blood vessels, mostly capillaries of continuous type with some arterioles. In right atrium and right ventricle, small arteries may superficially protrude from endocardial surfaces into the cardiac chambers.[76] Nerve fibers and branches of Purkinje cells are seen. This layer may also contain undifferentiated mesenchymal cells, fibroblasts, and macrophages. Adipose tissue may be noted in this layer, especially in the right ventricle. The subendocardium is continuous with the extracellular matrix that surrounds the myofibers in the myocardium.[77]

PERICARDIUM

The structure of the pericardium reflects its main functions: mechanical (compliance, ventricular interaction, and filling), membranous (immunologic and barrier), and ligamentous (stability of the heart in the chest).[78]

The pericardium is composed of two layers, the serosa and the fibrosa. The serosa is a mesothelial cell monolayer (see Fig. 2-13A) that covers the surface of the heart and the proximal great vessels and extends over the inner aspect of the remainder of the pericardial sac. The collagenous fibrosa anchors the heart to the sternum and extends to the diaphragm. Within the fibrosa are numerous nerves, blood vessels, and lymphatics.

The serosa and fibrosa layers over the surface of the heart have been termed the visceral pericardium or epicardium. The adipose tissue on the surface of the heart is commonly considered part of the epicardium. In contrast, some authors consider the epicardium to represent only the connective tissue layer containing nerves and blood vessels that lies under the mesothelial layer.[79] The serosa

and fibrosa not covering the heart surface have been termed the parietal pericardium[78]; the fibrosa of this portion of the pericardium is particularly thick. The adipose tissue surrounding the parietal pericardium may be up to 2 cm thick in normal adults.

Ultrastructurally, the serosal mesothelial cells possess rare cilia, microvilli, and intracytoplasmic filaments, chiefly cytokeratin and actin. The mesothelial cells are anchored with a basal lamina and desmosomes, and there is extensive interdigitation laterally with adjacent cells. The microvilli provide a friction-bearing surface and function in fluid and ion exchange. The fibrosa has collagen fibers and a smaller number of elastic fibers.[80] The collagenous nature of the parietal pericardium leads to inelasticity. With age, the collagen fibers of the pericardium straighten and become more stiff.[46]

VALVES

The valves of the heart are of two categories, the atrioventricular valves (mitral and tricuspid) and the semilunar valves (aortic and pulmonary). Their overall structural components are similar with minor variations.

Atrioventricular Valves

The valve leaflets have four layers, arranged from closest to atrium to closest to ventricle — the auricularis, the spongiosa, the fibrosa, and the ventricularis, respectively. The valve surfaces are covered with endothelial cells, which on the atrial surface are more plump and prominent with irregular nuclei.

The auricularis covers the spongiosa on the third of the leaflet closest to the annulus. It is composed of collagen, elastic fibers, and smooth muscle cells. The ventricularis is mainly composed of small elastic fibers that blend with the subendocardium of the adjacent ventricle. This layer extends only part of the distance to the leaflet free edge.

The fibrosa, the valves' central layer, is responsible for structural support and is composed of collagen and of elastic fibers that represent an extension of the annulus of the valve. On the ventricular aspect of the leaflets, this connective tissue extends into the chordae tendineae and the tips of the papillary muscles. The fibrosa layer extends the entire leaflet length to the free edge.

The spongiosa contains mainly proteoglycans, sparse elastic fibers, collagen, and connective tissue cells such as fibroblasts and primitive mesenchymal cells. The predominant glycosaminoglycans are hyaluronic acid, chondroitin sulfate B, chondroitin sulfate AC, and heparin.[81] In the mitral valve, the proximal third of the spongiosa also contains cardiac myocytes and capillaries, extending from the left atrial myocardium. The spongiosa, like the fibrosa, extends the entire length of the leaflet; therefore, the distal third of the atrioventricular valves is composed of only the fibrosa and the spongiosa.

A distinct type of cardiac interstitial cell is present in all valve layers. The cell has two morphologies — elongated and cobblestone. The interstitial cell is thought to secrete matrix and to participate in valve repair. These cells resemble smooth muscle cells and have gap junctions and cytoplasmic contractile elements.[82, 83] The valves also contain small nerves, both adrenergic and cholinergic, mostly at the valve base, and lymphatics.[84, 85]

The tricuspid valve is structurally similar to the mitral valve, with a few differences. The layers in the tricuspid valve are thinner, and no cardiac myocytes are present in the spongiosa. The auricularis on the posterior and septal leaflets is prominent and contains more smooth muscle cells.

The chordae tendineae are thin, tendon-like structures extending from the valve leaflet to the endocardial surface. They are composed mainly of parallel-arranged collagen fibers, with minor elastic elements. There is a thin covering of endocardium. Occasionally, they are thick and contain muscle, forming so-called chordae muscularis.

Semilunar Valves

The valve cusps of aortic and pulmonary valves are structurally similar to those of the atrioventricular valves, with minor variations. The cusps are covered with endothelial cells and comprise four layers, arranged from closest to ventricle to closest to aorta or pulmonary artery—the ventricularis, the spongiosa, the fibrosa, and the arterialis, respectively.[83]

The fibrosa is the major structural component of the cusps and contains dense collagen, elastic fibers in smaller amounts, and fibroblasts. The fibrosa blends into the valve commissures and the annulus of each valve, thus transferring some of the load created by the diastolic pressure gradient; it extends to the free edge of the valve cusps. At the base of the cusps, elastic fibers may aggregate and form an ill-defined superficial layer, the arterialis. Studies have indicated that the elastic fibers form a sponge-like network around the collagen fibers, giving the cusp great extensibility.[86] In the semilunar and atrioventricular valves, great deformations of the valve structure are necessary. This is made possible by the complicated interactions between collagen and elastin, which are only now being elucidated. Collagen is relatively inelastic, as previously discussed, and for fibers to slip over one another, macroscopic corrugations (surface rippling) and crimp (microscopic undulations of circumferentially arranged fibers) are necessary. Corrugations are thought to expand and flatten, allowing radial compliance, whereas crimp allows unfolding and is therefore responsible for circumferential compliance. Elastin interconnects and surrounds the collagen to provide a "return string mechanism," restoring the contracted configuration after each stretch of the valve. In the initial cusp stretch, elastin provides tension. After collagen is uncoiled and extended, it assumes the load and further limits extension. Elastin is then responsible for pulling back the collagen into its initial folded shape.[87] (See Chapter 13 for further discussion.)

The spongiosa lies between the ventricularis and the fibrosa. This layer is prominent only in the basal third of the cusp and does not extend to its edge; it is composed chiefly of proteoglycans, collagen, fibroblasts, and undifferentiated mesenchymal cells. This layer confers elasticity, dampens vibration and shock, and may allow shear to occur between the fibrosa and the ventricularis.[87]

The ventricularis layer represents a continuation of the ventricular endocardial layer; it contains prominent amounts of elastic fibers. This layer is thickened focally along the line of valve closure and forms local protuberances centrally on the cusp surfaces—the nodule of Arantius (nodulus Arantii) on the aortic cusps and the nodule of Morgagni (nodulus Morgagni) on the pulmonary cusps. The free edge of the valve contains only the fibrosa and ventricularis layers.

Age-related thickening of the valves occurs, most markedly at the posterior aortic cusp and the anterior cusp of the pulmonary valve.[88] Other age-related valvular lesions include Lambl's excrescences—small single or multiple fibroelastic papillary projections that form along the lines of valve closure[89]—and fibrous tags, which appear like Lambl's excrescences but project from valve free edges.

REFERENCES

1. Tennant M, McGeachie JK: Blood vessel structure and function: A brief update on recent advances. Aust N Z J Surg 60:747, 1990
2. Stary HC, Blackenhorn DH, Chandler AB, et al: A definition of the intima of human arteries and of its atherosclerois-prone regions: A report from the Committee on Vascular Lesions of the Council on Arteriosclerosis, American Heart Association. Circulation 85:391, 1992
3. Wolinsky H, Glagov S: A lamellar unit of aortic medial structure and function in mammals. Circ Res 20:99, 1967
4. Schlatmann TJM, Becker AE: Histologic changes in the normal aging aorta: Implications for dissecting aortic aneurysm. Am J Cardiol 39:13, 1977
5. Stefanadis C, Vlachopoulos C, Karayannacos P, et al: Effect of vasa vasorum flow on structure and function of the aorta in experimental animals. Circulation 91:2669, 1995
6. Barker SGE, Beesley JE, Baskerville PA, Martin JF: The influence of the adventitia on the presence of smooth muscle cells and macrophages in the arterial intima. Eur J Vasc Endovasc Surg 9:222, 1995
7. Zamir M, Silver MD: Vasculature in the walls of human coronary arteries. Arch Pathol Lab Med 109:659, 1985
8. van Son JAM, Smedts F, de Wilde PCM, et al: Histological study of the internal mammary artery with emphasis on its suitability as a coronary artery bypass graft. Ann Thorac Surg 55:106, 1993
9. Sims FH, Gavin JB, Vanderwee MA: The intima of coronary arteries. Am Heart J 118:32, 1989
10. Barger AC, Beeuwkes RI, Lainey LL, Silverman KJ: Hypothesis: Vasa vasorum and neovascularization of human coronary arteries: A possible role in the pathophysiology of atherosclerosis. N Engl J Med 310:175, 1984
11. Sims FH, Gavin JB: The early development of intimal thickening of human coronary arteries. Coron Artery Dis 1:205, 1990
12. Diaz-Flores L, Dominguez C: Relation between arterial intimal thickening and the vasa vasorum. Virchows Arch [Path Anat] 406: 165, 1985
13. Kumamato M, Nakashima Y, Sueishi K: Intimal neovascularization in human coronary atherosclerosis: Its origin and pathophysiological significance. Hum Pathol 26:450, 1995
14. Sims DE: Recent advances in pericyte biology: Implications for health and disease. Can J Cardiol 7:431, 1991
15. Orlidge A, D'Amore PA: Inhibition of capillary endothelial cell growth by pericytes and smooth muscle cells. J Cell Biol 105:1455, 1987
16. Antonelli-Orlidge A, Smith SR, D'Amore PA: Influence of pericytes

on capillary endothelial cell growth. Am Rev Respir Dis 140:1129, 1989

17. Harmon JV Jr, Edwards WD: Venous valves in subclavian and internal jugular veins: Frequency, position, and structure in 100 autopsy cases. Am J Cardiovasc Pathol 1:51, 1986

18. Leu HJ, Leu AJ: Phlebosclerosis, phlebothrombosis, and thrombophlebitis: A current perspective. Cardiovasc Pathol 5:183, 1996

19. Edwards WD: Pathology of pulmonary hypertension. Cardiovasc Clin 18:321, 1988

20. Burke AP, Farb A, Virmani R: The pathology of primary pulmonary hypertension. Mod Pathol 4:269, 1991

21. Vane JR, Anggard EE, Botting RM: Regulatory functions of the vascular endothelium. N Engl J Med 323:27, 1990

22. Tedgui A: Endothelial permeability under physiological and pathological conditions. Prostaglandins Leukot Essent Fatty Acids 54:27, 1996

23. Ghadially FN: Intracytoplasmic filaments. In: Ghadially FN (ed): Ultrastructural Pathology of the Cell and Matrix. 4th ed. Boston, Butterworth-Heinemann, 1997, p 887

24. Gotlieb AI: The role of endothelial cells in vascular integrity and repair. Cardiovasc Pathol 1:253, 1992

25. Vyalov S, Langille BL, Gotlieb AI: Decreased blood flow rate disrupts endothelial repair in vivo. Am J Pathol 149:2107, 1996

26. Weibel ER, Palade GE: New cytoplasmic components in arterial endothelia. J Cell Biol 23:101, 1961

27. Matsuda H, Sugiura S: Ultrastructure of "tubular body" in the endothelial cells of the ocular blood vessels. Invest Ophthalmol 9:919, 1970

28. Wagner DD, Olmsted JB, Marder VJ: Immunolocalization of von Willebrand protein in Weibel-Palade bodies of human endothelial cells. J Cell Biol 95:355, 1982

29. Staehelin LA: Structure and function of intercellular junctions. Int Rev Cytol 39:191, 1974

30. Chalcroft JP, Bullivant S: An interpretation of liver cell membrane and junction structure based on observation of freeze fracture replicas of both sides of the fracture. J Cell Biol 47:49, 1970

31. Wissler RW: The arterial medial cell—smooth muscle, or multifunctional mesenchyme? Circulation 36:1, 1967

32. Gabbiani G, Kocher O, Bloom WS, et al: Actin expression in smooth muscle cells of rat aortic intimal thickening, human atheromatous plaque, and cultured rat aortic media. J Clin Invest 73:148, 1984

33. Mayne R: Collagenous proteins of blood vessels. Arteriosclerosis 6:585, 1986

34. Ross R: The smooth muscle cell. II. Growth of smooth muscle in culture and formation of elastic fibers. J Cell Biol 50:172, 1971

35. Fernandez-Teran MA, Hurle JM: Myocardial fiber architecture of the human heart ventricles. Anat Rec 204:137, 1982

36. Fox CC, Hutchins GM: The architecture of the human ventricular myocardium. Hopkins Med J 130:289, 1972

37. Armour JA, Randall WC: Structural basis for cardiac function. Am J Physiol 218:1517, 1970

38. Lowe TE, Wartman WB: Myocardial infarction. Br Heart J 6:115, 1944

39. Bovendeerd PHM, Huyghe JM, Arts T, et al: Influence of endocardial-epicardial crossover of muscle fibers on left ventricular wall mechanics. J Biomech 27:941, 1994

40. Wang K, Gibson DG, Anderson RH: Architecture of atrial musculature in humans. Br Heart J 73:559, 1995

41. Tsang JC-C, Chiu RC-J: The phantom of "myocardial sinusoids": A historical reappraisal. Ann Thorac Surg 60:1831, 1995

42. Miller AJ: The lymphatics of the heart. Arch Intern Med 112:501, 1963

43. Szlavy L, Adams DF, Hollenberg NK, Abrams HL: Cardiac lymph and lymphatics in normal and infarcted myocardium. Am Heart J 100:323, 1980

44. Lannigan RA, Zaki SA: Ultrastructure of the myocardium of the atrial appendage. Br Heart J 28:796, 1966

45. Shozawa T, Okada E, Kawamura K, et al: Development of binucleated myocytes in normal and hypertrophied human hearts. Am J Cardiovasc Pathol 3:27, 1990

46. Kitzman DW, Edwards WD: Age-related changes in the anatomy of the normal human heart. J Gerontol 45:M33, 1990

47. Brodsky VY, Sarkisov DS, Arefyeva AM, et al: Polyploidy in cardiac myocytes of normal and hypertrophic human hearts: Range of values. Virchows Arch 424:429, 1994

48. Porter KR, Franzini-Armstrong C: The sarcoplasmic reticulum. Sci Am 212:72, 1965

49. Severs NJ: The cardiac gap junction and intercalated disc. Int J Cardiol 26:137, 1990

50. Saffitz JE: Myocyte interconnections at gap junctions and the development of anatomic substrates of ventricular arrhythmias. Cardiovasc Pathol 3:87, 1994

51. Spach MS: Changes in the topology of gap junctions as an adaptive structural response of the myocardium. Circulation 90:1103, 1994

52. Cohen C: The protein switch of muscle contraction. Sci Am 233:36, 1975

53. Hein S, Scholz D, Fujitani N, et al: Altered expression of titin and contractile proteins in failing human myocardium. J Mol Cell Cardiol 26:1291, 1994

54. Murray JM, Weber A: The cooperative action of muscle proteins. Sci Am 230:58, 1974

55. Huxley HE: The mechanism of muscular contraction. Sci Am 213:18, 1965

56. Tamura S, Takahashi M, Kawamura S, Ishihara T: Basophilic degeneration of the myocardium: Histological, immunohistochemical and immuno-electronmicroscopic studies. Histopathology 26:501, 1995

57. Ackermann DM, Edwards BS, Wold LE, Burnette JCJ: Atrial natriuretic peptide: Localization in the human heart. JAMA 256:1048, 1986

58. Edwards BS, Ackermann DM, Lee ME, et al: Identification of atrial natriuretic factor within ventricular tissue in hamsters and humans with congestive heart failure. J Clin Invest 81:82, 1988

59. Edwards BS, Rodeheffer RJ, Reeder GS, Burnett JC Jr: Expression of atrial natriuretic factor in the human ventricle is independent of chamber dilation. J Am Coll Cardiol 16:1589, 1990

60. Weber KT: Cardiac interstitium in health and disease: The fibrillar collagen network. J Am Coll Cardiol 13:1637, 1989

61. van Suylen RJ, van Bekkum EEC, Boersma H, et al: Collagen content and distribution in the normal and transplanted human heart: A postmortem quantitative light microscopic analysis. Cardiovasc Pathol 5:61, 1996

62. Ju H, Dixon IMC: Extracellular matrix and cardiovascular diseases. Can J Cardiol 12:1259, 1996

63. Caulfield JB, Borg TK: The collagen network of the heart. Lab Invest 40:364, 1979

64. Ghadially FN, Meachim G, Collins DH: Extra-cellular lipid in the matrix of human articular cartilage. Ann Rheum Dis 24:136, 1965

65. Ferrans VJ, Thiedemann K-U, Maron BJ, et al: Spherical microparticles in human myocardium: An ultrastructural study. Lab Invest 35:349, 1976

66. Foley DA, Edwards WD: Quantitation of leukocytes in endomyocardial tissue from 100 normal human hearts at autopsy: Implications for diagnosis of myocarditis from biopsy specimens of living patients. Am J Cardiovasc Pathol 2:145, 1988

67. Turlington BS, Edwards WD: Quantitation of mast cells in 100 normal and 92 diseased human hearts: Implications for interpretation of endomyocardial biopsy specimens. Am J Cardiovasc Pathol 2:151, 1988

68. Dembinski AS, Dobson JRI, Wilson JE, et al: Frequency, extent, and distribution of endomyocardial adipose tissue: Morphometric analysis of endomyocardial biopsy specimens from 241 patients. Cardiovasc Pathol 3:33, 1994

69. Caruso G, Frassanito F, Serio G, Pennella A: Is adipose tissue a normal component of the myocardium? Eur Heart J 10(suppl D):89, 1989

70. House AA, Walley VM: Right heart failure due to ventricular adiposity: "Adipositas cordis"—An old diagnosis revisited. Can J Cardiol 12:485, 1996

71. Shirani J, Berezowski K, Roberts WC: Quantitative measurement of normal and excessive (cor adiposum) subepicardial adipose tissue, its clinical significance, and its effect on electrocardiographic QRS voltage. Am J Cardiol 76:414, 1995

72. Grimley CE, Benbow EW, Stoddart RW: Epicardial lymphocytes: An autopsy study. Am J Cardiovasc Pathol 2:225, 1988

73. Walley VM, Kisilevsky R, Young ID: Amyloid and the cardiovascular system: A review of pathogenesis and pathology with clinical correlation. Cardiovasc Pathol 4:79, 1995

74. Singh S, Johnson PI, Lee RE, et al: Topography of cardiac ganglia in the adult heart. J Thorac Cardiovasc Surg 112:943, 1996

75. Melax H, Leeson TS: Fine structure of the endocardium in adult rats. Cardiovasc Res 1:349, 1967

76. Kolodziej AW, Lobo FV, Walley VM: Intra-atrial course of the right coronary artery and its branches. Can J Cardiol 10:263, 1994

77. Lannigan RA, Zaki SA: Ultrastructure of the normal atrial endocardium. Br Heart J 28:785, 1966

78. Spodick DH: Macrophysiology, microphysiology, and anatomy of the pericardium: A synopsis. Am Heart J 124:1046, 1992

79. Vaughan CM, D'Cruz IA: Applied anatomy of the pericardium: Echocardiographic interpretation. Prim Cardiol 19:56, 1993

80. Ishihara T, Ferrans VJ, Jones M, et al: Histologic and ultrastructural features of normal human parietal pericardium. Am J Cardiol 46:744, 1980

81. Baig MM: Acid mucopolysaccharides of congenitally defective, rheumatic, and normal human aortic valves. Am J Pathol 96:771, 1996

82. Zacks S, Rosenthal A, Granton B, et al: Characterization of cobble-stone mitral valve interstitial cells. Arch Pathol Lab Med 115:774, 1991

83. Mulholland DL, Gotlieb AI: Cell biology of valvular interstitial cells. Can J Cardiol 12:231, 1996

84. Su H, Mao Q, Zhang Y, et al: Distribution of peptide-containing nerves in the cardiac valves of rats of different ages. Cell Vision 2:40, 1995

85. Kawano H, Kawai S, Shirai T, Okada R: Morphological study on vagal innervation in human atrioventricular valves using histochemical method. Jpn Circ J 57:753, 1993

86. Scott M, Vesely I: Aortic valve cusp microstructure: The role of elastin. Ann Thorac Surg 60:S391, 1995

87. Schoen FJ: Aortic valve structure-function correlations: Role of elastic fibers no longer a stretch of the imagination. J Heart Valve Dis 6:1, 1997

88. Chida K, Ohkawa S, Watanabe C, et al: A morphological study of the normally aging heart. Cardiovasc Pathol 3:1, 1994

89. Boone SA, Campagna M, Walley VM: Lambl's excrescences and papillary fibroelastomas: Are they different? Can J Cardiol 8:372, 1992

Chapter 3

Age-related Cardiovascular Changes

Wanda M. Lester

Although the maximal lifespan has not apparently increased over time, the average life expectancy in the United States has increased from 47 years in 1900 to more than 78 years for women and 72 years for men today.[1] There has also been a rapid growth in the population of people older than 85 years of age, with expansion of this age group expected to continue.[2]

Aging may be defined in various ways. Broadly speaking, it refers to those changes occurring after maturity which decrease the probability of survival.[3, 4] It is important to distinguish between the changes that result from aging itself and those that are caused by disease, environment, or lifestyle.[3] For example, an increased heart weight in an elderly subject could be secondary to systemic hypertension or ischemic heart disease, or it could be caused by aging. Furthermore, there is much variation between individuals in the rate at which age-related changes in the cardiovascular system develop.[3] The theoretic mechanisms of aging include mutations in nuclear and mitochondrial DNA,[5] free radical toxicity, glycosylation of key proteins, changes in immune or neuroendocrine function, and other factors.[1, 3] Theories of aging have sometimes been divided into two types: one postulates that aging events occur randomly, accumulate over time, and are caused by factors external to the organism; the other proposes that aging events are genetically programmed.[6] Genetic mutations accumulate over time. It is also possible that genes that improve reproductive fitness may have adverse effects on longevity.[7] Caloric restriction has successfully extended the maximal lifespan in various animal models. A postulated mechanism for this effect is a lowering of free radical production within mitochondria,[8] which in turn would protect the mitochondria and their DNA from damage by free radicals.[9] Caloric restriction is likely be a less popular prescription for longevity than the provision of so-called youthful hormones such as growth hormone and androgens.[10] These active areas of research are not considered further here.

In this chapter, the effects of aging on the cardiovascular system are considered, with the exception of changes in the conduction system, which are found in Chapter 20. After discussions of autopsy studies, cardiovascular function in the elderly, and senile cardiovascular amyloidosis, the effect of aging on the endocardium, the individual heart valves, the myocardium, and the vasculature are presented. Information on progeria and Werner syndrome is included at the end of the chapter. (Note: Some age changes are also discussed in Chapter 2.)

AUTOPSY STUDIES OF ELDERLY SUBJECTS

Cardiovascular disease, including stroke, is an important cause of death in the elderly, accounting for 24% of deaths in 200 subjects older than 85 years of age in one series[11] and 52% of subjects older than 90 years in another.[12] There have been many reports of autopsy findings in elderly subjects,[11–18] but these studies offer no uniform definition of "elderly." Selection bias is an issue in all of them, because the percentage of subjects autopsied drops as the age at death increases.[2] Results from two recent autopsy studies[16, 17] of the hearts of nonagenarians are shown in Table 3-1; some entities listed in this table are discussed in more detail in a later section.

CARDIOVASCULAR FUNCTION IN THE AGED

Resting cardiac output has been reported either to decrease[19, 20] or to remain unchanged with aging.[21] One study suggested important but complex influences of gender on the effect of aging on cardiac performance.[22] Heart rate increases in response to exercise are impaired in the elderly,[19–21] so augmentation of stroke volume is vital to raise cardiac output. The maximal cardiac output response to exercise decreases with age.[19, 20, 22] Systolic ventricular performance is relatively well preserved, but left ventricular early diastolic filling is decreased in the elderly[23] and ventricular relaxation prolonged.[20, 23] Such abnormal diastolic function may result in higher left ventricular diastolic pressures.[20] Some age-related changes in hemodynamics may reflect impaired responses to adrenergic stimulation.[24] Inadequate compensatory responses to hemodynamic disturbances place elderly subjects at increased risk of syncope caused by hypotension, with the latter occurring in response to postural changes, food consumption, micturition, or defecation, and the risk is enhanced by concomitant diuretic therapy.[20, 25]

SENILE CARDIOVASCULAR AMYLOID

The general topic of cardiovascular amyloid is covered in Chapter 16. At least three types are found in the elderly: one involves the atria alone, derives from atrial natriuretic factor, and is termed isolated atrial amyloid; another involves both atria and ventricles, may be associ-

TABLE 3-1 • **Cardiac Findings at Autopsy in Nonagenarians**

Author	Lie[17]	Roberts[16]
Total cases	237	93
Males	93	51
Females	144	42
Percentage of deaths due to a cardiovascular cause	48	49
Heart weight in males (g)		
Range	235–640	260–660
Mean	405	436
Heart weight in females (g)		
Range	200–740	220–630
Mean	355	397
Percentage of cases with significant (>75% cross-sectional area narrowing) coronary artery disease involving		
0 vessels	57	37
1 vessel	18	21
2 vessels	14	32
3 vessels	6	10
4 vessels	5	0
Percentage of cases with mitral annular calcification	43	42
Percentage of cases with aortic valve calcific deposits	40	63
Percentage of cases with senile cardiac amyloid	65	17

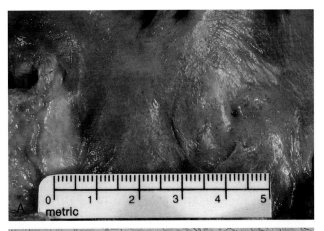

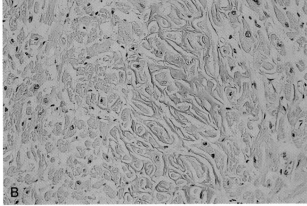

Figure 3-1 • Senile systemic cardiovascular amyloid. *A*, Small plaques are present in the atrial endocardium in some cases. *B*, Interstitial perimyocytic amyloid deposits are green with the sulphated Alcian blue stain.

ated with small deposits of amyloid in other organs, and derives from transthyretin; and the third type is senile aortic amyloid.[26, 27]

Isolated Atrial Amyloid

This is found in 80% of autopsied subjects who are older than 80 years of age. The deposits usually encircle cardiac myocytes. Their congophilia is resistant to potassium permanganate, and the amyloid does not contain tryptophan.[26] This type of amyloidosis appears to be more common in those who have cardiac disorders that are associated with increased plasma levels of atrial natriuretic factor, but it does not in itself seem to be clinically significant.[26]

Senile Systemic Cardiovascular Amyloid

Detected in 25% of people older than 80 years of age, it is occasionally associated with clinical cardiac dysfunction, specifically congestive heart failure and atrial fibrillation.[28, 29] The amyloid derives from transthyretin of normal composition, with the amyloid fibrils containing both intact and fragmented transthyretin. Deposits are found mainly in vessel walls of organs other than the heart, but within the heart they also occur between cardiac myocytes. They are found in both atria and ventricles (Fig. 3-1). There is less amyloid in the conduction system than in the rest of the myocardium.[26] Amyloid is also commonly present in pulmonary vessels and alveolar septa in these patients. Deposits are not observed within glomeruli, but lumps of amyloid are found in the renal medulla.[30] The congophilia of this amyloid is usually weaker than that of AA (derived from serum amyloid A protein) or AL (derived from light chain proteins) amyloidosis. It is resistant

to potassium permanganate and contains tryptophan.[26] Immunoperoxidase staining with an antibody to transthyretin can be used to establish the diagnosis. It is important to do this additional test when amyloid is detected on a heart biopsy, because senile systemic cardiovascular amyloid does not respond to alkylating agents.[29]

Aortic Amyloid

Amyloid deposits are present in the aortic media in 97% of patients older than 50 years of age, and intimal amyloid is found in 35% of them.[31] Adventitial amyloid, by contrast, occurs in fewer than 3% of such subjects, being present in the connective tissue and vasa vasora. The adventitial amyloid also derives from transthyretin and is similar to senile systemic amyloid. Aortic amyloid has no clinical consequences. It is more often observed in the thoracic than the abdominal aorta. The deposition of medial and intimal aortic amyloid develops independent of atrial or ventricular deposits. Medial aortic amyloid forms lumps and lines parallel to smooth muscle cells, sometimes appearing to be intracellular,[27] and can also be found in the media of the common carotid artery. This form of amyloid is weakly Congo red positive; it contains tryptophan, and its congophilia is resistant to potassium permanganate. Medial amyloid seems to be distinct from other known forms of amyloid and also from intimal amyloid.[31] It is associated with atheromas. Intimal aortic amyloid associated with atheromas derives from apolipoprotein A1.[32]

ENDOCARDIAL CHANGES WITH AGING

General Changes

With aging, the endocardium becomes thicker and more opaque. This is not a uniform change throughout the organ; it is most diffuse and prominent within the left atrium. Endocardial thickening is mildest in the right ventricle, with the most prominent opacity there usually involving the conus area near the pulmonary valve. The left ventricular endocardium becomes thickest at the base of the septum, near the mitral valve leaflets, and over the surface of papillary muscles. Histologically, the left atrial endocardium develops elastic tissue fragmentation and stratification, as well as collagen, smooth muscle cell, and focal adipose tissue accumulation.[33]

Friction Lesions

These linear endocardial plaques develop in relation to the chordae tendineae of tricuspid or mitral valves. Therefore, they have a linear arrangement parallel to chords. Histologically, they are composed of collagen and elastic tissue. Chords may adhere to them. They are not, strictly speaking, caused by aging but are more often found in older subjects. Right ventricular friction lesions develop adjacent to chords of the septal leaflet of the tricuspid valve. They are associated with left ventricular hypertrophy and are probably caused by an altered anatomic relationship between the chordae tendineae and the hypertrophied ventricular septum.[34] Left ventricular friction lesions are found on the ventricular wall deep to the

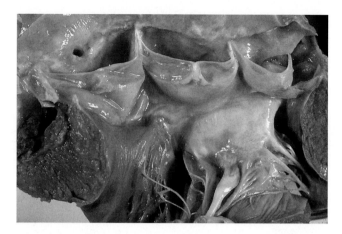

Figure 3-3 • Lines of closure and nodule of Arantius are evident on the central, rear coronary aortic valve cusp. Also, atheroma involves the anterior leaflet of the mitral valve, and there is a tiny fenestration near a commissure on the right cusp.

posterior mitral valve leaflet and are most often associated with a floppy mitral valve (Fig. 3-2).[35]

Jet Lesions

Jet lesions are fibroelastic thickenings that develop at sites where a high-pressure, jet-like stream of blood impinges on the endocardial surface (see Fig. 1-18). They may have a concavity directed toward the source of the jet if it strikes the endocardium obliquely. Platelets and fibrin are sometimes found on the surface of the lesion. If the jet stream contains microorganisms, a jet lesion may become infected. They are particularly associated with valvular regurgitation and small ventricular septal defects.[36]

THE AORTIC VALVE AND AGING

The nodules of Arantius (noduli Arantii) are small bumps of fibroelastic tissue found at the free margin and middle of the lines of closure of aortic valve cusps. In late fetal life, the semilunar lines on either side of the nodule are seen on gross examination. Subsequent thickening of the proximal portions of the cusps make both lines and nodules less obvious.[37] However, after age 20 years, the proximal portions of the cusps become opaque, rendering them clearly visible again (Fig. 3-3). The nodule on the noncoronary or posterior cusp is the most prominent. Both the lines of closure and nodules of Arantius form because of repetitive mechanical trauma on valve closure.

Cusp Thickening

A study in which the thickness of aortic valve cusps from 200 normal hearts was measured at three sites—the nodule of Arantius, the line of closure, and the midportion of the cusp—revealed no significant correlations between cusp thickness and an individual's height, weight, body surface area, or heart weight. The mean thickness at each site did not differ between males and females but

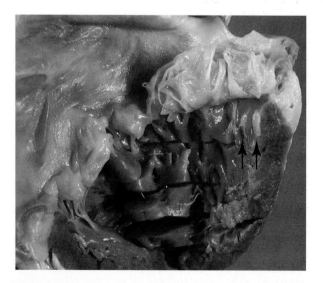

Figure 3-2 • Vertical friction lesions (arrows) located on the left ventricular wall deep to the posterior leaflet of the mitral valve in a case of floppy (myxomatous) valve.

did increase significantly with age. The nodule of Arantius was almost twice as thick as the valve along the line of closure; in turn, the closing edge was at least 25% thicker than the midportion of the cusp.[38] Histologically, there is thickening of the fibrosa and ventricularis layers of a cusp with aging.

Lipid Deposits

After age 30 years, atheromas are found in aortic valve cusps. They affect the arterialis and fibrosa layers, beginning at the basal and lateral portions of the cusp[37] and spreading toward the center.

Fenestrae

Fenestrae, which are small oval defects in the cusps usually near the commissures and above the lines of closure, are thought to be caused by wear and tear and are rarely found in persons younger than 1 year of age.[37] They are present in 12% of subjects between 10 and 45 years old[39] and do not increase in prevalence very much with increasing age (Figs. 3-3 and 3-4). They do not usually cause functional abnormality but may do so if they extend beyond the line of closure.

Lambl's Excrescences

Lambl's excrescences, which are filiform processes usually less than 0.5 cm long occurring on the ventricular side of aortic valve cusps, are most often located on the nodule of Arantius. They are found after the age of 40 years (Fig. 3-5). Lambl found them in 2% of 1000 autopsies.[40] They consist of fibrous tissue, sometimes contain elastic tissue, and probably derive from the organization of fibrin.[40] Lambl's excrescences are also discussed in Chapter 19.

Calcification

With aging, calcium deposits are laid down within the fibrosa layer of the aortic valve cusps. Although aortic

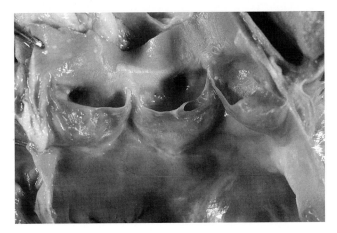

Figure 3-4 • Fenestrae, defects in the aortic valve cusp above the lines of closure, usually have no effect on valve function. In this illustration, they are best seen on the central, low, coronary cusp.

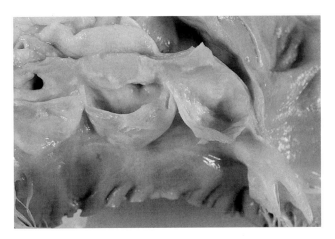

Figure 3-5 • Lambl's excrescences or whiskers protrude from the nodule of Arantius on two of these aortic valve cusps. Note lipid deposition and basal calcification on the sinus side of the cusp to the right of the photograph.

valve calcification is found in only 5% of subjects younger than 45 years, it has been reported in more than 20% of subjects older than 75 years of age.[39] This change tends to occur within a zone of oil red O–positive lipid present in the deep fibrosa layer near the spongiosa layer. The lipid deposits are distinct from the foam cell accumulation that occurs on the arterial side of the fibrosa and that is caused by atheromas. Ultrastructurally, the calcification is associated with debris derived from degenerated cells,[41] so aortic valve calcification is thought to be a degenerative change. It is suggested that subtle abnormalities of cusp shape and size may increase hemodynamic stresses in the valve and contribute to this process.[42] Further discussion of aortic valve calcific stenosis is found in Chapter 13.

Aortic Ring

After age 20 years, both the aorta and the aortic valve ring increase in circumference, almost linearly with age.[43] In subjects older than 90 years of age, the aortic valve circumference may be almost as large as that of the mitral valve.[44] Annular calcification may involve the anterior mitral valve leaflet and the atrioventricular node. This topic is discussed in a later section.

Aortic valve replacement can be performed successfully in octogenarians.[45]

THE MITRAL VALVE AND AGING

Leaflet Thickening

A study of mitral valve leaflet thicknesses in 200 normal adult hearts revealed no significant correlations with height, weight, body surface area, or heart weight and no significant difference related to gender. Mean valve thickness increased significantly with age. The closing edge of each leaflet is thicker than the clear zone, and along the closing edge the anterior leaflet is thicker than the posterior.[38]

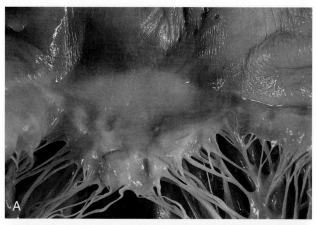

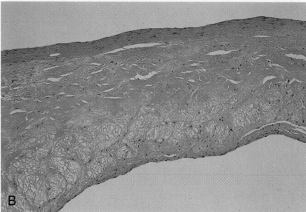

Figure 3-6 • *A,* Mitral valve atheroma on the anterior leaflet as viewed from the atrial side. Note the nodular thickening of the leaflets along the line of closure. *B,* Histologic section shows foam cells within the anterior leaflet along the ventricular side (H&E stain).

Thickening with the development of slight opacity begins at the base of the anterior mitral leaflet during late fetal life and subsequently progresses toward its free edges. Opacity of the posterior leaflet begins during the first 2 years of life.[37] The posterior leaflet is diffusely opaque in 17% of subjects between 10 and 45 years of age, with the prevalence of the change increasing with age.[39] Leaflet thickening is caused by thickening of the fibroelastic atrialis layer of the valve.[37]

Nodular thickening of mitral valve leaflets occurs on their atrial surface along the lines of closure (Fig. 3-6A). This change is present in all adults.[39] The nodules first appear overlying chordal insertions and then spread to areas between their insertions. They apparently are caused by the repetitive trauma of valve closure.[46] Histologically, they consist of fibroelastic tissue.[39] Hooding of portions of the leaflets between chordal attachments occurs because of left ventricular systolic pressure (Fig. 3-7). It is more prominent in the elderly and must be distinguished from a floppy mitral valve.[47]

Lambl's Excrescences

Lambl's excrescences are not restricted to the aortic valve. In a series of 250 consecutive autopsies, these filiform excrescences were identified on 85% of mitral valves.[40] They were not present in the hearts of subjects younger than 1 year, and they were found in all subjects older than 60 years of age. The lesions are best demonstrated by examination of the mitral valve under water in a strong light with a dark background, using a magnifying glass. They were found only on the atrial surface of the leaflets, usually along the line of closure, especially on the surfaces of nodules along that line. Histologic examination revealed connective tissue, sometimes including elastin, lined by endocardium. Lambl's excrescences may derive from superficial tears of the valve tissue or from organization of fibrin deposits, the latter condition being more likely.[40]

Lipid Deposits

The development of atheroma in the anterior leaflet of the mitral valve is an age-related phenomenon (see Figs. 3-3 and 3-6A). Thirty percent of females and 23% of males younger than 45 years of age lack this change, according to Pomerance,[39] whereas fewer than 1% of subjects older than 60 years do not have it.[48] Various patterns of gross involvement have been described,[48] ranging from a nodule in the central portion of the leaflet to a horizontal, bar-shaped deposit or diffuse involvement of the leaflet (see Figs. 3-6A and 3-6B). The deposits are found on the ventricular surface of the leaflet and rarely reach the zone of chordal attachment, although the chords themselves may be involved.[39] Histologically, the lipid is found both within macrophages and extracellularly (see Fig. 3-6B). The lesions are histologically similar to atheromas but do not develop the complications of ulceration, thrombosis, or dense calcification. Lipid deposits also occur in the posterior leaflet.

Annular Calcification

Calcification of the mitral annulus was found in 8.5% of autopsied patients older than 50 years of age in the

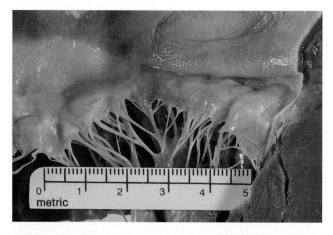

Figure 3-7 • Hooding of posterior mitral valve leaflet tissue extending toward the left atrium and caused by the effect of left ventricular systolic pressure on tissue between chordal attachments.

series of Pomerance,[49] being present in 4.6% of males and 11.5% of females. Prevalence increases with age, with calcification being present in 17% of men and 43.5% of women after 90 years. An echocardiographic study of subjects older than 62 years of age[50] revealed mitral annular calcification in 84% of those with calcified aortic valve cusps, in 70% of those with thickened aortic valve cusps or aortic root, and in only 33% of those with normal aortic valve cusps and root. Apart from aging, aortic stenosis, and female gender, other conditions associated with mitral annular calcification include hypertrophic cardiomyopathy,[51] hypertension, mitral valve prolapse, Marfan syndrome, Hurler syndrome, chronic renal failure,[52] and type II hyperlipidemia.[53] In some of these conditions there is, presumably, increased stress on the mitral valve ring which accelerates degenerative changes. For example, hypertension, aortic stenosis, and hypertrophic cardiomyopathy are all associated with increased left ventricular systolic pressure. The association with chronic renal failure reflects an abnormal calcium-phosphate metabolism.

Patients may have symptoms that are caused by conditions associated with mitral annular calcification or caused directly by the annular disease. Chest radiography is an insensitive technique for detection, but it can reveal a calcified C-, J-, U-, or, rarely, an O-shaped opacity in the mitral position.[52] Echocardiography reveals a bright band deep to the posterior leaflet.[52] Anterior displacement of the mitral valve and rigidity of the valve ring may mimic systolic anterior leaflet motion and require differentiation from that which occurs in hypertrophic cardiomyopathy. A Doppler echocardiographic study of 51 consecutive patients with an echocardiographic diagnosis of mitral annular calcification, patients with calcified mitral valve leaflets being excluded, revealed moderate to severe mitral regurgitation in 33% and significant mitral stenosis in 8%.[54] The mitral regurgitation is thought to result from leaflet displacement caused by the calcified annulus and its inability to decrease in size during ventricular systole.[54] Mitral stenosis is caused by impaired ability of the annulus to increase in size during diastole and physical narrowing of the valve orifice by the annular calcium deposits.[55] In some cases a hypertrophied, noncompliant left ventricle contributes to poor left ventricular filling.[56]

Complete heart block and other conduction defects may occur because calcification from the mitral ring extends into the conduction system or because of concomitant degeneration in the conduction tissue and mitral valve annulus. In one series, 76% of patients with mitral annular calcification had conduction defects, compared with 36% of age- and gender-matched controls. Atrial fibrillation has an increased frequency, probably reflecting left atrial enlargement.[52] A patient has been reported with a calcified nodule that extended from the calcified annulus into the left ventricular inferior wall, causing recurrent ventricular tachycardia.[57]

Mitral annular calcification was associated with a doubled risk of stroke in an 8-year follow-up study of subjects in the Framingham study,[58] with the risk independent of atrial fibrillation, congestive heart failure, or coronary heart disease. The stroke was thought to be embolic in two thirds of cases.[58] Instances of calcium emboli to the brain have been documented, but it is also possible that mitral annular calcification can form a substrate for thrombus deposition and subsequent embolization.[52] This may occur if the calcific mass erodes through the endocardium or the valve.[59]

Mitral annular calcification can be complicated by infection (Fig. 3-8). Three of 80 patients with mitral annular calcification developed endocarditis in one series.[59] A review of seven autopsied cases revealed *Staphylococcus aureus* as the causative organism in four. Only four patients had the diagnosis made during life. Vegetations tended to be smooth. Found at the base of the posterior mitral valve leaflet, they perforated the leaflet and were in continuity with mitral ring abscesses. Mitral valve chordal rupture was not present but can occur with or without infection. The abscesses spread directly through the myocardium to the pericardium in four of seven cases. Five individuals had myocardial abscesses. Systemic emboli were found in six cases.[60]

A case of left ventricular pseudoaneurysm apparently caused by left atrial and ventricular tearing by mitral annular calcification has been reported.[61]

Grossly, mitral annular calcification varies from a small nodule (Fig. 3-9) to a massive size. It is found deep to the posterior leaflet of the mitral valve. A spur of calcium projecting toward the left atrium may distort the overlying leaflet, and extensive deposits can form a subvalvular shelf.[49] Occasionally, the deposits extend across the ventricular surface of the anterior leaflet of the mitral valve, to form a complete "O" ring.[62] On section, the calcified ring sometimes shows a central softening, grossly resembling caseated material. The calcific material may ulcerate through the overlying leaflet, and associated

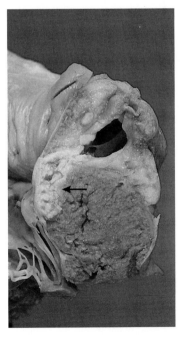

Figure 3-8 • Infected mitral annular calcification. A mass of infected calcified material (arrow) is present at the atrioventricular ring, deep to the posterior leaflet of the mitral valve.

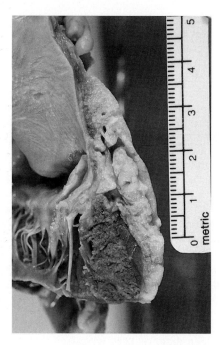

Figure 3-9 • Mitral annular calcification. A small nodule of calcification is present deep to the posterior leaflet of the mitral valve.

thrombi may be found (Fig. 14-8 provides further illustrations).

Histologic examination reveals amorphous basophilic material, occasionally with cartilage or bone formation, with surrounding fibrous tissue. Inflammation is common and usually mononuclear. Sometimes, foreign body giant cells are found. Palisading fibroblasts may occur in the absence of rheumatoid arthritis.[49]

Percutaneous mitral valvuloplasty[63] and mitral valve repair[64] surgery can be successfully performed in elderly patients.

THE PULMONARY VALVE AND AGING

This valve changes the least with age. The nodules of Morgagni at the center of the free edges of its cusps become more prominent with age. Pulmonary cusp fenestrae are found in up to 7% of hearts[39] but are rare before 10 years of age. The cusps become slightly opaque by age 50 years,[37] and the valve annulus dilates with increasing age.[44]

THE TRICUSPID VALVE AND AGING

The tricuspid valve rarely develops atheromatous plaques.[37] Tricuspid leaflets are translucent in most patients younger than 55 years of age and remain so in 20% of subjects older than 85 years. Nodular thickening along the line of closure is most prominent in the anterior leaflet and is more pronounced in subjects with pulmonary hypertension.[46] Calcification of the tricuspid annulus has been described in severe pulmonary hypertension[65] and hypercalcemia; it is not age related.

MYOCARDIAL CHANGES WITH AGE

Heart Weight and Size

Heart weight may be expressed as a raw weight or related to body weight, height, or surface area. The effect of age on heart weight in adults is controversial. Some authors[66, 67] concluded that there is no increase in heart weight with age if subjects with hypertension and other heart diseases are carefully excluded. Others[44] found an increase in mean heart weight in women between age 20 and 69 years but a stable heart weight in men over these years, with a decline in heart weight in both genders thereafter. In this study, the mean heart weight of women aged 20 to 29 years was 237 g, between 60 and 69 years it was 288 g, and from 90 to 99 years it was 238 g.[44] An autopsy study of 40 subjects older than 90 years of age revealed increased heart weight, defined as more than 350 g in women and more than 400 g in men, in 67%.[12] However, 22 of the 27 subjects with increased heart weight had a history of systemic hypertension during life. Of the remaining five with no such history, two had old transmural myocardial infarcts and one had amyloid deposits. These results suggest that few elderly subjects have an increased heart weight that cannot be explained by conditions other than aging.

Echocardiographically determined left ventricular mass increased with age in the Framingham study, but when subjects with cardiopulmonary disease, hypertension, or obesity were excluded, the left ventricular mass showed only minimal change. Only 12% of men and 15% of women from the Framingham group remained in this study after the rigorous exclusion criteria were applied.[68] An echocardiographic study of left ventricular free wall thickness disclosed a 30% increase in thickness between ages 25 and 44 years and between ages 65 and 84 years in active men without hypertension or cardiovascular disease. However, wall thicknesses were still within the normal limits in the older group.[19] Left ventricular chamber dimensions do not change with age in echocardiographic studies. This pattern of increased left ventricular wall thickness with unaltered chamber size may be caused by increased impedance due to age-related vascular changes.[19] Left atrial chamber size tends to increase with increasing age.[69]

Hypertension is an important variable in studies of heart weight, ventricular wall thicknesses, left ventricular hypertrophy, and myocardial morphology and biochemistry. The definition of hypertension in the elderly has changed.[70] It may be systolic, diastolic, or both. In the United States, 54% of all persons aged 65 to 74 years are hypertensive, and 72% of black patients in this age group are affected. However, age-related increases in blood pressure do not occur in all populations, there being important environmental influences such as diet.[71] Studies must also take account of the varying effects of antihypertensive drugs on left ventricular mass.[72]

A study of right ventricular heart biopsies taken from 15 patients aged 28 to 75 years (before commencement of chemotherapy) revealed correlations between myocyte diameter and age.[73] Myocyte nuclear area also increased with increasing age, but interstitial fibrous tissue was not increased in this study.[73] However, an autopsy study us-

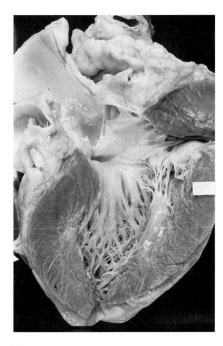

Figure 3-10 • Sigmoid septum. A smooth, prominent subaortic bulge of the septal wall into the left ventricular cavity gives the septum an "S" shape in the base-to-apex direction.

ing morphometric techniques revealed increased collagen in the subendocardial and subepicardial regions of the ventricular septum with aging.[74] Another autopsy study of hearts from subjects older than 80 years of age revealed myocardial interstitial fibrosis that was independent of hypertension, congestive heart failure, emphysema, and pulmonary or coronary artery disease. Interstitial fibrosis was more prominent in the atria than in the ventricles.[75] An increased size of right and left ventricular myocytes with aging has been demonstrated in some autopsy studies.[76, 77] In one,[77] left ventricular myocyte hypertrophy was confined to the inner two thirds of the myocardial wall. Myocyte nuclei in the subepicardial zone decreased in size with aging, whereas cell size did not change in that layer. Interstitial fibrosis in the elderly heart was most prominent in the subendocardium of the inferior left ventricle. A relative atrophy of subepicardial myocytes in the aging heart was reported by Okada and colleagues.[78]

The DNA content of the adult human ventricular myocardium, as analyzed biochemically, does not vary with age but does correlate with heart weight. Also, the degree of polyploidization of heart muscle nuclei, as determined by Feulgen cytophotometry, does not vary with age either.[79]

Sigmoid Septum

Autopsy study revealed that the thicknesses of the right and left ventricular free walls remain relatively constant during adulthood. An increase in ventricular septal thickness with age most likely reflects the development of a *sigmoid septum.*[44] This term defines a ventricular septum in which the base bulges toward the left ventricular cavity (Fig. 3-10). The condition is described only in hearts that are *not* hypertrophied, because hypertrophic

cardiomyopathy must not be confused with this condition. The development of a sigmoid septum may be secondary to a decrease in the long-axis dimension of the left ventricular chamber and a right shift of a dilated ascending aorta.[68] The sigmoid condition may be quantified by measuring the angle between a line drawn through the center of the ascending aorta and the plane of the mitral valve inlet.[80] When this method is used, the average age of subjects with an extremely sigmoid septum is 62 years, compared with 53 years in subjects with a straight septum.[80] A recent study[81] revealed a progressive increase in septal sigmoidity with increasing age and found it to be greater in men than in women. Sigmoidity of the septum did not correlate with patient height, weight, or cardiac mass. The condition is not thought to have clinical consequences, although the possibility that a caged-ball prosthetic valve in the mitral position might be more likely to impinge on a sigmoid septum was raised in the original study.[80]

Basophilic Degeneration

Basophilic degeneration is marked by the presence of perinuclear granular deposits within cardiac myocytes. They have a gray-blue appearance on hematoxylin and eosin staining (Fig. 3-11A), are found in 90[82] to 98%[83] of hearts, and increase in number with aging and in some

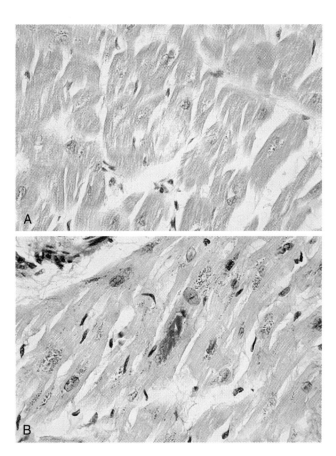

Figure 3-11 • Basophilic degeneration. *A,* A gray-blue deposit is present within a cardiac myocyte near the nucleus (H&E stain). *B,* The material is periodic acid–Schiff (PAS) positive (PAS-diastase stain).

forms of myofiber hypertrophy.[84] However, in these conditions only a few myocytes contain the deposits, whereas in hypothyroidism many are affected. The deposits are periodic acid–Schiff (PAS) positive (Fig. 3-11B) and resistant to 30 minutes of diastase exposure, but are lost after 48 hours exposure to diastase; amyloglucosidase and pectinase also abolish PAS positivity. The basophilic material is slightly positive with Alcian blue at pH 2.5. It is negative with the following stains: Feulgen, Mallory phosphotungstic acid hematoxylin, Congo red, crystal violet, Perls, Sudan IV, Mayer mucicarmine, toluidine blue, and Alcian blue at pH 1.0. The deposits do not autofluoresce.[82]

Ultrastructurally, basophilic degeneration consists of non–membrane-bound, short, 6- to 7-nm wide fibrils that lack periodicity and are randomly arranged, with interspersed 15-nm granules. The material found in basophilic degeneration is histochemically and ultrastructurally similar to amylopectin as found in type IV glycogen storage disease, to Lafora bodies, and to corpora amylacea, and it appears to derive from myocardial glycogen metabolism.[85] A monoclonal antibody raised to polyglycosan extracted from the myocardium of a patient with Lafora disease has been used to study basophilic degeneration. Immunoelectronmicroscopically, it specifically labeled fibrils within the deposits.[83]

Lipofuscin

These lipid-soluble, brown to yellow, granular autofluorescent pigments accumulate near the nucleus of cells (Fig. 3-12). Lipofuscin is thought to derive from the residue of lysosomal enzyme activity.[86] It is weakly acid-fast, PAS-positive diastase-resistant, and stains positively with Sudan black B, Nile blue sulphate, and Masson-Fontana stains. Ultrastructurally (Fig. 3-13), it consists of electron-dense granules of varying sizes, sometimes lamellar structures, and lipid.[87] Myocardial lipofuscin is said to be absent before the age of 10 years, and it accumulates linearly with age, being found in the hearts of all older individuals. Its accumulation does not seem to be altered by heart disease, heart size, or gender.[88] In a morphometric study of right ventricular biopsies, lipofuscin deposition increased with age and correlated weakly with systolic blood pressure.[73]

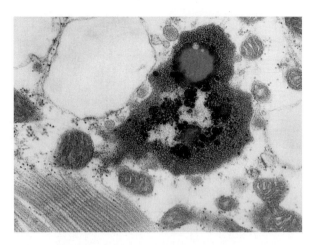

Figure 3-13 • Ultrastructure of lipofuscin. Electron-dense granules and lipid are shown.

Brown Atrophy

This term refers to the appearance of the heart in cachectic subjects, in whom the high lipofuscin content accounts for the brown appearance. This is not a specific age-related change.

EPICARDIAL AND PERICARDIAL CHANGES WITH AGING

The aging heart has an increased amount of subepicardial adipose tissue, especially involving the anterior right ventricle and the atrioventricular grooves.[69]

VASCULAR CHANGES WITH AGING

General

With aging, arteries develop thicker walls due to intimal and medial thickening. Elastin may be fragmented and partly replaced by collagen. Biochemical studies of the thoracic aorta of normotensive humans demonstrated absolute losses of collagen and elastin with aging, but their concentrations increased, suggesting that other components of the aortic wall are lost even more rapidly with aging.[89] Major arteries dilate with age,[90] and this must be taken into account when, for example, mass screening for abdominal aortic aneurysms is undertaken.[91] Dilation is more prominent in the proximal portions of arteries, whereas increased wall thickness is more pronounced distally.[92] Arteries become stiffer with age, and this change is manifested by increased systolic blood pressure, widening of the pulse pressure, and changes in pulse wave velocity and contour.[90] It has been suggested that oxidative modifications of glycated proteins such as collagen,

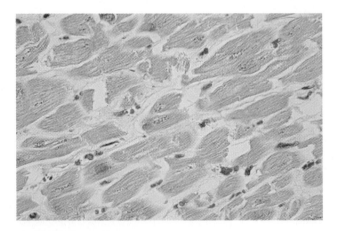

Figure 3-12 • Lipofuscin. Granular, golden-brown material is present near myocyte nuclei (H&E stain).

leading to accumulation of advanced glycation end products, may contribute to the increased stiffness of arteries that occurs with aging and diabetes.[93] The increased stiffness with aging occurs in the absence of clinically evident cardiovascular disease and is not different in men or women.[90] Changes in arterial stiffness with aging need not be homogeneously distributed about the arterial wall,[94] however, and the physics of arterial wall properties are complex.[95]

Aorta

As measured by classic pressure-volume measurement techniques, the human aorta becomes stiffer with age.[96] Studies using echocardiographic techniques to evaluate aortic blood flow[97, 98] and aortic root distensibility[99] have demonstrated that menopause and estrogen replacement have measurable effects on these aortic properties. The aorta also dilates with age.[100] Diffuse intimal thickening develops too and is more prominent in the distal than in the proximal aorta.[101] The thickness of the thoracic aortic media increases with age when measured on non–pressure-fixed material.[102] Schlatmann and Becker demonstrated that other histologic changes in the aorta, specifically formation of cystic spaces containing basophilic material, elastin fragmentation, medial fibrosis, and loss of smooth muscle cell nuclei, increase in severity with age[103] (see Chapter 5 also).

Coronary Arteries

The risk of clinical coronary heart disease events increases with age, and female resistance ends with menopause. This risk increases even in people who lack major risk factors for the disease. The percentage of events represented by angina pectoris decreases with age, whereas that represented by myocardial infarction increases. Furthermore, with increasing age, a higher percentage of myocardial infarctions are unrecognized clinically[104]; some are truly silent, and others are associated with atypical symptoms.[105] Elderly patients, especially hypertensive women with a first myocardial infarction, may be at increased risk of infarct rupture.[106] Also, they have a higher mortality rate with acute myocardial infarction—about 20 to 30% die in the first few weeks after the infarction, compared with fewer than 5% of patients younger than 55 years of age.[107] Elderly patients treated with thrombolytic therapy have an increased risk of intracerebral hemorrhage compared with that of younger patients[105]; however, pooled data from clinical trials indicate an overall benefit of this therapy in eligible elderly patients.[108] Successful use of direct percutaneous transluminal coronary angioplasty in octogenarians has been reported.[109] The mortality rate of coronary artery bypass grafting increases with increasing age.[105] A technical consideration in performing this surgery is the increased incidence of ascending aorta atherosclerosis and calcification in the elderly.[105] Clinical studies reveal that endothelial-dependent dilation of coronary arteries in response to acetylcholine decreases with age.[110] This is reversed by L-arginine.[111] Flow-mediated brachial artery dilation is stable until after age 40 in men and after the early 50s in women, declining thereafter in both genders.[112]

Studies evaluating the relationship between age and coronary arterial lumen size yield conflicting results.[113] In vivo angiographic studies of such relationships may be influenced by responses to stimuli such as nitroglycerin, in turn altered by age.[113] Some postmortem studies have not demonstrated an age-related increase in coronary artery diameters in the absence of atherosclerosis.[114] However, examination of non–pressure-fixed coronary arteries from 12,680 autopsies in the International Atherosclerosis Project did reveal a progressive increase in coronary artery lumen diameter with increasing age.[115] This was true regardless of whether cases with hypertension and/or coronary heart disease were excluded. The ratio of heart weight to coronary artery lumen area decreased with age in this study, suggesting an age-related increase in coronary artery size relative to myocardial mass.[115] Another study, in which coronary angiography and coronary fixation in distention were performed on 738 hearts, revealed increased coronary artery tortuosity with aging in 145 hearts free of coronary artery disease. Increased arterial diameter and tortuosity were associated.[116] The thickness of the coronary artery intima and media increase with aging.[117]

An autopsy study of the hearts of 100 men from each decade between 30 to 89 years, reported in 1950, did not find a linear relationship between degree of coronary atherosclerosis and age. Rather, the average severity of coronary atherosclerosis increased from age 30 to 49, was maximal from 50 to 59, and then was constant.[118] In the same year, a similarly designed study of women's hearts revealed an increase in the average severity of coronary atherosclerosis from 30 to 70 years of age, with plateauing thereafter.[119] Subjects older than 80 years of age reportedly have more multivessel coronary disease and more often have left main coronary disease than younger individuals.[106] Although a study of 40 autopsied nonagenarians revealed more than 75% cross-sectional area stenosis of one or more coronaries in 70% of cases,[12] another autopsy study of 237 nonagenarians revealed significant coronary disease in 43%.[17] In the latter study, 10% of subjects had significant disease of the left main coronary artery, 35% of the left anterior descending, 16% of the left circumflex, and 25% of the right coronary artery, a distribution thought similar to that in the general population.[15, 17]

Calcification

Microincineration methods demonstrated an increased coronary artery calcium content with age in a 1948 study. At that time, it was thought that the development of atheromas might be caused by calcification.[120] It is now recognized that coronary artery calcification is almost always associated with atheromatous plaques and is a secondary phenomenon. The role of osteocalcin, osteopontin, and bone morphogenetic protein-2 in the development of such calcification is under investigation.[121] Calcification of atherosclerotic plaques is not restricted to clinically significant lesions.[121] Hence, the prevalence of coronary artery calcification at any age is much higher than the expected incidence of coronary heart disease events at that age.[122] Age and gender are major risk factors for coronary artery calcification, which is found in 14% of subjects younger than 40 years of age but in more than 93% of men and 77% of women older than 70 years of age.[122] Autopsy studies of subjects age 90 years or older revealed calcific deposits in major coronary arteries in at least 92%.[12] The role of various new, sensitive tests for in vivo detection of coronary artery calcification is being defined.[122, 123]

DISORDERS OF PREMATURE AGING

Progeria or Hutchinson-Gilford Syndrome

The findings that characterize this condition are listed in Table 3-2. Most patients die of atherosclerotic coronary artery disease before reaching adulthood, although some adults with progeria have been described.[126] The mean age at death is 13.4 years, and death most often is caused by congestive heart failure or myocardial infarction, or both.[127] At autopsy, there is atherosclerosis of coronary and peripheral arteries and the aorta. Myocardial infarcts may be found. Cases of severe myocardial interstitial fibrosis in the absence of epicardial coronary artery disease have been described.[124] Intimal and medial thickening of small intramyocardial arteries also develops.[128] Lipofuscin may be found within cardiac myocytes but is not increased compared with that found in age-matched controls.[128] Calcification of the mitral annulus, atheroma deposition in the anterior mitral valve leaflet, and calcification of the aortic valve cusps are other common findings.[128] A patient with progeria who underwent percutaneous transluminal angioplasty and coronary artery bypass grafting at age 14 years has been reported.[127]

Progeria is either an autosomal recessive condition or has a sporadic autosomal dominant determination. Increased paternal age has been noted. Urinary hyaluronic acid secretion is increased. Abnormally low levels of insulin-like growth factor-I and a very high basal metabolic rate have been noted in some patients.[129, 130]

Werner Syndrome

Werner syndrome is an autosomal recessive condition in which stature is short because of an absence of the adolescent growth spurt. Graying and hair loss occur at about age 20 years, and loss of subcutaneous fat and connective tissue cause a "pinched" facial appearance.[131, 132] Other features of Werner syndrome are presented in Table 3-3.

Diagnosis of the syndrome is made in adulthood.

TABLE 3-2 • **Symptoms of Progeria or Hutchinson-Gilford Syndrome**[124,125]

Dwarfism
Abnormal facies (beak-like nose, exophthalmos, receding chin)
Marked loss of subcutaneous fat
Hypoplastic clavicles
Coxa valga
Horseriding stance
Normal intelligence

TABLE 3-3 • **Symptoms of Werner Syndrome**[131,132]

Ulcers of feet and legs
Calcinosis cutis
Osteoporosis
Diabetes mellitus
Hypogonadism
Abnormal voice due to laryngeal atrophy
Premature cataracts

Death occurs at a mean age of 47 years and is usually caused by malignancy or cardiovascular disease.[132] Hypercholesterolemia is not a usual part of the syndrome complex,[133] but evidence for a hypercoagulable state was found in some patients.[134] At autopsy, coronary and aortic atherosclerosis and calcification of the mitral annulus and aortic valve cusps are common findings.[133] Cultured skin fibroblasts from patients with Werner syndrome have a shortened lifespan and develop multiple chromosomal abnormalities,[131] suggesting the possibility of a chromosome breakage syndrome. Linkage of Werner syndrome to markers on chromosome 8 has been reported.[135]

REFERENCES

1. Knight JA: The process and theories of aging. Ann Clin Lab Sci 25:1, 1995
2. Waller BF: Hearts of the "oldest old." Mayo Clin Proc 63:625, 1988
3. Masoro EJ: Biology of aging: Facts, thoughts, and experimental approaches. Lab Invest 65:500, 1991
4. Partridge L, Barton NH: Optimality, mutation, and the evolution of aging. Nature 362:305, 1993
5. Sugiyama S, Hattori K, Hayakawa M, Ozawa T: Quantitative analysis of age-associated accumulation of mitochondrial DNA with deletion in human hearts. Biochem Biophys Res Commun 180:894, 1991
6. Troncale JA: The aging process: Physiologic changes and pharmacologic implications. Postgrad Med 99:111, 1996
7. Martin GM: The genetics of aging. Hosp Pract 32:47, 1997
8. Weindruch R: Caloric restriction and aging. Sci Am 274:46, 1996
9. Wallace DC: Mitochondrial genetics: A paradigm for aging and degenerative diseases? Science 256:628, 1992
10. Orlander PR, Nader S: Youthful hormones. Lancet 348(suppl II):6, 1996
11. Kohn RR: Cause of death in very old people. JAMA 247:2793, 1982
12. Waller BF, Roberts WC: Cardiovascular disease in the very elderly: Analysis of 40 necropsy patients 90 years or older. Am J Cardiol 51:403, 1983
13. Gross JS, Neufeld RR, Libow LS, et al: Autopsy study of the elderly institutionalized patient: Review of 234 autopsies. Arch Intern Med 148:173, 1988
14. McKeown F: Heart disease in old age. J Clin Pathol 16:532, 1963
15. Pomerance A: Pathology of the heart in the tenth decade. J Clin Pathol 21:317, 1968
16. Roberts WC: Ninety-three hearts ≥90 years of age. Am J Cardiol 71:599, 1993
17. Lie JT, Hammond PI: Pathology of the senescent heart: Anatomic observations on 237 autopsy studies of patients 90 to 105 years old. Mayo Clin Proc 63:552, 1988
18. Ishii T, Sternby NH: Pathology of centenarians. I. The cardiovascular system and lungs. J Am Geriatr Soc 26:108, 1978
19. Walsh RA: Cardiovascular effects of the aging process. Am J Med 82(suppl 1B):34, 1987
20. Wei JY: Age and the cardiovascular system. N Engl J Med 327:1735, 1992
21. Rodeheffer RJ, Gerstenblith G, Becker LC, et al: Exercise cardiac

output is maintained with advancing age in healthy human subjects: Cardiac dilatation and increased stroke volume compensate for a diminished heart rate. Circulation 69:203, 1984

22. Fleg JL, O'Connor F, Gerstenblith G, et al: Impact of age on the cardiovascular response to dynamic upright exercise in healthy men and women. J Appl Physiol 78:890, 1995
23. Crawford MH: Aging and left ventricular performance. West J Med 159:451, 1993
24. Xiao R-P, Lakatta EG: Deterioration of β-adrenergic modulation of cardiovascular function with aging. Ann N Y Acad Sci 673:293, 1992
25. Lipsitz LA: Orthostatic hypotension in the elderly. N Engl J Med 321:952, 1989
26. Cornwell GG III, Johnson KH, Westermark P: The age related amyloids: A growing family of unique biochemical substances. J Clin Pathol 48:984, 1995
27. Cornwell GG III, Westermark P, Murdoch W, Pitkänen P: Senile aortic amyloid: A third distinctive type of age-related cardiovascular amyloid. Am J Pathol 108:135, 1982
28. Olson LJ, Gertz MA, Edward WD, et al: Senile cardiac amyloidosis with myocardial dysfunction: Diagnosis by endomyocardial biopsy and immunohistochemistry. N Engl J Med 317:738, 1987
29. Kyle RA, Spittell PC, Gertz MA, et al: The premortem recognition of systemic senile amyloidosis with cardiac involvement. Am J Med 171:395, 1996
30. Pitkänen P, Westermark P, Cornwell GG III: Senile systemic amyloidosis. Am J Pathol 117:391, 1984
31. Mucchiano G, Cornwell GG III, Westermark P: Senile aortic amyloid: Evidence for two distinct forms of localized deposits. Am J Pathol 140:871, 1992
32. Westermark P, Mucchiano G, Marthin T, et al: Apolipoprotein A1-derived amyloid in human aortic atherosclerotic plaques. Am J Pathol 147:1186, 1995
33. McMillan JB, Lev M: The aging heart. I. Endocardium. J Gerontol 14:268, 1959
34. Goor D, Edwards JE: Friction lesions of the right ventricular endocardium: Relation to tricuspid chordae in cardiac hypertrophy. Arch Pathol 87:100, 1969
35. Salazar AE, Edwards JE: Friction lesions of ventricular endocardium: Relation to chordae tendineae of mitral valve. Arch Pathol 90:364, 1970
36. Edwards JE, Burchell HB: Endocardial and intimal lesions (jet impact) as possible sites of origin of murmurs. Circulation 18:946, 1958
37. McMillan JB, Lev M: The aging heart II: The valves. J Gerontol 19:1, 1964
38. Sahasakul Y, Edwards WD, Naessens JM, Tajik AJ: Age-related changes in aortic and mitral valve thickness: Implications for two-dimensional echocardiography based on an autopsy study of 200 normal human hearts. Am J Cardiol 62:424, 1988
39. Pomerance A: Aging changes in human heart valves. Br Heart J 29:222, 1967
40. Magarey FR: On the mode of formation of Lambl's excrescences and their relation to chronic thickening of the mitral valve. J Pathol 61:203, 1949
41. Kim KM, Valigorsky JM, Mergner WJ, et al: Aging changes in the human aortic valve in relation to dystrophic calcification. Hum Pathol 7:47, 1976
42. Roberts WC: The structure of the aortic valve in clinically isolated aortic stenosis: An autopsy study of 162 patients over 15 years of age. Circulation 42:91, 1970
43. Krovetz LJ: Age-related changes in the size of the aortic valve annulus in man. Am Heart J 90:569, 1975
44. Kitzman DW, Scholz DG, Hagen PT, et al: Age-related changes in normal human hearts during the first 10 decades of life. Part II (Maturity): A quantitative anatomic study of 765 specimens from subjects 20 to 99 years old. Mayo Clin Proc 63:137, 1988
45. Elayda MA, Hall RJ, Reul RM, et al: Aortic valve replacement in patients 80 years and older: Operative risks and long-term results. Circulation 88:11, 1993
46. Pomerance A: Pathogenesis of "senile" nodular sclerosis of atrioventricular valves. Br Heart J 28:815, 1966
47. Edwards JE: Floppy mitral valve syndrome. In: Waller BF (ed): Contemporary Issues in Cardiovascular Pathology. Philadelphia, FA Davis, 1988, p 249.
48. McManus JFA, Lupton CH Jr: Lipid deposits in the aortic cusp of the mitral valve. Arch Pathol 75:674, 1963
49. Pomerance A: Pathological and clinical study of calcification of the mitral valve ring. J Clin Pathol 23:354, 1970
50. Aronow WS, Schwartz KS, Koenigsberg M: Correlation of aortic cuspal and aortic root disease with aortic systolic ejection murmurs and with mitral anular calcium in persons older than 62 years in a long-term health care facility. Am J Cardiol 58:651, 1986
51. Motamed HE, Roberts WC: Frequency and significance of mitral anular calcium in hypertrophic cardiomyopathy: Analysis of 200 necropsy patients. Am J Cardiol 60:877, 1987
52. Nestico PF, Depace NL, Morganroth J, et al: Mitral annular calcification: Clinical, pathophysiology, and echocardiographic review. Am Heart J 107:989, 1984
53. Roberts WC: The senile cardiac calcification syndrome. Am J Cardiol 58:572, 1986
54. Labovitz AJ, Nelson JG, Windhorst DM, et al: Frequency of mitral valve dysfunction from mitral anular calcium as detected by Doppler echocardiography. Am J Cardiol 55:133, 1985
55. Osterberger LE, Goldstein S, Khaja F, Lakier JB: Functional mitral stenosis in patients with massive mitral annular calcification. Circulation 64:472, 1981
56. Hammer WJ, Roberts WC, de Leon AC Jr: "Mitral stenosis" secondary to combined "massive" mitral anular calcific deposits and small, hypertrophied left ventricles. Am J Med 64:371, 1978
57. Kelly RP, Kuchar DL, Thorburn CW: Subvalvular mitral calcium as a cause of surgically correctable ventricular tachycardia. Am J Cardiol 57:884, 1986
58. Benjamin EJ, Plehn JF, D'Agostino RB, et al: Mitral annular calcification and the risk of stroke in an elderly cohort. N Engl J Med 327:374, 1992
59. Fulkerson PK, Beaver BM, Auseon JC, Graber HL: Calcification of the mitral annulus: Etiology, clinical associations, complications, and therapy. Am J Med 66:967, 1979
60. Burnside JW, Desanctis RW: Bacterial endocarditis in calcification of the mitral anulus fibrosus. Ann Intern Med 76:615, 1972
61. Kiguchi H, Ishii T, Masuda S, et al: Cardiac pseudoaneurysm caused by mitral ring calcification. Cardiovasc Pathol 3:281, 1994
62. Roberts WC, Waller BF: Mitral valve "anular" calcium forming a complete circle or "O" configuration: Clinical and necropsy observations. Am Heart J 101:619, 1981
63. Tuzcu EM, Block PC, Griffin BP, et al: Immediate and long-term outcome of percutaneous mitral valvotomy in patients 65 years and older. Circulation 85:963, 1992
64. Jebara VA, Dervanian P, Acar C, et al: Mitral valve repair using Carpentier techniques in patients more than 70 years old: Early and late results. Circulation 86(suppl II):S53, 1992
65. Arnold JR, Ghahramani AR: Calcification of annulus of tricuspid valve (observation in two patients with congenital pulmonary stenosis). Chest 60:229, 1971
66. Hodkinson I, Pomerance A, Hodkinson HM: Heart size in the elderly: A clinicopathological study. J R Soc Med 72:13, 1979
67. Smith HL: The relation of the weight of the heart to the weight of the body and of the weight of the heart to age. Am Heart J 4:79, 1928
68. Dannenberg AL, Levy D, Garrison RJ: Impact of age on echocardiographic left ventricular mass in a healthy population (The Framingham Study). Am J Cardiol 64:1066, 1989
69. Waller BF, Bloch T, Barker BG, et al: The old-age heart: Aging changes of the normal elderly heart and cardiovascular disease in 12 necropsy patients aged 90 to 101 years. Cardiol Clin 2:753, 1984
70. Bennet NE: Hypertension in the elderly. Lancet 344:447, 1994
71. Whelton PK: Epidemiology of hypertension. Lancet 344:101, 1994
72. Schulman SP, Weiss JL, Becker LC, et al: The effects of antihypertensive therapy on left ventricular mass in elderly patients. N Engl J Med 322:1350, 1990
73. Unverferth DV, Baker PB, Arn AR, et al: Aging of the human myocardium: A histologic study based upon endomyocardial biopsy. Gerontology 32:241, 1986
74. Lenkiewicz JE, Davies MJ, Rosen D: Collagen in human myocardium as a function of age. Cardiovasc Res 6:549, 1972
75. Klima M, Burns TR, Chopra A: Myocardial fibrosis in the elderly. Arch Pathol Lab Med 114:938, 1990
76. Olivetti G, Melissari M, Capasso JM, Anversa P: Cardiomyopathy

of the aging human heart: Myocyte loss and reactive cellular hypertrophy. Circ Res 68:1560, 1991

77. Burns TR, Klima M, Teasdale TA, Kasper K: Morphometry of the aging heart. Mod Pathol 3:336, 1990

78. Okada R, Teragaki M, Fukuda Y: Histopathological study on the effects of aging in myocardium of hypertrophied hearts. Jpn Circ J 50:1018, 1986

79. Adler CP, Friedburg H: Myocardial DNA content, ploidy level and cell number in geriatric hearts: Post-mortem examinations of human myocardium in old age. J Mol Cell Cardiol 18:39, 1986

80. Goor D, Lillehei CW, Edwards JE: The "sigmoid septum." Variation in the contour of the left ventricular outlet. AJR Am J Roentgenol 107:366, 1969

81. Toth AB, Engel JA, McManus AM, McManus BM: Sigmoidity of the ventricular septum revisited: Progression in early adulthood, predominance in men, and independence from cardiac mass. Am J Cardiovasc Pathol 2:211, 1988

82. Rosai J, Lascano EF: Basophilic (mucoid) degeneration of myocardium: A disorder of glycogen metabolism. Am J Pathol 61:99, 1970

83. Tamura S, Takahashi M, Kawamura S, Ishihara T: Basophilic degeneration of the myocardium: Histological, immunohistochemical and immuno-electronmicroscopic studies. Histopathology 26:501, 1995

84. Haust MD, Rowlands DT, Garancis JC, Landing BH: Histochemical studies on cardiac "colloid." Am J Pathol 40:185, 1962

85. Yokota T, Ishihara T, Kawano H, et al: Immunological homogeneity of Lafora body, corpora amylacea, basophilic degeneration in heart, and intracytoplasmic inclusions of liver and heart in type IV glycogenosis. Acta Pathol Jpn 37:941, 1987

86. Koobs DH, Schultz RL, Jutzy RV: The origin of lipofuscin and possible consequences to the myocardium. Arch Pathol Lab Med 102:66, 1978

87. Hendy R: Electron microscopy of lipofuscin pigment stained by the Schmörl and Fontana techniques. Histochemie 26:311, 1971

88. Strehler BL, Mark DD, Mildvan AS, Gee MV: Rate and magnitude of age pigment accumulation in the human myocardium. J Gerontol 14:430, 1959

89. Cattell MA, Anderson JC, Hasleton PS: Age-related changes in amounts and concentrations of collagen and elastin in normotensive human thoracic aorta. Clin Chim Acta 245:73, 1996

90. Vaitkevicius PV, Fleg JL, Engel JH, et al: Effects of age and aerobic capacity on arterial stiffness in healthy adults. Circulation 88:1456, 1993

91. Grimshaw GM, Thompson JM: Changes in diameter of the abdominal aorta with age: An epidemiological study. J Clin Ultrasound 25:7, 1997

92. Learoyd BM, Taylor MG: Alterations with age in the viscoelastic properties of human arterial walls. Circ Res 20:354, 1967

93. Schleicher ED, Wagner E, Nerlich AG: Increased accumulation of the glycoxidation product N-(carboxymethyl) lysine in human tissues in diabetes and aging. J Clin Invest 99:457, 1997

94. Reneman RS, van Merode T, Brands PJ, Hoeks APG: Inhomogeneities in arterial wall properties under normal and pathological conditions. J Hyptens 10(suppl 6):S35, 1992

95. O'Rourke M: Arterial stiffness, systolic blood pressure, and logical treatment of arterial hypertension. Hypertension 15:339, 1990

96. Bader H: Dependence of wall stress in the human thoracic aorta on age and pressure. Circ Res 20:354, 1967

97. Pines A, Fisman EZ, Drory Y, et al: Menopause-induced changes in Doppler-derived parameters of aortic flow in healthy women. Am J Cardiol 69:1104, 1992

98. Pines A, Fisman EZ, Levo Y, et al: The effects of hormone replacement therapy in normal postmenopausal function: Measurements of Doppler-derived parameters of aortic flow. Am J Obstet Gynecol 164:806, 1991

99. Karpanou EA, Vyssoulis GP, Papakyriakou SA, et al: Effect of menopause on aortic root function in hypertensive women. J Am Coll Cardiol 28:1562, 1996

100. Bazett HC, Cotton FS, Laplace LB, Scott JC: The calculation of cardiac output and effective peripheral resistance from blood pressure measurements with an appendix on the size of the aorta in man. Am J Physiol 113:312, 1935

101. Movat HZ, More RH, Haust MD: The diffuse intimal thickening of the human aorta with aging. Am J Pathol 34:1023, 1958

102. Wellman WE, Edwards JE: Thickness of the media of the thoracic aorta in relation to age. Arch Pathol 50:183, 1950

103. Schlatmann JJM, Becker AE: Histologic changes in the normal aging aorta: Implications for dissecting aortic aneurysm. Am J Cardiol 39:13, 1977

104. Kannel WB, D'Agostino RB, Belanger AJ: Concept of bridging the gap from youth to adulthood. Am J Med Sci 310(suppl):S15, 1995

105. Keller NM, Feit F: Coronary artery disease in the geriatric population. Prog Cardiovasc Dis 38:407, 1996

106. Shirani J, Yousefi J, Roberts WC: Major cardiac findings at necropsy in 366 American octogenarians. Am J Cardiol 75:151, 1995

107. Sleight P: Is there an age limit for thrombolytic therapy? Am J Cardiol 72(suppl G):S30, 1993

108. Duncan AK, Vittone J, Fleming KC, Smith HC: Cardiovascular disease in elderly patients. Mayo Clin Proc 71:184, 1996

109. Laster SB, Rutherford BD, Giorgi LV, et al: Results of direct percutaneous transluminal coronary angioplasty in octogenarians. Am J Cardiol 77:10, 1996

110. Egashira K, Inou T, Hirooka Y, et al: Effects of age on endothelium-dependent vasodilation of resistance coronary artery by acetylcholine in humans. Circulation 88:77, 1993

111. Chauhan A, More RS, Mullins PA, et al: Aging-associated endothelial dysfunction is reversed by L-arginine. J Am Coll Cardiol 28:1796, 1996

112. Celermajer DS, Sorensen KE, Spiegelhalter DJ, et al: Aging is associated with endothelial dysfunction in healthy men years before the age-related decline in women. J Am Coll Cardiol 24:471, 1994

113. Johnson MR: A normal coronary artery: What size is it? Circulation 86:331, 1992

114. Hort W, Lichti H, Kalbfleisch H, et al: The size of human coronary arteries depending on the physiological and pathological growth of the heart, the age, the size of the supplying areas and the degree of sclerosis: A postmortem study. Virchows Arch [Pathol Anat] 397:37, 1982

115. Restrepo C, Eggen DA, Guzmán MA, Tejada C: Postmortem dimensions of the coronary arteries in different geographic locations. Lab Invest 28:244, 1973

116. Hutchins GM, Bulkley BH, Miner MM, Boitnot JK: Correlation of age and heart weight with tortuosity and caliber of normal human coronary arteries. Am Heart J 94:196, 1977

117. Ehrich W, de la Chapelle C, Cohn AE: Anatomical ontogeny B. Man I. A study of the coronary arteries. Am J Anat 49:241, 1931

118. White NK, Edwards JE, Dry TJ: The relationship of the degree of coronary atherosclerosis with age, in men. Circulation 1:645, 1950

119. Ackerman RF, Dry TJ, Edwards JE: Relationship of various factors to the degree of coronary atherosclerosis in women. Circulation 1:1345, 1950

120. Lansing AI, Blumenthal HT, Gray SH: Aging and calcification of the human coronary artery. J Gerontol 3:87, 1948

121. Demer LL, Watson KE, Boström K: Mechanism of calcification in atherosclerosis. Trends Cardiovasc Med 4:45, 1994

122. Wexler L, Brundage B, Crouse J, et al: Coronary artery calcification: Pathophysiology, epidemiology, imaging methods, and clinical implications. A statement for health professionals from the American Heart Association. Circulation 94:1175, 1996

123. Rumberger JA, Sheedy PF II, Breen JF, et al: Electron beam computed tomography and coronary artery disease: Scanning for coronary artery calcification. Mayo Clin Proc 71:369, 1996

124. Reichel W, Garcia-Bunuel R: Pathologic findings in progeria: Myocardial fibrosis and lipofuscin pigment. Am J Clin Pathol 53:243, 1970

125. Atkins L: Progeria: Report of a case with post-mortem findings. N Engl J Med 250:1065, 1954

126. Ogihara T, Hata T, Tanaka K, et al: Hutchinson-Gilford progeria syndrome in a 45-year-old man. Am J Med 81:135, 1986

127. Dyck JD, David TE, Burke B, et al: Management of coronary artery disease in Hutchinson-Gilford syndrome. J Pediatr 111:407, 1987

128. Baker PB, Baba N, Boesel CP: Cardiovascular abnormalities in progeria: Case report and review of the literature. Arch Pathol Lab Med 105:384, 1981

129. Spence AM, Herman MM: Critical re-examination of the prema-

ture aging concept in progeria: A light and electron microscopic study. Mech Ageing Dev 2:211, 1973

130. Brown WT: Progeria: A human-disease model of accelerated aging. Am J Clin Nutr 55(suppl):S1222, 1992

131. Duvic M, Lemak NA: Werner's syndrome. Dermatol Clin 13:163, 1995

132. Thweatt R, Goldstein S: Werner syndrome and biological aging: A molecular genetic hypothesis. Bioessays 15:421, 1993

133. Cohen JI, Arnett EN, Kolodny AL, Roberts WC: Cardiovascular features of the Werner syndrome. Am J Cardiol 59:493, 1987

134. Goto M, Kato Y: Hypercoagulable state indicates an additional risk factor for atherosclerosis in Werner's syndrome. Thromb Haemost 73:576, 1995

135. Goto M, Rubenstein M, Weber J, et al: Genetic linkage of Werner's syndrome to five markers on chromosome 8. Nature 355:735, 1992

Chapter 4

Atherosclerosis: Pathology and Pathogenesis

· · · · ·

Avrum I. Gotlieb • Malcolm D. Silver

Atherosclerosis is a chronic disease of elastic arteries and of large and medium-sized muscular ones. Intimal cells in the vessel wall interact with serum constituents to play a central role in forming cellular intimal lesions that ultimately become human fibrofatty plaques.[1] Growth of a plaque results in eventual reduction of lumen size and encroachment on the media. Clinical disease, which may manifest as myocardial infarction, stroke, peripheral vascular disease, or aortic aneurysm with or without rupture, is caused by several complications of plaque formation: reduction of blood flow to an end organ, thromboembolic and/or atheroembolic events, and localized complications in the vessel wall itself, especially plaque hemorrhage and rupture.

Atherosclerosis is to be distinguished from arteriosclerosis, which describes degenerative diseases of arteries, including Mönckeberg medial calcific sclerosis (see later discussion) and arteriosclerosis of the peripheral arteries of the lower limbs characterized by intimal thickening and medial fibrosis. Small arteries usually do not develop atherosclerosis except as described later in this chapter, but they do show intimal and medial hyperplasia, hypertrophy, and fibrosis in such conditions as systemic hypertension and diabetes mellitus (see Chapter 6). Veins develop phlebosclerosis (see Chapter 2) but not atherosclerosis, with the exception of a yellow plaque in the vena cava at the junction of this vein and the left common iliac veins,[2] or if a vein is placed in the arterial circulation—for example, a saphenous vein graft used in coronary artery bypass surgery. A form of arteriosclerosis develops rapidly in organ transplants (see Chapter 23). Such lesions are circumferential and involve small arteries and arterioles as well. It is likely that the pathogenesis of this accelerated or graft arteriosclerosis differs from atherosclerosis in general in that immune reactions related to alloantigens in the graft wall result in smooth muscle cell hyperplasia and matrix deposition leading to intimal thickening.[3, 4]

Although mortality rates associated with atherosclerosis have decreased substantially,[5, 6] the challenge for both medical practitioners and researchers is to unravel the multifactorial etiology of the disease, the prime cause of death in North America and Europe. Because atherosclerosis-associated diseases consume a substantial part of health care budgets,[7] investment in research to study its pathogenesis and develop strategies to prevent it can reap huge benefits. The incidence of atherosclerotic lesions may change over time in a given population.[8, 9] In addition, for those who have the disease, new medical and surgical treatments are being devised to treat symptoms, arrest the process, and promote regression of the vascular lesions. The usefulness of specific treatment regimens can now be studied using the direct end point of regression or lack of progression of fibrofatty plaques.[10] Presently these techniques are invasive, but imaging technologies for the eventual noninvasive assessment of plaque size and composition are being developed.[11, 12]

For 150 years, pathologists have carefully studied morphologic changes in the human vascular wall to understand the initiation and evolution of fibrofatty plaques. Using this knowledge, animal models were developed to study the pathogenesis of these lesions.[13] In addition, the production of genetic variants of common laboratory species that develop atherosclerosis spontaneously or develop abnormalities in responsiveness to atherogenic challenges has been very useful[14]; several transgenic animal models are available. Surgical and autopsy pathology studies have been important in assessing new clinical treatments. Powerful morphologic techniques have appeared, including use of monoclonal antibodies in immunohistochemistry[15] and the molecular biology technique of in situ hybridization,[16] that provide sensitive methods to study the composition of the cells and the matrix of lesions, the activation of genes, and the localization of gene products. Based on a solid foundation of traditional morphology, modern cell and molecular biology studies provide physicians with knowledge of the dynamic interactions that occur in the vessel wall and in the plaque during atherogenesis.

This chapter provides a current perspective of pathology and cellular and molecular biology of atherosclerosis, focusing on the pathogenesis of the atherosclerotic plaque.

OVERVIEW: UNIFYING CLINICOPATHOLOGIC THEORY

The overall paradigm to consider in providing a unifying theory for clinicopathologic issues is that of the three stages of atherogenesis: the initiation/formation stage; the adaptation stage; and the clinical stage (Fig. 4-1). In all three, dynamic events that determine a plaque's structure, the vessel wall response to its presence, and its clinical outcomes are continuously occurring within the plaque and the vessel.

Initiation/Formation Stage

1. Intimal lesions initially occur at sites predisposed to lesion formation as a result of endothelial dysfunction and/or accumulation of smooth muscle cells. The latter

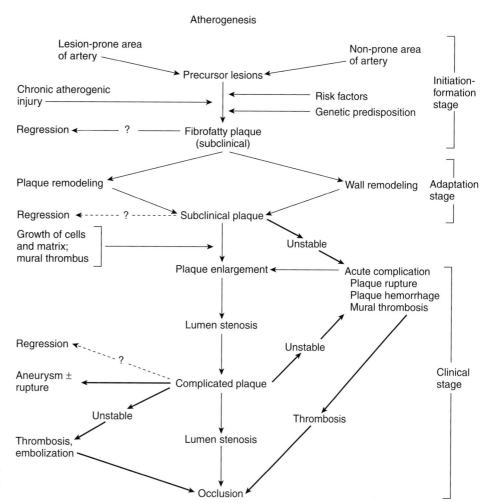

Figure 4-1 • Three stages of atherogenesis and its clinical complications.

occurs in an intimal cell mass or at arterial branch points. In individuals at increased risk for atherosclerosis, lesions also occur in nonpredisposed areas.

2. Lipid accumulation at these foci depends on disruption of the integrity of the endothelial barrier. Modified low-density lipoproteins (LDLs) are internalized by intimal smooth muscle cells via scavenger receptors. The types of connective tissue synthesized by the cells in the intima render these sites prone to lipid accumulation. Oxidized LDLs may induce cell injury through the formation of reactive oxygen species. This leads to further disruption of the integrity of the endothelial barrier and accumulation of macrophages by upregulation of leukocyte adhesion molecules. The macrophages accumulate modified lipids via scavenger receptors and become foam cells, as do intimal smooth muscle cells.

3. The activated macrophages release growth factor and cytokines, which promote further entry of macrophages. Fibroblast growth factor and platelet-derived growth factor (PDGF) are involved. Smooth muscle cell proliferation is stimulated. Oxidized lipoproteins promote tissue damage, including cell necrosis and/or apoptosis and further macrophage accumulation.

4. Endothelial injury leads to a reduction in the anticoagulant and fibrinolytic properties of the vessel wall,

predisposing it to mural thrombosis. This stimulates the release of growth factors and further accelerates smooth muscle proliferation and the secretion of matrix components. The thrombus becomes organized and is incorporated into the plaque. The intima is thickened so that its deeper parts are poorly nourished and undergo necrosis, an event augmented by proteolytic enzymes released by macrophages and tissue damage caused by oxidized LDL and other agents. The fibrofatty plaque is formed, and angiogenesis promotes vascularization of the plaque. The plaque becomes heterogenous with respect to smooth muscle cell localization, inflammatory cell infiltration, and matrix organization. Plaques show low levels of smooth muscle cell proliferation and apoptosis, suggesting that cell turnover does occur although the change in cell number is regulated.[17-19]

Adaptation Stage

1. The artery wall adapts to the presence of an atherosclerotic plaque. As the plaque encroaches on the vessel lumen (e.g., in coronary arteries), the vessel undergoes remodeling to maintain normal lumen size. Hemodynamic shear stress is an important regulator of this process. It is likely that cell proliferation, apopto-

sis, and both matrix synthesis and degradation are important modulating factors. Apoptosis occurs in the remodeling of normal arteries in neonatal lambs, suggesting that it too is an important process for vascular remodeling.[20] It is also likely that the plaque itself undergoes remodeling and that apoptosis may be an important process, because factors associated with its regulation are found in plaques.[18] Once a plaque encroaches on about 45% of the lumen, compensatory remodeling can not maintain lumen size and it narrows (stenosis). Abnormalities of vasoactive substances may disrupt the adaptive process—for example, as might occur with decreased synthesis of nitric oxide (NO) by endothelial cells or reduced responsiveness of smooth muscle cells to NO-induced relaxation.

2. Plaques continue to grow as a dynamic process involving smooth muscle cells, macrophages, lymphocytes, matrix synthesis, matrix degradation, and neovascularization. Surface thrombi may develop and be incorporated into the plaque. Hemorrhage arising from new, fragile vessels within the plaque may also increase plaque size. As noted in the next section, plaque rupture may occur during this stage in mild and moderate lesions and produce a sudden clinical event.

Clinical Stage

1. Plaque complications appear, including surface ulceration, fissure formation, calcification, and aneurysm formation. Continued plaque growth leads to severe luminal stenosis. The catastrophic event of plaque rupture with ensuing thrombosis and occlusion of the lumen usually occurs in advanced plaques and may produce the first sign or symptom of clinical disease. However, angiographic studies suggest that plaques causing even less than 50% stenosis may rupture. Therefore, a plaque's instability may not be related to size or duration of existence but to active biologic processes present within it. Conditions believed to promote plaque rupture include endothelial denudation with ulceration or fissure formation, hemodynamic shear stress at the plaque shoulder, a thin fibrous cap, inflammatory activity at the interface between an area of lipid deposition and fibrous tissue, and the presence of metalloproteinases most often released by macrophages that digest connective tissue matrix. Brown and Fuster presented the hypothesis that intensive lipid-lowering therapy promotes plaque stabilization and is important in the substantial reduction in clinical events seen with such regimens.[21]

2. Severe luminal stenosis (greater than 75% in the coronary arteries) or vascular occlusion leads to clinical complications in atherosclerosis, including ischemic heart disease (angina pectoris, sudden death, acute myocardial infarction), stroke, and peripheral vascular disease. Severe weakening of the artery wall can cause aneurysm with eventual rupture.

3. The potential exists for atherosclerotic plaques to regress as a result of alterations in risk factors and lifestyle and use of medication to lower specific factors such as hyperlipidemia.[21] In animal studies, lipid-induced lesions do show regression after a few years if diet is restored to normal.[22, 23] The regressed lesions show a marked reduction of lipid with a persisting fibrous plaque.[24] Coronary angiographic studies in humans have shown reduction in plaque size.[21] These studies await confirmation by methods that can accurately assess plaque size and plaque composition in vivo.

EPIDEMIOLOGY AND RISK FACTORS

Epidemiologic research has identified environmental and genetic factors that increase the likelihood of developing atherosclerosis.[25, 26] About 300 variables have been reported as risk factors for coronary artery disease. After review of the associations with respect to their strength, independence, dose-responsiveness, consistency, mechanistic plausibility, temporal sequence, and reversibility, only about 20 are considered major ones. They include cigarette smoking (more than 10 cigarettes per day), systemic hypertension, dyslipidemia, a family history of premature coronary artery disease characterized by myocardial infarction or sudden death before the age of 55 years in a parent or sibling, diabetes mellitus, and a high concentration of LDL cholesterol. Age-matched men are at greater risk for developing atherosclerosis than premenopausal women. In the postmenopausal period, women catch up to men in risk.[27] Estrogen use in women is associated with reduced cardiovascular disease.[28] Estrogen replacement therapy improves the risk factors of high LDLs and low high-density lipoproteins (HDLs).[29] Having more than one major risk factor is particularly hazardous because of their additive or synergistic effects.[27, 30] Atherosclerosis also increases with increasing age.[31] Additional risk factors include obesity (more than 30% overweight), lack of exercise, and stressful psychosocial factors including the type A personality lifestyle.[32] Increased levels of total plasma homocysteine are also considered a risk factor,[23–26] as are elevated plasma fibrinogen levels.[37] Data on risk factors support the concept of a multifactorial process in the pathogenesis of atherosclerosis.

Role of Risk Factors in Pathogenesis

The ability to accurately predict progression of atherosclerosis in a given individual with risk factors is still limited; in addition to the known population risk factors, still other etiologic ones are likely to be identified in the future. Studies now focus on how risk factors work at the cellular and molecular levels, both independently and synergistically.

Cigarette Smoking

Aortic and coronary artery lesions were positively associated with cigarette smoking in autopsied men from 25 to 64 years of age.[38] The mechanisms are not known, although endothelial damage, hypoxia, and a link to thrombosis[39] have been implicated. Cessation of smoking produces a dramatic reduction in cardiovascular death.[40]

Hypertension

Studies in animals and humans suggest that atherosclerotic lesions do not commonly develop as a result of hypertension per se; alone, it does not cause an intimal accumulation of lipid. Hypertension accelerates atherogenesis in the Watanabe heritable hyperlipidemic (WHHL) rabbit, which spontaneously develops hypercholesterolemia as a result of LDL receptor deficiencies. In this animal, most early lesions occur just distal to a branch orifice, whereas in the hypertensive WHHL rabbit they are more diffuse, indicating that hypertension does more than increase the severity of indigenous lesions. Hypertension promotes an increase in intracellular microfilaments in aortic endothelial cells; this is thought to be causally related to an associated increase in vessel wall permeability.[41] There is also an increase in adhesion and deposition of macrophages on/in the intima.[42] Hypertension also promotes hypertrophy of medial smooth muscle cells in experimental animals. Its treatment has a beneficial effect, although elevated systolic blood pressure is probably a more potent risk factor.[43]

Lipoproteins

LDL contains much of the total circulating cholesterol and is positively related to coronary disease.[44–46] Familial hypercholesterolemia is a genetic trait that predisposes to severe hypercholesterolemia and coronary atherosclerosis. The regulation of cholesterol and lipoprotein receptor metabolism were elucidated by Brown and Goldstein,[47] who were subsequently awarded a Nobel prize. In homozygotes, totally defective or absent receptor activity for LDL exists, resulting in severe complicated atherosclerosis in the first and second decades of life. In heterozygotes, there is 50% abnormal receptor activity and less severe hypercholesterolemia.[48, 49] Interest has also focused on the role of lipoprotein polymorphisms, which increase the risk of cardiovascular disease[50] during high cholesterol intake. The LDL cholesterol concentration was significantly increased in persons with apolipoprotein E3 (Apo E3) and E4 phenotype but not in those with Apo E2.[51] Apo E4 predisposes to the development of atherosclerosis.[52] Conversely, HDL is inversely related to cardiovascular death.[53] Very low-density lipoprotein (VLDL) is correlated with triglyceride levels, and both VLDL and triglyceride are not independently associated with cardiovascular disease.[54] However, there is evidence that increased triglycerides may be associated with coronary artery disease.[55, 56] High serum levels of the lipoprotein Lp(a) correlate with coronary heart disease.[57–60] Lp(a) is found in the arterial wall and accumulates at that location in patients with coronary heart disease.[61] Lp(a) is present at sites of vascular injury induced by balloon angioplasty in nonhuman primates.[62]

HDL levels increase in response to exercise and weight loss, especially the subfraction HDL_2.[63, 64] Obesity is associated with decreased HDL levels. Postmenopausal estrogen supplementation results in significantly higher HDL and HDL_2.[65] These hormones induce changes in lipoprotein metabolism.[66] However, postmenopausal estrogen use is associated with the development of endometrial carcinoma.[67] Oral contraceptive agents have been reported not to raise the incidence of cardiovascular disease in women.[68] Dubey and associates have suggested that the cardiovascular protection obtained from hormone replacement therapy in postmenopausal women depends in part on the affinity of the estrogen for estrogen receptors in the vascular smooth muscle cells[68a] (see also Chapter 17).

Moderate alcohol consumption (two or fewer drinks a day) causes an increase in HDL levels.[69] The incidence of coronary artery disease increases when more than two drinks a day are consumed.[69] No advising group currently advocates use of alcoholic beverages to promote increased HDL, because it is not known whether such HDL elevations protect against coronary atherosclerosis and because alcohol consumption can have other serious adverse effects. The role of the molecule resveratrol, previously implicated in the protective effect of some wines against ischemic heart disease,[70] requires further studies.[71]

Diabetes Mellitus

Diabetes mellitus is an independent as well as an associated risk factor for atherosclerosis.[72] Hypertension and hyperlipidemia are factors that increase the risk in association with diabetes mellitus.[73] Diabetic women lose their protection from atherosclerosis and have a prevalence rate of atherosclerotic disease similar to that of diabetic men. This may be a result of the greater effects, in women, of higher triglyceride and lipoprotein cholesterol serum concentrations.[74] Diabetes accelerates coronary atherosclerosis[75]; the initial severity of diabetes is an important determinant of long-term survival in those undergoing aortocoronary artery bypass surgery.[76] Factors associated with diabetes can cause smooth muscle cell proliferation.[77] It has been suggested that advanced glycosylation end products promote activation of endothelial cells and release of growth factors that may stimulate smooth muscle cell proliferation.[78] These end products induce monocyte/macrophage-directed transendothelial migration and secretion of PDGF, both processes that are important in atherogenesis.[79] LDL modification by advanced glycosylation end products may have a role in atherogenesis, possibly by impairing LDL-receptor–mediated clearance mechanisms.[80] Studies support the concept that hyperglycemia can cause vascular dysfunction by activating the diacylglycerol (DAG)–protein kinase C pathways.[81] (Diabetic microangiopathy is discussed in Chapter 16.)

Homocysteine

Elevated plasma total homocysteine (tHcy) is a risk factor for atherosclerotic disease.[36] Possible mechanisms include endothelial damage, enhanced thrombosis, and both the inhibition of endothelial cell growth and stimulation of smooth muscle cell growth leading to intimal thickening.[82] Folic acid supplementation usually lowers tHcy levels; however, multivitamin use, methylenetetrahydrofolate reductase genotypes, and initial tHcy and vitamin levels are involved in the variable responsiveness to folic acid[83] (see also Chapter 16).

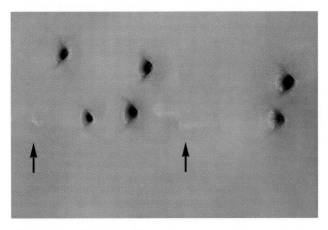

Figure 4-2 • Gross photograph of fatty streaks (arrows) in the thoracic aorta.

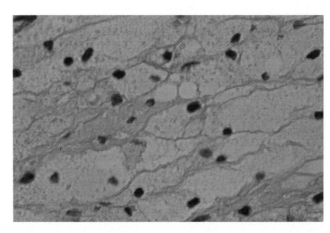

Figure 4-3 • Histologic section of a fatty streak lesion from the thoracic aorta showing foam cells (H&E stain).

Risk Management

Several international groups have adopted specific guidelines based on the management of risk factors[84-86] to prevent coronary heart disease. Dietary modification, modification of lifestyle, and hypolipidemic drug therapy, mostly aimed at treating hypercholesterolemia,[87, 88] reduce the incidence of coronary artery disease,[45, 46, 89, 90] and both arrest progression and promote regression of fibrofatty plaques.[91] There is no uniform opinion concerning dietary regulation in the pediatric age group. The management of disorders of plasma lipid and lipoprotein metabolism in this cohort has been addressed,[92] as have educational programs to modify risk factors in school-age children.[93, 94] Results of the Pathobiological Determinants of Atherosclerosis in Youth study[95] suggest that primary prevention with risk factor modification should be extended to young people, both male and female.[96] Moreover, risk factor reduction may require different management strategies in the geriatric population.[97] For instance, a correlation between coronary heart disease and serum cholesterol level does not persist beyond the age of 60 years.[98] Many physicians, however, promote risk factor reduction for elderly patients.[99]

LESIONS

The vasculature is modified early in life, with resultant changes that predispose individuals to atherosclerotic plaque formation. For instance, within the first few months, the intima of the left anterior descending coronary artery has the same thickness as the media.[100] Atherogenesis also seems to start very early in life.[101] Through human autopsy studies, specific intimal lesions that are considered to be early or precursor lesions to plaque have been identified. They include fatty streaks[102-104] and intimal thickening. Gelatinous lesions are much less understood, and mural microthrombi are currently not considered to be precursor lesions.[105] Aortic fatty streaks are observed in early childhood and even in neonates; however, in the coronary artery they start at about 10 years of age.[106] Fibrous plaques are found in a high proportion of young adults in populations that have a high incidence of atherosclerosis.[107, 108] All these lesions are silent and produce no clinical symptoms, but they do predispose the individual to future clinical disease.

Fatty Streaks

Fatty streaks are flat or slightly elevated and vary in size from 3 to 5 mm (Fig. 4-2). They consist of a large number of lipid-laden foam cells (Fig. 4-3) that contain cholesteryl esters and a variable amount of extracellular lipid (Fig. 4-4). These cells, found in the intima, are derived from smooth muscle cells of the vessel wall (myogenic foam cells)[109, 110] and from blood monocytes.[111] Modified LDL is ingested by macrophages through the scavenger receptor–mediated pathway.[112] There is no fibrotic component to these lesions. Women between the ages of 15 and 34 years have more extensive fatty streaks than men but the same extent of raised plaques.[106] Fatty streaks are reversible and are seen to the same extent in the aortas of the young in populations that do and do not develop atherosclerosis in later life.[88, 113] This has been

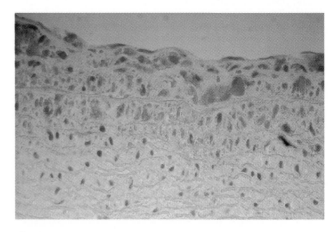

Figure 4-4 • Histologic section of fatty streak lesion stained with oil red O to show both intracellular and extracellular lipid.

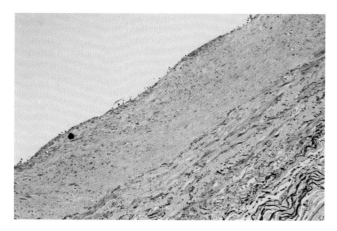

Figure 4-5 • Fibromuscular intimal thickening of the aorta (Movat stain).

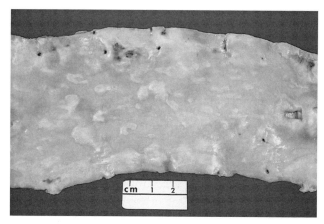

Figure 4-6 • Fibrofatty plaques in the thoracic aorta.

documented quantitatively in the coronary artery and aorta in various geographic populations.[114] At present, there is no marker that enables differentiation between those fatty streaks that will become fibrofatty plaques and those that regress. Therefore, it is likely that other factors interact with the fatty streak to promote progression toward a fibrofatty plaque. Stary and Letson provided evidence that fatty streaks progress to advanced lesions in areas of eccentric intimal thickening, probably related to hemodynamic forces.[115]

Intimal Thickening

Diffuse intimal thickening (Fig. 4-5) is a site of predilection for fibrofatty plaques[116] (see also Chapter 8). Haust and More[110] and Geer and colleagues[117] described the presence of smooth muscle cells in these thickenings. Morphologic studies show that fibroplastic intimal thickening begins in the aorta during childhood and progresses throughout life.[118] Stary and coworkers described intimal thickening and suggested that eccentric thickening predisposes individuals to plaque formation.[119, 120] Atheronecrosis appears in most cases in which the intima is more than 300 μm thick.[121]

Gelatinous Lesions

Gelatinous lesions or elevations, 2 to 4 mm in diameter, are characterized by edematous swellings of the intima that demonstrate reduced metachromasia in sections stained with toluidine blue, compared with those in the normal vessel wall. The connective tissue is separated, and there is a decreased cellularity in the lesion relative to normal tissue.[105] Smith and Ashall[122] proposed that gelatinous lesions were soft, translucent thickenings containing little or no lipid that underwent transition to fibrous plaques. These lesions have not been extensively studied and are not referred to in many of the current theories of atherogenesis.

Mural Microthrombi

The presence of fresh mural microthrombi has been described.[105] These microthrombi contained fibrin and

platelets and were present overlying morphologically normal endothelium or an early lesion. Very occasional microthrombi could be seen incorporated into the vessel wall. Jorgensen[123] referred to several papers that showed a single platelet or an aggregate of platelets in contact with a normal endothelial cell. It is very unlikely that these rare findings indicated any pathobiologic effect, because there was no evidence that the contact promoted functional changes in either platelet or endothelial cell. Recent findings suggest that endothelial dysfunction may promote microthrombus formation.[123a]

Fibrofatty Plaque

The atherosclerotic lesion (plaque) is often termed a fibrofatty plaque (Fig. 4-6), although it is clear, as Table 4-1 indicates, that there is much more present in a plaque than just fibrous tissue and lipid. The term *atherosclerotic plaque*, coined by Marchand, a pathologist from Leipzig[11] (from the Greek *athero*, meaning gruel or porridge, referring to the central necrotic material found in many plaques, and *sclerosis*, meaning fibrosis), is still much used but conveys little information about the nature of a

TABLE 4-1 • **Important Components of Fibrofatty Plaque**

Cells
    Endothelial
    Foam
    Smooth muscle
    Macrophages
    Lymphocytes

Matrix
    Collagen
    Proteoglycans
    Elastin
    Glycoproteins

Lipids and lipoproteins

Serum proteins

Platelet and leukocyte products

Necrotic debris

Microvessels

Hydroxyapatite crystals

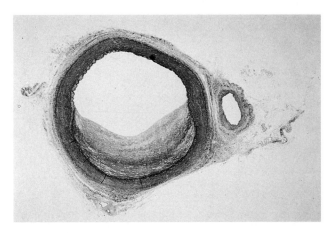

Figure 4-7 • Cross section of an atherosclerotic coronary artery with dilation of the artery to maintain lumen size (Movat stain).

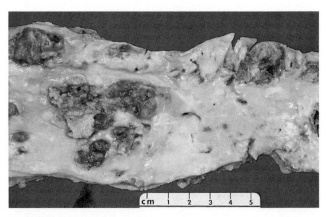

Figure 4-8 • Complicated aortic fibrofatty plaques showing fusion of plaques, ulceration, fissures, and mural thrombi.

plaque. Tracey and Kissling[118, 121] reported that aortic fibrous plaques could be classified histologically as either atheronecrotic or fibroplastic, depending on the presence or absence of a necrotic core. A detailed histologic classification of atherosclerotic lesions has been proposed by the American Heart Association.[120, 123b] Virmani and colleagues have proposed a simpler classification based on a descriptive morphology focusing on the state of the fibrous plaque.[123c] For plaque to form, a critical thickness of 250 to 400 μm is required in the aortic intima and 100 to 200 μm in the intima of the coronary arteries.[118, 121] The specific dysfunctions leading to a necrotic core have not been identified, but a disruption of the diffusion of nutrients is probably important.

Human plaques tend to be morphologically similar in all populations studied.[124, 125] Beginning at age 15 years and continuing to age 24 years, the coronary arteries of men have twice as many plaques as those of women.[126] Adults with increased serum cholesterol levels show the same type of fibrofatty plaques as those who are normocholesterolemic. Populations in which the rate of atherosclerosis is low do not have plaques that differ qualitatively from those in populations with high rates of atherosclerosis. Although diabetes enhances the rate of development of clinical atherosclerosis, plaques from diabetics have the same morphology as do those from nondiabetics.[72] Therefore, a variety of risk factors result in the same type of pathologic lesion in the vessel wall. In addition, atherosclerotic plaques that develop in surgically implanted saphenous vein bypass grafts have typical fibrofatty features,[127, 128] except that some are more friable because they contain less fibrous tissue. Stary and coworkers classified atherosclerotic lesions into six categories based on light microscopic morphology.[129]

Location

Some arteries are largely spared, whereas some, such as the coronary vessels, the infrarenal aorta, major vessels supplying the lower extremities, and the carotids at their bifurcations, are at greater risk. Plaques are often found in areas affected by increased[130] or decreased[131] hemodynamic shear stress or other hemodynamic factors.[132] Shear stress affects endothelial shape, endothelial actin micro-

filament organization,[133, 134] prostacyclin and histamine synthesis and secretion, and both vascular permeability and endothelial repair.[135] Several mechanisms are postulated by which endothelial cells sense changes in shear stress, including effects of shear sensors on their luminal membrane and effects on force sensors associated with cell-cell junctions, basal adhesion sites, and the cell cytoskeleton.[136]

Gross Morphology

A simple plaque is an elevated, white/yellow, smooth-surfaced lesion that is focal in distribution and irregular in shape albeit with reasonably well-defined borders (see Fig. 4-6). Fibrofatty plaques are oval, with their largest diameter being 8 to 12 mm, and are mostly oriented in the direction of blood flow. At aortic branch points and in smaller vessels such as the coronary or cerebral arteries, the plaque is often eccentric (Fig. 4-7). Plaques fuse when lesions progress, and in more advanced stages they can cover an area of several square centimeters (Figs. 4-8 and 4-9). In epicardial coronary arteries, it is believed that a significant clinical stenosis occurs when more than 75% of the lumen is narrowed, because at that point distal flow is reduced.[137]

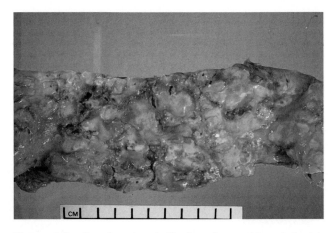

Figure 4-9 • Complicated aortic fibrofatty plaques with marked calcification.

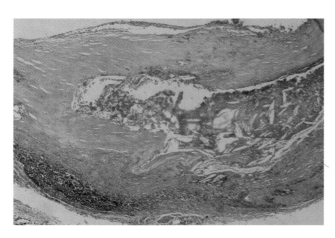

Figure 4-10 • Atherosclerotic plaque showing the fibrous cap and central area of necrosis (Movat stain).

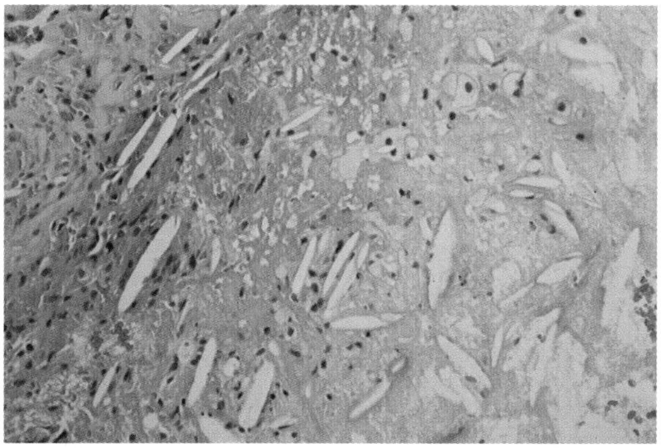

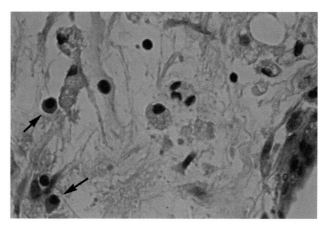

Figure 4-12 • Atherosclerotic plaque showing clefts of lipid crystals and associated foreign body giant cells (H&E stain).

Microscopic Morphology

Initially, the plaque is covered by endothelium. The lesion involves the intima and only very little of the superficial media. Its composition is heterogeneous from area to area. The tissue between the vascular lumen and the necrotic core is called the fibrous cap (Fig. 4-10); it contains smooth muscle cells, macrophages, lymphocytes, foam cells, and connective tissue components. Modified smooth muscle cells are often found in an ellipsoid space in the connective tissue[138] and throughout the plaque's matrix (Fig. 4-11). The central core consists of necrotic debris (Fig. 4-12). Lipid crystals and associated foreign body giant cells may be present in association with the necrotic areas (see Fig. 4-12) and also within the fibrous tissue. There are often foam cells in this area, as well as in focal groups within the tissue matrix; they are of macrophage origin or are smooth muscle cells that have taken up lipids (Fig. 4-13). Experimental studies in vitro demonstrate this clearly.[117, 139] The macrophages are derived from blood monocytes[102, 140–142] that adhere to the endothelium and then enter the wall between endothelial cells, perhaps under the influence of chemotactic factors.[143] Other mechanisms for foam cell development have been

suggested by studies showing that platelets or substances shed from activated platelets, or substances shed from both, mediate the accumulation of macrophage cholesteryl ester.[144]

Numerous chronic inflammatory and immune cells are present within the plaque (Fig. 4-14). In the past, morphologic criteria were used to identify these cells, but histochemical markers have enhanced identification.[145] Antibodies, especially of monoclonal type, are used not only in frozen tissue but also in routinely fixed paraffin-embedded tissue (Fig. 4-15). T cells have been observed in surgically removed internal carotid artery plaques[146] and in the subendothelial intimal space in areas with an increased predilection to develop plaques.[147] Chronic inflammatory cells are also seen in the adventitia, especially with prominent plaque involvement of the media.

Neovascularization has a very important role in plaque growth and subsequent plaque pathology (see Fig. 4-14).[148] Although much is known about the regulation of angiogenesis,[149] the pathogenesis of plaque neovascularization is not understood. It is postulated that vessel ingrowth occurs from vasa vasorum. The vasa vasorum of the human aorta are described by Okuyama.[150, 151] They are rare in healthy coronary arteries but plentiful in

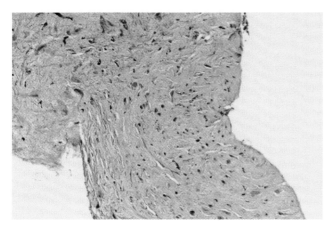

Figure 4-11 • Atherosclerotic plaque showing smooth muscle cells within the plaque matrix (Movat stain).

Figure 4-13 • Atherosclerotic plaque showing pigmented macrophages (arrows) in areas of loose fibrosis (H&E stain).

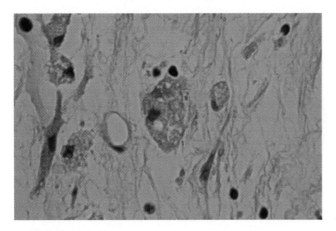

Figure 4-14 • Atherosclerotic plaque showing neovascularization and focal lymphocytes (H&E stain).

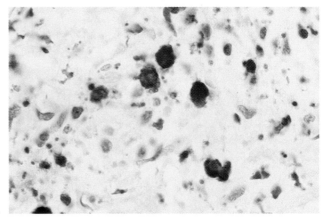

Figure 4-15 • Atherosclerotic plaque showing macrophages stained with an antibody specific for macrophages.

atherosclerotic ones. Angiographic examinations of the latter have confirmed this finding and have shown direct flow from the vessel lumen via branches to the vasa vasorum that then feed into plaques.[152] Newly formed vessels are fragile and may rupture, resulting in an acute expansion of the plaque as a consequence of hemorrhage.[153] Hemosiderin-laden macrophages, often present in focal areas of the plaque, indicate remote hemorrhage (see Fig. 4-13) or a healed focal rupture of the fibrous cap, or both.[154]

If a plaque occupies 45% or less of the potential lumen area, chronic dilation of the artery through remodeling occurs so that lumen size remains unchanged[155] (see Fig. 4-7). Beyond 45% stenosis, the artery is unable to compensate, and arterial enlargement no longer keeps pace with increased plaque size.

Complicated Plaques

The term *complicated plaque* is used to describe the following conditions: erosion, ulceration, or fissuring of a plaque's surface; plaque hemorrhage; mural thrombosis; calcification; and aneurysm. Fissuring may lead to intraintimal thrombosis. Platelets and coagulation factors enter the plaque via the fissure, and the point of entry may then be sealed by thrombosis.[156] Erosion, ulceration, and fissuring probably occur after focal denudation of the surface endothelium (see Figs. 4-8 and 4-9). Focal denudation can be repaired,[157] but repeated injury results in a chronic loss of surface endothelium. Endothelial cells are also lost, at least in part, as a result of a reduction or dysfunction of the large actin microfilament bundles, which are important in their adhesion to the substratum[158] or to alterations in the subendothelial matrix.

The intensity and type of inflammatory reaction found in complicated plaques varies considerably. One may contain relatively few chronic inflammatory cells, whereas another may reveal a florid reaction in which giant cells, often related to crystalline material and both polymorphs and eosinophils, are found. Again, the intensity of adventitial collection of chronic inflammatory cells, mainly lymphocytes that sometimes have germinal centers, may vary.

Calcification occurs both in areas of necrosis and elsewhere in the plaque (Fig. 4-16). The calcium compounds in aortic tissue are hydroxyapatite-like and consist of calcium, phosphate, and carbonate. The crystals are often deposited in and on collagen fibrils, oriented in the same direction as the fibril. Calcium concentration increases with age in the normal aorta (see also Chapter 3). The initiating factors for aortic mineralization are not known, although several have been postulated. Membrane vesicles derived from necrotic tissue were thought to be a nidus for crystal formation. Alteration in tissue pH, in proteoglycan structure and organization, or in collagen organization, are possible factors in promoting plaque mineralization.[158] Calcification of atherosclerotic plaques is currently being investigated as an active process related, at least in part, to processes of bone mineralization. This is because osteoblastic differentiation factors[159] and calcium-binding proteins[160, 161] are found in plaques. In addition, clones of cells that undergo bone formation have been identified in vessels[162] (calcification occurring in valvular heart disease is discussed in Chapter 13). Bone marrow metaplasia is not rare in complicated plaques.

Mural thrombosis occurs as a result of disrupted blood flow around the plaque, at the site of its protrusion into

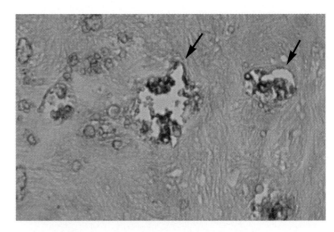

Figure 4-16 • An atherosclerotic plaque showing focal calcification (arrows) (H&E stain).

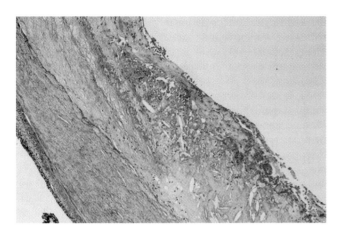

Figure 4-17 • An atherosclerotic plaque showing ulceration and fissuring (Movat stain).

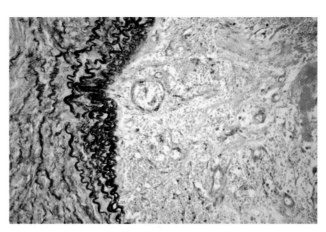

Figure 4-19 • Organized thrombus within arterial lumen with neovascularization (elastic-trichrome stain).

the lumen. The flow disturbance causes damage to the endothelial lining; it may become locally denuded and no longer form an effective thromboresistant surface, or the endothelial cells may become dysfunctional and promote prothrombotic activities such as procoagulant processes, platelet activation, or antifibrinolysis. In addition, the necrotic plaque debris released from ulcerated or fissured plaques is thrombogenic (Fig. 4-17). Figure 4-18 shows an acute thrombus. Thrombi may become organized (Fig. 4-19), or they may lyse, grow, and/or embolize.

Plaque rupture is under intense study as an important process leading to acute occlusion of the vascular lumen (Figs. 4-20 and 4-21).[163] Because there is much evidence from biologic studies that plaques are dynamic in nature and undergo continuous remodeling, it is hypothesized that interactions of physical hemodynamic forces with degradative processes in the fibrous cap lead to a weakening of the plaque, especially at the interface of normal artery and plaque. Proteolytic activity promotes extracellular matrix degradation, which leads to weakening of the wall. It is believed that some ruptures heal without producing an acute clinical event.

CELLS

The cells of a plaque include endothelial cells, both on the lumen surface and in new vessels (neovascularization), smooth muscle cells, macrophages, and lymphocytes. These cells are exposed to the physical forces of blood flow and blood pressure and to molecules from the blood, from the vessel wall, and from the cells themselves through either paracrine or autocrine pathways. The key events are that endothelial cells become dysfunctional; monocytes enter the vessel wall and, as resident macrophages, provide elements for chronic inflammatory processes; lymphocytes enter the wall and are activated, regulating unknown immunologic events; smooth muscle cells undergo phenotypic modulation to provide much of the plaque's matrix; and angiogenesis occurs to promote new blood vessel growth. These events, which occur in the initial formation stage and during adaptation, result in remodeling. They continue to orchestrate the dynamic events leading to complicated plaques and acute or chronic clinical disease.

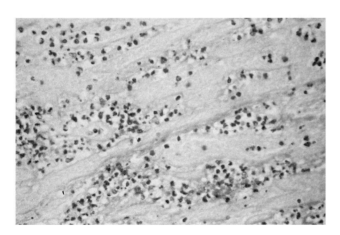

Figure 4-18 • Acute thrombus with polymorphonuclear leukocytes, platelets, and fibrin (H&E stain).

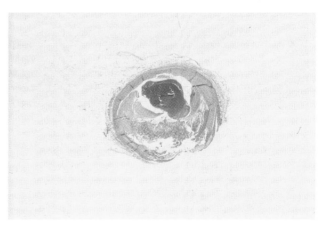

Figure 4-20 • Atherosclerotic plaque rupture with luminal thrombosis (H&E stain).

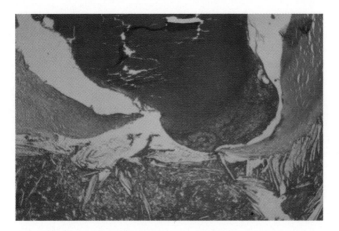

Figure 4-21 • Atherosclerotic plaque with rupture of the fibrous cap and acute luminal thrombosis caused by contact of blood with necrotic debris of plaque (H&E stain).

Endothelial Cells

Endothelial cells form a macromolecular barrier separating the vessel wall from the blood.[132, 164] The actin cytoskeleton (Fig. 4-22), in association with intercellular tight and adherens junctions (Fig. 4-23), forms a tight monolayer that can be disrupted by a variety of mechanisms, leading to exposure of the vessel wall to high levels of plasma constituents.[165] Figure 4-22B shows that the actin cytoskeleton is much more prominent at sites of increased hemodynamic shear stress, whereas the filaments become very thin in endothelial cells covering the surface of experimental atherosclerotic plaques (Fig. 4-22C).

Since cell culture techniques have been applied to the study of pure populations of large vessel endothelial[50, 166, 167] and smooth muscle cells,[168] their role in the development and subsequent growth of fibrofatty plaques has been extensively investigated.[167] Vascular endothelial cells are not inert lining cells; rather, they are metabolically active and interact with important physiologic processes at the blood–vascular wall interface, including coagulation, fibrinolysis, platelet aggregation,[168] and both leukocyte adherence, and migration. It is apparent that the endothelium can subserve diametrically opposite functions in many instances, and it is the regulation of these functions that defines its state at any given time (Table 4-2). Endothelial cells modulate smooth muscle cell function within the vessel wall by releasing locally acting polypeptides and glycoproteins and by direct intercellular communication. Indeed, smooth muscle cell proliferation as well as vasodilation and vasoconstriction are affected by such endothelial–smooth muscle cell interactions. Endothelin, a potent vasoconstrictor,[169] and NO, a potent vasodilator,[170] are secreted by endothelial cells and act via paracrine pathways to regulate smooth muscle cell function.

Endothelial cells also effect thrombosis by producing many substances that regulate blood coagulation. They

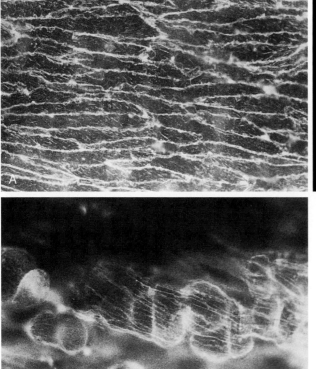

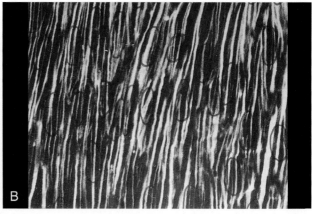

Figure 4-22 • Actin microfilament bundles localized with the use of fluorescence microscopy for rhodamine phalloidin, in endothelial cells of aorta. *A*, Bundles are shown in an area of normal blood flow; *B*, in an area of high hemodynamic shear stress; and *C*, on the surface of a macrophage-rich experimental atherosclerotic plaque.

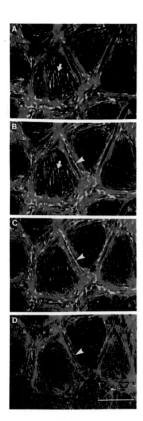

Figure 4-23 • Double immunofluorescence labeling of an in vitro confluent monolayer of endothelial cells. Actin microfilament bundles were localized with the use of rhodamine phalloidin, and vinculin with antibodies. Dense peripheral bands of actin microfilaments, short central microfilament bundles, and vinculin-containing adhesion junctions form structures that keep the monolayer together. A–D, Optical slices through the cell (top (D) to bottom (A) of cell) obtained by confocal laser microscopy.

can be induced to express tissue factor (TF), a cell surface glycoprotein that serves as a cofactor for factor VIIa and forms a complex with it to initiate coagulation. The cells produce factors VIII[171] and V[172] and have procoagulant activity.[173–175] They secrete prostacyclin (PGI_2) and NO, which are potent inhibitors of platelet aggregation.[176, 177] After vascular injury with endothelial damage, von Willebrand factor, synthesized by endothelial cells and megakaryocytes, provides one of the links between platelets and the subendothelial extracellular matrix.[178]

Endothelial cells have a surface receptor, thrombomodulin. In the presence of thrombin, thrombomodulin activates protein C,[179] an anticoagulant that inactivates factors V and VIII. In addition, the cells secrete protein S, a vitamin K–dependent cofactor of activated protein C[180]; both are powerful anticoagulants.[175] Anticoagulant activity is also expressed by the binding of thrombin to antithrombin III complexed with heparin-like glycosaminoglycans of the endothelial cell membrane.

Endothelial cells have a very prominent role in fibrinolysis. They produce different forms of plasminogen activator, including both a urokinase-like and a tissue-type plasminogen activator (tPA).[181–183] There is specific and functional binding of plasminogen and tPA to human endothelial cells.[184, 185] These cells also produce plasminogen activator inhibitor (PAI) and antiactivators that inhibit the activities of plasminogen activators.[186, 187] PAI binds to extracellular matrix that is produced by endothelial cells and may stabilize PAI against spontaneous loss of activity.[188] There appears to be an independent regulation of PAI, whose secretion may be influenced by many factors, including interleukin-1 (IL-1), dexamethasone, and phorbol myristate acetate.[189] In addition, activated protein C stimulates the fibrinolytic activity of endothelial cells and decreases antiactivator activity.[190] The net fibrinolytic state is a consequence of the balance among these various components.

Smooth Muscle Cells

These are the most important cells in the plaque because they are prevalent, secrete much of the plaque matrix, and may become foam cells. The normal function of the cell in the media is to maintain vascular tone. The myofilaments that regulate tone consist of actin and myosin filaments. There are also actin-associated proteins in smooth muscle, including α-actinin, filamin, and tropomyosin. Actin filaments insert into cytoplasmic densities (dense bodies),[191] both in the cytoplasm and along the cytoplasmic side of the cell membrane, where they appear as very prominent bands or patches. Force transmission, from the contractile apparatus to the cell membrane, appears to be mediated by actin filaments that insert into dense bodies along the cell membrane.

Apart from various neural and hormonal signals, blood vessel contractility is regulated by local mechanisms. Those in larger arteries, especially coronary arteries, have been successfully investigated in the last few years. PGI_2 was the first discovered vasoactive substance produced within the vessel wall.[177] Another important event was the recognition by Furchgott and associates of an endothelial-derived relaxing factor (EDRF).[192, 193] These investigators showed that acetylcholine and other factors cause relaxation with an intact endothelium and arterial contraction when the endothelium is denuded. Pharmacologic and biochemical studies indicate that EDRF is identical to nitrous oxide (NO).[169] There may be other relaxing factors, such as endothelium-derived hyperpolarizing factor,[194] and other chemicals that can fulfill similar criteria as a biologic agent (e.g., lysolecithins).[195]

The cyclic guanosine monophosphate (cGMP) and the cyclic adenosine monophosphate (cAMP) systems underlie the actions of NO and PGI_2, respectively. Both agents regulate not only vascular tone but also platelet–vessel

TABLE 4-2 • **Endothelial Functions in Health and Disease**

Selective impermeability	Enhanced permeability
Platelet resistance	Platelet adhesion
Procoagulation	Anticoagulation
Fibrinolysis	Antifibrinolysis
Leukocyte resistance	Leukocyte adhesion
Quiescence	Migration/proliferation
Growth inhibition	Growth promotion
Vasodilation	Vasoconstriction

wall interactions and, therefore, could be important in adaptive mechanisms that protect the wall from atherogenesis. Evidence shows that endothelial-dependent relaxation is impaired in atherosclerotic vessels,[196, 197] although there is substantial flow-dependent coronary artery dilation in human vessels that are diseased.[198] Therefore, the loss of relaxation favors vasospasm and local thrombosis.

Endothelial cells also have a prominent role in vasoconstriction,[198] especially release of endothelin, a very potent 21-residue peptide that causes long-lasting constriction.[170, 199] Peptides of the endothelin gene family are also involved in mitogenesis and vascular remodeling.[200] In addition, noradrenalin, thrombin, neuropeptide Y, calcium ionophore A23187, arachidonic acid, hypoxia, stretch, and increased mural pressure all cause vasoconstriction that is dependent on or enhanced by an intact endothelium.

The Vascular Matrix

The arterial media is structured of relatively discrete lamellar units that resolve into "musculoelastic fascicles." These consist of elongated smooth muscle cells demarcated by elastic fibers oriented in the same direction as the cells. The cells are surrounded by a matrix consisting of the basal lamina and a fine meshwork of collagen fibrils, extending from the basal lamina to extracellular collagen and elastin. The microarchitecture of these subunits reflects the distribution and magnitude of local tensile stresses.[201] The resting adult smooth muscle cells produce types I, III, IV, and V collagen.[202, 203] The interstitial stroma of the media contains types I, III, V,[204] VI,[205] and VIII collagen[206] and a variety of glycoproteins including fibronectin, the 220,000-D glycoprotein that mediates cell–matrix adhesion. Collagen type VIII has been identified, immunohistochemically,[207] especially in the subendothelial intimal matrix of elastic arteries. Smooth muscle cells also produce heparan sulfate, chondroitin sulfate, and dermatan sulfate proteoglycans.[208] Elastin is produced from proelastin[209] in young aortic smooth muscle cells but not in cells of the normal adult artery.

Endothelial cells are associated with an abluminal basement membrane, which consists of type IV collagen, laminin, heparan sulfate proteoglycans, and nidogen (entactin). Of importance is the process by which endothelial cells adhere to the substratum. Type IV collagen forms the scaffold of the basement membrane (to which other constituents are attached) and supplies mechanical support. Laminin, a glycoprotein involved in cell attachment, forms stable complexes with nidogen/entactin and can bind to heparan sulfate chains and also to heparin.[210] Heparan sulfate proteoglycans are strongly negatively charged and control filtration through the basement membrane.[211] Two laminin-specific cell membrane receptors have been identified.[212] The Arg-Gly-Asp (RGD) sequence responsible for cell membrane–fibronectin interaction is also found in laminin as well as other basement membrane components.[213] Secreted protein that is acidic and rich in cysteine (SPARC), a glycoprotein secreted by endothelial cells after injury, binds to the basement membrane and extracellular matrix components and is probably involved in the regulation of extracellular calcium by binding Ca^{2+} ions.[214]

It now appears that through complex interactions the extracellular matrix modulates, and is itself modulated by, a variety of cell processes important in vascular repair. With respect to proliferation, epidermal growth factor (EGF)–like repeats are present both in the core protein of heparan sulfate proteoglycan and in laminin.[215] Heparan sulfate proteoglycans may have a role in the storage of basic fibroblast growth factor (bFGF) (see later discussion) under physiologic and pathologic circumstances.[216] Decorin binds transforming growth factor-β (TGF-β), a growth factor that also regulates collagen synthesis.[217] Both collagen and proteoglycan metabolism are altered during migration and proliferation of endothelial cells.[218, 219] Heparan sulfate proteoglycan, which may modulate cell adhesion,[220] is reduced markedly at the tips of growing capillaries.[221] Therefore, it is possible that changes in this proteoglycan facilitate cell migration. Proteoglycan metabolism of aortic smooth muscle cells is modulated by collagen in contact with the cells.[222]

During atherogenesis, the profile of the proteoglycans produced is changed. Dermatan sulfate is most prominent in atheromas,[223, 224] although others are found, mainly chondroitin sulfate and heparan sulfate.[225, 226] Yla-Herttuala and associates[227] reported that in normal coronary arteries the contents of dermatan sulfate and chondroitin sulfates A and C increased significantly with age, but not as much as the very large increases seen in atherosclerotic vessels. Proteoglycans have the ability to interact with β-lipoproteins[228] and may be important in trapping lipids and promoting their accumulation in the plaque.[228] In fact, proteoglycan synthesis is greater in the aortas of susceptible animals compared with nonsusceptible ones,[229] and proteoglycan synthesis increases early during the proliferative response to injury to the endothelium and media.[230]

Matrix synthesis and degradation is regulated by cytokines, growth factors, and matrix degradation agents, which include matrix metalloproteinases, serine proteases, and cysteine proteases. Smooth muscle cells and macrophages are predominantly the source of these molecules. They act via paracrine and autocrine pathways. Matrix metalloproteins (there are more than 12 to date) act at neutral pH in the extracellular matrix on preferred substrates, since more than one may digest any given matrix component. They are released in inactive precursor forms, and naturally occurring inhibitors, called tissue inhibitors of metalloproteinases (TIMPs), are present.[231]

PATHOBIOLOGIC PROCESSES THAT OCCUR IN THE LESION

Many physiologic processes that occur during the initiation and development of an atherosclerotic plaque are normal cellular events (see Table 4-2); however, when they occur inappropriately in time or place, they are considered pathobiologic. In general, much is known about several of these processes but less is known about how they interact in plaque development.

Plaque Thrombosis

The evidence that fibrofatty plaques are initiated by microthrombi[232] is less compelling than it used to be. Careful studies indicate that areas of endothelial denudation are not present in normal endothelium. The concept that atherosclerosis is initiated by endothelial denudation followed by platelet adherence to subendothelial collagen and microfibrils is not tenable. Moreover, it is likely that even if single cell denudation occurred, it would be rapidly repaired.[157, 233]

There is no question, however, that plaques do grow as a result of mural thrombosis and that a plaque, by its very nature, may promote thrombosis. Damage to surface endothelium and flow disturbances are initiating factors. For example, endothelial dysfunction characterized by activation of coagulation factors (e.g., tissue factor) or reduction in fibrinolytic and anticoagulation factors, or both, promotes thrombosis. Mural thrombi may be occlusive, or they may be mural and nonocclusive. Physiologic organizational processes recanalize a thrombus or incorporate it into the vessel wall, or both. Often, layers of connective tissue of varying maturation and cellularity are present within a plaque, showing a varying extent of organization, with the most recent closest to the lumen.

Role of Growth Factors

Studies on atherosclerotic plaques removed by atherectomy or at surgery show a low rate of smooth muscle cell proliferation. This does not negate the important role proliferation has in plaque growth, especially during the initiation/formation stage.[234] For instance, insulin[235, 236] and insulin-like growth factor[237] are mitogenic to smooth muscle cells, whereas a somatostatin analog inhibits accelerated transplant atherosclerosis.[238] Insulin, insulin-like growth factor-1, and PDGF interact additively in the induction of the protooncogene c-*myc* and in the stimulation of smooth muscle proliferation.[77]

Platelet-Derived Growth Factor

PDGF was the first growth factor linked with atherogenesis. It was postulated that in the early stages PDGF, released by platelets adherent to the vessel wall at sites of denuded endothelium, had chemotactic and mitogenic effects on vessel wall smooth muscle cells. PDGF is a 27- to 31-kD glycoprotein dimer composed of two polypeptide chains, termed A and B, linked by disulfide bridges. PDGF-B is structurally identical to the p28[sis] translation product encoded by the c-*sis* oncogene. All three possible dimeric isoforms of PDGF, the homodimers AA and BB and the heterodimer AB, have been identified.[239] The two chains may undergo transcriptional and post-translational changes as well. Possibly there are three transmembrane PDGF receptors of 170 to 185 kD with an α and β subunit, which form three different dimeric receptors with different PDGF isoform specificities.[240] According to this

model, PDGF-AA binds only to the $\alpha\alpha$ receptor, PDGF-AB binds to the $\alpha\alpha$ and $\alpha\beta$ forms, and PDGF-BB binds to all three. The biologic effects of PDGF do not appear to be caused by a single molecule but rather by several molecules of a family.

In vitro, PDGF elicits a chemotactic response in smooth muscle cells,[241] monocytes,[242] and fibroblasts.[243] All PDGF isoforms can elicit a mitogenic response, as shown by Hosang and Rouge.[244] The receptor subtype composition of a target cell determines the mitogenic and chemotactic efficacy of the various PDGF isoforms. Any of the three can mediate mitogenesis, and at least two, but probably all three, induce chemotaxis and phosphoinositide breakdown.[244] Oxidized LDL induces PDGF-A chain expression in smooth muscle cells[245] and stimulates mitogen-activated protein kinase.[246]

In vivo, PDGF is believed to have an important role in the formation of proliferative atherosclerotic lesions and in medial hypertrophy associated with hypertension.[247] Rat arterial smooth muscle cells and smooth muscle cells from diseased human arteries expressed PDGF-A gene and secreted PDGF-like activity into the medium when grown in culture.[248–250] Human vascular smooth muscle cells derived from healthy human vessels express at least two PDGF receptors in vitro. They secrete PDGF-AA and can potentially regulate their growth in an autocrine and paracrine manner.[244] Furthermore, PDGF stimulates collagen and collagenase production by fibroblasts[251] and is a potent vasoconstrictor.[252] Fish oils inhibit PDGF production,[253] and that may be a mechanism by which they are antiatherogenic.

PDGF messenger ribonucleic acid (mRNA) has been detected in human atherosclerotic plaques.[16] Because macrophages,[254] endothelial cells,[255] and even arterial smooth muscle cells[256] produce PDGF, it is likely that plaque PDGF has several sources.

Examination of human carotid atherosclerotic plaques obtained by endarterectomy revealed an excess expression of PDGF-B mRNA in lesions, compared with the normal vessel wall.[257] A study of dissected carotid artery plaques (fibrous cap, main body, and core) indicated that PGDF-A mRNA was highly correlated with smooth muscle α-actin, whereas PGDF-B mRNA was correlated with the macrophage colony-stimulating factor-1 receptor (fms) and, to a lesser extent, with mRNA for von Willebrand factor, an endothelial cell marker. The level of PDGF-A mRNA was higher in atherosclerotic plaques than in normal vessels. PDGF-A was found in the cap and core; PDGF-B was present in all parts but in decreasing amounts from cap to core. Furthermore, the signal intensity of tumor necrosis factor (TNF) was related to fms and PDGF-B. Therefore, in atherosclerotic plaques, PDGF-B mRNA is probably almost completely a product of macrophages[258] and endothelial cells, whereas PDGF-A is a product of smooth muscle cells. Non–smooth muscle cells observed in atherosclerotic plaques include T lymphocytes and macrophages.[146] Communication among the cellular components of the plaque is realized via growth factors and cytokines. In human atherosclerotic plaques, PDGF-A and -B chains have been detected at the mRNA level by in situ hybridization.[259]

The stimulus for growth of plaque vessels is not known. However, several possibilities exist, including hypoxia and release of angiogenic factors from platelets, endothelial cells, smooth muscle cells, and/or macrophages.[149] Fibroblast growth factors and vascular endothelial growth factor (VEGF) are the best characterized factors that stimulate angiogenesis.[260, 261] Other growth factors involved are TGF-α[262] and TGF-β,[263] TNF-α,[264] and angiogenin.[265] Platelet-derived endothelial cell growth factor specifically stimulates endothelial cell growth.[266] EGF domains have been identified in multidomain extracellular matrix proteins such as laminin, tenascin, and thrombospondin. Such extracellular matrix proteins play an important role in tissue repair by promoting cell growth. Thrombospondin has an autocrine growth supportive action on smooth muscle cells and acts synergistically with EGF. For a review of EGF-like domains in extracellular matrix proteins and their role in growth and differentiation, see Engel.[267]

Fibroblast Growth Factors

There are nine different isoforms of fibroblast growth factors (FGFs). Basic fibroblast growth factor (bFGF, pI 9.6) and acidic fibroblast growth factor or endothelial cell growth factor (aFGF, ECGF, pI 5.6) have multiple functions. They stimulate proliferation and induce or delay differentiation. The oncogene *int-2* product is closely related to FGF.[268] Both bFGF and aFGF bind to the same receptor, but not to other growth factor receptors, nor do other growth factors bind to the FGF receptor.[269] Four species of FGF receptors exist. They probably differ in their degree of glycosylation. The 145-kD receptor species has a higher affinity for bFGF than for aFGF; in contrast, aFGF displays a higher affinity for the 125-kD receptor species than does bFGF.[270] These differences might explain the different biologic effects of bFGF and aFGF.

Rapid changes in the structure of the cytoskeleton are induced by bFGF.[271, 272] Furthermore, bFGF has a role in regulating the cellular oncogenes c-*fos* and c-*myc*, which are involved in cell differentiation and proliferation.[273] In endothelial cell cultures, bFGF also downregulates production of PDGF-B mRNA and PDGF-B chain synthesis.[274] bFGF is detected in macrophages and could play a crucial role in wound healing, because it stimulates the proliferation of endothelial cells, vascular smooth muscle cells, and fibroblasts.[260, 275] In vivo, bFGF is a potent angiogenic factor, as demonstrated in several animal models. The effect of FGF on endothelial cell proliferation and neovascularization may imply importance in wound healing and atherogenesis.

aFGF, in combination with heparin, inhibits collagen production but stimulates proteoglycan synthesis in confluent smooth muscle cell cultures.[276] The mitogenic effect of aFGF is potentiated by heparin.[277] Depending on the cell type, aFGF is 30- to 100-fold less potent than bFGF.[273] However, when potentiated by heparin, the mitogenic effect of aFGF is as powerful as that induced by bFGF.

Both aFGF and bFGF lack the classic signal peptide sequence and are supposedly released to the cell exterior in combination with extracellular matrix components, most likely heparin and heparin-related proteoglycans such as heparan sulfate proteoglycan. Heparin, heparan sulfate, and heparan sulfate–degrading enzymes release extracellular matrix–bound bFGF.[278] In addition, FGF may be released from injured endothelial cells and bind to the extracellular matrix.[279, 280] Depending on the cell type, the mitogenicity of FGFs can be inhibited or stimulated by TGF-β.

Transforming Growth Factor

There are two transforming growth factors, TGF-α and TGF-β. TGF-α shows 35% homology with epidermal growth factor (EGF) and binds to the same receptor. TGF-α, a mitogen for mesenchymal cells, promotes angiogenesis and inhibits proliferation of most epithelial cells and lymphocytes.[262] TGF-β has been isolated from platelets[281] and from other transformed or nontransformed cells. This provides a way by which the factor could interact with a plaque. TGF-β isolated from human platelets is a 25-kD homodimer composed of disulfide-linked 12.5-kD peptides.[282] Three forms of TGF-β have been characterized TGF-β1, -β2, and -β3. They are encoded by three distinct genes. These different molecules show a 70 to 80% homology of their amino acid sequence. TGF-β signaling pathways have been identified involving the Smad proteins as TGF-β signal transducers.[283] TGF-β delays re-endothelialization.[284] Activated T lymphocytes and macrophages produce TGF-β, which is also chemotactic for monocytes. This might be a mechanism for continued macrophage recruitment into the vessel wall. In general, TGF-β regulates production of extracellular matrix components by increasing the transcription of collagen, fibronectin, and proteoglycan genes. TGF-β does not enhance smooth muscle cell fibronectin synthesis.[285] TGF-β is a cell-specific regulator in the manufacture of two types of chondroitin sulfate proteoglycans by smooth muscle cells.[286] The synthesis of receptors for matrix proteins such as integrins is also increased by TGF-β. Increased synthesis of protease inhibitors such as PAI and TIMP by TGF-β inhibits matrix degradation. The overall effect is to increase matrix constituents and receptors for cell-matrix interaction.[287] Direct transfer of the TGF-β gene into arteries promotes fibrocellular hyperplasia.[288] Human connective growth factor is markedly overexpressed in atherosclerotic lesions and may represent downstream effectors for TGF-β.[289] TNF-α secreted by activated macrophages is a potent angiogenetic factor.[264] TGF-β is strongly chemotactic for monocytes and can induce their expression of angiogenic activity[290]; this may be a mechanism for promoting angiogenesis within a plaque.

Lipids and Plaque

Sixty percent of the dry weight of advanced lesions consists of cholesterol, cholesteryl esters, and phospholipids[290]; in addition, lipoproteins can also be identified. The fatty acid composition esterified to cholesterol in plaque corresponds to the fatty acid composition of the diet.[291] Most plaque cholesterol is able to exchange with plasma cholesterol monohydrate, but some cholesterol bound to collagen cannot do so.[291]

Studies in many species have focused on the specific role of lipids in the response to injury. As noted previously, lipoproteins may be injurious to endothelial cells. In general, total vascular tissue cholesterol correlates with serum cholesterol concentration.[292] Variability in the response of plasma cholesterol to dietary cholesterol does exist in nonhuman primates, and across other species as well. Lesions in animals made hypercholesterolemic are of the fatty streak type, but some do develop full fibrofatty characteristics. The initial localization of intraarterial LDL is at sites in the aorta most prone to early atherosclerotic lesions. This occurs before significant accumulation of lipid-filled foam cells.[293] The number of macrophages relative to smooth muscle cells may be changed by dietary manipulation. Diets rich in oleic acid promote macrophage collection, whereas diets rich in peanut oil result in a plaque containing more smooth muscle cells.[284, 285] A comparative study between two different models of hypercholesterolemia—the WHHL rabbit and the hypercholesterolemia fat-fed rabbit—showed no difference either in the initial responses of the arterial wall to hypercholesterolemia or in the expansion and maturation of the fatty streak lesion.[43] Therefore, an absence of LDL receptor in the WHHL rabbit and the difference in cholesterol distribution between the two models did not alter the morphology of atherosclerotic lesions. However, the documented differing sensitivities of different parts of the arterial tree (i.e., aorta vs. coronary arteries) to diet-induced lesions suggest that it is not lipids alone that promote atherogenesis and that other factors, such as vessel wall properties, local hemodynamic factors,[296] and cellular and molecular constituents of the blood cell, have important roles in pathogenesis.

However, lesions similar to those found in humans may occur in normocholesterolemic rabbits, especially if endothelium has been subjected to chronic injury.[297] Lesions generated in this model are generally associated with platelet and fibrin deposits. Accumulation of lipid in endothelium-denuded aortas of normocholesterolemic animals occurs preferentially in areas that have become re-endothelialized. Lipid deposition in the vessel wall may, in part, be its response to injury and repair. Changes in the composition of extracellular matrix due to repair may be involved in trapping of lipids.[298] In addition, studies show that platelet-mediated cholesteryl ester lipid droplet accumulation in macrophages and vascular smooth muscle cells may be caused, in part, by cholesterol release from activated platelets. The vessel wall may have a limited way of responding to injury during atherogenesis. Therefore, lipid accumulation within a lesion does not necessarily imply a direct causal relation between serum lipid and the presence of lipids in a plaque.

In many instances, in both diet-induced and injury-induced experimental lesions, the lipid component regresses prominently.[299–301] The role of macrophages and of HDL in reverse cholesterol transport has been considered.[302]

THEORIES ON THE PATHOGENESIS OF ATHEROSCLEROSIS

The pathogenesis of atherosclerosis is probably multifactorial and lesions probably evolve in stages. Four important points are noted in Table 4-3. There are many theories, each stressing one event. It is more likely that not all plaques arise through the same sequence of events and that many steps are involved in the development of each. Several cellular processes are involved in atherogenesis (Table 4-4).

Theories of pathogenesis can be divided into those that suggest that the primary event is some form of endothelial damage or dysfunction (e.g., the response to injury hypothesis) and those that hypothesize that smooth muscle cell dysfunction is a primary event (the monoclonal theory).

Monoclonal Theory

The monoclonal theory proposed that the inciting agent was a mutagen and highlighted the importance of smooth muscle as the target cell.[303] Studies showed that some small aortic atherosclerotic plaques are derived from one or a few cells. Others suggested that the monoclonality of plaques is not universal and is unlikely to be important in their growth to cause clinical disease.[304] However, the monoclonality of some plaques deserves consideration. It is possible that there are environmental agents that promote plaque growth. Marek disease, caused by a herpes-type DNA virus, induces fatty lesions in chickens[305] and promotes accumulation of cholesterol and cholesteryl ester in cultured arterial smooth muscle cells.[306] High levels of cytomegalovirus antibodies have been demonstrated in patients undergoing vascular surgery for atherosclerosis.[307] The presence of DNA virus in the vessel wall probably has no direct role in atherosclerosis, because of the large number (55%) of arterial wall specimens, both atherosclerotic and nonatherosclerotic, that contain cytomegalovirus nucleic acids.[308] It is also possible that a form of selection occurs that promotes monoclonality. Some smooth muscle cells in the intima may be more likely to proliferate in the microenvironment of early lesions (e.g., hypercholesterolemia). Several studies show that smooth muscle cells of the vessel wall are heterogenous, at least with respect to a variety of phenotypic markers.

Response to Injury Hypothesis

The response to injury hypothesis, described by Ross, is useful in formulating testable hypotheses.[247] It brings

---

TABLE 4-3 • **Atherogenesis**

Initiation and growth of a plaque is a slowly evolving dynamic process with superimposed acute events.

Risk factors accelerate progression.

Pathogenesis is multifactorial; the relative importance of specific genetic and external factors varies in individuals.

Interactions between cellular and matrix component of the vessel wall and serum constituents, leukocytes, platelets, and physical forces regulate the formation of the fibrofatty plaque.

TABLE 4-4 • **Important Cellular Processes in the Pathogenesis of the Atherosclerotic Plaque**

Angiogenesis (neovascularization)

Cell-cell and cell-substrate adhesion

Cell-cell communication
    Soluble factors
    Junctions

Cell contractility

Cell death; necrosis and apoptosis

Cell injury, reactive oxygen species

Cell-matrix interactions

Cell migration and chemotaxis

Cell proliferation

Inflammation and immune reactions

Matrix synthesis and degradation

Mineralization

Modulation of coagulation, fibrinolysis, and platelet activation

Phenotypic modulation

Interaction of physical forces with cells

Thrombosis

Vasomotor activity

together several observations related to endothelial integrity, macrophage and smooth muscle cell function, lipids, and thrombus formation. The theory describes several pathways that lead to the formation of a fibrofatty plaque. In one, endothelium or blood monocytes, or both, may be altered to allow the latter to penetrate the endothelium and become resident foam cell macrophages in the subendothelial space. Growth factors released from the cells and the lipids themselves then stimulate smooth muscle cell proliferation leading, over time, to plaque formation. In addition, in some cases subsequent surface thrombosis may occur at sites where endothelium is denuded or retracted over the foam cell lesions. This augments plaque growth as platelets release growth factors and thrombi organize and become incorporated into the plaque. Another pathway focuses on the role of endothelial dysfunctional injury that promotes activation of endothelial cells. One result may be the release from endothelial cells of growth factors that act on smooth muscle cells. This theory stresses the importance of macrophages and smooth muscle cells and emphasizes growth factor activity as an important variable in plaque growth. The need for actual endothelial denudation, platelet adhesion, and release of PDGFs as primary early events has been removed from the theory, as noted later. This is a major change from the hypothesis advanced in 1976.[309]

Endothelial Injury

Endothelial injury is thought to be caused by a variety of agents, including hypercholesterolemia, hemodynamic stress, microorganisms (*Chlamydia*),[310] viral injury,[311-313]

and constituents of cigarette smoke. The proposed mechanisms attempt to explain how injury occurs and leads to the initiation of foam cell deposition in the vessel wall. Studies indicate that endothelial cells may be injured by oxidized LDLs in the artery wall, because lipid peroxides damage cell membranes. In this case, oxidative modification can be achieved by macrophages,[314] smooth muscle cells, and endothelial cells.[315] Oxidized LDL is toxic to endothelial cells and at the same time recruits monocytes and inhibits their migration from the vessel wall.[268, 316] It has also been suggested that serum immunoglobulin G interacts with dead endothelial cells to trigger the complement system and an ensuing inflammatory reaction characterized by monocytes.[317]

Endothelial injury, resulting in frank denudation and exposure of subendothelial connective tissue, was believed to be a major initiating step in fibrofatty plaque development. This concept was important in the older version of the response to injury hypothesis.[309] The denudation supposedly allowed platelets both to adhere to the vessel wall and to degranulate, releasing a PDGF that stimulated medial smooth muscle cells to migrate into the intima and proliferate. It is now apparent that much of the endothelial denudation reported by scanning electron microscopic studies represented artifacts of fixation and tissue preparation. Improved techniques do not confirm such frank denudation.[63, 318] Even in conditions in which there is an increased turnover of endothelial cells, which in itself indicates cell loss, rapid repair processes prevent denudation. However, once a lesion appears and becomes elevated, even as a prominent fatty streak lesion, endothelial cell denudation may occur as a result of the stretching and subsequent retraction of cells from each other. In an advanced, complicated, fibrofatty plaque, frank denudation is associated with plaque ulceration, fissures, and mural thrombosis.

Endothelial Repair

How do rapid endothelial repair processes work? Because large areas of denuded nonatherosclerotic aortic endothelium are not common, it is likely that rapid spreading of adjacent endothelial cells covers small areas of desquamation.[318-320] Small in vitro wounds (three to five cells wide) re-endothelialize within 8 hours and before any cell proliferation. The speed of closure is reduced by hemodynamic shear stress[321, 322] and is more rapid in those wounds where cells are required to change their shape as little as possible.

Although complete re-endothelialization occurs after small denuding wounds, in some cases in which medial injury accompanied endothelial injury the endothelial cells did not completely regrow after widespread denudation.[323] This may be a result of the loss of bFGF in the latter stages of repair of a severe injury. It is apparent that growth factors are important in regulating repair. bFGF is a potent mitogen that enhances endothelial migration and proliferation during repair. Endothelial cells are also affected by other growth factors, such as TGF-β, which is released by platelets and inhibits early endothelial cell re-endothelialization.[281] The substances of the subendothelial matrix, including proteins such as fibronectin and various types of collagens, have a profound effect on endothelial cell shape and proliferative behavior.[219]

A series of intracellular events occur during repair[233] and are characterized by specific changes in the endothelial cytoskeleton, which consists of three dynamic fibrous protein systems, microfilaments, microtubules, and intermediate filaments. The microfilaments and microtubules regulate cell shape and motility, processes important in repair. Filamentous actin microfilaments are present both centrally and at the cell periphery as a dense peripheral band (DPB) (see Fig. 4-23). Endothelial cells contain paranuclear centrosomes, which are microtubule organizing centers. Initially, adjacent endothelial cells attempt to repair an area of denudation by rapidly extruding cell processes, called lamellipodia, into the denuded area. An intact microfilament system, including the DPB, is necessary for this to occur. If repair is incomplete after 1 hour, a second set of events occurs, marked by a redistribution of the centrosome toward the front of the cell and cell elongation in preparation for translocation. DPB breakdown ensues, and directed migration occurs to re-endothelialize the small wound. Within a few hours after closure centrosomes lose their polarity and become randomly distributed around the nucleus; the DPB reappears a few hours later, reestablishing the resting state of the confluent monolayer. If the cells are treated with a drug that prevents microfilament formation, re-endothelialization occurs but at a much slower rate. In contrast, when cells are treated with a drug that prevents microtubule formation, neither centrosome reorientation nor cell migration occurs. These results suggest that microtubules may be the cytoskeleton system that limits reestablishment of an endothelial monolayer.

The role of cell proliferation is also important.[324, 325] However, it occurs after the onset of migration[326] and not until 16 to 20 hours after injury; therefore, it is not a rapid process. Small wounds are initially repaired independent of cell proliferation; however, proliferation may occur later. Large wounds require cell proliferation for initial repair as a means of reestablishing the monolayer.

Thrombin may enhance the rate of repair by promoting rapid reversible microfilament reorganization similar to the pattern present during migration.[327] It is possible that atherogenic agents act by delaying repair through perturbation of the endothelial cytoskeleton and by inhibiting growth- and migration-enhancing factors.

The concept of functional endothelial injury has been introduced to explain functional imbalances in a variety of cellular activities that may promote atherogenesis initiation.[328] Imbalances have been suggested in the coagulation-anticoagulation-fibrinolysis systems, in platelet activation, in regulation of permeability, and in those endothelial cell activities that regulate smooth muscle cell growth and macrophage activation (see Table 4-2). Activation of endothelial cells by cytokines such as IL-1 and TNF induce procoagulant activity and leukocyte adhesion[329] and may predispose to the initiation of atherosclerosis. Injured endothelial cells appear to regulate neointimal formation through enhanced smooth muscle cell proliferation[330] by release of PDGF and fibroblast growth factor. Endothelial cells exposed to mild elevations in hemodynamic shear stress respond by developing prominent actin microfilament bundles, which probably allow better adhesion of the cell to the subendothelium.[134] This may induce endothelial dysfunction characterized by reduced actin in the cell periphery. Because peripheral actin is associated with junctions that keep cells together, endothelial integrity may be disrupted. Agents such as thrombin, a central player in coagulation and platelet physiology, also promote similar rearrangements of actin away from the periphery of the cell and toward its center.[327] In hypertension, acute changes in endothelial cells are characterized by an increase in actin microfilament bundles that are associated with enhanced endothelial permeability.[41] In all of these instances, endothelial cells undergo structural changes leading to dysfunction without any frank denudation.

There is still much to be learned about endothelial injury. The list of agents that promote it is incomplete. Furthermore, the processes by which these agents may injure the endothelial cell are not well known. Synergistic actions among agents have not been addressed. Studies of dysfunctional injuries are in their infancy, especially as they relate to the maintenance of endothelial integrity, regulation of smooth muscle cell growth, platelet function, and coagulation and fibrinolysis. Understanding of both the processes that promote endothelial cell injury and the ways in which injury disrupts vessel wall homeostasis are important to develop rational methods in preventing and treating atherosclerosis.

Smooth Muscle Cell Modulation

Vascular smooth muscle cells show phenotypic modulation between a contractile state and a synthetic state.[331] Synthetic-state cells demonstrate characteristics of fibroblast-like cells, with few myofilaments, intermediate filaments, and a large amount of rough endoplasmic reticulum, Golgi apparatus, and free ribosomes. Contractile-state cells contain myofilaments, intermediate filaments, and dense bodies with fewer other organelles[332]; a basal lamina is present, the cell membrane exhibits many caveolae, which increase its surface area by about 70%, and both adherens-type junctions and gap junctions are present between cells. Synthetic-phenotype muscle cells respond to mitogens, but contractile-phenotype cells do not.[333] Macrophages stimulate the phenotypic change from contractile to synthetic type in vascular smooth muscle cell cultures.[334] A proposed mechanism is release of an endoglycosidase that degrades heparan sulfate in the basement membrane of the smooth muscle cell. In addition to derivation from macrophages, endoglycosidase is also released by platelets and T lymphocytes.

Vascular smooth muscle cells contain a predominance of α-actin, some β-actin, and very little γ-actin.[335] However, smooth muscle cells of the neointima formed in response to vascular injury undergo a change to a secretory (synthetic) phenotype and show both a decrease in the amount of actin and a change in the isotypes. β-actin becomes the predominant type, α-actin decreases, and there is a significant increase in γ-actin.[335] These cells migrate and proliferate, so the change of actin isotype may be related to a change in cell functions. In addition, a change in the 10-nm intermediate filaments of smooth muscle cells occurs. Most cells contain vimentin, and some contain both vimentin and desmin.[336] After vascular injury, the smooth muscle cells of the thickened intima contain increased amounts of vimentin and decreased amounts of desmin.[335] The functional significance of these findings is not known; however, it is possible that vimentin-rich medial cells are the ones that migrate to the intima and proliferate.

Trauma to the vascular wall is followed by a complex repair process that involves interactions between blood cells and other blood constituents, endothelial cells, and smooth muscle cells. Smooth muscle cells exhibit a proliferative response in which a subpopulation undergoes significant ultrastructural modulation, migrates to the intima, and replicates. This "response to injury" mechanism, characterized by both proliferation and a concomitant synthesis of extracellular matrix, is a fundamental component in the restoration of vessel integrity. Migration of smooth muscle cells into the intima has been observed only in models in which there is prominent endothelial loss and medial damage.[7] The medial proliferation was thought to be caused by the release of PDGF from adhering aggregating platelets. Initially, it was considered that endothelial denudation alone would not produce smooth muscle proliferation,[337] but even mild denuding injury does promote it. However, proliferation is limited and does not lead to intimal thickening.[338] Platelets alone may not be totally responsible, because proliferation continues for weeks after endothelial–smooth muscle cell injury,[339] whereas a massive interaction of platelets with the intima of the denuded vessel is transient.[340]

Endothelin stimulates vascular smooth muscle cell proliferation in tissue culture and induces expression of c-*fos* and c-*myc* protooncogenes.[341] The trophic effect of endothelin on vascular wall smooth muscle cells suggests that it may be involved in the pathophysiology of atherosclerosis. Thrombin, TGF-β, and increased shear stress stimulate endothelin production; these stimuli are likely to be present at a site of endothelial damage.[342]

Other factors, including LDL from hypercholesterolemic animals,[343] macrophage-derived growth factor,[344] and interferon,[345] are mitogenic for smooth muscle cells. In addition, heparin-like products from endothelial cells,[340] exogenous heparin,[346] and heparan sulfate proteoglycans synthesized by postconfluent smooth muscle cells have potent antiproliferative activity.[347] Inhibition of angiotensin-converting enzyme suppresses the proliferative response of smooth muscle cells in vascular injury. The latter finding further suggests that these cells may regulate their own growth.

Kinetic studies of smooth muscle proliferation after balloon catheter injury[339] showed that 4 days after injury, such cells had migrated into the intima and were actively proliferating. Only the innermost continued to replicate after 4 weeks, but cell turnover continued for at least 12 weeks and possibly arrested if and when the endothelium recovered. Intimal cell numbers did not increase despite this persistent replication (i.e., cell replication was matched by cell loss); nonetheless, intimal thickening continued through synthesis of connective tissue.[339] A follow-up study demonstrated that only 50% of cells that initially migrated participated in the intimal proliferative response.[348] Nonproliferating cells were ultimately greatly outnumbered by their dividing neighbors, but their existence raises questions concerning regulation of cell proliferation and the heterogeneity of smooth muscle cells that did migrate. Smooth muscle cells from undisturbed vessels are more heterogeneous in proliferative behavior than those from the neointima of an injured vessel.[349] All these studies have a direct bearing on understanding the intimal thickening that occurs in bypass venous grafts and in postangioplasty arteries, as well (see Chapter 22).

Inflammation

The immunoinflammatory component of plaques has been studied.[317] Using specific antibodies to both monocytes (CD14 antigen cluster) and smooth muscle–specific actin (anti–α-actin antibodies), the cellular composition of lipid core and fibrous cap can be elucidated. Immunohistochemical studies showed that 60% of the lipid foam cells react with antibodies to CD14 antigen cluster and are monocytes or cells derived from them (resident macrophages). In contrast, the fibrous cap consists of only 20% cells of monocyte origin.[350]

About 20% of the cells in the fibrous cap are T lymphocytes (CD3-positive cells). B cells and natural killer cells are almost completely absent.[146] CD4-positive T lymphocytes are more frequent in early plaques and fatty streaks. CD8+ cells, which contain most of the cytotoxic T-cell activity, are possibly involved in the initiation of a lesion. CD4 cells induce antibody production and regulate cell-mediated immune responses.[317] Plaque T lymphocytes express activation markers (e.g., human lymphocyte antigen-DR and IL-2 receptors), suggesting that they may be activated by antigens in the plaque. In turn, the activated T lymphocytes secrete bioactive lymphokines that may participate in local regulation of smooth muscle cell growth and differentiation either directly or indirectly via plaque macrophages.[351] Understanding the intricate and complex interactions of cells in the plaque may provide new avenues of prevention and therapy. Chapter 8 provides some discussion of the adventitial inflammatory lesions associated with atherosclerotic plaques.

In accelerated or graft arteriosclerosis, it is proposed that activated lymphocytes stimulated by alloantigens in the graft vessel wall induce macrophages to secrete growth factors that induce smooth muscle cell proliferation and matrix secretion, leading to prominent intimal thickening (see Chapter 23).

Another inflammatory condition that may be important in the pathogenesis of atherosclerosis is that induced by microorganisms. Although there is evidence that bacteria and viruses may play a role in the pathogenesis of plaque, further studies are required to link microorganisms to inflammatory pathways and to clinical disease, the latter through clinical trials using antibiotics to treat specific infections.[312, 313]

COMPLICATIONS OF AORTIC ATHEROSCLEROSIS

Stenosis, Thrombosis, and Aneurysms of Aortic Branches

When atherosclerosis affects the ostia of major aortic branches, the disease can be limited to a vessel's orifice or its proximal portion. Complications include stenosis or thrombosis and distal embolization, with the potential that distal organs become atrophic (Fig. 4-24), ischemic, or infarcted.

The clinical significance of ostial disease depends on the presence of collateral vessels, especially in the mesenteric circulation. Atherosclerotic lesions are common at the ostia of celiac and mesenteric arteries at autopsy. However, the clinical incidence of mesenteric ischemia is low, and symptoms generally occur when all three vessels are affected.[352] This is explained by the existence of collateral circulation between celiac and superior mesenteric arteries (pancreaticoduodenal artery) and superior and inferior mesenteric arteries (arc of Rioland, artery of Drummond). See Chapter 8 for a discussion of coronary artery ostial stenosis.

Atherosclerotic aneurysms only rarely affect aortic branches, being observed particularly in renal (Fig. 4-25), splenic, and hepatic arteries.[353] They have also been reported in the pancreatic, mesenteric,[354] and celiac arteries.[355]

Penetrating Atherosclerotic Ulcer

In progression, atherosclerotic plaques extend into the media. In some vascular beds they may extend to the adventitia, with accumulation of lipid there—so-called "collar stud" lesions seen in cerebral vessels. Plaques also ulcerate, releasing their contents into the blood stream to cause distal embolization. The depth of deficit produced in the vessel wall by this process depends, in part, on the severity of the atherosclerosis and how far it extends into the media. An ulcer may extend a short distance into the

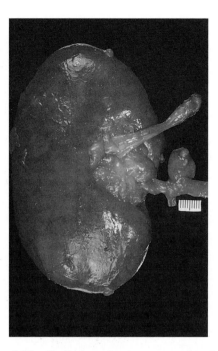

Figure 4-25 • Small atherosclerotic aneurysm of renal artery.

media, producing a smooth-surfaced crater that does not distend the external surface of the vessel. Such lesions are seen frequently in the abdominal aorta at autopsy. They may occlude as a result of thrombosis. However, if the ulcerated atherosclerotic plaque extensively damages the media and extends far into the vessel wall, initial ulceration or subsequent expansion of the resultant deficit leads to a saccular aneurysm that is small initially but expands (Fig. 4-26). Its lumen is filled with thrombus. Such lesions are not associated with intramural hematomas, because associated fibrosis in the vessel wall related to the atherosclerotic plaque inhibits that development.

Reports[356, 357] originating mainly from surgical or imaging units describe "penetrating atherosclerotic aortic ulcers" that the authors believe result from ulceration of an atheromatous plaque with extension deep into the aortic media. The frequency of these lesions is not known, but they seem to be uncommon. The authors suggest that the lesions may precipitate a localized intramedial dissection or rupture into the adventitia to form a pseudoaneurysm. The lesion is thought to be progressive and potentially serious. Surgical resection has been recommended, but that viewpoint is not unanimous. These reported lesions may, in at least some instances, be produced by a spontaneous intimal tear and a localized dissection (see Chapter 5 for further discussion).

Embolic Disease

The atheromatous aorta can be a source of both peripheral and visceral emboli. This complication has been extensively reported in the literature, but its exact incidence is not known; discordance exists between clinical impressions and pathologic findings.[358, 359] For example, atheromatous emboli may be clinically unrecognized if

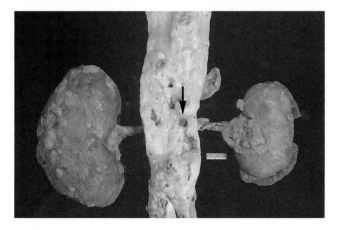

Figure 4-24 • Ostial stenosis of left renal artery (arrow) with atrophy of that organ.

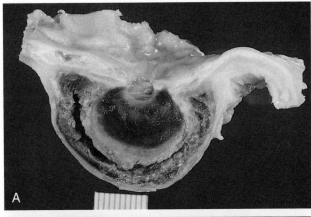
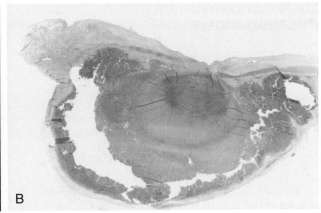
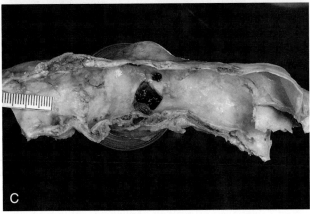

Figure 4-26 • Plaque eroding through aortic media producing saccular aneurysm. *A,* Early gross lesion with atheromatous material in outer wall and thrombus in aneurysm lumen. *B,* Histology of *A* (H&E stain). *C,* Small intimal ostium leading into larger saccular aneurysm bulging beyond aortic wall.

the vessels they affect are small and collateral circulation prevents infarction, yet their effects, marked by occluded vessels, are recognized at autopsy. Alternatively, emboli may induce clinical signs and symptoms of infarction but, if thrombotic, may be lysed by the time of a pathologic examination.

Types of Emboli

Essentially, two types of emboli occur. The first is composed of crystalline and lipid material variably admixed with platelet clumps or small amounts of fibrin (atheroemboli). The second type originates from thrombi formed on ulcerated aortic plaques or, more often, from those found in the lumen of atherosclerotic aneurysms. They are generally larger and tend to occlude major aortic branches, particularly those in the lower limbs.

Clinical Syndromes Caused by Emboli

Different clinical syndromes are caused by the two types of emboli. Atheroemboli are small, often multiple, and characteristically lodge in arteries 100 to 200 μm in diameter.[360] They are probably caused by either spontaneous ulceration of aortic plaques or intimal trauma after surgical manipulation in a patient with a severely diseased aorta or during invasive diagnostic procedures.[361–363] They generally cause widespread vessel occlusion, which may result in either peripheral or visceral lesions. Large emboli, on the other hand, usually appear with large, single-vessel occlusion and sudden ischemia of the lower limbs.

Dahlberg and colleagues[364] reported on 22 patients with histologically proven cholesterol embolism. Twenty had one or more identifiable precipitating factors, including warfarin administration, angiography, angioplasty, intra-aortic balloon pump placement, vascular surgery, aortitis, or cardiopulmonary resuscitation. In this series, clinical symptoms were related to both peripheral and visceral involvement and were often associated with laboratory abnormalities (leukocytosis, eosinophilia, hypocomplementemia, elevated sedimentation rate). Peripheral symptoms included the "blue toe syndrome," characterized by cutaneous bluish-red and painful lesions, generally on ankles or toes, with palpable pedal pulses. Livedo reticularis or small areas of cutaneous gangrene were observed. In those cases, the source of peripheral embolism was usually the infrarenal aorta or more distal vessels.[365] Histologic examination of skin or muscle biopsy specimens revealed crystalline emboli in small arteries, establishing the diagnosis.

Visceral symptoms were variable, depending on the organ or organs involved. In Dahlberg's series, they included abdominal pain, flank or back pain, gross hematuria, accelerated hypertension, deteriorated renal function, a single case of spinal cord infarction, and one case of penile gangrene. Specific organ involvement was identified from clinical laboratory studies, surgical specimens, or autopsies. Renal embolism was clinically recognized in 14 patients, whereas 4 had symptoms of bowel infarction.

Splenic infarction was a common finding at autopsy but caused clinical symptoms in only one patient. Rarer sites of atheromatous embolization in their series were the adrenal (symptomatic in only one of three patients), the spinal cord, and the penis.

Systemic Arterial Involvement

Renal Involvement

Atheromatous embolism sometimes produces multiple small renal infarcts and may be a cause of progressive renal failure after 50 years of age or of hypertension. Its frequency as a clinical entity is apparently low, although in postmortem studies atheromatous emboli are found in 4.7 to 15% of cases.[366, 367] The atheromatous material, in which crystals are the prominent feature, is found in arteries of lobular or, less often, arcuate size (Fig. 4-27). The lesion is unlikely to be confused with local atherosclerotic disease because atherosclerosis in such small arteries is uncommon and is usually devoid of crystalline lipid deposits. Lack of attachment to the arterial wall and the presence of intact red blood cells at the periphery of the embolus characterize the acute lesion. With subsequent organization, the crystalline clefts become surrounded by fibrous tissue containing occasional multinucleate giant cells (see Fig. 4-27).

Meyrier and colleagues[368] reported 32 cases of chronic renal failure in patients with widespread atherosclerotic disease. In 22, renal insufficiency was caused by atheromatous stenosis of renal arteries; in 8 it was caused by both atheromatous embolism and renal artery stenosis; and in 2 cases atheromatous embolism alone was found on renal biopsy. The authors used the term "atheromatous renal disease" to describe this kind of renal failure and suggested that renal angiography and/or renal biopsy can confirm the diagnosis.

Intestinal Involvement

The incidence of intestinal complications of cholesterol embolism is not well defined. Kealy[367] reviewed 2126 necropsies of patients older than 60 years of age and found evidence of such emboli in 0.79% of cases. In 18% of his cases, sections from the bowel were available. In

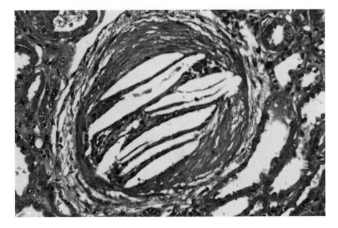

Figure 4-27 • Atherosclerotic emboli to kidney. Note lipid clefts and fibrous tissue organization about them (H&E stain).

four, he found atheromatous emboli in the submucosal vessels of small and large bowels, but there was no evidence of infarction except for one case, in which ulceration and perforation of the ileum occurred. On the other hand, Dahlberg[364] reported four cases of bowel infarction, but did not specify the intestinal segment involved.

Cerebral Involvement

Cases of cerebral infarction due to atheromatous emboli from the aorta are described[369] (see Chapter 15).

Lower Limbs

Acute limb ischemia is often a consequence of large emboli that originate from aortic atherosclerotic aneurysms, or, less commonly, from ulcerated infrarenal plaques. Peripheral vessels in lower limbs excised for ischemic complications show atheromatous emboli also. A shower of atheromatous emboli may sometimes trigger the final acute ischemic event leading to amputation.

Abdominal Aneurysm

An aneurysm is a segmental dilation of an artery, a vein, or the heart wall. This definition implies that the aneurysm wall includes part of the thinned native structure and establishes a difference between a "true" and a "false" aneurysm. The latter is formed after rupture of a vessel or the heart. In that case, the resultant hematoma becomes confined by connective tissue, not vessel or heart wall components, and is connected to the lumen through the ostium at the rupture site (see also Chapters 5 and 18). False aneurysms of the aorta resulting from atherosclerotic disease are uncommon and are usually caused by leakage associated with an aortic graft. In this section, the term aneurysm refers to a true aneurysm.

Abdominal aortic aneurysms are very common.[370] Their rupture is the 13th most common cause of death in the United States.[364] Most are single, but multiple aneurysms may occur.

In the past, thoracic aneurysms were predominantly caused by syphilitic aortic disease. Their diminishing number is explained by measures taken in to prevent and treat syphilis. The incidence of thoracic aneurysms, as reported by Bickerstaff and associates,[371] is 5.9 per 100,000 persons per year. The most common cause of thoracic aneurysm is a localized dissection that occurs spontaneously or after trauma (see Chapter 5). Nondissecting aneurysms are rare; when they do occur, they are generally caused by atherosclerosis.

The majority of abdominal aortic aneurysms, on the other hand, are atherosclerotic; it is estimated that at least 40 of every 1000 persons older than 50 years of age harbor such lesions.[372] Often, they are asymptomatic until they rupture with catastrophic consequences and a low operative survival rate.[373] Elective surgery, on the other hand, has a low operative mortality rate and produces excellent long-term results. Therefore, the early clinical detection and identification of prognostic factors that herald rupture are critical.

Men are affected by atherosclerotic abdominal aneurysms more often than women, in ratio of 3.8:1 to 6:1.[370, 374] Halpert and Williams found that aortic aneurysms gradu-

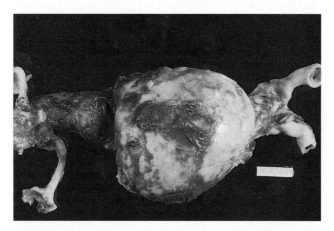

Figure 4-28 • Fusiform atherosclerotic aneurysm in distal aorta; incidental finding at autopsy.

ally increase in frequency with age (from 6% in the sixth decade to 14% in the ninth decade).[375] Women with aneurysms are generally 2 to 8 years older than men who have them. Both the incidence of lesions and the mortality caused by them are significantly lower in blacks than in whites.[376] Among risk factors are systemic hypertension and a long history of cigarette smoking.

Studies suggest a familial tendency for abdominal atherosclerotic aneurysms.[377, 378] Increased collagenase and elastase activity has been recorded in tissues from aneurysmal aorta, compared with atherosclerotic nonaneurysmal aorta.[379, 380] Cigarette smokers who are at risk have increased serum levels of pancreatic elastase after a physiologic stimulus. The results, although controversial, suggest that a variety of pathologic processes may help aneurysm formation.[381]

Rate of Aneurysm Expansion

Data about the rate of expansion of atherosclerotic abdominal aneurysms and the risk of their rupture are incomplete and contradictory. Nennhaus and colleagues[382] reviewed ultrasound examinations performed sequentially on a group of patients. They calculated that the diameter of aneurysms increased by a median rate of 0.21 cm/year. The risk of rupture over 5 years was calculated as 0% for aneurysms smaller than 5 cm in diameter and 25% for those with a diameter greater than 5 cm. These data contrast with previous studies that estimated a higher risk of rupture for aneurysms less than 5 cm in diameter.[383]

Pathology

Atherosclerotic aneurysms result from a structural weakening of the arterial wall caused by extension of the disease into the media with its destruction. They commonly affect the infrarenal aortic segment and are rare in the ascending or thoracic aorta. Their dimensions are extremely variable; generally, they range from 5 to 10 cm in diameter. A clinical diagnosis of abdominal aortic aneurysm is unlikely unless the diameter of the infrarenal aortic segment is at least 1.5 times normal, which in patients older than 50 years is about 2.5 cm.[384]

Gross Morphology

On gross examination, two types of aneurysms can be distinguished: fusiform (cylindric) and saccular (Fig. 4-28; see Fig. 4-26C). In the more common fusiform variety, the dilation involves the entire circumference of the aortic segment, with the aneurysmal segment gradually emerging from and returning to normal luminal diameter (see Fig. 4-28). Usually, the entire lesion is confined between the origin of the renal arteries and the aortic bifurcation, but it may extend to involve one or both iliac arteries or the celiac trunk, or, rarely, to form an abdominothoracic aneurysm. Saccular aneurysms, in contrast, form a sharply delineated dilation affecting only a portion of the aortic circumference; usually they communicate with the main arterial lumen by a neck that is smaller than the diameter of the saccular protrusion. These aneurysms occur in the thoracic and abdominal regions.

When opened, almost all aneurysms, regardless of their size or shape, contain laminated, old, yellow-brown thrombus and, near the lumen, recently deposited thrombus (Fig. 4-29). The characteristic laminated "lines of Zahn" are caused by successive episodes of mural thrombosis (Fig. 4-30). In a fusiform aneurysm, the intra-aneurysmal lumen approximates that of the natural aortic channel. In rare instances, thrombus in a saccular aneurysm completely seals off its ostium.

Histology

Histologically, the aorta adjacent to the aneurysm usually shows severe atherosclerosis. In the wall of the aneurysm, depending on its size, the atherosclerotic process extends a variable distance into or through the media and destroys it by attenuating elastic lamellae and causing atrophy of smooth muscle cells. Sometimes, lipid associated with atherosclerosis extends into the adventitia. Con-

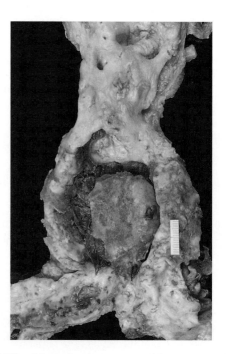

Figure 4-29 • Atherosclerotic aneurysm of the aorta opened to show aneurysmal sac filled with thrombus.

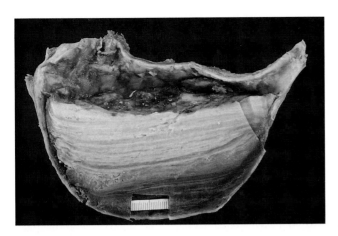

Figure 4-30 • Transected atherosclerotic aneurysm reveals fresh thrombus near the lumen and laminated old thrombus proceeding peripherally toward the aneurysm wall.

nective tissue stains usually reveal medial remnants in the wall, but if the atherosclerotic process is severe they may not be obvious at the greatest curvature of the aneurysm wall. Medial remnants may calcify and, in rare instances, show bony metaplasia with evidence of hematopoiesis. The expanding lesion compresses the surrounding adventitia, which usually shows fibrosis and a mild chronic inflammatory reaction. The latter may extend into the medial remnants, but this is not common. Again, medial remnants may show increased vascularization.

The thrombus in the lumen of the aneurysm is of varying age, depending on its nearness to the lumen. The most recent deposits show platelet aggregates, fibrin, and polymorphonuclear leukocytes. Proceeding peripherally, the morphologic changes caused by loss of cellular structure produce a homogenous hyaline appearance. Areas of calcification and lipid material containing crystal caused by thrombus breakdown are not uncommon findings in the outer layers. Organization of the thrombus is almost never seen. Recent hemorrhage or thrombus may be found in the outer layers of the thrombus, giving indication of aneurysm expansion.

Because of current methods of treating aneurysms surgically, it is usual to receive only the luminal thrombus in surgical pathology. This may be intact and present a cast of the aneurysm lumen with a central passage marking the intra-aneurysmal lumen. More often, the excised thrombus is in many fragments. If lipid degeneration in the old thrombus is marked, the yellowish appearance of the outer surface of the excised thrombus may suggest that pieces of atherosclerotic vessel wall are attached to it. However, connective tissue stains reveal that this is not so. Indeed, it is most uncommon to find such vascular attachments.

If an aneurysm has ruptured, histologic findings depend on whether the patient came to autopsy or tissue was received in surgical pathology. In the former instance and near the rupture site (usually posterolaterally), hemorrhage is found in the outer layers of the luminal thrombus and extending through the aneurysm wall at the site of rupture to fill and expand periadventitial tissue. From there, it may rupture into a body cavity, usually the abdo-

men. In some instances, there may be evidence of an earlier "sentinel leak," marked by old blood and pigment-filled macrophages extending into or through the wall of the aneurysm. Sometimes, there is evidence of repair at the site of a previous hemorrhage. In surgical pathology, fragments of thrombus and pieces of vessel or aneurysmal wall are received and show the changes described for nonruptured aneurysms. If old and severe hemorrhage is identified in adventitia or periadventitial tissue, then it can be assumed that rupture did occur previously.

Pathogenesis

The pathogenesis of abdominal aortic aneurysms is well reviewed in a monograph edited by Tilson and Boyd.[385] The basis of aneurysm formation is a progressive medial weakening and attenuation. Atherosclerosis causes progressive atrophy of musculolamellar medial units and their replacement by fibrous tissues. The weakened vascular segment then becomes susceptible to dilation by systolic blood pressure. Once arterial dilation develops, it gradually progresses according to the principles of Laplace and Bernoulli, and medial atrophy parallels dilation until the aneurysm wall consists only of fibrous connective tissue surrounded by residual adventitia. As mentioned previously, augmented collagenolytic and elastolytic activity is observed in the aortic wall in abdominal aneurysmal disease. Smooth muscle apoptosis has been identified in abdominal aortic aneurysms in associated with p53, a potential mediator of cell cycle arrest and programmed cell death.[386] These findings, as well as evidence for a genetic predisposition for aortic aneurysms, suggest that different pathogenetic mechanisms may exist in different persons.[387]

Why most atherosclerotic aneurysms are found in the abdominal aorta is not well understood. Several factors may be implicated. Aortic systolic pressure and pulse wave are increased in that segment of the vessel owing to its decreased cross-sectional area and the presence of a pulse wave reflected from the bifurcation.[388] Apparently, the proportion of pulse wave reflected is determined by the ratio of the sum of the cross-sectional area of the branches to the cross-sectional area of the parent vessel. With aging, the aortic wall becomes stiffer in its abdominal section owing to fragmentation of medial elastic fibers.

Complications

Complications of abdominal aortic aneurysms are essentially related to rupture, infection, and embolization. Occlusive thrombosis of an aneurysm may also occur but is rare.

Embolization

Peripheral embolization from an aneurysm has already been discussed.

Rupture and "Contained" Rupture

Rupture of an abdominal aortic aneurysm is a frequent and often lethal event. It usually occurs in a previously asymptomatic patient 2 to 5 cm distal to the origin of renal arteries and on the left lateral aortic wall. Most frequently, the resultant hemorrhage extends into the retroperitoneal space. However, an aneurysm may rupture into the pleural space, gastrointestinal tract, inferior vena cava, or left renal vein. In published series, the incidence of rupture is variable; however, its occurrence appears to be related to aneurysm size,[382, 384] with risk of rupture increasing dramatically after an aneurysm exceeds 5 cm in diameter.[382, 383, 389]

Hemorrhage from the rupture site may rapidly extend into the peritoneal cavity and cause hypovolemic shock. In this case, the patient usually presents with a triad of symptoms: abdominal or back pain, hypotension, and a tender, pulsatile abdominal mass. Such findings strongly suggest rupture and mandate immediate surgical repair. However, this clinical presentation is not frequent, and signs of hypovolemic shock occur in only about one half the patients.[390] More frequently, the hemorrhage that follows a rupture remains "contained" by periaortic soft tissues for an unpredictable time.[391] In that case, symptoms of severe abdominal pain occur, in the absence of profound hemorrhagic shock. The pain can mimic other causes of acute or chronic disease, such as renal colic, intra-abdominal abscess,[389] obstructive jaundice,[392] acute diverticulitis, appendicitis, or femoral neuropathy,[393] depending on the site and progression of the hematoma. Gastrointestinal symptoms of nausea and vomiting occur frequently at the onset of aneurysm rupture and are attributed to irritation of the sympathetic and parasympathetic nervous system.[394, 395] In patients with vague abdominal symptoms, the clinical diagnosis of a ruptured abdominal aneurysm may be difficult.

Emergency surgery in patients who were believed to have an acute rupture, but did not, resulted in a fourfold increase in operative mortality in one series.[396] Studies emphasize the value of computed tomographic (CT) scans in the early detection of periaortic hematomas.[397–399] Furthermore, investigators have observed CT-scan findings of "contained" aneurysmal rupture in stable and sometimes asymptomatic patients—findings that have been present for months or, in some cases, even years before surgical treatment.[400, 401] The criteria for identifying chronic contained rupture, as described by Jones and coworkers,[402] are known abdominal aortic aneurysm, previous symptoms of pain that may have resolved, stable condition and normal hematocrit, a CT scan showing retroperitoneal hematoma, and pathologic confirmation of organized hematoma.[402] The incidence of contained rupture of aortic aneurysm seen at surgery varies. Jones and associates[402] reported an incidence of 35%; Flynn and colleagues[403] reported 4.6% in 260 patients studied over a 1-year period. Identification of the lesion may avoid emergency laparotomy for all patients with suspected but unproved ruptured aneurysm, permitting adequate preoperative preparation with a reduction of mortality rate.[304]

Aortoenteric Fistula

Rupture into the gastrointestinal tract is a rare but potentially lethal complication of both treated and untreated atherosclerotic aneurysm.[405] Aortoenteric fistulas can be classified as primary or secondary. Primary fistulas arise de novo as a result of direct erosion of an existing atherosclerotic aortic aneurysm into the adjacent bowel,

usually the third portion of the duodenum.[406] However, fistulas may involve other segments of the gastrointestinal tract, such as the ileum or even the large bowel. They are a consequence of progressive stretching or compression of the intestinal wall by an enlarging aortic aneurysm.

Aortocaval Fistula

Rupture into the inferior vena cava is a rare complication. Its incidence varies from 0.3 to 3% in patients undergoing surgery for abdominal aortic aneurysm and from 3 to 4% in surgical patients with ruptured aneurysm.[407, 408]

Rupture into the Left Renal Vein

Rupture into the left renal vein is the rarest type of rupture of an abdominal aortic aneurysm into the vascular tree. It is associated with an anomalous retroaortic position of the left renal vein, which enters the inferior vena cava distal to its usual position. A distinctive sign is a continuous bruit heard especially on the left side of the abdomen.[409]

Infection

Secondary bacterial infection of an atherosclerotic aortic aneurysm is a rare complication, although ulcerated lesions may provide a portal of entry for microorganisms. The infection usually begins in the mural thrombus. Moreover, the extensive thrombus may render an infected focus inaccessible to antibiotic therapy.

Microorganisms frequently responsible for aneurysm infection include *Salmonella*[410, 411] and *Staphylococcus*,[411a] but other agents[410] such as *Escherichia coli*[412] and *Bacteroides* are becoming increasingly common pathogens. An infection may arise by hematogenous spread from other sites; however, in most reported cases, an obvious source of bacteremia could not be identified. Inoculation of an aneurysm wall may occur during medical procedures that require arterial or venous catheterization. Infective microorganisms can be isolated from blood cultures or from the arterial wall or thrombus in patients with an infected aneurysm. However, positive cultures from abdominal aortic aneurysm contents are not always associated with aneurysmal infection.[413–415]

Histologically, both vessel wall and mural thrombus may show an acute inflammatory reaction with necrosis. Microorganisms are demonstrable with special stains.

Inflammatory Aneurysm

Walker and associates[416] introduced the term "inflammatory aneurysm of the abdominal aorta" to describe aneurysms characterized by marked periaortic inflammation and fibrosis. Their incidence varies from 2.5 to 15% of all abdominal aortic aneurysms.

Most inflammatory aneurysms are situated between the renal arteries and aortic bifurcation. However, they can be found on the thoracoabdominal aorta.[417] Men seem affected more often than women (ratio, 9:1), and a high percentage of smokers is noted among patients with these aneurysms. Most are found in persons in their 50s and 60s, and the reported average age at the time of surgery varies from 62.2 to 69 years.[416, 418–421]

The inflammatory aneurysm wall appears extremely thickened (up to 3 cm) and is both firm and pinkish or gray-white, owing to intense surrounding fibrosis. The fibrous tissue may appear "juicy." In most instances, fibrous tissue extends from the aortic wall to involve adjacent organs, especially the duodenum, inferior vena cava, left renal vein, or veins, and they may become firmly adherent to the aneurysm wall. Ureteral stenosis and/or displacement as a result of the fibrosis are also frequently documented. Such changes may induce hydronephrosis, uremia, and death.[422-424] Occasionally, adventitial fibrous tissue extends to encase the sigmoid colon, the small bowel, or even the pancreas or stomach. On section, the diameter of the aneurysm varies from 4 to 14 cm. The fibrous thickening is almost always confined to the antero-lateral wall, whereas the posterior one tends to be normal or slightly attenuated; a frequent complication is erosion of the posterior wall into the adjacent lumbar vertebrae.

Microscopically, there is severe atherosclerotic disease, with complicated lesions often associated with mural thrombosis and medial atrophy with loss of smooth muscle cells and rarefaction of elastic lamellae. Adventitial endarteritis is a common finding. Striking features are a marked lymphoplasmacytic inflammatory cell infiltrate and granulation tissue or fibrous tissue proliferation in the adventitia (see Fig. 5–29). The inflammatory infiltrate is occasionally organized into lymphoid follicles with germinal centers; small granulomas with multinucleated giant cells may be found.

Inflammatory aneurysms are prone to the same complication as "classic" atherosclerotic aneurysms, including rupture, embolism, and thrombosis. However, rupture occurs much less frequently in inflammatory aneurysms; when it does happen, it is usually through the posterior wall.[425]

The most common presenting signs and symptoms are abdominal pain, weight loss, raised erythrocyte sedimentation rate, and abdominal tenderness.[426] Imaging is especially helpful in making the preoperative diagnosis. A CT scan reveals the "ring" of thickened tissue surrounding the aorta, and magnetic resonance imaging delineates the lesion. The condition must be distinguished from retroperitoneal fibrosis, in which no associated abdominal aneurysm exists.[427, 428]

The marked periaortic fibrosis in this condition may make surgery extremely difficult or impossible. The most serious complications result from surgical dissection of adherent structures. When surgery is contraindicated, therapy with steroids may provide benefit, but this treatment is controversial.[429]

The cause of an inflammatory aneurysm is not known. A commonly held opinion is that it is a variant of an atherosclerotic aneurysm that demonstrates a particular response, perhaps immune-mediated, to a component of the atherosclerotic plaque.[421, 430] Ceroid has been suggested as that component. Hypotheses have been formulated to explain both the inflammatory infiltrate and the fibrosis. Gaylis[431] postulated that these aneurysms are a response to lymph stasis caused by obstruction of lymph vessels around an enlarging atherosclerotic aneurysm. Other theories hold that release of platelet products and lipids from atherosclerotic plaques protruding into the periaortic tissue might play a role.[432] On the other hand, the finding in some cases of an association between inflammatory aortic aneurysm, coronary arteritis, and aortitis makes some authors consider the inflammatory aneurysm a localized manifestation of systemic vasculitis.[433] That inflammatory aneurysm and retroperitoneal fibrosis could have a common pathogenetic mechanism is suggested by the overlap of clinical and histologic features of these lesions[434] (see also Chapter 5).

Complications of Aneurysm Surgery

Since the first successful graft replacement of an abdominal aortic aneurysm in 1951 by Du Bost and colleagues,[435] who used an aortic allograft, the effectiveness of surgical treatment has been verified by many reports.[436-438] Cloth grafts are now employed (see Chapter 22, where the healing of endovascular grafts is also discussed).

Intraoperative Complications

Intraoperative complications include hemorrhage secondary to arterial clamping or rupture of the calcified aneurysmal wall during surgical manipulations. Venous and other lacerations may occur, owing to fibrous adhesions to the aneurysmal sac.

Early Postoperative Complications

Complications occurring soon after surgery include acute renal failure, pulmonary embolism or atelectasis, myocardial infarction, and hemorrhage, the latter usually from the interstices of the graft. A small hemorrhage (50 to 150 ml) is not uncommon after surgery in patients dying of other causes. Ischemia of the extremities, ischemic colitis, and cerebrovascular accidents also occur. Ischemia of the spinal cord with paraplegia is now a rare complication except in the presence of ruptured aneurysm.[439] It is a consequence of the interruption of arteria radicularis magna in the absence of a collateral blood flow from lower lumbar arteries.

Acute Renal Failure

Regarding the complications of aortic surgery, Wittenstein[440] found acute renal failure the most common and a major cause of postoperative death; it is usually a result of hypoperfusion, especially in patients with ruptured aneurysm, or of myoglobinuria occurring after declamping of the iliac arteries.[441]

Acute Lower Limb Ischemia

This is a significant contributing factor to postoperative morbidity and mortality. In a series of 262 patients reported by Strom and colleagues,[442] the incidence was 10.3%. The authors observed that postoperative limb ischemia was more frequent in patients with combined aortic aneurysm and aortoiliac occlusive disease. The causes are distal embolization from the aneurysm or from atheromatous plaques of the common iliac arteries (44%); coagulopathies (including antithrombin III deficiency), abnormal platelet aggregation, and inadequate heparinization (26%); raised intimal flaps (18%); inadequate outflow (8%); and congestive heart failure (4%).[442]

Late Postoperative Complications

Late postoperative complications can be related to the status of the graft or to changes secondary to operative procedures. The more common complications are colonic ischemia, secondary aortoenteric fistulas, recurrent aortic and anastomotic aneurysms, false aneurysms, graft infections, sexual dysfunction in men, and ureteral damage.

Colonic Ischemia

The incidence of colonic ischemia after surgery varies in different series from 1 to 10%.[443–446] It is usually associated with severe morbidity and mortality rates of 40 to 100%. The complication is especially likely in repair of a ruptured abdominal aneurysm.[447, 448]

In 75% of cases, colonic ischemia follows ligation of the inferior mesenteric artery during aneurysmectomy. If that occurs, collateral circulation derives mostly from the superior mesenteric artery, through the arc of Riolan and the left marginal artery. However, the arc of Riolan is absent in 20 to 33% of the normal population, and the superior mesenteric artery is often severely stenosed by atherosclerotic plaques. Identification of an unusually large inferior mesenteric artery at surgery may suggest a deficient, collateral circulation. In that setting, impairment to blood flow after inferior mesenteric artery ligation cannot be compensated, and ischemic damage may result. This is especially common at the splenic flexure and the descending colon. Other factors influencing the extent and pattern of bowel lesions include the bacterial population within the lumen, tryptic digestion of the mucosa, and possible immune mechanisms leading to focal reactions such as the Arthus and Shwartzman phenomena.[449]

There are essentially two manifestations of colonic ischemia: ischemic colitis and gangrene. In ischemic colitis, the mucosa shows linear ulceration and hemorrhage (corresponding to the radiographic appearance of thumbprinting). Histologic changes are confined to the mucosa and submucosa and consist of hemorrhage edema and necrosis accompanied by a diffuse leukocyte infiltrate. Intracapillary fibrin thrombi present in small vessels of both the mucosa and submucosa are characteristic of this condition. The muscularis mucosa is generally spared. In the reparative phase, submucosal granulation tissue may be so exuberant that it causes segmental stenosis (ischemic stricture of the colon); hemosiderin-laden macrophages are generally abundant within granulation tissue.

When full-thickness necrosis is present, the bowel appears dilated and markedly congested, and a fibrinous peritoneal reaction is almost always present. The bowel wall is extremely thinned and friable and can easily perforate, causing diffuse peritonitis and fatal sepsis.

Typical clinical presentation is with acute pain in the left iliac fossa; nausea and vomiting are followed by bloody diarrhea. Fever and leukocytosis are also common. Barium enema and endoscopy are used to confirm the diagnosis. Ischemic bowel disease can also occur intraoperatively during aneurysm surgery, soon after ligation of an inferior mesenteric artery; in this case, the mesenteric artery must be reimplanted on the graft.

Another manifestation of ischemic bowel disease is ischemic proctitis. It occurs particularly in patients with occlusive disease of the internal iliac arteries and is a consequence of a reduced blood flow to the rectum via the middle hemorrhoidal arteries.

Secondary Aortoenteric Fistula

Secondary aortoenteric fistula is a complication of aortic aneurysm surgery.[450] Secondary fistulas are more frequent than primary ones (see earlier discussion). They occur from the first postoperative week to years after surgery, with a mean interval, reported by Champion and coworkers,[451] of 36 months. Their reported incidence in different series varies from 0.36 to 2%. Such fistulas generally develop between the proximal aortoprosthetic anastomosis and the third portion of the duodenum, but they may involve the stomach, jejunum, ileum, or colon. Multiple fistulas have been described. Rarely, they pass between a femoral anastomosis of a Y graft and the appendix, cecum, or sigmoid colon. Aortoenteric fistulas may extend directly between the aortic and the intestinal lumen, with or without an interposed false aneurysm. Less commonly, a paraprosthetic sinus may develop between the graft body and bowel.[440]

The pathogenesis of secondary aortoenteric fistulas seems to be related to both mechanical and infectious processes. Local ischemic injury to the bowel during the original operation may also be a predisposing factor. Another possible mechanism is dehiscence of a suture line as a primary event, followed by a false aneurysm that subsequently erodes into the bowel lumen.

The clinical presentation mirrors that of a primary aortoenteric fistula (see previous discussion). The mortality rate in untreated patients is 100%; death occurs from sepsis or massive gastrointestinal hemorrhage.

Recurrent and Anastomotic Aneurysm

After aortic surgery, "recurrent aneurysms" may develop in an aortic segment close to or remote from the graft, although their occurrence seems rare. Yao and colleagues[452] suggested that thoracic aneurysms developing after abdominal aortic surgery were probably already present at operation. Aneurysms of the iliac, femoral, or popliteal arteries may also occur after graft replacement of an abdominal aortic aneurysm.[453]

Anastomotic false aneurysms occur at 0.2% of aortic and 1.2% of iliac anastomoses. They are more common at femoral anastomoses.[454] Various explanations have been offered for this complication. They include systemic hypertension, graft dilation, failure of suture material,[455] endarterectomy at the site of anastomosis, and varying compliance between graft and arterial wall.[456, 457] Anastomotic false aneurysms can occur even years after operation. When detected, they require surgical management, because if they rupture the outcome is often poor.

Treiman and colleagues[458] reported a series of anastomotic false aneurysms of the abdominal aorta and iliac arteries. The mean age of their patients was 69 years, and the male-female ratio was 2:1. Systemic hypertension was a common finding. When present, symptoms and signs of a ruptured false aneurysm included an intra-abdominal pulsatile mass, abdominal pain, an occluded graft, or evidence of a coexistent femoral false aneurysm in patients with aortobifemoral bypass. Aneurysm size (as detected by angiography and CT scan) ranged from 2 to 18 cm.

Infection

Infection of a vascular graft is a rare but serious complication; it requires an aggressive surgical approach, with removal of the prosthetic material followed by an extra-anatomic bypass.[459] However, the mortality rate and the frequency of limb amputation are extremely high in such cases. In a series of 2411 arterial reconstructions performed during a 4-year period, Lorentzen and coworkers[460] found a 2.6% incidence of graft infection. Gram-positive cocci were the most common pathogens. Although aortic grafts may become infected years after implantation, most infections occurred in the early postoperative period. Factors implicated include faulty aseptic technique, groin incision, skin wound infection, hematogenous spread from remote septic foci, emergency aneurysm repair, perigraft hematoma, and infected intestinal bag contents.

Bacterial colonization of an aortic aneurysm wall or of luminal contents was also implicated as a possible source of graft infection. The reported incidence of positive bacterial cultures in aortic aneurysms repaired on an elective basis is 10 to 16%, but the origin of such bacteria and their clinical importance are as yet undetermined.

Sexual Dysfunction

The frequency of sexual impotence and retrograde ejaculation in men after aneurysm surgery has been reported to be as high as 25 to 50%.[461] These complications are caused by bilateral disruption of the sympathetic chain at the L1-L2 level (leading to impotence)[461] and interruption of the presacral and hypogastric plexuses near the aortic bifurcation (leading to retrograde ejaculation).

Ureteral Involvement

Late ureteral obstruction with consequent hydronephrosis is usually caused by ureteral involvement by reactive periaortic fibrosis. The reported frequency of this complication varies in different series from 2 to 20%. In one case described by Sacks and Miller,[462] a patient developed a ureteral stricture 12 days after placement of an aortic bifurcation graft.

Other Complications

Rarer late complications include duodenal obstruction resulting from perigraft collagenous adhesions,[463] vertebral osteomyelitis resulting from contiguous paraprosthetic aortic abscess,[464] aneurysm of an arterial prosthesis caused by an intense foreign body reaction against the graft,[465] chylous ascites,[466] and perigraft seroma.

Endovascular Treatment of Abdominal Aortic Aneurysms

Abdominal aortic aneurysms are now being treated at some centers by the endovascular insertion of a woven Dacron arterial graft passed through the common femoral artery and secured in place both above and below the aneurysm by a variety of means. Treiman and Bernhard[469] have discussed this form of therapy. The criteria for such grafts are evolving. Potential advantages include reduced operative time, cardiac stress, blood loss, duration of aortic cross-clamping, pain, duration of hospitalization, and cost of hospitalization. In addition, the risk of such operatively induced complications as impotence, aortoenteric fistula, and intra-abdominal adhesions with subsequent bowel obstruction should be eliminated; other complications can be expected to be reduced, as well. Furthermore, the endovascular insertion of a graft may allow treatment in patients for whom the risks associated with a standard resection are great because of associated medical conditions. Complications include technical problems associated with graft deployment, the systemic effects of both anesthesia and surgery, and specific problems related to device reliability during follow-up (see Chapter 22 also). Current results indicate this is an effective and safe method of treatment of abdominal aortic aneurysms in the short term. However, further long-term studies and comparison with concurrent controls are needed to establish efficacy. The use of endovascular grafts to treat aneurysms at other locations is also under investigation.

Surgical treatment has improved greatly in recent decades, with diminishing morbidity and mortality rates. An "acceptable" mortality rate for an unruptured abdominal aortic aneurysm is 2%. However, complications still occur during surgery, in the early postoperative period or later.

Thoracic Aneurysms

The etiology of thoracic aneurysms has changed during the past 50 years. Atherosclerosis is a common cause when an aneurysm is not associated with an intimal tear and its complications.[467, 468] Traumatic and mycotic thoracic aneurysms are much less common, and syphilitic aneurysms very rare.

Atherosclerotic aneurysms are predominantly found just distal to the left subclavian artery, but they are also reported in the ascending aorta, although dissecting aneurysms are much more common at that site. The aneurysms have the same gross and microscopic appearance as abdominal atherosclerotic aneurysms.

Men are generally affected more often than women, but the risk of rupture seems higher in women. The mean age of patients with atherosclerotic thoracic aneurysm reported by Pressler and McNamara[468] was 69 years (range, 42 to 94 years); patients with dissecting aneurysms tend to be younger (mean age, 61; range, 26 to 90). The natural history and clinical behavior of thoracic atherosclerotic aneurysms are similar to those of their abdominal counterparts.

Almost all thoracic aneurysms expand and eventually rupture. In the series of Pressler and McNamara,[468] 76 patients had atherosclerotic aneurysms; among this group, rupture accounted for 25 (44%) of 57 deaths. Thoracic atherosclerotic aneurysms are often asymptomatic and are discovered on routine chest radiography or during examination for other diseases. They are also found incidentally at autopsy, but this is uncommon.

ATHEROSCLEROSIS OF PERIPHERAL ARTERIES

Marchand[470] introduced the term atherosclerosis in 1904 to replace arteriosclerosis and even included Mönckeberg medial calcification in the definition; nowadays, the term atherosclerosis is used to indicate the lesions of atheroma only. Most chronic occlusive lesions of peripheral arteries are caused by atherosclerosis. It commonly affects large and medium-sized vessels (e.g., aorta, iliac, femoral, popliteal, tibial) and involves smaller vessels to a lesser extent.[471] It is an important cause of disability and death in aging Western populations. The morphologic alterations caused by atherosclerosis are often superimposed on those of senile arteriosclerosis or Mönckeberg calcification. Contrary to popular belief, atherosclerosis is also an established problem in the indigenous population of Africa.[472]

Lower Limb Arteries

Atherosclerosis appears to be more common in lower than upper limb vessels. Certain anatomic peculiarities may determine the site of atherosclerosis in peripheral arteries. For example, the superficial femoral artery is most frequently occluded at the level of the adductor hiatus, where it is susceptible to repeated local injury by the tough, tendinous arch of the adductor magnus muscle. The profunda femoris is usually spared.[473, 474] The severity of the lesions in peripheral arteries in any given patient correlates well with the degree of atherosclerosis in the aorta and coronary arteries.[475] There have been no systemic studies of the natural history of atheromas of the lower extremities.[476] Although atherosclerosis often shows a diffuse pattern of involvement in peripheral arteries, complicating occlusive thrombosis frequently occurs at certain preferential sites[477]:

1. Thrombosis of the aortic bifurcation (Leriche syndrome). This produces intermittent claudication, sexual impotence, and sometimes rest pain or peripheral gangrene.
2. Iliac artery thrombosis. This causes claudication at different sites according to the artery involved—gluteal muscle claudication (internal iliac artery); buttock, thigh, or calf claudication (common iliac); and calf and thigh claudication (external iliac). Occlusion of these vessels and of the aorta may cause gangrene of the toes.
3. Thrombosis of the femoropopliteal arteries. This is the most common site of peripheral artery thrombosis. It produces intermittent claudication, and sometimes rest pain or gangrene.
4. Thrombosis of arteries of the leg. The arteries of the calf may thrombose individually. If coexistent femoral and popliteal thrombosis is present, distal gangrene is likely.
5. Thrombosis of the small arteries of the hands and feet. This occurs in both atherosclerosis and Buerger's disease. The vessels are too small for direct surgical intervention. Thrombosis of digital arteries may cause ischemia or even gangrene. Thrombosis of the plantar arch imperils the whole forefoot.

Popliteal Artery Aneurysm

The popliteal artery is the most common site of an aneurysm affecting limb arteries. Of all aneurysms, those of the popliteal artery are second in frequency to abdominal aortic aneurysms.[478] Atherosclerosis is the usual cause, but some are produced by medial degeneration[479] (see Chapter 6). Popliteal aneurysms are often bilateral and may be related to trauma. Many patients have complications on first presentation; the most common is distal thromboembolism, which leads to limb loss in 20% of cases.

Carotid and Vertebral Arteries

See Chapter 15.

Intestinal Vasculature

The vasculature of the abdominal viscera is another circulatory unit that has been neglected in systematic pathologic investigation.

Small Bowel Ischemia

Recurrent mesenteric ischemia (abdominal angina) is usually associated with severe stenosis or occlusion at their aortic ostia of two of the three mainstream arteries, notably including the superior mesenteric.[480] Usually, the total cross-sectional area of the celiac and mesenteric arteries is reduced by more than two thirds. Slowly developing stenosis due to atherosclerosis is the basis of the anginal syndrome, whereas sudden blockage by thromboembolism or acute thrombosis is a more likely cause of intestinal infarction. Local thrombosis and thromboembolism may be difficult to distinguish. Finding emboli at other sites favors a diagnosis of thromboembolism as the cause of an intestinal infarction. (Atheromatous embolism is discussed earlier in this chapter.) Bowel infarction may also occur in patients with a narrowed superior mesenteric artery if there is a reduction of blood flow due to heart failure or to splanchnic vasoconstriction.

Colonic Ischemia

Because of good collaterals, ischemic changes seldom occur after acute occlusion of the inferior mesenteric artery. The nongangrenous form of the disease is about 10 times more common than gangrenous ischemic colitis.[481, 482] The usual manifestation is an acute ischemic colitis that sometimes goes on to infarction. Poor circulatory perfusion is of greater importance than luminal occlusion in the pathogenesis of colonic ischemia. Ischemic lesions in the colon occur frequently in the so-called "watershed area" near the splenic flexure, at the junction between superior and inferior mesenteric blood supplies.

Transient Intestinal Ischemic Attack

According to Coligado and Flesher,[483] occlusion of branches of the inferior mesenteric artery may result in transient ischemia of a segment of the colon, appearing as ischemic colitis. The mucosa is the most vulnerable layer, and infarction leads to ulceration, often complicated by coliform bacterial infection. Healing may lead to stricture. The submucosa and the muscle coat are more resistant to hypoxia and are kept alive by the collateral circulation. Occlusion of a small branch of the superior mesenteric artery may produce similar consequences in the small bowel, but in this case, secondary infection is less likely.

MÖNCKEBERG MEDIAL CALCIFICATION

Mönckeberg medial calcification (Mönckeberg sclerosis), is characterized by dystrophic medial calcification, usually associated with aging, that is commonly found in the arteries of the extremities, head, and neck. The lesion is also common in thyroid vessels and in those of the uterus of older women. Calcification may be confined to and may replace the internal elastic lamella or the medial smooth muscle; extensive replacement is associated with pale-staining, acellular, hyalinized fibrous tissue. Because the process involves the media only, it does not cause luminal narrowing. Nevertheless, peripheral arteries that show severe atherosclerosis histologically often have concomitant Mönckeberg medial calcification.

REFERENCES

1. Wissler RW: The arterial medial cell: Smooth muscle of multifunctional mesenchyme? Atherosclerosis 8:201–213, 1968
2. Gereinger E: Venous atheroma. Arch Pathol 48:410, 1949
3. Shi C, Lee W, He Q, et al: The immunological basis of transplant-associated arteriosclerosis. Proc Natl Acad Sci U S A 93:4051–4056, 1996
4. Fyfe AI, Rosenthal A, Gotlieb AI: Immunosuppressive agents and endothelial repair: Prednisolone delays migration and cytoskeletal rearrangement in wounded porcine aortic monolayers. Arterioscler Thromb Vasc Biol 15:1166–1171, 1995
5. Gillum RF, Folsom A, Luepker RV, et al: Sudden death and acute myocardial infarction in a metropolitan area, 1970–1980: The Minnesota heart survey. N Engl J Med 309:1353–1358, 1983
6. Stern MP: Recent decline in ischemic heart disease mortality. Ann Intern Med 91:630–640, 1979
7. American Heart Association: Position statement on diagnosis and treatment of primary hyperlipidemia in childhood. Arteriosclerosis 6:685A–692A, 1986
8. Newman WP, Guzman MA, Strong JP, et al: Secular trends in atherosclerotic lesions: Comparison of two studies of autopsied men conducted in different time periods. Mod Pathol 1:109–113, 1988
9. Newman WP, Strong JP, Johnson WD, et al: Community pathology of atherosclerosis and coronary heart disease in New Orleans: Morphologic findings in young black and white men. Lab Invest 44:496–501, 1981
10. Brensike JF, Levy RI, Kelsey SF, et al: Effects of therapy with cholestyramine on progression of coronary arteriosclerosis: Results of the NHLBI Type III Coronary Intervention Study. Circulation 69:313–324, 1984
11. Hoeg JM, Feuerstein IM, Tucker EE: Detection and quantification of calcific atherosclerosis by ultrafast computed tomography in children and young adults with homozygous familial hypercholesterolemia. Arterioscler Thromb 14:1066–1074, 1994
12. Martin AJ, Ryan LK, Gotlieb AI, et al: Arterial imaging: Comparison of high resolution US and MR imaging with histologic correlation. Imaging Ther Technol 17:189–202, 1997
13. Ross R, Fuster V: The pathogenesis of atherosclerosis. In: Fuster V, Ross R, Topol EJ (eds): Atherosclerosis and Coronary Artery Disease. Philadelphia, Lippincott-Raven, 1996, pp 441–461
14. Dammerman M, Breslow JL: Genetic basis for lipoprotein disorders. Circulation 91:505–512, 1995
15. Tsukada T, Rosenfield M, Ross R, Gown AM: Immunocytochemical analysis of cellular components in atherosclerotic lesions: Use of monoclonal antibodies with the Watanabe and fat-fed rabbit. Arteriosclerosis 6:601–613, 1986
16. Wilcox JN, Smith KM, Williams LT, et al: Platelet-derived growth factor mRNA detection in human atherosclerotic plaques by in situ hybridization. J Clin Invest 82:1134–1143, 1988
17. Bennett MR, Evan GI, Schwartz SM: Apoptosis of human vascular smooth muscle cells derived from normal vessels and coronary atherosclerotic plaques. J Clin Invest 95:2266–2274, 1995
18. Geng Y-J, Libby P: Evidence of apoptosis in advanced human atheroma: Co-localization with interleukin-1β-converting enzyme. Am J Pathol 147:251–266, 1995
19. Isner JM, Kearney M, Bortman S, Passeri J: Apoptosis in human atherosclerosis and restenosis. Circulation 91:2703–2711, 1995
20. Cho A, Courtman DW, Langille BL: Apoptosis (programmed cell death) in arteries of the neonatal lamb. Circ Res 76:168–175, 1995
21. Brown BG, Fuster V: Impact of management in stabilization of coronary disease. In: Fuster V, Ross R, Topol EJ (eds): Atherosclerosis and Coronary Artery Disease. Philadelphia, Lippincott-Raven, 1996, pp 191–203
22. Armstrong MC, Megan MB: Lipid depletion of atheromatous coronary arteries in rhesus monkeys after regression diets. Circ Res 30:675–680, 1972
23. Clarkson TB, Bond MG, Bullock BC, Marzetta CA: A study of atherosclerosis regression in Macaca mulatta. IV. Changes in coronary arteries from animals with atherosclerosis induced for 19 months and then regressed for 24 or 48 months at plasma cholesterol concentrations of 300 or 200 mg/dl. Exp Mol Pathol 34:345–368, 1981
24. Armstrong MC, Megan MB: Arterial fibrous protein in cynomolgus monkeys after atherogenic and regression diets. Circ Res 36:256–261, 1975
25. Kannel WB, McGee D, Gordon T: A general cardiovascular risk profile: The Framingham study. Am J Cardiol 38:46–51, 1976
26. Keys A: Seven Countries: A Multivariate Analysis of Death and Coronary Heart Disease. Cambridge, MA, Harvard University Press, 1980
27. Castelli WP: Epidemiology of coronary heart disease: The Framingham Study. Am J Med 76(suppl 2A):4–12, 1984
28. Stampfer MJ, Colditz GA, Willett WC, et al: Postmenopausal estrogen therapy and cardiovascular disease: Ten year follow-up from the nurses' health study. N Engl J Med 325:756–762, 1991
29. Nabulsi AA, Folsom AR, White A, et al: Association of hormone replacement therapy with various risk factors in postmenopausal women. N Engl J Med 328:1069–1075, 1993
30. Criqui MH, Barret-Connor E, Holdbrook MJ, et al: Clustering of cardiovascular disease risk factors. Prev Med 9:525–535, 1980
31. Weingand KW, Clarkson TB, Adams MR, Bostrom AD: Effects of age and/or puberty on coronary artery atherosclerosis in cynomolgus monkeys. Atherosclerosis 62:137–144, 1986
32. Manuck SB, Kaplan JR, Matthews KA: Behavioral antecedents of coronary heart disease and atherosclerosis. Arteriosclerosis 6:2–14, 1986
33. Harker LA, Ross R, Slichter SJ, Scott CR: Homocystine-induced arteriosclerosis: The role of endothelial cell injury and platelet response in its genesis. J Clin Invest 58:731–741, 1976
34. Harker LA, Slichter SJ, Scott CR, Ross R: Homocystinemia: Vascular injury and arterial thrombosis. N Engl J Med 291:537–543, 1974
35. Mayer EL, Jacobsen DW, Robinson K: Homocysteine and coronary atherosclerosis. J Am Coll Cardiol 27:517–527, 1996
36. Verhoef P, Kok FJ, Kruyssen DACM, et al: Plasma total homocysteine, B vitamins and risk of coronary atherosclerosis. Arterioscler Thromb Vasc Biol 17:989–995, 1997
37. Levenson J, Giral P, Megnien JL, et al: Fibrinogen and its relations to subclinical extracoronary and coronary atherosclerosis in hypercholesterolemic men. Arterioscler Thromb Vasc Biol 17:45–50, 1997
38. Strong JP, Richards ML: Cigarette smoking and atherosclerosis in autopsied men. Atherosclerosis 23:451–476, 1976
39. Wilhelmsen L, Svardsudd K, Korsan-Bergsten K, et al: Fibrinogen as a risk factor for stroke and myocardial infarction. N Engl J Med 311:501–505, 1984
40. Gordon T, Kannel WB, McGee D: Death and coronary attacks in men after giving up cigarette smoking: A report from the Framingham Study. Lancet 2:1345–1348, 1974
41. Huttner I, Boutet M, Rona G, More RH: Studies of protein passage through arterial endothelium. III. Effect of blood pressure

levels on the passage of fine structure protein tracers through rat arterial endothelium. Lab Invest 29:536–546, 1973

42. Chobanian AV, Lichtenstein AH, Nilakhe V, et al: Influence of hypertension on aortic atherosclerosis in the Watanabe rabbit. Hypertension 14:203–209, 1989

43. Rosenfield ME, Tsukada T, Gown AM, Ross R: Fatty streak initiation in Watanabe heritable hyperlipemic and comparably hypercholesterolemic fat fed rabbits. Arteriosclerosis 7:9–23, 1987

44. Keys A (ed): Coronary heart disease in seven countries. Circulation 41(suppl I):I1–I211, 1970

45. Lipid Research Clinics Program: The lipid research clinics coronary primary prevention trial results. I. Reduction in incidence of coronary heart disease. JAMA 251:351–364, 1984

46. Lipid Research Clinics Program: The lipid research clinics coronary primary prevention trial results: II. The relationship of reduction in incidence of coronary heart disease to cholesterol lowering. JAMA 251:365–374, 1984

47. Brown MS, Goldstein JL: A receptor-mediated pathway for cholesterol homeostasis. Science 232:34–47, 1986

48. Miller NE: Associations of high-density lipoprotein subclasses and apolipoproteins with ischemic heart disease and coronary atherosclerosis. Am Heart J 113:589–597, 1987

49. Motulsky AG: Genetic aspects of familial hypercholesterolemia and its diagnosis. Arteriosclerosis 9(suppl 1):I3–I7, 1989

50. Breslow JL: Genetic basis of lipoprotein disorders. J Clin Invest 84:373–380, 1989

51. Gylling H, Kontula K, Koivisto U-M, et al: Polymorphisms of the gene encoding apoproteins A-I, B, C-III, and E and LDL receptor, and cholesterol and LDL metabolism during increased cholesterol intake. Arterioscler Thromb Vasc Biol 17:38–44, 1997

52. Davignon J, Gregg RE, Sing CF: Apolipoprotein E polymorphism and atherosclerosis. Arteriosclerosis 8:1–21, 1988

53. Wilson PWF, Myers RH, Larson MG, et al: Apolipoprotein E alleles, dyslipidemia, and coronary heart disease: The Framingham Offspring Study. JAMA 272:1666–1671, 1994

54. Gordon T, Castelli WP, Hjortland MC, et al: High-density lipoprotein as a protective factor against coronary heart disease: The Framingham Study. Am J Med 62:707–714, 1977

55. Hulley SB, Rosenman RH, Bawol RD, Brand RJ: Epidemiology as a guide to clinical decisions: The association between triglyceride and coronary disease. N Engl J Med 302:1383–1389, 1980

56. Whayne TF, Alaupovic P, Curry MD, et al: Plasma apolipoprotein B and VLDL-, LDL-, and HDL-cholesterol as risk factors in the development of coronary artery disease in male patients examined by angiography. Atherosclerosis 39:411–424, 1981

57. Dahlen GH, Guyton JR, Attar M, et al: Association of levels of lipoprotein Lp(a), plasma lipids, and other lipoproteins with coronary artery disease documented by angiography. Circulation 74:758–765, 1986

58. Hoff HF, Beck JG, Skibinski CI, et al: Serum Lp(a) level as a predictor of vein graft stenosis after coronary artery bypass surgery in patients. Circulation 77:1238–1244, 1988

59. Rhoads GG, Dahlen G, Berg K, et al: Lp(a) lipoprotein as a risk factor for myocardial infarction. JAMA 256:2540–2544, 1986

60. Schriewer H, Assmann G, Sandkamp M: The relationship of lipoprotein (a) [Lp(a)] to risk factors of coronary heart disease. J Clin Chem Clin Biochem 22:591–596, 1984

61. Rath M, Niendorf A, Reblin T, et al: Detection and quantification of lipoprotein (a) in the arterial wall of 107 coronary bypass patients. Arteriosclerosis 9:579–592, 1989

62. Ryan MJ, Emig LL, Hicks GW, et al: Localization of lipoprotein (a) in a monkey model of rapid neointimal growth. Arterioscler Thromb Vasc Biol 17:181–187, 1997

63. Haffner S, Appelbaum-Bowden D, Hoover J, Hazzard W: Association of high-density lipoprotein cholesterol 2 and 3 with Quetelet, alcohol, and smoking: The Seattle Lipid Research Clinic population. CVD Epidemiol Newsletter 31:20, 1982

64. Nye ER, Carlson K, Kirstein P, Rossner S: Changes in high density lipoprotein subfractions and other lipoproteins induced by exercise. Clin Chim Acta 113:51–57, 1981

65. Krauss RM: Regulation of high density lipoprotein levels. Med Clin North Am 66:403–430, 1982

66. Henriksson P, Stamberger M, Erikkson M, et al: Oestrogen-induced changes in lipoprotein metabolism: Role in prevention of atherosclerosis in the cholesterol-fed rabbit. Eur J Clin Invest 19:395–403, 1989

67. The Writing Group of PEPI Trial: Effects of estrogen or estrogen/progestin regimens on heart disease risk factors in postmenopausal women. JAMA 273:199–208, 1995

68. Stampfer MJ, Willett WC, Colditz GA, et al: A prospective study of past use of oral contraceptive agents and risk of cardiovascular diseases. N Engl J Med 319:1313–1317, 1988

68a. Dubey RK, Jackson EK, Gillespie DG, et al: Clinically used estrogens differentially inhibit human aortic smooth muscle cell growth and mitogen-activated protein kinase activity. Arterioscler Thromb Vasc Biol 20:964–972, 2000

69. Kagan A, Yanok K, Rhoads GC, McGee DL: Alcohol and cardiovascular disease: The Hawaiian experience. Circulation 64(suppl III):27–31, 1981

70. Soleas GJ, Diamandis EP, Goldberg DM: Wine as a biologic fluid: History, production, and role in disease prevention. J Clin Lab Anal 11:287–313, 1997

71. Soleas GJ, Diamandis EP, Goldberg DM: Resveratrol: A molecule whose time has come? and gone? Clin Biochem 30:91–113, 1997

72. Steiner G: Diabetes in atherosclerosis: An overview. Diabetes 30(suppl 2):1–7, 1981

73. Kannel WB, McGee DL: Diabetes and cardiovascular disease: The Framingham Study. JAMA 241:2035–2038, 1979

74. Walden CE, Knopp RH, Wahl PW, et al: Sex differences in the effect of diabetes mellitus on lipoprotein triglyceride and cholesterol concentrations. N Engl J Med 311: 953–959, 1984

75. Garcia MJ, McNamara PM, Gordon T, Kannell WD: Morbidity and mortality in diabetics in the Framingham population. Diabetes 23:105–111, 1974

76. Lawrie GM, Morris GC, Glaeser DH: Influences of diabetes mellitus on the results of coronary bypass surgery. JAMA 256:2967–2971, 1986

77. Banskota NK, Taub R, Zellner K, King GL: Insulin, insulin-like growth factor I and platelet-derived growth factor interact additively in the induction of the protooncogene c-myc and cellular proliferation in cultured bovine aortic smooth muscle cells. Mol Endocrinol 3:1183–1190, 1989

78. Brownlee M, Cerami A, Vlassara H: Advanced glycosylation end products in tissue and the biochemical basis of diabetic complications. N Engl J Med 318:1315–1321, 1988

79. Kirstein M, Brett J, Radoff S, et al: Advanced protein glycosylation induces transendothelial human monocyte chemotaxis and secretion of platelet-derived growth factor: Role in vascular disease of diabetes and aging. Proc Natl Acad Sci U S A 87:9010–9014, 1990

80. Bucala R: Lipoprotein modification by advanced glycosylation end-products (AGEs): Role in atherosclerosis. Trends Cardiovasc Med 7:39–47, 1997

81. Kunisaki M, Fumio U, Nawata H, King GL: Vitamin E normalizes diacylglycerol-protein kinase C activation induced by hyperglycemia in rat vascular tissue. Diabetes 45:S117–S119, 1996

82. Tsai JC, Perrella MA, Yoshimuzi M, et al: Promotion of vascular smooth muscle cell growth by homocysteine: A link to atherosclerosis. Proc Natl Acad Sci U S A 91:6369–6373, 1994

83. Malinow MR, Nieto FJ, Kruger WD, et al: The effects of folic acid supplementation on plasma total homocysteine are modulated by multivitamin use and methylenetetrahydrofolate reductase genotypes. Arterioscler Thromb Vasc Biol 17:1157–1162, 1997

84. Assmann G, Schulte H: European lipid guidelines: Therapeutic recommendations. Am J Cardiol 63:53H–55H, 1989

85. Canadian consensus conference on the prevention of heart and vascular disease by altering serum cholesterol and lipoprotein risk factors. Can Med Assoc J 139(suppl):1, 1988

86. NIH Consensus Development Conference: Lowering blood cholesterol to prevent heart disease. JAMA 253:2080–2086, 1985

87. Leaf A: Management of hypercholesterolemia: Are preventative interventions advisable? N Engl J Med 321:680–684, 1989

88. Report of the National Cholesterol Education Program expert panel on detection, evaluation and treatment of high blood cholesterol in adults. Arch Intern Med 148:36–69, 1988

89. Frick MH, Elo O, Happa K, et al: Helsinki heart study: Primary-prevention trial with gemfibrozil in middle-aged men with dyslipidemia. Safety of treatment, changes in risk factors, and incidence of coronary heart disease. N Engl J Med 317:1237–1245, 1987

90. Manninen V, Elo MO, Frick MK, et al: Lipid alterations and decline in the incidence of coronary heart disease in the Helsinki Heart Study. JAMA 260:641–651, 1988

91. Blankenhorn DH, Kramsch DM: Reversal of atherosis and sclerosis: The two components of atherosclerosis. Circulation 79:1–7, 1989

92. American Heart Association: 1989 Heart Facts. Dallas, American Heart Association, 1989

93. Walter HJ, Hofman A, Vaughan, RD, Wynder EL: Modification of risk factors for coronary heart disease: Five-year results of a school-based intervention trial. N Engl J Med 318:1093–1100, 1988

94. Williams CL, Wynder EL: Hyperlipidemia in childhood and the development of atherosclerosis. Ann N Y Acad Sci 263:1–482, 1991

95. PDAY Research Group: Relationship of atherosclerosis in young men to serum lipoprotein cholesterol concentrations and smoking. JAMA 264:3018–3024, 1990

96. McGill HC Jr, McMahan A, Malcom GT, et al, for the PDAY Research Group: Effects of serum lipoproteins and smoking on atherosclerosis in young men and women. Arterioscler Thromb Vasc Biol 17:95–106, 1997

97. Hazzard WR: Atherosclerosis and aging: A scenario in flux. Am J Cardiol 63:20H–24H, 1989

98. Castelli WP, Garrison RJ, Wilson PW, et al: Incidence of coronary heart disease and lipoprotein cholesterol levels: The Framingham study. JAMA 256:2835–8, 1986

99. Gordon DJ, Rifkind BM: Treating high blood cholesterol in the older patient. Am J Cardiol 63:48H–52H, 1989

100. Stary HC: Evolution and progression of atherosclerotic lesions in coronary arteries of children and young adults. Arteriosclerosis 9(suppl I):I-19, 1989

101. Nicklas TA, Farris RP, Smoak CG, et al: Dietary factors relate to cardiovascular risk factors in early life: Bogalusa Heart Study. Arteriosclerosis 8:193–199, 1988

102. Faggiotto A, Ross R: Studies of hypercholesterolemia in the nonhuman primate. II. Fatty streak conversion to fibrous plaque. Arteriosclerosis 4:341–356, 1984

103. Robertson WB, Geer JC, Strong JP, McGill HC Jr: The fate of the fatty streak. Exp Mol Pathol Suppl 1:28–39, 1963

104. Walker LN, Reidy MA, Bowyer DE: Morphology and cell kinetics of fatty streak lesion formation in the hypercholesterolemic rabbit. Am J Pathol 125:450–459, 1986

105. Movat HZ, Haust MD, More RH: The morphologic elements in the early lesions of arteriosclerosis. Am J Pathol 35:93–101, 1959

106. McGill HC Jr: Fatty streaks in the coronary arteries and aorta. Lab Invest 18:560–564, 1968

107. Enos WF, Holmes RH, Beyer J: Coronary disease among United States soldiers killed in action in Korea: Preliminary report. JAMA 152:1090–1093, 1953

108. McNamara JJ, Molot MA, Stremple JF, Cutting RT: Coronary artery disease in combat casualties in Vietnam. JAMA 216:1185–1187, 1971

109. Haust MD: Morphogenesis and fate of potential and early atherosclerotic lesions in man. Hum Pathol 2:1–29, 1971

110. Haust MD, More RH: Significance of the smooth muscle cell in atherogenesis. In: Jones RL (ed): Evolution of the Atherosclerotic Plaque. Chicago, University of Chicago Press, 1963, p 51

111. Geer JC: Fine structure of human aortic intimal thickening and fatty streaks. Lab Invest 14:1764–1783, 1965

112. Steinberg D, Parthasarathy S, Carew TE, et al: Beyond cholesterol: Modifications of low density lipoprotein that increases its atherogenicity. N Engl J Med 320:915–924, 1989

113. Restrepo C, Montenegro MR, Solberg LA: Atherosclerosis in persons with selected diseases. Lab Invest 18:552–559, 1968

114. Tejada C, Strong JP, Montenegro MR, et al: Distribution of coronary and aortic atherosclerosis by geographic location, race, and sex. Lab Invest 18:509–526, 1968

115. Stary HC, Letson GD: Morphometry of coronary artery components in children and young adults. Arteriosclerosis 3:A485, 1983

116. Velican C, Velican D: Intimal thickening in developing coronary arteries and its relevance to atherosclerotic involvement. Atherosclerosis 23:345–355, 1976

117. Geer JC, McGill HC Jr, Strong JP: The fine structure of human atherosclerotic lesions. Am J Pathol 38:263–287, 1961

118. Tracey RE, Kissling GE: Age and fibroplasia as preconditions for atheronecrosis in human coronary arteries. Arch Pathol Lab Med 3:957–963, 1987

119. Stary HC, Blankenhorn DH, Chandler AB, et al: A definition of the intima of human arteries and of its atherosclerosis-prone regions: A report from the Committee on Vascular Lesions of the Council on Arteriosclerosis, American Heart Association. Special Report. Circulation 85:391–405, 1992

120. Stary HC, Chandler AB, Glagov S, et al: A definition of initial, fatty streak, and intermediate lesions of atherosclerosis: A report from the Committee on Vascular Lesions of the Council on Arteriosclerosis, American Heart Association. Special report. Arterioscler Thromb 14:840–856, 1994

121. Tracey R, Kissling GE: Age and fibroplasia as preconditions for atheronecrosis in the human thoracic aorta. Arch Pathol Lab Med 109:651–658, 1985

122. Smith EB, Ashall C: Compartmentalization of water in human atherosclerotic lesion. Arteriosclerosis 4:21–27, 1984

123. Jorgensen L: Platelets and endothelial cell injury. In: Carlson LA (ed): International Conference on Atherosclerosis. New York, Raven Press, 1978

123a. Crawley J, Lupu F, Westmuckett AD, et al: Expression, localization and activity of tissue factor pathway inhibitor in normal and atherosclerotic human vessels. Arterioscler Thromb Vasc Biol 20:1362–1373, 2000

123b. Stary HC, Chandler AB, Dinsmore RE, et al: A definition of advanced types of atherosclerotic lesions and a histological classification of atherosclerosis: A report from the Committee on Vascular Lesions of the Council on Arteriosclerosis, American Heart Association. Arterioscler Thromb Vasc Biol 15:1512–1531, 1995

123c. Virmani R, Kolodgie FD, Burke AP, et al: Lessons from sudden coronary death: A comprehensive morphological classification scheme for atherosclerotic lesions. Arterioscler Thromb Vasc Biol 20:1262–1275, 2000.

124. Restrepo C, Tracey RE: Variations in human aortic fatty streaks among geographic locations. Atherosclerosis 21:179–193, 1975

125. Tracey RE, Kissling GE: Comparisons of human populations for histologic features of atherosclerosis. Arch Pathol Lab Med 112:1056–1065, 1988

126. Strong JP, Restrepo C, Guzman M: Coronary and aortic atherosclerosis in New Orleans. II. Comparisons of lesions by age, sex and race. Lab Invest 939:364–369, 1978

127. Neitzel GF, Barboriak JJ, Pintar K, Qureshi I: Atherosclerosis in aortocoronary bypass grafts: Morphologic study and risk factor analysis 6 to 12 years after surgery. Arteriosclerosis 6:594–600, 1986

128. Smith SH, Geer JC: Morphology of saphenous vein-artery bypass grafts: Seven to 116 months after surgery. Arch Pathol Lab Med 107:13, 1983

129. Stary HC, Chandler AB, Dinsmore RE, et al: A definition of advanced types of atherosclerotic lesions and a histological classification of atherosclerosis: A report from the Committee on Vascular Lesions of the Council on Arteriosclerosis, American Heart Association. Arterioscler Thromb Vas Biol 15:1512–1531, 1995

130. Cornhill JF, Roach MR: A quantitative study of the localization of atherosclerotic lesions in the rabbit aorta. Atherosclerosis 23:489–501, 1976

131. Zarins CK, Giddens DP, Bharadavaij BK, et al: Carotid bifurcation atherosclerosis: Quantitation of plaque localization with flow velocity profiles and wall shear stress. Circ Res 53:502–514, 1983

132. Gotlieb AI, Langille BL: The role of rheology in atherosclerotic coronary artery disease. In: Fuster V, Ross R, Topol EJ (eds): Atherosclerosis and Coronary Artery Disease. Philadelphia, Lippincott-Raven, 1996, pp 595–606

133. Kim DW, Gotlieb AI, Langille BL: In vivo modulation of endothelial F-actin microfilaments by experimental alterations in shear stress. Arteriosclerosis 9:439–445, 1989

134. Kim DW, Langille BL, Wong MKK, Gotlieb AI: Patterns of endothelial microfilament distribution in the rabbit aorta in situ. Circulation Res 64:21–31, 1988

135. Vyalov S, Langille BL, Gotlieb AI: Decreased blood flow rate disrupts endothelial repair in vivo. Am J Pathol 149:2107–2118, 1996

136. Cowan DB, Langille BL: Cellular and molecular biology of vascular remodeling. Curr Opin Lipidol 7:94–100, 1996

137. Rodbard S: Vascular caliber. Cardiology 60:4–49, 1975
138. Ross R, Wight TN, Standness E, Thiele B: Human atherosclerosis. I. Cell constitution and characteristics of advanced lesions of the superficial femoral artery. Am J Pathol 114:79–93, 1984
139. Goldstein JL, Hoff HF, Ho JK, et al: Stimulation of cholesterylester synthesis in macrophages by extracts of atherosclerotic human aortas and complexes of albumin/cholesteryl esters. Arteriosclerosis 1:210–226, 1981
140. Faggiotto A, Ross R, Hacker L: Studies of hypercholesterolemia in the nonhuman primate. I. Changes that lead to fatty streak formation. Arteriosclerosis 4:323–340, 1984
141. Gerrity RG: The role of the monocyte in atherogenesis. I. Transition of blood-borne monocytes into foam cells in fatty lesions. Am J Pathol 103:181–190, 1981
142. Gerrity RG: The role of the monocyte in atherogenesis. II. Migration of foam cells from atherosclerotic lesion. Am J Pathol 103:191–200, 1981
143. Gerrity, RC, Gross JA, Soby L: Control of monocyte recruitment by chemotactic factor(s) in lesion-prone areas of swine aorta. Arteriosclerosis 5:55, 1985
144. Curtiss LK, Black AS, Takagi Y, Plow EF: New mechanism for foam cell generation in atherosclerotic lesions. J Clin Invest 80:367–373, 1987
145. Gown AM, Tsukada T, Ross R: Human atherosclerosis. II. Immunocytochemical analysis of the cellular composition of human atherosclerotic lesions. Am J Pathol 125:191–207, 1986
146. Jonasson L, Holm J, Skalli O, et al: Regional accumulations of T cells, macrophages, and smooth muscle cells in the human atherosclerotic plaque. Arteriosclerosis 6:131–138, 1986
147. Emeson EE, Robertson AL: T lymphocytes in aortic and coronary intimas: Their potential role in atherogenesis. Am J Pathol 130:369–376, 1988
148. Schutte HE: Changes in the vasa vasorum of the atherosclerotic aortic wall. Angiologica 5:210–222, 1968
149. Pepper MS: Manipulating angiogenesis: From basic science to the bedside. Arterioscler Thromb Vasc Biol 17:605–619, 1997
150. Okuyama K, Yaegashi H, Takahashi T, et al: The three-dimensional architecture of vasa vasorum in the wall of the human aorta: A computer-aided reconstruction study. Arch Pathol Lab Med 112:726–730, 1988
151. Okuyama K, Yaginuma G, Takahashi T, et al: The development of vasa vasorum of the human aorta in various conditions: A morphometric study. Arch Pathol Lab Med 112:721–725, 1988
152. Barger AC, Beeuwkes R, Lainey LL, Silverman KJ: Hypothesis: Vasa vasorum and neovascularization of human coronary arteries. A possible role in the pathophysiology of atherosclerosis. N Engl J Med 310:175–177, 1984
153. Falk E: Plaque rupture with severe pre-existing stenosis precipitating coronary thrombosis: Characteristics of coronary atherosclerotic plaques underlying fatal occlusive thrombi. Br Heart J 50:127–134, 1983
154. Freidman M: The pathogenesis of coronary plaques, thromboses, and hemorrhages: An evaluative review. Circulation 52(suppl 6):III34–III40, 1975
155. Glagov S, Weisenberg E, Zarins CK, et al: Compensatory enlargement of human atherosclerotic coronary arteries. N Engl J Med 316:1371–1375, 1987
156. Davies MJ, Thomas AC: Plaque fissuring: The cause of acute myocardial infarction, sudden ischemic death, and crescendo angina. Br Heart J 53:363–373, 1985
157. Wong MKK, Gotlieb AI: In vitro reendothelialization of single cell wound: Role of microfilament bundles in rapid lamellipodia-mediated wound closure. Lab Invest 51:75–81, 1984
158. Glimcher MJ: Mechanism of calcification: Role of collagen fibrils and collagen-phosphoprotein complexes in vitro and in vivo. Anat Rec 224:139–153, 1989
159. Bostrom K, Watson KE, Horn S, et al: Bone morphogenetic protein expression in human atherosclerotic lesions. J Clin Invest 91:1800–1809, 1993
160. Giachelli CM, Bae N, Almeida M, et al: Osteopontin is elevated during neointima formation in rat arteries and is a novel component of human atherosclerotic plaques. J Clin Invest 92:1686–1696, 1993
161. Shanahan CM, Cary NRB, Metcalfe JC, Weissberg PL: High expression of genes for calcification-regulating proteins in human atherosclerotic plaques. J Clin Invest 93:2393–2402, 1994
162. Watson KE, Boström K, Ravindranauth R: TGF-b1 and 25-hydroxycholesterol stimulate osteoblast-like vascular cells to calcify. J Clin Invest 93:2106–2113, 1994
163. Lee RT, Libby P: The unstable atheroma. Arterioscler Thromb Vasc Biol 17:1859–1867, 1997
164. Van Hinsbergh VWM: Endothelial permeability for macromolecules: Mechanistic aspects of pathophysiological modulation. Arterioscler Thromb Vasc Biol 17:1018–1023, 1997
165. Ettenson DS, Gotlieb AI: Centrosome dependent endothelial wound repair requires early transcription following injury. Arterioscler Thromb 13:1270–1281, 1993
166. Gimbrone MA, Cotran RS, Folkman J: Human vascular endothelial cells in culture: Growth and DNA synthesis. J Cell Biol 60:673–684, 1974
167. Jaffe EA, Nachman RL, Becker CG: Culture of human endothelial cell derived from umbilical veins: Identification of morphologic criteria. J Clin Invest 52:2745–2758, 1973
168. Prescott SM, McIntyre TM, Zimmerman GA: The role of platelet-activating factor in endothelial cells. Thromb Haemost 64:99–103, 1990
169. Palmer RMJ, Ferrige AG, Moncada S: Nitric oxide release accounts for the biological activity of endothelium-derived relaxing factor. Nature 327:524–526, 1987
170. Yanagisawa M, Kurihara H, Kimura S, et al: A novel potent vasoconstrictor peptide produced by vascular endothelial cells. Nature 332:411–415, 1988
171. Jaffe EA: Cell biology of endothelial cells. Hum Pathol 18:234–239, 1987
172. Cerveny TJ, Fass DN, Mann KG: Synthesis of coagulation factor V by cultured aortic endothelium. Blood 63:1467–1474, 1984
173. Bevilaqua MP, Pober JS, Majeau R, et al: Interleukin (IL 1) induces biosynthesis and cell surface expression of procoagulant activity in human vascular endothelial cells. J Exp Med 160:618–623, 1984
174. Stern DM, Drillings M, Kisiel W, et al: Activation of factor IX bound to cultured bovine aortic endothelial cells. Proc Natl Acad Sci U S A 31:913–917, 1983
175. Stern DM, Nawroth PP, Harris K, Esmon CT: Cultured bovine aortic endothelial cells promote activated protein C-protein-S-mediated inactivation of factor Va. J Biol Chem 261:713–718, 1986
176. Hawiger J: Formation and regulation of platelet and fibrin hemostatic plug. Hum Pathol 18:111–122, 1987
177. Moncada S, Vane JR: Pharmacology and endogenous roles of prostaglandin endoperoxides, thromboxane A$_2$ and prostacyclin. Pharmacol Rev 30:293–331, 1979
178. Titani K, Walsh KA: Human von Willebrand-factor: The molecular glue of platelet plugs. Trends Biochem 13:94–97, 1988
179. Esmon NL, Owen WG, Esmon CT: Isolation of a membrane-bound cofactor for thrombin catalyzed activation of protein C. J Biol Chem 257:859–864, 1982
180. Fair DS, Marlar RA, Levin EG: Human endothelial cells synthesize protein S. Blood 67:1168–1171, 1985
181. Laug WE: Secretion of plasminogen activators by cultured bovine endothelial cells: Partial purification, characterization and evidence for multiple forms. Thromb Haemost 45:219–224, 1981
182. Levin EG, Loskutoff DJ: Cultured bovine endothelial cells produce both urokinase and tissue type plasminogen activators. J Cell Biol 94:631–636, 1982
183. Levin EG, Loskutoff DJ: Serum-mediated suppression of cell-associated plasminogen activator activity in cultured endothelial cells. Cell 22:701–707, 1980
184. Hajjar KA, Hamel NM, Harpel PC, Nachman RL: Binding of tissue plasminogen activator to cultured human endothelial cells. J Clin Invest 80:1712–1719, 1987
185. Hajjar KA, Harpel PC, Jaffe EA, Nachman RL: Binding of plasminogen to cultured human endothelial cells. J Biol Chem 261:11656–11662, 1986
186. Loskutoff DJ, Van Mourik JA, Erickson LA, Lawrence DA: Detection of an unusually stable fibrinolytic inhibitor produced by bovine endothelial cells. Proc Natl Acad Sci U S A 80:2956–2960, 1983

187. Van Mourik JA, Lawrence DA, Loskutoff DJ: Purification of an inhibitor of plasminogen-activator (anti-activator) synthesized by endothelial cells. J Biol Chem 259:4914–4921, 1984

188. Mimuro J, Loskutoff DJ: Binding of type 1 plasminogen activator inhibitor to the extracellular matrix of cultured bovine endothelial cells. J Biol Chem 264:5058–5063, 1989

189. Schleef RR, Wagner NV, Loskutoff DJ: Detection of both type 1 and type 2 plasminogen activator inhibitors in human cells. J Cell Physiol 134:269–274, 1988

190. Sakata Y, Curriden S, Lawrence D, et al: Activated protein C stimulates the fibrinolytic activity of cultured endothelial cells and decreases antiactivator activity. Proc Natl Acad Sci U S A 82:1121–1125, 1985

191. Bond M, Somlyo AV: Dense bodies and actin polarity in vertebrate smooth muscle. J Cell Biol 95:403–413, 1984

192. Furchgott RF, Vanhoutte PM: Endothelium-derived relaxing and contracting factors. FASEB J 3:2007–2018, 1989

193. Furchgott RF, Zawadzki JR: The obligatory role of endothelial cells in the relaxation of arterial smooth muscle by acetylcholine. Nature 288:373–376, 1980

194. Feletou M, Vanhoutte PM: Endothelium-dependent hyperpolarization of canine coronary smooth muscle. Br J Pharmacol 93:515–524, 1988

195. Saito T, Wolf A, Menon NK, et al: Lysolecithins as endothelium-dependent vascular smooth muscle relaxants that differ from endothelium-derived relaxing factor (nitric oxide). Proc Natl Acad Sci U S A 85:8246–8250, 1988

196. Bossaller C, Habib GB, Yamamoto H, et al: Impaired muscarinic endothelium-dependent relaxation and cyclic guanosine 5′-monophosphate formation in atherosclerotic human coronary artery and rabbit aorta. J Clin Invest 79:170–174, 1987

197. Verbeuren TJ, Jordaens FH, Zonnekeyn LL: Effect of hypercholesterolemia on vascular reactivity in the rabbit. 1. Endothelium-dependent and endothelium-independent contractions and relaxations in isolated arteries of control and hypercholesterolemic rabbits. Circ Res 58:552–564, 1986

198. Drexler H, Zeiher AM, Wollschlager H, et al: Flow-dependent coronary artery dilatation in humans. Circulation 80:466–474, 1989

199. Clozel M, Fischli W: Human cultured endothelial cells do secrete endothelin-1. J Cardiovasc Pharmacol 13(suppl 5):S-229–231, 1989

200. Simonson MS, Dunn MJ: Cellular signaling by peptides of the endothelin gene family. FASEB J 4:2989–3000, 1990

201. Clark JM, Seymour G: Transmural organization of the arterial media: The lamellar unit revisited. Arteriosclerosis 5:19–34, 1985

202. Jander R, Rauterberg J, Glanville RW: Further characterization of the three polypeptide chains of bovine and human short-chain collagen (intima collagen). Eur J Biochem 133: 39–46, 1983

203. Mayne R: Collagenous proteins of blood vessels. Arteriosclerosis 6:585–593, 1986

204. Morton LF, Barnes MJ: Collagen polymorphism in the normal and diseased blood vessel wall. Atherosclerosis 42:41–51, 1982

205. Von der Mark H, Aumailley M, Wick G, et al: Immunochemistry, genuine size and tissue localization of collagen VI. Eur J Biochem 142:493–502, 1984

206. Sage H, Trueb B, Bornstein P: Biosynthetic and structural properties of endothelial cell type VIII collagen. J Biol Chem 258: 13391–13401, 1983

207. Kittelberger R, Davis PF, Greenhill NS: Immunolocalization of type VIII collagen in vascular tissue. Biochem Biophys Commun 159:414–419, 1989

208. Berenson GS, Radhakrishnamurthy B, Srinivasan SR, et al: Carbohydrate-protein macromolecules and arterial wall integrity: A role in atherogenesis. Exp Mol Pathol 41:267–287, 1984

209. Ross R: The smooth muscle cell. II. Growth of smooth muscle in cell culture and formation of elastic fibres. J Cell Biol 50:172–186, 1971

210. Skubitz APN, McCarthy JB, Charonis AS, Furcht LT: Localization of three distinct heparin-binding domains of laminin by monoclonal antibodies. J Biol Chem 263:4861–4868, 1988

211. Timpl R: Structure and biological activity of basement membrane proteins. Eur J Biochem 180:487–502, 1989

212. Aumailley M, Nurcombe V, David E, et al: The cellular interactions of laminin fragments: Cell adhesion correlates with two fragment-specific high affinity binding sites. J Biol Chem 262:11532–11538, 1987

213. Ruoslahti E: Fibronectin and its receptors. Annu Rev Biochem 57: 375–413, 1988

214. Sage H, Decker J, Funk S, Chow M: SPARC: A Ca^{2+}-binding extracellular protein associated with endothelial cell injury and proliferation. J Moll Cell Cardiol 21(suppl 1):13–22, 1989

215. Panayotou G, End P, Aumailley M, et al: Domains of laminin with growth factor activity. Cell 56:93–101, 1989

216. Folkman J, Klagsburg M, Sasse J, et al: A heparin-binding angiogenic protein-basic fibroblast growth factor is stored within basement membrane. Am J Pathol 130:393–400, 1988

217. Wight TN: The vascular extracellular matrix. In: Fuster V, Ross R, Topel E (eds): Atherosclerosis and Coronary Artery Disease. Philadelphia, Lippincott-Raven, 1996, pp 421–440

218. Kinsella MG, Wight TN: Modulation of sulfated proteoglycan synthesis by bovine aortic endothelial cells during migration. J Cell Biol 102:679–687, 1986

219. Madri JA, Stenn KS: Aortic endothelial cell-migration. 1. Matrix requirements and composition. Am J Pathol 106:180–186, 1982

220. Rapraeger AC, Berfield M: Heparan sulfate proteoglycans of mouse mammary epithelial cells: A putative membrane proteoglycan associates quantitatively with lipid vesicles. J Biol Chem 258: 3632–3636, 1983

221. Ausprunk DH, Boudreau CL, Nelson DA: Proteoglycans in the microvasculature. I. Histochemical localization in microvessels of the rabbit eye. Am J Pathol 103:353–366, 1981

222. Lark MW, Wight TN: Modulation of proteoglycan metabolism by aortic smooth muscle cell growth on collagen gels. Arteriosclerosis 6:638–650, 1986

223. Kumar V, Berenson GS, Ruiz H, et al: Acid mucopolysaccharides of human aorta. III. Variations of atherosclerotic involvement. J Atheroscler Res 7:583, 1967

224. Stevens RL, Colombro M, Gonzales JJ, et al: The glycosaminoglycans of the human artery and their changes in atherosclerosis. J Clin Invest 58:470–481, 1976

225. Klynstra FB, Bottcher CJF, Van Melsen JA, Van der Laan EJ: Distribution and composition of acid mucopolysaccharides in normal and atherosclerotic human aortas. J Atheroscler Res 7:301–309, 1967

226. Toledo OMS, Mourao PAS: Sulfated glycosaminoglycans of human aorta: Chondroitin 6-sulfate increase with age. Biochem Biophys Res Commun 89:50–55, 1979

227. Yla-Herttuala S, Sumuvuori H, Karkola K, et al: Glycosaminoglycans in normal and atherosclerotic human coronary arteries. Lab Invest 54:402–407, 1986

228. Alavi MZ, Richardson M, Moore S: The in vitro interactions between serum lipoproteins and proteoglycans of the neointima of rabbit aorta after a single balloon catheter injury. Am J Pathol 134:287, 1989

229. Wight TN: Differences in the synthesis and secretion of sulfated glycosaminoglycan by aorta explant monolayer cultured from atherosclerosis-susceptible and -resistant pigeons. Am J Pathol 101: 127–141, 1980

230. Helin P, Lorenzen I, Garbarsch G: Repair in arterial tissue: Morphological and biochemical changes in rabbit aorta after a single dilation injury. Circ Res 29:542–554, 1971

231. Birkedal-Hansen H: Proteolytic remodelling of extracellular matrix. Curr Opin Cell Biol 7:728–735, 1995

232. Duguid JB: Thrombosis as a factor in the pathogenesis of aortic atherosclerosis. J Pathol Bacteriol 60:57–61, 1948

233. Wong MKK, Gotlieb AI: Repair of small endothelial wound: A two step process. J Cell Biol 107:1777–1783, 1988

234. Folkman J, Klagsburg M: A family of angiogenic peptides. Nature 329:671–672, 1987

235. Pfeifle B, Ditschuneit H: Effect of insulin on growth of cultured human arterial smooth muscle cells. Diabetologia 20:155–158, 1981

236. Stout RW: Overview of the association between insulin and atherosclerosis. Metabolism 34(suppl 1):7–12, 1985

237. King GL, Goodman DA, Buzney S, et al: Receptors and growth-promoting effects of insulin and insulin-like growth factors on cells from bovine retinal capillaries and aorta. J Clin Invest 75: 1028–1036, 1985

238. Foegh ML, Khirabadi BS, Chambers E, Ramwell PW: Peptide inhibition of accelerated transplant atherosclerosis. Transplant Proc 21:3674–3676, 1989

239. Johnsson A, Heldin C-H, Wasteson A, et al: The c-sis gene encodes a precursor of the B chain of PDGF. EMBO J 3:921–928, 1984

240. Seifert RA, Hart CE, Phillips PE, et al: Two different subunits associate to create platelet-derived growth factor receptors. J Biol Chem 264:8771–8778, 1989

241. Grotendorst GR, Chang T, Seppa HEJ, et al: Platelet-derived growth factor is chemoattractant for vascular smooth muscle cells. J Cell Physiol 113:261–266, 1982

242. Deuel TF: Polypeptide growth factors: Roles in normal and abnormal cell growth. Annu Rev Cell Biol 3:443–492, 1987

243. Seppa H, Grotendorst G, Seppa S, et al: Platelet-derived growth factor is chemotactic for fibroblasts. J Cell Biol 92:584–588, 1982

244. Hosang M, Rouge M: Human vascular smooth muscle cells have at least two distinct PDGF receptors and can secrete PDGF-AA. J Cardiovasc Pharmacol 14(suppl 6):S22–S26, 1989

245. Zwijsen RM, Japenga SC, Heijen AM, et al: Induction of platelet-derived growth factor chain A gene expression in human smooth muscle cells by oxidized low density lipoproteins. Biochem Biophys Res Commun 186:1410–1416, 1992

246. Kusuhara M, Chait A, Cader A, Berk BC: Oxidized LDL stimulates mitogen-activated protein kinases in smooth muscle cells and macrophages. Arterioscler Thromb Vasc Biol 17:141–148, 1997

247. Ross R: The pathogenesis of atherosclerosis: An update. N Engl J Med 314:488–500, 1986

248. Libby P, Warner SJC, Salmon RN, Birinyi LK: Production of EDGF-like mitogen by smooth muscle cells from human atheroma. N Engl J Med 318:1493–1498, 1988

249. Majesky MW, Benditt EP, Schwartz SM: Expression and developmental control of PDGF-A chain and B chain/Sis genes in rat aortic smooth muscle cells. Proc Natl Acad Sci U S A 25:1524–1528, 1988

250. Sejersen T, Betsholz C, Sjolund M, et al: Rat skeletal myoblasts and arterial smooth muscle cells express the gene for the A chain but not the B chain (c-cis) of EDGF and produce a PDGF-like protein. Proc Natl Acad Sci U S A 83:6844–6848, 1986

251. Deuel TF, Seniar RM, Huang JS, Griffin GL: Chemotaxis of monocytes and neutrophils to platelet-derived growth factor. J Clin Invest 69:1046–1049, 1982

252. Berk BC, Alexander RW, Brock TA, et al: Vasoconstriction: A new activity of platelet derived growth factor. Science 232:87–90, 1986

253. Fox PL, DiCorleto PE: Fish oils inhibit endothelial cell production of platelet-derived growth factor-like protein. Science 241:453–456, 1988

254. Shimokado K, Raines EW, Madtes DK, et al: A significant part of macrophage-derived growth factor consists of at least two forms of PDGF. Cell 43:277–286, 1985

255. Jaye M, McConathy E, Drohan W, et al: Modulation of the sis gene transcript during endothelial cell differentiation in vitro. Science 228:882–885, 1985

256. Seifert RA, Schwartz SM, Bowen-Pope DF: Developmentally regulated production of platelet-derived growth factor-like molecules. Nature 311:669–671, 1984

257. Barrett TB, Benditt EP: Platelet-derived growth factor gene expression in human atherosclerotic plaques and normal artery wall. Proc Natl Acad Sci U S A 85:2810–2814, 1988

258. Barrett TB, Benditt EP: Sis (platelet-derived growth factor B chain) gene transcript levels are elevated in human atherosclerotic lesions compared to normal artery. Proc Natl Acad Sci U S A 84:1099–1103, 1987

259. Gordon D, Schwartz SM, Benditt EP, Wilcox JN: Growth factors and cell proliferation in human atherosclerosis. Transplant Proc 21:3692–3694, 1989

260. Gospodarowicz D, Neufeld G, Schweigerer L: Molecular and biological characterization of fibroblast growth factor: An angiogenic factor which also controls the proliferation and differentiation of mesoderm and neuroectoderm-derived cells. Cell Differ 19:1–17, 1986

261. Lobb RR, Harper JW, Fett JW: Purification of heparin binding growth factors. Anal Biochem 154:1–14, 1986

262. Schreiber AB, Winkler ME, Derynch R: Transforming growth factor-α: A more potent angiogenic mediator than epidermal growth factors. Science 232:1250–1253, 1986

263. Roberts AB, Sporn MB, Assoian RK, et al: Transforming growth factor type-beta: Rapid induction of fibrosis and angiogenesis in vivo and stimulation of collagen formation. Proc Natl Acad Sci U S A 83:4167–4171, 1986

264. Leibovich SJ, Polverini PJ, Shepard HM, et al: Macrophage-induced angiogenesis is mediated by tumour necrosis factor-α. Nature 329:630–632, 1987

265. Fett JW, Strydom DJ, Lobb RR, et al: Isolation and characterization of angiogenin, an angiogeneic protein from human carcinoma cells. Biochemistry 24:5480–5486, 1985

266. Ishikawa F, Miyazono K, Hellman U, et al: Identification of angiogenic activity and the cloning and expression of platelet-derived endothelial cell growth factor. Nature 338:557–562, 1989

267. Engel J: EGF-like domains in extracellular matrix proteins: Localized signals for growth and differentiation? FEBS Lett 251:1–7, 1989

268. Smith R, Peters G, Wichson C: Multiple RNAs expressed from the int-2 gene in mouse embryonal carcinoma cell-lines encode a protein with homology to fibroblast growth factors. EMBO J 7:1013–1022, 1988

269. Gospodarowicz D, Ferrara N, Schweigerer L, Neufeld G: Structural characterization and biological functions of fibroblast growth factor. Endocr Rev 8:1–10, 1987

270. Neufeld G, Gospodarowicz D: Basic and acidic fibroblast growth factor interact with the same cell surface receptor. J Biol Chem 261:5631–5637, 1986

271. Wong MKK, Gotlieb AI: Endothelial monolayer integrity: Perturbation of F-actin filaments and the DPB vinculin network. Arteriosclerosis 10:76–84, 1990

272. Ettenson DS, Gotlieb AI: Basic fibroblast growth factor is a signal for the initiation of centrosome redistribution to the front of migrating endothelial cells, at the edge of an in vitro wound. Arterioscler Thromb Vasc Biol 15:515–521, 1995

273. Gospodarowicz D, Neufeld G, Schweigerer L: Fibroblast growth factor: Structural and biological properties. J Cell Physiol Suppl 5: 15–26, 1987

274. Kourembanas S, Faller DV: Platelet-derived growth factor production by human umbilical vein endothelial cells is regulated by basic fibroblast growth factor. J Biol Chem 264:4456–4459, 1989

275. Daley SJ, Gotlieb AI: Fibroblast growth factor receptor 1 expression is associated with neointimal formation in vitro. Am J Pathol 148:1193–1202, 1996

276. Tan EML, Levine E, Sorger T, et al: Heparin and endothelial cell growth factor modulate collagen and proteoglycan production in human smooth muscle cells. Biochem Biophys Res Commun 163: 84–92, 1989

277. Thornton SC, Mueller SN, Levine EM: Human endothelial cells: Use of heparin in cloning and long-term serial cultivation. Science 222:623–625, 1983

278. Bashkin P, Doctrow S, Klagsbrun M, et al: Basic fibroblast growth factor binds to subendothelial extracellular matrix and is released by heparatinase and heparin-like molecules. Biochemistry 28: 1737–1743, 1989

279. Gajdusek CM, Carbon S: Injury-induced release of basic fibroblast growth factor from bovine aortic endothelium. J Cell Physiol 139: 570–579, 1989

280. Vlodavsky I, Folkman J, Sullivan R, et al: Endothelial cell-derived fibroblast growth factor: Synthesis and deposition into subendothelial extracellular matrix. Proc Natl Acad Sci U S A 84:2292–2296, 1987

281. Sporn MB, Roberts AB, Wakefield LM, Crombrugghe B: Some recent advances in the chemistry and biology of transforming growth factor-beta. J Cell Biol 195:1039–1045, 1987

282. Assoian RK, Komoriya A, Meyers CA, et al: Transforming growth factor-beta in human platelets. J Biol Chem 258:7155–7160, 1983

283. Massague J, Hata A, Liu F: TGF-β signalling through the Smad pathway. Trends Cell Biol 7:187–192, 1997

284. Heimark RL, Twardzik DR, Schwartz SM: Inhibition of endothelial regeneration by type-beta transforming growth factor from platelets. Science 233:1078–1080, 1986

285. Majack RA: Beta-type transforming growth factor specifies organizational behavior in vascular smooth muscle cell cultures. J Cell Biol 105:465–471, 1987

286. Chen J-K, Hoshi H, McKeehan WL: Transforming growth factor type β specifically stimulates synthesis of proteoglycan in human adult arterial smooth muscle cells. Proc Natl Acad Sci U S A 84: 5287–5291, 1987

287. Sporn MB, Roberts AB: Transforming growth factor-β: Multiple actions and potential clinical applications. JAMA 262:938–941, 1989

288. Nabel EG, Shum L, Pompili VJ, et al: Direct transfer of transforming growth factor β1 gene into arteries stimulates fibrocellular hyperplasia. Proc Natl Acad Sci U S A 90:10759–10763, 1993

289. Oemar BS, Lüscher TF: Connective tissue growth factor: Friend or foe? Arterioscler Thromb Vasc Biol 17:1483–1489, 1997

290. Loomis CR, Shipley GG, Small DM: The phase behavior of hydrated cholesterol. J Lipid Res 20:525–535, 1979

291. Small DM: Progression and regression of atherosclerotic lesions: Insights from lipid physical biochemistry. Arteriosclerosis 8:103–129, 1988

292. Steinberg D, Parthasarathy S, Carew TE: In vivo inhibition of foam cell development by probucol in Watanabe rabbits. Am J Pathol 62:6B–12B, 1988

293. Schwenke DC, Carew TE: Initiation of atherosclerotic lesions in cholesterol-fed rabbits. I. Focal increases in arterial LDL. Arteriosclerosis 9:895–907, 1989

294. Alderson ML, Hayes KC, Nicolosi RJ: Peanut oil reduces diet-induced atherosclerosis in cynomolgus monkeys. Arteriosclerosis 6:465–474, 1986

295. Vesselinovitch O, Wissler RW, Schaffner TJ, Borensztajn J: The effect of various diets on atherogenesis in rhesus monkeys. Atherosclerosis 35:189–207, 1980

296. Roach MR: The effects of bifurcations and stenoses on arterial disease. In: Hwang NHC, Norman NA (eds): Cardiovascular Flow Dynamics and Measurements. Baltimore, University Park Press, 1977, pp 489–539

297. Moore S: Dietary atherosclerosis and arterial wall injury. Lab Invest 60:733–736, 1989

298. Bihara-Varga M, Gruber E, Rotheneder M, et al: Interaction of lipoprotein Lp(a) and low density lipoprotein with glycosaminoglycans from human aorta. Arteriosclerosis 8:851–857, 1988

299. Armstrong ML, Warner ED, Connor WE: Regression of coronary atheromatosis in rhesus monkeys. Circ Res 27:59–72, 1970

300. Clarkson TB, Bond MG, Bullock BC, et al: A study of atherosclerosis regression in *Macaca mulatta*. V. Changes in abdominal aorta and carotid and coronary arteries from animals with atherosclerosis induced for 38 months and then regressed for 24 or 48 months at plasma cholesterol concentrations of 300 or 200 mg/dl. Exp Mol Pathol 41:96–118, 1984

301. Vesselinovitch D, Wissler RW, Hughes R, Borensztajn J: Reversal of advanced atherosclerosis in rhesus monkeys. Part 1. Light microscopic studies. Atherosclerosis 23:155–176, 1976

302. Kashyap ML: Basic considerations in the reversal of atherosclerosis: Significance of high-density lipoprotein in stimulating reverse cholesterol transport. Am J Cardiol 63:56H–59H, 1989

303. Benditt EP, Benditt JM: Evidence for a monoclonal origin of human atherosclerotic plaque. Proc Natl Acad Sci U S A 70:1753–1756, 1973

304. Thomas WA, Kim DN: Atherosclerosis as a hyperplastic and neoplastic process. Lab Invest 48:245–255, 1983

305. Fabricant CG, Fabricant J, Litrenta MM, Minick RC: Virus-induced atherosclerosis. J Exp Med 148:335–340, 1978

306. Fabricant CG, Hajjar DP, Minick RC, Fabricant J: Herpesvirus infection enhances cholesterol and cholesteryl ester accumulation in cultured arterial smooth muscle cells. Am J Pathol 105:176–184, 1981

307. Adams MR, Clarkson TB, Kaplan JR, Koritnik DR: Experimental evidence in monkeys for beneficial effects of estrogen on coronary artery atherosclerosis. Transplant Proc 21:3662–3664, 1989

308. Hendrix MGR, Dormans PHJ, Kitslaar P, et al: The presence of cytomegalovirus nucleic acids in arterial walls of atherosclerotic and nonatherosclerotic patients. Am J Pathol 134:1151–1157, 1989

309. Ross R, Glomset JA: The pathogenesis of atherosclerosis. N Engl J Med 295:369–377,420–425, 1976

310. Chiu B, Viira E, Tucker W, Fong IW: *Chlamydia pneumoniae*, cytomegalovirus and herpes simplex virus in atherosclerosis of the carotid artery. Circulation 96:2144–2148, 1997

311. Cunningham MJ, Pasternak RC: The potential role of viruses in the pathogenesis of atherosclerosis. Circulation 77:964–969, 1988

312. Ridker P: Inflammation, infection and cardiovascular risk: How good is the clinical evidence? Circulation 97:1671, 1998

313. Kol A, Libby P: The mechanisms by which infectious agents may contribute to atherosclerosis and its clinical manifestations. Trends Cardiol Med 8:191, 1998

314. Parthasarathy S, Printz DJ, Boyd D, et al: Macrophage oxidation of low density lipoprotein generates a modified form recognized by the scavenger receptor. Arteriosclerosis 6:505–510, 1986

315. Parthasarathy S, Wieland E, Steinberg D: A role of endothelial cell lipoxygenase in the oxidative modification of low density lipoprotein. Proc Natl Acad Sci U S A 86:1046–1050, 1989

316. Steinberg D: Lipoproteins and atherosclerosis: A look back and a look ahead. Arteriosclerosis 3:283–301, 1983

317. Hansson GK, Jonasson L, Seifert PS, Stemme S: Immune mechanisms in atherosclerosis. Arteriosclerosis 9:567–578, 1989

318. Taylor KE, Glagov S, Zarins CK: Presentation and structural adaptation of endothelium over experimental foam cell lesions: Quantitative ultrastructural study. Arteriosclerosis 9:881–894, 1989

319. Hansson GK, Schwartz SM: Endothelial cell dysfunction without cell loss. In: Cryer A (ed): Biochemical Interactions at the Endothelium. New York, Elsevier Sciences, 1983, pp 343–361

320. Reidy MA, Schwartz SM: Endothelial injury and regeneration IV. Endotoxin: A nondenuding injury to aortic endothelium. Lab Invest 48:25–34, 1983

321. Reidy MA, Schwartz SM: Endothelial regeneration. III. Time course of intimal changes after small defined injury to rat aortic endothelium. Lab Invest 44:301–306, 1981

322. Langille BL, Adamson SL: Relationship between blood flow direction and endothelial cell orientation at arterial branch sites in rabbits and mice. Circ Res 48:481–488, 1981

323. Lindner V, Reidy MA, Fingerle J: Regrowth of arterial endothelium: Denudation with minimal trauma leads to complete endothelial cell regrowth. Lab Invest 61:556–563, 1989

324. Haudenschild CC, Schwartz SM: Endothelial regeneration. II. Restitution of endothelial continuity. Lab Invest 41:407–418, 1979

325. Schwartz SM, Gajdusek CM, Selden SC III: Vascular wall growth control: The role of the endothelium. Arteriosclerosis 1:107–126, 1981

326. Coomber BL, Gotlieb AI: In vitro endothelial wound repair interaction of cell migration and proliferation. Arteriosclerosis 10:215–222, 1990

327. Wong MKK, Gotlieb AI: Endothelial monolayer integrity: Perturbation of F-actin filaments and the dense peripheral band-vinculin network. Arteriosclerosis 10:76–84, 1990

328. Werns SW, Walton JA, Hsia HH, et al: Evidence of endothelial dysfunction in angiographically normal coronary arteries of patients with coronary artery disease. Circulation 79:287–291, 1989

329. Cotran RS: New roles for the endothelium in inflammation and immunity. Am J Pathol 129:407–413, 1987

330. Koo EWY, Gotlieb AI: Endothelial stimulation of intimal cell proliferation in a porcine aortic organ culture. Am J Pathol 134:497–503, 1989

331. Campbell GR, Campbell JH, Manderson JA, et al: Arterial smooth muscle: A multifunctional mesenchymal cell. Arch Pathol Lab Med 112:977–986, 1988

332. Gabella G: Structural apparatus for force transmission in smooth muscles. Physiol Rev 64:455–477, 1984

333. Chamley-Campbell JH, Campbell GR, Ross R: Phenotype-dependent responses of cultured aorta smooth muscle to serum mitogens. J Cell Biol 89:379–83, 1981

334. Campbell GR, Campbell JH, Remick R, et al: The influence of endothelial cells and macrophages on smooth muscle phenotype and proliferation. Atherosclerosis 7:389–393, 1986

335. Kocher O, Skalli O, Bloom WS, Gabbiani G: Cytoskeleton of rat aortic smooth muscle cells: Normal conditions and experimental intimal thickening. Lab Invest 50:645–652, 1984

336. Schmid E, Osborn M, Rungger-Bradle E, et al: Distribution of vimentin and desmin filaments in smooth muscle tissue of mammalian and avian aorta. Exp Cell Res 137:329–340, 1982

337. Reidy MA, Silver M: Endothelial regeneration. VII. Lack of intimal proliferation after defined injury to rat aorta. Am J Pathol 118:173–177, 1985

338. Fingerle J, Johnson R, Couser W, et al: Effects of thrombocytopenia on smooth muscle proliferation and intima formation in injured rat carotid. FASEB J:A1007, 1988

339. Clowes AW, Reidy MA, Clowes MM: Mechanisms of stenosis after arterial injury. Lab Invest 49:208–215, 1983

340. Groves H, Kinlough-Rathbone RL, Richardson M, et al: Thrombin generation and fibrin formation following injury to rabbit neointima: Studies of vessel wall reactivity and platelet survival. Lab Invest 46:605–612, 1982

341. Komuro I, Kurihara H, Sugiyama T, et al: Endothelin stimulates c-fos and c-myc expression and proliferation of vascular smooth muscle cells. FEBS Lett 238:249–252, 1988

342. Yanagisawa M, Tomoh M: Endothelin, a novel endothelium-derived peptide. Biochem Pharmacol 38:1877–1883, 1989

343. Fischer-Dzoga K, Fraser R, Wissler RW: Stimulation of proliferation in stationary primary cultures of monkey and rabbit aortic smooth muscle cells. I. Effects of lipoprotein fractions of hyperlipemic serum and lymph. Exp Mol Pathol 24:346, 1976

344. Martin BM, Gimbrone MA, Unanue ER, Cotran RS: Stimulation of nonlymphoid mesenchymal cell proliferation by a macrophage-derived growth factor. J Immunol 126:151–1515, 1981

345. Hansson GK, Jonasson L, Holm J, et al: γ-Interferon regulates vascular smooth muscle proliferation and Ia antigen expression in vivo and in vitro. Circ Res 63:712–719, 1988

346. Castellot JJ, Beeler DL, Rosenberg RD, Karnovsky MJ: Structural determinants of the capacity of heparin to inhibit the proliferation of vascular smooth muscle cells. J Cell Physiol 120:315, 1984

347. Fritze LMS, Reilly CF, Rosenberg RD: An antiproliferative heparan sulfate species produced by postconfluent smooth muscle cells. J Cell Biol 100:1041, 1985

348. Clowes AW, Clowes MM, Fingerle J, Reidy MA: Kinetics of cellular proliferation after arterial injury. V. Role of acute distension in the induction of smooth muscle proliferation. Lab Invest 60:360–364, 1989

349. Haudenschild CC, Grunwald J: Proliferative heterogeneity of vascular smooth muscle cells and its alteration by injury. Exp Cell Res 157:364–370, 1985

350. Hansson GK, Jonasson L, Holm J, Bondjers G: Cellular composition of the human atherosclerotic plaque. Fed Proc 43:786, 1984

351. Stemme S, Jonasson L, Holm J, Hansson GK: Immunologic control of vascular cell growth in arterial response to injury and atherosclerosis. Transplant Proc 24:3697–3699, 1989

352. Marston A: Vascular Disease of the Gastrointestinal Tract: Pathophysiology, Recognition and Management. Baltimore, Williams & Wilkins, 1986

353. Smith JA, Macleish DG, Collier NA: Aneurysms of visceral arteries. Aust N Z J Surg 59:329, 1988

354. Le Bas P, Batt M, Gagliardi JM, et al: Aneurysm of the inferior mesenteric artery associated with occlusion of the celiac axis and superior mesenteric artery. Ann Vasc Surg 1:254, 1986

355. Kazui T, Babe M, Komatsu S: Aneurysm of the celiac artery. J Cardiovasc Surg 29:567, 1988

356. Hussain S, Glover JL, Bree R, Bendick P: Penetrating atherosclerotic ulcers of the thoracic aorta. J Vasc Surg 9:710, 1989

357. Stanson AW, Kazmier FJ, Jollier LH, et al: Penetrating atherosclerotic ulcers of the thoracic aorta: Natural history and clinicopathologic correlations. Ann Vasc Surg 1:15, 1986

358. Bickerstaff LK, Hollier LH, Van Peenen JH, et al: Abdominal aortic aneurysm: The changing natural history. J Vasc Surg 1:6, 1984

359. Lord JW Jr, Rossi G, Dalema M, et al: Unsuspected abdominal aortic aneurysm as the cause of peripheral arterial occlusive disease. Ann Surg 177:767, 1973

360. Anderson WR, Richards AM: Evaluation of lower extremity muscle biopsies in the diagnosis of atheroembolism. Arch Pathol 86:535, 1968

361. Ramires G, O'Neill WM, Lambert R, Loomer HA: Cholesterol embolism: A complication of angiography. Arch Intern Med 138:1430, 1978

362. Scully RE, Mark EJ, McNelly BV: Case records of the Massachusetts General Hospital: Case 6-1987. N Engl J Med 316:321, 1987

363. Tilley WS, Siami G, Stone WJ: Renal failure due to cholesterol emboli following PTCA. Am Heart J 110:1301, 1985

364. Dahlberg PHF, Frecentese DR, Cogbill TH: Cholesterol embolism: Experience with 22 histologically proven cases. Surgery 105:737, 1989

365. Fisher DF Jr, Clagett GP, Brigham RA, et al: Dilemmas in dealing with the blue toe syndrome: Aortic versus peripheral source. Am J Surg 148:836, 1984

366. Chomette G, Auriol M, Trantaloc P, et al: Les embolies cholesteroliques: Incidence anatomique et expressions cliniques. Ann Med Interne (Paris) 131:17, 1980

367. Kealy WF: Atheroembolism. J Clin Pathol 31:984, 1978

368. Meyrier A, Bechet P, Simon P, et al: Atheromatous renal disease. Am J Med 85:139, 1988

369. Winter W Jr: Atheromatous emboli: A cause of cerebral infarction. Arch Pathol 64:137, 1957

370. Bengtsson H, Sonesson B, Bergqvist D: Incidence and prevalence of abdominal aortic aneurysms, estimated by necropsy studies and population screening by ultrasound. Ann N Y Acad Sci 800:1–24, 1996

371. Bickerstaff LK, Pairolero PC, Hollier LH, et al: Thoracic aortic aneurysms: A population-based study. Surgery 92:1103, 1982

372. Santiago F. Screening for abdominal aortic aneurysm: The U-boat in the belly (letter). JAMA 258:1932, 1987

373. Wolinsky H, Galgov S: Structural basis for the static mechanical properties of the aortic media. Circ Res 14:400, 1964

374. Gore E, Hirse AE: Atherosclerotic aneurysm of the abdominal aorta: A review. Prog Cardiovasc Dis 16:113, 1973

375. Halpert B, Williams RK: Aneurysms of the aorta: An analysis of 249 necropsies. Arch Pathol 74:163, 1962

376. Lilienfeld DE, Grumbersom PE, Sparfka JH, et al: Epidemiology of aortic aneurysm: First mortality trends in the United States, 1951–1981. Arteriosclerosis 7:637, 1987

377. Cole CW, Barber GG, Bouchard AG, et al: Abdominal aortic aneurysm: Consequences of a positive family history. Can J Surg 32:117, 1989

378. Johansen K, Koepsell T: Familial tendency for abdominal aortic aneurysm. JAMA 256:1934, 1986

379. Busuttil RW, Abou-zamzam AM, Machleder HI: Collagenase activity of the human aorta: A comparison of patients with and without abdominal aortic aneurysm. Arch Surg 115:1373, 1980

380. Campa JS, Greenhalgh RM, Powell JT: Elastin degradation in abdominal aortic aneurysms. Atherosclerosis 65:13, 1987

381. Tilson MD: A perspective on research in abdominal aortic aneurysm disease, with a unifying hypothesis. In: Yao JST (ed): Aortic Surgery. Philadelphia, WB Saunders, 1989, p 27

382. Nennhaus HH, Javid H: The distinct syndrome of spontaneous aorto-caval fistulae: An unknown complication of abdominal aortic aneurysm. Br J Surg 59:461, 1972

383. Crawford ES, Hess KR: Abdominal aortic aneurysm. N Engl J Med 321:1040, 1989

384. Cronenwett JL, Murphy TF, Zelonoch GB, et al: Actuarial analysis of variables associated with rupture of small abdominal aortic aneurysm. Surgery 98:472, 1985

385. Tilson MD, Boyd CD (ed): The abdominal aortic aneurysm. Ann N Y Acad Sci 80:1–298, 1996

386. Lopez-Candales A, Holmes DR, Liao S, et al: Decreased vascular smooth muscle cell density in medial degeneration of human abdominal aortic aneurysms. Am J Pathol 150:993–1007, 1997

387. Verloes A, Sakalihasan N, Limet R, Koulischer L: Genetic aspects of abdominal aortic aneurysm. Ann N Y Acad Sci 800:44–55, 1996

388. Blakemore AH, Voorhees AB Jr: Aneurysms of the aorta: A review of 365 cases. Angiology 5:209, 1954

389. Szilagyi DE, Smith RS, Maxwell AJ, et al: Expanding and rupturing abdominal aneurysms. Arch Surg 83:83, 1961

390. May AG, De Weese JA, Frank I, et al: Surgical treatment of abdominal aortic aneurysm. Surgery 663:711, 1968

391. Donaldson NC, Rosenberg JM, Buckman CA: Factors affecting survival after ruptured abdominal aortic aneurysm. J Vasc Surg 2:564, 1985

392. Liebermann DA, Keefer EB, Rahatzad N, et al: Ruptured abdominal aortic aneurysm causing obstructive jaundice. Dig Dis Sci 28:88, 1983

393. Merchant RF, Cafferata HT, de Palma RG: Ruptured aortic aneurysm seen initially as acute femoral neuropathy. Arch Surg 117:811, 1982

394. Karabin GA: Retroperitoneal hemorrhage. Am J Surg 56:471, 1942
395. Loewenthal J, Milton GW, Shead GU: Differential diagnosis of leaking retroperitoneal aneurysm. Med J Aust 2:137, 1959
396. Razzuk MA, Lington RR, Darling RC: Femoral neuropathy secondary to rupturous abdominal aortic aneurysm with false aneurysms. JAMA 201:139, 1967
397. Johnson WC, Dale ME, Gerzog SG, et al: The role of computer tomography in asymptomatic aortic aneurysm. Surg Gynecol Obstet 162:49, 1986
398. Senapati A, Hurst PAE, Thomas MD, et al: Differentiation of ruptured aortic aneurysm from acute expansion by computerized tomography. J Cardiovasc Surg 27:719, 1986
399. Weinbaum SE, Dubner S, Tuner JW: The accuracy of computer tomography in the diagnosis of retroperitoneal blood in the presence of abdominal aortic aneurysm. J Vasc Surg 6:11, 1987
400. Carruthers R, Sauerbrei E, Gutelius J, Brown P: Sealed abdominal aortic aneurysm imitating metastatic carcinoma. J Vasc Surg 4:529, 1986
401. Rosenthal D, Clark MD, Stanton PE, Lamis PA: "Chronic-contained" rupture abdominal aortic aneurysm: Is it real? J Cardiovasc Surg 27:723, 1986
402. Jones CS, Reilly K, Dowsing MC, Glover JL: Chronic contained rupture of abdominal aortic aneurysm. Arch Surg 121:542, 1986
403. Flynn WR, Courtney DS, Yao JST, Bergan J: Contained rupture of aortic aneurysm. In: Bergan JJ, Yao JST (eds): Aortic Surgery. Philadelphia, WB Saunders, 1989
404. Johnson J, McDevitt NB, Procter HS, et al: Emergence or elective operation for symptomatic abdominal aortic aneurysm. Arch Surg 110:654, 1975
405. Brennann BH, Sheppard AD, Ernst CB: Aortoenteric and caval fistulae. In: Bergan JJ, Yao JST (eds): Aortic Surgery. Philadelphia, WB Saunders, 1989, p 497
406. Sweeney MS, Gadacz TR: Primary aortoduodenal fistula: Manifestations, diagnosis and treatment. Surgery 96:492, 1984
407. Baker WH, Sharrer LA, Ehrenhaf JL: Aortocaval fistula as a complication of abdominal aortic aneurysm. Surgery 72:933, 1972
408. Dardik J, Dardik I, Strom MG: Intravenous rupture of arteriosclerotic aneurysms of the abdominal aorta. Surgery 647, 1976
409. Yashar JJ, Hallman GL, Colley DA: Fistula between aneurysm of aorta and left renal vein: Report of a case. Arch Surg 86:51, 1969
410. Perry MO: Infected aortic aneurysms. J Vasc Surg 2:597, 1985
411. Zak KG, Strauss L, Saphra I: Rupture of diseased large arteries in the course of enterobacterial (*Salmonella*) infections. N Engl J Med 258:824, 1958
411a. Jarrett F, Darling RC, Munolth ED, et al: Experience with infected aneurysms of the abdominal aorta. Arch Surg 110:1281, 1975
412. McNamara MF, Finnegan MO, Bakshy KR: Abdominal aortic aneurysms infected by *Escherichia coli*. Surgery 98:87, 1985
413. McAuley CE, Steed DL, Webster MMV: Bacterial presence in aortic thrombus at elective aneurysm resection: Is it clinically significant? Am J Surg 147:322, 1984
414. Schwartz JA, Powell TW, Burnham SH, Johnson G: Culture of abdominal aortic aneurysm contents. Arch Surg 122:777, 1987
415. Sommerville RL, Allen EV, Edwards JE: Bland and infected arteriosclerotic abdominal aortic aneurysms: A clinicopathologic study. Medicine (Baltimore) 38:207, 1959
416. Walker DI, Bloor K, Williams G, Gillie I: Inflammatory aneurysms of the abdominal aorta. Br J Surg 59:609, 1972
417. Crawford, JL, Stowe CL, Safi JH, et al: Inflammatory aneurysms of the aorta. J Vasc Surg 2:113, 1985
418. Feiner HD, Raghavendra BN, Phelps R, et al: Inflammatory abdominal aortic aneurysms: Report of six cases. Hum Pathol 15:454, 1984
419. Gaylis H, Isaacson C: Abdominal aortic inflammatory aneurysms. In: Bergan JJ, Yao JST (eds): Aortic Surgery. Philadelphia, WB Saunders, 1989, p 267
420. Savarese RP, Rosenfeld JC, De Laurentis DA: Inflammatory abdominal aortic aneurysm. Surg Gynecol Obstet 162:405, 1986
421. Sterpetti A, Hunter WJ, Feldhaus RJ, et al: Inflammatory aneurysm of the abdominal aorta: Incidence, pathological and etiologic considerations. J Vasc Surg 9:643, 1989
422. Darke SG, Glass RE, Eadie DA: Abdominal aortic aneurysm: Perianeurysmal fibrosis and ureteric obstruction and deviation. Br J Surg 64:649, 1977
423. James TGI: Uraemia due to aneurysm of the abdominal aorta. Br J Urol 7:157, 1935
424. Labardini MM, Ratcliff RK: The abdominal aortic aneurysm and the ureter. J Urol 98:590, 1967
425. Szilagyi DE, Elliott JP, Smith RF: Clinical fate of the patient with asymptomatic abdominal aneurysm and unfit for surgical treatment. Arch Surg 104:600, 1972
426. Pennell RC, Hollier LH, Lie JT, et al: Inflammatory abdominal aortic aneurysms: A 30 year review. J Vasc Surg 2:859, 1983
427. Cullenward MJ, Scalan KA, Pozniak MA, Archer CA: Inflammatory aortic aneurysm (periaortic fibrosis): Radiologic imaging. Radiology 159:75, 1986
428. Ramires AA, Riles TS, Imparato AM, Meighbow AJ: CAT scans of inflammatory aneurysms: A new technique for preoperative diagnosis. Surgery 91:390, 1982
429. Clyne CAC, Abercrombi GF: Perianeurysmal retroperitoneal fibrosis: Two cases responding to steroid. Br J Urol 49:463, 1977
430. Rose AG, Dent DM: Inflammatory variant of abdominal atherosclerotic aneurysm. Arch Pathol Lab Med 105: 4049, 1981
431. Gaylis H: Pathogenesis of anastomotic aneurysms. Surgery 90:509, 1981
432. Mitchinson MJ: The pathology of idiopathic retroperitoneal fibrosis. J Clin Pathol 23:681, 1970
433. Cole SD, Lie JT: Inflammatory aneurysm of the aorta, aortitis and coronary arteritis. Arch Pathol Lab Med 112:1121, 1988
434. Serra RM, Engle JE, Jones RE, et al: Perianeurysmal retroperitoneal fibrosis: A universal case of renal failure. Am J Med 68:149, 1980
435. Du Bost C, Allary M, Oeconomos N: Resection of an aneurysm of the abdominal aorta: Re-establishment of the continuity by a preserved human arterial graft, with results after five months. Arch Surg 64:405, 1952
436. De Bakey ME, Crawford ES, Cooley DA, et al: Aneurysm of abdominal aorta: Analysis of results of graft replacement therapy one to eleven years after operation. Ann Surg 160:622, 1964
437. Hicks GL, Eastland MW, de Weese JA, et al: Survival improvement following aortic aneurysm resection. Ann Surg 181:654, 1975
438. Thompson JE, Hollier LH, Patman RD, Person AV: Surgical management of abdominal aneurysms: Factors influencing mortality and morbidity in a 20-year experience. Ann Surg 181:654, 1975
439. Golden GT, Sears HF, Wellows HA Jr, et al: Paraplegia complicating resection of aneurysms of the infrarenal abdominal aorta. Surgery 73:91, 1973
440. Wittenstein GJ: Complications of aortic aneurysm surgery: Prevention and treatment. Thorac Cardiovasc Surg 35, Spec No 2:136, 1987
441. Bane AE, McClerkin WW: A study of shock: Acidosis and the declamping phenomenon. Ann Surg 161:41, 1965
442. Strom JA, Bernhard VB, Towne JB: Acute limb ischemia following aortic reconstruction: A preventable cause of the overall increased mortality. Arch Surg 119: 420, 1984
443. Fry PD: Colonic ischemia after aortic reconstruction. Can J Surg 31:162, 1988
444. Johnson WC, Nabseth DC: Visceral infarction following aortic surgery. Ann Surg 180:312, 1974
445. Schroeder T, Christoffersen JK, Andersen J, et al: Ischemic colitis complicating reconstruction of abdominal aorta. Surg Gynecol Obstet 160:299, 1985
446. Welling RE, Roeder Sheiner LR, Arbaugh JJ, et al: Ischemic colitis following repair of ruptured abdominal aortic aneurysm. Arch Surg 120:1368, 1985
447. Ernst CB: Prevention of intestinal ischemia following abdominal aortic construction. Surgery 93:102, 1983
448. Kim MW, Hundahl SA, Dang CR, et al: Ischemic colitis after aortic aneurysmectomy. Am J Surg 145:392, 1983
449. Goldgraber MB, Kirsner B: The Arthus phenomenon in the colon of rabbits. Arch Path 667:566, 1959
450. Vollman JF, Kogel H: Aorto-enteric fistulas as postoperative complication. J Cardiovasc Surg 28:473, 1987
451. Champion MC, Sullivan SN, Coles JC, et al: Aortoenteric fistula: Incidence, presentation, recognition and management. Ann Surg 195:314, 1982
452. Yao JST, Flinn WR, Rizzo RJ, et al: Recurrent aortic and anastomotic aneurysms. In: Bergan JJ, Yao JST (eds): Aortic Surgery. Philadelphia, WB Saunders, 1989

453. Plate G, Hollier LA, O'Brien P, et al: Recurrent aneurysms and late vascular complications following repair of abdominal aortic aneurysms. Arch Surg 120:590, 1985

454. Szilagyi DE, Smith RF, Elliott JP, et al: Anastomotic aneurysm after vascular reconstruction. Surgery 78:800, 1975

455. Moore WS, Hall AD: Late suture failure in the pathogenesis of anastomotic false aneurysms. Ann Surg 172:1064, 1970

456. Clagett GP, Salander JM, Eddlemann WL, et al: Dilation of knitted Dacron aortic prosthesis and anastomotic false aneurysms: Etiologic consideration. Surgery 110:153, 1983

457. Gaylis H: Etiology of abdominal aortic inflammatory aneurysms: Hypothesis (letter). J Vasc Surg 23:643, 1985

458. Treiman GS, Weaver FA, Crossman DV, et al: Anastomotic false aneurysms of the abdominal aorta and the iliac arteries. J Vasc Surg 8:268, 1988

459. O'Hara PJ, Hertzer NR, Beven EG, Krajewski LP: Surgical management of infected abdominal aortic grafts: Review of a 25-year experience. J Vasc Surg 3:725, 1986

460. Lorentzen JE, Nielsen OM, Arendrup H, et al: Vascular graft infection: An analysis of sixty-two graft infections in 2411 consecutively implanted synthetic vascular grafts. Surgery 98:81, 1985

461. Weinstein MH, Machleder HI: Sexual function after aorto-iliac surgery. Ann Surg 191:787, 1975

462. Sacks D, Miller J: Ureteral leak around bifurcation graft: A complication of ureteral stenting. J Urology 140:1526, 1988

463. Lord RD, Nankivell C, Graham AR, Tracy GD: Duodenal obstruction following abdominal aortic reconstruction. Ann Vasc Surg 1: 597, 1987

464. Delen D, Volckaer A, Van Der Brande P, Stadmik P: Spinal osteomyelitis: An unusual complication in aortic graft surgery. J Cardiovasc Surg 28:743, 1987

465. Bak S, Gravgaard E: Aneurysm of an arterial prosthesis. A case report. Acta Chir Scad 152:763, 1986

466. Brandham RR, Gregoire HB, Wilson R: Chylous ascetis following resection of an abdominal aortic aneurysm. Ann Surg 36:238, 1970

467. Morse DE: Embryology, anatomy and histology of the aorta. In: Lindsay J Jr, Jurst JW (eds). The Aorta. Orlando, FL, Grune & Stratton, 1979, p 15

468. Pressler V, McNamara JJ: Thoracic aortic aneurysms: Natural history and treatment. J Thorac Cardiovasc Surg 79:489, 1980

469. Treiman GS, Berhnard VM: Endovascular treatment of abdominal aortic aneurysms. Annu Rev Med 49:363–373, 1998

470. Marchand F: Uber arteriosklerose (atherosclerose). Ver Kongr Inn Med 21:23, 1904

471. Kakkar VV: Peripheral vascular disease. Medicine (Baltimore) 24/27:95, 1978

472. Robbs JV: Atherosclerotic peripheral arterial disease in blacks: An established problem. S Afr Med J 67:797, 1985

473. Lindbom A: Arteriosclerosis and arterial thrombosis in the lower limb: A roentgenological study. Acta Radiol (suppl):1–80, 1950

474. Rodda R: Arteriosclerosis in the lower limbs. J Pathol 65:315, 1953

475. Wagner M, Taitel A: A correlated anatomic study of degenerative disease at the bifurcations of the abdominal aorta and the common carotid arteries. Angiology 13: 284, 1962

476. Schenk EA: Pathology of occlusive disease of the lower extremities. Cardiovasc Clin 5:287–310, 1973

477. Kinmonth JB, Rob CG, Simeone FA: Vascular Surgery. London, Edward Arnold, 1962

478. Gaylis H: Popliteal artery aneurysms: A review of analysis of 55 cases. S Afr Med J 48:75, 1974

479. Pickering G: Arteriosclerosis and atherosclerosis. Am J Med 34:7, 1963

480. Reiner L: Mesenteric vascular occlusion studied by postmortem injection of the mesenteric arterial circulation. In: Sommers SC (ed): Cardiovascular Pathology Decennial: 1966–1975. East Norwalk, CT, Appleton-Century-Crofts, 1975, p 315

481. Marston A: Vascular diseases of the alimentary tract. Clin Gastroenterol 1:3, 1973

482. Marston A: Intestinal Ischeamia. London, Edward Arnold, 1977

483. Coligado EY, Fleshler B: Reversible vascular occlusion of the colon. Radiology 89:432, 1967

Nonatherosclerotic Diseases of the Aorta and Miscellaneous Diseases of the Main Pulmonary Arteries and Large Veins

Renu Virmani • Allen P. Burke

In the Western world, the most important disease of the aorta and its major branches is atherosclerosis, which often results in abdominal aortic aneurysms and peripheral vessel stenoses. Perhaps even more frequent than atherosclerosis are degenerative changes of aging, which are usually asymptomatic, but may lead to annular dilatation and aortic insufficiency. Aortic dissections, which have various causes, are less frequent but often produce catastrophic illness. Inflammatory conditions of the aorta are likewise uncommon. They are a diverse group that include infections, collagen vascular or autoimmune diseases, and idiopathic conditions. The aorta, a high-pressure conduit, is especially prone to trauma, most often manifest by lethal rupture or formation of pseudoaneurysms of the descending thoracic aorta (see Chapter 18). Although rare, primary thrombosis of the vessel may occur in the absence of atherosclerotic plaques.

With the exception of atherosclerosis, which is discussed in Chapter 4, the major pathologic conditions of the aorta are discussed in this chapter. Additional topics include sarcomas of the great vessels and a variety of thrombotic, inflammatory, and congenital processes involving the main branches of both the pulmonary arteries and the venae cavae. Diseases of the pulmonary circulation, including the distal tree, are presented in Chapter 7.

AGING CHANGES OF THE AORTA

The aorta was called "the greatest artery" by the ancients. This designation is appropriate because the aorta absorbs the impact of 2.3 to 3 billion heartbeats a year while delivering roughly 200 million liters of blood to the various parts of the body.[1] The vessel absorbs the impact of systole by distending. During diastole, the aortic wall recoils, helping to propel the blood distally. Therefore, its elastic properties are essential in maintaining this pumping function. Because loss of elasticity in soft tissue is a function of senescence, it is not surprising that advanced age changes aortic hemodynamics. Histologically, the aging aorta demonstrates fragmentation of elastin with a concomitant increase in collagen, resulting in an increased collagen/elastin ratio and leading to a loss in its distensibility.[2] The degeneration of elastin produces increased wall stiffness, leading to an increased pulse wave velocity.[3–5] It has been shown that interruption of the vasa vasorum may also lead to an acutely decreased distensibility in the ascending aorta.[6] The changes in elastic tissue incurred as a result of old age are reflected in further gross and microscopic abnormalities. The aorta becomes tortuous because of an increase in its length, and its intimal surface doubles between the second and sixth decades. The vessel's circumference likewise increases with age, with the largest increase occurring in the ascending portion and the smallest in the abdominal aorta.[7] Medial thickness does not change significantly, whereas intimal thickness increases with age, the greatest increase occurring in the abdominal aorta. Age changes are also discussed in Chapter 3.

Hypertension and atherosclerosis greatly affect the extent of age-related aortic changes. Hypertension accentuates age-related increase in abdominal aortic circumference. Hypertension and atherosclerosis both have a marked effect by increasing abdominal aortic circumference and intimal thickness.[7]

ANNULOAORTIC ECTASIA

Definition

Annuloaortic ectasia, a term used principally by surgeons, was introduced in 1961 to denote aneurysmal dilatation of the ascending aorta with pure aortic valve regurgitation.[8] In the broadest sense, the term is employed when specific conditions, such as Takayasu disease, cause aortic aneurysm with valvular insufficiency.[9] However, the term is generally restricted to cases of idiopathic medial degeneration of the aorta,[10] in patients with or without Marfan syndrome. The percentage of patients with extracardiac manifestations of Marfan syndrome varies from 16 to 22% at the low end[11, 12] to more than 50%[13] at the high end.

Clinical Findings

Idiopathic annuloaortic ectasia is more common in men than in women and typically appears in the fourth, fifth, and sixth decades. Patients with Marfan syndrome are diagnosed at a much younger age with symptoms of aortic root dilatation often occurring in their third and fourth decades, and they are more likely to have a family history of aortic disease. The tendency to group together idiopathic annuloaortic ectasia and Marfan syndrome comes from the difficulty in clearly separating the two entities. Annuloaortic ectasia in patients with and without

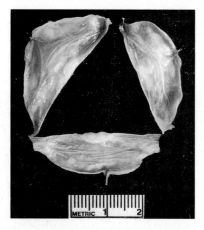

Figure 5-1 • Aortic insufficiency secondary to aortic root dilatation. The three valve cusps are relatively normal except for their increased annular circumference. This 51-year-old man had idiopathic aortic root dilatation. (From Virmani R, Burke AP, Farb A [eds]: Atlas of Cardiovascular Pathology. Philadelphia, WB Saunders, 1996, p 56.)

Marfan syndrome forms a continuum, because a family history can often be elicited from patients without manifestations of the syndrome.[11] The specific cardiovascular features of Marfan syndrome are discussed later, as is aortic dissection, the second most common complication of annuloaortic ectasia after aortic insufficiency.

Aortic root dilatation accounts for more than 50% of aortic valve replacements for pure aortic regurgitation, and, in the majority of patients, the cause is idiopathic[14] (Fig. 5-1). The remaining patients have known defects such as Marfan syndrome, inflammatory aortic disease, osteogenesis imperfecta, operated congenital heart disease, or intrinsic valve disease.

Pathogenesis and Pathologic Findings

The cause of annuloaortic ectasia is unknown and may be partly due to age-related degenerative changes. However, inherited genetic defects certainly have a causative role, as demonstrated by the presence of aortic root dilatation in first-degree relatives of more than 50% of patients.[11] The precise nature of the genetic defects in patients without Marfan syndrome has yet to be determined.

Grossly, the proximal aorta is dilated, resulting in a pear-shaped, symmetric enlargement. Aortic valve incompetence is secondary to dilatation of the aortic wall at the commissural level, so that cusps are effectively shortened and cannot converge during systole. The aneurysmal process may involve the entire ascending aorta but generally spares the arch. Dissections may occur within the ectatic aorta and be incidentally discovered during surgery. However, the majority of acute aortic dissections occur in the absence of a root aneurysm.[15]

Histologic findings are nonspecific and include cystic medial degeneration of the aortic wall, which may be a causative factor in aortic weakness. The affected aortic wall is prone to dissection and aortic rupture without dissection.[12] It has been suggested that dissections, when they occur, are usually small, circumscribed, and limited to the ascending aorta.[1] The elastic composition of the aorta in patients with annuloaortic ectasia is decreased in some cases and associated with fibrosis and elastin fragmentation histologically. This decrease does not, however, correlate with family history or degree of aortic root dilatation.[16]

Pathologic changes in the aortic valve result from the inability of its cusps to close during diastole. Secondary changes may follow from increased tension and bowing of the cusps. These include thickening and retraction of the cusps, which increase the valves' inability to close and intensify aortic regurgitation.[17] Reduced aortic distensibility may also contribute to gradual left ventricular dilatation and dysfunction observed in patients with chronic aortic regurgitation.[18]

ANEURYSM OF THE SINUS OF VALSALVA

Aneurysm of the sinus of Valsalva was first described in 1839.[1] An aneurysm results from a weakness in the sinus wall leading to a dilatation, or blind pouch (diverticulum), forming in one wall, usually the right.

Most aneurysms are congenital and have a strong association with a ventricular septal defect (VSD). Other congenital anomalies associated with sinus of Valsalva aneurysms include coarctation of the aorta and the bicuspid aortic valve. This congenital aneurysm may result from a lack of fusion between the elastica of the aortic media and the heart at the fibrous annulus of the aortic valve. Infective endocarditis and syphilis, which destroy tissue in this area, currently account for the majority of acquired aneurysms of the sinus of Valsalva. The latter represent fewer than 20% of total cases.

Patients' ages at which congenital aneurysms appear range from 11 to 67 years, with a mean of 34 years. Asians and men seem more susceptible to aneurysms than Caucasians and women.[19] In a clinical review of 377 cases, the majority of aneurysms were located in the right sinus (81%) and were equally divided between those associated with VSD (46%) and those without VSD (54%). The next most frequent site was the noncoronary sinus (17%); at this site, only 6% of lesions were associated with VSD. Only 2% were reported in the left coronary sinus.[20]

The clinical course before rupture is silent. In patients with associated VSD, heart failure and mitral regurgitation may occur. Rupture of the aneurysm results in symptoms that depend upon the amount of blood that flows through the rupture site and the chamber of flow. In those patients, cardiovascular collapse and even sudden death occurs. In those who survive the initial rupture, cardiomegaly is usual.[21] Aortic regurgitation is present in one third of patients and right-or left-sided heart failure occurs in 80%. Chest pain is usually absent. The aneurysmal sac may obstruct the right ventricular tract and (rarely) cause coronary occlusion; conduction disturbances are also reported.

Location of an aneurysm within the right sinus of Valsalva predicts its site of rupture. Those in the left portion of the right sinus protrude toward, and rupture into, the right ventricular outflow tract near the pulmonary valve; VSD is frequently associated with this partic-

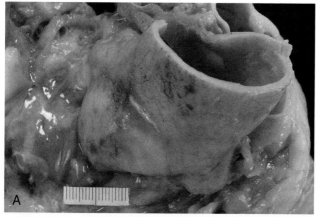

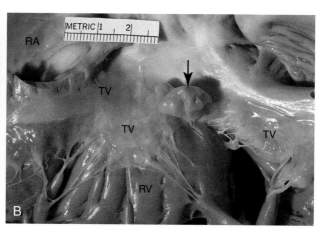

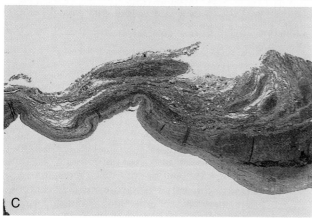

Figure 5-2 • *A*, Left sinus of Valsalva aneurysm projecting into pericardial cavity 1.0 cm beyond aortic wall. Incidental finding in a 74-year-old man who died of ischemic heart disease. (Courtesy of Dr. M.D. Silver). *B*, Eighteen-year-old male with incidental sinus of Valsalva aneurysm affecting the noncoronary sinus, who died of dehiscence of a repaired coarctation of the aorta. Note the aneurysm bulging into the right atrium (arrow). (TV = tricuspid valve, RA = right atrium, and RV = right ventricle). *C*, This 51-year-old man had sudden onset of congestive heart failure. A diagnosis of sinus of Valsalva aneurysm ruptured into the right ventricle was made, and the patient underwent surgical repair. A portion of the sinus of Valsalva and the aneurysmal wall were submitted for histology. Note the atrophied wall of the sinus (right) and replacement by smooth muscle cells in a proteoglycan matrix and collagen in aneursym wall (left) with absence of elastic tissue (Movat stain).

ular anomaly. Those that arise in the mid-right sinus protrude and rupture into the body of the right ventricle; associated VSD is uncommon. When an aneurysm originates from the posterior portion of the right sinus, it protrudes toward the plane of the tricuspid valve and rupture usually occurs into the right atrium.[22] Other reported sites of rupture of aneurysms located in the right or left sinuses are left ventricle and atrium, pericardium, pulmonary artery, and superior vena cava. (See discussion of annular abscesses in Chapter 14.)

The diameter of the rupture site at the base of the sinus ranges from 0.4 to 1.1 cm (mean 0.7 cm) (Fig. 5-2*A*, *B*, *C*). The wall of the aneurysm is thin and consists of smooth muscle cells in a proteoglycan matrix; usually, no elastic fibers are identified.

AORTIC DISSECTION

Aortic dissection, the passage of the blood within the media, occurs infrequently, but when it does, consequences are often catastrophic. The incidence in the United States is 2000 cases per year.[23] Mortality is high and has been estimated at 1% per hour if the condition is untreated. Aortic dissections occur more frequently in men than in women (2 or 3 : 1), and, in the absence of Marfan syndrome, usually occur in individuals older than 60 years of age. There is often a history of long-standing systemic hypertension, which explains the high prevalence of aortic dissections in African Americans. The

majority of dissections arise because of an acquired or inherited weakness of the aortic media that is manifested by cystic medial necrosis. Rare causes include aortitis and medial dysplasia, which can be diagnosed only by histologic examination. Advanced atherosclerosis is rarely observed in individuals with aortic dissection, although mild to moderate disease may be present. Dissections that occur in those with atherosclerosis-induced mural hematoma (so-called penetrating atherosclerotic ulcer) are, by definition, limited in extent. (These ulcers are also discussed in Chapter 4.)

Classification

Of the three classifications of aortic dissection in use, the most frequently employed is that of DeBakey (Fig. 5-3). In a type I DeBakey dissection, the tear is located in the ascending aorta, with the dissection extending to the descending aorta (Figs. 5-3, 5-4*A*). It is the most common dissection, which occurs in 54% of cases.[24] In type II dissections (21% of the total), the intimal tear is also located in the ascending aorta, but the dissection is limited to that part of the vessel (Figs. 5-3, 5-4*B*). The remaining 25% are type III dissections, which differ fundamentally from other types, because the intimal tear is in the descending or transverse aorta, usually in the distal arch or the proximal descending vessel (Figs. 5-3, 5-5*A*, *B*). Type III dissections are further classified into type IIIa (dissection extending retrograde into the ascending

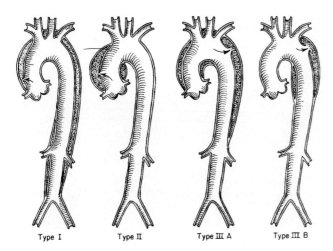

Type I   Type II   Type III A   Type III B

Figure 5-3 • DeBakey classification of aortic dissections showing sites of intimal tears and extent of dissections. (From Isselbacher EM, Eagle KA, Desanctis RW: Diseases of the aorta. In: Braunwald E [ed]: Heart Disease. A Textbook of Cardiovascular Medicine. Philadelphia, WB Saunders, 1997, p 1555.)

aorta, which accounts for 9% of the total) and type IIIb (dissection confined to the transverse arch or the descending aorta, which accounts for 16% of total).

The Stanford classification is based on the site of dissection, with type A signifying involvement of the ascending aorta irrespective of its site of origin, and type B not involving the ascending aorta. A simplified classification that is functionally nearly identical to the Stanford is based simply on the site of the intimal tear (proximal vs. distal). Because the etiologic bases for aortic dissections vary with the site of the intimal tear, this simplified classification is best when discussing pathogenesis; however, clinically, the DeBakey classification is used widely.

Proximal dissections are likely to result in death or life-threatening symptoms, and are, therefore, usually at an acute stage, at autopsy, or in surgical specimens. Distal dissections are more often chronic, demonstrating organized thrombus within the dissection plane and adventitial scarring.

Associated Conditions and Etiologic Factors

Cystic medial degeneration of the aorta is the usual histologic change underlying most types of aortic dissection. The most common associated pathologic conditions are hypertension, bicuspid aortic valve, and Marfan syndrome (Table 5-1). In approximately 20% of patients, no known associations exist other than idiopathic aortic root dilatation (annuloaortic ectasia) in those with proximal dissections.

Hypertension

Hypertension is present in 80% of patients with type III dissections and in about half of those with types I and II dissections (see Table 5-1). The mechanism of medial degeneration in these patients is not known. Because hypertension is far more prevalent than aortic dissection, there are likely additional factors that predispose hypertensive patients with aortic dissection to their aortic disease. There appears to be little interrelationship between hypertension and other major associated conditions because it is present in only 2 to 9% of Marfan patients with aortic dissection and in 2 to 8% of those with bicuspid aortic valve and dissection. The peak incidence of aortic dissection in hypertensive patients is in their sixth and seventh decades, with men affected twice as often as women.

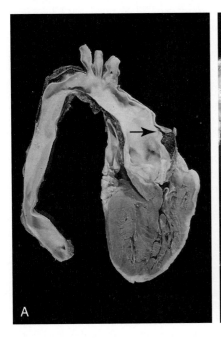
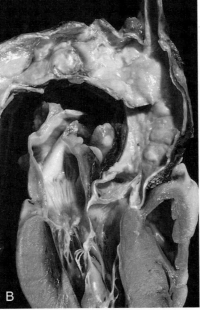

Figure 5-4 • *A*, Aortic dissection, idiopathic, type I. A 61-year-old man had a sudden onset of anterior chest pain and died within 1 hour. He had no history of systemic hypertension. At autopsy, there was hemopericardium and an aortic tear located 2.5 cm distal to the aortic valve (arrow). The dissection extended the entire length of the aorta. *B*, Aortic dissection, related to hypertension, type II. A 42-year-old man with a history of remote myocardial infarction and hypertension had severe substernal chest pain radiating to the back and right arm. He died soon after admission to the hospital. At autopsy, there was hemopericardium and a transverse tear of the ascending aorta 4 cm distal to the aortic valve, which had three cusps. The dissection extended to involve the arch vessels but did not go into the abdominal aorta. Note moderate atherosclerosis without plaque ulceration. No cystic medial necrosis was present in histologic sections of the aorta.

Figure 5-5 • *A,* Aortic dissection, related to hypertension, type III. A 71-year-old man with systemic hypertension, dead after rupturing a dissecting saccular aneurysm into the left pleural cavity. A healed dissection was present in the descending thoracic aorta and extended just distal to the left renal artery (not shown). There was organizing thrombus in the large aneurysm near the left subclavian artery. Note fibrous tags in the false lumen at sites of intercostal artery origin. The probe entered the site of the tear and extended into the large false lumen. (From Virmani R, Burke AP, Farb A [eds]: Atlas of Cardiovascular Pathology. Philadelphia, WB Saunders, 1996, p 130.) *B,* Aortic transverse sections from the descending aorta of a 75-year-old black woman who had abdominal pain and an abdominal bruit. Chest computed tomographic scans (CT) and magnetic resonance imaging (MRI) demonstrated a thoracic aortic aneurysm. Transesophageal echocardiography showed a type III dissection. The patient was treated medically for hypertension and congestive heart failure but died suddenly 48 hours after admission. Note the site of dissection in an area of atherosclerotic plaque (arrow) and the dissection extending distally. There is early organization of the thrombus in the false lumen (F).

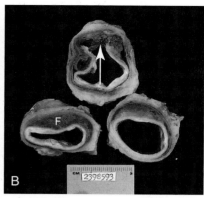
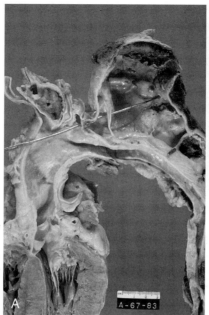

Bicuspid and Unicuspid Aortic Valve

The association between a congenitally malformed aortic valve and aortic dissection was first reported by Abbott in 1927. It was subsequently demonstrated that this association is present only in type I and type II dissections.[24] Of 551 cases reported from four autopsy series, a bicuspid valve was present in 54 (10%),[24–27] which was more than fivefold the rate of occurrence of bicuspid valves in the general population. A population-based study demonstrated that the relative risk for aortic dissection in patients with a congenital bicuspid valve was 9 times greater than that in normal subjects, and 18 times greater in those with a congenital unicuspid valve.[24] This increased relative risk was reflected in a higher frequency

of bicuspid (10 times greater) and unicuspid valves (22 times greater) in patients with types I and II aortic dissection, compared with the general autopsy population. In contrast, the incidence of congenital bicuspid valve in type III dissections was not increased.[24] The mechanism of aortic dissection in patients with bicuspid aortic valve appears to be independent of hemodynamic alterations secondary to aortic stenosis, because significant valvular stenosis was observed in only 38%[24] (Fig. 5-6). It remains to be documented whether aortic cystic medial change is associated with bicuspid aortic valve in the absence of aortic dissection.

Marfan Syndrome

Marfan syndrome accounts for 6 to 9% of all aortic dissections. Conversely, aortic dissections occur in over one third of patients with this syndrome. Of 16 patients with Marfan syndrome in Larson and Edwards' population-based study, 7 (44%) had aortic dissections,[24] 3 had type I dissection, 3 had type II dissection, and 1 had type III dissection.

Miscellaneous Conditions

In addition to hypertension, Marfan syndrome, and congenitally malformed aortic valves, other conditions underlie, or are associated with, aortic dissection. A link between pregnancy and aortic dissection has been postulated but not corroborated in some studies.[24] Over half the aortic dissections in women occur among those who are 40 years of age or younger, with some occurring during pregnancy, usually in the third trimester and rarely in the postpartum period. Increases in blood pressure, blood volume, and cardiac output have been implicated as causa-

TABLE 5-1 • **Frequency of Factors Predisposing to Aortic Dissection From Published Reprints**

	Hypertension (%)	Marfan Syndrome (%)	Bicuspid AV (%)	None (%)
Type I/II	52[1]	5[1]	14–16[1, 3]	27[1]
Type III	75–83[1, 2]	2[1]	0–2[1, 3]	15–21[1, 2, 6]
Total	63–69[4, 5]	5–9[4, 5]	2–8[3, 4]	26[4]

1. Larson EW, Edwards WD: Risk factors for aortic dissection: A necropsy study of 161 cases. Am J Cardiol 53:849–855, 1984
2. Roberts CS, Roberts WC: Aortic dissection with the entrance tear in the descending thoracic aorta. Analysis of 40 necropsy patients. Ann Surg 213:356–368, 1991
3. Roberts CS, Roberts WC: Dissection of the aorta associated with congenital malformation of the aortic valve. J Am Coll Cardiol 17:712–716, 1991
4. Nakashima Y, Kurozumi T, Sueishi K, Tanaka K: Dissecting aneurysm: A clinicopathologic and histopathologic study of 111 autopsied cases. Hum Pathol 21:291–296, 1990
5. Wilson SK, Hutchins GM: Aortic dissecting aneurysms: Causative factors in 204 subjects. Arch Pathol Lab Med 106:175–180, 1982
6. Some distal dissections may be precipitated by rupture of calcified atheromas
AV, aortic valve.

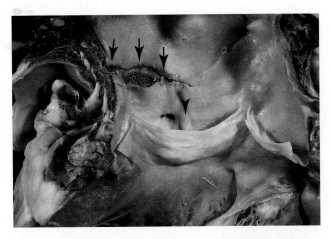

Figure 5-6 • Aortic dissection associated with bicuspid aortic valve. A 32-year-old hypertensive white man had a history of headaches for 2 weeks. He experienced severe pain in midchest, right shoulder, and neck and cardiac arrest 3 hours later in the emergency room. He had a hemopericardium at autopsy. The heart weighed 550 g, and a transverse tear (arrows) was noted 1 cm distal to the sinotubular junction distal to the right coronary ostium. The aortic valve was congenitally bicuspid, with the commissures located anterior and posteriorly and a raphe (arrowhead) in the right coronary sinus. The ascending aorta was dilated to 11 cm in circumference. The dissection extended to the arch vessels. Histologic sections showed focal mild medial degeneration in the aortic wall.

tive factors, but a clear link between pregnancy and aortic dissection has yet to be documented.

Familial dissections in the absence of Marfan syndrome have been reported with increasing frequency.[28] To date, it is uncertain whether these patients have a forme fruste of Marfan syndrome with a similar genetic defect.

Cardiac surgery is associated with an increased risk of aortic dissection, usually occurring at an anastomotic site (aortotomy or site of saphenous vein grafting) or at the site of cross-clamping. The most common surgical procedure complicated by aortic dissection is aortic valve replacement. A majority of these iatrogenic dissections are discovered during the operation and repaired, but 20% are discovered in the early postoperative period. A few occur as a late complication. Rarely, aortic dissections are observed after cardiac catheterization or intra-aortic balloon pump insertion and are thought to result from direct trauma to the intima. It is unclear whether patients with iatrogenic dissections are at increased risk because of inherent weakness in their aortas. In such cases, careful histologic evaluation for the presence of cystic medial change is warranted.

Uncommon conditions associated with aortic dissection include Noonan and Turner syndromes as well as coarctation of the aorta. An association with cocaine abuse has been postulated, but it is unclear whether this is mediated by catecholamine-induced hypertension. Blunt trauma has also been implicated, but aortic rupture with pseudoaneurysm is a much more common complication of chest trauma (see later).

Histologic confirmation of aortic dissection is mandatory because, occasionally, the cause is inflammatory rather than degenerative, the most common being giant cell aortitis. Takayasu disease and syphilis may induce

aortic rupture, but dissection is exceptional in these conditions. Fibromuscular dysplasia, a common cause of dissections of muscular arteries, rarely involves the aorta but may induce it to dissect.[29, 30]

Gross Pathologic Findings

Acute Lesions

In most series, an intimomedial entry tear is found in virtually all cases.[24, 27, 31, 32] Rare exceptions have been described in which no entry or exit has been located. In clinical series, the absence of an entry tear, as documented by imaging studies, is relatively common in patients with aortic dissections (so-called intramural hematoma). It is possible that imaging studies are relatively insensitive in detecting entry tears, explaining their greater frequency in autopsy studies. The existence of aortic dissections without entry tears has relevance to the pathogenesis of the disease (see later).

The site of the intimal tear in type I or type II dissection is usually 1 to 3 cm distal to the sinotubular junction (Figs. 5-3, 5-4B, 5-6). The tear is usually transverse, located over the right and noncoronary cusps, and involves less than 50% of the aortic circumference. However, a tear may be longitudinal (see Fig. 5-15), diagonal, or irregular and occasionally involve nearly the entire circumference of the vessel. Murray and Edwards described the pathologic sequelae of an aortic intimal tear.[33] Occasionally, the intimal tear may heal without associated dissection.[34] Most spontaneous type I or type II dissection occur in an area of aneurysmal dilatation, occasionally accompanied by dilatation of the aortic root. The splitting of the wall by the dissecting hematoma in the media may produce acute aneurysmal dilatation of the aorta, aortic insufficiency, and a false lumen in the vessel wall.

Type III Lesion

In contrast to proximal dissections, those of type III are frequently silent and show evidence of healing in more than 50% of cases (Figs. 5-5A, B). The appearance of a healed dissection differs from that of an acute one, with the lining of the false channel being wrinkled, dull, and whitish-gray secondary to organization. The degree of preexisting aneurysmal dilatation is generally minimal in distal dissections, but the false lumen may be markedly dilated. There may be multiple entry and exit tears, resulting in luminal webs connecting true and false lumens. These webs are anatomic landmarks that help radiologic diagnosis of acute and chronic dissections.[35] Entry tears are often of different ages; grossly, the appearance of a false lumen's lining may suggest the age of the dissection and whether it is acute or chronic. The connections between the true or false lumen and the major aortic branches should be documented at autopsy to correlate pathologic findings with a clinical history of renal or mesenteric obstruction. Occasionally, the pathologist encounters dissections in patients with previous surgical bypass procedures, further complicating anatomic dissection.

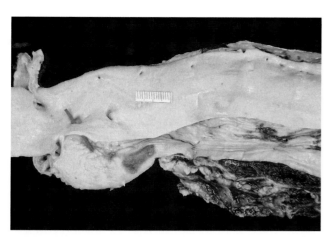

Figure 5-7 • Healed old medial dissection (type III) with marker defining the intimal tear leading to the false channel. Note its thickened, wrinkled surface and brown thrombi attached to it. (Courtesy of Dr. M.D. Silver.)

Old Dissection

If an old dissection is present, the medial false channel is lined with a wrinkled gray "pseudointima" that may have thrombi attached to it and show atherosclerotic changes (Fig. 5-7). Alternatively, linear scar may be found in the media (see later).

Histologic Findings

The hallmark of histologic change in aortic dissection not secondary to aortitis is medial degeneration, so-called cystic medial necrosis. Medial degeneration has been defined as the pooling of proteoglycans and the appearance of cyst-like structures in the media, and medionecrosis as an apparent loss of nuclei in the media.[36] These conditions may be present to a mild degree in normal aortas. Histologic changes are best evaluated if the vessel is sectioned in the transverse plane. The site of block collection is important; we usually section the aorta at or near the site of dissection, as well as at some distance from it in an area of intact aorta. Although an elastic van Gieson stain demonstrates elastic fibers, Movat pentachrome stain is preferable, as it defines proteoglycans, an important component of cystic medial necrosis, and smooth muscle cells, which are lost in areas of degeneration.

Schlatmann and Becker graded the extent of cystic medial necrosis into three categories based on the extent of cystic change, elastic fragmentation, fibrosis and medionecrosis, or loss of nuclei within the media.[2] The most dramatic cystic medial necrosis is seen in patients with Marfan syndrome and forms of idiopathic annuloaortic ectasia. The severe form is characterized by pools of proteoglycans in the aortic wall with fragmentation and loss of elastic lamellae (Fig. 5-8A, B). However, in many cases of aortic dissection, including those of Marfan syndrome, only mild medial changes are noted (Fig. 5-9). In these instances, there is a minimal increase in proteoglycans with focal mild elastic tissue loss. In other cases, loss of elastic lamellae is marked by minimal proteoglycan deposition (Figs. 5-10, 5-11A).

Severe cystic medial necrosis is observed in 44% of Marfan patients, compared with only 18% of patients without the syndrome.[24] It has been suggested that severe medial degenerative changes are more pronounced in pa-

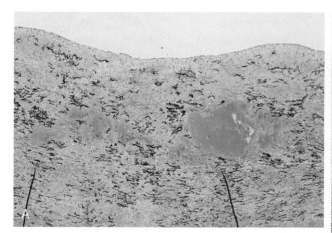

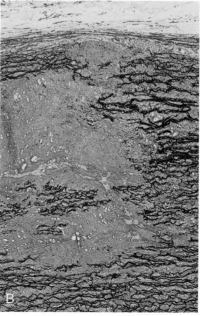

Figure 5-8 • *A*, Histologic section of the aorta from a patient with aortic dissection secondary to Marfan syndrome. There is marked loss of elastic lamellae and focal extensive proteoglycan deposition (cystic medial change). Movat stain. (From Virmani R, Burke AP, Farb A [eds]: Atlas of Cardiovascular Pathology. Philadelphia, WB Saunders, 1996, 129.) *B*, Idiopathic dissection with cystic medial change. This patient had a healed aortic dissection with areas of extensive cystic medial change and loss of elastic lamellae and focal pools of proteoglycans within the aortic wall (Movat stain).

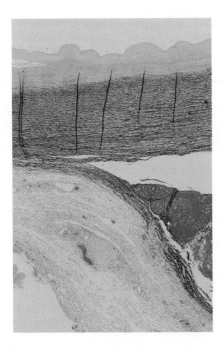

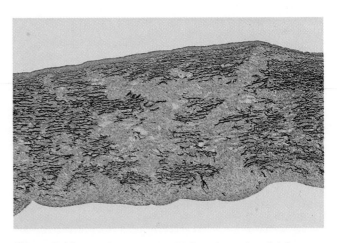

Figure 5-10 • Marfan syndrome, old dissection and medial degeneration. Note the loss of elastic fibers without proteoglycan deposition. The intima is seen at the top of the figure, and organized lining of the false lumen is at the bottom of the field. Areas of elastic lamellae are replaced by smooth muscle cells, but no increase in proteoglycan deposition is observed. (Movat stain.)

Figure 5-9 • Marfan syndrome with mild to no cystic medial change. A 40-year-old woman died suddenly after a short period of chest pain radiating to the neck and back. At autopsy, gross features of Marfan syndrome were obvious. Note the acute aortic dissection involving the outer third of the aortic wall and minimal cystic medial change. (Movat stain.)

tients with Marfan syndrome and proximal type I dissections. In seven aortic dissections in Marfan patients reported by Larson and Edwards, three aortas had severe cystic medial necrosis; the other four, with either type II or III dissections, had mild medial degenerative changes.

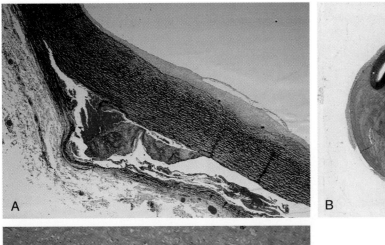

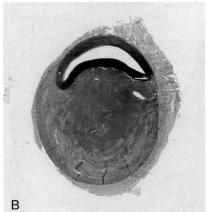

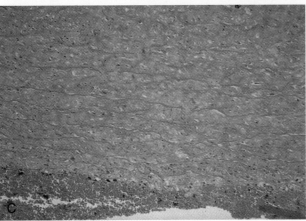

Figure 5-11 • Acute aortic dissection. Note dissection plane close to the medial/adventitial border. No atherosclerotic plaque is identified on the intimal surface. There is only mild cystic medial necrosis noted in the inner media. (Movat stain.) (From Sekosan M, Farolan MJ, Burke A, Ronan SG: Pathology of vascular disease. In: Eton D [ed]: Vascular Disease: A Multi-Specialty Approach. Austin, TX, Landes Bioscience, 1997.) B, Extension of the dissection into the carotid artery. (Movat stain.) C, Histology of acute dissection—false channel containing blood at base of photograph. Note polymorphs in adjacent media and loss of nuclei in overlying media (H&E stain).

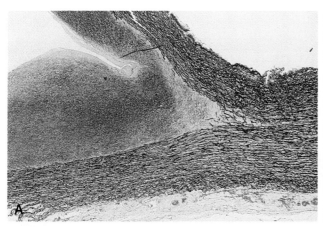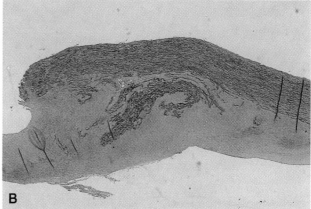

Figure 5-12 • *A*, A transverse histologic section of the descending thoracic aorta shows the true lumen on the right and a false lumen on the left. Note the extensive elastosis in tissue lining the false channel of this healed dissection. (Movat stain.) (From Virmani R, Burke AP, Farb A [eds]: Atlas of Cardiovascular Pathology. Philadelphia, WB Saunders, 1996, p 130.) *B*, Transverse section adjacent to an intimal tear showing healed dissection in the ascending aorta of a patient with a congenitally bicuspid aortic valve. Note in the tissue lining the false channel, the tags of elastic lamellae separated by areas of smooth muscle cells in a proteoglycan matrix and without elastic fibers; compare with Figure 5-11*A* (Movat stain).

The plane of hemorrhagic dissection is usually between the inner two thirds and the outer third of the aortic media (Figs. 5-8, 5-10), or less commonly, at the junction between the media and the adventitia (Fig. 5-11*A*, *B*). The age of the dissection may be estimated by evaluating the lining of the medial false channel. In an acute dissection, blood fills the lumen; the adjacent medial walls have flecks of fibrin attached to them and often show an acute inflammatory exudate (Figs. 5-9, 5-11*C*). In an old or healed dissection, the false channel is lined by thickened fibromuscular tissue with or without a dif-

fuse deposit of fine elastic tissue (Figs. 5-10, 5-12*A*, *B*); organizing mural thrombus may be seen along with atherosclerotic deposits. Fragments of elastica damaged in the original dissection curve into this tissue (Fig. 5-12*B*), and the media superficial to the dissection may show marked medionecrosis, possibly a secondary effect caused by the dissection interference with vasa vasorum. A dissection of intermediate age shows granulation tissue in the false channel's lining. Remember that a dissection may heal, obliterating the false channel and leaving a linear scar in the outer media (Fig. 5-13).

Ultrastructural Findings

The three-dimensional architecture of the aorta revealed by scanning electron microscopy after hot formic acid or sodium hydroxide digestion demonstrates a decreased number of interlaminar elastic fibers, which are irregular in arrangement and shape (Fig. 5-14*A*–*D*). The resulting rarefaction of interconnections between elastic laminae weakens the aortic wall, leading to the initiation and progression of a dissection.[37]

Pathogenesis

There is controversy concerning the initiating event. One theory proposes that the intimal tear exposes the medial layer to the driving force of the blood (or pulse pressure), splitting the diseased media. The blood then passes into the space between the dissection planes, resulting in a false lumen that distends with blood. The pressure in the false lumen directs blood back into the true lumen via a reentry tear, or causes the false lumen to rupture the thin layer of outer media and adventitia.

A second theory suggests that the entry of blood into the dissection plane occurs via ruptured vasa vasorum within the aortic media. Accordingly, intimal tears would be secondary or not occur at all. Although pathologic studies usually document the presence of an intimal tear

Figure 5-13 • Greenish connective tissue marked by a bar containing numerous blood vessels marking the site of a healed dissection in the outer media. Greenish adventitial fibrosis seen at base of photograph (Movat stain).

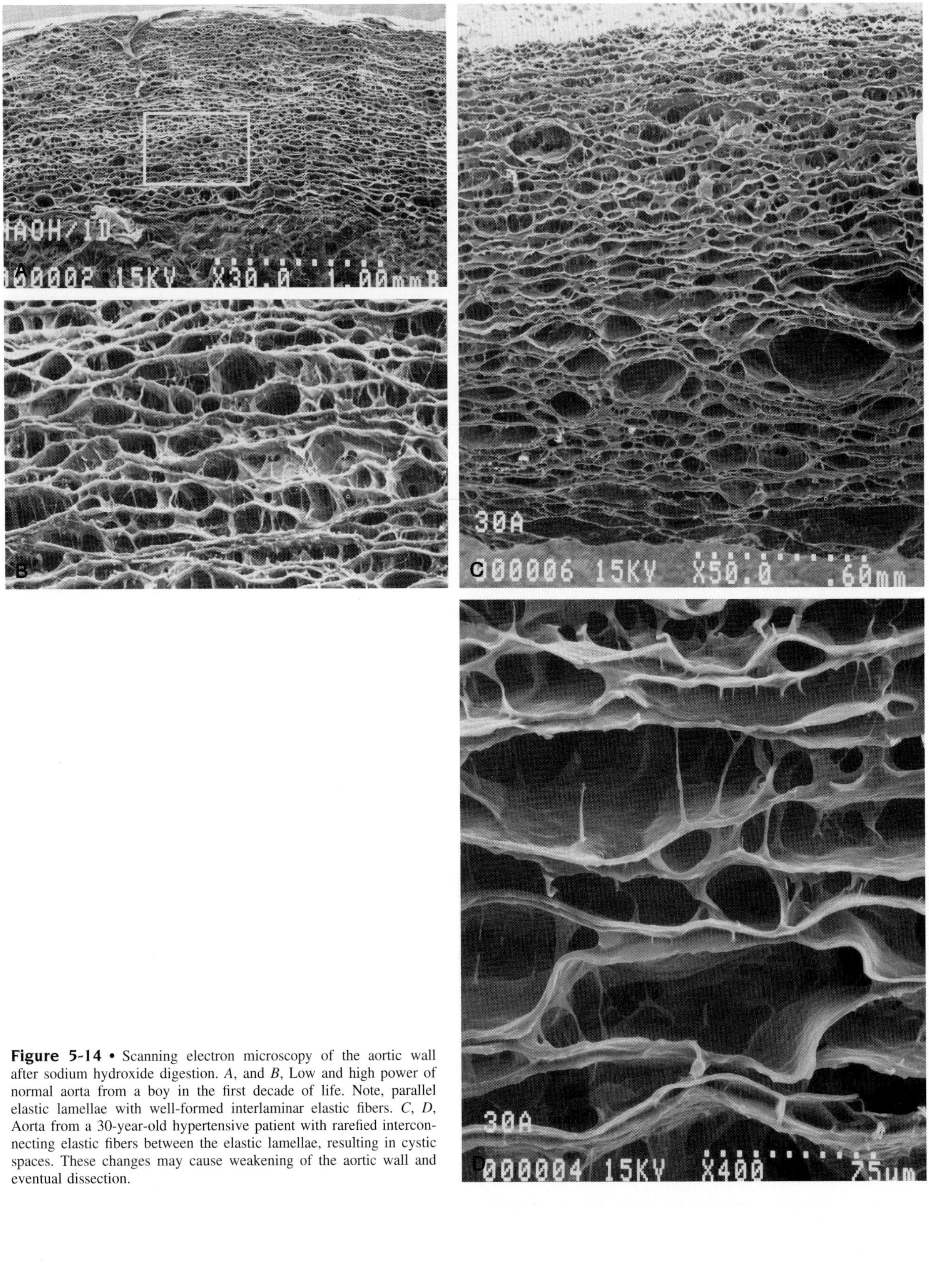

Figure 5-14 • Scanning electron microscopy of the aortic wall after sodium hydroxide digestion. *A,* and *B,* Low and high power of normal aorta from a boy in the first decade of life. Note, parallel elastic lamellae with well-formed interlaminar elastic fibers. *C, D,* Aorta from a 30-year-old hypertensive patient with rarefied interconnecting elastic fibers between the elastic lamellae, resulting in cystic spaces. These changes may cause weakening of the aortic wall and eventual dissection.

in the majority of aortic dissections (which is also our experience), Wilson and Hutchins were unable to detect them in 13% of 204 cases.[38]

Clinical Presentation

Severe pain, the most common initial symptom, is reported by 74 to 90% of patients and its typically described as "tearing," "ripping," or "stabbing." Pain that migrates along the lines of dissection is present in 70% of cases.[39] Its location usually coincides with the site of dissection: anterior chest pain occurring in ascending aortic dissections (type II) and interscapular chest pain in descending thoracic aortic dissections (types I and III). Less frequent symptoms include congestive heart failure, syncope, cerebrovascular accident, ischemic peripheral neuropathy, paraplegia, and sudden death.

Physical examination may help to establish the diagnosis and the site of dissection. A pulse deficit between the arms, the murmur of aortic insufficiency, and neurologic signs generally indicate a proximal dissection. Hypotension often indicates a rupture of the false lumen, causing cardiac tamponade or intrapleural or retroperitoneal hemorrhage.

Complications and Cause of Death

The two major direct complications of aortic dissection are rupture of the false lumen and compression of the true lumen or arterial branches. Ninety percent of proximal dissections rupture into the pericardium; the majority of the remaining 10% into the left pleural cavity; rare sites of rupture include the mediastinum and right pleural space. In distal dissections, rupture of the false lumen occurs into the left pleural cavity in 60% of patients, and into the right cavity in 24% (Table 5-2). Rarely, the false lumen ruptures into the pericardium, the mediastinum, or the retroperitoneum.[32]

Sustained loss of a peripheral pulse occurs in 24% of patients with aortic dissection; 8% experience impaired renal perfusion; 5% have compromised visceral perfusion; 3% suffer stroke; and 3% develop paraplegia.[40] Rarely, cerebral ischemia may be the initial symptom in patients with aortic dissection.[41] Compression of coronary ostia, arch vessels, and branches of the abdominal aorta cause myocardial ischemia, stroke, and renal or mesenteric insufficiency, respectively. Compression caused either by

intimal flaps or webs, or dilatation of the false lumen can squash the true lumen. Repair of aortic dissections that extend into the abdominal aorta may include fenestration of intimal flaps or replacement of a segment of the aorta, with revascularization of renal arteries.[42]

In an autopsy series of 505 patients with dissecting aortic aneurysms, 8% had direct extension into a coronary artery. Both ostia were involved in 18 cases (46%), the right ostium only in 15 cases (38%), and the left in 5 cases (13%).[43]

The cause of death in hospitalized patients with aortic dissection is rupture of the false lumen (62%), followed by causes unrelated to the dissection (15%), heart failure (9%), renal failure (7%), myocardial infarct (4%), and shock without false luminal rupture (3%).[37] The cause of sudden death in aortic dissection is almost always false lumen rupture. However, in approximately 5% of patients, no rupture of the false lumen is found to explain a sudden death.

Imaging Studies

An enlarged aortic knob or widening of the aortic silhouette on chest radiograph may help to support the diagnosis of proximal aortic dissection. Diagnostic techniques include aortography, contrast-enhanced computed tomography (CT), magnetic resonance imaging (MRI), and transthoracic or transesophageal echocardiography. Depending upon the site of dissection, each has its advantage and disadvantage in evaluating a patient.[34, 44]

Abdominal Aortic Dissections

Abdominal aortic dissections are rare, accounting for 1% of all aortic dissections.[45] A total of 26 cases with autopsy confirmation have been published. The mean age of the patients, 18 of whom were men, was 62 years. The incidence of rupture of the false lumen was only 50%, lower than that of other types of aortic dissection. For this reason, it has been suggested that the chance of healing the false lumen is directly proportional to the distance of the intimal tear from the aortic root (sinotubular junction).

MARFAN SYNDROME

Marfan syndrome is an autosomal dominant disorder characterized by abnormalities of eyes, skeleton, and cardiovascular system. Eye changes include myopia, retinal detachment, elongated globe, and ectopia lentis. Skeletal changes are joint hypermobility, tall stature, pectus excavatum, reduced thoracic kyphosis, scoliosis, arachnodactyly, dolichostenomelia, pectus carinatum, and erosion of the lumbosacral vertebrae from dural ectasia.

Classically, the diagnosis is made on clinical criteria, including history of a close family relative with the syndrome as well as ocular and skeletal changes. Suspicion is supported by noting mutations in the gene that encodes fibrillin-1 on chromosome 15. Sporadic cases of Marfan

TABLE 5-2 • **Site of False Lumen Rupture, Aortic Dissections**

	Types I and II (%)	Type III (%)	All (%)
Pericardium	90	6	70
Mediastinum	2	6	3
Left pleural cavity	6	59	19
Right pleural cavity	2	23	7
Retroperitoneum	0	6	1

Adapted from Nakashima Y, Korozumi T, Sueishi K, Tanaka K: Dissecting aneurysm: A clinicopathologic and histopathologic study of 111 autopsied cases. Hum Pathol 21:291–296, 1990.

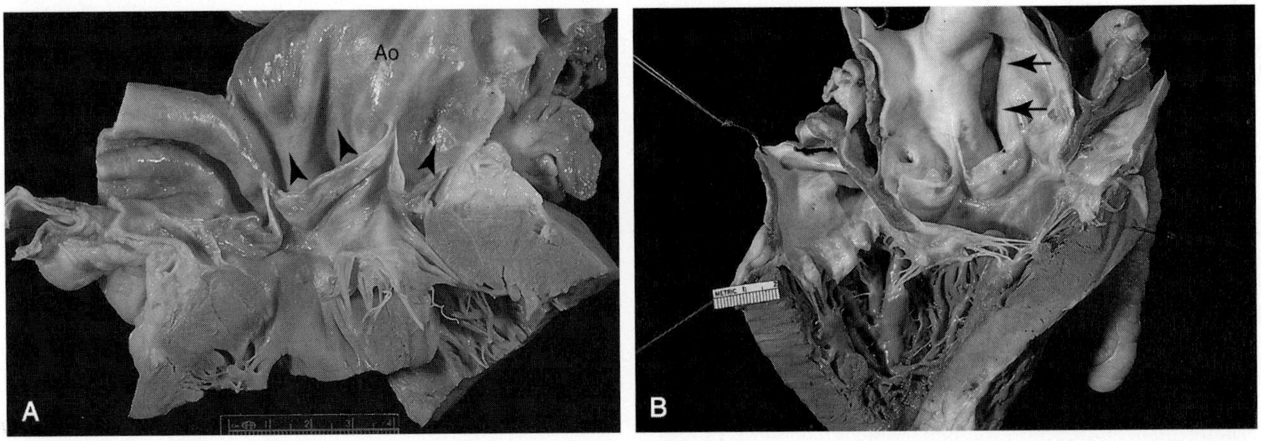

Figure 5-15 • *A*, Marfan syndrome with annuloaortic ectasia in the absence of dissection. This 32-year-old man died suddenly. At autopsy, there were classic features of Marfan syndrome, and the aortic root was markedly dilated with involvement of the aortic sinuses (arrowheads), the annulus, and the ascending aorta. The aortic root was 55 mm in diameter, and the aortic valve was insufficient. Ao, aorta. *B*, Marfan syndrome, annuloaortic ectasia with dissection in a 23-year-old man who died suddenly. At autopsy, there were classic features of Marfan syndrome. Note the annuloaortic ectasia with a longitudinal intimal tear (arrows). (From Virmani R, Burke AP, Farb A [eds]: Atlas of Cardiovascular Pathology. Philadelphia, WB Saunders, 1996, p 128.)

syndrome with that mutation have been reported in patients without a family history. To confirm the diagnosis in these patients, there should be documented manifestations in the skeletal, cardiovascular, and one other system.

Cardiovascular abnormalities are detected in most patients with the syndrome; their frequency depends on criteria used for diagnosis. Cardiovascular involvement is manifested by aortic root dilatation (39%) (Fig. 5-15A), aortic dissections (36%) (Fig. 5-15B), mitral valve prolapse (without other cardiac involvement) (21%), and miscellaneous other cardiovascular manifestations including aneurysms of the sinus of Valsalva and peripheral aneurysms. Although isolated aneurysms of Valsalva are relatively uncommon, aortic root dilatation is believed to begin in the sinuses and may be manifest soon after birth.[1]

Because of the likelihood of aortic dissection and aortic insufficiency, patients with Marfan syndrome should be followed for aortic root dilatation. Yearly transesophageal echocardiography is performed. If the aortic root is 1.5 times greater than the expected mean diameter (based on height and weight of patient), more frequent observations are required.[46, 47] Aortic regurgitation generally occurs when aortic diameter exceeds 50 to 60 mm, but there are no absolute echocardiographic guidelines that predict the onset of symptoms or dissection. Aortic dissection usually does not occur in adults until the ascending aortic diameter is 55 mm. For this reason, many patients undergo elective composite graft repair if the aortic root approaches that diameter.

Mitral valve prolapse in patients with Marfan syndrome occurs with advancing age. Women are more often affected than men. By sensitive two-dimensional echocardiography, as many as 60 to 80% of them have mitral insufficiency. The rate of mitral valve prolapse documented at autopsy in these patients is probably lower; gross findings include elongated, redundant anterior and posterior mitral valve leaflets, with mitral annular calcification in 10%.[48] Marfan syndrome is also discussed in Chapter 16.

EHLERS-DANLOS SYNDROME

Ehlers-Danlos syndrome (EDS) is marked by hypermobility of joints, hyperextensibility of skin, and fragile tissues prone to dystrophic scarring and easy bruising. Body stature and habitus are usually normal, in contrast to patients with Marfan syndrome.

At least nine different forms of the disease have been recognized, many showing considerable clinical and pathologic overlap. Cardiac complications are limited to type IV EDS, caused by defects in type III collagen. At the molecular level, the defect is heterogeneous, with several different mutations resulting in the clinical phenotype. Pathologic manifestations of EDS IV include rupture of the aorta or the large elastic arteries without dissection, frequently resulting in sudden death. The most frequently involved sites are the abdominal aorta and its branches, the great vessels of the aortic arch, and the large arteries of the limbs.[49] Characteristically, there are multiple rupture sites in the aorta (Fig. 5-16). See Chapter 16 for further discussion.

TRAUMA

Traumatic rupture of the aorta is usually the result of blunt chest trauma. Death frequently occurs at the site of an accident, or within an hour thereafter. A minority of aortic ruptures heal, producing pseudoaneurysms that may not be diagnosed for years.[50]

The most common site of injury, seen in 65% of cases, is in the descending aorta, within 1 cm of the origin of the subclavian artery at the insertion of the ligamentum arteriosum (65%) (Fig. 5-17). Fewer are located in the ascending aorta (14%), in the distal descending thoracic aorta (12%), or in the abdominal aorta (9%). Complete transections occur in two thirds of all cases, and usually if the tear site is adjacent to the left subcla-

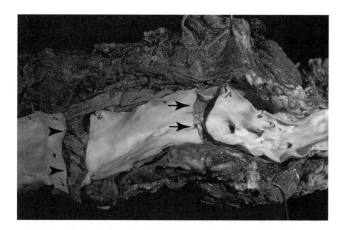

Figure 5-16 • Ehlers-Danlos syndrome, type IV, affecting a 14-year-old black boy who complained of chest and abdominal pain while lifting weights; emergency computed tomographic (CT) scan showed an aortic dissection and rupture, and the patient expired shortly afterward. He had a history of easy bruising and poor wound healing, was 6'1" tall and weighed 123 lbs. At autopsy, he had a hemothorax and the aorta was transected transversely just distal to the left subclavian artery origin (arrows) and just proximal to the celiac artery (arrowheads). (From Sekosan M, Farolan MJ, Burke A, Ronan SG: Pathology of vascular disease. In: Eton D [ed]: Vascular Disease A Multi-Specialty Approach. Austin, TX, Landes Bioscience, 1997.)

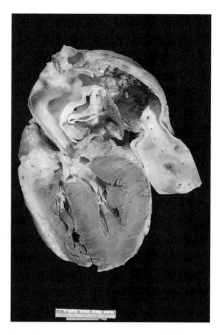

Figure 5-17 • Traumatic aneurysm. Heart and attached ascending, transverse, and descending thoracic aorta from a young woman with a history of chest trauma 5 years before death, showing a localized aneurysm in the descending thoracic aorta just distal to the ligamentum arteriosum. (From Virmani R, Burke AP, Farb A [eds]: Atlas of Cardiovascular Pathology. Philadelphia, WB Saunders, 1996, p 139.)

vian artery. The remaining third of aortic ruptures are associated with incomplete intimomedial tears and dissection, with two thirds of these developing in the ascending aorta. The tears are usually transverse, and are multiple in approximately 10% of cases.

It is estimated that 10 to 20% of patients live long enough to undergo surgical repair of a traumatic aneurysm. Rarely, a traumatic pseudoaneurysm or aneurysm is asymptomatic, and the history of chest trauma may be remote or nearly forgotten.[51] In such patients, the aneurysm may be discovered on a routine chest radiograph. Occasionally, there may be rupture into an adjacent structure, such as the esophagus.[52] Grossly and histologically, there is a sharp demarcation between the normal media and the fibrous lining of a pseudoaneurysm. With time, the lining surface shows an organized hematoma or calcification. Aneurysms occurring after incomplete intimomedial tears, or after localized dissection of the aortic wall, may have remnants of medial elastic tissue in their outer lining. They are discussed in Chapter 17.

AORTITIS

Aortitis is an inflammation of the aortic wall, with or without disruption of elastic fibers, aortic wall necrosis, or fibrosis. The definition implies an absence of underlying conditions that secondarily result in chronic inflammation. The most important of these is atherosclerosis, which is characterized by chronic inflammation of the intima, often with involvement of the media and even the adventitia. Moreover, because atherosclerosis may be superimposed on aortitis, making a distinction between atherosclerosis and aortitis as a primary diagnosis is sometimes difficult. This distinction is usually facilitated, however, by considering the distribution of the process and the clinical data.

Aortitis may be classified as infectious or noninfectious (Table 5-3). The most important causes are Takayasu disease (especially in younger patients), syphilis, and giant cell aortitis (especially in older patients). Because there are no pathognomonic histologic features of the three major types of aortitis, evaluation of clinical and pathologic data is important to arrive at a final diagnosis.

The connective tissue diseases that may involve the aorta are rheumatoid arthritis, ankylosing spondylitis, Reiter syndrome, and Behçet disease, all discussed later. Tuberculous aortitis is currently rare in developed countries; it involves the thoracic or abdominal aorta with equal frequency and is usually the result of contiguous spread

---

TABLE 5-3 • **Classification of Aortitis**

Noninfectious

Takayasu arteritis

Giant cell arteritis

Aortitis of collagen vascular disease
  Rheumatoid arthritis
  Ankylosing spondylitis
  Reiter syndrome
  Behçet disease
  Systemic lupus erythematosus

Inflammatory aneurysms of the abdominal aorta

Sarcoidosis

Infectious

Syphilitic aortitis

Tuberculosis

Pyogenic (bacterial or fungal [mycotic aneurysm]) aortitis

from a tuberculoma of the lung or an infected periaortic lymph node. Extremely rarely, the aorta may be involved by sarcoid, which tends to affect small and medium-sized arteries of the lung. Because tuberculous and sarcoid involvements of the aorta are rare, they are not further discussed.

Takayasu Arteritis

The Japanese ophthalmologist, Takayasu,[53] first described this arteritis in 1908 in a 21-year-old woman with ocular changes. However, it was not until 1951 that Shimizu and Sano[54] detailed the clinical features of this disorder, which, in 1954, was named Takayasu arteritis. Takayasu disease has many synonyms, including aortic arch syndrome, pulseless disease, reversed coarctation, occlusive thromboaortopathy, and young female arteritis. Aortitis in patients without the clinical history of the acute phase of the disease, but with pathologic features of Takayasu aortitis, is sometimes termed "nonspecific aortoarteritis."

Clinical Manifestations

Takayasu disease affects women more frequently than men in a ratio of 8 to 1. The incidence in North American and European populations is approximately 2 per million per year. The majority of cases reported have been in Asian and African patients, but the disease has a worldwide distribution.[55–57] The age at diagnosis ranges from 3.5 to 66 years, with a mean of 20 to 50 years.

The acute phase of the disease is characterized by malaise, weakness, fever, arthralgias, myalgias, weight loss, pleuritic pain, and anorexia. This phase may vary widely in severity and often precedes the occlusive phase by weeks to months, or an asymptomatic period may intervene for 6 to 8 years. Coronary artery involvement may result in myocardial infarction and cardiac arrest.[58]

Symptoms of the late phase include diminished or absent pulses in 96% of patients, bruits in 94%, hypertension in 74%, and heart failure in 28%.[55] In addition to stenotic lesions, aneurysmal dilatations may cause palpable pulsatile masses, and embolisms from mural thrombi occur. Rarely, sudden death results from rupture of a rapidly expanding aneurysm. Although stenotic lesions generally dominate, the incidence of aneurysmal lesions is estimated to be greater than 30%; indeed, aneurysms may be the sole clinical manifestation.[59] Involvement of the aortic root and the aortic valve occurs in 10 to 20% of patients and may lead to aortic insufficiency.[60]

Ueda and associates subdivided Takayasu disease into three types.[61] Type I has involvement of the aortic arch and the brachiocephalic vessels; in type II, the descending thoracic and abdominal aorta are affected without arch involvement, whereas in type III, lesions are located at the arch and at both thoracic and abdominal aorta. Lupi-Herrera suggested an additional variant (type IV), denoting involvement of the pulmonary arteries as well[55] (Fig. 5-18).

Abnormalities of laboratory tests in Takayasu disease are most severe in the acute phase of the illness and

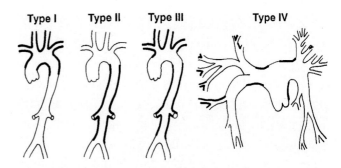

Figure 5-18 • Classification of Takayasu arteritis modified by Lupi-Herrera and colleagues.[55] Type I: Disease limited to the aortic arch and its branches. Type II: Lesions affect the descending thoracic and abdominal aorta without involving the arch. Type III: Extensive lesions involve the arch as well as the thoracic and abdominal aorta. Type IV: The features of types I, II, and III are present, as is pulmonary artery involvement. Thickened lines represent areas of inflammation. (From Virmani R, Lande A, McAllister HA: Pathologic aspects of Takayasu arteritis. In: Lande A, Berkmen YM, McAllister HA [eds]: Aortitis, Clinical, Pathologic and Radiographic Aspects. New York, Raven Press, 1986, p 587.)

include an elevated sedimentation rate, which is usually normal in the chronic phase, a low-grade, and a mild normochromic normocytic anemia. Elevated serum immunoglobulin IgG and IgM levels develop, and immune complexes are frequently present. There is an association with HLA B5, Bw52, and Dw12 antigens in patients with severe inflammation and a rapidly progressive course.[62]

Pathology

The acute phase is characterized by edema, patchy necrosis, chronic inflammation, and scattered giant cells in the outer two thirds of the media, adventitia, adventitial fat, and vasa vasorum (Fig. 5-19A–C). The vasa vasorum may show intimal proliferation with obliteration but no fibrinoid necrosis.

The late phase is characterized by marked intimal and adventitial thickening of the vessels (Fig. 5-20A, B). Medial scarring with replacement of areas of elastic lamellae and revascularization gives rise to the coarse "tree bark" appearance of the intima seen in the gross morphology that is characteristic of this form of aortitis. Stenotic lesions are produced by a circumferentially thickened intima with a glossy, gray, or myxoid appearance on cut surface. Multisegmental involvement with normal areas between affected segments are characteristic, although there may be diffuse involvement of the aorta and isolated disease of individual arteries. In a series of patients from the United States, the most frequently affected arteries after the aorta were the subclavian (90%), carotid (45%), vertebral (25%), and renal (20%).[63] Detailed autopsies have shown that subclavian arteries, mesenteric arteries, and abdominal aorta were histologically involved in nearly 80% of patients.[56]

In the late phase, the intima is hypocellular with scattered smooth muscle cells and fibroblasts (Fig. 5-21A). Medial elastic laminae are disorganized or focally absent and replaced by collagen and granulation tissue (Fig. 5-

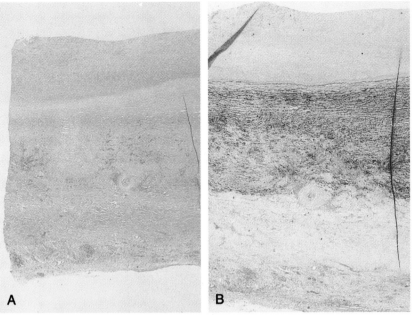

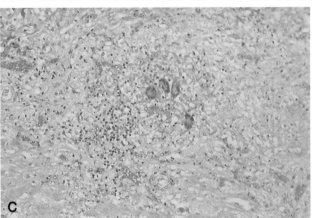

Figure 5-19 • Takayasu aortitis. *A*, Low-power view of the thoracic aorta showing marked thickening of the adventitia (bottom half) and intimal thickening (top half). The media shows focal destruction and inflammation (H&E stain). *B*, Movat-stained higher magnification of the section shown in Figure 5-19*A*, demonstrating the medial disruption by inflammatory infiltrate and both fibrointimal and adventitial thickening, commonly observed in this disease. Note endarteritis obliteration of the vasa vasorum. *C*, High-power view of Figure 5-19*A* demonstrating destruction of the media and marked inflammation consisting of lymphocytes, macrophages, and giant cells (H&E stain).

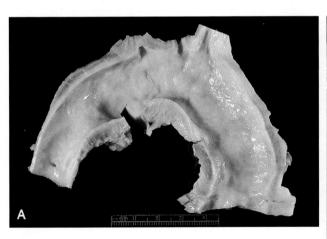

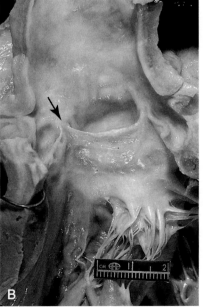

Figure 5-20 • *A*, Takayasu aortitis causing stenotic lesions. A 51-year-old white female had severe congestive heart failure. Physical examination revealed aortic incompetence and pericarditis. Coronary angiography showed bilateral ostial stenosis. At autopsy, there was marked thickening of the ascending aorta, the arch vessels, and a portion of the descending thoracic aorta (to right of photograph). Note the normal thickness of the distal thoracic aorta (to left of photograph). *B*, Same patient as in Figure 5-20*A* showing thickened and fibrotic aortic valve cusps but no commissural fusion. Instead, there is widening of the commissures (arrow). Also note the markedly thickened ascending aortic wall. (*A*, From Virmani R, Burke AP, Farb A [eds]: Atlas of Cardiovascular Pathology. Philadelphia, WB Saunders, 1966, p 139.)

121

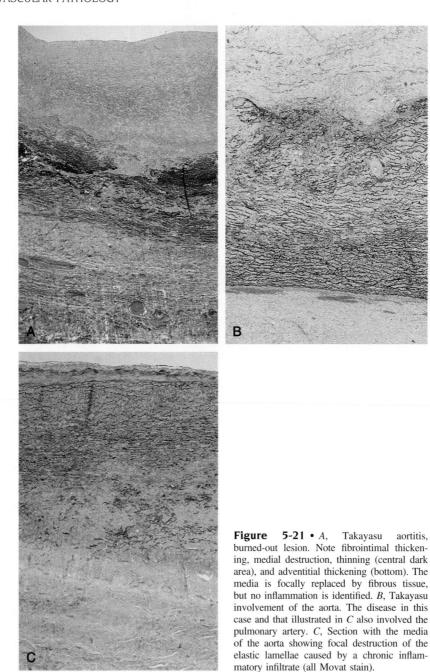

Figure 5-21 • *A*, Takayasu aortitis, burned-out lesion. Note fibrointimal thickening, medial destruction, thinning (central dark area), and adventitial thickening (bottom). The media is focally replaced by fibrous tissue, but no inflammation is identified. *B*, Takayasu involvement of the aorta. The disease in this case and that illustrated in *C* also involved the pulmonary artery. *C*, Section with the media of the aorta showing focal destruction of the elastic lamellae caused by a chronic inflammatory infiltrate (all Movat stain).

21*B*, *C*). Areas of necrosis with giant cell infiltrates occasionally persist into the late phase. Areas of scarring may demonstrate dystrophic calcification of media and adventitia.

Coronary artery involvement occurs in 15% of patients, typically limited to the ostia or proximal segments (see Fig. 5-20*A*). Rarely, it is the sole manifestation of the disease. Diffuse involvement of the entire epicardial coronary artery system has been reported.[64–69] Sequelae of coronary artery involvement include angina, myocardial infarction, and sudden death.

Giant Cell Arteritis

Giant cell arteritis is a systemic panarteritis that predominantly affects elderly patients and is manifested by focal granulomatous inflammation of large and medium-sized arteries, especially the temporal artery. The aorta and its major branches are affected in 15% of cases.[18] The incidence in the United States is 15 to 30 cases per year per 100,000 persons among those older than 50 years.[70] The disease occurs predominantly in women, with a high incidence in persons of Northern European descent. Its etiology is unknown but may be a manifestation of autoimmunity or infection.[71, 72] Ten to 15% of patients with giant cell arteritis and temporal artery involvement also have aortic disease; they often have polymyalgia rheumatica.

Clinical Manifestations

Symptoms of giant cell arteritis that suggest aortic involvement are claudication of upper or lower extremi-

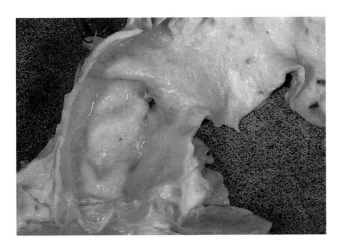

Figure 5-22 • Giant cell aortitis. Aneurysm formation in the ascending aorta. Note the intimal "tree-bark" appearance with focal thinning and a tear in the ascending aorta. The patient, a 72-year-old white woman, manifested sudden chest pain and collapse. She had a hemopericardium at autopsy.

ties, parasthesias, Raynaud phenomenon, abdominal angina, coronary ischemia, transient ischemic attacks, and aortic arch and great vessel "steal" syndromes.[73] Aortic aneurysms with aortic valve regurgitation or aortic dissection are being recognized more frequently in patients with this type of arteritis.[74, 75] Unlike Takayasu arteritis, renal artery involvement is rare, and hypertension is not a characteristic complication of giant cell aortitis.[73]

Laboratory tests reveal a very high sedimentation rate, elevated acute phase reactants, hypergammaglobulinemia, and increased serum C_3 and C_4 complement levels, the latter often reflecting disease activity. Angiography may demonstrate aortic root dilatation; aortic insufficiency; and long, smooth, tapering stenoses with areas of dilatation in subclavian, axillary, and brachial arteries.

Pathology

The aorta typically demonstrates aortic root dilatation, with medial dissection in occasional cases of aortic rupture. The intima is wrinkled, demonstrating a tree-bark appearance similar to that seen in other inflammatory aortic diseases (Fig. 5-22). Histologically, the inflammatory infiltrate is mononuclear, consisting of lymphocytes, plasma cells, and histiocytes (Fig. 5-23). There is disruption of the internal elastic lamina with fragmentation and a giant cell reaction of the Langhan type (Fig. 5-23B). The disruption may be accompanied by a significant degree of necrosis. The finding of a large number of giant cells is helpful but not considered a prerequisite for diagnosis because, in some cases, only a few are found either in the temporal or other arteries at autopsy. In healed lesions, intimal fibrosis predominates and minimal cellular reaction remains; however, elastic tissue stains demonstrate extensive disruption of the elastic fibers.

It is usually the combination of clinical features and microscopic findings that helps to separate giant cell arteritis from other arteritic diseases.[76] Features of giant cell aortitis that help distinguish it from Takayasu disease are patient age older than 70 years, intimal scarring that is only mild or moderate, and lack of adventitial scarring and inflammation with endarteritis obliterans. In some cases, a definitive distinction cannot be made, and a nonspecific diagnosis of aortitis is given.

Syphilitic Aortitis

Cardiovascular syphilis once accounted for 5 to 10% of all cardiovascular deaths; today, however, in North America only occasional cases are seen at autopsy. Cardiac complications occur in approximately 10% of untreated individuals. The latent period varies from 5 to 40 years, with a usual time frame of 10 to 25 years. Syphilis is caused by an infection with *Treponema pallidum.* At present, this organism cannot be cultured continuously in vitro, hindering studies on its virulence and pathogenic mechanisms. Now, however, its genome has been sequenced.[77] Future analysis of the metabolic pathways the spirochete uses should aid its culture, further understanding of its pathology and pave the way for potential vaccines.

Syphilitic heart disease can be divided into four categories: (1) syphilitic aortitis; (2) syphilitic aortic aneu-

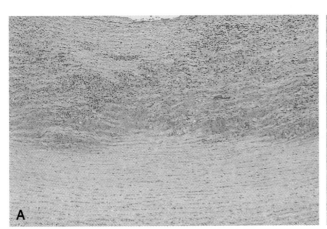

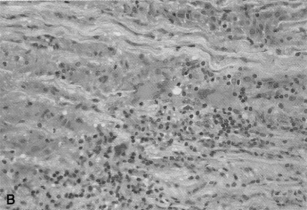

Figure 5-23 • *A,* Giant cell aortitis. Histologic section showing extensive destruction of the inner half of the media (bluish area). *B,* Higher magnification demonstrating lymphocytes, macrophages, and Langhan-type giant cells in the media (both H&E stain).

rysm; (3) syphilitic aortic valvulitis with aortic regurgitation; and (4) syphilitic coronary ostial stenosis. Of 126 patients reported by Heggtveit, 42 (33%) had only syphilitic aortitis and 84 (67%) had one or more of the major complications of aneurysm, aortic regurgitation, and coronary ostial stenosis.[78] A clinical diagnosis of syphilis was made in only 20% of these cases.

Pathology

Syphilitic aortitis involves the proximal aorta and does not extend distal to the renal arteries, probably because the rich vascular and lymphatic circulation in the vessel's wall is limited to the thoracic aorta. However, well-documented cases of syphilitic aneurysms of the abdominal aorta exist.[79, 80] The aortic intima has a fine tree-bark appearance with focal areas of intimal thickening that are white and shiny (Fig. 5-24A). In late stages, the gross intimal lesions are often obscured by superimposed atherosclerosis (Fig. 5-24B). The aortic wall may be thickened in early stages, with subsequent aneurysmal thinning and calcification. Aortic rupture may occur, but dissections are unusual.[78, 81, 82] Because of aortic root involvement and superimposed intimal thickening, there may be coronary ostial narrowing.

The initial histologic lesion is a multifocal lymphoplasmacytic infiltrate around adventitial vasa vasorum with extension into the media (Fig. 5-25A). Occasional giant cells may occur. The lesion is not specific, however, because endarteritis obliterans also occurs in Takayasu aortitis and ankylosing spondylitis, and plasma cells and even giant cells are observed in all types of aortic inflammation, including atherosclerosis (Table 5-4).[83] The inflammation causes medial destruction. With time, it is replaced by scar tissue, resulting in intimal wrinkling. The inflammation may extend into the aortic root, producing aortic regurgitation from dilatation of the aortic annulus. Microgummas may occur within the aortic media. They have a central area of necrosis, showing a faint outline of dead cells and surrounding palisading macrophages, lymphocytes, and plasma cells (Fig. 5-25B, D).

Treponemas are usually scant in these gummas and are difficult to demonstrate.

Syphilitic aneurysms may be saccular or fusiform. Their frequency in various sites is as follows: sinus of Valsalva, less than 1%; ascending aorta, 46%; transverse arch, 24%, descending arch, 5%; descending thoracic aorta, 5%; abdominal aorta, 7%; and multiple sites, 4%.[77] The most common complications of syphilitic aneurysms are aortic insufficiency and rupture. Uncommon complications include superior vena cava syndrome, bony erosion of sternum or vertebrae,[84] aortopulmonary fistula,[85] paraparesis,[82] dissection,[81] and stroke.[86]

Differential Diagnosis. Because the histologic appearance of syphilitic aortitis may mimic that of noninfectious aortitis, especially Takayasu disease and ankylosing spondylitis, we do not advise making a diagnosis of syphilitic aortitis based only upon histology in the absence of serologic evidence of the disease. In general, massive aortic root dilatation with thinning of the aortic wall is most likely the result of syphilis, but lesser degrees of aneurysm formation are currently more typical of Takayasu aortitis or giant cell aortitis.

A history of syphilis is needed to diagnose syphilitic aortitis; other manifestations of tertiary disease are seen in 10 to 30% of patients with cardiovascular syphilis. In the absence of a clinical history, positive serology, which may be performed on postmortem serum, is a prerequisite for diagnosis. In the late stages of tertiary syphilis, nontreponemal tests may be negative, requiring confirmation by such tests as *Treponema pallidum* immobilization or fluorescent treponemal antibody (FTA-ABS) absorption. However, it must be remembered that an isolated positive FTA-ABS is not diagnostic, as false positives may occur in collagen vascular diseases that also cause aortitis.

Rheumatoid Aortitis

Rheumatoid involvement of the heart is well recognized and produces symptomatic disease. Histologic features of aortitis are present in approximately 10% of

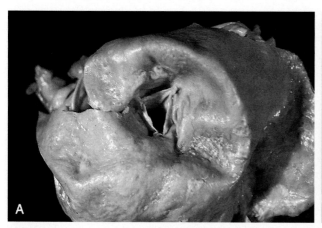
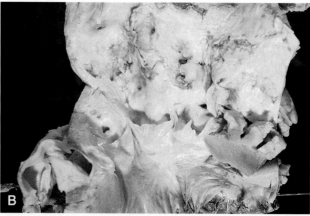

Figure 5-24 • *A*, Syphilitic aortic aneurysm. A localized ascending aortic aneurysm with mild dilatation of the aortic sinuses and aortic valve incompetence from a middle-aged man with a history of syphilis. Note wrinkling of the intima without superimposed atherosclerosis. *B*, Ascending aorta, aortic valve, and left ventricular outflow tract from another 58-year-old man with a positive Venereal Disease Research Laboratory (VDRL) test result. Note the focal intimal wrinkling; however, the characteristic appearance has been obscured by superimposed atherosclerosis.

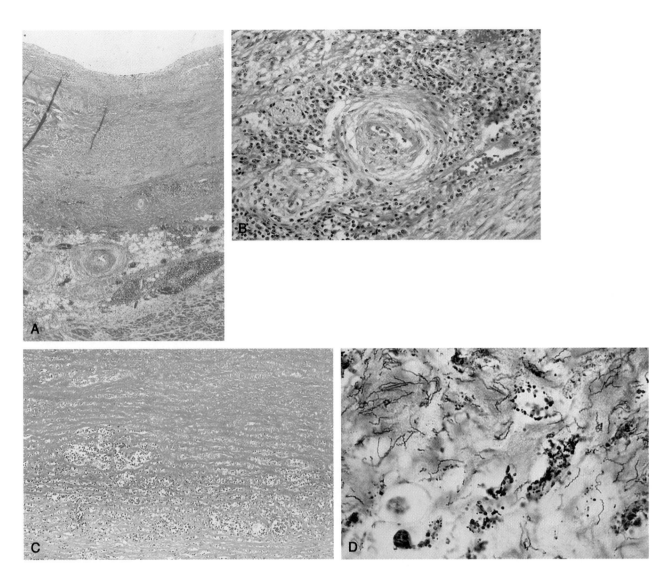

Figure 5-25 • Syphilitic aortitis. *A*, Histologic section of the ascending aorta showing adventitial (bottom of photograph) and medial chronic inflammatory infiltrate. *B*, Higher magnification from the adventitia, demonstrating endarteritis obliterans and perivascular cuffing by lymphocytes and plasma cells. *C*, Microgumma in the wall of the ascending aorta. Note predominantly acute inflammatory infiltrate within the medial wall and intima. There is no nuclear staining of the surrounding media (upper field), but elastic lamellae can still be clearly discerned (*A*, *B*, and *C*, H&E stain). *D*, In rare cases, *Treponema pallidum* organisms (thin, coiled structures) may be identified in the aortic tissues. The photograph was taken from a section stained by Warthin-Starry silver technique. (From Virmani R, Burke AP, Farb A [eds]: Atlas of Cardiovascular Pathology. Philadelphia, WB Saunders, 1996, p 145.)

TABLE 5-4 • **Pathologic Differential Diagnosis of Aortitis**

Feature	Giant Cell	Takayasu	Syphilitic	Collagen-vascular*
Aortic aneurysms	+++	+/−	+++	++
Luminal narrowing	−/+	+++	−	−
Coronary ostial stenosis	+	++	++	+
Aortic valve involvement	−	++	−	+++
Arch involvement	++	+++	++	−/+
Skip areas	−	+++	+/−	+/−
"Tree barking"	+++	+++	+++	+
Site in aorta	throughout	thoracic +/− abd	ascending +/− abd	ascending
Dissection	+/−	−	−	−
Aortic annular dilatation	+	−	++−+++	++
Luminal thrombosis	+/−	+++	+/−	−
Superimposed atherosclerosis	++	+/−	+++	+/−
Endarteritis obliterans	+/−	++	+++	++
Giant cells	+++	+/++	+/−	+
Plasma cells	+	+/++	+++	++
Medial necrosis	+/−	+	+/++	+

* Includes rheumatoid and seronegative spondyloarthropathies (ankylosing spondylitis/Reiter syndrome). In rheumatoid aortitis, characteristic necrobiotic nodules may be present in some cases.

abd, abdominal.

125

autopsied cases and are usually not related to clinical symptoms.[87, 88] Gravallese and colleagues reported clinically significant aortitis in 3 of 188 consecutive autopsies of patients with rheumatoid arthritis,[87] two of whom had aortic insufficiency and heart failure, and the third of whom had a ruptured abdominal aortitic aneurysm.

The mean duration of rheumatoid aortitis is 10 years, and there is no sex predilection. Pathologically, the vessel wall is thickened with focal necrosis; aneurysms may develop in the thoracic or abdominal aorta. Microscopically, well-formed rheumatoid nodules are found in approximately 50% of cases (Fig. 5-26); in the remainder, there is a lymphoplasmacytic infiltrate, predominantly in the media and adventitia, accompanied by necrosis of smooth muscle cells and loss of medial elastic fibers.[87] In the absence of rheumatoid nodules, the histologic features demonstrate considerable overlap with Takayasu disease, syphilis, and ankylosing spondylitis; a clinical history is generally adequate for establishing the diagnosis. In contrast to ankylosing spondylitis, the severity of aortitis in patients with rheumatoid arthritis appears closely associated with the severity of the disease, rather than its duration.

Ankylosing Spondylitis

Ankylosing spondylitis is an idiopathic inflammatory disorder of young men, marked by progressive bilateral sacroiliitis, peripheral arthritis, and uveitis. The etiology of the disease is uncertain, although the demonstration of HLA-B27 antigen in as many as 95% of affected patients and in 50% of their first-degree relatives provides overwhelming evidence of a genetic linkage.[89] Aortic disease in ankylosing spondylitis has been described since the 1950s.[90] Symptomatic aortic involvement affects from 1 to 10% of patients and is usually related to the duration of the disease, although aortic involvement may precede arthritis. Evidence of aortic insufficiency is found in one third of men with the disease, and transesophageal echocardiography demonstrates thickened subaortic structures in a high proportion of these patients.[91]

Pathologically, there is inflammation and scarring of the sinus of Valsalva and several centimeters of the proximal tubular aorta. In the active phase, endarteritis obliterans is seen along with perivascular infiltration by lymphocytes and plasma cells (Fig. 5-27A, B). In the chronic phase, fibrosis involves adventitia, media, and intima; calcification may be present. The coronary ostia may be narrowed, and the aortic valve is invariably thickened. Fibrosis extends into the membranous and muscular septum and onto the anterior leaflet of the mitral valve, resulting in a characteristic "bump" seen at autopsy[92, 93] (Fig. 5-28).

The clinical manifestations of aortic involvement reflect the pathologic extent of inflammation and fibrosis. Aortic valve disease results in aortic regurgitation, and extension of the fibrotic process into the membranous and muscular septa may induce heart block, conduction defects, or sudden death.

Reiter Syndrome

Patients with Reiter syndrome manifest the triad of nongonococcal urethritis, conjunctivitis, and polyarthritis. Young men are most often affected, and the arthritis is typically located in the sacroiliac joint. Cardiovascular involvement is uncommon and is remarkably similar to that found in ankylosing spondylitis. Two to 5% of patients develop an aortitis with dilatation of the aortic root and aortic regurgitation. Other cardiovascular manifestations include pericarditis, myocarditis, and various conduction delays.[94] The latter are likely secondary to aortic root inflammation extending into the area of the atrioventricular node. Like ankylosing spondylitis, aortic involvement is limited to the ascending aorta. Microscopically, there is disruption of elastic tissue and infiltration by chronic inflammatory cells.[76, 92] Note that further discussion of rheumatoid arthritis, ankylosing spondylitis, and Reiter syndrome appears in Chapter 16.

Behçet Disease

Behçet disease is a recurring illness manifested by aphthous stomatitis, genital ulceration, and uveitis.[95] It occurs worldwide, but most patients are from the Mediterranean region, the Middle East, Japan, and Korea. Its etiology is unknown, although viral, bacterial, and chemical factors have been implicated.

A patient's age ranges from 31 to 56 years at appearance of the disease and there is a male predominance among those affected. Large-vessel involvement occurs in 2 to 20% of patients.[96, 97] Pathologic findings include peripheral arterial aneurysms that grossly resemble mycotic aneurysms,[98] aneurysms of the sinus of Valsalva,[99] abdominal aortic aneurysms,[100, 101] arterial occlusions, arterial dissections, and large-vein thrombophlebitis. Arterial aneurysms are more frequent than arterial occlusions,

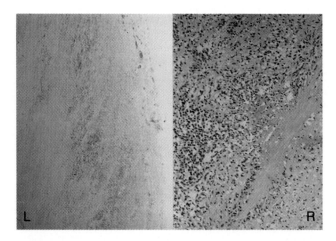

Figure 5-26 • Rheumatoid arthritis. A 57-year-old woman with long-standing rheumatoid arthritis, myocardial infarction, and congestive heart failure died of cardiac complications. At autopsy, rheumatoid nodules were found in the aortic, mitral, and tricuspid valves, the left ventricle, the coronary arteries, and the aorta. Note the rheumatoid nodule in the adventitial medial interface (left panel) and at higher power (right panel) (both H&E stain). (From Virmani R, Burke AP, Farb A [eds]: Atlas of Cardiovascular Pathology. Philadelphia, WB Saunders, 1996, p 142.)

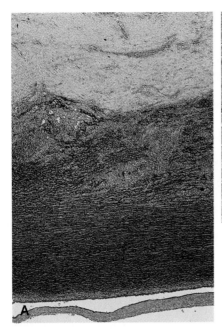
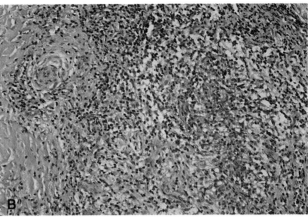

Figure 5-27 • A 62-year-old man with ankylosing spondylitis, scleritis, episcleritis, and a sudden onset of congestive heart failure from aortic valve incompetence. Laboratory tests showed HLA-B27 positivity, intermittent (ESR) elevation, and negative antinuclear antibody (ANA) and rheumatoid factor (RF). Patient underwent aortic valve replacement with a piece of aorta submitted for histologic examination. *A,* The aorta at low power shows granulomatous inflammation involving the outer media with loss of elastic lamellae and thickened adventitia. (Movat stain) *B,* Higher magnification in the area of inflammation showing granulomatous inflammation consisting of histiocytes and rare giant cells with marked lymphocytic infiltration. Also note thickened vasa vasorum (H&E stain).

although the two may occur together in the same patient. The abdominal aorta is most commonly involved by aneurysm, followed by the iliac, common femoral, superficial femoral, popliteal, subclavian, carotid, and posterior tibial arteries.[102]

Aortitis in Behçet disease can be divided into active and scar stages. In the former, intense round cell inflammatory infiltrate occurs in the media and adventitia, with a predominance of inflammatory cells around proliferating vasa vasorum. Rarely, giant cells are seen.[96] In late stages, there is fibrous thickening of the intima and adventitia, with mild perivascular inflammatory infiltrate and proliferation of vasa vasorum. Endarteritis obliterans of vasa vasorum may progress to luminal obliteration. The histologic features are similar to those of Takayasu disease and ankylosing spondylitis.[103]

Inflammatory Aneurysm of the Abdominal Aorta

Inflammatory aneurysm of the aorta as a distinct entity was first described by Walker and associates in 1972.[104] Its incidence is 11% of all operated abdominal aortic aneurysms. The male to female ratio is 9 to 1, similar to that of atherosclerotic abdominal aneurysm. The etiology of inflammatory aneurysm is unknown, although there may be pathogenetic similarities to retroperitoneal fibrosis.[105] The condition is sometimes considered a variant of aortic atherosclerotic aneurysm and occurs in a similar location, generally the abdominal aorta.[106] An association with coronary arteritis suggests a localized manifestation

of a systemic vasculitis or an autoimmune disease.[107] A genetic risk determinant has been mapped to the HLA-DR B1 locus.[108]

Clinically, patients often manifest abdominal pain, a mass, or both. In some, there is an elevated erythrocyte sedimentation rate. CT and ultrasonographic scans demonstrate an area of soft tissue density surrounding an atherosclerotic portion of the aneurysmal wall; this density corresponds pathologically to the marked fibrosis and perianeurysmal inflammation.[105] At surgery, this inflamed

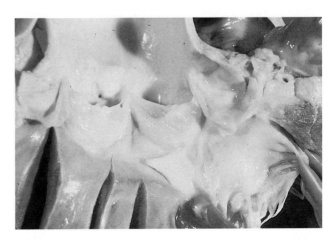

Figure 5-28 • Ankylosing spondylitis. This 58-year-old man manifested chest pain. Note marked thickening of the aortic valve and a fibrous "bump" over the membranous sputum and the anterior mitral leaflet. Note sections have been made in the septal wall. (Courtesy of Dr. W. C. Roberts.)

fibrotic process distinguishes inflammatory aneurysms from pure atherosclerotic aneurysms, and is recognized as a thick wall extending into the retroperitoneum. There is occasionally displacement and obstruction of ureters, duodenum, jejunum or ileum, sigmoid colon, renal artery or vein, and inferior vena cava. Spontaneous aortic rupture is unusual.

Grossly, the luminal wall of the aneurysm consists of atherosclerotic plaque, and there is no clear demarcation between plaque, attenuated media, and periadventitial fibrous tissue.[92] Microscopically, the aneurysmal aortic wall consists of complex atherosclerotic plaque with the media attenuated, fragmented, or replaced by fibrous tissue (Fig. 5-29A). The adventitia is also replaced by a dense connective tissue almost in direct continuity with the atherosclerotic plaque. The fibrous tissue extends beyond the adventitia and entraps fat, nerves, ganglia, and lymph nodes (Fig. 5-29B). Within the fibrous tissue is either a focal or diffuse heavy lymphocytic and plasma cell inflammatory infiltrate (see also Chapter 4).

Pyogenic Aortitis and Infectious Aneurysm

Nontreponemal infections of the aorta generally result in saccular, or less commonly, fusiform aneurysms. The original designation "mycotic aneurysm" is gradually being replaced by the more accurate term "infectious aneurysm." There are four routes of bacterial invasion. These are by: (1) implantation on the intimal surface; (2) embolization of bacteria into vasa vasorum; (3) direct extension of infection from a contiguous extravascular site; and (4) traumatic inoculation of contaminated material into the vessel wall. Contiguous inoculation is generally a complication of vertebral osteomyelitis,[109] and surface inoculation is often a complication of recent or remote infective endocarditis. In some cases of intimal inoculation, the site of infection is an atherosclerotic plaque.[110] Aneurysm formation may evolve rapidly over the course of days after initiation of the aortitis.[111]

The femoral artery is the most common site of these aneurysms (56%), followed by the abdominal (18%) and the thoracic aorta (15%), and the mesenteric and peripheral arteries (11%).[112] Before the advent of antibiotics, streptococcal species, including pneumococcal, staphylococcal, and gonococcal organisms were the most common pathogens.[110] Recently, *Salmonella* species have been isolated more frequently.[111, 113] In a review, the organisms cultured from infectious aneurysms were *Staphylococcus aureus* (46%), *Salmonella* species (15%), streptococci (8%), *Escherichia coli* (8%), no organisms detected (9%), in miscellaneous (13%).[112]

Grossly, infectious aneurysms are often saccular outpouchings measuring up to 5 cm in diameter (Fig. 5-30). There is typically marked edema and inflammation of the adventitia, which result in a characteristic soft tissue swelling on CT scan or MRI. Histologically, there are numerous neutrophils in the vessel wall with extension into the adventitia. It should be remembered that chronic inflammation with occasional neutrophils are typically seen in atherosclerosis; infected atherosclerotic plaques should be suspected only if there is a pyogenic reaction and if the history suggests sepsis.

AORTIC THROMBOSIS

Thrombi are associated with ulcerated atherosclerotic plaques, and mural thrombi are a constant finding in atherosclerotic abdominal aortic aneurysms. In some patients, aortic thrombosis may occur in the absence of severe atherosclerosis (Fig. 5-31), and be a result of coagulation disorders[114] or thrombocytosis.[115] Idiopathic thrombosis of the aorta occurs in neonates.[116] Unusual causes of aortic thrombosis in adults include metastatic tumors and infections.[117, 118] Intimal sarcoma of the aorta should be considered in the differential diagnosis of an aortic mural thrombus (see later).

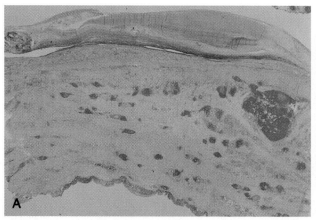
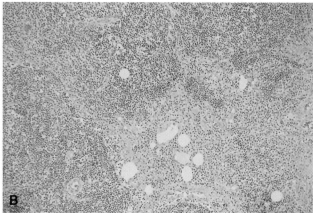

Figure 5-29 • Inflammatory aneurysm. A 73-year-old white female with a painful pulsatile abdominal aortic aneurysm. On magnetic resonance imaging (MRI) study the aneurysm showed hyperintensity of the aortic wall on T2-weighted images with enhancement after gadolinium injection, suggestive of an inflammatory process. Patient had a history of smoking and hypertension. A, Histology (lower power) revealed a markedly thickened adventitia with focal collections of chronic inflammatory cells and entrapped nerves. The media is markedly attenuated and the intimal surface shows atherosclerotic involvement (Movat stain). B, Higher power. Note entrapped fat, marked scarring, and chronic inflammatory process, with lymphoid follicles in adventitia (H&E stain).

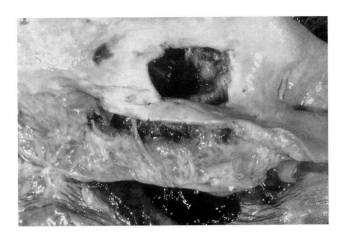

Figure 5-30 • Pyogenic aortitis (inflammatory aneurysm). Note large hemorrhagic aneurysm through which a probe could be passed into the aortic lumen. The aneurysm was located in the descending thoracic aorta. (From Sekosan M, Farolan MJ, Burke A, Ronan SG: Pathology of vascular disease. In: Eton D [ed]: Vascular Disease: A Multi-Specialty Approach. Austin, TX, Landes Bioscience, 1997.)

SARCOMAS OF THE GREAT VESSELS

Sarcomas of the Aorta

The majority of aortic sarcomas are located predominantly within the lumen, suggesting that they are derived from intimal cells, endothelial cells, and smooth muscle cells.[119-121] Consistent with this hypothesis, most are of myofibroblastic phenotype, with angiosarcomas a close

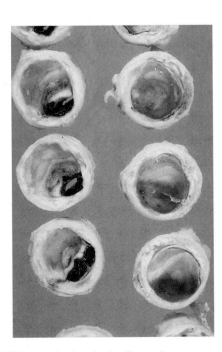

Figure 5-31 • Aortic thrombosis. The patient was a middle-aged woman given heparin for suspected pulmonary embolism. Thrombocytopenia with multiple arterial thrombi, including aortic thrombosis, occurred in response to antiheparin antibodies. Multiple sections of aorta with acute thrombosis in lumen. (From Virmani R, Burke AP, Farb A [eds]: Atlas of Cardiovascular Pathology. Philadelphia, WB Saunders, 1996, p 205.)

second. They are rare tumors; fewer than 250 have been reported in the literature.

Clinical Findings

Patients are usually middle-aged adults; mean age is approximately 60 years and there is no sex predilection[122] (see Table 5-5). Clinical symptoms are often caused by embolization to lower extremities or mesenteric arteries. Indeed, the diagnosis may first be made upon removal of embolic implants in the mesenteric arteries or arteries of the lower extremities.[121, 122] Other symptoms include back pain, shock from rupture of an aneurysm formed by the tumor, and malignant hypertension. On occasion, the tumor is first diagnosed at repair of an abdominal aortic aneurysm, and rare aortic sarcomas have developed at the anastomotic site of dacron grafts.[121] The clinical course may be influenced by metastatic lesions, which most frequently occur in bone, peritoneum, liver, and mesenteric lymph nodes.[121, 123]

Pathologic Findings

Approximately 70% of aortic sarcomas arise in the abdominal aorta and 30% appear in the descending thoracic portion or aortic arch.[119, 124] Usually, in the gross the lumen is nearly filled with a soft necrotic mass (Fig. 5-32A, B) prone to embolization. Occasionally, the tumor may produce an aneurysmal dilatation of the aorta, imparting a gross morphology like that of an atherosclerotic aneurysm.

Intimal sarcomas have a variety of histologic appearances; the majority are spindle cell sarcomas demonstrating myofibroblastic differentiation, expressing smooth-muscle and muscle-specific actin and vimentin. The luminal surface is often stratified into a cellular layer, which overlies a second layer of dense fibrous tissue.

TABLE 5-5 • **Clinicopathologic Features of 21 Aortic Intimal Sarcomas[1]**

Mean age, years	63 ± 10
Male : female ratio	12 : 9
Aortic site	
Ascending	2
Descending thoracic	7
Abdominal	12
Diagnostic procedure	
Aneurysm repair	8
Embolectomy	6
Aortectomy	3
Autopsy	3
Graft revision	1
Histologic appearance	
Myofibroblastic sarcoma/MFH	13[2]
Angiosarcoma, typical	3
Angiosarcoma, epithelioid	4[3]
Osteosarcoma/chondrosarcoma, myxoid	1

[1] Tumors reviewed by the authors. Includes 11 previously published cases. From Burke AP, Virmani R: Sarcomas of the great vessels. A clinicopathologic study. Cancer 71:1761–1773, 1993.
[2] Two of these had prominent myxoid areas.
[3] Three of these focally expressed cytokeratin.
MFH, malignant fibrous histiocytoma.

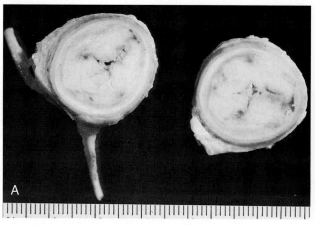
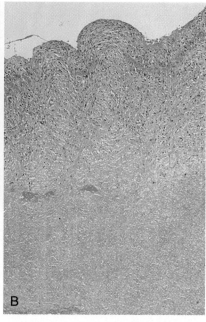

Figure 5-32 • Aortic sarcoma. *A,* Two transected segments of the abdominal aorta with lumen filled with necrotic tumor. *B,* Histologically, the luminal surface (above) is cellular, relative to the hyalinized portion of the tumor (below) (H&E stain). (From Virmani R, Burke AP, Farb A [eds]: Atlas of Cardiovascular Pathology. Philadelphia, WB Saunders, 1996, p 156.)

Epithelioid and myxoid areas may be present, and foci, especially in areas of extraluminal growth, may resemble those of malignant fibrous histiocytoma. The second most common histologic variant is an angiosarcoma (Fig. 5-33), which may have epithelioid characteristics reflected by tumor cells expressing cytokeratin. Rarely, osteo- or chondrosarcoma may be present.

The differential diagnosis is from metastatic carcinoma. A clinical history and careful exclusion of primary epithelial neoplasms help to exclude carcinoma, which rarely grows into the aortic lumen. Embolic myxoma may be confused with aortic sarcomas that have a myxoid matrix; however, myxoma cells are absent in a sarcoma, and an echocardiogram does not demonstrate an atrial mass.

Treatment

Resection of the involved segment with aortic grafting is usually performed at diagnosis, although occasionally diagnosis is made initially by biopsy.[125] Tumor recurrence at the anastomotic site has been documented in several cases.[119, 124] The prognosis is usually dismal, and most patients die within months. However, an occasional patient survives for years after initial surgery.[121, 122]

Sarcomas of the Pulmonary Artery

Sarcomas of the pulmonary artery are similar to aortic sarcomas in that the majority are presumed derived from the intima.[121, 122] They are only slightly more common that aortic sarcomas and appear in somewhat younger patients than those with aortic sarcomas, approximately at the age of 45 years (Table 5-6). The most common initial symptom is dyspnea, and the initial clinical diagnosis is almost always that of pulmonary embolism.[126] Rarely, the tumor may rupture and cause hemopericardium.[127] With MRI and CT scanning, a preoperative diagnosis of intraluminal tumor may be made,[128] and the pathologic diagnosis may be established by performance of endarterectomy or after pneumonectomy. However, most patients carry a diagnosis of recurrent pulmonary embolism for

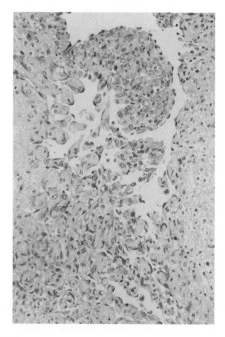

Figure 5-33 • Aortic angiosarcoma. Note the anastomosing vascular tufts lined by atypical endothelial cells (H&E stain).

TABLE 5-6 • **Clinicopathologic Features of 30 Pulmonary Artery[1] Intimal Sarcomas**

Mean age, years	46 ± 18
Male : female ratio	19 : 11
Pulmonary artery site	
Pulmonary trunk	14
Right pulmonary artery	8
Left pulmonary artery	8
Diagnostic procedure	
Biopsy	3[2]
Embolectomy with endarterectomy	9
Pneumonectomy/lobectomy	10
Autopsy	8
Histologic appearance	
Myofibroblastic (MFH)	16
Myxoid chondrosarcoma/osteosarcoma	6
Myxoid myofibroblastic (MFH)	4
Leiomyosarcoma	3
Angiosarcoma	1

[1] Tumors reviewed by the authors. Includes 16 previously published cases. From Burke AP, Virmani R: Sarcomas of the great vessels. A clinicopathologic study. Cancer 71:1761–1773, 1993.
[2] Two open biopsies, one fine-needle aspiration (transthoracic).
MFH, malignant fibrous histiocytoma.

months before a sarcoma is suspected, and diagnosis is often made first at autopsy.[122, 129]

Grossly, the tumor is a soft, necrotic, often mucoid mass distending the arterial lumen (Fig. 5-34*A, B*). Sites of involvement include pulmonary trunk (80%), left pulmonary artery (58%), right pulmonary artery (57%), both pulmonary arteries (37%), pulmonary valve (29%), and right ventricle (8%).[129] Distal luminal extension is common, and distal pulmonary parenchymal masses are frequently present.

Histologically, more than 50% are spindle cell sarcomas of presumed myofibroblastic derivation,[130] and are commonly classified as malignant fibrous histiocytoma. Other histologic types include leiomyosarcoma (20%), chondro- or osteosarcoma (7%), angiosarcoma (7%), rhabdomyosarcoma (6%),[131] malignant mesenchymoma (6%), malignant fibrous histiocytoma (3%), and liposarcoma (1%).[129]

Metastatic sites include kidneys, brain, lymph nodes, and skin. Survival of more than 2 years without metastases or treatment is common, but few patients live 5 years after diagnosis. It has been emphasized that treatment is often delayed because the diagnosis is not suspected early in the course of disease,[131] and that with early resection, prognosis might improve.[132]

Sarcomas of the Inferior Vena Cava

In contrast to sarcomas of the aorta and the pulmonary artery, sarcomas of the inferior vena cava are usually well-differentiated leiomyosarcomas that arise from the vessel wall. Such a site of origin of a bulky tumor may not be evident preoperatively in a patient with a retroperitoneal leiomyosarcoma. The majority of venous leiomyosarcomas arise in the inferior caval vein, although rare examples of origin from the pulmonary vein (which may be difficult to distinguish from left atrial sarcomas), the superior vena cava, and the femoral vein have been reported.[122]

Most patients with sarcomas of the inferior vena cava are women.[133] The mean age for appearance is the sixth decade (Table 5-7). The initial symptoms depend on the site of the tumor in the caval vein and whether it is inferior or superior to the hepatic vein. With luminal compromise, patients develop Budd Chiari syndrome if the tumor is near the hepatic vein, and inferior vena cava syndrome or recurrent pulmonary emboli occur. Distal tumors are more likely to appear with abdominal pain or metastatic disease. Metastases have been reported in lungs, kidneys, pleura, chest wall, liver, and skeleton.

Grossly, 34% of caval leiomyosarcomas are infrarenal, 42% arise in the midportion of the inferior vena cava, and 24% arise between the liver and the heart.[133] They are usually large, with a mean diameter of 10 cm. The tumors are firmly attached to the inferior vena cava and are discrete, firm, whorled masses that extend into the retroperitoneum. More than 75% are attached to the ves-

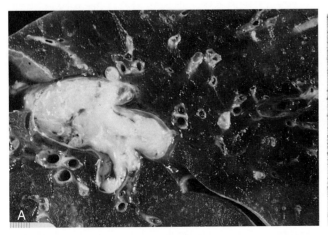

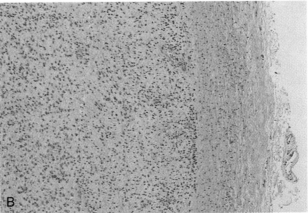

Figure 5-34 • Pulmonary artery sarcoma. *A,* The tumor resembles a mucoid clot, filling the proximal pulmonary artery. (From Virmani R, Burke AP, Farb A [eds]: Atlas of Cardiovascular Pathology. Philadelphia, WB Saunders, 1996, p 157.) *B,* Histologically, the tumor is a myxoid spindle cell proliferation present within the lumen of the vessel (media seen at the right) (H&E stain).

TABLE 5-7 • **Twenty-six Sarcomas of Large Veins**[1]

Mean age, years	50 ± 19
Male:female ratio	10:16
Site	
IVC inferior to hepatic vein	12
IVC involving hepatic vein	7
IVC between hepatic vein and atrium	4
Femoral vein	2
Superior vena cava	2
Pulmonary vein	2
Diagnostic procedure	
Resection	16
Biopsy	4
Resection with vein graft	3
Embolectomy with endarterectomy[2]	2
Autopsy	1
Histologic appearance	
Leiomyosarcoma	24
Angiosarcoma	1
Myofibroblastic sarcoma	1

[1] Tumors reviewed by the authors. Includes 16 previously published cases. From Burke AP, Virmani R: Sarcomas of the great vessels. A clinicopathologic study. Cancer 71:1761–1773, 1993.
[2] Two tumors were predominantly luminal.
IVC, inferior vena cava.

sel wall, and the remainder are primarily intraluminal. Microscopically, most are relatively well-differentiated leiomyosarcomas (Fig. 5-35), composed of fascicles of spindle cells oriented at acute angles to one another; the cells possess blunt-ended nuclei, occasional cytoplasmic perinuclear vacuoles, and fuchsinophilic intracytoplasmic fibers. Intracytoplasmic desmin is identified by immunohistochemistry in about 50% of cases. Tumor giant cells are occasionally present.

The prognosis of leiomyosarcomas of the inferior vena cava is better than that of intimal sarcomas of the aorta or the pulmonary artery. With complete excision, long-term survival is possible; the 10-year survival has been estimated at 14%.[133]

MISCELLANEOUS DISEASES OF THE LARGE VEINS

Thrombosis of the Superior Vena Cava

Thrombosis of the superior vena cava and its tributaries results in superior vena cava syndrome, characterized by reduced venous outflow from head, neck, and upper extremities. Symptoms are facial edema, cyanosis, dyspnea, and prominent neck veins. The most common causes are thoracic neoplasms including lung carcinomas, lymphomas, and metastatic disease. Unusual causes are fibrosing mediastinitis, indwelling catheters, pacemakers, LeVeen shunts, administration of megestrol acetate,[134] aortic dissections and aneurysms, rupture of a bronchial artery aneurysm,[135] and Behçet disease.[136]

Thrombosis of the Inferior Vena Cava

Obstruction of the inferior vena cava is most often a complication of thrombotic occlusion related to neoplasms growing within the lumen or those causing external compression.[137] The neoplasms are usually renal,[138–140] adrenal, hepatic,[141] or testicular.[142] Idiopathic forms of diffuse thrombosis of the inferior vena cava have been reported.[143] An uncommon complication of orthotopic liver transplant is thrombosis of the inferior vena cava. It can be successfully treated surgically.[144] Tumor-induced thrombosis may be treated with placement of a filter to prevent pulmonary embolism, similar to treatment for recurrent thromboembolism from leg veins.[145] Neonatal thrombosis of the inferior vena cava may be the result of renal vein thrombosis and cause fibrous obstruction of the vein and duodenal varices in adulthood.[146]

Thrombosis of the hepatic veins (Budd Chiari syndrome) may be complicated by obstruction of the inferior vena cava. Symptoms of hepatic vein thrombosis include ascites, jaundice, gastrointestinal bleeding, hepatomegaly, leg edema, varicose veins, and venous collaterals over the abdominal and chest wall. The most common known cause is thrombosis secondary to myeloproliferative diseases.[147] Other causes include abdominal trauma, hepatic tumors, pregnancy, and oral contraceptive use.

Obstruction of distal hepatic veins and inferior vena cava by membranous webs is a form of Budd Chiari syndrome associated with similar symptoms. Membranous obstruction of the inferior vena cava is sometimes considered congenital, and sometimes is a sequel of repeated thrombosis.[148] The simultaneous occurrence of myeloproliferative syndromes and membranous obstruction of the inferior vena cava supports the latter view and corroborates the link between hepatic vein thrombosis and membranous obstruction.[149]

Mortality is high in the acute phase of hepatic vein obstruction, but prognosis is good if the initial phase is survived. Treatment includes anticoagulation, measures to control ascites and bleeding, portocaval shunts, and orthotopic liver transplants if there is severe liver failure. Membranes in the inferior vena cava may be lysed by percutaneous angioplasty.

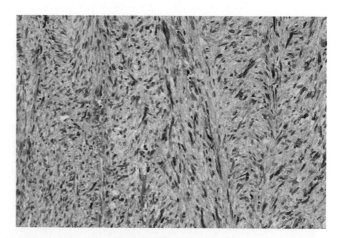

Figure 5-35 • Leiomyosarcoma, inferior vena cava. Histologically, fascicles of spindle cells are oriented at acute angles to one another. The cells have blunt-ended nuclei and abundant eosinophilic cytoplasm (H&E stain).

Venous Aneurysms

Venous aneurysms are often the result of increased flow and turbulence adjacent to arteriovenous malformations, or as complications of surgery. Congenital venous aneurysms are rare and have been described in jugular, portal, superior mesenteric, splenic, femoral, popliteal, saphenous, and axillary veins, as well as venae cavae.[150–153] Symptoms of aneurysms of the inferior vena cava include deep venous thrombosis, pulmonary embolism, retroperitoneal hemorrhage after rupture, and abdominal mass. Aneurysms of the inferior vena cava may complicate membranous obstruction at the level of the hepatic veins.[154] There are few pathologic descriptions of venous aneurysms; in our experience, the aneurysm wall is composed of focally thinned and disorganized smooth muscle, with luminal thrombosis in some cases.

MISCELLANEOUS DISEASES OF THE PROXIMAL PULMONARY ARTERIES

Pulmonary Artery Thrombosis

Thrombosis of elastic arteries is almost always caused by thromboembolism.[155] In situ thrombosis of elastic pulmonary arteries is rare and may be associated with the antiphospholipid syndrome,[156] Behçet disease,[157, 158] Takayasu disease, and other forms of vasculitis affecting the pulmonary arteries.[159, 160] Pulmonary artery thrombosis is an uncommon complication of right-sided heart catheterization.[161] In situ thrombosis of medium-sized muscular pulmonary arteries is a frequent finding in pulmonary hypertension; more distal thrombi are usually the result of a showering of pulmonary emboli.[155]

Vasculitis of the Main Pulmonary Arteries

The vasculitic syndrome with the most frequent involvement of the main pulmonary arteries is Takayasu disease. Abnormalities of pulmonary arteries are seen in as many as 70% of patients in whom angiography is performed.[162] The angiographic lesions are occlusions (67%), stenoses (32%), and, rarely, aneurysms (1%).[160] Lesions occur in the entire course of the pulmonary arteries, but are most numerous in segmental and subsegmental branches. Histologically, the arteries show disruption of the elastic layers with thinning of the media and pronounced fibrosis of the adventitia. Occlusions, which are more common distally, are characterized by marked intimal fibrosis and eccentric intimal fibrotic thickening.[162] Behçet disease involves the pulmonary tree in about 10% of patients, manifesting as aneurysms and thrombosis (see later). Giant cell arteritis rarely involves the proximal pulmonary arteries. It causes thrombotic occlusion and medial granulomas.[163, 164]

Pulmonary Artery Aneurysms

Most aneurysms of the pulmonary artery are noninflammatory. They are usually found in patients with severe pulmonary hypertension that is idiopathic, secondary, or caused by congenital or acquired heart disease or pulmonary disease.[165, 166] Inflammatory pulmonary aneurysms are found in 1% of patients with Behçet disease,[136, 158, 167–169] and, rarely, in patients with syphilis.[165] Pseudoaneurysms of the pulmonary artery are usually the result of catheter-induced trauma.[170] Presumed congenital (idiopathic) pulmonary artery aneurysms have been described in patients without predisposing factors.[165, 171] There is an association between pulmonary aneurysm and pregnancy,[172] and spontaneous rupture of the pulmonary artery without aneurysm has been reported.[173] Pulmonary artery aneurysm is a rare manifestation of Marfan syndrome.[165]

Grossly, pulmonary artery aneurysms may be fusiform or saccular.[174] Aneurysmal dilatation of the pulmonary root is defined as a diameter of 4 cm or greater.[165] The histologic findings of hypertension-induced pulmonary artery aneurysms include medial degeneration in the fusiform types and atherosclerosis in the saccular forms.[166] Behçet aneurysms show inflammatory infiltrates in all layers of arteries and veins,[167] leading to thrombosis, destruction of the elastic laminae, and arteriobronchial fistula.[158] The major complication of hypertension-induced pulmonary aneurysms is dissection[172, 175] and rupture.

FIBROMUSCULAR DYSPLASIA OF THE GREAT ARTERIES

Fibromuscular dysplasia is generally a disease of muscular arteries. There are scattered reports of its producing aortic and iliac dissections,[29, 30, 176] thoracic coarctation,[177, 178] and abdominal aortic aneurysm.[179] Medial dysplasia of the pulmonary arteries has been described in association with pulmonary hypertension.[180, 181]

The opinions or assertions contained herein are the private views of the authors and are not to be construed as official or as reflecting the views of the Department of the Army or Navy or the Department of Defense.

REFERENCES

1. Isselbacher EM, Eagle KA, Desanctis RW: Disease of the aorta. In: Braunwald E, (ed): Heart Disease: A Textbook of Cardiovascular Medicine. Philadelphia, WB Saunders, 1997, pp 1546–1581
2. Schlatmann T, Becker A: Pathogenesis of dissecting aneurysm of aorta. Comparative histopathologic study of significance of medial changes. Am J Cardiol 39:21–26, 1977
3. O'Rourke MF: Arterial Function in Health and Disease. London, Churchill Livingstone, 1982
4. Cliff WJ: Aging in the arterial wall. In: van Haher H (ed): Interdisciplinary Topics in Gerontology. Vol. 11. Basel, Karger, 1977 pp 89–99
5. Meyer WW, Walsh SZ, Ling J: Functional Morphology of human arteries during fetal and postnatal development. In: Schwartz CJ, Werthessen NT, Wolf S (eds): Structure and Function of the Circulation. Vol. 1. New York, Plenum Press, 1980, pp 95–379
6. Stefanadis C, Vlachopoulos C, Karayannacos P, et al: Effect of vasa vasorum flow on structure and function of the aorta in experimental animals. Circulation 91:2669–2678, 1995
7. Virmani R, Avolio AP, Mergner WJ, et al: Effect of aging on aortic morphology in populations with high and low prevalence of

hypertension and atherosclerosis. Comparison between occidental and Chinese communities. Am J Pathol 139:1119–1129, 1991

8. Ellis RP, Cooley DA, DeBakey ME: Clinical considerations and surgical treatment of annulo-aortic ectasia. J Thorac Cardiovasc Surg 42:363–369, 1961

9. Shimokawa H, Koiwaya Y, Kaku T: Annuloaortic ectasia in a case of Takayasu arteritis associated with Hashimoto's disease. Br Heart J 49:94–97, 1983

10. Cooley DA: Annuloaortic ectasia. Ann Thorac Surg 28:303–304, 1979

11. Savunen T: Cardiovascular abnormalities in the relatives of patients operated upon for annulo-aortic ectasia. A clinical and echocardiographic study of 40 families. Eur J Cardiothorac Surg 1:3–9; discussion 9–10, 1987

12. Savunen T, Inberg M, Niinikoski J, et al: Composite graft in annulo-aortic ectasia. Nineteen years' experience without graft inclusion. Eur J Cardiothorac Surg 10:428–432, 1996

13. Painvin GA, Weisel RD, David TE, et al: Surgical treatment of annuloaortic ectasia. Can J Surg 23:445–449, 1980

14. Dare AJ, Veinot JP, Edwards WD, et al: New observations on the etiology of aortic valve disease: A surgical pathologic study of 236 cases from 1990. Hum Pathol 24:1330–1338, 1993

15. Kirklin JW, Barratt-Boyes BG: Aortic valve disease. In: Kirklin JW, Barratt-Boyes BG (eds): Cardiac Surgery. New York, Churchill Livingstone, 1993, pp 491–571

16. Halme T, Savunen T, Aho H, et al: Elastin and collagen in the aortic wall: Changes in the Marfan syndrome and annuloaortic ectasia. Exp Mol Pathol 43:1–12, 1985

17. Dare AJ, Veinot JP, Edwards WD, et al: New observations on the etiology of aortic valve disease: Of the clinical history, operative details, and functional state of the valve. Hum Pathol 24:1286–1293, 1993

18. Wilson RA, McDonald RW, Bristow JD, et al: Correlates of aortic distensibility in chronic aortic regurgitation and relation to progression to surgery. J Am Coll Cardiol 19:733–738, 1992

19. Perloff J: Congenital heart disease in adults. In: Braunwald E (ed): Heart Disease: A Textbook of Cardiovascular Medicine. Philadelphia, WB Saunders, 1997, pp 963–87

20. Xu Q, Peng Z, Rahko PS: Doppler echocardiographic characteristics of sinus of Valsalva aneurysms. Am Heart J 130:1265–1269, 1995

21. Boutefeu JM, Moret PR, Hahn C, Hauf E: Aneurysm of the sinus of Valsalva. Report of seven cases and review of the literature. Am J Med 65:18–24, 1978

22. Sakakibara S, Konno S: Congenital aneurysms of the sinus of Valsalva: Anatomy and classification. Am Heart J 63:405–424, 1962

23. Wheat MW Jr: Acute dissecting aneurysms of the aorta. Diagnosis and treatment—1979. Am Heart J 99:373–387, 1980

24. Larson EW, Edwards WD: Risk factors for aortic dissection: A necropsy study of 161 cases. Am J Cardiol 53:849–855, 1984

25. Gore I, Seiwert VJ: Dissecting aneurysm of the aorta: Pathologic aspects. An analysis of eighty-five fatal cases. Arch Pathol 53:121–141, 1952

26. Edwards WD, Leaf DS, Edwards JE: Dissecting aortic aneurysm associated with congenital bicuspid aortic valve. Circulation 57:1022–1025, 1978

27. Roberts CS, Roberts WC: Dissection of the aorta associated with congenital malformation of the aortic valve. J Am Coll Cardiol 17:712–716, 1991

28. Nicod P, Bloor C, Godfrey M, et al: Familial aortic dissecting aneurysm. J Am Coll Cardiol 13:811–819, 1989

29. Gatalica Z, Gibas Z, Martinez-Hernandez A: Dissecting aortic aneurysm as a complication of generalized fibromuscular dysplasia. Hum Pathol 23:586–588, 1992

30. Heggtveit HA: A case of fibromuscular dysplasia and aortic dissection. Hum Pathol 23:1438–1440, 1992

31. Roberts WC: Aortic dissection: Anatomy, consequences, and causes. Am Heart J 101:195–214, 1981

32. Roberts CS, Roberts WC: Aortic dissection with the entrance tear in the descending thoracic aorta. Ann Surg 213:356–368, 1991

33. Murray CA, Edwards JE: Spontaneous laceration of ascending aorta. Circulation 47:848–858, 1973

34. Silver MD: The healed and sealed aortic intimomedial tear. Cardiovasc Pathol 6:315–320, 1997

35. Williams DM, Joshi A, Dake MD, et al: Aortic cobwebs: An anatomic marker identifying the false lumen in aortic dissection—imaging and pathologic correlation. Radiology 190:167–174, 1994

36. Sariola H, Viljanen T, Luosto R: Histological pattern and changes in extracellular matrix in aortic dissections. J Clin Pathol 39:1074–1081, 1986

37. Nakashima Y, Shiokawa Y, Sueishi K: Alterations of elastic architecture in human aortic dissecting aneurysm. Lab Invest 62:761–760, 1990

38. Wilson SK, Hutchins GM: Aortic dissecting aneurysms: Causative factors in 204 subjects. Arch Pathol Lab Med 106:175–180, 1982

39. Spittell PC, Spittell JA Jr, Joyce JW, et al: Clinical features and differential diagnosis of aortic dissection: Experience with 236 cases (1980 through 1990). Mayo Clin Proc 68:642–651, 1993

40. Fann JI, Sarris GE, Mitchell RS, et al: Treatment of patients with aortic dissection presenting with peripheral vascular complications. Ann Surg 212:705–713, 1990

41. Veyssier-Belot C, Cohen A, Rougemont D, et al: Cerebral infarction due to painless thoracic aortic and common carotid artery dissections. Stroke 24:2111–2113, 1993

42. Laas J, Heinemann M, Schaefers HJ, et al: Management of thoracoabdominal malperfusion in aortic dissection. Circulation 84:III20–III24, 1991

43. Hirst AE, Johns VJ, Kime SW: Dissecting aneurysm of the aorta: A review of 505 cases. Medicine 37:217–239, 1958

44. Yamada E, Matsumura M, Kyo S, Omoto R: Usefulness of a prototype intravascular ultrasound imaging in evaluation of aortic dissection and comparison with angiographic study, transesophageal echocardiography, computed tomography, and magnetic resonance imaging. Am J Cardiol 75:161–165, 1995

45. Roberts CS, Roberts WC: Aortic dissection with the entrance tear in abdominal aorta. Am Heart J 121:1834–1835, 1991

46. Pyeritz RE: Marfan syndrome: Current and future clinical and genetic management of cardiovascular manifestations. Semin Thorac Cardiovasc Surg 5:11–16, 1993

47. Godfrey M: The Marfan syndrome. In: Beighton P (ed): McKusick's Heritable Disorders of Connective Tissue, 5th ed. St. Louis, Mosby, 1993, pp 51–136

48. Roberts WC, Honig HS: The spectrum of cardiovascular disease in Marfan syndrome: A clinicopathologic study of 18 necropsy patients. Am Heart J 104:115–135, 1982

49. Byers PH: Disorders of collage biosynthesis and structure. In: Scriver CR, Beaudet AL, Sly WA, Valle D (eds): The Metabolic and Molecular Bases of Inherited Diseases. New York, McGraw-Hill, 1995, p 4029

50. Prat A, Warembourg H Jr, Watel A, et al: Chronic traumatic aneurysms of the descending thoracic aorta (19 cases). J Cardiovasc Surg (Torino) 27:268–272, 1986

51. Jensen BT: Fourteen years' survival with an untreated traumatic rupture of the thoracal aorta. Am J Forensic Med Pathol 9:58–59, 1988

52. Swanson S, Gaffey M: Traumatic false aneurysm of descending aorta with aortoesophageal fistula. J Forensic Sci 33:816–822, 1988

53. Takayasu M: Case with unusual changes of the central vessels in the retina. Acta Soc Ophthalmol Jpn 112:554–561, 1908

54. Shimizu K, Sano K: Pulseless disease. J Neuropathol 1:37–47, 1951

55. Lupi-Herrera E, Sanchez-Torres G, Marcushamer J, et al: Takayasu arteritis. Clinical study of 107 cases. Am Heart J 93:94–103, 1977

56. Hall S, Barr W, Lie JT: Takayasu arteritis. A study of 32 North American patients. Medicine 64:89–99, 1985

57. Morooka S, Saito Y, Nonaka Y, et al: Clinical features and course of aortitis syndrome in Japanese women older than 40 years. Am J Cardiol. 53:859–861, 1984

58. Basso C, Baracca E, Zonzin P, Thiene G: Sudden cardiac arrest in a teenager as first manifestation of Takayasu disease. Int J Cardiol 43:87–89, 1994

59. Matsumura K, Hirano T, Takeda K, et al: Incidence of aneurysms in Takayasu arteritis. Angiology 42:308–315, 1991

60. Ueda H, Sugiura M, Ito I, et al: Aortic insufficiency associated with aortitis syndrome. Jpn Heart J 8:107–120, 1967

61. Ueda H, Morooka S, Ito I, et al: Clinical observations on 52 cases of aortitis syndrome. Jpn Heart J 10:277–288, 1969

62. Numano F, Ohta N, Sasazuki T: HLA and clinical manifestations in Takayasu disease. Jpn Circ J 46:184–189, 1982
63. Shelhamer JH, Volkman DJ, Parrillo JE, et al: Takayasu arteritis and its therapy. Ann Intern Med 103:121–126, 1985
64. Amano J, Suzuki A: Coronary artery involvement in Takayasu arteritis. Collective review and guideline for surgical treatment. J Thorac Cardiovasc Surg 102:554–560, 1991
65. Nishimura T, Uehara T, Hayashida K, Kozuka T: Coronary arterial involvement in aortitis syndrome: Assessment by exercise thallium scintigraphy. Heart Vessels 7(suppl):106–110, 1992
66. Noma M, Sugihara M, Kikuchi Y: Isolated coronary ostial stenosis in Takayasu arteritis: Case report and review of the literature. Angiology 44:839–844, 1993
67. Panja M, Kar AK, Dutta AL, et al: Cardiac involvement in non-specific aorto-arteritis. Int J Cardiol 34:289–295, 1992
68. Seguchi M, Hino Y, Aiba S, et al: Ostial stenosis of the left coronary artery as a sole clinical manifestation of Takayasu arteritis: A possible cause of unexpected sudden death. Heart Vessels 5: 188–191, 1990
69. Talwar KK, Kumar K, Chopra P, et al: Cardiac involvement in nonspecific aortoarteritis (Takayasu arteritis). Am Heart J 122: 1666–1670, 1991
70. Huston KA, Hunder GG, Lie JT, et al: Temporal arteritis: A 25-year epidemiologic, clinical, and pathologic study. Ann Intern Med 88:162–170, 1978
71. Hellmann DB: Immunopathogenesis, diagnosis, and treatment of giant cell arteritis, temporal arteritis, polymyalgia rheumatica, and Takayasu arteritis. Curr Opin Rheumatol 5:25–32, 1993
72. Odeh M, Oliven A: Temporal arteritis associated with acute Q fever. A case report. Angiology 45:1053–1057, 1994
73. Klein RG, Hunder GG, Stanson AW, Sheps SG: Large artery involvement in giant cell (temporal) arteritis. Ann Intern Med 83: 806–812, 1975
74. Evans JO, Fallon WM, Hunder GG: Increased incidence of aortic aneurysm and dissection in giant cell (temporal) arteritis. A population-based study. Ann Intern Med 122:502–507, 1995
75. Costello JJ, Nicholson WJ: Severe aortic regurgitation as a late complication of temporal arteritis. Chest 98:875–877, 1990
76. Virmani R, Burke AP: Pathologic features of aortitis. Cardiovasc Pathol 3:205–216, 1994
77. Fraser CM, Norris SJ, Weinstock GM, et al: Complete genome sequence of *Treponema pallidum* the syphilis spirochete. Science 281:375–388, 1998
78. Heggtveit HA: Syphilitic aortitis. A clinicopathologic autopsy study of 100 cases, 1950–1960. Circulation 29:346–355, 1964
79. Costa M, Robbs JV: Abdominal aneurysms in a black population: Clinicopathological study. Br J Surg 73:554–558, 1986
80. Marconato R, Inzaghi A, Cantoni GM, et al: Syphilitic aneurysm of the abdominal aorta: Report of two cases. Eur J Vasc Surg 2: 199–203, 1988
81. Chauvel C, Cohen A, Albo C, et al: Aortic dissection and cardiovascular syphilis: Report of an observation with transesophageal echocardiography and anatomopathologic findings. J Am Soc Echocardiogr 7:419–421, 1994
82. Kellett MW, Young GR, Fletcher NA: Paraparesis due to syphilitic aortic dissection. Neurology 48:221–223, 1997
83. Beckman EN: Plasma cell infiltrates in atherosclerotic abdominal aortic aneurysms. Am J Clin Pathol 85:21–24, 1986
84. Fulton JO, Zilla P, De Groot KM, Von Oppell UO: Syphilitic aortic aneurysm eroding through the sternum. Eur J Cardiothorac Surg 10:922–924, 1996
85. Pessotto R, Santini F, Bertolini P, et al: Surgical Treatment of an aortopulmonary artery fistula complicating a syphilitic aortic aneurysm. Cardiovasc Surg 3:707–710, 1995
86. Nakane H, Okada Y, Ibayashi S, et al: Brain infarction caused by syphilitic aortic aneurysm. A case report. Angiology 47:911–917, 1996
87. Gravallese EM, Corson JM, Coblyn JS, et al: Rheumatoid aortitis: A rarely recognized but clinically significant entity. Medicine (Baltimore). 68:95–106, 1989
88. Reimer KA, Rodgers RF, Oyasu R: Rheumatoid arthritis with rheumatoid heart disease and granulomatous aortitis. JAMA 235: 2510–2512, 1976
89. Brewerton DA, James DC: The histocompatibility antigen (HL-A 27) and disease. Semin Arthritis Rheum 4:191–207, 1975
90. Ansell BM, Bywaters EGL, Doniach I: The aortic lesions of ankylosing spondylitis. Br Heart J 20:507–515, 1958
91. Arnason JA, Patel AK, Rahko PS, Sundstrom WR: Transthoracic and transesophageal echocardiographic evaluation of the aortic root and subvalvular structures in ankylosing spondylitis. J Rheumatol 23:120–123, 1996
92. Virmani R, McAllister HA: Pathology of the aorta and major arteries. In: Lande A, Borkman YM, McAllister HA (eds): Aortitis: Clinical, Pathologic, and Radiographic Aspects. New York, Raven Press, 1986, pp 7–53
93. Bulkley BH, Roberts WC: Ankylosing spondylitis and aortic regurgitation. Description of the characteristic cardiovascular lesion from study of eight necropsy patients. Circulation 48:1014–1027, 1973
94. Paulus HE, Pearson CM, Pitts W Jr: Aortic insufficiency in five patients with Reiter's syndrome. A detailed clinical and pathologic study. Am J Med 53:464–472, 1972
95. Chajek T, Fainaru M: Behçet's disease. Report of 41 cases and a review of the literature. Medicine (Baltimore) 54:179–196, 1975
96. Matsumoto T, Uekusa T, Fukuda Y: Vasculo-Behçet's disease: A pathologic study of eight cases. Hum Pathol 22:45–51, 1991
97. Humza M: Large artery involvement in Behçet's disease. J Rheumatol 14:554–559, 1987
98. Bastounis E, Maltezos C, Giambouras S, et al: Arterial aneurysms in Behçet's disease. Int Angiol 13:196–201, 1994
99. Koh KK, Lee KH, Kim SS, et al: Ruptured aneurysm of the sinus of Valsalva in a patient with Behçet's disease. Int J Cardiol 47: 177–179, 1994
100. Tuzuner A, Uncu H: A case of Behçet's disease with an abdominal aortic aneurysm and two aneurysms in the common carotid artery. A case report. Angiology 47:1173–1180, 1996
101. Roeyen G, Van Schil PE, Vanmaele RG, et al: Abdominal aortic aneurysm with lumbar vertebral erosion in Behçet's disease. A case report and review of the literature. Eur J Vasc Endovasc Surg 13:242–246, 1997
102. Tuzun H, Besirli K, Sayin A, et al: Management of aneurysms in Behçet's syndrome: An analysis of 24 patients. Surgery 121:150–156, 1997
103. Seo JW, Park IA, Yoon DH, et al: Thoracic aortic aneurysm associated with aortitis—case reports and histological review. J Korean Med Sci 6:75–82, 1991
104. Walker DI, Bloor K, Williams G, Gillie I: Inflammatory aneurysms of the abdominal aorta. Br J Surg 59:609–614, 1972
105. Feiner HD, Raghavendra BN, Phelps R, Rooney L: Inflammatory abdominal aortic aneurysm: Report of six cases. Hum Pathol 15: 454–459, 1984
106. Rose AG, Dent DM: Inflammatory variant of abdominal atherosclerotic aneurysm. Arch Pathol Lab Med 105:409–413, 1981
107. Cohle SD, Lie JT: Inflammatory aneurysm of the aorta, aortitis, and coronary arteritis. Arch Pathol Lab Med 112:1121–1125, 1988
108. Rasmussen TE, Hallett JW Jr, Metzger RL, et al: Genetic risk factors in inflammatory abdominal aortic aneurysms: Polymorphic residue 70 in the HLA-DR B1 gene as a key genetic element. J Vasc Surg 25:356–364, 1997
109. Rubery PT, Smith MD, Cammisa FP, Silane M: Mycotic aortic aneurysm in patients who have lumbar vertebral osteomyelitis. A report of two cases. J Bone Joint Surg Am 77:1729–1732, 1995
110. Worrell JT, Buja LM, Reynolds RC: Pneumococcal aortitis with rupture of the aorta. Report of a case and review of the literature. Am J Clin Pathol 89:565–568, 1988
111. Carreras M, Larena JA, Tabernero G, et al: Evolution of salmonella aortitis towards the formation of abdominal aneurysm. Eur Radiol 7:54–56, 1997
112. Blebea J, Kempczinski RF: Mycotic aneurysms. In: Yao JST, Pearce WH (eds): Aneurysms. New Findings and Treatments. Norwalk, CT, Appleton and Lange, 1994 pp 389–410
113. Huppertz HI, Sandhage K: Reactive arthritis due to Salmonella enteritidis complicated by carditis. Acta Paediatr 83:1230–1231, 1994
114. Hohlfeld J, Schneider M, Hein R, Barthels M, et al: Thrombosis of the terminal aorta, deep vein thrombosis, recurrent fetal loss, and antiphospholipid antibodies. Case report. Vasa. 25:194–199, 1996
115. Josephson GD, Tiefenbrun J, Harvey J: Thrombosis of the descending thoracic aorta: A case report. Surgery 114:598–600, 1993

116. Kawahira Y, Kishimoto H, Lio M, et al: Spontaneous aortic thrombosis in a neonate with multiple thrombi in the main branches of the abdominal aorta. Cardiovasc Surg 3:219–222, 1995

117. Steffen CM, Thursby PF: Neoplastic obstruction of the abdominal aorta. Aust N Z J Surg 65:136–137, 1995

118. Sanchez-Gonzalez J, Garcia-Delange T, Martos F, Colmenero JD: Thrombosis of the abdominal aorta secondary to Brucella spondylitis. Infection 24:261–226, 1996

119. Nanjo H, Murakami M, Ebina T, et al: Aortic intimal sarcoma with acute myocardial infarction. Pathol Int 46:673–681, 1996

120. Raaf HN, Raaf JH: Sarcomas related to the heart and vasculature. Semin Surg Oncol 10:374–382, 1994

121. Burke A, Virmani R: Sarcomas of the great vessels. Cancer 71:1761–1773, 1993

122. Burke A, Virmani R: Tumors of the great vessels. Tumors of the Heart and Great Vessels. Vol. 16. Washington, DC, Armed Forces Institute of Pathology, 1996, pp 211–226

123. Ruijter ET, Ten Kate FJ: Metastasising sarcoma of the aorta. Histopathology. 29:278–281, 1996

124. Sekine S, Abe T, Seki K, et al: Primary aortic sarcoma: Resection by total arch replacement. J Thorac Cardiovasc Surg 110:554–556, 1995

125. Ronaghi AH, Roberts AC, Rosenkrantz H: Intraaortic biopsy of a primary aortic tumor. J Vasc Interv Radiol 5:777–780, 1994

126. Kruger I, Borowski A, Horst M, et al: Symptoms, diagnosis and therapy of primary sarcomas of the pulmonary artery. Thorac Cardiovasc Surg 38:91–95, 1990

127. al-Robaish A, Lien DC, Slatnik J, Nguyen GK: Sarcoma of the pulmonary artery trunk: Report of a case complicated with hemopericardium and cardiac tamponade. Can J Cardiol 11:707–709, 1995

128. Kauczor HU, Schwickert HC, Mayer E, et al: Pulmonary artery sarcoma mimicking chronic thromboembolic disease: Computed tomography and magnetic resonance imaging findings. Cardiovasc Intervent Radiol 17:185–189, 1994

129. Nonomura A, Kurumaya H, Kono J, et al: Report of two autopsy cases studied by immunohistochemistry and electronmicroscopy, and review of 110 cases reported in the literature. Acta Pathol Jpn 38:883–896, 1998

130. Johansson L, Carlen B: Sarcoma of the pulmonary artery: Report of four cases with electron microscopic and immunohistochemical examinations, and review of the literature. Virchows Arch 424:217–224, 1994

131. Emmert-Buck MR, Stay EJ, et al: Pleomorphic rhabdomyosarcoma arising in association with the right pulmonary artery. Arch Pathol Lab Med 118:1220–1222, 1994

132. Anderson MB, Kriett JM, Kapelanski DP, et al: Primary pulmonary artery sarcoma: A report of six cases. Ann Thorac Surg 59:1487–1490, 1995

133. Mingoli A, Feldhaus R, Cavallaro A, Stipa S: Leiomyosarcoma of the inferior vena cava: Analysis and search of world literature on 141 patients and report of three new cases. J Vasc Surg 14:688–699, 1991

134. Abulafia O, Sherer DM: Recurrent transient superior vena cava-like syndrome possibly associated with megestrol acetate. Obstet Gynecol 85:899–901, 1995

135. Hoffmann V, Ysebaert D, De Schepper A, et al: Acute superior vena cava obstruction after rupture of a bronchial artery aneurysm. Chest 110:1356–1358, 1996

136. Tunaci A, Berkmen YM, Gokmen E: Thoracic involvement in Behçet's disease: Pathologic, clinical, and imaging features. AJR Am J Roentgenol 164:51–56, 1995

137. Didier D, Racle A, Etievent JP, Weill F: Tumor thrombus of the inferior vena cava secondary to malignant abdominal neoplasms: US and CT evaluation. Radiology 162:83–89, 1987

138. Ashleigh RJ, Sambrook P. Case report: Unilateral hydronephrosis following obstruction of the inferior vena cava by tumour thrombus. Clin Radiol 44:130–131, 1991

139. Leder RA: Genitourinary case of the day. Angiomyolipoma of the kidney with fat thrombus in the inferior vena cava. AJR Am J Roentgenol 165:198–199, 1995

140. Federici S, Galli G, Ceccarelli PL, et al: Wilms' tumor involving the inferior vena cava: Preoperative evaluation and management. Med Pediatr Oncol 22:39–44, 1994

141. Ohwada S, Tanahashi Y, Kawashima Y, et al: Surgery for tumor thrombi in the right atrium and inferior vena cava of patients with recurrent hepatocellular carcinoma. Hepatogastroenterology 41:154–157, 1994

142. Adsan O, Muftuoglu YZ, Suzer O, Beduk Y: Thrombosis of the inferior vena cava by a testicular tumour. Int Urol Nephrol 27:179–182, 1995

143. Arao M, Ogura H, Ino T, et al: Unusual inferior vena cava obstruction causing extensive thrombosis: An intravascular endoscopic observation. Intern Med 32:861–864, 1993

144. Brouwers MA, de Jong KP, Peeters PM, et al: Inferior vena cava obstruction after orthotopic liver transplantation. Clin Transplant 8:19–22, 1994

145. Brenner DW, Brenner CJ, Scott J, et al: Suprarenal Greenfield filter placement to prevent pulmonary embolus in patients with vena caval tumor thrombi. J Urol 147:19–23, 1992

146. Zhou H, Janssen D, Gunther E, Pfeifer U: Fatal bleeding from duodenal varices as a late complication of neonatal thrombosis of the inferior vena cava. Virchows Arch A Pathol Anat Histopathol 420:367–370, 1992

147. Valla D, Benhamou JP: Obstruction of the hepatic veins or suprahepatic inferior vena cava. Dig Dis 14:99–118, 1996

148. Kage M, Arakawa M, Kojiro M, Okuda K: Histopathology of membranous obstruction of the inferior vena cava in the Budd-Chiari syndrome. Gastroenterology 102:2081–2090, 1992

149. Sevenet F, Deramond H, Hadengue A, et al: Membranous obstruction of the inferior vena cava associated with a myeloproliferative disorder: A clue to membrane formation? Gastroenterology 97:1019–1021, 1989

150. Levesque H, Cailleux N, Courtois H, et al: Idiopathic saccular aneurysm of the inferior vena cava: A new case. J Vasc Surg 18:544–545, 1993

151. van Ieperen L, Rose AG: Idiopathic aneurysm of the inferior vena cava. A case report. S Afr Med J 77:535–536, 1990

152. Sweeney JP, Turner K, Harris KA: Aneurysms of the inferior vena cava. J Vasc Surg 12:25–27, 1990

153. Gradman WS, Steinberg F: Aneurysm of the inferior vena cava: Case report and review of the literature. Ann Vasc Surg 7:347–53, 1993

154. Augustin N, Meisner H, Sebening F: Combined membranous obstruction and saccular aneurysm of the inferior vena cava. Thorac Cardiovasc Surg 43:223–226, 1995

155. Wagenvoort CA: Pathology of pulmonary thromboembolism. Chest 107:10S–17S, 1995

156. Luchi ME, Asherson RA, Lahita RG: Primary idiopathic pulmonary hypertension complicated by pulmonary arterial thrombosis. Association with antiphospholipid antibodies. Arthritis Rheum 35:700–705, 1992

157. Barbas CS, de Carvalho CR, Delmonte VC, et al: Behçet's disease: A rare case of simultaneous pulmonary and cerebral involvement. Am J Med 85:576–578, 1988

158. Raz I, Okon E, Chajek-Shaul T: Pulmonary manifestations in Behçet's syndrome. Chest 95:585–589, 1989

159. Naschitz JE, Zuckerman E, Sharif D, et al: Case report: Extensive pulmonary and aortic thrombosis and ectasia. Am J Med Sci 310:34–37, 1995

160. Roche-Bayard P, Rossi R, Mann JM, et al: Left pulmonary artery thrombosis in chlorpromazine-induced lupus. Chest 98:1545, 1990

161. Connors AF Jr, Castele RJ, Farhat NZ, Tomashefski JF Jr: Complications of right heart catheterization. A prospective autopsy study. Chest 88:567–572, 1985

162. Yamada I, Shibuya H, Matsubara O, et al: Pulmonary artery disease in Takayasu arteritis: Angiographic findings. AJR Am J Roentgenol 159:263–269, 1992

163. Glover MU, Muniz J, Bessone L, et al: Pulmonary artery obstruction due to giant cell arteritis. Chest 91:924–925, 1987

164. Ladanyi M, Fraser RS: Pulmonary involvement in giant cell arteritis. Arch Pathol Lab Med. 111:1178–1180, 1987

165. Barbour DJ, Roberts WC: Aneurysm of the pulmonary trunk unassociated with intracardiac or great vessel left-to-right shunting. Am J Cardiol 59:192–194, 1987

166. Butto F, Lucas RV Jr, Edwards JE: Pulmonary arterial aneurysm. A pathologic study of five cases. Chest 91:237–241, 1987

167. Hamuryudan V, Yurdakul S, Moral F, et al: Pulmonary arterial

aneurysms in Behçet's syndrome: A report of 24 cases. Br J Rheumatol 33:48–51, 1994

168. Jerray M, Benzarti M, Rouatbi N: Possible Behçet's disease revealed by pulmonary aneurysms. Chest 99:1282–1284, 1991

169. Numan F, Islak C, Berkmen T, et al: Behçet disease: Pulmonary arterial involvement in 15 cases. Radiology 192:465–468, 1994

170. Karak P, Dimick R, Hamrick KM, et al: Immediate transcatheter embolization of Swan-Ganz catheter-induced pulmonary artery pseudoaneurysm. Chest 111:1450–1452, 1997

171. Fukai I, Masaoka A, Yamakawa Y, et al: Rupture of congenital peripheral pulmonary aneurysm. Ann Thorac Surg 59:528–530, 1995

172. Hankins GD, Brekken AL, Davis LM: Maternal death secondary to a dissecting aneurysm of the pulmonary artery. Obstet Gynecol 65:45S–48S, 1985

173. Steingrub J, Detore A, Teres D: Spontaneous rupture of pulmonary artery. Crit Care Med 15:270–271, 1987

174. Coard KC, Martin MP: Ruptured saccular pulmonary artery aneurysm associated with persistent ductus arteriosus. Arch Pathol Lab Med 116:159–161, 1992

175. Masuda S, Ishii T, Asuwa N, et al: Concurrent pulmonary arterial dissection and saccular aneurysm associated with primary pulmonary hypertension. Arch Pathol Lab Med 120:309–312, 1996

176. Patel KS, Wolfe JH, Mathias C: Left external iliac artery dissection and bilateral renal artery aneurysms secondary to fibromuscular dysplasia: A case report. Neth J Surg 42:118–120, 1990

177. Vuong PN, Janzen J, Bical O, Susa-Uva M: Fibromuscular dysplasia causing atypical coarctation of the thoracic aorta: Histological presentation of a case. Vasa 24:194–198, 1995

178. Sumboonnanonda A, Robinson BL, Gedroyc WM, et al: Middle aortic syndrome: Clinical and radiological findings. Arch Dis Child 67:501–505, 1992

179. Matsushita M, Yano T, Ikezawa T, et al: Fibromuscular dysplasia as a cause of abdominal aortic aneurysm. Cardiovasc Surg 2:615–618, 1994

180. Wagenvoort CA: Medial defects of lung vessels: A new cause of pulmonary hypertension. Hum Pathol 17:722–726, 1986

181. Fukuhara H, Kitayama H, Yokoyama T, Shirotani H: Thromboembolic pulmonary hypertension due to disseminated fibromuscular dysplasia. Pediatr Cardiol 17:340–345, 1996

Disease of Medium- and Small-Caliber Vessels Including Small Arteries, Arterioles, and Capillaries

. . . . .

Avrum I. Gotlieb • Alan G. Rose

The observation that specific diseases characteristically involve medium- and/or small-caliber vessels was made more than 50 years ago as a result of morphologic studies in cases of diabetes mellitus and vasculitis. In 1941, Allen[1] postulated that the glomerular lesions of diabetic glomerulosclerosis, described by Kimmelstiel and Wilson[2] 5 years previously, originated from an abnormality of glomerular capillary basement membranes. Within a few years, microaneurysms of the retinal microcirculation were recorded[3] and hypersensitivity vasculitis, which primarily affects small vessels, was classified as a separate entity, distinct from classic polyarteritis nodosa, which mainly involves medium-size arteries.[4] Table 6-1 lists diseases of medium- and small-caliber vessels. Small vessel vasculitis is reviewed by Jennette and Falk.[4a]

GENERAL VASCULAR CHANGES OCCURRING IN MEDIUM- AND SMALL-VESSEL DISEASE

Specific structural and functional characteristics of medium and small vessels predispose them to a variety of vascular injuries.

Endothelial Cells

Because the luminal diameters of these vessels (especially capillaries and arterioles) are small, endothelial cell swelling, proliferation, or both may narrow them sufficiently to produce local tissue ischemia and infarction. Activation of surface adhesion molecules causes the binding and subsequent migration of leukocytes through the endothelium.[5, 6] Disruption of adhesion and/or tight junctions between endothelial cells increases vascular permeability,[7, 8] whereas dysfunction of cell-substratum adhesion can promote endothelial cell loss and focal denudation.[6]

Basement Membrane

Thickening and/or disarrangement of the basement membrane may alter vascular permeability.[9] The signifi-

cance of basement membrane thinning in myotonic dystrophy is not known.[10]

Vessel Wall

Hemorrhage and Microaneurysms

Because small vessel walls are thin, hemorrhage develops easily. Aneurysm formation and rupture are also important sequelae of some small vessel diseases. Glomerular capillary microaneurysms are thought to be caused by the separation of the capillary basement membrane from the mesangium at anchor points.[11] Mesangiolysis may be noted in bone marrow transplant recipients after irradiation and/or cytotoxic therapy and thus may lead to aneurysmal ectasia of capillary loops. Retinal and other microaneurysms develop in weakened, thin-walled, vessels, probably because of pericyte loss and changes in the media of larger vessels.[12, 13]

Deposits in the Wall

Various substances may be deposited in the walls of small-caliber vessels. Localization of immune complexes in a thin vessel wall has a profound effect because of the inflammatory reaction induced by complement. Subintimal deposition of ultrastructural, finely granular material occurs in some conditions, including thrombotic microangiopathies. In the kidney, it is proposed that the material represents either nonspecific proteinaceous fluid resulting from ischemia-mediated altered vascular permeability[14] or from an intramural deposit of fibrin.[15] Organization of the latter deposits in renal arterioles and arteries may be an important mechanism in the luminal narrowing of both malignant hypertension and sclerodema.[15] Experimentally, focal insudation of blood components, including fibrin, into the media can be induced in arterioles as a response to a chronic irritative stimulus.[16] Amyloid may also deposit in arterioles and cause mural thickening.

Intimal Medial Changes

Intimal proliferation and/or thickening that narrows the lumen of medium and small arteries or arterioles can promote ischemia. In many conditions, this proliferation/thickening evolves in the same manner as in larger

TABLE 6-1 • **Diseases of Medium- and Small-Caliber Vessels**

Congenital Caliber-persistent artery Congenital arteriovenous fistula	Plague Whipple disease Leptospirosis Schistosoma

Familial
Neurofibromatosis
Pseudoxanthoma elasticum
Myotonic dystrophy
Friedreich ataxia
Sickle cell disease
	Toxic
	Drug-induced
	
	Coagulopathies
	Thrombotic microangiopathies
	  Thrombotic thrombocytopenic purpura
	  Hemolytic uremic syndrome
	Disseminated intravascular coagulation (DIC)

Endocrine—metabolic Diabetes mellitus Hypothyroidism Homocystinuria	**Hypertension** Benign hypertension Accelerated (malignant) hypertension

Immunologic
Idiopathic hypersensitivity (leukocytoclastic) vasculitis
  Serum sickness/serum–sickness-like reactions
  Henoch-Schönlein purpura
  Hypocomplementemic vasculitis
Small vessel vasculitis associated with
  Mixed cryoglobulinemia
  Collagen vascular disease
  Malignancy
  Other miscellaneous disorders
Other vasculitides
  Isolated angiitis of the central nervous system
  Behçet disease
  Radiation vasculitis
Wegener granulomatosis
Lymphomatoid granulomatosis
Thromboangiitis obliterans
Vascular allograft rejection
	Neoplastic
	Intravascular lymphomatosis
	Endovascular papillary angioendothelioma
	Intravascular papillary endothelial hyperplasia
	Other
	
	Miscellaneous
	Fibromuscular dysplasia
	Amyloidosis
	Emboli
	Idiopathic intimal hyperplasia of small arteries and arterioles
	Erythromelalgia
	Dermal microangiopathy associated with end-stage renal failure
	Small vessel disease isolated to individual organs
	Progressive arterial occlusive disease (Köhlmeier-Degos)
	Cystic adventitial disease
	Moyamoya syndrome
	Arterial endofibrosis

Infectious Rickettsia *Meningococcus* *Pseudomonas* Syphilis Fungi	**Mucoid Vasculopathy** **Mediolytic Vasculopathy (segmental mediolytic arteriopathy)**

vessels.[14] Smooth muscle cells, especially in small arteries, undergo hyperplasia leading to medial thickening. They also migrate through the internal elastic membrane and proliferate in the intima. Intimal thickening is attributable not only to increased numbers of cells but also to enhanced collagen, elastin, and matrix production. Fibrointimal thickening in both renal and myocardial arterioles is significantly greater in cigarette smokers than in nonsmokers.[17, 18]

Lumen

Any changes in plasma viscosity, red blood cell aggregation,[19] or abnormalities of platelet aggregation[20] are likely to affect small vessel function. For example, platelet aggregates are considered an important factor in sudden cardiac death by some authors[21] (see Chapter 8 for an alternative viewpoint). Intravascular occlusion occurs in conditions of hyperviscosity (e.g., macroglobulinemia, polycythemia rubra vera), in thrombotic coagulopathies, and secondary to the presence of microemboli. Intravascular thrombotic occlusion, frequently seen in small-

vessel vasculitides, can often be related to endothelial damage and/or reduced blood flow.

SPECIFIC MEDIUM- AND SMALL-CALIBER VESSEL DISEASES

Congenital

Caliber-Persistent Artery

The term *caliber-persistent artery*[21a, b] describes an arterial branch (usually in the gastric mucosa) that lacks a normal arterial branching pattern and thus produces an oversized vessel in an unusual location (e.g., gastric mucosa [Fig. 6-1], jejunum, lip). Erosion of such a vessel in the stomach may lead to fatal hemorrhage, the origin of which may be difficult to localize not only for the surgeon but also for the pathologist in biopsy material or at autopsy (see Fig. 6-1). The condition is underdiagnosed and has often been referred to as Dieulafoy erosion or as idiopathic gastric hemorrhage.[21c]

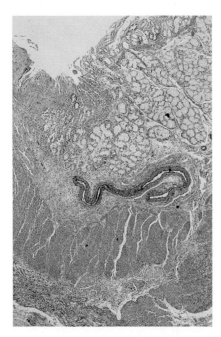

Figure 6-1 • Histologic section of edge of gastric ulcer (top left) showing a caliber-persistent artery in the submucosa adjacent to the muscularis mucosae. Erosion of such an artery may produce fatal hemorrhage (elastic van Gieson stain).

Congenital Arteriovenous Fistula

Arteries and veins arise from the same embryonic vascular plexus and differentiate later, into distinctive and different structures. Arteriovenous (AV) anastomoses are a normal development in certain sites in the body (e.g., palms, soles, terminal phalanges, nose, ears, eyelids, tongue tip). Failure of differentiation of the embryonic vascular plexus may lead to the formation of a macroscopically obvious congenital arteriovenous malformation containing numerous connections between arteries and veins. Associated hemangiomas are a frequent finding.[21d] Congenital AV fistulas may be localized or diffuse. The diffuse form is more common and may lead to hypertrophy of the affected portion of the body. Congenital AV fistulas may occur at any site (e.g., lower limbs, head [Fig. 6-2] neck, chest wall, abdominal cavity, heart). Idiopathic cardiomegaly in infancy is occasionally caused by unsuspected (e.g., intracranial) congenital AV fistulas. However, the shunt in most such fistulas does not produce heart failure.

Familial

Neurofibromatosis

Vascular abnormalities, particularly those involving stenotic lesions of small renal arteries, are relatively common in neurofibromatosis or von Recklinghausen disease.[22–24] Arterial changes include focal nodular proliferation of the intima, intimal and medial fibrosis, fragmentation of the elastica, and occasional microaneurysm formation. Venous aneurysms are rare.[25] Although it was suggested that Schwann cell proliferation caused intimal thickening, an ultrastructural study identified the major constituent as smooth muscle cells undergoing differentiation.[22] Similar small-vessel alterations have been described in the central nervous system of patients with neurofibromatosis,[24] and neurofibromatosis type I is associated with intracranial aneurysms[25a] (see Chapter 16 also).

Pseudoxanthoma Elasticum

Peripheral vascular calcification associated with degeneration of the elastica is the most common vascular complication of pseudoxanthoma elasticum.[26, 27] Although small arteries are affected, involvement of large and medium-sized arteries, including those of the extremities and the splanchnic, coronary, or renal circulations, is more significant clinically[28] (see Chapter 16 also). Calciphylaxis, a rare condition, has been reported to lead to the elasticum-like changes[28a] of microscopic pseudoxanthoma.

Myotonic Dystrophy

Olsen and associates[10] reported a unique finding of significant thinning of muscle capillary basement membrane in patients with myotonic dystrophy. A fluorescein angiographic study of the anterior segment of the eye consistently revealed microvascular tortuosity and leakage of fluorescein into the iris among this group. These changes did not occur in controls or patients with other neuromuscular diseases.[29] The significance of the findings is uncertain (see Chapter 10 also). Annane and coworkers reported impaired coronary reserves in relation to DNA mutation size in symptom-free patients with normal large coronary arteries and ventricular dimensions.[29a] They hypothesized that vascular smooth muscle cells were impaired.

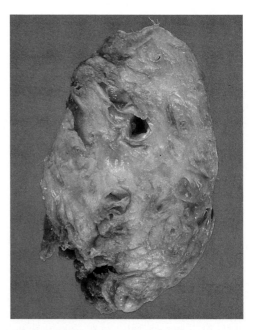

Figure 6-2 • Congenital arteriovenous fistula (cirsoid aneurysm) removed from the scalp of an adult. A few large arteries and veins are visible on the cut surface, but most vessels comprising the lesion could only be identified microscopically.

Friedreich Ataxia

Patients with this hereditary disease often have cardiac involvement.[30–32] Stenosis of small coronary arteries secondary to fibrointimal proliferation, focal fibromuscular dysplasia, and either subintimal or medial deposits of (PAS)-positive material have all been described. The role of such abnormalities in the pathogenesis of Friedreich ataxia is not yet established.[33] In a case report, small pulmonary arteries exhibited histologic features similar to those seen in small coronary arteries[34] (see Chapter 10 also).

Sickle Cell Disease

Sickle cell disease is a hereditary hemoglobinopathy in which blood flow through the microcirculation is impaired because of decreased deformability of red blood cells.[35] The propensity for sickled red blood cells to adhere to vascular endothelium abnormally[36] predisposes to microvascular occlusion and tissue infarction.[37–37b] Histopathologic and morphometric features of neovascular lesions in human proliferative sickle cell retinopathy have been described[37c] (see Chapter 16 also).

Endocrine/Metabolic

Diabetes Mellitus

See Chapter 16.

Hypothyroidism

The pathologic effects of hypothyroidism on the cardiovascular system are discussed in Chapter 16. Baker and Hamilton[38] used 0.5 cm PAS-stained paraffin sections and Silver and associates[39] used electron microscopy to show that small intramyocardial vessels of patients with myxedema have thickened basement membranes. The increased amount of PAS-positive material, also seen within the media, is considered a vascular manifestation of the accumulation of carbohydrate material within connective tissues throughout the body.[40]

Homocystinuria

Widespread vascular abnormalities are characteristic of homocystinuria (see Chapter 16). Changes found in small arteries and arterioles include intimal swelling and proliferation, vacuolization of endothelial cells, increased amount of ground substance within the media, and proliferation of perivascular connective tissue[41–43] (see Chapters 6 and 16).

Inflammatory/Immunologic

The term *vasculitis* describes clinicopathologic processes marked by inflammation and blood vessel necrosis. Vessels of one or many organs may be affected as a primary process, or changes may occur as a secondary, sometimes minor component, of another major systemic disorder. Generally, vasculitis is believed to be immunologic in nature. However, for the most part, etiologic agents have not been identified.

The vasculitides may be classified according to a variety of parameters, including size of vessel affected; or the type, location, or nature of inflammatory cell infiltrate. The Zeek classification of necrotizing vasculitis[44, 45] encompassed five distinct entities: hypersensitivity angiitis, allergic granulomatous angiitis, rheumatic arteritis, periarteritis nodosa, and temporal arteritis. Fauci and associates[46, 47] expanded the classification to include other entities, such as Wegener and lymphomatoid granulomatosis, thromboangiitis obliterans, mucocutaneous lymph node syndrome, and Behçet disease. Apart from the common vasculitides, other, less common vasculitis also occurs in childhood.[47a]

Attempts were made to categorize vasculitis according to specific etiologic factors and immunopathogenetic mechanisms. Although a specific associative factor is occasionally found (e.g., chronic hepatitis B infection),[48, 49] no such association is apparent in most cases. Alarcon-Segovia[50] proposed a working classification of necrotizing vasculitis based on putative pathogenetic mechanisms. This classification divided the immunologic vasculitides into four subcategories:[51] immune complex diseases,[52] anaphylaxis-allergy,[53] cellular hypersensitivity, and undetermined.[50] Among clinicians managing patients with vasculitides, the Fauci classification,[46, 47] or modified versions of it, has been the most popular. A comprehensive classification that would encompass both immunopathogenetic mechanisms and clinicopathologic entities and that would achieve wide acceptance is still awaited.

Two new systems for the classification of the primary vasculitides have been proposed: (1) the 1990 American College of Rheumatology (ACR) classification criteria,[53a] which were provided in both traditional and tree formats, and (2) the 1992 Chapel Hill Consensus Conference (CHCC) definitions.[53b] Bruce and Bell[53c] compared both systems in the same cohort of patients with primary systemic vasculitis and found significant discordance between the criteria set in them. Because the ACR criteria set does not include microscopic polyangiitis, Wegener granulomatosis tends to be overdiagnosed. The CHCC definitions are biopsy dependent, and surrogate features for their defining histology are required to allow practical application.

In this chapter, discussion is restricted to the major vasculitides, which primarily affect medium-sized and small vessels (Table 6-2). However, it is important to realize that although some forms of vasculitis, such as polyarteritis nodosa, may affect small vessels, the major clinical or pathologic manifestations are usually attributable to involvement of medium-sized vessels. In a minority of primary vasculitic syndromes, the extent of mixed small and medium-sized vessel involvement is such that the designation "polyangiitis overall syndrome"[53d] is most appropriate.

Polyarteritis Nodosa

Classic polyarteritis nodosa is an acute necrotizing vasculitis that usually affects medium-sized and smaller arteries but occasionally involves larger arteries. The characteristic lesion is patchy in distribution along a vessel, is no more than a millimeter in length, and may

TABLE 6-2 • **Vasculitic Disease Affecting Medium and Small Vessels**

Medium Vessels

Polyarteritis nodosa group of systemic necrotizing vasculitis
    Classic polyarteritis nodosa
    Allergic angiitis and granulomatosis (Churg-Strauss variant)
    "Overlap syndrome" of systemic angiitis
Kawasaki disease
Giant cell arteritis (temporal arteritis)

Small Vessels

Idiopathic hypersensitivity (leukocytoclastic) vasculitis
    Serum sickness/serum–sickness-like reactions
    Henoch-Schönlein purpura
    Hypocomplementemic vasculitis
Small vessel vasculitis associated with
    Mixed cryoglobulinemia
    Collagen vascular disease
    Malignancy
    Other miscellaneous disorders
Isolated angiitis of the central nervous system
Behçet disease
Radiation vasculitis
Wegener granulomatosis
Lymphomatoid granulomatosis
Buerger disease (thromboangiitis obliterans)
Vascular allograft rejection

involve either the entire circumference of a vessel or only part of it. The most prominent morphologic feature is an area of fibrinoid necrosis in which medial muscle and adjacent tissues are fused into a structureless eosinophilic mass that stains for fibrin. A prominent acute inflammatory response extends through all layers of the vessel wall in the area of necrosis, with prominent adventitial involvement. Neutrophils, lymphocytes, plasma cells, and macrophages are present in varying proportions, and eosinophils are often conspicuous (Fig. 6-3A). Characteristically, different arteries may show lesions of different ages. In a particular vessel, acute necrotizing and healing lesions coexist. Polyarteritis nodosa is frequently associated with perinuclear antineutrophilic cytoplasmic antibodies (see later). As a result of luminal thrombosis in the affected segment, infarcts are common in distal organs (Fig. 6-3B) including bowel, liver, pancreas, and brain. Injury to medium-sized arteries produces aneurysms that are usually less than 0.5 cm in diameter and occur particularly along branches of the renal, coronary (Fig. 6-3C), and cerebral arteries. These may rupture. Lungs are affected in 5 to 10% of cases. After some months, the vascular lesions heal, especially in response to corticosteroid therapy. Necrotic tissue and inflammatory exudates are resorbed. The affected vessel then shows medial fibrosis and a prominent loss of elastic laminae (Fig. 6-3D).

Microscopic polyarteritis, also termed *microscopic polyangiitis,* is distinguished from classic polyarteritis nodosa by involvement of small arteries and arterioles and the microcirculation (e.g., vessels of renal glomeruli).

Allergic Granulomatosis and Angiitis (Churg-Strauss Syndrome)

This is a systemic vasculitis with prominent eosinophilia that occurs in young persons with asthma or al-

lergy.[53e, f] It is strongly associated with antineutrophilic cytoplasmic antibodies ([C]-ANCA) (see later). Necrotizing lesions of small and medium-sized arteries, arterioles, and veins are found in many organs, including lungs, spleen, kidney, heart, liver, and central nervous system. They show granulomas and a prominent eosinophilic infiltrate in and around blood vessels. Because fibrinoid necrosis, thrombosis, and aneurysm formation may simulate polyarteritis nodosa, Churg-Strauss syndrome is sometimes regarded as an "overlap syndrome" of polyarteritis nodosa. However, it appears to be a distinct entity. The disease must also be distinguished from other eosinophilic syndromes, such as parasitic and fungal infestations, Wegener granulomatosis, eosinophilic pneumonia (Loeffler syndrome), and drug vasculitis. Untreated persons with allergic granulomatosis and angiitis have a poor prognosis, but corticosteroid therapy in such patients is now almost always successful.

Kawasaki Disease (Mucocutaneous Lymph Node Syndrome)

Kawasaki disease, an acute disease of infancy and early childhood, appears clinically with a high fever, rash, conjunctival and oral lesions, and lymphadenitis.[54] An acute necrotizing vasculitis, similar to that of polyarteritis nodosa, affects coronary arteries with aneurysm formation (Fig. 6-4A, B) and occurs in as many as 70% of patients, causing death in 1 to 2% of cases. The coronary artery aneurysm may be a cause, subsequently, of sudden death (see Chapter 11). The condition is associated with activation of T cells and macrophages, resulting in elevated levels of several cytokines.[54a] Like many childhood viral diseases, Kawasaki disease is usually self-limited, and although an infectious cause has been sought, none has been proved conclusively.[54b] Persistent endothelial dysfunction has been identified during long term follow-up[54c] in epicardial coronary arteries of patients who have had Kawasaki disease.

Giant Cell Arteritis (Temporal Arteritis, Granulomatous Arteritis)

Giant cell arteritis is a focal, segmental, chronic, granulomatous inflammation of large, medium-sized, and small arteries, but the disease most often affects the temporal artery. The average age at onset is 70 years, and the disease is rare in persons younger than age 50 years. Giant cell arteritis is usually benign clinically and self-limited, with symptoms subsiding within 6 to 12 months. Patients have headache and throbbing temporal pain, with or without constitutional symptoms including malaise, fever, and weight loss, accompanied by generalized muscular aching or stiffness in the shoulders and hips (polymyalgia rheumatica).[54d] The skin overlying the temporal artery may be swollen, tender, and red. Visual symptoms occur in almost half of patients and may proceed from transient to permanent blindness in one or both eyes. Occasionally, by involving other vessels, the disease gives rise to infarcts in myocardium, brain, or gastrointestinal tract, any of which may be fatal.

The affected temporal artery, on either or both sides, is cord-like and exhibits nodular thickening. The lumen is

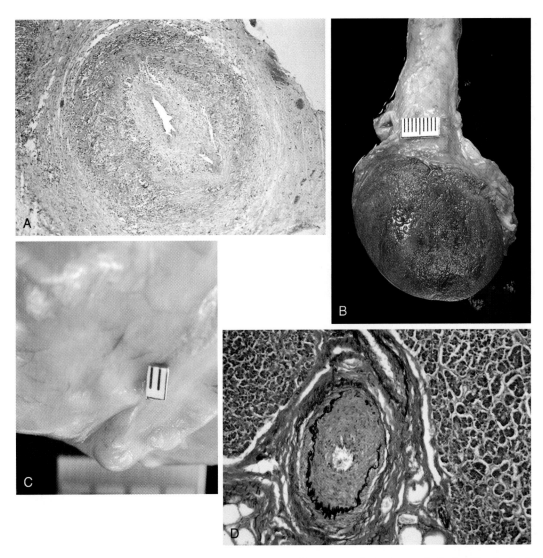

Figure 6-3 • Polyarteritis nodosa. *A*, Causing inflammation affecting part of an artery wall. *B*, Resulting in focal testicular infarction; *C*, Causing aneurysms of the left anterior descending coronary artery near the heart apex in a 22-year-old male IV drug abuser who developed hepatitis B. *D*, From a patient who survived polyarteritis nodosa shows healed lesion in pancreas with replacement of intimal elastic lumina in a part of the vessel circumference and intimal thickening (*A*, H&E stain; *D*, Verhoeff elastic stain).

reduced to a slit or may be obliterated by thrombus (Fig. 6-5*A*). Microscopic examination reveals granulomatous inflammation of the media and intima consisting of aggregates of histocytes, lymphocytes, and plasma cells, with varying admixtures of eosinophils and neutrophils. Giant cells are usually prominent but they vary widely in number and tend to be distributed in the area of the internal elastic lamina (Fig. 6-5*B*). Their cytoplasm may contain fragments of elastica. Foci of necrosis are characterized by changes in the internal elastica, which becomes swollen, irregular, and fragmented. Foci may completely disappear in advanced lesions. Macrophages containing 92-kD gelatinase (MMP-2) were identified and localized primarily to regions of disruption of the internal elastic lamina.[54e] In late stages, the intima is thickened and the media is fibrotic (see Chapter 5 also). Thrombosis may obliterate the lumen, after which organization and canalization occur (Fig. 6-5*C*). Similar changes are observed when vessels in other organs are affected.

The etiology of giant cell arteritis is obscure, and no bacterial or viral cause has been demonstrated. The morphologic alterations suggest an immunologic reaction, and data suggest that this is a T cell-dependent disease[54f] and that persistent macrophage activation and cytokine production are important features.[54g] Degradation of elastin by leukocyte elastase may provide peptides that act as autoimmune targets for T cells.[54h]

Temporal artery biopsy may not disclose the disease in as many as 50% of patients with otherwise classic manifestations. The response to corticosteroid therapy is usually dramatic, with symptoms subsiding in a matter of days.

Takayasu Disease

Another inflammatory disease of yet unknown etiology but with immunologic characteristics that affects large arteries (e.g., aorta) (Fig. 6-6) and their major branches is

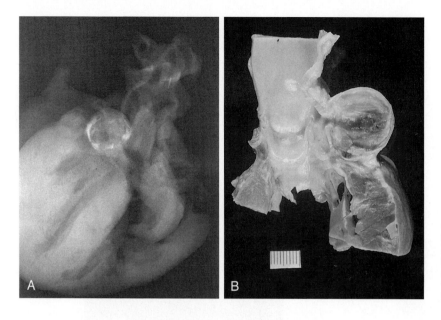

Figure 6-4 • Aneurysm on the left anterior descending coronary artery of a 4-year-old boy who died suddenly. He had symptoms compatible with Kawasaki disease 2 years earlier. *A,* Postmortem radiograph revealed calcification in aneurysm wall. *B,* Gross specimen: note fibrosis in adjacent left ventricular wall. (Specimen courtesy of Dr. M.D. Silver.)

Takayasu arteritis.[55a] This disease causes focal destruction of the internal elastic lamina and has few giant cells as well as luminal thrombosis, intimal thickening, and a more pronounced medial granulomatous inflammation (see Chapter 5; Figs. 5-18 and 5-21 demonstrate histologic changes caused by the disease in the aorta).

Hypersensitivity Vasculitis and Its Subtypes

Although the skin alone is most commonly affected in primary hypersensitivity vasculitis, virtually any organ may be involved. The classic clinical presentation is that of palpable purpura, a result of inflammation and extrava-

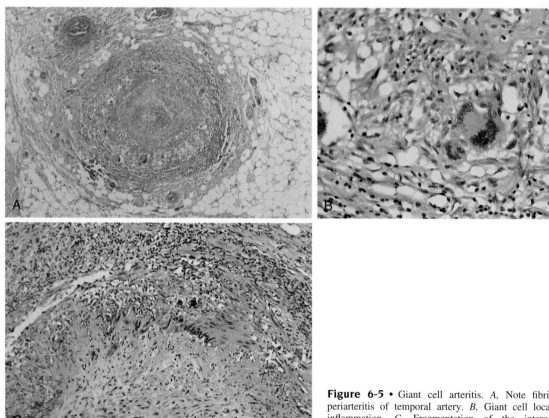

Figure 6-5 • Giant cell arteritis. *A,* Note fibrinoid necrosis and periarteritis of temporal artery. *B,* Giant cell located in an area of inflammation. *C,* Fragmentation of the internal elastic lamina (*A, B,* H&E stain; *C,* Verhoeff elastic stain).

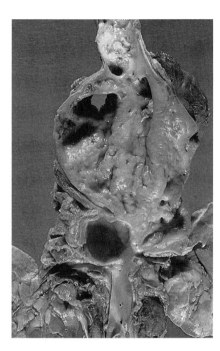

Figure 6-6 • Diffuse involvement of the thoracic and abdominal aorta to the origin of the renal arteries by Takayasu disease has caused many saccular aneurysms of varying sizes.

sation of red blood cells.[56] Urticarial lesions also occur as a manifestation of small-vessel vasculitis. The latter presentation is called urticarial vasculitis.[51, 57] No specific laboratory test is diagnostic. Raised levels of circulating antigen related to factor VIII have been reported in systemic forms of necrotizing vasculitis such as polyarteritis and Wegener granulomatosis but not in cutaneous small-vessel vasculitis.[58, 59] Lockwood and colleagues[60] identified autoantibodies to normal neutrophil constituents in patients with Wegener granulomatosis and hypersensitivity vasculitis and suggested that such a test might help both to identify and to follow up patients with these conditions. Antineutrophilic cytoplasmic antibodies (ANCA) have been demonstrated in the serum of patients with some vasculitides.[60a] Two types of staining are seen: perinuclear (P)-ANCA and cytoplasmic (C)-ANCA.[60b] The former occurs in polyarteritis nodosa, idiopathic glomerulonephritis, Churg-Strauss vasculitis, and systemic necrotizing vasculitis overlap syndromes, and is against myeloperoxidase. The latter, seen predominantly in Wegener granulomatosis, recognizes proteinase-3, a leukocyte protease.

A definitive diagnosis rests on histopathologic study of affected tissues.[61] A systematic approach in establishing tissue diagnosis includes review of previously biopsied tissue, care in the choice of biopsy site, and use of open or multiple biopsies to obtain adequate tissue.[62] In hypersensitivity vasculitis, a tissue diagnosis is usually accomplished easily because of frequent cutaneous involvement.

The most common histologic pattern is a polymorphonuclear leukocytic infiltrate of postcapillary venules[63] associated with leukocytoclasia (hence, the sometimes used designation "leukocytoclastic vasculitis"[64, 65]) and evi-

dence of vascular damage such as endothelial cell swelling, fibrinoid necrosis of the vessel wall, and extravasation of red blood cells[55, 66] (Fig. 6-7). Although diagnosis is readily made if all or most of these histopathologic features are present, opinions differ as to the minimal criteria required.[67] Most authors agree that a perivenular inflammatory cell infiltrate alone does not warrant a diagnosis, and other features indicating vascular injury are required.[66–68] In contrast to the lesions of polyarteritis nodosa, those of hypersensitivity vasculitis are usually all at the same stage of development at any given time, in keeping with a specific immunologic event precipitating vascular injury.

Two distinct patterns of leukocytic infiltration are described.[66, 69] In patients with serum hypocomplementemia, a predominant neutrophilic infiltrate is found, whereas in those with normal serum complement levels, lymphocytes, including activated forms, predominate. This may represent a difference in the type of immunologic mechanism at work. Studies by Tosca and associates[70] indicated that in neutrophilic-predominant vasculitis, the delayed hypersensitivity response was readily elicited, whereas it was reduced in lymphocytic-predominant vasculitis. Experimental evidence in the autoimmune MRL/Mp mouse strain suggests that mononuclear (lymphocytic) vasculitis is a distinct form of vascular inflammation that may subsequently evolve into a neutrophilic-predominant vasculitis.[71] However, not all authors agree that so-called "lymphocytic vasculitis" is a specific clinicopathologic entity.[72]

In one report, the severity of dermatopathologic changes predicted clinical severity,[65] whereas in another,[73]

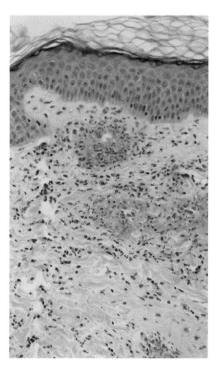

Figure 6-7 • Hypersensitivity leukocytoclastic vasculitis in skin. Note inflammatory infiltrate with fibrinoid necrosis of vessel wall, prominent infiltrate of polymorphonuclear leukocytes, and extravasation of erythrocytes (H&E stain).

vasculitis that involved the deep dermis, or subcutaneous tissue, was more likely to be associated with an underlying systemic disease. In general, prognosis in hypersensitivity vasculitis is good, with or without therapy, especially if the disease is restricted to the skin.[55, 64] Extracutaneous sites of involvement include joints, kidneys, lung, gastrointestinal tract and peripheral nervous system.[55, 74] Small-vessel angiitis of internal organs may produce microinfarcts. Generally, these do not cause major organ dysfunction. However, in a few patients, renal failure may threaten life.[55]

Subtypes of hypersensitivity vasculitis are all characterized by an immunologically mediated, small-vessel necrotizing angiitis, but they are distinguished by clinical presentation, specific laboratory findings, or the presence of an underlying systemic disorder.

Serum Sickness

Serum sickness is a clinical syndrome that results from the injection of heterologous serum or serum proteins into an individual. Because heterologous serum is rarely used today, classic serum sickness is now uncommon. However, reactions to non–protein-containing drugs, which are similar to those of serum sickness, are relatively common (see Chapter 17).

Henoch-Schönlein Purpura

Henoch-Schönlein purpura, or anaphylactoid purpura, is a systemic small-vessel vasculitis. It appears as a clinical syndrome of nonthrombocytopenic purpura, arthritis, gastrointestinal bleeding, and renal disease, the latter usually caused by focal or diffuse glomerulonephritis. Among suspected precipitating events leading to immune complex deposition in this disease are viral and streptococcal infections, drug administration, and ingestion of certain foods.[55] The characteristics of Henoch-Schönlein purpura differ from those of classic hypersensitivity vasculitis in that IgA is principally detected as part of circulating immune complexes and/or immune deposits within dermal vessels and renal glomeruli.[75] Plasma von Willebrand factor (vWF) appears to be a good marker of vascular inflammation and endothelial damage in Henoch-Schönlein purpura.[76]

Hypocomplementemic Vasculitis

This is an entity in which differences in the early components of the classic complement pathway are associated with cutaneous leukocytoclastic vasculitis that manifests as chronic urticaria.[77] Diagnostic criteria were proposed by Schwartz and coworkers,[78] who noted an enhanced predilection for it to develop in patients with chronic obstructive pulmonary disease. Although renal involvement is relatively common, it is rarely severe.[79]

Vasculitis Associated With Mixed Cryoglobulinemia

Diagnosis of this condition is established by the concurrent demonstration of a cryoglobulinemia, usually of the mixed monoclonal/polyclonal type, and of a small-vessel necrotizing vasculitis.[77] In a case report of monoclonal IgM λ-cryoglobulinemia with vasculitis, the cryoglobulin was bound to procollagen type I within interstitial connective tissue.[80]

Vasculitis Associated With Other Systemic Diseases

The association of necrotizing small-vessel vasculitis and a variety of collagen vascular diseases, including systemic lupus erythematosis (SLE),[81, 82] rheumatoid arthritis,[83, 84] systemic sclerosis,[85] and Sjögren syndrome[86, 87] is well recognized (see Chapter 16). Necrotizing small-vessel vasculitis has also been described in an array of *neoplastic conditions* including myeloproliferative disorders,[88] hairy cell leukemia,[89–91] lymphoproliferative disorders,[92, 93] multiple myeloma,[94] and a variety of carcinomas.[95–98] The association of other *miscellaneous entities* with small-vessel vasculitis has been reviewed by Gilliam and Smiley.[99] Described associations include those with celiac disease,[100] inflammatory bowel disease,[101] sarcoidosis,[102] and primary biliary cirrhosis.[103]

Pathogenesis

Most authors believe that hypersensitivity vasculitis is an immune complex disease in which circulating complexes, composed of soluble antigens bound to antibodies, deposit within blood vessels and activate complement,[47, 104–106] which, in turn, attracts neutrophils to bind to endothelial cells, to become activated, and to release both lysosomes and oxygen free radicals, resulting in vascular damage. Monocytes also bind by upregulation of endothelial adhesion molecules and promote release of cytokines from themselves and adjacent endothelial cells.

The Arthus reaction and both acute and chronic serum sickness reactions in animals have long been used as models to study the pathogenesis of immune–complex-mediated vascular damage.[107] Serum sickness is a localized acute vasculitic reaction that develops in the skin of animals after the local injection of an antigen to which the animal has been sensitized. Using this model, Cochrane[108] demonstrated that immune complexes, identified by immunofluorescence early in the reaction, became undetectable after 24 to 48 hours. Serum sickness reactions are initiated in experimental animals by injecting heterologous serum proteins and thereby producing a syndrome of arthritis, glomerulonephritis, endocarditis, and vasculitis involving vessels of varying size. Histamine-induced increased vascular permeability plays an important role in this condition by allowing circulating immune complexes to enter the vessel wall.[109, 110] An in vivo model of small-vessel lymphocytic vasculitis was produced by injecting mice with lymphocytes sensitized to smooth muscle antigens.[111]

The observations and experimental evidence in humans that immune complexes have an important role in the various forms of vasculitis, including that involving small vessels, are compelling.[104–106, 112] Individual susceptibility is associated with hepatitis B or hepatitis C virus infection in 10 to 30% of patients with polyarteritis nodosa.[112a] As previously noted, human vasculitis often develops in a number of systemic diseases that are considered immunologically mediated (e.g., SLE, rheumatoid arthritis). Also, elevated levels of immune complexes are detected in the serum of patients with active vasculitis, providing presumptive evidence that they are involved in pathogenesis.[113–115] Again, immunoglobulin and complement components are demonstrable by immunofluorescence techniques in vessels with histologic evidence of necrotizing vasculitis when lesions are 24 hours of age but not older.[116, 117] Both Braverman[116] and Gower[117] showed that immune complex deposition occurred before the onset of the neutrophilic inflammatory cell reaction, suggesting that they initiated the vasculitis. The presence of electron-dense deposits within blood vessel walls has been confirmed ultrastructurally[116, 117] as has their presence in the histologically normal renal arterioles of a patient with hypersensitivity vasculitis.[118]

It is important to emphasize that in an individual case, the localization of immunoglobulin in a vessel wall by immunofluorescence does not necessarily mean that there has been immunologic damage, because such deposits may be related to nonspecific trapping.[112, 119, 120] To make a definitive immunofluorescent diagnosis, McCluskey and associates[119] advanced strict criteria. They concluded that (1) the antigen be in the same location as the immunoglobulin; (2) antigen staining is abolished by absorption of antisera with purified putative antigen and (3) the putative antigen is not found in other diseases in which immunoglobulin deposition occurs, thus reducing the likelihood that the antigen was trapped in the tissue nonspecifically. In most cases, necrotizing vasculitis is not associated with any specifically identifiable antigen; therefore, the above criteria cannot be fulfilled. Nonetheless, an inability to clearly demonstrate specific antigens in individual patients with primary vasculitis should not detract from the strong evidence that supports a role for immune complexes in pathogenesis.

The putative antigens implicated in human vasculitis have been reviewed by Savage and Ng.[106] The best known, associated with both medium- and small-vessel vasculitis, is the hepatitis B virus.[48, 49, 120] If hepatitis B infection is associated with polyarteritis nodosa, both circulating and in situ vascular deposits of hepatitis B surface antigen-antibody complexes are found.[121] Other infections associated with vasculitis include herpes simplex,[122] herpes zoster,[122] cytomegalovirus,[123] hepatitis A,[124] parvovirus,[125] streptococcus,[126] cryptococcus,[127] Mediterranean spotted fever,[128] and infectious mononucleosis.[129] Small-vessel vasculitis has also been reported after influenza vaccination.[130] Reference was made earlier to neoplastic diseases and autoimmune connective tissue disorders that are also associated with vasculitis. Drug-induced vasculitis is discussed in Chapter 17.

Although the concept of immune–complex-mediated mechanisms of vascular damage is popular, Alexander[71] has proposed an alternative model in which cell-mediated mechanisms are important. This was based on both experimental observations in the MRL/Mp strain of autoimmune mice and on clinicoimmunopathologic studies in patients with primary Sjögren syndrome. A small number of the latter group showed a transition from mononuclear to neutrophilic inflammation, suggesting that neutrophilic vasculitis may be secondary in this setting.

Other Vasculitides Primarily Involving Small Vessels

Small-vessel involvement may be prominent in a small number of other vasculitic syndromes that are not usually grouped as part of the hypersensitivity vasculitic spectrum.

Dermatomyositis

Complement-mediated cytotoxic antibodies against capillaries elicit a perivascular inflammatory cellular response in skin and skeletal muscle. There may be an association with an increased risk of visceral malignancy. Anti-histidyl-t-RNA-synthetase (Jo-1) antibodies may be detected in the patient's serum (see Chapter 16 also).

Isolated Angiitis of the Central Nervous System

This entity, also known as granulomatous angiitis, is of unknown etiology and is characterized by a vasculitis usually of granulomatous nature, restricted to vessels of the central nervous system.[131–133] Arterioles are most commonly affected. Some authors consider it a nonspecific inflammatory reaction because it may be perceived as associated with a variety of conditions such as Hodgkin disease and herpetic infections.[134]

Treatment with steroids or cyclophosphamide has been effective in some patients.[134a]

Behçet Disease

This systemic illness was originally defined by recurrent aphthous ulcers of the oral and genital mucosa and ocular inflammation.[135] More extensive involvement, including that of the central nervous, genitourinary, gastrointestinal, and cardiovascular systems, is now recognized.[136] Cardiac lesions are rare, but involvement of arteries and veins is not. In some cases, the latter involvement may prove fatal.[137]

The underlying pathologic lesion is a small-vessel vasculitis that predominantly affects venules.[138] Although destructive panarteritis of larger vessels is found occasionally,[139] these changes may be secondary to vasculitic involvement of intramural capillaries and venules.[137] Biopsies of mucocutaneous lesions show a perivascular infiltration by lymphocytes, monocytes, and occasional plasma cells, affecting arterioles and venules. Endothelial cell swelling and proliferation may develop, but frank necrosis of small vessels is uncommon.[139, 140] Cutaneous vasculitis in Behçet disease appears mainly as a venulitis or phlebitis.[140a] It is suggested that the entity represents a delayed type of hypersensitivity reaction to an unknown antigenic stimulus.[141] There is a primary association of HLA-B51 with Behçet disease.[141a, 141b]

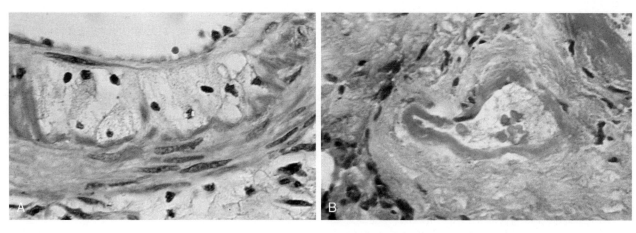

Figure 6-8 • *A,* Small artery shows postirradiation ballooning degeneration of intimal cells, which also show some nuclear atypism. *B,* A larger dose of radiation has induced fibrinoid necrosis of the wall of this small artery. No thrombus has yet formed at this stage (*A, B,* H&E stain).

Radiation Vasculitis

Acute radiation vasculitis injury is marked by endothelial damage, ballooning degeneration of intimal cell (Fig. 6-8A), and smooth muscle cell necrosis (Fig. 6-8B) with or without thrombosis of small arteries and arterioles. In the chronic phase, fibrous or mucoid intimal thickening (or both) is seen[142] (see Chapter 18 also).

Wegener Granulomatosis

A systemic necrotizing vasculitis of unknown etiology, Wegener granulomatosis manifests granulomatous lesions of the respiratory tract, including nose, sinuses, and lungs (see Chapter 7 also), as well as renal glomerular disease. Men are affected more often than women and usually in their fifth and sixth decades. Studies demonstrate (C)-ANCA in the blood of most patients. It is suggested that (C)-ANCA activate circulating neutrophils that injure endothelial cells.

The lesions of Wegener granulomatosis are marked by parenchymal necrosis, vasculitis, and granulomatous inflammation composed of neutrophils, lymphocytes, plasma cells, macrophages, and eosinophils. Individual lung lesions may be as large as 5 cm in diameter and may cavitate. Thus, they must be distinguished from lesions caused by tuberculosis. Vasculitis involving small arteries and veins occurs most frequently in the respiratory tract, the kidney, and the spleen. Vasculitis is characterized principally by chronic inflammation; however, acute inflammation, necrotizing and non-necrotizing granulomatous inflammation, and fibrinoid necrosis are frequently present. Medial thickening and intimal proliferation are common and often result in narrowing or obliteration of the vascular lumen. Other vasculitis syndromes producing vasculitis of the lung have been reviewed by Travis and Fleming.[142a]

Most patients with Wegener granulomatosis have symptoms referable to the respiratory tract, particularly pneumonitis and sinusitis. The kidney initially exhibits focal necrotizing glomerulonephritis, which progresses to crescentic glomerulonephritis. Hematuria and proteinuria are common, and the glomerular disease can induce renal failure. Rashes, muscular pains, joint involvement, and neurologic symptoms occur. Untreated Wegener granulomatosis carries a very high mortality. However, patients treated with cyclophosphamide experience a striking improvement in prognosis; complete remission and substantial disease-free intervals are induced.

Lymphomatoid Granulomatosis

Lymphomatoid granulomatosis[143] is a neoplastic proliferation of B cells infected with Epstein-Barr virus and associated with a prominent T-cell reaction and vasculitis.[143a] Angiocentric and angiodestructive infiltrates consisting of mature lymphocytes, activated lymphocytes, plasma cells, histiocytes, and immunoblasts are histologic features. The cellular nodules surround and infiltrate small arteries and veins. Lymphomatoid granulomatosis is a lymphoma that mainly involves the lungs (see Chapter 7 also), but the skin, the central nervous system, and the kidneys may also be involved. The condition is identical pathologically to polymorphic reticulosis[144] and to nonhealing midline granuloma of the Stewart type.[145] Unlike Wegener granulomatosis, granulomas in polymorphic reticulosis are absent or poorly formed. Multidrug chemotherapy induces complete remission in 50% of patients.

Thromboangiitis Obliterans (Buerger Disease Syndrome)

Thromboangiitis obliterans produces occlusive disease of arteries in the arms and legs.[145a] It occurs almost exclusively in young and middle-aged men who smoke heavily. Cessation can be followed by remission, and resumption of smoking by exacerbation. Yet, the mechanism of action of tobacco smoke is obscure. An increased prevalence of HLA-A9 and HLA-B5 haplotypes among victims lends credence to the idea that genetically controlled hypersensitivity to tobacco is involved in the disease's pathogenesis. Studies have indicated that endothelium-dependent vasodilatory responses in nondiseased forearm vessels are dysfunctional in patients with throm-

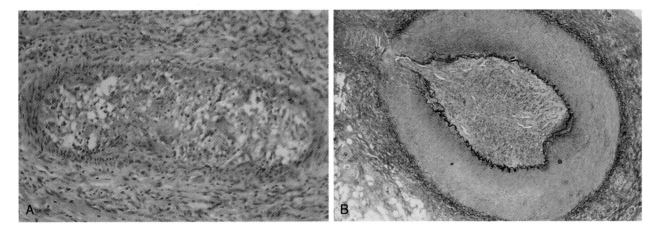

Figure 6-9 • *A*, Acute lesion of Buerger syndrome characterized by a hypercellular, organizing thrombus with giant cells filling the lumen of this small peripheral artery (H&E stain). *B*, Late stage shows total occlusion of the popliteal artery by organized thrombus, intact internal elastic lamina, and minimal recanalization (elastic van Gieson stain).

boangiitis obliterans, suggesting a systemic impairment and the possible importance of endothelial dysfunction in initiating thrombotic arterial lesions.[145b]

Buerger disease begins with an acute occlusive thrombosis of the peripheral arteries and veins, which evokes an inflammatory cellular infiltrate involving the entire neurovascular bundle. Small microabscesses within the thrombus feature a central area of neutrophils accompanied by scanty Langhans or foreign body giant cells (Fig. 6-9A). The early lesions often become severe enough to cause gangrene of the extremity. Late in the course of the disease, luminal thrombi are completely organized (Fig. 6-9B) and partly recanalized. The internal elastic lamina is usually preserved.

Vascular Rejection of Allografts

Homologous or allogeneic transplantation of heart, kidney, liver, heart-lung, and pancreas in humans results in lesions in large, medium, and small vessels caused by immunologically mediated transplant rejection. In many cases, allograft biopsies are used to aid diagnosis and assess rejection reaction. The pathology of cardiac transplantation is presented in detail elsewhere (Chapter 23). In this section, discussion is limited to vascular changes, particularly those involving small vessels in noncardiac transplants.

Kidney

Clinical renal allograft rejection has been very extensively studied.[146]

Hyperacute Rejection

Hyperacute rejection usually develops during or immediately after surgery and is marked by severe leukocytic infiltration of glomerular capillaries, fibrinoid necrosis of arterioles and capillaries, and intravascular platelet thrombosis leading to tissue necrosis.[146] It is mediated by preexisting antibodies that bind to endothelium and activate complement.

Acute Rejection

Acute rejection occurs anywhere from between 1 and 2 weeks to several months after transplantation. Two patterns occur in the kidney. In the interstitial form, inflammation occurs primarily within the interstitium and affects the tubules, whereas the glomeruli and vessels are relatively spared. Immunohistochemical techniques indicate that T cells account for about 80% of the infiltrating inflammatory cells, with the remainder being B cells, killer cells, and macrophages.[147] In acute vascular rejection, vessels of all sizes, including arterioles and venules, show changes that include endothelial swelling and leukocytic infiltration of the subendothelial space. More severe cases show frank fibrinoid necrosis of the vascular wall and intravascular thrombosis. Proliferation of smooth muscle cells and lipid-containing foam cells leads to intimal thickening, vascular compromise, and secondary ischemic damage.

Chronic Rejection and Graft Arteriopathy

Chronic rejection can occur in a progressive manner starting about 8 weeks after transplantation and eventually producing renal insufficiency. There is no clear-cut distinction between the vascular changes of acute and chronic rejection, and the two may occur together. Graft arteriopathy is characterized by luminal narrowing primarily caused by marked concentric intimal fibrosis with or without intimal foam cells. The internal elastic lamina is multilayered or fragmented, and there is medial fibrosis. Intravascular thrombosis may also occur. Immunofluorescence studies usually show IgM, IgG, C3, and fibrin present in the vessel wall in both acute and chronic rejection. Vascular rejection in the transplanted kidney must be differentiated from the arteriopathy associated with cyclosporin treatment, another frequent cause of allograft failure.[148]

Liver

In the rejection of hepatic allografts, a spectrum of vascular lesions is seen.[149, 150] Mononuclear inflammatory cell infiltrates are present in and around both central and portal vein branches. Arteriolar changes, including intimal fibrosis and hyperplasia, are often subtle, whereas lesions of medium-sized vessels similar to those seen in renal allografts are easier to identify. Although somewhat less extensive than in renal allografts, antibody deposition is found particularly in the peripheral arteries of transplanted livers with chronic rejection.[151]

Lung

Pulmonary vascular findings in the transplanted lungs of patients who have had a *heart-lung transplant* include accelerated intimal hyperplasia of elastic and muscular arteries as well as arterioles and veins.[152] It is suspected that subclinical episodes of rejection cause this vascular damage, but this is unproved. Transbronchial lung biopsies have been advocated to distinguish rejection, characterized in part by the presence of dense perivascular lymphocytic infiltrates from opportunistic infections.[153]

Pancreas

Vascular lesions including acute endovasculitis, with or without fibrinoid necrosis of the vessel wall and chronic fibrointimal proliferation, are also part of the rejection reaction in pancreatic allografts. The role of pancreatic graft biopsy in this setting has yet to be established.[154]

Infectious

Microorganisms may produce inflammation of small vessels. In some instances, the resultant vasculitis is important in initiating the primary pathologic lesion, whereas, in others, it is secondary to direct extension of an adjacent infectious focus. In the latter case, vessel involvement may exacerbate the primary infective process by inducing tissue necrosis resulting from vascular occlusion or by providing a pathway for hematogenous spread. Organisms can produce vasculitis directly by their presence, by a toxic effect, or by an immune–complex-mediated mechanism. The degree of acute vascular damage is variable. Sequelae of infectious vasculitides includes luminal narrowing resulting from fibrointimal thickening and microaneurysm formation.

Discussion in this section is limited to infections that induce prominent small-vessel involvement. Diseases in which small-vessel involvement occurs as a minor or clinically insignificant component of the infectious process are excluded. For example, in tuberculosis, small-vessel arteritis, which may be nongranulomatous,[155] does occur but tends to be clinically unimportant when compared with erosion of moderate and large vessels.[156] In leprosy, arterioles, capillaries, and venules close to the lesions may show organisms in swollen endothelial cells that are associated with perivascular cuffing by mononuclear leukocytes, but vascular damage is usually not severe.[157]

Rickettsia

The rickettsiae are obligate intracellular parasites that produce a vasculitis that primarily involves the microcirculation.[158] Its extent and severity vary with the type of rickettsial infection. In general, organisms disseminate from the entry site via the blood stream and invade endothelial and medial smooth muscle cells of small vessels to induce severe vasculitis. Rickettsiae can be detected in thin paraffin sections using the Wolbach modification of the Giemsa stain.[159] Immunofluorescence tests also detect rickettsiae in the skin lesions of Mediterranean and Rocky Mountain spotted fevers.[160, 161]

Rocky Mountain Spotted Fever

This condition, which accounts for more than 90% of human rickettsial diseases, is caused by the tick-borne *Rickettsia rickettsii*. Capillaries, arterioles, and venules (but not lymphatics) of many organs, including skin, kidney, heart, brain, liver, and testes, are involved to a varying extent. The necrotizing arterial lesions are most prominent in the skin and testes, whereas capillary damage is found in all organs.[162] In the acute phase, necrosis of the vessel wall is associated with a polymorphonuclear leukocytic infiltration, but in older lesions, mononuclear inflammatory cells, which extend into the perivascular areas, predominate. Necrotizing arteritis is frequently associated with occlusive thrombi and secondary hemorrhagic necrosis of tissue. Walker and Mattern[158] showed that, in the kidney, the distribution of *R. rickettsii* organisms correlated with that of the perviascular interstitial inflammatory cell infiltrates. In the heart, the predominant vascular lesion is a mild focal monuclear infiltration of small veins sometimes associated with intraluminal thrombosis.[163] Experimentally, in guinea pigs, vascular damage was found before identification of rickettsial organisms or circulating antibodies against them, suggesting that the vasculitis was induced by a toxin.[164] In vitro studies show a fourfold increase in the adherence of platelets to cultured human endothelial cells infected with *R. rickettsii* as compared with uninfected controls, providing a possible mechanism for the thrombocytopenia seen clinically.[165]

Epidemic Typhus

In epidemic typhus, endothelial swelling and proliferation in arterioles, capillaries, and venules with luminal narrowing and thrombosis also occur, as does perivascular inflammation. Vascular necrosis is, however, less prominent than in *R. rickettsii* infection.

Scrub Typhus

In contrast to both Rocky Mountain spotted fever and epidemic typhus, vascular damage tends to be slight in scrub typhus caused by *Rickettsia tsutsugamushi*.[163] The skin macules show a mononuclear, leukocytic, perivascular cuffing, and only very rarely is a necrotizing arteritis seen. Systematically, capillaries, venules, and veins demonstrate endothelial and subendothelial edema, and, occasionally, focal necrosis of the intima and mononuclear cell infiltration of the vessel wall are observed. Thrombi occur less frequently than in the epidemic typhus and spotted fever groups.

Q Fever

Q fever, caused by *Coxiella burnetii,* is usually a self-limiting, acute disease involving lungs, liver, and bone marrow. The most distinctive pathologic finding is that of fibrin-ring granulomas, but small-vein vasculitis can also be found in the liver.[166]

Rickettsial infection has also been the postulated cause of an outbreak of an acute febrile vasculitic syndrome that involved small cerebral vessels.[167]

Meningococcus

In acute meningococcemia, there is involvement of the small vessels, especially of the skin, producing a hemorrhagic or vesicular skin rash. Histologically, perivascular cuffing of small vessels by neutrophils, macrophages, and occasional lymphocytes, with or without microthrombi, are seen. Suppurative necrosis of the vessel wall with hemorrhage into the dermis may develop. The gram-negative diplococci of *Neisseria meningitidis* can sometimes be identified histologically within the vessel wall, within thrombi, or in perivascular tissue. Adrenal hemorrhage, which may occur in acute meningococcemia (Waterhouse-Friderichsen syndrome), is associated with fibrin microthrombi within the microcirculation of the adrenal cortex.

Pseudomonas

Pseudomonas aeruginosa, a gram-negative bacillus, produces severe systemic infection in susceptible hosts such as patients with extensive burns, hematologic malignancies, or immune deficiency. Capillaries, arterioles, and venules, as well as larger vessels, are affected. Infiltration of the vessel wall is seen on hematoxylin stain, as a marked basophilia, the closely clustered bacteria obscuring features of the underlying wall. There is usually no associated intramural inflammatory response, but a mixed inflammatory cell infiltrate may be seen in cases of *ecthyma gangrenosum,* a cutaneous *P. aeruginosa* infection.[168] Thrombosis does occur, but intraluminal colonies of bacteria are generally not observed, suggesting that septic embolization is not an important pathogenetic phenomenon. Associated with these vascular lesions are foci of hemorrhagic, nonsuppurative tissue necrosis.[169]

The pathogenesis of *P. aeruginosa* vasculitis is multifactorial, with the organism exhibiting both locally invasive and toxigenic properties.[170] Early experimental studies in the rat[171] suggested that vessels were invaded from without rather than through intimal permeation. However, Margaretten and colleagues[172] argued that, because vessel wall invasion could be found with little or no bacterial infection in surrounding tissue, hematogenous spread had to be important. Although various enzymes secreted by *P. aeruginosa* are considered to act locally, toxins (e.g., exotoxin A) and phospholipase are primarily responsible for systemic manifestations.[173] A possible experimental model of Kawasaki disease has been produced by injecting immunodeficient mice and guinea pigs with supraliminal doses of *Pseudomonas* bacilli.[174]

Syphilis

In all tissue affected by syphilis, small arteries and arterioles show endothelial swelling and a concentric intimal cell proliferation that eventually obliterate the lumen and lead to local tissue necrosis. Surrounding the vessels is a characteristic perivascular cuff of lymphocytes and plasma cells. Proliferation of pericytic cells has been seen on ultrastructural examination of syphilitic chancres.[175] In tertiary nasal syphilis, abnormalities of arterioles and capillaries were more prominent than those of venules.[176] The pathogenesis of tissue damage in syphilis is likely related to immediate or delayed hypersensitivity reactions, or to both.[177]

Fungi

Systemic fungal infections are a serious problem in current medical practice, primarily because of an increased number of immunosuppressed patients.[178, 179]

Mucormycosis[180] and aspergillosis[181] are two systemic fungal infections in which dissemination and tissue destruction are related in part to the ability of these fungi to invade both small and larger blood vessels. The vascular invasion often induces thrombosis with secondary ischemic necrosis of tissue. *Scedosporium apiospermum (Pseudallescheria boydii)* mimics *Aspergillus* spp. and *Fusarium* spp., both clinically and histopathologically. Imidazoles such as miconazole, but not amphotericin B, are considered the therapeutic compounds of choice.[181a] Mucormycosis is caused by fungi of the genera *Rhizopus, Mucor,* and *Absidia,* all of which have broad nonseptate hyphae that branch at different angles up to 90 degrees. In contrast, *Aspergillus* has thinner septate hyphae that branch at more acute angles, generally 45 degrees or less. Although vessel involvement is usually not seen in superficial *candidiasis,* it is a feature in about one third of cases of deep organ or systemic infection.[182]

The morphologic diagnosis of deep mycotic infections in tissue sections has been reviewed.[183] The use of special stains such as Grocott methenamine silver to demonstrate fungi is considered essential[184] but does not replace microbiologic cultures required for definitive typing of the organism.

Plague

Yersinia pestis is a bacterium that causes severe necrosis of tissue.[185] The small vessels in areas of suppuration become necrotic and thrombosed, further extending the area of tissue destruction. The disease offers an example of a virulent organism that increases its pathologic effect by invading small vessels and inducing thrombosis.

Whipple Disease

Whipple disease, a multisystem illness, has as its pathologic hallmark the finding of macrophages laden with PAS-positive, rod-shaped bacilli.[186] The bacilli are found in the arterial vessels of the small intestine[187] and the liver[188] as well as in endothelial and free cells in the medial layer of small arteries of the heart, the kidneys, and spleen.[189] Arteritis may be seen, with bacilli having been described both in areas of active arteritis and in noninflamed segments showing fibrointimal hyperplasia.[189] A molecular phylogenetic approach showed that the Whipple bacillus is a member of the actinomycete taxon of bacteria.[190] Schoedon and colleagues[190a] have successfully propagated the causative organs, *Tropheryma whippeli,* in cell culture.

Leptospirosis

Leptospirosis, an acute infectious disease, affects many organs, including liver, kidney, lung, and skeletal muscles. An important clinical feature is a hemorrhagic diathesis. In an experimental study using guinea pigs, vascular damage was mainly restricted to capillaries and associated with a paucity of microorganisms in the vicinity, in keeping with a toxic pathogenesis.[191]

Schistosoma

Bilharzial *(Schistosoma)* infection may be associated with a local necrotizing arteritis,[192] probably an allergic reaction to the ovum or its products. Usually, the ovum penetrates the arterial wall to form a granuloma alongside the artery.

Toxic

Certain drugs may cause necrotizing vasculitis of medium-sized and small arteries via a direct toxic effect. In analgesic nephropathy, luminal narrowing of small vessels of the urinary tract and skin, caused by deposition of hyaline-like material within the vessel wall, is one of the characteristic findings.[52, 53] Cocaine may produce arterial thrombosis and arteriolar intimal thickening.[192a] These and other drug-induced vascular diseases are discussed in Chapter 17.

Coagulopathic Disorders

In this section, conditions in which intravascular thrombosis appears to be a primary event are discussed.

Thrombotic Thrombocytopenic Purpura

In thrombotic thrombocytopenic purpura (TTP), a patient has thrombocytopenic purpura, hemolytic anemia, and widespread hyaline platelet-fibrin thrombin in arterioles and capillaries.[193, 194] The syndrome may be associated with other entities such as connective tissue diseases, pregnancy, or use of drugs such as cyclosporin A or oral contraceptives. In the majority of cases, however, TTP develops without an identifiable cause or associated factor.[193] The diagnosis may be confirmed histologically by gingival or bone marrow biopsy, but the yield is low.[195]

The thrombi found in TTP are bland, are often occlusive, and show varying degrees of organization. Associated findings include endothelial cell swelling and proliferation and dilation of both arterioles and capillaries with microaneurysm formation.[196, 197] Ultrastructurally, granular and fibrillar material is seen in the subendothelial regions of small arteries, arterioles, capillaries, and veins, whereas the lumen contains mostly platelets and a small amount of fibrin.[196]

In a review of proposed pathogenetic mechanisms, Lian[198] concluded that in some patients, platelet thrombus formation appeared triggered by a specific platelet-agglutinating factor, whereas in others, endothelial cell damage was followed by platelet adhesion and aggregation. A rat model of von Willebrand–factor-mediated thrombotic thrombocytopenia that uses botrocetin injections has been developed. This may provide further insight into pathogenesis.[199]

Hemolytic Uremic Syndrome

Hemolytic uremic syndrome (HUS) shares with TTP features of microangiopathic hemolytic anemia, thrombocytopenia, and microvascular thrombosis; it differs, however, because thrombosis is usually limited to the kidneys. The disease occurs in any age group but classically affects infants and small children, who appear to have a better prognosis than older patients.

On gross examination, the kidneys in HUS are swollen and pale with "flea-bite" hemorrhages. Histologically, in addition to thrombosis, small arteries and arterioles show mucinous and onion-skin types of intimal thickening, with varying degrees of luminal narrowing. Fibrinoid necrosis of the vessel wall and focal areas of tissue infarction may also occur.[14] Glomerular capillary walls are thickened and splitting, or reduplication of basement membranes can be demonstrated with silver stains. Ultrastructurally, granular or fibrillar electron-dense material is found within the subendothelial space of glomerular capillaries, and it may be associated with mesangial cell interposition.[200] Morel-Margoer and associates[201] found that adults with HUS who had a good outcome had significantly less intimal hyperplasia in small arterial vessels in comparison with those who did not. The authors suggested that a renal biopsy performed early in the course of this illness might help to establish a prognosis.

Renal morphologic features are not specific and may be observed in toxemia of pregnancy, malignant hypertension, scleroderma, and acute renal allograft rejection.[44] Rarely, microthrombi are observed within the glomerular capillaries of patients with metastatic carcinoma,[202, 203] but pulmonary microvascular abnormalities in this group seem to be a more important cause of their hemolytic anemia.[202] A small subset of patients with clinical features of HUS, but without evidence of microangiopathy, have also been described.[204]

Clinically, HUS is associated with a number of factors, including viral and bacterial infections, drugs such as oral contraceptives or cyclosporin,[205] and pregnancy.[206] A classification based on causes includes classic, postinfectious, hereditary, immune-mediated, and pregnancy-related forms.[207] Current hypotheses regarding the complex pathogenesis of HUS were reviewed by Drummond.[207] They include (1) the uncovering of new antigens (e.g., Thomsen-Friedenreich cryptantigen) on the surfaces of endothelial cells, platelets, and red blood cells by bacterial or viral neuraminidases; (2) an inherited or acquired abnormality in prostacyclin metabolism; and (3) endothelial cell damage secondary to exotoxins, such as vero-cell cytotoxin produced by *Escherichia coli* or to endotoxins such as that produced in *Shigella dysenteriae.*[208] In each case, damage to endothelial cells appears to be crucial. With verotoxin-1, a direct and dose-dependent cytotoxic effect on cultured human endothelial cells has been demonstrated.[209] Verotoxin-1 also increases platelet-aggregating activity in plasma.[210] Endothelial apoptosis has been identified as a significant process in the pathobiology of TTP and of sporadic HUS.[210a]

Disseminated Intravascular Coagulation (DIC)

Disseminated intravascular coagulation (DIC) occurs as an acute, often life-threatening epiphenomenon in a spectrum of clinical settings including septicemia, shock, trauma, and pregnancy. A subacute or chronic counterpart may be seen associated with malignancies, vascular disorders, and liver disease.[211] Histologically, DIC is diagnosed by the presence of fibrin thrombi, usually restricted to small vessels.[212] Despite widespread clinical manifestations, a diligent search is often necessary to find the microscopic fibrin thrombi at autopsy. Even in clinically confirmed cases, such a search may be unsuccessful. Alternatively, clinically unsuspected DIC may be found during a postmortem examination.[213] The kidneys, the liver, and the lungs are the most frequently affected organs. Shimamura and colleagues[214] attempted to correlate the distribution of microthrombi (i.e., hepatic, hepatorenal, renal, and undetermined) with the temporal course of DIC. Thrombi in aneurysmally dilated arterioles, previously considered pathognomonic of TTP, are observed in DIC.[212] Perivascular hemorrhage is also a feature, but the thrombosed vessels are inflamed, in contrast to the hemorrhagic vasculitis of meningococcemia. Skin biopsy may help to establish a definitive diagnosis for cases in which the clinical diagnosis is equivocal.[215] Cutaneous lesions that are 2 or 3 days old show epidermal necrosis secondary to local ischemia.

Intravascular thrombosis in DIC results from release of tissue factors into the circulation or because of widespread endothelial cell injury. Consumption of platelets and coagulation factors occurs concurrently with activation of the fibrinolytic system, thus predisposing to hemorrhages. A rat model of DIC that uses dexamethasone-prepared E. coli has been developed.[216]

Systemic Hypertension

Systemic hypertension has been classified as idiopathic primary hypertension (essential) or secondary hypertension (nonessential). The latter disorder represents about 10% of cases in which a specific cause is found. These include renal parenchymal diseases, renal vessel diseases, or both; hormonal conditions, including pheochromocytoma; Cushing syndrome, primary aldosteronism (Conn syndrome); and hyperthyroidism and coarctation of the aorta, whether congenital or acquired after aortitis. Hyperthyroidism elevates systolic pressure only. The likely cause of essential hypertension is a dysfunction of the renin-angiotensin-aldosterone system resulting in increased peripheral resistance and blood volume. Some genetic conditions have been identified that disrupt the system and are associated with hypertension. The vascular changes in hypertensive patients may promote further hyperplasia by altering vascular resistance.

In "benign" hypertension, the primary lesion, which is found in small arteries and arterioles, is a hyaline deposition. It occurs in most body organs and is important in promoting hypertensive glomerulonephrosclerosis. Similar changes develop in systemic arteries with aging in the absence of hypertension. The vascular media is hypertrophied with increased elastin fibers and hyperplasia of smooth muscle cells, and the intima is hyperplastic (Fig. 6-10A). In accelerated or "malignant" hypertension characterized by a blood pressure that rapidly increases with diastolic pressures of 110 to 130 mm Hg or more, there is a more marked vascular change characterized by mucinous and onion-skin intimal thickening, primarily of small arteries (Fig. 6-10B), as well as fibrous intimal thickening of larger arteries.[14] Arteriolar necrosis is a striking feature, with fibrinoid necrosis present in small arteries (Fig. 6-10C) and arterioles often associated with intravascular thrombosis. The lumens of arterioles are narrowed. It should be noted that benign hypertension is present in most cases of aortic arch dissections and is associated with cerebral hemorrhage. The existence of Charcot-Bouchard aneurysms is controversial,[216a] and arteriolar twists and coils (Fig. 6-11) may be mistaken for aneurysms. Fibrinoid necrosis of small arteries has been postulated as a cause of hypertensive cerebral haemorrhage.[216b]

Severe pulmonary hypertension is marked by fibrinoid necrosis of small and medium-sized arterial walls, thrombosis, and the formation of plexiform lesions[217] (see Chapter 7).

Neoplastic

Tumor invasion of small vessels is a very common, probably ubiquitous, occurrence in malignant neoplasms of all types. In this section, discussion is limited to a few neoplastic processes in which small-vessel involvement is a major pathologic feature.

Intravascular Lymphomatosis

This rare, almost invariably fatal, condition is marked histologically by a proliferation of atypical mononuclear cells within the lumens of small vessels. The disease appears most commonly with central nervous system involvement. At autopsy, small collections of intravascular neoplastic cells are found in most organs, but because meningeal vessels are often extensively involved, meningeal biopsy is proposed as a method of obtaining an antemortem diagnosis.[218]

In the past, many investigators[218–221] considered this entity a neoplasm derived from endothelial cells. This is reflected in alternate nomenclature (e.g., malignant angioendotheliomatosis, neoplastic angioendotheliosis, angioendoliomatosis proliferans). Several studies using immunohistochemical techniques indicated that the malignant intravascular cells are actually of lymphoid origin.[222–225]

Endovascular Papillary Angioendothelioma

Endovascular papillary angioendothelioma (Dabska tumor) is an uncommon cutaneous vascular tumor of childhood defined histologically by an intravascular proliferation of cells with immunohistochemical staining properties suggesting postcapillary high endothelial cell differentiation.[226] This is consistent with the presence of

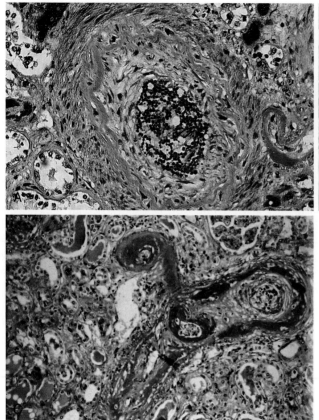

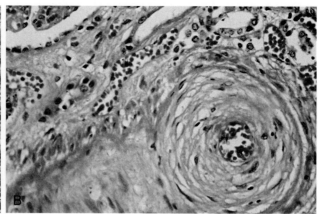

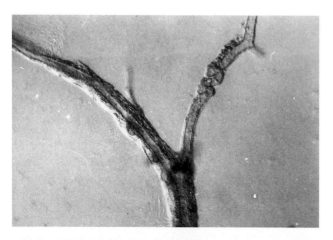

Figure 6-10 • Hypertension. *A*, Intimal hyperplasia in renal arteriole in patient with benign nephrosclerosis. *B*, Onionskin type of pattern of intimal and medial arterial hyperplasia. *C*, Kidney with arteriolar fibrinoid necrosis in malignant hypertension (H&E stain).

intravascular lymphocytes often associated with the endothelium, which itself is often epithelioid in nature. Although locally aggressive, the prognosis is almost invariably very good.

Intravascular Papillary Endothelial Hyperplasia

Intravascular papillary endothelial hyperplasia,[227] also known as Masson vegetant intravascular hemangioendo-thelioma,[228] is an exuberant intravascular proliferation of endothelial cells that form intravascular papillary fronds (Fig. 6-12) and may mimic angiosarcoma. The lack of cellular pleomorphism and significant mitotic activity of this intravascular lesion distinguishes it from angiosarcoma. Although originally regarded as a true neoplasm, it is now generally accepted as an unusual form of organizing thrombus.[229]

Other tumors characterized by a proliferation of small

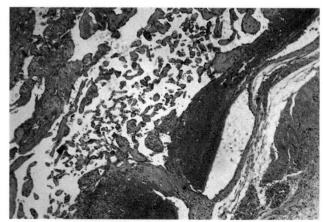

Figure 6-11 • Charcot-Bouchard pseudoaneurysm. Anteriolar branch (top right) of small intracerebral artery shows a focal aneurysm-like configuration resulting from localized kinking of the elongated vessel (Nomarski differential interference contrast technique).

Figure 6-12 • Intravascular papillary endothelial hyperplasia (so-called Masson vegetant intravascular hemangioendothelioma) shows intravascular papillary fronds covered by endothelial cells evolving from a bland organizing thrombus (H&E stain).

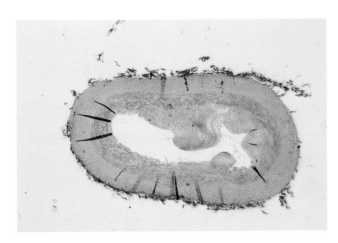

Figure 6-13 • Renal artery dysplasia with focal intimal hyperplasia protruding into the artery lumen (Masson trichrome stain).

vessels include capillary hemangiomas, epithelioid hemangioma (angiolymphoid hyperplasia with eosinophilia), pyogenic granuloma (lobular capillary hemangioma), Kaposi's sarcoma, and some intramuscular hemangiomas, epithelioid hemangioendotheliomas, and angiosarcomas. These are beyond the scope of this chapter, and the reader is referred to standard skin and soft tissue pathology texts for details.[229a]

Miscellaneous

Fibromuscular Dysplasia

Fibromuscular dysplasia is a noninflammatory, non-necrotic thickening of large and medium muscular arteries, including renal, carotid, vertebral, and splanchnic vessels. Its cause is not known, but it is considered a developmental anomaly. The luminal stenosis it produces in renal arteries may cause renovascular hypertension. Fibromuscular dysplasia can appear at any age, even in childhood; however, it occurs most often in young women. In most cases, the distal two thirds of the renal artery and its primary branches display several segmental stenoses caused by fibrous and muscular ridges projecting into the lumen with a disorderly arrangement and proliferation of smooth muscle cell in the vessel wall. About 95% of cases have medial hyperplasia, and some smooth muscle is replaced by fibrous tissue and myofibroblasts. In some instances, intimal fibroplasia predominates (Fig. 6-13), and in unusual cases, connective tissue encircles the adventitia. Other than renal hypertension, the major complication of fibromuscular dysplasia is medial dissection with aneurysm and potential rupture of affected vessels.

Amyloidosis

Amyloid may deposit within small vessels throughout the body (see Chapter 16). The pathology of amyloid as it involves the kidney and its microvasculature and in cerebral amyloid angiopathy have been described.[230–232] Involvement of small intramyocardial arteries by various types of amyloid is observed in endomyocardial biopsies, including a subset of patients exhibiting echocardio-

graphic evidence of interventricular septal thickening.[223] In rare cases of systemic amyloidosis, involvement is exclusively vascular, with tissue parenchyma being spared.[234, 235]

Emboli

Small-caliber vessels of both the systemic and pulmonary circulations are the site of embolization of many substances that originate both intravascularly and extravascularly. These include the following:

1. Systemic bland thromboemboli may originate from the aorta and the large arteries, endocardium of the left side of the heart in conditions such as atrial fibrillation, myocardial infarction and cardiomyopathy, or heart valves in nonbacterial thrombotic endocarditis.[236] Prosthetic heart valves are also a source (see Chapter 21). The deep veins of the lower limb remain the most common source of pulmonary thromboemboli (Fig. 6-14) (see Chapter 7). Sources from pelvic plexuses should be sought in autopsied cases.
2. Septic thromboemboli usually derive from infective endocarditis of native or prosthetic heart valves[237] (see Chapter 14), but they may also originate from heart and vascular septic mural thrombi.
3. Tumor emboli are usually derived from tumor infiltration of pulmonary veins or left-sided cardiac tumors, mainly myxoma.
4. Lipid crystal/atheromatous emboli arise from complicated atherosclerotic plaques in the aorta and other major arterial vessels[238] (Fig. 6-15). The emboli occur either spontaneously or develop as a complication of vascular surgery or angioplasty.[239] The diagnosis is often confirmed by skin biopsy.[240, 241] The significance of atheromatous emboli within mural capillaries of carotid endarterectomy specimens[242] has yet to be defined.
5. Bone marrow/fat emboli are usually related to trauma with closed chest massage in resuscitation, a common cause of such emboli found at postmortem examination.
6. Gaseous emboli occur as a complication of surgery,

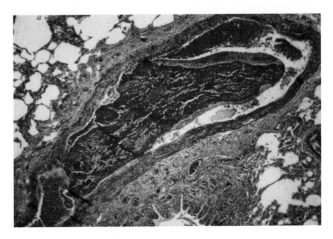

Figure 6-14 • Thromboembolism lodged in a pulmonary artery (H&E stain).

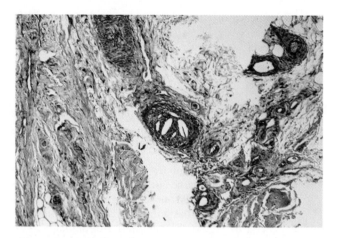

Figure 6-15 • Cholesterol emboli in lower limb arterioles from a patient with severe atherosclerosis of the abdominal aorta (Masson trichrome stain).

intravascular catheterization, trauma,[243, 244] and diving accidents (sudden decompression).

7. Amniotic fluid embolism[245-247] is associated with childbirth.

8. Calcific fragments embolized from ulcerated, calcified mitral annuli occur in older patients.[248] Emboli related to small coronary vessels and secondary to cardiovascular surgery are discussed in Chapter 21.

9. Brain and myocardium are uncommon emboli, with their occurrence usually related to trauma.

10. Various foreign materials present after instrumentation or surgery can form emboli. Walley and colleagues[249] published a compendium to aid their identification.

All of these emboli can occlude small-caliber vessels and cause local ischemia and infarction. Emboli may also undergo fibrinolysis or organization with recanalization (Fig. 6-16). Localized abscesses may result from septic emboli.

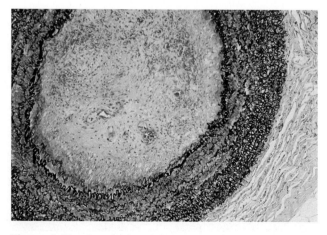

Figure 6-16 • Organization of thrombus in elastic artery. Note neovascularization throughout the fibrous tissue occluding the lumen (H&E stain).

Idiopathic Intimal Hyperplasia of Small Arteries/Arterioles

Rarely, widespread occlusive intimal hyperplasia of small arterial vessels has been observed in the absence of an underlying identifiable cause such as vasculitis.[250] Although the vascular lesions are histologically similar to those seen in malignant atrophic papulosis, there is none of the skin involvement characteristic of the latter entity.

Erythromelalgia

Erythromelalgia, which presents clinically as a syndrome of redness and burning pain in the extremities, may be associated with chronic myeloproliferative disorders or may occur as a primary entity.[250a] The skin from involved areas shows arteriolar inflammation histologically with fibromuscular intimal proliferation and thrombotic occlusion.[251] Erythromelalgia is distinguished from primary erythromelalgia by the presence of fibromuscular intimal proliferation and occlusive thrombi.[251a] Michiels and associates[252] postulated that platelet activation and aggregation that occurred preferentially within arterioles were the underlying primary process causing the clinical presentation, but not all authors have agreed with that opinion.[253]

Dermal Microangiopathy Associated With End-Stage Renal Failure

Ichimaru and Horie[254] reported a series of 63 patients with end-stage renal failure who had subepidermal capillary basement membrane thickening with multilamination of the basal lamina ultrastructurally. In many cases, a chronic inflammatory cell infiltrate with a mast cell and eosinophil component was found. A uremic toxic pathogenesis for these microvascular changes has been postulated.

Small-Vessel Diseases Isolated to the Testes

Arteriolar hyalinosis is an uncommon lesion characterized by hyalinization and luminal narrowing of testicular arterioles. It affects patients with infertility or cryptorchidism, and, rarely, normal young males. Ultrastructurally, granular material is found in the subendothelial zone as well as extending between medial smooth muscle cells.[255] The etiology and significance of this lesion are not known.

Alterations confined to small venules in the testes of infertile men with varicoceles have also been reported.[256] These include vascular wall and perivascular fibrosis, myoepithelial cell proliferation, and perivascular lymphocytic infiltrates. The etiology of the vascular changes is unknown, but they may contribute to male infertility.

Progressive Arterial Occlusive Disease (Malignant Atrophic Papulosis)

In progressive arterial occlusive disease (Köhlmeier-Degos), small and medium-sized arteries undergo a progressive occlusive fibrosis leading to tissue infarction.[257-259] The skin and gastrointestinal tract are the most commonly involved sites. Köhlmeier in 1941[260] interpreted the multiple intestinal perforations in his patient as a result of mesenteric thromboangiitis obliterans, but Degos and associates in 1942[261] considered the pathology distinct and gave it the name "atrophic papulosquamous dermatitis."

The characteristic feature of this disease is the deposition of intimal fibrous tissue in arterioles or small and medium arteries, leading to progressive vascular occlusions in many organs (e.g., skin, gastrointestinal tract, genitourinary tracts, retroperitoneum, adrenals, pericardium, myocardium, brain, conjunctiva). The lesion contains ectatic and congested vessels, thrombotic occlusions, and, often, lymphocytic infiltrates, either perivascular, vascular, or both. Rarely, there is evidence, usually in arterioles, of vasculitis and of the intima and media being infiltrated by lymphocytes, histiocytes, and neutrophils. There is male predominance, and the average duration of the disease is 2 years. Diagnosis is usually suggested by distinctive skin lesions consisting of a central porcelain-white area surrounded by an erythematous halo, together with unique vascular changes. Veins and lymphatics were not primarily affected.

Other authors[257, 258] have pointed out that progressive arterial occlusive disease is easily distinguished from polyarteritis nodosa, which involves the full thickness of the vessel wall in an inflammatory process with scarring of the media as well. Aneurysm formation occurs in polyarteritis but not in this condition. The etiology of this fatal disorder is unknown.[262] Rosenberg[263] commented on the striking resemblance between the vascular lesions in Köhlmeier-Degos progressive arterial occlusive disease and those occurring in systemic arterial disease resulting from chronic arsenicism. All therapy has been unsuccessful.

Cystic Adventitial Disease

In cystic adventitial disease, an adventitial cyst narrows or occludes the arterial lumen. This rare condition (one in 1200 cases of claudication) was first reported by Atkins and Key in 1947[264]; by 1973, more than 54 cases had been reported.[265] Only 8 of 59 recorded cases occurred in women.[266]

The patient usually manifests a sudden onset of calf cramp and severe intermittent claudication. In men, symptoms appear in the fourth and fifth decades, whereas women are not affected until the sixth decade.[266] Full flexion of the knee may produce temporary acute ischemia. There is an absence of generalized arterial changes, and the condition comes into the differential diagnosis of Buerger disease. Most patients have been manual workers.

Ischemia is the result of stenosis and/or occlusion of the artery by an intramural cyst that forms between the media and adventitia. The cyst is either uni- or multiloculated and filled under pressure with clear fluid or gelatinous material. It usually lacks an epithelial lining, but, occasionally, one has been present.[267] The cyst contents (mainly mucoproteins) and wall structure suggest mucinous degeneration, such as occurs in a ganglion[268] (Fig. 6-17).

Arteriography distinguishes this condition from Buer-

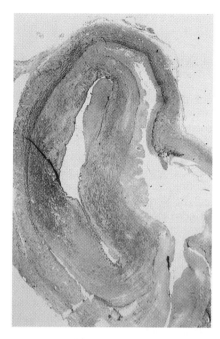

Figure 6-17 • Histology of resected segment of popliteal artery from a man with cystic adventitial disease shows an intra-adventitial cyst (right) lined by fibrous tissue apart from scanty mesothelial-like cells (top). Mural, organizing fibrin thrombus is present within the lumen of the artery (top) (elastic van Gieson stain).

ger disease by showing that the artery is intrinsically normal. The obstruction is seldom complete, and bilateral involvement is not seen. Occasionally, the arterial caliber is normal, but the cyst prevents the usual increase of blood flow associated with exercise.[267]

Cystic adventitial disease usually involves the popliteal artery at, or just above, the upper level of the femoral condyles. Other arteries are sometimes affected (e.g., external iliac, common femoral, radial, ulnar). Cystic adventitial disease has also been reported in veins.

The three theories of causation are as follows[266]:

1. Repeated trauma. This seems unlikely, because the condition has been encountered in children.
2. Mucin-secreting cells derived from an adjacent joint or tendon sheath become included in the arterial adventitia as a developmental anomaly. Subsequent mucin production leads to cyst formation and arterial compression. Although this theory is attractive, the absence of cells within the inner portions of almost all reported cysts makes it an unlikely explanation.
3. Schramek and Hashmonai[265] suggested that intramural hemorrhage may have had a role in the pathogenesis of some cases.

Treatment includes aspiration of the cyst or resection with graft interposition.[269]

Arterial Endofibrosis

This is an exercise-related condition reported in competition cyclists.[270] Iliac arterial stenosis occurs in arteries showing fibrosis of the intimal wall with no inflammatory lesions or atherosclerosis. The pathogenesis of the condition is unknown.

Moyamoya Syndrome

Patients with moyamoya syndrome develop multiple occlusions of their cerebral circulation, with an unusual net-like system of collaterals.[271] The condition is generally diagnosed by arteriography, and most reports have been of Japanese patients. There is narrowing of the distal internal carotid artery and the proximal portions of its major branches, together with multiple occlusions.[272] The changes are often bilateral, with more severe involvement of one side. The vertebrobasilar system may also be affected. Four necropsy cases[273, 274] revealed intimal thickening of affected arteries without any abnormalities of the media or adventitia and with no inflammation. A case with carotid arterial atherosclerosis was also reported. Cerebral hemorrhage that derives from the overgrown collateral arteries in the brain is an important complication of the condition.[275] After exclusion of cases in which an etiology can be found, there remain many characterized by bilateral involvement of the terminal portions of the internal carotid arteries and by onset in early childhood resulting from unknown etiology. The cases of "spontaneous occlusion of the circle of Willis" form part of moyamoya syndrome.[275] Increased medial thickness in the vertebrobasilar system is related to the severity of the occlusive changes in the carotid system rather than to systemic hypertension.[276] However, some cases of moyamoya syndrome have been associated with renovascular hypertension.[277, 277a] Suggested causes of the condition are many and include primary vascular malformation, response to trauma or inflammation, autoimmune disease, or hypertension. The high level of fibroblast growth factor-2 in the cerebrospinal fluid or moyamoya patients may be a factor in the development of stenosis of intracranial major arteries and angiogenesis of collateral circulation.[277b] Findings from some studies suggest that abnormal regulation of extracellular matrix metabolism related to elastin may be important in pathogenesis.[277c]

Mucoid Vasculopathy

Sandhyamani[278, 279] described a nonatherosclerotic, noninflammatory vascular disorder characterized by a general thickening of blood vessels in more than 44% of autopsies in southern India, mainly among males of lower socioeconomic status. The condition affects arteries, veins, and vasa nervosa; vessels are firm yet rubbery. Concentric thickening of both intima and media leads to diffuse luminal narrowing. Histologically, vessel changes include abnormally large deposits of intimal mucopolysaccharide, accompanied by hypercellularity of vessel wall elements. Dystrophic mineralization of internal elastic laminae and of medial mucopolysaccharide material are features in some cases.

Similarity to certain experimental nutritional deficiencies[280] has been suggested. Mucoid vasculopathy also resembles, in some respects, the vascular changes seen in cases of idiopathic peripheral limb gangrene observed in Central Africa.[281-284] It should be noted that organization of an arterial thrombus may lead to a lesion similar to those described as mucoid vasculopathy. Mucoid vascu-

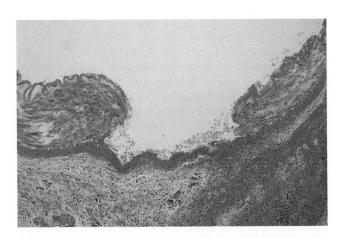

Figure 6-18 • Segmental mediolytic arteriopathy led to acute focal medial rupture of a small intra-abdominal artery. The ends of the ruptured media have retracted. A fibrin deposit lines the inner aspect of the remaining adventitia, which is the only layer maintaining the integrity of the vessel. The rupture has evoked an inflammatory cellular response in the surrounding tissues (H&E stain).

lopathy as an entity has not yet been reported from several major centers in South Africa despite active efforts to identify the lesion (Cooper K, personal communication, 1998).

Mediolytic Vasculopathy (Segmental Mediolytic Arteriopathy)

Segemental mediolytic arteriopathy (SMA) is a very rare vascular disease that usually appears as a sudden intra-abdominal hemorrhage. Although abdominal arteries such as the hepatic artery,[285] mesenteric arteries,[286] and splenic artery[287] are most often affected, other arteries in the body, such as the epicardial coronary arteries,[288] may also be affected. Slavin and colleagues[288] suggested that SMA may result from vasospasm, and the organization of uncomplicated SMA lesions could lead to a picture resembling some forms of fibromuscular dysplasia.

Slavin and colleagues[289] also proposed that SMA might occur in two clinical settings: (1) in abdominal muscular arteries and arterioles of mainly elderly patients who manifested either ischemic bowel disease or shock, and (2) in the coronary arteries of neonates who had suffered severe hypoxemia. Both of these situations are associated with severe vasospasm of the affected vascular beds. Electron microscopy reveals that SMA is initiated by transformation of the arterial smooth muscle cytoplasm into a maze of dilated, fluid-filled vacuoles. With vacuolar rupture, the smooth muscle cells are disrupted and mediolysis is completed. This is followed by fibrin deposition and hemorrhage at the adventitial-medial junction and within the media. Transmural mediolysis leads to arterial wall gaps—that is, defects in the vessel wall bounded on the outside by the weak serofibrinous layer and the outer adventitial zone (Fig. 6-18).

Eskenasy-Cottier and associates[290] reported the case of a young woman with intracerebral arterial involvement by SMA complicated by dissection. It has been suggested that immune complexes may be deposited in the walls of affected arteries[291] and that this finding supports the role of autoimmune disorders in the pathogenesis of SMA. In fact, some cases have been associated with immune disorders such as microscopic polyarteritis nodosa[292] and SLE.[293]

Other organ changes noted in patients with SMA have included the following[294]: mesangial hyperplasia of glomeruli, histocytic infiltrates and scanty Aschoff-like bodies in the heart, and capsular inflammation of the spleen.

REFERENCES

1. Allen AC: So-called intercapillary glomerulosclerosis: A lesion associated with diabetes mellitus. Morphogenesis and significance. Arch Pathol 32:33, 1941
2. Kimmelstiel P, Wilson G: Intercapillary lesions in the glomeruli of the kidney. Am J Pathol 12:83, 1936
3. Ballantyne AJ, Lowenstein AV: Diseases of the retina. I. The pathology of diabetic retinopathy. Trans Ophthal Soc UK 63:95, 1943
4. Zeek PM, Smith CC, Weeter JC: Studies on periarteritis nodosa III. The differentiation between the vascular lesions of periarteritis nodosa and of hypersensitivity. Am J Pathol 24:889, 1948
4a. Jennette JC, Falk RJ: Small vessel vasculitis. N Engl J Med 337:1512, 1997
5. Walpola PL, Gotlieb AI, Cybulsky MI, Langille BL: VCAM-1 expression and monocyte adherence in arteries exposed to altered shear stress. Arterioscler Thromb Vasc Biol 15:2, 1995
6. Walpola PL, Gotlieb AI, Langille BL: Monocyte adhesion and changes in endothelial cell number, morphology, and F-actin distribution elicited by low shear stress in vivo. Am J Pathol 142:1392, 1993
7. Williamson JR, Kilo C: Basement-membrane thickening and diabetic microangiopathy. Diabetes 25(suppl 2):925, 1976
8. Ettenson D, Gotlieb AI: The role of endothelial cells in vascular integrity and repair in atherosclerosis. Adv Pathol Lab Med 6:285, 1993
9. Alpert JS, Coffman JD, Balodimos MC, et al: Capillary permeability and blood flow in skeletal muscles of patients with diabetes mellitus and genetic prediabetes. N Engl J Med 286:454, 1972
10. Olson ND, Nuttall FQ, Sinha A, et al: Thin muscle capillary basement membranes in myotonic dystrophy. Diabetes 28:686, 1979
11. Bloodworth Jr JMB: A re-evaluation of diabetic glomerulosclerosis 50 years after the discovery of insulin. Hum Pathol 9:439, 1978
12. Bloodworth Jr JMB: Diabetic microangiopathy. Diabetes 12:99, 1963
13. Factor SM, Okun EM, Minase T: Capillary microaneurysms in the human diabetic heart. N Engl J Med 302:384, 1980
14. Sinclair RA, Antonovych TT. Mostofi FK: Renal proliferative arteriopathies and associated glomerular changes: A light and electron microscopic study. Hum Pathol 7:565, 1976
15. Kincaid-Smith P: Participation of intravascular coagulation in the pathogenesis of glomerular and vascular lesions. Kidney Int 7:242, 1975
16. Cuenoud HF, Joris I, Langer RS, Majno G: Focal arteriolar insudation: A response of arterioles to chronic non-specific irritation. Am J Pathol 127:592, 1987
17. Black HR, Zeevi GR, Silten RM, Walker Smith GJ: Effect of heavy cigarette smoking on renal and myocardial arterioles. Nephron 34:173, 1983
18. Naeye RL, Truong LD: Effect of cigarette smoking on intramyocardial arteries and arterioles in man. Am J Clin Pathol 68:493, 1977
19. McMillan DE: Plasma protein changes, blood viscosity, and diabetic microangiopathy. Diabetes 25(suppl 2):858, 1976
20. Halushka PV, Lurie D, Colwell JA: Increased synthesis of prostaglandin-E-like material by platelets from patients with diabetes mellitus. N Engl J Med 297:1306, 1977
21. Davies MJ, Thomas AC, Knapman PA, Hangartner JR: Intramyocardial platelet aggregation in patients with unstable angina suffering sudden ischemic cardiac death. Circulation 73:418, 1986
21a. Krasznai G, Szokoly V: Congenital vascular malformation (caliber persistence) as a pathogenetic factor of lethal gastric hemorrhage. Acta Chir Acad Sci Hung 9:137, 1968
21b. Molnar P, Miko T: Multiple arterial caliber persistence resulting in hematomas and fatal rupture of the gastric wall. Am J Surg Pathol 6:83, 1982
21c. Miko TL, Thomazy VA: The caliber persistent artery of the stomach: A unifying approach to gastric aneurysm, Dieulafoy's lesion, and submucosal arterial malformation. Hum Pathol 19:914, 1888
21d. Cross FS, Glover DM, Simeone FA, Oldenburg FA: Congenital arteriovenous aneurysms. Ann Surg 148:649, 1958
22. Greene JF, Fitzwater JE, Burgess J: Arterial lesions associated with neurofibromatosis. Am J Clin Pathol 62:481, 1974
23. Zachos M, Parkin PC, Babyn PS, Chait P: Neurofibromatosis type 1 vasculopathy associated with lower limb hypoplasia. Pediatrics 100:395, 1997
24. Rubinstein LJ: The malformative central nervous system lesions in the central and peripheral forms of neurofibromatosis: A neuropathological study of 22 cases. Ann NY Acad Sci 486:14, 1986
25. Nopajaroonsri C, Lurie AA: Venous aneurysm, arterial dysplasia, and near-fatal hemorrhage in neurofibromatosis type 1. Hum Pathol 27:982, 1996
25a. Schievink WI: Genetics of intracranial aneurysms. Neurosurgery 40:651, 1997
26. Neldner KH: Pseudoxanthoma elasticum. Clin Dermatol 6:61, 1988
27. Van Soest S, Swart J, Tijmes N, et al: A locus for autosomal recessive pseudoxanthoma elasticum, with penetrance of vascular symptoms in carriers, maps to chromosome 16p13.1. Genome Res 7:830, 1997
28. Mendelsohn G, Bulkley BH, Hutchins GM: Cardiovascular manifestations of pseudoxanthoma elasticum. Arch Pathol Lab Med 102:298, 1978
28a. Nikko AP, Dunningan M, Cockerell CJ: Calciphylaxis with histologic changes of pseudoxanthoma elasticum. Am J Dermatopathol 18:396, 1996
29. Stern LZ, Cross HE, Crebo AR: Abnormal iris vasculature in myotonic dystrophy: An anterior segment angiographic study. Arch Neurol (Chicago) 35:224, 1978
29a. Annane D, Merlet P, Radvanyi H, et al: Blunted coronary reserve in myotonic dystrophy. An early and gene-related phenomenon. Circulation 94:973, 1996
30. Child JS, Perloff JK, Bach PM, et al: Cardiac involvement in Friedreich's ataxia: A clinical study of 75 patients. J Am Coll Cardiol 7:1370, 1986
31. Lorenz TH, Kurtz CM, Shapiro HH: Cardiopathy in Friedreich's ataxia (spinal form of hereditary sclerosis). Arch Intern Med 86:412, 1950
32. Unverferth DV, Schmidt WR, Baker PB, Wooley CF: Morphologic and functional characteristics of the heart in Friedreich's ataxia. Am J Med 82:5, 1987
33. James TN, Cobbs BW, Coghlan HC, et al: Coronary disease, cardioneuropathy, and conduction system abnormalities in the cardiomyopathy of Friedreich's ataxia. Br Heart J 57:446, 1987
34. James TN, Fisch C: Observations on the cardiovascular involvement in Friedreich's ataxia. Am Heart J 66:164, 1963
35. Embury SH: The clinical pathophysiology of sickle cell disease. Annu Rev Med 37:361, 1986
36. Hebbel RP, Schwartz RS, Mohandas N: The adhesive sickle erythrocyte: Cause and consequence of abnormal interactions with endothelium, monocytes/macrophages and model membranes. Clin Hematol 14:141, 1985
37. Hebbel RP: Adhesive interactions of sickle erythrocytes with endothelium. J Clin Invest 99:2561, 1997
37a. Kaul DK, Fabry ME, Nagel RL: The pathophysiology of vascular obstruction in the sickle syndromes. Blood Rev 10:29, 1996
37b. Ballas SK, Mohandas N: Pathophysiology of vaso-occlusion. Hematol Oncol Clin North Am 10:1221, 1996
37c. McLeod DS, Merges C, Fukushima A, et al: Histopathologic features of neovascularization in sickle cell retinopathy. Am J Ophthalmol 124:455, 1997
38. Baker SM, Hamilton JD: Capillary changes in myxoedema. Lab Invest 6:218, 1957
39. Silver MD, Huckell VF, Lorber M: Basement membranes of small cardiac vessels in patients with diabetes and myxoedema: Preliminary observations. Pathology 9:213, 1977
40. Berenson GS, Radhakrishnamurthy B, Srinivasan SR, Dalferes ER Jr: Macromolecules in the arterial wall in relation to injury and repair: A survey. Angiology 25:649, 1974

41. Baumgartner R, Wick H, Ohnacker H, et al: Vascular lesions in two patients with congenital homocystinuria due to different defects of remethylation. J Inherit Metab Dis 3:101, 1980

42. McCully KS: Vascular pathology of homocysteinemia: Implications for the pathogenesis of arteriosclerosis. Am J Pathol 56:111, 1969

43. Schimke RN, McKusick VA, Huang T, Pollack AD: Homocystinuria: Studies of 20 families with 38 affected members. JAMA 193:87, 1965

44. Zeek PM: Periarteritis nodosa: A critical review. Am J Clin Pathol 22:777, 1952

45. Zeek PM: Periarteritis and other forms of necrotizing angiitis. N Engl J Med 248:764, 1953

46. Cupps TR, Fauci AS: The Vasculitides: Major Problems in Internal Medicine. Vol. 13. Philadelphia, WB Saunders, 1981, p 1

47. Fauci AS, Haynes BF, Katz P: The spectrum of vasculitis: Clinical, pathologic, immunologic and therapeutic considerations. Ann Intern Med 89:660, 1978

47a. Dillon MJ: Rare vasculitic syndromes. Ann Med 29:175, 1997

48. Gocke DJ, Morgan C, Lockshin M, et al: Association between polyarteritis and Australia antigen. Lancet 2:1149, 1970

49. Sergent JS, Lockshin MD, Christian CL, Gocke DJ: Vasculitis with hepatitis B antigenemia. Medicine (Baltimore) 56:1, 1976

50. Alarcon-Segovia D: The necrotizing vasculitides: A new pathogenetic classification. Med Clin North Am 61:241, 1977

51. Aboobaker J, Greaves MW: Urticarial vasculitis. Clin Exp Dermatol 11:436, 1986

52. Abrahams C, Furman KI, Salant D: Dermal micro-angiopathy in patients with analgesic nephropathy. S Afr Med J 54:393, 1978

53. Abrahams C, Van Tonder H, Hesse VE: Abnormal vessels in the urinary tract following analgesic abuse in men. Arch Pathol Lab Med 100:630, 1976

53a. Hunder GG, Arend WP, Bloch DA, et al: The American College of Rheumatology 1990 criteria for the classification of vasculitis. Arthritis Rheum 33:1065, 1990

53b. Jennette JC, Falk RJ, Andrassy K, et al: Nomenclature of systemic vasculitides. Arthritis Rheum 37:187, 1994

53c. Bruce IN, Bell AL: A comparison of two nomenclature systems for primary systemic vasculitis. Br J Rheumatol 36:453, 1997

53d. Leavitt RY, Fauci AS: Polyangiitis overlap syndrome: Classification and prospective clinical experience. Am J Med 81:79, 1986

53e. Eustace JA, Nadasdy T, Choi M: Disease of the month: The Churg Strauss syndrome. J Am Soc Nephrol 10:2048, 1999

53f. Cottin V, Cordier JF: Churg-Strauss syndrome. Allergy 54:535, 1999

54. Onouchi Z, Kawasaki T: Overview of pharmacological treatment of Kawasaki disease. Drugs 58:813, 1999

54a. Choi IH, Chwae YJ, Shim WS, et al: Clonal expansion of CD8+ T cells in Kawasaki disease. J Immunol 159:481, 1997

54b. Culora GA, More IE: Kawasaki disease, Epstein-Barr virus and coronary artery aneurysm. J Clin Pathol 50:161, 1997

54c. Mitani Y, Okuda Y, Shimpo Y, et al: Impaired endothelial function in epicardial coronary arteries after Kawasaki disease. Circulation 96:454, 1997

54d. Hayreh SS, Podhajsky PA, Raman R, Zimmerman B: Giant cell arteritis: Validity and reliability of various diagnostic criteria. Am J Ophthalmol 123:392, 1997

54e. Nikkari ST, Hoyhtya M, Isola J, Nikkari T: Macrophages contain 92-kD gelatinase (MMP-9) at the site of degenerated internal elastic lamina in temporal arteritis. Am J Pathol 149:1427, 1996

54f. Brack A, Rittner HL, Younge BR, et al: Glucocorticoid-mediated repression of cytokine gene transcription in human arteritis-SCID chimeras. J Clin Invest 99:2842, 1997

54g. Brack A, Geisler A, Martinez-Taboada VM, et al: Giant cell vasculitis is a T cell-dependent disease. Mol Med 3:530, 1997

54h. Gillot JM, Masy E, Davril M, et al: Elastase derived elastin peptides: Putative autoimmune targets in giant cell arteritis. J Rheumatol 24:677, 1997

55. Pantanowitz D, Immelman EJ, Rose AG, et al: Arteritis: Part II. Takayasu disease. A roundtable discussion. Cardiovasc J South Afr 4:74, 1993

55a. Rizzi R, Bruno S, Stellacci C, Dammacco R: Takayasu's arteritis: A cell mediated large vessel vasculitis. Int J Clin Lab Res 29:8, 1999

56. Winkelmann RK, Ditto WB: Cutaneous and visceral syndromes of necrotizing or allergic angiitis: A study of 38 cases. Medicine (Baltimore) 43:59, 1964

57. Soter NA: Urticarial vasculitis. In: Wolff K, Winkelmann RK (eds): Vasculitis. Philadelphia, WB Saunders, 1980, p 183

58. Belch JJF, Zoma AA, Richards IM, et al: Vascular damage and factor VIII-related antigen in the rheumatic diseases. Rheumatol Int 7:107, 1987

59. Woolf AD, Wakerlely G, Wallington TB, et al: Factor VIII related antigen in the assessment of vasculitis. Ann Rheum Dis 46:441, 1987

60. Lockwood CM, Bakes D, Jones S, Savage COS: Auto-immunity and systemic vasculitis. Contrib Nephrol 61:141, 1988

60a. Harper L, Savage CO: Pathogenesis of ANCA-associated systemic vasculitis. J Pathol 190:349, 2000

60b. Savige J, Gillis D, Benson E, et al: International consensus statement on testing and reporting of antineutrophil cytoplasmic antibodies (ANCA). Am J Clin Pathol 111:507, 1999

61. Winkelmann RK: Pathology of vasculitis. In: Wolff K, Winkelmann RK (eds): Vasculitis. Philadelphia, WB Saunders, 1980, p 31

62. Haynes BF, Allen NB, Fauci AS: Diagnostic and therapeutic approach to the patient with vasculitis. Med Clin North Am 70:355, 1986

63. Copeman PWM, Ryan RJ: The problem of classification of cutaneous angiitis with reference to histopathology and pathogenesis. Br J Dermatol 82(suppl 5):2, 1970

64. Ekenstam Ea, Callen JP: Cutaneous leukocytoclastic vasculitis: Clinical and laboratory features of 82 patients seen in private practice. Arch Dermatol 120: 484, 1984

65. Hodge SJ, Callen JP, Ekenstam E: Cutaneous leukocytoclastic vasculitis: Correlation of histopathological changes with clinical severity and course. J Cutan Pathol 14:279, 1987

66. Soter NA: Cutaneous necrotizing venulitis. In Wolff K, Winkelmann RK (eds): Vasculitis. Philadelphia, WB Saunders, 1980

67. Jones RE: Questions to the editorial board and other authorities. Am J Dermatopathol 7:181, 1985

68. Jones RR, Eady RAJ: Endothelial cell pathology as a marker for urticarial vasculitis: A light microscopic study. Br J Dermatol 110: 139, 1984

69. Soter NA, Mihm MC, Gigli I, et al: Two distinct cellular patterns in cutaneous necrotizing angiitis. J Invest Dermatol 66:344, 1976

70. Tosca A, Hatzis J, Kyriakis K et al: Delayed hypersensitivity and differences of histologic pattern in allergic cutaneous vasculitis. Angiology 39:360, 1988

71. Alexander EL: Immunopathologic mechanisms of inflammatory vascular disease in primary Sjögren's syndrome: A model. Scand J Rheumatol (suppl)61:280, 1986

72. Massa MC, Su WPD: Lymphocytic vasculitis: Is it a specific clinicopathologic entity? J Cutan Pathol 11:132, 1984

73. Sanchez NP, Van Hale HM, Su WPD: Clinical and histopathologic spectrum of necrotizing vasculitis. Arch Dermatol 121:220, 1985

74. Leavitt RY, Fauci AS: Pulmonary vasculitis. Am Rev Respir Dis 134:149, 1986

75. Giangiacomo J, Tsai CC: Dermal and glomerular deposition of IgA in anaphylactoid purpura. Am J Dis Child 131:981, 1977

76. Soylemezoglu O, Sultan N, Gursel T, et al: Circulating adhesion molecules ICAM-1, E-selectin, and von Willebrand factor in Henoch-Schönlein purpura. Arch Dis Child 75:507, 1996

77. Cupps TR, Fauci AS: The Vasculitides. Major Problems in Internal Medicine. Vol 13. Philadelphia, WB Saunders, 1981, p 151

78. Schwartz HR, McDuffie FC, Black LF, et al: Hypocomplementemic urticarial vasculitis: Association with chronic obstructive pulmonary disease. Mayo Clin Proc 57:231, 1982

79. Ramirez G, Sabiha SR, Espinoza L: Hypocomplementemic vasculitis and renal involvement. Nephron 45:147, 1987

80. Clemmensen I, Jensen BA, Holund B, et al: Circulating monoclonal IgM lambda cryoglobulin with collagen type I affinity in vasculitis. Clin Exp Immunol 64:587, 1986

81. Ansari A, Larson PH, Bates HD: Vascular manifestations of systemic lupus erythematosus. Angiology 37:423, 1986

82. Callen JP, Kingman J: Cutaneous vasculitis in systemic lupus erythematosus. A poor prognostic indicator. Cutis 32:433, 1983

83. Schneider HA, Yonker RA, Katz P, et al: Rheumatoid vasculitis: Experience with 13 patients and review of the literature. Semin Arthritis Rheum 14:280, 1985

84. Soter NA, Austen KF, Gigli I: The complement system in necro-

tizing angiitis of the skin: Analysis of complement component activities in serum of patients with concomitant collagen-vascular disease. J Invest Dermatol 63:219, 1974

85. Oddis CV, Eisenbeis Jr CH, Reidboard HE, et al: Vasculitis in systemic sclerosis: Association with Sjögren's syndrome and the CREST syndrome variant. J Rheumatol 14:942, 1987

86. Alexander E, Provost TT: Sjögren's syndrome: Association of cutaneous vasculitis with central nervous system disease. Arch Dermatol 123:801, 1987

87. Tsokos M, Lazarou SA, Moutsopoulos HM: Vasculitis in primary Sjögren's syndrome: Histologic classification and clinical presentation. Am J Clin Pathol 88:26, 1987

88. Longley S, Caldwell JR, Panush RS: Paraneoplastic vasculitis: Unique syndrome of cutaneous angiitis and arthritis associated with myeloproliferative disorders. Am J Med 80:1027, 1986

89. Farcet J-P, Weschsler J, Wirquinn V, et al: Vasculitis in hairy-cell leukemia. Arch Intern Med 147:660, 1987

90. Gabriel SE, Conn DL, Phyliky RL, et al: Vasculitis in hairy cell leukemia: Review of the literature and consideration of possible pathogenic mechanisms. J Rheumatol 13:1167, 1986

91. Spann CR, Callen JP, Yan LT, Apgar JT: Cutaneous leukocytoclastic vasculitis complicating hairy cell leukemia (leukemic reticuloendotheliosis). Arch Dermatol 122:1057, 1986

92. Kesseler ME, Slater DN: Cutaneous vasculitis: A presenting feature in Hodgkin's disease. J R Soc Med 79:485, 1986

93. Mor F, Leibovici L, Wysenbeek AJ: Leukocytoclastic vasculitis in malignant lymphoma: Case report and review of the literature. Isr J Med Sci 23:829, 1987

94. McMillen JJ, Krueger SK, Dyer GA: Leukocytoclastic vasculitis in association with immunoglobulin A myeloma. Ann Intern Med 105:709, 1986

95. Callen JP: Cutaneous leukocytoclastic vasculitis in a patient with an adenocarcinoma of the colon. J Rheumatol 14:386, 1987

96. Hoag GN: Renal cell carcinoma and vasculitis: Report of two cases. J Surg Oncol 35:35, 1987

97. Miyachi H, Akizuki M, Yamagata H, et al: Hypertrophic osteoarthropathy, cutaneous vasculitis and mixed-typed cryoglobulinemia in a patient with nasopharyngeal carcinoma. Arthritis Rheum 30:825, 1987

98. Vincent D, Dubas F, Hauw JJ, et al: Nerve and muscle microvasculitis in peripheral neuropathy: A remote effect of cancer? J Neurol Neurosurg Psychiatry 49:1007, 1986

99. Gilliam JN, Smiley JD: Cutaneous necrotizing vasculitis and related disorders. Ann Allergy 37:328, 1976

100. Simla S, Kokkonen J, Kallioinen M: Cutaneous vasculitis as manifestation of coeliac disease. Acta Paediatr Scand 71:1051, 1982

101. Newton JA, McGibbon DH, Marsden RA: Leukocytoclastic vasculitis and angio-oedema associated with inflammatory bowel disease. Clin Exp Dermatol 9:618, 1984

102. Johnston C, Kennedy C: Cutaneous leukocytoclastic vasculitis associated with acute sarcoidosis. Postgrad Med J 60:549, 1984

103. Diederichsen H, Sorensen PG, Mickley H, et al: Petechiae and vasculitis in asymptomatic primary biliary cirrhosis. Acta Derm Venereol (Stockh) 65:263, 1985

104. Pierson KK: Leukocytoclastic vasculitis viewed as a phase of immune-mediated vasculopathy. Semin Thromb Hemost 10:196, 1984

105. Sams WM: Human hypersensitivity angiitis, an immune complex disease. J Invest Dermatol 85(suppl):144s, 1985

106. Savage COS, Ng YC: The aetiology and pathogenesis of major systemic vasculitides. Postgrad Med J 62:627, 1986

107. Mannik M: Experimental models for immune-complex-mediated vascular inflammation. Acta Med Scand 715(suppl):145, 1987

108. Cochrane CG, Weigle WO, Dixon FJ: The role of polymorphonuclear leukocytes in the initiation and cessation of the Arthus vasculitis. J Exp Med 110:481, 1959

109. Cochrane CG: Studies on localization of circulating antigen antibody complexes and other macromolecules in vessels. I. Structural studies. J Exp Med 118:489, 1963

110. Cochrane CG: Studies on localization of circulating antigen antibody complexes and other macromolecules in vessels. II. Pathogenetic and pharmacodynamic studies. J Exp Med 118:503, 1963

111. Hart MN, Tassell SK, Sadewasser KL, et al: Autoimmune vasculitis resulting from in vitro immunization of lymphocytes to smooth muscles. Am J Pathol 119:448, 1985

112. McCluskey RT, Feinberg R: Vasculitis in primary vasculitides, granulomatoses and connective tissue diseases. Hum Pathol 14:305, 1983

112a. Lie JT: Biopsy diagnosis in rheumatic disease. The vasculitides. New York, Igaku-Shoin, 1997, pp 61–113

113. Kammer GM, Soter NA, Schur PH: Circulating immune complexes in patients with necrotizing vasculitis. Clin Immunol Immunopathol 15:658, 1980

114. Mackel SE, Tappenier G, Brumfield H, Jordan RE: Cutaneous vasculitis: Detection with C1q and monoclonal rheumatoid factor. J Clin Invest 64:1652, 1979

115. Yancey KM, Lawley TJ: Circulating immune complexes: Their immunohistochemistry, biology and detection in selected dermatologic and systemic diseases. J Am Acad Dermatol 10:711, 1984

116. Braverman IM, Yen A: Demonstration of immune complexes in spontaneous and histamine-induced lesions and in normal skin of patients with leukocytoclastic angiitis. J Invest Dermatol 64:105, 1975

117. Gower RG, Sams Jr WM, Thorne EG, et al: Leukocytoclastic vasculitis: Sequential appearance of immunoreactants and cellular changes in serial biopsies. J Invest Dermatol 68:477, 1977

118. Montoliu J, Torras A, Revert L: Electron-dense deposits in the renal arterioles of two patients with hypersensitivity vasculitis. Hum Pathol 15:390, 1984

119. McCluskey RT, Hall CL, Colvin RB: Immune complex mediated diseases. Hum Pathol 9:71, 1978

120. Thorne EG, Grower R, Claman N: Hepatitis B surface antigen and leukocytoclastic vasculitis. J Invest Dermatol 68:243, 1977

121. Trepo CG, Zuckerman AJ, Bird RC, Prince AM: The role of circulating hepatitis B antigen/antibody immune complexes in the pathogenesis of vascular and hepatic manifestations in polyarteritis nodosa. J Clin Pathol 27:863, 1974

122. Cohen C, Trapuck DS: Leukocytoclastic vasculitis associated with cutaneous infection by herpesvirus. Am J Dermatopathol 6:561, 1984

123. Curtis JL, Egbert BM: Cutaneous cytomegalovirus vasculitis: An unusual clinical presentation of a common opportunistic pathogen. Hum Pathol 13:1138, 1982

124. Inman RD, Hodge M, Johnston MEA, et al: Arthritis, vasculitis and cryoglobulinemia associated with hepatitis A virus infection. Ann Intern Med 105:700, 1986

125. Li Loong TC, Coyle PV, Anderson MJ, et al: Human serum parvovirus associated vasculitis. Postgrad Med J 62:493, 1986

126. Ingelfinger JR, McCluskey RT, Schneeberger EE, Grupe WE: Necrotizing arteritis in acute post-streptococcal glomerulonephritis. Pediatrics 91:1228, 1977

127. Shrader SK, Watts JC, Dancik JA, Band JD: Disseminated cryptococcosis presenting as cellulitis with necrotizing vasculitis. J Clin Microbiol 24:860, 1986

128. De Micco C, Raoult D, Benderitter T, et al: Immune complex vasculitis associated with Mediterranean spotted fever. J Infect 14:163, 1987

129. Hoffman GS: Franck WA: Infectious mononucleosis, autoimmunity and vasculitis: A case report. JAMA 241:2735, 1979

130. Blumberg S, Bienfang D, Kantrowitz FG: A possible association between influenza vaccination and small-vessel vasculitis. Arch Intern Med 140:847, 1980

131. Cupps TR, Fauci AS: The Vasculitides: Major Problems in Internal Medicine. Vol. 13. Philadelphia, WB Saunders, 1981, p 123

132. Cupps TR, Moore PM, Fauci AS: Isolated angiitis of the central nervous system: Prospective diagnostic and therapeutic experience. Am J Med 74:97, 1983

133. Launes J, Livanainen M, Erkinjuntti T, et al: Isolated angiitis of the central nervous system. Acta Neurol Scand 74:108, 1986

134. Younger DS, Hays AP, Brust JCM, Rowland LP: Granulomatous angiitis of the brain: An inflammatory reaction of diverse etiology. Arch Neurol 45:514, 1988

134a. Moore PM: Vasculitis of the central nervous system. Semin Neurol 14:307, 1994

135. Behçet H: Über rezidivierende, aphthose, aurch ein virus veruschte Geschwure am mund, am Ange und an den Gentalien. Derm Wschr 105:1152, 1937

136. Lakhanpal S, Tani K, Lie JT, et al: Pathologic features of Behçet's syndrome: A review of Japanese autopsy registry data. Hum Pathol 16:790, 1985

137. Shimizu T, Ehrlich GE, Inaba G, Hayashi K: Behçet disease (Behçet syndrome). Semin Arthritis Rheum 8:223, 1979

138. Clausen J, Bierring F: Involvement of post-capillary venules in Behçet disease: An electron microscopic study. Acta Derm Venereol (Stockh) 63:191, 1983

139. Reza MJ, Demanes DJ: Behçet's disease: A case with hemoptysis, pseudotumour cerebri and arteritis. J Rheumatol 5:320, 1978

140. Lehner T: Pathology of recurrent oral ulceration and oral ulceration in Behçet syndrome: Light, electron and fluorescence microscopy. J Pathol 97:481, 1969

140a. Chen KR, Kawahara Y, Miyakawa S, Nishikawa T: Cutaneous vasculitis in Behçet's disease: A clinical and histopathologic study of 20 patients. J Am Acad Dermatol 36:689, 1997

141. Bang D, Honma T, Saito T, et al: The pathogenesis of vascular changes in erythema nodosum-like lesions of Behçet's syndrome: An electron microscopic study. Hum Pathol 18:1172, 1987

141a. Kilmartin DJ, Finch A, Acheson RW: Primary association of HLA-B51 with Behçet's disease in Ireland. Br J Ophthalmol 81:649, 1997

141b. Mizuki N, Inoko H, Ohno S: Pathogenic gene responsible for the predisposition of Behçet's disease. Int Rev Immunol 14:33, 1997

142. Churg J, Churg A: Idiopathic and secondary vasculitis: A review. Mod Pathol 2:144, 1989

142a. Travis WD, Fleming MV: Vasculitis of the lung. Pathology 4:23, 1996

143. Liebow AA, Carrington CRB, Friedman PJ: Lymphomatoid granulomatosis. Hum Pathol 3:457, 1972

143a. Guinee D Jr, Jaffe E, Kingma D, et al: Pulmonary lymphomatoid granulomatosis. Evidence for a proliferation of Epstein-Barr virus infected B-lymphocytes with a prominent T-cell component and vasculitis. Am J Surg Pathol 18:753, 1994

144. De Remee RA, Weiland LH, McDonald RJ: Polymorphic reticulosis, lymphomatoid granulomatosis. Two diseases or one? Mayo Clin Proc 53:634, 1978

145. Stewart JP: Progressive lethal granulomatous ulceration of the nose. J Laryngol Otol 48:657, 1933

145a. Lie JT: Thromboangiitis obliterans (Buerger's disease) revisited. Pathol Annu 23:257, 1988

145b. Makita S, Nakamura M, Murakami H, et al: Impaired endothelium-dependent vasorelaxation in peripheral vasculature of patients with thromboangiitis obliterans (Buerger's disease). Circulation 94:II-211, 1996

146. Busch GJ, Garovoy MR, Tilney NL: Variant forms of arteritis in human renal allografts. Transplant Proc 11:100, 1979

147. Sako H, Nakane Y, Okino K, et al: Immunohistochemical study of the cells infiltrating human renal allografts by the ABC and IGSS method using monoclonal antibodies. Transplant 44:43, 1987

148. Sommer BG, Innes VT, Whitehurst RM, et al: Cyclosporine-associated renal arteriopathy resulting in loss of allograft function. Am J Surg 149:756, 1985

149. Demetris AJ, Lasky S, van Thiel DH, et al: Pathology of hepatic transplantation: A review of 62 adult allograft recipients immunosuppressed with a cyclosporine/steroid regimen. Am J Pathol 118:151, 1985

150. Porter KA: The pathology of rejection in human liver allografts. Transplant Proc 20(suppl 1):483, 1988

151. Demetris AJ, Markus BH, Burnham J, et al: Antibody deposition in liver allografts with chronic rejection. Transplant Proc 19(suppl 5):121, 1987

152. Yousem SA, Burke CM, Billingham ME: Pathologic pulmonary alterations in long-term human heart-lung transplantation. Hum Pathol 16:911, 1985

153. Higenbottam T, Stewart S, Penketh A, Wallwork J: Transbronchial lung biopsy for the diagnosis of rejection in heart-lung transplant patients. Transplant 46:532, 1988

154. Sutherland DER, Casanova D, Sibley RK: Role of pancreas graft biopsies in the diagnosis and treatment of rejection after pancreas transplantation. Transplant Proc 19:2329, 1987

155. Lipper S, Watkins DL, Kahn LB: Nongranulomatous septic vasculitis due to miliary tuberculosis: A pitfall in diagnosis for the pathologist. Am J Dermatopathol 2:71, 1980

156. Baumgarten EC, Cantor MO: Tuberculous mesarteritis with aneurysm of the femoral artery. JAMA 100:1918, 1933

157. Fite GL: Leprosy from the histologic point of view. Arch Pathol 35:611, 1943

158. Walker DH, Mattern WD: Rickettsial vasculitis. Am Heart J 100:896, 1980

159. Wolbach SB: Studies on Rocky Mountain spotted fever. J Med Res 41:1, 1919

160. Brezina R: Diagnosis and control of rickettsial diseases. Acta Virol (Praha) 29:338, 1985

161. De Micco C, Raoult D, Toga M: Diagnosis of Mediterranean spotted fever by using an immunofluorescence technique. J Infect Dis 153:136

162. Peterson JC, Overall JC, Shapiro JL: Rickettsial diseases of childhood: A clinical pathological study of tick typhus, Rocky Mountain spotted fever, murine typhus, and endemic typhus. J Pediatrics 30:495, 1947

163. Allen AC, Spitz S: A comparative study of the pathology of scrub typhus (Tsutsugamushi disease) and other rickettsial diseases. Am J Pathol 21:603, 1945

164. Moe JB, Mosher DF, Kenyon RH, et al: Functional and morphologic changes during experimental Rocky Mountain spotted fever in guinea pigs. Lab Invest 35:235, 1976

165. Silverman DJ: Adherence of platelets to human endothelial cells infected by *Rickettsia rickettsii*. J Infect Dis 153:694, 1986

166. Srigley JR, Geddie WR, Vellend H, et al: Q fever: The liver and bone marrow pathology. Am J Surg Pathol 9:752, 1985

167. Wenzel RP, Hayden FG, Groschel DHM, et al: Acute febrile cerebrovasculitis: A syndrome of unknown, perhaps rickettsial, cause. Ann Intern Med 104:606, 1986

168. Greene SL, Su WPD, Miller SA: Ecthyma gangrenosum: Report of clinical histopathologic and bacteriologic aspects of eight cases. J Am Acad Dermatol 11:781, 1984

169. Markley K, Gurmendi G, Chavez PM, Bazan A: Fatal *Psuedomonas* septicemias in burned patients. Ann Surg 145:175, 1957

170. Vasil ML: *Pseudomonas aeruginosa*: Biology, mechanisms of virulence, epidemiology. J Pediatr 108:800, 1986

171. Teplitz C: Pathogenesis of *Pseudomonas* vasculitis and septic lesions. Arch Pathol 80:297, 1965

172. Margaretten W, Nakai H, Landing BH: Significance of selective vasculitis and the "bone marrow" syndrome in *Pseudomonas* septicemia. N Engl J Med 265:773, 1961

173. Pollak M: The virulence of *Pseudomonas aeruginosa*. Rev Infect Dis 6(suppl 3): S617, 1984

174. Keren G, Wohman M: Can *Pseudomonas* infection in experimental animals mimic Kawasaki's disease? J Infect 9:22, 1984

175. Wrzolkowa T, Kozakiewicz J: Ultrastructure of vascular and connective tissue changes in primary syphilis. Br J Vener Dis 56:137, 1980

176. Toppozada H, Talaat M, Elwany S: The human respiratory nasal mucosa in nasal syphilis: An ultramicroscopic study. Acta Otolaryngol (Stockh) 99:272, 1985

177. Myrvik QN, Pearsall NN, Weiser RS (eds): Fundamentals of Medical Bacteriology and Mycology for Students of Medicine and Related Sciences. Philadelphia, Lea & Febiger, 1974

178. Hawkins C, Armstrong D: Fungal infections in the immunocompromised host. Clin Hematol 13:599, 1984

179. Holmberg K, Meyer RD: Fungal infections in patients with AIDS and AIDS-related complex. Scand J Infect Dis 18:179, 1986

180. McBride RA, Corson JM, Dammin GJ: Mucormycosis: Two cases of disseminated disease with cultural identification of *Rhizopus*. Review of literature. Am J Med 28:832, 1960

181. Young RC, Bennett JE, Vogel CL, et al: Aspergillosis: The spectrum of the disease in 98 patients. Medicine (Baltimore) 49:147, 1970

181a. Lopez FA, Crowley RS, Wastila L, et al: *Scedosporium apiospermum (Pseudallescheria boydii)* infection in a heart transplant recipient: A case of mistaken identity. J Heart Lung Transplant 17:321, 1998

182. Parker Jr JC, McCloskey JJ, Knauer KA: Pathobiologic features of human candidiasis: A common deep mycosis of the brain, heart and kidney in the altered host. Am J Clin Pathol 65:991, 1976

183. Schwarz J: The diagnosis of deep mycoses by morphologic methods. Hum Pathol 13:519, 1982

184. Grocott RG: A stain for fungi in tissue sections and smears using Giomori's methenamine silver nitrate technique. Am J Clin Pathol 25:975, 1955

185. Girard G: Plaque. Ann Rev Microbiol 9:253, 1955

186. Weiner SR, Utsinger P: Whipple disease. Semin Arthritis Rheum 15:157, 1986

187. Greenberger NJ, DeLor CH, Fisher J, et al: Whipple's disease. Characterization of anaerobic corynebacteria and demonstration of bacilli in vascular endothelium. Am J Dig Dis 16:1127, 1971

188. Haubrich WS, Watson JHL, Sieracki JC: Unique morphologic features of Whipple's' disease: A study by light and electron microscopy. Gastroenterology 39:454, 1960

189. James TN, Haubrich WS: De subitaneis mortibus XIV. Bacterial arteritis in Whipple's disease. Circulation 52:722, 1975

190. Helman DA, Schmidt TM, MacDermott RP, Falkow S: Identification of the uncultured bacillus of Whipple's disease. N Engl J Med 327:293, 1992

190a. Schoedon G, Goldenberger D, Forrer R, et al: Deactivation of macrophages with IL-4 is the key to the isolation of *Tropheryma whippelli*. J Infect Dis 176:672, 1997

191. De Brito T, Bohm GM, Yasuda PH: Vascular damage in acute experimental leptospirosis of the guinea pig. J Pathol 128:177, 1979

192. Rupe CE: Inflammation of arteries. In: Gifford R (guest ed), Brest AN (ed): Peripheral Vascular Disease. Cardiovascular Disease. Cardiovascular Clinics. Philadelphia, FA Davis, 1971, p 141

192a. Hoang MP, Lee EL, Anand A: Histologic spectrum of arterial and arteriolar lesions in acute and chronic cocaine-induced mesenteric ischemia. Am J Surg Pathol 22:1404, 1998

193. Machin SJ: Thrombotic thrombocytopenic purpura. Br J Haematol 56:191, 1984

194. Ruggenenti P, Remuzzi G: The pathophysiologoy and management of thrombotic thrombocytopenic purpura. Eur J Haematol 56:191, 1996

195. Berkowitz LR, Dalldorf FG, Blatt PM: Thrombotic thrombocytopenic purpura: A pathology review. JAMA 241:1709, 1979

196. Feldman JD, Mardiney MR, Unanue ER, Cutting H: The vascular pathology of thrombotic thrombocytopenic purpura: An immunohistochemical and ultrastructural study. Lab Invest 15:927, 1966

197. Orbison JL: Morphology of thrombotic thrombocytopenic purpura with demonstration of aneurysms. Am J Pathol 28:129, 1952

198. Lian EC-Y: Pathogenesis of thrombotic thrombocytopenic purpura. Semin Hematol 24:82, 1987

199. Sanders WE, Read MS, Reddick RL, et al: Thrombotic thrombocytopenia with von Willebrand factor deficiency induced by botrocetin: An animal model. Lab Invest 59:443, 1988

200. Vitsky BH, Suzuki Y, Strauss L, Churg J: The hemolytic-uremic syndrome: A study of renal pathologic alterations. Am J Pathol 57:627, 1969

201. Morel-Maroger L, Kanfer A, Solez K, et al: Prognostic importance of vascular lesions in acute renal failure with microangiopathic hemolytic anemia (hemolytic uremic syndrome): Clinicopathologic study in 20 adults. Kidney Int 15:548, 1979

202. Antman KH, Skarin AT, Mayer RJ, et al: Microangiopathic hemolytic anemia and cancer: A review. Medicine (Baltimore) 58:377, 1979

203. Laffay DL, Tubbs RR, Valenzuela R: Chronic glomerular microangiopathy and metastatic carcinoma. Hum Pathol 10:433, 1979

204. Bohle A, Grabensee B, Fischer R, et al: On four cases of hemolytic-uremic syndrome without microangiopathy. Clin Nephrol 24:88, 1985

205. Case records of the Massachusetts General Hospital: Weekly clinicopathological exercises. N Engl J Med 318:1047, 1988

206. Hayslett JP: Postpartum renal failure. N Engl J Med 312:1556, 1985

207. Drummond KN: Hemolytic uremic syndrome—then and now. N Engl J Med 312:116, 1985

208. Koster F, Levin J, Walker L, et al: Hemolytic uremic syndrome after shigellosis: Relation to endotoxemia and circulating immune complexes. N Engl J Med 298:297, 1978

209. Obrig TG, Del Vecchio PJ, Karmali MA, et al: Pathogenesis of haemolytic uraemic syndrome (letter). Lancet II 19:687, 1987

210. Rose PE, Armour JA, Williams CE, Hill EGH: Verotoxin and neuraminidase induced platelet aggregating activity in plasma: Their possible role in the pathogenesis of haemolytic uraemic syndrome. J Clin Pathol 38:438, 1985

210a. Mitra D, Jaffe EA, Weksler B, et al: Thrombotic thrombocytopenic purpura and sporadic hemolytic-uremic syndrome plasmas induce apoptosis in restricted lineages of human microvascular endothelial cells. Blood 89:1224, 1997

211. Fruchtman S, Aledort LM: Disseminated intravascular coagulation. J Am Coll Cardiol 8:159B, 1986

212. Robboy SJ, Colman RW, Minna JD: Pathology of disseminated intravascular coagulation (DIC): Analysis of 26 cases. Hum Pathol 3:327, 1972

213. Kim H-S, Suzuki M, Lie JT, Titus JL: Clinically unsuspected disseminated intravascular coagulation (DIC): An autopsy survey. Am J Clin Pathol 66:31, 1976

214. Shimamura K, Oja K, Nakazawa M, Kojima M: Distribution patterns of microthrombi in disseminated intravascular coagulation. Arch Pathol Lab Med 107:543, 1983

215. Robboy SJ, Mihm MC, Colman RW, Minna JD: The skin in disseminated intravascular coagulation. Br J Dermatol 88:221, 1973

216. Lopez-Garrido J, Galera-Davidson H, Redina IO, et al: Dexamethasone-prepared *Escherichia coli*-induced disseminated intravascular coagulation: Animal model. Lab Invest 56:534, 1987

216a. Challa VR, Moody DM, Bell MA: The Charcot-Bouchard aneurysm controversy: Impact of a new histologic technique. J Neuropathol Exp Neurol 51:264, 1992

216b. Rosenblum WI: The importance of fibrinoid necrosis as the cause of cerebral hemorrhage in hypertension. Commentary. J Neuropathol Exp Neurol 52:11, 1993

217. Wagenvoort CA, Wagenvoort N: Pathology of Pulmonary Hypertension. New York, John Wiley, 1977

218. Petito CK, Gottlieb GJ, Dougherty JH, Petito FA: Neoplastic angioendotheliosis: Ultrastructural study and review of the literature. Ann Neurol 3:393, 1978

219. Fulling KH, Gersell DJ: Neoplastic angioendotheliomatosis: Histologic, immunohistochemical and ultrastructural findings in two cases. Cancer 51:1107, 1983

220. Kitagawa M, Matsubara O, Song S-Y, et al: Neoplastic angioendotheliosis: Immunohistochemical and electron microscopic findings in three cases. Cancer 56:1134, 1985

221. Wick MR, Banks PM, McDonald TJ: Angioendotheliomatosis of the nose with fatal systemic dissemination. Cancer 48:2510, 1981

222. Bhawan J, Wolff SM, Ucci AA, Bhan AK: Malignant lymphoma and malignant angioendotheliomatosis—one disease. Cancer 55:570, 1985

223. Carroll TJ, Schelper RL, Goeken JA, Kemp JD: Neoplastic angioendotheliomatosis: Immunopathologic and morphologic evidence for intravascular malignant lymphomatosis. Am J Clin Pathol 85:169, 1986

224. Ferry JA, Harris NL, Picker LJ, et al: Intravascular lymphomatosis (malignant angioendotheliomatosis): A B-cell neoplasm expressing surface homing receptors. Mod Pathol 1:444, 1988

225. Wick MR, Mills SE, Scheithauer BW, et al: Reassessment of malignant "angioendotheliomatosis": Evidence in favor of its reclassification as "intravascular lymphomatosis." Am J Surg Pathol 10:112, 1986

226. Manivel JC, Wick MR, Swanson PE, et al: Endovascular papillary angioendothelioma of childhood: A vascular lesion possibly characterized by "high" endothelial cell differentiation. Hum Pathol 17:1240, 1986

227. Kreutner A, Smith RM, Trefny FA: Intravascular papillary endothelial hyperplasia. Cancer 42:2304, 1978

228. Kuo TT, Sayers CP, Rosai J: Masson's vegetant intravascular hemangioendothelioma. Cancer 38:1227, 1976

229. Enzinger RM, Weiss SW: Soft Tissue Tumors. 2nd ed. St. Louis, CV Mosby, 1988

229a. Rosai J: Skin tumors and tumor-like conditions. In: Ackerman's Surgical Pathology. St. Louis, Mosby, 1996, pp 106–222

230. Watanabe T, Saniter T: Morphological and clinical features of renal amyloidosis. Virchows Arch A 366:125, 1975

231. Mandybur TI: Cerebral amyloid angiopathy: The vascular pathology and complications. J Neuropathol Exp Neurol 45:79, 1986

232. Vinters HV: Cerebral amyloid angiopathy: A critical review. Stroke 18:311, 1987

233. Frenzel H, Schwartzkopff B, Kuhn H, et al: Cardiac amyloid deposits in endomyocardial biopsies: Light microscopic, ultrastructural and immunohistochemical studies. Am J Clin Pathol 85:674, 1986

234. Jennette JC, Sheps DA, McNeill DD: Exclusively vascular sys-

temic amyloidosis with visceral ischemia. Arch Pathol Lab Med 106:323, 1982

235. Ng LL, Gresham GA: Paraproteinaemia and small vessel amyloidosis. J R Soc Med 79:111, 1986

236. Lopez JA, Ross RS, Fishbein MC, Seigel RJ: Non-bacterial thrombotic endocarditis: A review. Am Heart J 113:773, 1987

237. Arnett EN, Roberts WC: Prosthetic valve endocarditis: Clinicopathologic analysis of 22 necropsy patients with comparison observations in 74 necropsy patients with active infective endocarditis involving natural left-sided cardiac valves. Am J Cardiol 38:281, 1976

238. Kaufman JL, Stark K, Brolin RE: Disseminated atheroembolsim from extensive degenerative atherosclerosis of the aorta. Surgery 102:63, 1987

239. Weitz Z, Gafter U, Chagnac A, Levi J: Cholesterol emboli in atherosclerotic patients: Reports of four cases occurring spontaneously or complicating angioplasty and aortorenal bypass. J Am Geriatr Soc 35:357, 1987

240. Falanga V, Fine MJ, Kapoor WN: The cutaneous manifestations of cholesterol crystal embolization. Arch Dermatol 122:1194, 1986

241. McGowan JA, Greenberg A: Cholesterol atheroembolic renal disease: Report of 3 cases with emphasis on diagnosis by skin biopsy and extended survival. Am J Nephrol 6:135, 1986

242. Elisevich K, Kaufmann JCE: Atheromatous emboli in mural capillaries of carotid endarterectomy specimens. Surg Neurol 21:141, 1984

243. King MW, Aitchison JM, Nel JP: Fatal air embolism following penetrating lung trauma: An autopsy study. J Trauma 24:753, 1984

244. O'Quinn RJ, Lakshminarayan S: Venous air embolism. Arch Intern Med 142:2173, 1982

245. Mulder JI: Amniotic fluid embolism: An overview and case report. Am J Obstet Gynecol 152:430, 1985

246. Price TM, Baker VV, Cefalo RC: Amniotic fluid embolism: Three case reports with a review of the literature. Obstet Gynecol Surv 40:462, 1985

247. Scofield GF, Beaird JB: Fatal embolism by amniotic fluid in the lungs. Am J Clin Pathol 28:400, 1957

248. Lin C-S, Schwartz IS, Chapman I: Calcification of the mitral annulus fibrosus with systemic embolization: A clinicopathologic study of 16 cases. Arch Pathol Lab Med 111:411, 1987

249. Walley VM, Stinson WA, Upton C et al: Foreign materials found in the cardiovascular system after instrumentation or surgery (including a guide to their light microscopy identification). Cardiovasc Pathol 2:157, 1993

250. Rao RN, Hilliard K, Wary CH: Widespread intimal hyperplasia of small arteries and arterioles. Arch Pathol Lab Med 107:254, 1983

250a. Kalgaard OM, Seem E, Kvernebo K: Erythromelalgia: A clinical study of 87 cases. J Intern Med 242:191, 1997

251. Michiels JJ, ten Kate FWJ, Vuzevski VD, Abels J: Histopathology of erythromelalgia in thrombocythaemia. Histopathology 8:669, 1984

251a. Drenth JP, Vuzevski V, Van Joost T, et al: Cutaneous pathology in primary erythromelalgia. Am J Dermatopathol 18:30, 1996

252. Michiels JJ, Abels J, Steketee J, et al: Erythromelalgia caused by platelet mediated arteriolar inflammation and thrombosis in thrombocytopenia. Ann Intern Med 102:466, 1985

253. Priollet P, Bruneval P, Lazareth I, et al: Erythromelalgia without arteriolar changes (letter). Ann Intern Med 103:639, 1985

254. Ichimaru K, Horie A: Microangiopathic changes of subepidermal capillaries in end-stage renal failure. Nephron 46:144, 1987

255. Frei D, Hedinger C: Arteriolare hyalinose in hodenbiopsien. Virchows Arch A Pathol Anat Histopathol 381:269, 1979

256. Andres TL, Trainer TD, Lapenas DJ: Small vessel alterations in the testes of infertile men with varicocele. Am J Clin Pathol 76:378, 1981

257. Strole WE Jr, Clark WH Jr, Isselbacher KJ: Progressive arterial occlusive disease (Köhlmeier-Degos). A frequently fatal cutaneous disorder. N Engl J Med 276:195, 1967

258. Strole WE Jr, Clark WH, Isselbacher KJ: Progressive arterial occlusive disease (Köhlmeier-Degos). N Engl J Med 276:195, 1967

259. McFarland HR, Wood WG, Drowns BV, Meneses ACO: Papulosis atrophicans maligna (Köhlmeier-Degos disease): A disseminated occlusive vasculopathy. Ann Neurol 3:388, 1978

260. Kohlmeier W: Multiple Hautnekrosen bei trobangiitis obliterans. Arch Dermatol Syph 181:783, 1941

261. Degos R, Delort J, Tricot R: Dermatite papulosquameuse atrophiante. Bull Soc Fr Dermatol Syph 49:148, 1942

262. Molenaar WM, Rosman JB, Donker AJM, Houthoff AJ: The pathology and pathogenesis of malignant atrophic papulosis (Degos' disease): A case study with reference to other vascular disorders. Pathol Res Pract 182:98, 1987

263. Rosenberg HG: Systemic arterial disease and chronic arsenicism in infants. Arch Pathol 97:360, 1974

264. Atkins HJB, Key JA: A case of myxomatous tumor arising in the adventitia of the left external iliac artery. Br J Surg 34:426, 1947

265. Schramek A, Hashmonai M: Subadventitial haematoma of the popliteal artery. J Cardiovasc Surg 14:447, 1973

266. Bergan JJ: Adventitial cystic disease of the popliteal artery. In: Rutherford RB (ed): Vascular Surgery. Philadelphia, WB Saunders, 1977, p 569

267. Lambley DG: Intermittent claudication due to cystic degeneration of popliteal artery. Br Med J 2:849, 1963

268. Leaf G: Amino acid analysis of protein present in a popliteal artery cyst. Br Med J 3:415, 1967

269. Terry JT, Schenken JR, Lohff MR, Neiss DD: Cystic adventitial disease. Hum Pathol 12:639, 1981

270. Abraham P, Saumet JL, Chevalier JM: External iliac artery endofibrosis in athletes. Sports Med 24:221, 1997

271. Goldberg HJ: "Moyamoya" associated with peripheral vascular occlusive disease. Arch Dis Child 49:964, 1974

272. Halonen H, Halonen V, Donner M, et al: Occlusive disease of intracranial main arteries with collateral networks in children. Neuropadiatrie 4:187, 1973

273. Isler W: Multiple occlusions with unusual net-like collaterals ("Moyamoya" disease). In: Acute Hemiplegias and Hemisyndromes. Childhood Clinics in Developmental Medicine. London, Heinemann, Vols. 41, 42, 1971, p 50

274. Oka Y, Yamashita M, Sodoshima S, Tanaka K: Cerebral haemorrhage in moyamoya disease at autopsy. Virchows Arch A Pathol Anat Histopathol 392:247, 1981

275. Hosoda Y: Pathology of so-called "spontaneous occlusion of the circle of Willis." Pathol Annu 19:231, 1984

276. Ohtoh T, Iwasaki Y, Namiki T, et al: Hemodynamic characteristics of the vertebrobasilar system in moyamoya disease. Hum Pathol 19:465, 1988

277. Yamashita M, Tanaka, Kishikawa T, Yokota K: Moyamoya disease associated with renovascular hypertension. Hum Pathol 15:191, 1984

277a. Choi Y, Kang BC, Kim KJ, Cheong HI, Hwang YS, Wang KC, Kim IO: Renovascular hypertension in children with moyamoya disease. J Pediatr 131:258, 1997

277b. Yoshimoto T, Houkin K, Takahashi A, Abe H: Angiogenic factors in moyamoya disease. Stroke 27:2160, 1996

277c. Yamamoto M, Aoyagi M, Tajima S, et al: Increase in elastin gene expression and protein synthesis in arterial smooth muscle cells derived from patients with moyamoya disease. Stroke 28:1733, 1997

278. Sandhyamani S: Mucoid vasculopathy of unknown etiology. Angiology, 42:48, 1991

279. Sandhyamani S: Mucoid vasculopathy: Vascular lesions in an autopsy study. Mol Pathol 6:333, 1993

280. Sriramachari S, Gopalan C: Aortic changes in induced malnutrition. Indian J Med Sci (Bombay) 11:405, 1957

281. Steiner OL, Hutt MSR: Vascular changes in the idiopathic peripheral gangrene of the tropics. Trop Geogr Med 24:219, 1972

282. Gelfand M: Symmetrical gangrene in the African. Br Heart J 1:847, 1947

283. Turpie AGG, Forbes CD, McNicol GP: Idiopathic gangrene in African children. Br Med J 3:646, 1967

284. Lowenthal MN: Peripheral gangrene in infancy and childhood. Br Med J 2:700, 1967

285. Nagashima Y, Taki A, Misugi K, et al: Segmental mediolytic arteries (sic): A case report with review of the literature. Pathol Res Pract 194:643, 1998

286. Kato K, Yamada K, Akiyama Y, et al: Cardiovasc Surg 4:644, 1996

287. Chan RJ, Goodman TA, Artez TH, Lie JT: Segmental mediolytic arteriopathy of the splenic and hepatic arteries mimicking systemic necrotizing vasculitis. Arthritis Rheum 41:935, 1998

288. Slavin RE, Saeki K, Bhagavan B, Maas AE: Segmental arterial

mediolysis: A precursor to fibromuscular dysplasia? Mod Pathol 8: 287, 1995

289. Slavin RE, Cafferty L, Cartwright J Jr: Segmental mediolytic arteritis. A clinicopathologic and ultrastructural study of two cases. Am J Surg Pathol 13:558, 1989

290. Eskenasy-Cottier AC, Leu HJ, Bassetti C, et al: A case of dissection of intracranial cerebral arteries with segmental mediolytic "arteritis." Clin Neuropathol 13:329, 1994

291. Juvonen T, Rasanen O, Reinila A, et al: Segmental mediolytic arteritis—electron microscopic and immunohistochemical study. Eur J Vasc Surg 8:70, 1994

292. Ito MR, Ohtani H, Nakamura Y, et al: An autopsy case of segmental mediolytic arteritis (SMA) accompanied with microscopic polyarteritis nodosa. Ryumachi 35:693, 1995

293. Juvonen T, Niemela O, Reinila A, et al: Spontaneous intraabdominal haemorrhage caused by segmental mediolytic arteritis in a patient with systemic lupus erythematosus—an underestimated entity of autoimmune origin? Eur J Vasc Surg 8:96, 1994

294. Slavin RE, Gonzalez-Vitale JC: Segmental mediolytic arteritis: A clinical pathologic study. Lab Invest 35:23, 1976

Chapter 7

Diseases of the Pulmonary Circulation

. . . . .

Alan G. Rose

The primary function of the pulmonary circulation is to provide the entire circulation of blood to and through the lungs for gaseous exchange (oxygen intake and carbon dioxide excretion). During its passage, the blood is also filtered of particulate matter and bacteria; the loss of carbon dioxide also serves to maintain a normal blood pH.

Normally, the pulmonary vascular bed has a low resistance because of its prominent elastic tissue component. Thus, pulmonary vascular resistance decreases passively with increased flow. Recruitment of additional blood vessels, particularly in the upright position, also contributes to the drop in vascular resistance that characterizes increased flow through the pulmonary circuit.

Like the liver, the lung has a dual blood supply, namely the pulmonary and bronchial arteries. The latter are able to nourish much of the lung parenchyma if the pulmonary circulation is compromised. Congestive heart failure negates the benefit of this double arterial supply (see later).

The pulmonary vascular endothelial cells keep the encompassing vascular smooth muscle cells in a state of relaxation.[1] As in the systemic circulation, pulmonary vascular endothelial cells promote relaxation or contraction of adjacent smooth muscle through elaboration of endothelium-derived relaxing factor (EDRF) and endothelin, respectively. Secretion of EDRF may be lost with endothelial cell dysfunction resulting from a variety of causes (e.g., shear stress).[1]

NORMAL PULMONARY CIRCULATION AND AGE-RELATED CHANGES INCLUDING ATHEROSCLEROSIS

Normal Pulmonary Circulation in the Fetus

The placenta is the source of oxygen for the fetus. Oxygenated blood leaving the placenta is directed via the ductus venosus and inferior vena cava to the right atrium. From here, most of this blood crosses the patent foramen ovale to reach the left atrium, followed by the left ventricle and the ascending aorta. The right ventricle and the pulmonary artery receive a little blood from the inferior vena cava, and almost all from the superior vena cava. Most of this blood enters the ductus arteriosus because of the high pulmonary vascular resistance, leaving only 10 to 15% of the right ventricular stroke volume to enter the pulmonary circulation.

Neonatal Transition in the Pulmonary Circulation

Gravanis and associates[2] summarized changes in the human cardiovascular system that occur with the transition to extrauterine life. (1) Pulmonary vascular resistance falls dramatically in association with lung expansion and increased alveolar PO_2, which markedly decrease pulmonary arterial vasoconstriction. By 2 months of age, smooth muscle begins to disappear from pulmonary arterioles. (2) Elimination of the low-resistance placental circulation is associated with a significant rise in systemic vascular resistance. (3) Abolition of umbilical venous return leads to reduced blood flow to the right atrium. (4) The abrupt increase in pulmonary blood flow is promptly reflected in a raised left atrial volume and pressure. (5) The two previous events (3) and (4) lead to functional closure of the valve of the foramen ovale. Over time, complete anatomic closure occurs in about 75% of individuals. (6) The ductus arteriosus completely constricts functionally within 12 hours of birth because of an increased systemic arterial PO_2 and the effect of various prostaglandins.[3] Physiologic patency of the ductus may last for up to 3 days postnatally and anatomic closure of its lumen takes 4 weeks or longer (see Chapter 1 also).

Persistent Fetal Pulmonary Circulation

Persistent fetal pulmonary circulation (i.e., persistent pulmonary hypertension) is a term used to describe the failure of the previously described normal physiologic process that causes the pulmonary vascular resistance to drop postnatally. Pulmonary arterial pressure remains high, pulmonary blood flow is low, and blood is shunted through the ductus arteriosus and/or foramen ovale into the systemic circulation. Pathologic lesions that may lead to persistent fetal pulmonary circulation include (1) patent ductus arteriosus, (2) respiratory distress syndrome, (3) pulmonary hypoplasia, and (4) misalignment of lung vessels. Inhaled nitrous oxide improves systemic oxygenation in infants with persistent pulmonary hypertension and may reduce the need for more invasive treatment.[4]

Normal Pulmonary Circulation in the Adult

As noted earlier, the lungs have a dual blood supply. They receive systemic venous blood via the pulmonary artery and arterial blood via the bronchial circulation.

Since some bronchial veins drain into pulmonary veins, the bronchial circulation constitutes a physiologic right-to-left shunt. The resulting desaturation of left atrial blood is usually trivial, because the bronchial circulation comprises about 1% of cardiac output. In some forms of lung disease (e.g., severe bronchiectasis), the bronchial circulation may be markedly increased by up to 30% of left ventricular output and produce a significant right-to-left shunt with resultant arterial desaturation. In cyanotic congenital heart disease, the bronchial blood is not fully oxygenated; it may participate in gas exchange and improve systemic oxygenation.[4]

The presence of a dual circulation renders the lungs, like the liver, resistant to infarction. If a portion of the pulmonary circulation is occluded by a thromboembolus, the bronchial circulation may be able to maintain the viability of pulmonary tissue. However, cardiac failure cancels the advantage of having a dual circulation and favors the establishment of a pulmonary infarct.

The bronchial arteries run in close apposition to the subdivisions of the major bronchi and bronchioles and supply their walls. Because of the higher systemic pressure in these arteries, they tend to have thicker walls than corresponding pulmonary arteries. At times, these vessels may present a greatly thickened dysplastic-looking media.

Pulmonary arteries within the lung parenchyma accompany the lobar and segmental ramifications of the bronchial tree. They all have an elastic media right down to a diameter of 0.5 mm. At this level, the muscular pulmonary arteries, which have internal and external elastic laminae, arise and accompany the smaller bronchi and bronchioles until they give origin to arterioles. At the level of the alveolar ducts, most arterioles give rise to alveolar capillaries.

Within the lung parenchyma it is not easy to distinguish venules from small pulmonary arteries, because the latter normally possess a thin media. The only site in the lung where pulmonary veins and venules are confidently identified is within interlobular fibrous septa, because arteries are not found at this site. Serial sectioning is used sometimes to trace a parenchymal venule into a septal vein. It is a caveat that elastic-stained sections are essential for proper histologic examination of the pulmonary vasculature. (See Chapter 2 for further discussion of pulmonary vessel histology.)

The pulmonary circulation is one of low resistance because of the large amount of elastic tissue present in the pulmonary arteries and the underutilized vascular reserve of this portion of the circulation. Gravity plays a role in the distribution of blood in the lungs. In the upright position, blood vessels in their upper portions are less well perfused than those at the bases (e.g., in the normal right lung there is a nine times difference in blood flow between apex and base). In the supine position or with exercise, this difference is abolished because of the opening of vessels in the upper portions of the lungs. This "recruitment" of blood vessels explains why pulmonary blood flow can rise considerably on effort with only a small increase in pulmonary pressure (i.e., pulmonary vascular resistance decreases on effort). A similar recruitment occurs in patients with moderately large septal defects or if moderate mitral stenosis is present.

Aging and the Pulmonary Circulation

Pulmonary arterial pressure and vascular resistance increase with advanced age,[1] as does systemic vascular resistance. This may result from reduced pulmonary vascular bed compliance secondary to intimal fibrosis or increased mural thickness in muscular pulmonary arteries as well as reduced left ventricular filling compliance, which has a direct effect on the pulmonary vascular bed.[5] Although the topic of pulmonary hypertension is dealt with later, it should be noted that about 13% of individuals up to 45 years of age and 28% of those up to 75 years of age have mild pulmonary hypertension.[6] Age-related changes in the peripheral pulmonary veins will be dealt with in a subsequent section of this chapter.

Atherosclerosis of the Pulmonary Artery

Although atherosclerosis (Fig. 7-1) of the main pulmonary artery or its major branches may be encountered

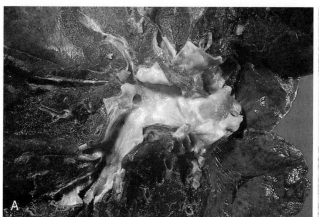
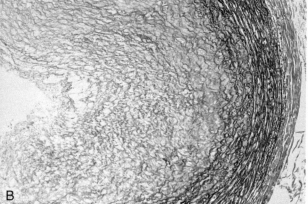

Figure 7-1 • *A,* Pale (yellow at post mortem examination) atherosclerotic plaques in the right main pulmonary artery and its major branches from a patient with pulmonary arterial hypertension. The arterial walls are thicker than normal. *B,* Histologic appearance of the intimal atherosclerosis (Elastic van Gieson stain).

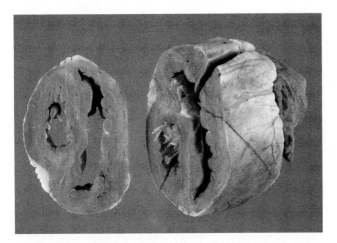

Figure 7-2 • Transverse section through both cardiac ventricles shows the right ventricle relatively more hypertrophied and dilated than the left because of pulmonary hypertension.

with advanced age, the commonest cause of such a morphologic change is pulmonary hypertension. The observation of pulmonary arterial atherosclerosis in conjunction with right-sided chamber hypertrophy, with or without dilation (Fig. 7-2), is a commonly used and reliable gross indicator of pulmonary hypertension at autopsy. In such patients, the right ventricle appears disproportionately hypertrophied compared with the left.

CONGENITAL CARDIAC ANOMALIES THAT MAY AFFECT THE ADULT PULMONARY CIRCULATION

Atrial Septal Defect

Those with an atrial septal defect may survive to old age despite the hazards posed by the development of associated pulmonary hypertension (see later), tricuspid incompetence, atrial fibrillation, paradoxic thromboembolism, or stroke.[7] The insertion of transvenous atrial septal closure devices per catheter now allows closure without surgery.

Ebstein Anomaly

Patients with a downward displacement of deformed tricuspid valve leaflets (Ebstein anomaly) (Fig. 7-3; also see Fig. 14-23), often survive to adulthood without surgical correction of the anomaly.[8] Right-sided heart failure is commonly present.

Morphologic Right Ventricle Supporting the Systemic Circulation

A morphologic right ventricle is unable to support the systemic circulation for a normal lifespan and usually fails after two or three decades of life. The cause of progressive right ventricular dysfunction is unknown but may include long-term myocardial ischemia, chronic pres-

sure overload, and, perhaps, differences in contraction. The right ventricle shows myocyte hypertrophy and diffuse fibrosis. An atrial baffle procedure (e.g., Mustard operation), has been used to correct the hemodynamic abnormality in patients with transposition of the great arteries. After the atrial baffle procedure, the morphologic right ventricle continues to support the aorta and the systemic circulation. A similar situation exists in corrected transposition. In the Damus-Kaye-Stansel procedure, which is currently used to treat patients with complete transposition of the great arteries, the proximal pulmonary trunk is connected to the ascending aorta in an end-to-side anastomosis, and there is a conduit from the right ventricle to the distal pulmonary trunk. In the Rastelli procedure, which is used for pulmonary atresia with ventricular septal defect (VSD), persistent truncus arteriosus, or complete transposition, the VSD is closed in such a way that blood from the left ventricle is directed into the aorta; a conduit links the right ventricle to the distal pulmonary trunk.

Surgically Created Shunts

Nowadays, patients with cyanotic heart disease often reach adulthood owing to shunts that were created or inserted surgically to alleviate a low pulmonary blood flow. The shunts not only improve flow but also encourage pulmonary artery growth.[9] They include (1) Potts shunt, a side-to-side anastomosis of the descending thoracic aorta to the left pulmonary artery; (2) Waterston shunt, a side-to-side anastomosis of the ascending aorta to the right pulmonary artery; and (3) Blalock-Taussig shunt, joining the subclavian artery to a pulmonary artery, in classic form—an end-to-side anastomosis—or in modified form—an interposed synthetic graft. These shunts may induce kinking or thrombosis of the pulmonary artery, and pulmonary vascular disease results from large shunts. Previous thoracotomy prevents these patients from receiving a lung transplant.

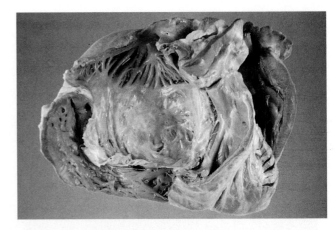

Figure 7-3 • Severe Ebstein anomaly of a tricuspid valve. The valve ring is distally displaced into the right ventricle, and the excessive dysplastic leaflet tissue is attached to the underlying endocardium, resulting in severe tricuspid insufficiency.

SPECIFIC CONGENITAL ANOMALIES AFFECTING THE PULMONARY CIRCULATION

The lesions dealt with in this section are listed in Table 7-1.

TABLE 7-1 • **Specific Congenital Anomalies Affecting the Pulmonary Circulation**

Coronary artery arising from pulmonary artery
Anomalous origin of either coronary artery from the contralateral or "wrong" sinus of Valsalva
Pulmonary artery stenosis
Unilateral absence of pulmonary artery
Congenital pulmonary valve stenosis
Congenital absence of pulmonary valve
Scimitar syndrome
Hemangioma of lung
Pulmonary arteriovenous fistula

Coronary Artery Arising From the Pulmonary Artery

One or both coronary arteries may arise from the pulmonary artery because of a disturbance in the normal development of the proximal truncus arteriosus whereby a surrounding coronary vascular network unites with coronary buds arising from the septating truncus. In the fetus, the higher pulmonary flow is sufficient to maintain a forward flow of blood in the anomalous coronary artery. Because of the low postnatal pulmonary arterial pressure, the supplied myocardium is inadequately perfused; indeed, slight retrograde flow may occur, and myocardial infarction may ensue. Longer survival with development of collaterals between left and right coronary arteries may lead to high flow in the malconnected artery and significant retrograde flow into the pulmonary artery (Fig. 7-4).

Origin of the Left Coronary Artery From the Pulmonary Artery

Bland-White-Garland syndrome is the commonest form of this anomaly.[10, 11] The left coronary artery usually originates from the posterior sinus of the pulmonary artery. Neonatal myocardial necrosis may result from underperfusion of the subendocardium, particularly underperfusion of the left ventricle. Only about 25% of these patients survive to adolescence or adulthood, and they often have coexistent mitral regurgitation, angina pectoris, or congestive cardiac failure.[12] Sometimes, clinical features of myocardial ischemia become evident only in adult life.[13, 14] In the 53-year-old asymptomatic woman reported by Suzuki and associates,[15] marked right coronary arterial predominance and hypoplastic circumflex branch of the left coronary artery contributed to her long survival.

Origin of the Right Coronary Artery From the Pulmonary Artery

This occurs much less frequently than anomalous origin of the left coronary artery from the site.

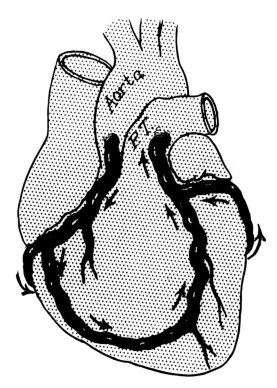

Figure 7-4 • Schematic portrayal of the circulation in anomalous origin of the left coronary artery from the pulmonary trunk. Fully saturated blood in the right coronary artery is diverted into the anomalous left coronary artery, and thence into the pulmonary trunk. Because of the arteriovenous type of arrangement, the myocardium is deprived of adequate blood pressure and oxygen. (From Edwards, JE: Anomalous coronary arteries with special reference to arteriovenous-like communications. Circulation 17:1001, 1958.)

Origin of Both Coronary Arteries From the Pulmonary Artery

An extremely rare occurrence, it is a much more serious condition than either of the above variants of this condition.

Origin of Either Coronary Artery From the Contralateral or "Wrong" Sinus of Valsalva

Origin of the left coronary artery (LCA) from the right sinus of Valsalva or from the proximal right coronary artery (RCA) may cause the LCA to pass between the aorta and the pulmonary artery/right ventricular outflow tract. In this situation, the artery may be compressed by a "hemodynamic vise," which in some individuals leads to sudden death during or shortly after exercise. The mechanism of the resultant myocardial ischemia is not completely understood. It may be caused by the slit-like orifice of the aberrant coronary artery with its acute angle takeoff and/or compression of this vessel against the main pulmonary artery by expansion of the aortic root as a result of an exertion-associated increase in intraaortic pressure.[15] Most patients are males (89%).[16] Why the condition causes fatal cardiac arrest in some young individuals and allows a normal lifespan in others remains unexplained.[17] A similar abnormality involving the RCA appears less dangerous.[15, 18] (See further discussion in Chapter 11 and Figs. 11-11, 11-13, and 11-14.)

Pulmonary Artery Stenosis

Congenital stenoses may occur anywhere along the course of the pulmonary artery or its smaller branches. Branch pulmonary artery stenosis may be associated with tetralogy of Fallot, pulmonary atresia after occlusion of the ductus arteriosus, single ventricle, isolated congenital pulmonary stenosis, and various types of cyanotic congenital heart disease in patients treated by a Blalock-Taussig shunt. These conditions may respond to high-pressure balloon dilation. Sometimes, even if a large patch is used to correct the stenosis, it may recur because of failure of the affected arterial segment to grow pari passu with the child.

Gentles and colleagues[19] reported an improved rate of successful dilation of stenotic peripheral pulmonary arteries with high-pressure balloons. Intravascular stents have also been successfully implanted in patients with congenital and acquired branch pulmonary stenosis; significant restenosis is rare (3%).[20] The long-term results of balloon dilation and stenting are still unknown. Percutaneous balloon valvuloplasty has also been used to treat neonates with critical congenital pulmonary stenosis.[21]

Unilateral Absence of Pulmonary Artery

In this rare congenital anomaly, the pulmonary artery fails to bifurcate and runs as a single vessel to supply only one lung. The deprived lung is supplied by a branch from the aorta (i.e., unilateral absence of a pulmonary artery[22]) and is associated with systemic blood supply to the lung lacking a pulmonary artery. Many cases are associated with ventricular septal defects and an early onset of pulmonary hypertension followed by right-sided heart failure. The result is that few of these patients reach adulthood. Histology of the lung supplied by the systemic artery varies according to the caliber of the supplying systemic artery. If the latter vessel is stenosed, the small pulmonary arteries in that lung may appear atrophic and thin-walled. Pulmonary hypertension may also occur in the lung supplied by the systemic artery; therefore, in some instances, hypertensive pulmonary vascular lesions are found in both lungs.[23, 24] Absence of a right pulmonary artery is often associated with patent ductus arteriosus, but not with tetralogy of Fallot, and the systemic artery may arise from the ascending aorta in some cases. Absence of a left pulmonary artery is often associated with tetralogy of Fallot, and the systemic arterial supply is not derived from the ascending aorta.

Congenital Pulmonary Valve Stenosis

Pulmonary stenosis comprises about 7% of congenital cardiac disease.[23, 25] Pulmonary valve stenosis may be associated with a dome- or funnel-shaped valve, a bicuspid one, or a dysplastic valve. Familial, congenital, pulmo-

nary valve stenosis with autosomal dominant inheritance has been reported.[26] Carcinoid heart disease typically results in pulmonary stenosis and tricuspid incompetence[25] (see Chapter 13). Balloon dilation appears less successful in treatment of patients with carcinoid pulmonary valve stenosis than in those who have the congenital form.[27]

Congenital Absence of the Pulmonary Valve

Congenital absence of the pulmonary valve is a rare cardiac anomaly[28] that may be associated with other significant abnormalities (e.g., pulmonary arterial stenosis).

Pulmonary Sequestration

Pulmonary sequestration is a congenital anomaly characterized by the development of a hamartomatous-like mass of nonfunctioning, sometimes cystic, lung tissue supplied by one or more systemic arteries. The mass lies either within normal lung—*intralobar sequestration*—or as accessory tissue on the external, often the left, aspect of the lung—*extralobar sequestration.* Hypertensive changes may develop within the vessels of the sequestration. Some "hybrid" arteries within a sequestration may have a structure intermediate between pulmonary and bronchial arteries. One report raises the possibility of a genetic predisposition in some cases.[29]

Scimitar Syndrome

This malformation affects heart, lungs, and both pulmonary arteries and veins in the following manner. The heart shows dextroposition and dextrorotation; a hypoplastic right lung is bilobed and may show bronchiectasis; the right pulmonary artery is either small, or absent, and one or more large systemic pulmonary arteries may originate from the descending aorta to supply the right lung. The major feature is a partial, anomalous, pulmonary venous drainage from the right lung or its lower lobe to the abdominal inferior vena cava via a single scimitar-shaped venous trunk that penetrates the diaphragm as noted by radiography. Pulmonary hypertension rarely occurs.

Hemangioma of the Lung

This type of hemangioma may be capillary or cavernous in nature, or a mixture of the two (Fig. 7-5). The lesions, which may be single or multiple, occur in any part of the lung. A capillary hemangioma is composed of aggregates of small, capillary-sized blood vessels, whereas its cavernous counterpart shows larger, blood-filled, endothelial-lined spaces separated by fibrous septa. The condition may be associated with hemangiomas in other organs (e.g., liver, kidneys). Such a hemangioma is probably a hamartoma rather than a true neoplasm. A hemangioma should not be confused with a sclerosing hemangioma of a lung, which has also been called papillary or sclerosing pneumocytoma.[30, 31]

Pulmonary embolism (see later, and Fig. 7-5B) has

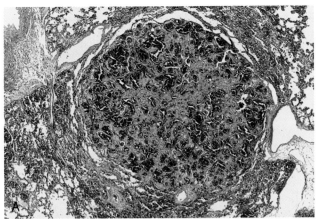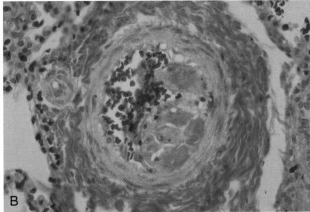

Figure 7-5 • *A,* Mixed cavernous-capillary hemangioma of the lung. *B,* Small pulmonary artery in same patient contains microspheres (empty vacuoles, top) and histiocytes within its lumen after therapeutic embolization of a liver hemangioma (both Masson trichrome stain).

resulted from therapeutic embolization of a nonpulmonary (e.g., facial) hemangioma with fibrin glue.[32] Oshika and associates[30] successfully performed angiographic embolization of a right bronchial artery that supplied a hemangioma of the right middle lobe.

Pulmonary Arteriovenous Fistula

These appear as vascular malformations composed of pulmonary arteries that connect directly with pulmonary veins in the absence of an intervening capillary bed. The lesion may be confined to one lobe; it is often subpleural and found in the lower lobe. Multiple pulmonary arterial arteriovenous fistulas are encountered in patients affected by familial telangiectasia (Rendu-Osler-Weber disease). Pulmonary arteriovenous malformations complicate some forms of cavopulmonary anastomosis.[33] Their causes are not known, but they may be related to the absence of pulsatile blood flow or the presence or absence of unknown circulating factors. Srivastava and colleagues[33] postulated that arteriovenous malformations were related to the diversion of normal hepatic venous flow from the pulmonary circulation and may be analogous to those associated with liver disease, which have been found to resolve after liver transplantation. Complications of pulmonary arteriovenous malformation include cerebral abscess and thrombosis, systemic hypoxia, severe pulmonary hemorrhage, and infective endocarditis. Pulmonary hypertension does not occur.

CLASSIFICATION AND CAUSES OF PULMONARY HYPERTENSION

Definition of Pulmonary Hypertension

Pulmonary blood pressure is normally one eighth of systemic blood pressure. In practice, a pulmonary blood pressure of 30/15 mm Hg or higher, with a mean pressure greater than 20 mm Hg, diagnoses pulmonary hypertension.

Classification of Pulmonary Hypertension

If a cause for pulmonary hypertension can be identified, the patient falls into the group of those with secondary pulmonary hypertension. Primary or idiopathic pulmonary hypertension comprises the remaining patients in whom no cause for pulmonary hypertension is found. It is usually taken for granted in speaking of pulmonary hypertension that it denotes a persistent hypertensive state that has been present for months or years. This is in contradistinction to short-lived, acute pulmonary hypertension of a duration ranging from minutes to hours, days, or weeks. Possible causes of the latter state include massive, acute pulmonary (e.g., saddle) thromboembolism, which is usually rapidly fatal, or raised intracranial pressure, sudden exposure to high altitude, or iatrogenic inadvertent pulmonary embolotherapy.

Etiology and Mechanisms of Production of Secondary Pulmonary Hypertension

It should be noted that in an individual with secondary pulmonary hypertension more than one mechanism (Table 7-2) may operate (e.g., in emphysema, there is both obliteration and compression of blood vessels as well as vasoconstriction of small pulmonary arteries). Hypoxia-induced vasoconstriction appears to be the more important mechanism and is more evident in so-called "blue bloaters," who suffer from bronchiolitis-induced centrilobular emphysema. Hypoxic vasoconstriction also explains why an attack of acute bronchitis in patients with chronic

TABLE 7-2 • **Mechanisms of Production of Secondary Pulmonary Hypertension**

Passive or venous pulmonary hypertension
Hyperkinetic pulmonary hypertension
Obstructive or obliterative pulmonary hypertension
Vasoconstrictive pulmonary hypertension

cor pulmonale (see later) produces pulmonary hypertensive heart failure so readily.

Passive or Venous Pulmonary Hypertension

Passive or venous pulmonary hypertension occurs with any condition that elevates left atrial pressure[34, 35]; for example, mitral stenosis (Fig. 7-6), mitral incompetence or left ventricular failure resulting from systemic hypertension, myocardial infarction, valvular heart disease, or cardiomyopathy, among other conditions. Pulmonary hypertension is common in patients with left ventricular dysfunction but is unrelated to the severity of left ventricular systolic dysfunction. It closely correlates with diastolic dysfunction and the degree of severity of mitral regurgitation. All of these conditions are associated with an elevation of blood pressure in pulmonary veins, which have no valves. This is the only one of the four mechanisms of pulmonary hypertension that leads to intimal sclerotic changes in pulmonary venules in addition to prominent arterial changes.

Hyperkinetic Pulmonary Hypertension

The operative mechanism is increased blood flow through the lungs with a normal or reduced vascular resistance. Once pulmonary blood flow has increased more than three times normal, 15 L/minute in an adult, a state of maximum vasodilation is established and no further reduction in resistance is possible. From that point, pulmonary blood pressure increases in proportion to increased flow. Possible causes include (1) acyanotic con-

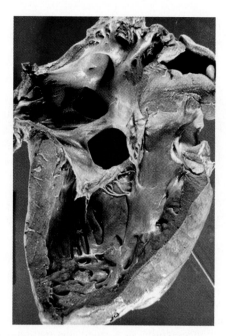

Figure 7-7 • View of the right heart in a 40-year-old woman with large ostium primum and ostium secundum atrial septal defects who died of pulmonary hypertension.

genital heart disease (e.g., atrial septal defect [Fig. 7-7], ventricular septal defect, patent ductus arteriosus); and (2) cyanotic congenital heart disease (e.g., single atrium, single ventricle, complete transposition of the great arteries).

If the shunt is large, early surgical closure is recommended, because there is danger of severe, irreversible sclerotic changes developing in small pulmonary arteries. Once established, such changes may be progressive.

In a personal communication (1973), J.E. Edwards noted that individuals with pulmonary hypertension from birth (i.e., caused by a large septal defect), fail to show the usual postnatal involution of the pulmonary arterial media that occurs in normal individuals (Fig. 7-8A). Such an individual with congenital pulmonary hypertension has a pulmonary arterial media that looks just like an aortic media, both macroscopically (Fig. 7-8B) and with regard to its lamellar unit pattern (i.e., the well-developed elastic tissue lamellae show no evidence of fragmentation [Fig. 7-8C]).

Obstructive or Obliterative Pulmonary Hypertension

This mechanism operates if more than two thirds of the pulmonary vascular cross-sectional area is blocked or destroyed. Thus, a single pneumonectomy does not produce pulmonary hypertension.

Obstructive Pulmonary Hypertension

This state results most commonly from a blockage of the lumen of the pulmonary arteries by widespread, repeated peripheral pulmonary thromboemboli (Fig. 7-9A–C). The veins of the lower leg (Fig. 7-9D) are the commonest source of such thromboemboli, with venous

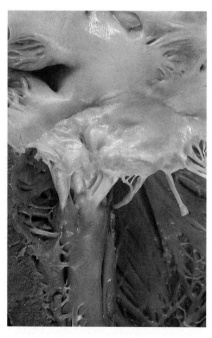

Figure 7-6 • Severe postrheumatic mitral stenosis and incompetence, an important cause of passive venous pulmonary hypertension. (From Rose AG: Pathology of natural heart valves and indications for heart valve replacement. In: Pathology of Heart Valve Replacement. Lancaster, United Kingdom. MTP Press Limited [with kind permission from Kluwer Academic Publishers Group], 1987.)

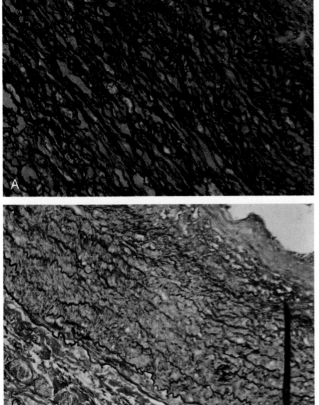

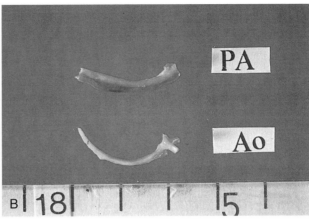

Figure 7-8 • *A,* Normal pulmonary artery in an adult. Note the fragmented medial elastin. *B,* The pulmonary artery (PA) is thicker than the aorta (Ao) in this 25-year-old patient with pulmonary hypertension caused by a large congenital ventricular septal defect. *C,* Pulmonary artery histology in this patient resembles that of a normal aorta and shows nonfragmented medial elastic lamellae (*A* and *C,* elastic van Gieson stain).

stasis as the major predisposing factor.[36, 37] Obstructed pulmonary arteries may contain recanalized channels within their original lumens (so-called "colander appearance"), may show concentric or eccentric intimal thickening, sometimes with hemosiderin deposits, or they may have fresh thromboemboli in their lumens. Elastic pulmonary arteries may contain webs of fibrous tissue traversing the lumen (Fig. 7-10). Arterioles may also be involved because of small emboli or impaction-gendered fragmentation of larger emboli. The majority of emboli are thrombotic in nature.

The risk for recurrent thromboembolic events is significantly higher in carriers of factor V Leiden than in patients without this disorder.[38] The molecular basis for this highly prevalent thrombophilic condition is substitution of glutamine for arginine at amino acid 506 in the factor V gene. The product, factor V, resists inactivation by activated protein C. Approximately 3% of many populations are heterozygous for the defect. Patients who are homozygous appear to be more severely affected clinically.[39] Large trials assessing the risk-benefit ratio of long-term anticoagulation in carriers of the mutation who have had a first episode of venous thromboembolism are still awaited. Other disorders favoring development of venous thrombosis include hyperhomocysteinemia, which is, in part, genetically determined. High-plasma homocysteine levels are a risk factor for deep vein thrombosis in the general population.[40] Patients with concurrent hereditary homocystinuria and factor V Leiden can have an increased risk of thrombosis.[41]

Other forms of embolism that may lead to chronic pulmonary hypertension include embolization of talcum or starch particles to the pulmonary arterioles in narcotic addicts who inject intravenously various drugs intended for oral use. They produce granulomas in small vessels, resulting in fatal pulmonary hypertension.[23] Pulmonary schistosomiasis is usually associated with liver involvement by the same parasite. Pulmonary hypertension results either from the liver disease or from the embolism of the schistosomal ova to the lungs, with resultant granulomatous inflammation (Fig. 7-11) and plexiform lesion formation.[42] A new animal model to study *Schistosoma hematobium* infection has been introduced.[43]

In patients with malignant disease, tumor emboli to the lungs are common but are usually not widespread enough to produce pulmonary hypertension. Such patients tend to die of their disease before pulmonary hypertension develops. Extremely rarely, extensive tumor emboli (derived most often from metastatic breast [40%], stomach [15%] and lung [10%] carcinomas) lead to subacute pulmonary hypertension.[44] Most such patients have a mixture of tumor and thrombotic microemboli followed by predominantly tumor microemboli, and, least frequently of all, by a combination of neoplastic microemboli and large, fatal tumor emboli.

Pulmonary emboli that may be encountered histologically and which do not cause chronic pulmonary hypertension include fat, bone marrow after resuscitation, and other tissue and cells (e.g., bone marrow megakaryocytes in pulmonary capillaries are common). Trauma may lead

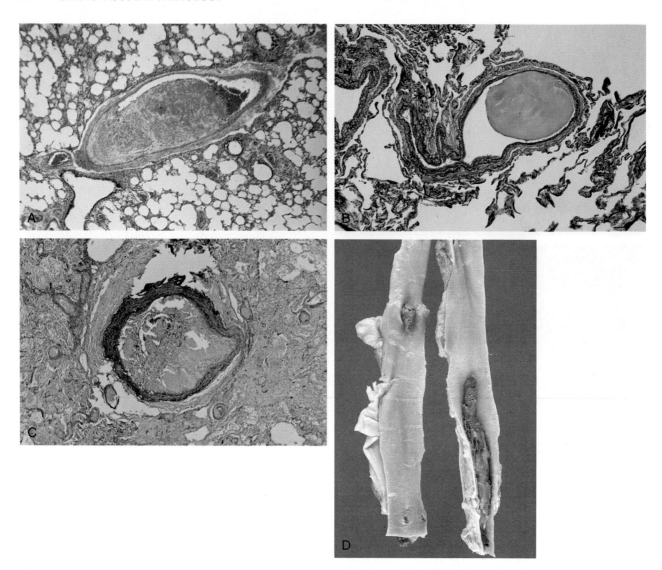

Figure 7-9 • Histology of pulmonary thromboembolism. *A,* Recent thromboembolus in a small pulmonary artery shows early organization. Initial vasospasm of the artery following impaction of the embolus, followed by later relaxation, led to the reappearance of an elliptic, slit-like lumen (top) (H&E stain). *B,* Old, eccentric, organized thromboembolus within a small pulmonary artery. *C,* Recanalized thromboembolus has yielded a colander-like appearance to the pulmonary arterial lumen. *D,* Bilaterally thrombosed iliofemoral venous segments in a patient who died of pulmonary thromboembolism. Thrombus on the left side embolized, leaving scanty thrombus protruding from the ostium of a venous tributary (*B* and *C,* Elastic van Gieson stain).

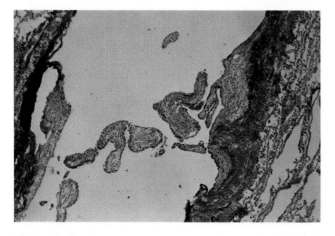

Figure 7-10 • Fibrous band resulting from a previously organized, large thromboembolus spans the lumen of an elastic pulmonary artery (Elastic van Gieson stain).

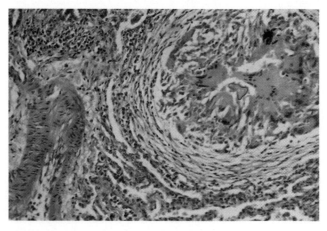

Figure 7-11 • Perivascularly extruded schistosome ovum (pulmonary bilharziasis) has evoked a granulomatous inflammatory response alongside a small pulmonary artery (H&E stain).

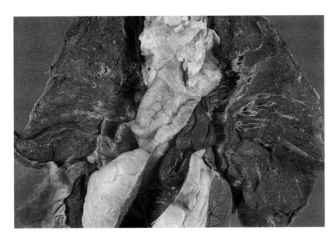

Figure 7-12 • Massive pulmonary thromboembolism from leg veins led to the sudden death of this patient. Note coiled appearance of thromboembolus.

to emboli of liver, brain, or adipose tissue. Amniotic fluid embolism, which produces a disseminated intravascular coagulopathy, is a risk in pregnant women. Included also are air and gas emboli; infected vegetations from right-sided infective endocarditis; other foreign body emboli, including iatrogenic material such as sclerosants injected into esophageal varices,[45] cyanoacrylate used to occlude arteriovenous malformations,[46] and vascular hemostatic material (e.g., Vasoseal,[47] microspheres [see Fig. 7-5*B*]); and embolism by nematodes. In addition, a massive saddle thromboembolus (Fig. 7-12) in the pulmonary artery leads to sudden death, but not chronic pulmonary hypertension, by inducing acute right-sided heart failure, hypotension, and circulatory collapse. A cardiac myxoma situated in the right atrium or the right ventricle has the potential to give rise to tumor-thrombus emboli to the lungs. Usually, there are insufficient emboli to lead to secondary pulmonary hypertension.

In situ pulmonary thrombosis is a rare cause of obstructive pulmonary hypertension, but it may occur with heparin-associated thrombocytopenia/thrombosis, pulmonary hypertension (see later), or pulmonary atherosclerosis.[48] Pulmonary hypertension may reverse the pressure difference between left and right atria. Because at least one of four adults has a patent flap valve at the fossa ovalis, the latter may open and paradoxic embolism may occur (Fig. 7-13) (i.e., a right-sided embolus may pass from the right atrium via the patent foramen ovale into the left atrium and thus reach the systemic circulation).

Obliterative Pulmonary Hypertension

This also results from destruction and/or compression of pulmonary blood vessels and may be caused by emphysema, arteritis (e.g., bilharzial arteritis, polyarteritis nodosa) or pulmonary fibrosis from any cause (sarcoidosis, silicoanthracosis, idiopathic pulmonary fibrosis, rheumatoid arthritis, systemic sclerosis). In emphysema, bullous formation leads to widespread destruction of the microcirculation. This partially explains why pulmonary hypertension is present at a stage when the pulmonary arteries show less advanced morphologic changes than expected. Vasoconstriction also contributes to the pulmonary hypertension of emphysema.

Vasoconstrictive Pulmonary Hypertension

Hypoxic Pulmonary Hypertension

This results from vasoconstriction of pulmonary arteries that is induced by a reduced alveolar P_{O_2}. Pulmonary arteries differ from systemic ones in that they constrict rather than dilate in response to hypoxia. The small muscular pulmonary arteries, which are about $100\ \mu$ in diameter, are the major site of hypoxic pulmonary vasoconstriction.[49] This response is advantageous in situations of localized poor ventilation in the lung, because pulmonary blood flow is directed away from such zones to

Figure 7-13 • A paradoxic embolus in transit. *A*, Thromboembolus in right atrium is passing through a patent flap valve at the fossa ovalis. *B*, Left atrial view in the same heart shows that the larger portion of the thromboembolus has already crossed the atrial septum. This is one mechanism of paradoxic embolism.

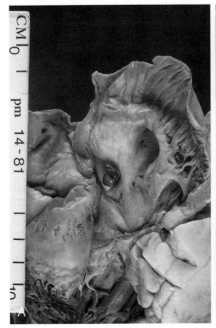
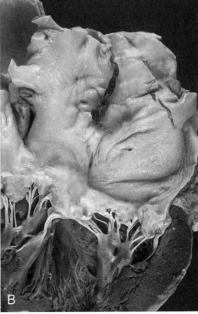

those with adequate oxygenation. The response is disadvantageous if both lungs are totally hypoxic because of high altitude, or if diseases such as kyphoscoliosis, obstructive sleep apnea/obesity hypoventilation (also termed the pickwickian syndrome), or chronic obstructive airway disease with emphysema are present (Fig. 7-14A, B).

In normal adults, pulmonary arterioles smaller than 80 μ in external diameter contain no medial muscle; their walls consist of a single elastic lamina. In chronic hypoxic pulmonary hypertension, there is extension of smooth muscle into arterioles as small as 20 μ in diameter, yielding a distinct tunica media with internal and external elastic laminae. The muscle is believed to originate from intermediate precursor cells located deep to the endothelium of the nonmuscularized arteriole.[49] Another characteristic feature of hypoxic pulmonary hypertension is the development of eccentric, longitudinally arranged smooth muscle within the intima of small muscular pulmonary arteries (Fig. 7-14B) and arterioles.[50] Venules may show medial hypertrophy and intimal changes similar to those found in arterioles.

Chronic pulmonary hypertension is induced in rats by exposing them to intermittent hypoxia for only 4 hours per day.[51] The induced morphologic changes regress only if the animals are treated with continuous normoxia; intermittent normoxia of 16 hours per day is ineffective.[52]

Chronic alveolar hypoxia in humans occurs in a wide variety of unrelated conditions, all of which result in decreased oxygen tension of alveolar gas.[53] In high-altitude residents, the cause lies outside the body. Lung diseases such as chronic air flow obstruction are often associated with chronic alveolar hypoxia, but they may also occur in obstructive sleep apnea syndrome (OSAS) and kyphoscoliosis. Sleep-disordered breathing is a continuum—from chronic snoring to obstructive sleep apnea to severe OSAS—associated with progressively increasing clinical consequences. Few reports of the pathology of OSAS have been published.[54, 55] Patients with the condition stop breathing intermittently during sleep because of upper airway obstruction.[56] The condition is common and affects 7.8% of men and 2.3% of women in the United States.[49] Ahmed and colleagues[55] presented findings in OSAS, namely pulmonary hemosiderosis and capillary proliferation. They suggested that chronic left ventricular failure contributed to pulmonary hypertension. The degree of pulmonary siderosis was disproportionate to the severity of morphologic abnormalities in the left ventricle. However, a hemodynamic study of OSAS noted that pulmonary hypertension became much worse during maximal exercise[57] in association with some left ventricular dysfunction. As Kay[49] pointed out, the pathogenesis of OSAS may be more complex than previously thought, and factors other than the effect of chronic hypoxia on pulmonary vascular smooth muscle may be significant. In view of limitations in current data about its associations and the effectiveness of treatment, the United States National Institutes of Health has funded a long-term, multicenter, prospective study to examine the cardiovascular and cerebrovascular mortality and morbidity associated with sleep-disordered breathing.[58, 59] Another author[60] hypothesized that sleep apnea may be a predisposing factor for tobacco use, because nicotine decreases both somnolence and obesity, the main symptoms of OSAS, and also reduces the frequency and duration of apneas. Other effects of cigarette smoking on the lung are well known. Patients with severe emphysema also have a vasoconstrictive element to their pulmonary hypertension because of a low alveolar partial pressure of oxygen and a high carbon dioxide level.

Reactive Pulmonary Hypertension

Whenever there is increased pulmonary blood pressure or increased pulmonary arterial blood flow, a pulmonary

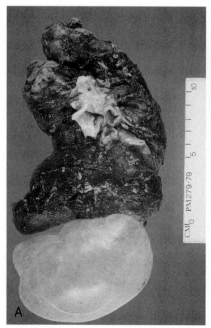
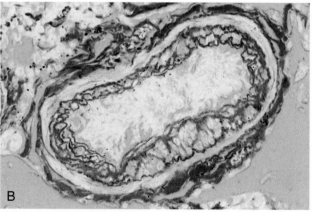

Figure 7-14 • *A,* Emphysema of right lung with a very large basal bulla. *B,* Longitudinal muscle within thickened intima of a small muscular pulmonary artery is prominent in emphysema (Elastic van Gieson stain).

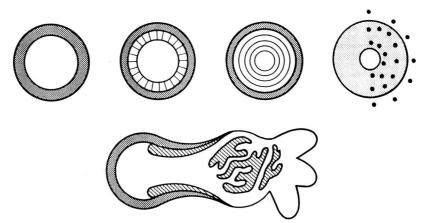

Figure 7-15 • Diagrammatic summary of arterial changes occurring in plexogenic pulmonary arteriopathy/Heath-Edwards grading. Top (left to right) shows arteries with medial hypertrophy (grade 1); intimal cellular proliferation (grade 2); concentric-laminar intimal fibrosis (grade 3), and fibrinoid necrosis with or without arteritis (grade 6). A plexiform lesion (grade 4) is shown at the bottom. Angiomatoid/dilation lesion is not illustrated. (From Wagenvoort CA, Wagenvoort N: Pathology of Pulmonary Hypertension. New York, John Wiley & Sons, 1977. Reprinted by permission of John Wiley & Sons, Inc.)

vasoconstrictive response is elicited, (i.e., secondary to passive venous or hyperkinetic pulmonary hypertension).

Histologic Grading of Plexogenic Pulmonary Arteriopathy and Subsequent Modifications

Donald Heath and Jesse Edwards developed a grading scheme for the sequential analysis of pulmonary vascular alterations encountered in congenital heart disease. The hallmark of the Heath-Edwards classification[61] is the plexiform lesion, which indicates irreversible pulmonary hypertension. Correction of a congenital cardiac lesion leading to overperfusion of the lungs in such cases usually causes the patient's death because of severe, irreversible pulmonary hypertension. This is because in the late stage of the disease the patient has very high pulmonary arterial pressure that leads to shunt reversal, and the congenital defect acts as a safety valve. Further experience has shown that severe intimal fibrosis of small pulmonary arteries may lead to similar fatal results. Increased understanding of the pathogenesis of vascular lesions has also led to modification of the original classification.

Originally, the plexiform lesion was thought to be spe-

cific for the shunting of blood through the lungs that is associated with congenital heart disease, but it may also occur in about 85% of cases of primary (idiopathic) pulmonary hypertension[1] (see later). Some authors[62] have suggested that a subset of patients with primary pulmonary hypertension have thrombotic lesions either per se or associated with plexogenic arteriopathy. This raises, once again, the problem of deciding whether one is dealing with thromboemboli or in situ thrombosis. In most instances, this is a distinction that the pathologist is unable to make. The lack of an apparent source of thromboembolism does not exclude its possibility.

At present, and for several reasons, pathologists are less likely to be called upon to interpret lung biopsies for grading pulmonary hypertension than in the past. Firstly, there is greater accuracy in the clinical assessment of the severity of pulmonary hypertension. Secondly, open lung biopsy-induced pleural adhesions may preclude subsequent lung transplantation. Thirdly, the classic Heath-Edwards[61] histologic grading system (Fig. 7-15; see Table 22-5) applies only to advanced pulmonary arteriopathy in hypertension that is caused by the hyperkinetic mechanism or idiopathic plexogenic pulmonary hypertension. The grading system should *not* be applied to other forms of pulmonary hypertension because they are not associated with the development of plexiform lesions. Fourthly, lung biopsy produces a significant morbidity and mortality in young patients with congenital heart disease.

With these reservations, the following modification of the original Heath-Edwards grading system is offered (Table 7-3). The arterial changes described later are most apparent in smaller (approximately 300 μ in diameter) muscular pulmonary arteries. The earlier, milder changes consist of medial hypertrophy of small arteries and arteriolar muscularization, grade 1 (Fig. 7-16); intimal cellular proliferation, grade 2 (Fig. 7-17); and intimal fibrosis, grade 3 (Fig. 7-18). Grades 4, 5, and 6 are now known to be nonsequential and are lumped together as a combined grade 456, which indicates severe, usually irreversible, pulmonary hypertension. The plexiform lesion, grade 4 (Fig. 7-19), is an expanded portion of a small artery immediately distal to a severely narrowed zone of the same vessel. Its pathogenesis is still unknown. Theories include (1) presence of previous fibrinoid necrosis (Fig. 7-20) of the artery with secondary thrombosis and recan-

---

TABLE 7-3 • **Modified Heath-Edwards Grading of Pulmonary Arterial Lesions in Pulmonary Hypertension, Including Plexiform Lesions**

Grade 1:	Medial hypertrophy of muscular pulmonary arteries Muscularization of pulmonary arterioles
Grade 2:	Cellular intimal proliferation plus all of the above
Grade 3:	Intimal fibrosis plus all of the above 3a: less than 30% narrowing of the lumen by intimal fibrosis

Borderline between reversible and irreversible lesions

	3b: more than 30% narrowing of the lumen by intimal fibrosis
Grade 456:	Plexiform lesions ⎫ Angiomatoid lesions ⎬ plus all of the above Fibrinoid necrosis/arteritis ⎭

Modified from Heath D, Edwards, JE: The pathology of hypertensive pulmonary vascular disease. A description of six grades of structural changes in the pulmonary arteries with special reference to congenital cardiac septal defects. Circulation 18:533, 1958.

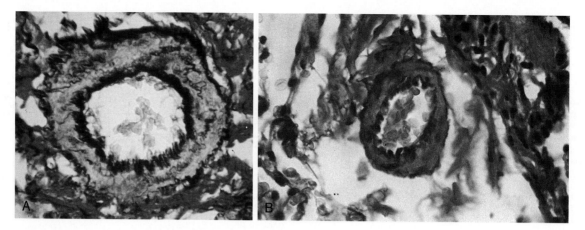

Figure 7-16 • Grade 1 pulmonary hypertension. *A*, Medial hypertrophy in a small muscular pulmonary artery from a patient with a patent atrial septal defect and pulmonary hypertension. *B*, Arteriole contains medial smooth muscle (both Elastic van Gieson stain).

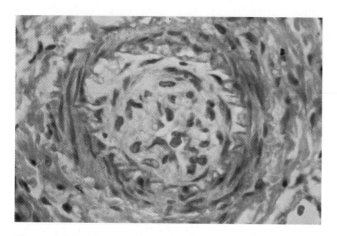

Figure 7-17 • Grade 2 pulmonary hypertension demonstrated by intimal cellular proliferation (H&E stain).

alization attempts, grade 6 lesion, or (2) reactive endothelial cell hyperplasia induced by a jet lesion[63] produced by the narrowed, more proximal arterial segment. (3) Edwards, in a personal communication, (J.E. Edwards, 1995) stated his belief that the plexiform lesion represents an arteriovenous communication. Developing this concept further, I suggest that the angiomatoid/dilation lesion, grade 5 (Fig. 7-21), which has the appearance of a conglomeration of dilated venous channels, may truly represent dilated veins with a single elastic lamina and a thin media connected directly to an artery and forming an arteriovenous communication, rather than representing altered arteries mistaken for veins as suggested by other authors.[64] The intimate relationship between, and essential coexistence of, plexiform and angiomatoid/dilation lesions supports this suggestion. Schistosomiasis may produce pulmonary plexiform and dilation lesions. Defaria[65] interpreted such plexiform lesions as arteriovenous anastomoses.

Rabinovitch and colleagues[66, 67] proposed a grading system that aimed to assess more subtle pulmonary hy-

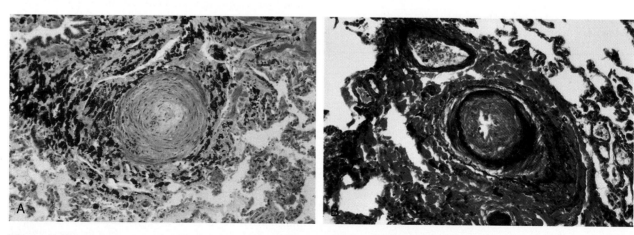

Figure 7-18 • Grade 3 pulmonary hypertension. *A*, The lumen of this small muscular pulmonary artery is more than 75% narrowed by concentric laminar intimal fibrosis (grade 3b of the modified grading) (H&E stain). *B*, Elastic van Gieson stain of a similarly affected artery confirms dense intimal fibrosis.

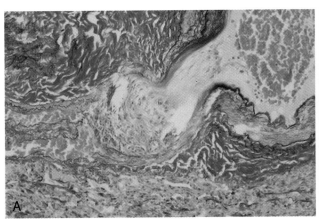
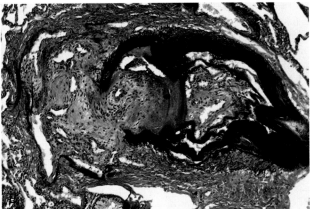

Figure 7-19 • Grade 4 pulmonary hypertension. *A*, A plexiform lesion is present within a small branch of a muscular pulmonary artery just distal to a zone of intimal fibrosis. This appearance supports the theory that a jet lesion is important in its pathogenesis. *B*, Another plexiform lesion shows evidence of focal destruction of the arterial wall at its site, supporting the concept that previous arterial necrosis is its precursor (both elastic van Gieson stain).

pertensive changes than the Heath-Edwards grading. In the Rabinovitch grading system, grade A shows extension of smooth muscle into smaller and more peripheral arteries than normal; pulmonary blood flow is increased, but pulmonary artery pressure is normal. Grade B features medial hypertrophy plus the changes in A. Pulmonary artery pressure is increased. In grade C, in addition to the changes noted, there is a reduction in the number of small pulmonary arteries, and pulmonary vascular resistance is increased. The number of arteries is counted in relation to the number of alveoli. In the neonate, the alveolar/arterial ratio is 20:1, at 2 years of age, it is 12:1, and in the adult, 6:1. A typical finding in a young child with a VSD could be a ratio of 25:1. This grading system proved of less value than the Heath-Edwards grading, possibly due to problems with improper fixation or lack of adequacy of lung biopsy samples. Nonspecific changes that may be encountered in lungs with pulmonary hypertension include cholesterol granulomas and focal calcification or ossification.

Clinical Idiopathic or Primary Pulmonary Hypertension: Six Possible Histologic Types

In 1% of patients with cor pulmonale, the cause of the high pulmonary artery pressure remains clinically unclear.[68] The underlying severe, and mostly progressive, pulmonary vascular disease with unknown etiology is defined as idiopathic or primary pulmonary hypertension, IPH. The World Health Organization (WHO)[69] defines it as "pulmonary arterial hypertension of unknown cause." At autopsy or on lung biopsy such clinical IPH takes one of six pathologic forms (see numbered headings later).

The management of primary pulmonary hypertension has been revolutionized by the finding that long-term intravenous prostacyclin improves survival and the quality of life for patients with this disorder. Familial pulmonary hypertension has a chromosomal locus at 2q31–q32. All effective treatments,[70] such as intravenous prostaglandins, endarterectomy, or atrial septostomy, increase systemic

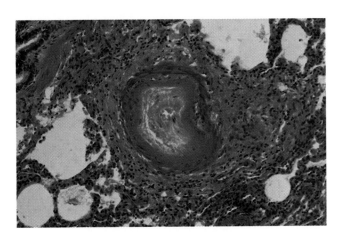

Figure 7-20 • Fibrinoid necrosis (grade 6 lesion). Early fibrinoid necrosis of the outer intimal layer of a severely narrowed small pulmonary artery (H&E stain).

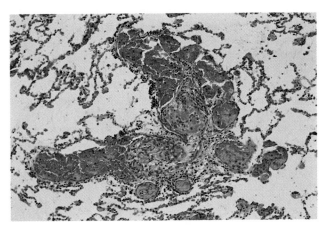

Figure 7-21 • An angiomatoid or dilation lesion (grade 5) shows dilated, thin-walled vascular channels surrounding a plexiform lesion. The channels may either represent dilated arterial collaterals or dilated venular components of an arteriovenous fistula (H&E stain).

blood flow and prevent intravascular pulmonary thrombosis that might otherwise occur with low flow. Improved systemic flow also leads to increased myocardial perfusion and prevention of right ventricular failure. Despite potentially serious complications, long-term prostacyclin may be especially helpful in seriously ill patients awaiting transplantation.[71]

1. Thromboembolic or Obstructive Pulmonary Arterial Lesions

Clinically unsuspected and repeated peripheral thromboembolism of the lungs is the commonest pathologic basis for clinically diagnosed IPH. The term thromboembolus was originally introduced to describe a thrombotic mass within a blood vessel that pathologically cannot be distinguished from a local thrombosis or one formed elsewhere in the circulation and transported there via the blood stream. Some authors question whether all cases represent unsuspected microthromboembolism and suggest that in situ muscular arterial thrombosis may develop in some cases.[72] Pietra and associates[62] proposed that many of these cases represent primary in situ thrombosis of small pulmonary arteries or thrombotic pulmonary arteriopathy with recanalization, characterized by colander-type luminal lesions.

2. Primary Plexogenic Arteriopathy

The development of plexogenic pulmonary arteriopathy may result from congenital heart disease with a left-to-right shunt or be associated with hepatic injury (i.e., cirrhosis or schistosomiasis of the liver or portal vein thrombosis). Plexogenic pulmonary arteriopathy associated with IPH has also been observed in patients with human immunodeficiency virus (HIV) infection.[73, 74] The pathogenesis of the plexogenic arteriopathy that develops with HIV is unknown, but patients with acquired immunodeficiency syndrome (AIDS) may produce a growth factor that stimulates pulmonary arterial endothelial proliferation.[74] The condition tends to be diagnosed earlier in these patients because of their close medical scrutiny, but survival rates appear no better than those IPH patients without HIV infection. Routine tests for HIV may be recommended in patients who manifest IPH. This association raises the question of viral involvement in the pathogenesis of IPH in general.

Primary or idiopathic plexogenic pulmonary arteriopathy may develop in the absence of any cardiac or hepatic disease. Women are affected two to three times more often than men. It mainly affects children and young adults. At death, not all patients have plexiform lesions, and the pulmonary arteriopathy may be limited to variations of grades 1 to 3 of the Heath-Edwards grading system. An epidemic of pulmonary hypertension in Europe in the 1960s appeared related to the use of the slimming drug aminorex fumarate.[75] The ingestion of "bush tea" has had a similar affect. It has been suggested that such substances may cause subtle injury to the endothelium. The United States Food and Drug Administration approved the use of other amphetamine-like anorexic agents, namely fenfluramine and its d-isomer, dexfenfluramine. There are now reports that these drugs may also induce IPH in susceptible subjects[76, 77] by inhibiting potassium current, causing membrane depolarization and resultant pulmonary arterial vasoconstriction.[78] The drug, and its major metabolite nordexfenfluramine, also releases serotonin from platelets and decreases postsynaptic uptake of serotonin in the brain. Serotonin contracts pulmonary arteries[79] and exerts mitogenic effects on arterial smooth muscle.[80] In addition to pulmonary hypertension, combination therapy with the two anorectic agents, fenfluramine and phentermine, has been associated with valvular heart disease[81–83] that shows features similar to those seen in carcinoid or ergotamine-induced valve disease. Both drugs (fenfluramine and phentermine) have since been withdrawn from the market (see Chapter 17 also).

3. Pulmonary Venoocclusive Disease

Pulmonary venoocclusive disease (PVOD) is a rare pathologic form of clinical IPH. It accounts for about 5% of such cases.[1] The pulmonary venules (Fig. 7-22) show features suggestive of prior thrombotic obstruction with organization as evidenced by considerable, eccentric fibrous intimal thickening.[84] This condition may occur at all ages. The major vascular occlusion lies in the pulmonary venules, which may appear arterialized; the pulmonary arteries show only lesser secondary changes. Capillary congestion, hemorrhage and pulmonary siderosis may also be observed. PVOD is discussed in further detail below.

4. Capillary Hemangiomatosis

In capillary hemangiomatosis,[85, 86] there is a patchy overgrowth of portions of the lung parenchyma (alveolar spaces and walls), plus perivascular and peribronchial interstitium by a proliferation of capillary-sized vessels (Fig. 7-23). Even where this proliferation is less marked, the alveolar septa contain more than only a single capillary. The proliferated vessels appear to contain little if any blood, raising the question of whether the vessels are in continuity with the pulmonary circulation.

Repeated bleeding, inducing associated hemosiderin and calcific deposits, may lead to the clinical symptom of

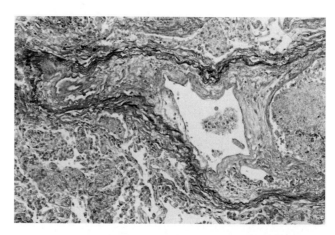

Figure 7-22 • Pulmonary venule within interlobular septum shows severe fibrous intimal thickening characteristic of pulmonary venoocclusive disease (Elastic van Gieson stain).

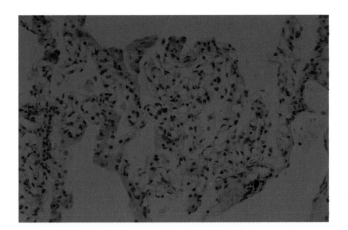

Figure 7-23 • Capillary hemangiomatosis demonstrates an obliterative proliferation of capillary-sized blood vessels within the lung. In this area, the proliferation occupies alveolar airspace (H&E stain).

hemoptysis. Both clinically and microscopically, the condition may mimic pulmonary siderosis and pulmonary venoocclusive disease. The mode of production of IPH is uncertain. The proliferation of capillary-sized vessels may compress venules, and there may be secondary thrombotic obstruction of them. This may lead to medial hypertrophy and intimal thickening in medium-sized pulmonary arteries. The diagnosis of capillary hemangiomatosis is seldom made before death.

In the case reported by Wagenvoort and colleagues,[86] the angiomatous, vasoformative tissue infiltrated vascular walls and regularly destroyed the media and fibrotic intima of the pulmonary veins in the interlobular septa; occasionally, it also affected the pulmonary arteries. Pulmonary hypertension was believed to have resulted from occlusion of pulmonary veins and venules by the invading capillaries.[87] The endothelial nuclei of the capillary channels showed hyperchromasia and pleomorphism. Abundant iron and calcium incrustations were noted in the fibrosed lung.

5. Malalignment of Lung Vessels and Alveolar Capillary Dysplasia

Malalignment of lung vessels[88, 89] is a rare congenital abnormality that leads to persistent neonatal IPH. The syndrome comprises malalignment of lung vessels, impaired maturity of lung tissue with interstitial fibrosis, and persistent neonatal pulmonary hypertension. The pulmonary veins lie immediately adjacent to the pulmonary arteries, sometimes having a common adventitia. In their subsequent course, the veins connect with larger veins in the interlobular septa (Fig. 7-24). The diagnosis is seldom made before death, and it may be missed even after death unless special attention is paid to pulmonary veins. The exact mode of production of the pulmonary hypertension awaits elucidation. Arteriovenous shunting in this form of pulmonary angioplasia cannot be excluded.

6. Isolated Pulmonary Arteritis

In isolated pulmonary arteritis, the pathologic findings of an active or healed arteritis are limited to the pulmo-

nary arteries. No plexiform lesions are detected, but the pulmonary arteries may show varying degrees of medial hypertrophy, intimal fibrosis, and thrombotic lesions.[62] Many patients are children.[90]

Miscellaneous Causes of IPH

A miscellaneous group of conditions, some of which are idiopathic themselves, may lead to pulmonary hypertension. Thus, it is difficult to classify them as IPH or secondary pulmonary hypertension. Various forms of *arteritis* (see later) may be associated with pulmonary hypertension. To avoid duplication, these conditions are not dealt with here.

Pulmonary Vascular Amyloid

Pulmonary vascular amyloid may also produce pulmonary hypertension.[91] Three earlier cases reported in the literature were associated with myeloma, primary amyloidosis, and familial Mediterranean fever. Amyloid-associated pulmonary hypertension may have an insidious clinical onset, and contribute to both morbidity and mortality. Diffuse infiltration of pulmonary arteries by amyloid or light chains may lead to arterial luminal narrowing and, rarely, pulmonary hypertension.[92] The amorphous intramural deposits replace the normal musculoelastic tissue and may mimic healed arteritis on routine sections. Pulmonary vascular amyloidosis is most frequently seen in the diffuse alveolar septal variant of pulmonary amyloidosis; it occurs most often in the setting of primary amyloidosis (AL). In some cases, the vascular deposits are the

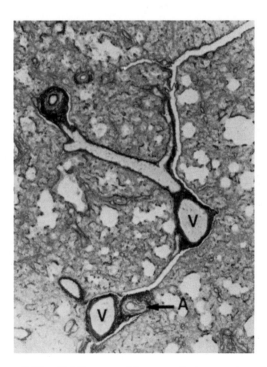

Figure 7-24 • Malalignment of lung vessels in a newborn infant. Pulmonary veins (V) lie adjacent to pulmonary arteries (A) and also merge with larger interlobular septal veins (elastic van Gieson stain). (From Wagenvoort CA, Wagenvoort N: In: Silver MD [ed]: Cardiovascular Pathology, 2nd ed. New York, Churchill Livingstone, 1991.)

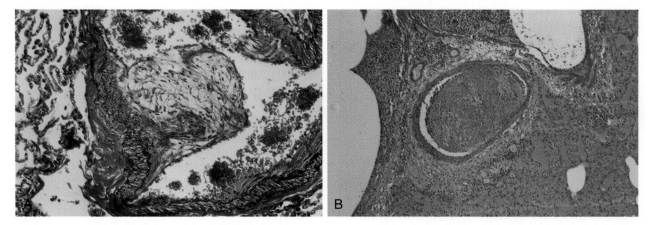

Figure 7-25 • Pulmonary arterial disease caused by percutaneous paraquat absorption. *A,* Eccentric intimal thickening of a small pulmonary artery, probably caused by organized thrombus, in a lung biopsy from a vineyard worker. *B,* Pulmonary arterial thrombosis and subinfarction of the lung in a rat treated with cutaneous applications of paraquat (both H&E stain).

dominant feature. The usual special stains (e.g., sulfated alcian blue, Congo red, thioflavine T, methyl violet, and peroxidase-labeled antibodies to kappa and lambda light chains) are useful to demonstrate amyloid. Patients with amyloidosis also develop pulmonary hypertension secondary to restrictive amyloid heart disease or recurrent pulmonary thromboembolism.

With aging, all breeds of dogs develop vascular amyloid deposits confined to the intima and media of medium-sized pulmonary arteries; such deposits are not detected in other tissues.[93] Apolipoprotein AL-derived pulmonary vascular deposits were detected in 22% of dogs aged 10 years or older. In humans, multiorgan amyloidosis associated with rheumatoid arthritis has led to the formation of plexiform lesions in blood vessels of the brain.[94]

Cocaine Abuse

A single patient has been reported[95] with fatal plexogenic pulmonary hypertension, which was attributed to chronic intravenous abuse of cocaine, unassociated with recurrent thromboembolism or foreign body granulomatous disease of the lung.

Percutaneous Absorption of Paraquat

Absorption of paraquat percutaneously, in amounts insufficient to cause acute, severe pathologic changes, can induce pulmonary damage, both vascular and interstitial, in both humans and experimental animals.[96] Vascular changes include intraarterial thrombi (Fig. 7-25), medial hypertrophy of small arteries, and muscularization of arterioles. Paraquat is not the first toxin known to induce pulmonary arterial changes in animals. Two pyrrolidine alkaloids, monocrotaline and fulvine,[23] both contained in Jamaican bush tea, cause arterial lesions in rats. Bush tea toxicity causes hepatic venoocclusive disease in humans, but the pulmonary arteries are not affected.

Complications of Pulmonary Hypertension

The most serious complication of pulmonary hypertension is death resulting from either (1) right-sided cardiac failure, (2) ventricular fibrillation, or (3) terminal thrombotic occlusion of the right and left pulmonary arteries (Fig. 7-26). Severe pulmonary hypertension can lead to shunt reversal when pulmonary blood pressure exceeds the systemic pressure (so-called Eisenmenger syndrome) (Fig. 7-27). Both true and dissecting aneurysms[97] may complicate pulmonary hypertension (see later). Pulmonary arterial rupture without dissection may also occur.

Cor Pulmonale

The term "cor pulmonale" has been used in a general sense to mean involvement of the heart secondary to lung disease. It is also used to describe hypertrophy or failure of the right ventricle secondary to involvement of the

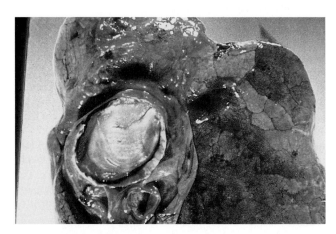

Figure 7-26 • Terminal thrombotic occlusion of an aneurysmal, atherosclerotic left pulmonary artery in a patient with right heart failure from pulmonary hypertension.

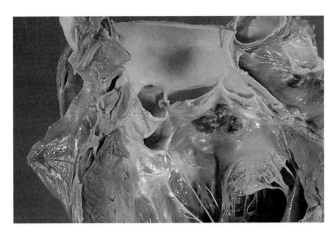

Figure 7-27 • Left ventricular view of a perimembranous ventricular septal defect situated immediately proximal to the aortic valve. Severe pulmonary hypertension led to shunt reversal (Eisenmenger syndrome). The jet lesion on the anterior mitral leaflet (and portion of aortic valve) subsequently became infected and is obscured by infected vegetations.

pulmonary circulation by lung disease. Some authors have suggested that the term be abandoned because it has no precise meaning.[98] According to a WHO definition,[99] cor pulmonale is a "hypertrophy of the cardiac right ventricle resulting from diseases affecting the structure and/or function of the lung, except where these pulmonary alterations are the result of diseases that primarily affect the left side of the heart" (e.g., mitral stenosis); therefore, this definition excludes lung diseases secondary to left-sided cardiac disease.

Cor pulmonale is about five times more common in men than women and three quarters of patients are older than 50 years of age. Known causes of cor pulmonale include the obstructive/obliterative mechanism as well as the vasoconstrictive mechanism described above. The passive venous and hyperkinetic mechanisms of production of pulmonary hypertension do not operate in cor pulmonale. IPH also causes it.

THROMBOSIS OF SMALL PULMONARY ARTERIES

In Conditions of Pulmonary Underperfusion

Congenital heart conditions associated with underperfusion of the lungs (e.g., Fallot tetralogy, pulmonary atresia), favor thrombosis of small pulmonary arteries due to stasis. Coexistent cyanosis may lead to polycythemia, which further increases the risk of thrombosis due to increased blood viscosity. Multiple thrombi may occur, but pulmonary hypertension is usually absent.

Due to Acute Graft-Versus-Host Disease

Lysis of endothelial cells, occurring preferentially in pulmonary blood vessels, has been observed in some bone marrow transplantation recipients with acute graft-versus-host disease.[99a, 99b] The condition produces small pulmonary nodules and fever.

PULMONARY ARTERITIDES

The term arteritis[100] encompasses a heterogeneous group of disorders characterized by inflammatory destruction of the blood vessel wall, i.e., an acute or chronic inflammatory disease that results in structural damage, such as necrosis, fibrosis, elastopathy, or neovascularization of the intima and/or media. The latter changes constitute the final common pathway by which any artery responds to a wide variety of noxious stimuli (see Chapter 6 also).

Affecting Major Pulmonary Arteries

Infectious Arteritis

Pulmonary infectious processes (e.g., tuberculosis) may impinge on a pulmonary artery, but arterial integrity is usually maintained. Infected emboli may weaken the arterial wall from within, and sometimes an infectious (mycotic) aneurysm results.

Noninfectious Arteritis

Takayasu Disease

Takayasu disease commonly affects the major pulmonary arteries[101] (44.2% of the patients described by Ishikawa[102]) in addition to its more usual involvement of the aorta. Others[103] have stated that the pulmonary artery is only occasionally involved. Rarely, isolated pulmonary artery involvement can occur, the so-called type IV in the Ueda classification of Takayasu disease[104–106] as modified by Lupi-Herrera and colleagues.[107] It should be noted that the Nasu classification, which is more commonly used in Japan than the Ueda classification,[105] does not include pulmonary artery involvement separately. The American College of Rheumatology has defined diagnostic criteria for Takayasu disease.[108]

The macroscopic and microscopic changes in elastic pulmonary arteries (Fig. 7-28A) are identical to those observed in the aorta (i.e., a medial granulomatous inflammatory response to focal necrosis of the media with subsequent healed mesoaortitis and reactive fibrotic thickening of both intima and adventitia). A patient with right-sided pulmonary artery stenosis and pulmonary valve stenosis resulting from Takayasu arteritis has been reported.[109] In another case, occlusion of the right upper lobe pulmonary artery produced left circumflex coronary steal and myocardial ischemia.[110] Koyabu and associates[111] encountered a 52-year-old man with Takayasu disease and recurrent pulmonary hemorrhage in whom angiography revealed occlusion of many branches of the pulmonary artery. They were filled via collateral circulation from coronary, intercostal, and internal mammary arteries. Pulmonary hypertension and right-sided heart failure caused by Takayasu arteritis has also been re-

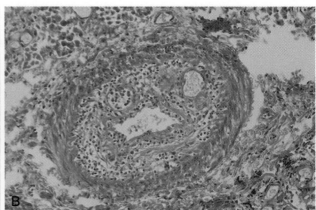

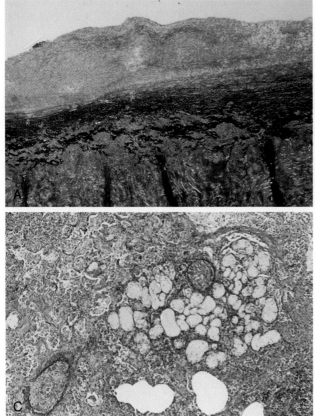

Figure 7-28 • Pulmonary arteriopathy in Takayasu disease. *A,* Scarring of main pulmonary artery; note adventitial fibrosis (bottom), outer medial destruction (middle), and intimal fibrous thickening (top). *B,* Microscopic pulmonary arteriopathy. *C,* Dilation lesion (top right) surrounds a plexiform-like lesion. (*A* and *C,* elastic van Gieson stain; *B,* H&E stain). (From Rose AG, Halper J, Factor SM: Primary anteriopathy in Takayasu's disease. Arch Pathol Lab Med 108:644, 1984. Copyrighted 1984, American Medical Association.)

ported.[112] The patient in question had no pulmonary perfusion of the left lung.

Over many years, 7% of a large series of patients with Takayasu disease encountered at Groote Schuur Hospital, Cape Town, South Africa, had pulmonary arterial involvement.[105] This was probably an underestimation of frequency because sophisticated clinical means of evaluating the pulmonary circulation were not available during the first 20 years of the series.

Giant Cell Arteritis

Pulmonary involvement is rare in giant cell arteritis.[113] Pulmonary disease is said to be present in 9% of patients but has seldom been studied pathologically.[114] Manifestations include interstitial infiltrates, pulmonary nodules, pulmonary arterial vasculitis, and granuloma formation in elastic and muscular pulmonary arteries. Giant cell arteritis may lead to pulmonary artery obstruction[115] and even lung infarction after superimposed thrombosis.[116] Surgical intervention to relieve pulmonary arterial obstruction caused by giant cell arteritis may be useful at times.[117]

Behçet Disease

Behçet disease is a systemic vasculitis exhibiting the triad of uveitis and both oral and genital ulceration. Large pulmonary artery vasculitis is a frequent finding. Pulmonary arterial aneurysm may result.[118, 119] Small vessel vasculitis and capillaritis are rarer and have been attributed to immune complex deposition.[120] The aorta may develop saccular or dissecting aneurysms, and large venous thrombophlebitis is also a feature.[121]

Affecting Small Pulmonary Arteries

Infectious Arteritis

Small pulmonary arterial branches may span the lumen of tuberculous cavities in the lung. Certain fungal elements which have an affinity for blood vessels, e.g. Aspergillus or Mucormycosis, may infect pulmonary arteries. Immunosuppressed patients are particularly prone to pulmonary fungal infections.

Noninfectious Arteritis

Takayasu Disease

Takayasu disease may also affect small intrapulmonary vessels producing a unique, little recognized form of pulmonary arteriopathy[122] (Fig. 7-28*B* and *C*) that is characterized by focal deficiencies in the outer media, with a granulation tissue type of capillary ingrowth both here and in the thickened, fibrosed intima. Depending on the stage of the arteriopathy, there may be a mononuclear cell arteritis and widespread focal angiomatoid-like (dilation) lesions in the lung. A similar form of arteriopathy was observed in a major coronary artery in one of three patients reported by Rose and colleagues.[122]

Sarcoidosis

The etiology of sarcoidosis is unknown, but the pulmonary pathology is consistent with an inhaled causative agent. The true incidence of large proximal pulmonary artery involvement in sarcoidosis is unknown, but it has

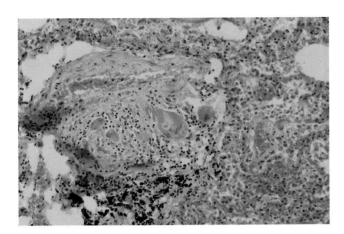

Figure 7-29 • Pulmonary sarcoidosis. An active granuloma involves the wall of a small pulmonary artery. One giant cell contains a typical asteroid body (H&E stain).

been reported occasionally.[123] The disease is the commonest cause of granulomatous pulmonary angiitis affecting small vessels. Other causes include active tuberculosis, necrotizing sarcoid granulomatosis, Wegener granulomatosis, bilharziasis, foreign body embolization, and chronic berylliosis. Granulomatous angiitis is present in 69% of open lung biopsies from patients with sarcoidosis.[124, 125] Transbronchial lung biopsies are less helpful diagnostically. Sarcoid granulomas (Fig. 7-29) preferentially affect the upper two thirds of both lungs. Elastic stains aid the detection of small vessel involvement. In biopsies, the disease is more common in pulmonary venules (92%) compared with its incidence in small pulmonary arteries (39%). In the study of positive biopsy samples by Rosen and associates,[125] 31% had both arterial and venous granulomas, 61% had venous granulomas alone, and 8% had arterial granulomas only. Most granulomas appear to arise intravascularly, and, depending on the stage at which they are seen, may be limited to the vascular intima.[124] Other granulomas lie extravascularly and impinge on a blood vessel as a granuloma expands in size. The relationship between sarcoidal granulomatous angiitis and the subsequent development of pulmonary hypertension is not clear-cut. Salazar and colleagues[126] reported the second case of sarcoidosis with combined portal and pulmonary hypertension.

In this era of organ transplantation, it should be noted that normal organs transplanted into recipients with preexisting sarcoidosis are likely to develop sarcoid granulomas, whereas organs from donors with known sarcoidosis given to "normal" recipients do not appear to develop significant or progressive disease.[127]

Necrotizing Sarcoid Granulomatosis

The relationship of necrotizing sarcoid granulomatosis (NSG) to sarcoidosis is unknown.[128] The terminology begs the question of whether the disease represents necrotizing angiitis with a sarcoid reaction, or sarcoidosis with necrosis of granulomas and inflamed blood vessels, arteries, and veins. At present, NSG is regarded as a variant of sarcoidosis, because clinical and radiologic features suggest it is the histologic substratum of a variety of sarcoidosis termed "nodular sarcoidosis."[129] Necrosis in NSG is strongly correlated with the presence of severe vasculitis.[130]

Wegener Granulomatosis

Wegener granulomatosis[131] (WG) is a multisystemic disorder characterized by the triad of (1) necrotizing vasculitis and aseptic necrosis of the upper respiratory tract, nose, and sinuses; (b) usually multiple, bilateral pulmonary lesions caused by vasculitis with necrotizing granuloma formation and (3) focal, segmental glomerulitis that may progress to crescentic glomerulonephritis. Variants, with involvement of other organs, or sparing of one or two of the classic sites, are encountered. The pathologic manifestations of pulmonary WG[132] can be divided into the following three major criteria: (1) vasculitis-producing arteritis (Fig. 7-30), venulitis, and capillaritis, which can be acute, chronic, necrotizing granulomatosis, non-necrotizing granulomatosis, and/or that associated with fibrinoid necrosis and cicatricial changes; (2) parenchymal necrosis as microabscesses or geographic necrosis; and (3) granulomatous inflammation with a mixed inflammatory cellular response, scattered giant cells, palisaded histiocytes, and poorly formed granulomas. Vasculitis is often found in blood vessels situated within the nodular inflammatory lesions of WG. Only about 10% of open lung biopsy specimens show vasculitis away from such inflammatory lesions. WG is only one of many potential causes of diffuse pulmonary hemorrhage associated with vasculitis.

The cause of the disease is not known, but a hypersensitivity reaction to an unknown antigen has been postulated to lead to necrotizing vasculitis. The granulomatous, pseudotuberculous inflammatory response around vessels includes scattered neutrophils, occasionally microabscesses, and both eosinophils and lymphocytes. The vasculitis is easy to overlook. The nodular mass lesions in the lungs may cavitate. The histology correlates poorly with a serum antineutrophil cytoplasmic antibody (ANCA).

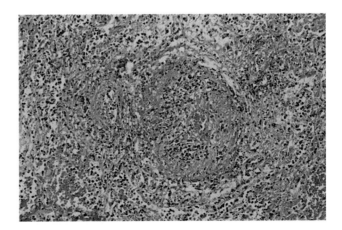

Figure 7-30 • Acute pulmonary microvasculitis in Wegener granulomatosis of the lung (H&E stain).

Mixed Connective Tissue Disease

Mixed connective tissue disease (MCTD) is the term used to describe patients who clinically have coexistent features suggestive of systemic lupus erythematosus (SLE), polymyositis, and systemic sclerosis, often with the presence of nuclear ribonucleoprotein antibody and the absence of antibodies to DNA and Sm antigen that categorize SLE. About 80% of patients are females. Pulmonary hypertension is one of the leading causes of death in MCTD.[133] Watanabe and associates[134] reported that in clinically stable women, delivery of a baby may lead to pulmonary thromboembolism and secondary pulmonary hypertension. The pathogenesis of the pulmonary hypertension is unknown, but it is claimed by some authors that autoantibodies might cause derangement of endothelial cells and lead to a proliferative vasculopathy characteristic of pulmonary hypertension in MCTD.[135] Others have specifically implicated anticardiolipin antibodies in the development of the pulmonary hypertension.[133] Its evolution appears to correlate with diffuse involvement by arteries greater than 200 μ in diameter.[136] The endothelial damage in the early stage, followed by microthrombi and proliferation of intimal myocytes, seems to progress to severe pulmonary vascular disease with pulmonary hypertension. Recovery from pulmonary hypertension of an adolescent with MCTD treated with vasodilator and antiinflammatory drugs has been reported.[137] As MCTD evolves, some patients develop features of a specific collagen disease.

Classic Polyarteritis Nodosa

The pathology of polyarteritis nodosa (PAN) is that of a necrotizing arteritis of medium-sized and small arteries in various organs.[138] Crops of lesions of differing ages occur. Pulmonary artery involvement has been considered rare. Previously, it was also thought that patients with PAN do not have interstitial pneumonitis and fibrosis. A detailed pathologic study[139] of the lungs of 10 autopsied patients revealed that 70% had bronchial arteritis and 50% diffuse alveolar damage (DAD) involving all lobes bilaterally; DAD was acute in two patients and organizing in three. In the latter, fibrosis was more severe in the lower lobes. DAD and interstitial fibrosis are complications of PAN. Nevertheless, pulmonary arteries are seldom affected. Cases of "polyarteritis nodosa" in which asthma, blood eosinophilia, and pulmonary infiltrates are found are most likely examples of allergic granulomatosis or Churg-Strauss syndrome.[140, 141] It consists of granulomas with associated eosinophils in patients with a background of a severe allergy such as asthma, allergic rhinitis, or, occasionally, drug sensitization.

Microscopic Polyangiitis (Microscopic Form of Polyarteritis Nodosa)

Microscopic polyarteritis was alternatively named microscopic polyangiitis.[142] Akikusa and colleagues[143] reported that necrotizing alveolar capillaritis was detected in about half of their 25 microscopic polyangiitis autopsy cases that exhibited early stage systemic vasculitis. Pulmonary arteritis, which correlated positively with necrotizing alveolar capillaritis, was observed in 16% of cases. The latter lesion may lead to diffuse intrapulmonary hemorrhage. Pulmonary capillaritis and necrotizing alveolar capillaritis have been described in various diseases, including the collagen vascular disorders.[144]

Systemic Lupus Erythematosus

Defined previously, SLE is the most common connective tissue disorder and may affect any organ in the body. Pleuropulmonary manifestations (e.g., pleuritis with or without an effusion) occur in 50% of cases. More serious lesions in the lung include acute or chronic lupus pneumonitis, pulmonary sepsis, and pulmonary hypertension.[145] There is an association between SLE and the antiphospholipid syndrome leading to venous thrombosis and pulmonary embolism. Leg vein thrombosis is part of the antiphospholipid syndrome that in turn is not limited to patients with SLE.[146] However, the pulmonary hypertension that occurs in about 14% of patients with SLE[147] is of the plexogenic arteriopathy type.[148] Some patients with SLE may have coexistent sarcoidosis or pneumoconiosis.

Other Connective Tissue Diseases

Pulmonary hypertension has been reported in association with dermatomyositis[149] and in systemic sclerosis as well as in its CREST syndrome variant[150] (*c*alcinosis, *R*aynaud phenomenon, *e*sophageal dysfunction, *s*clerodactyly, and *t*elangiectasia). Approximately 9 to 50% of patients with CREST syndrome have pulmonary hypertension. Overall, about one third of patients with systemic sclerosis have pulmonary hypertension with pulmonary arteries showing intimal fibrosis and medial hypertrophy without plexiform lesions. Vasculitis is decidedly uncommon. Rheumatoid arthritis rarely produces pulmonary hypertension. When the latter occurs it is characterized by necrotizing arteritis of small pulmonary arteries. Plexiform lesions are not seen.[151]

Segmental Mediolytic Arteriopathy

Segmental mediolytic arteriopathy (SMA) is a newly described, rare variant of arterial fibromuscular dysplasia that mainly affects visceral small and medium-sized arteries[152–154] (see Chapter 6). The condition may manifest at any age. Myolytic dysplasia of the arterial media with associated intramural dissection, thrombosis, or rupture of aneurysms can cause visceral hemorrhage or infarction. Due to aneurysm formation, the condition may be clinically misdiagnosed as polyarteritis nodosa. Lie[153] reported involvement of the pulmonary arteries by SMA (Fig. 7-31A).

Chemical Arteritis

Aspiration of gastric contents into the bronchial tree and alveoli may induce a chemical arteritis (Fig. 7-31B) affecting small pulmonary arteries in the field of aspiration and digestion of the lung parenchyma. The arterial damage may evoke a polymorphonuclear inflammatory cellular response if the patient does not die immediately. As far as I am aware, this form of arteritis has not yet been documented in the literature. The inhalation of kerosene by children may produce similar pulmonary damage.

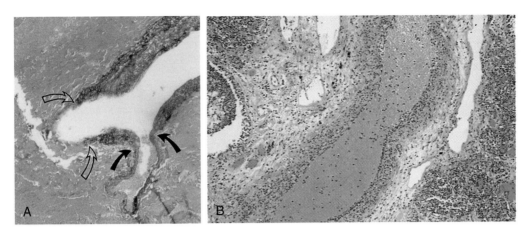

Figure 7-31 • *A,* Pulmonary artery with segmental mediolysis (defined by arrows) surrounded by diffuse lung hemorrhage. (From Lie JT: Systemic, cerebral, and pulmonary segmental mediolytic arteriopathy: Villainous masquerades of vasculitis. Cardiovasc Pathol 5:305, 1996.) *B,* Small pulmonary artery within an area of recent aspiration of gastric contents shows numerous neutrophils infiltrating all layers of its wall induced by chemical (acidic) digestion. (Both H&E stain.)

ANEURYSMS OF THE MAIN PULMONARY ARTERY AND ITS MAJOR BRANCHES

True Aneurysm

Any condition that either weakens the wall of the pulmonary artery or leads to pulmonary hypertension may favor the formation of pulmonary arterial aneurysms (see Chapter 5 also). Thoracic Behçet syndrome is characterized by thrombosis of the superior vena cava and the formation of characteristic aneurysms of the pulmonary arteries.[155]

True aneurysms of the pulmonary artery[156] are more common in the left and right main pulmonary vessels than in the pulmonary trunk (Fig. 7-32), despite the relative frequency of poststenotic dilation of the pulmonary artery in pulmonary valvar stenosis. Such pulmonary artery aneurysms (PAA) tend to be more often saccular than fusiform, bland rather than infective or mycotic, and associated with pulmonary hypertension or congenital heart disease, particularly patent ductus arteriosus, rather than being congenital[157] or idiopathic in nature, per se. Aneurysms associated with patent ductus arteriosus may be either bland and related to elevated pressure; less often, they are mycotic and caused by infective endocarditis.[158] Surgical ligation of a patent ductus arteriosus may also be followed by formation of an aneurysm.[159] PAA have also been associated with IPH, mitral valve disease, and other forms of pulmonary hypertension.[23] Marfan syndrome as well as its forme fruste may predispose the patient to pulmonary artery aneurysm caused by the medionecrotic-like changes in the pulmonary arterial media. Some cases of so-called idiopathic dilation of the pulmonary artery may be related to forme fruste of Marfan syndrome. Rupture of a pulmonary arterial aneurysm has been reported.[160]

Dissecting Aneurysm

Dissecting aneurysms[161] of the pulmonary arteries are rare. Segmental mediolytic arteriopathy, which may predispose to dissection of peripheral pulmonary arterial branches, is discussed earlier. Rupture of a dissecting aneurysm of the pulmonary artery in a 27-year-old pregnant woman with an uncorrected patent ductus arteriosus and severe pulmonary hypertension has been reported.[162] The wall of the affected pulmonary artery showed atherosclerosis and cystic medionecrosis. A dissecting aneurysm of the thoracic aorta may also impinge on the major pulmonary arteries (i.e., the right pulmonary artery may be totally occluded by an acute dissecting aneurysm of the ascending aorta[163]).

Air Dissection of Pulmonary Artery Branches

Interstitial emphysema of the lungs, which usually complicates positive pressure ventilation of the lungs, especially in infants, may lead to tracking of air both

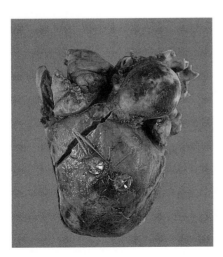

Figure 7-32 • Aneurysmal pulmonary artery in a young child who had surgical correction of a common atrioventricular canal defect. Severe pulmonary hypertension was present.

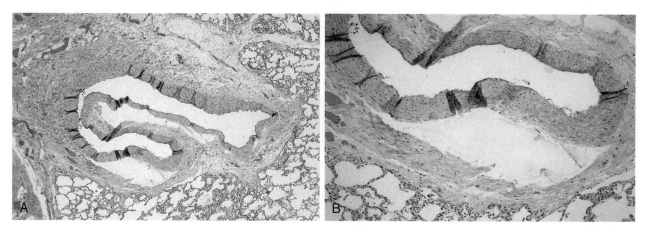

Figure 7-33 • *A*, Pulmonary interstitial emphysema led to dissection of air between the media and the adventitia (lower) of an intrapulmonary branch of the pulmonary artery. Additional air is present in a similar situation between the two branches (center). *B*, High-power view of lower branch of the pulmonary artery shown in *A* shows air separating media (top) from adventitia (bottom). (Both H&E stain.).

around and sometimes within the walls of the pulmonary arteries and veins. Although prolonged survival after the onset of interstitial emphysema may lead to a giant cell response around the edge of the air bubbles, no such response is noted if the patient does not survive for long after the event. The dissection of the air usually occurs either external to or within the adventitia or separates the adventitia from the media of the affected pulmonary vessels (Fig. 7-33). Such dissection is often overlooked at autopsy. The major complication of interstitial air is related to its splinting effect, which causes loss of lung elasticity and compression both of blood vessels and mediastinum by air bubbles. "Air block" is a rare phenomenon in which the hilar arteries and veins are compressed and occluded by the dissecting air.[164]

Gas Embolism

This may arise rarely as a complication of the air block syndrome. Rupture of alveolar walls may allow air (or therapeutically administered oxygen) to escape into the pulmonary veins and eventually into the systemic arteries and veins when the intraalveolar pressure exceeds that of the veins. Since oxygen may diffuse out of the vasculature after death,[165] one may encounter a situation in which radiography at the time of death may reveal gas in the heart and great vessels, but no gas may be evident in the major vessels on repeat radiography before autopsy a day later.

False Aneurysm

I have encountered a false aneurysm (Fig. 7-34) of the pulmonary artery that complicated bronchoscopy in a patient with a bronchogenic carcinoma. The instrument passed through necrotic hilar tumor tissue and disrupted the wall of a major pulmonary arterial branch. Death followed delayed rupture of the unorganized wall of the communicating hematoma.

Infectious (Mycotic) Aneurysm

A septic embolus that lodges within a branch of the pulmonary artery, or a pulmonary parenchymal inflamma-

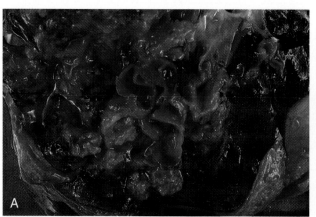
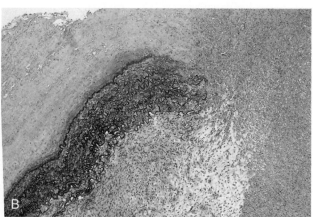

Figure 7-34 • False aneurysm of left pulmonary artery. *A*, Aneurysm (center) abuts on pulmonary artery branch (top right) to left lower lobe of lung. Friable tumor surrounds the aneurysm. *B*, Site of traumatic disruption of the pulmonary artery (Elastic van Gieson stain).

tory process, may lead to a mycotic aneurysm. A Rasmussen aneurysm is a special type of mycotic aneurysm encountered on a pulmonary artery branch spanning a tuberculous cavity within the lung.

TUMORS OF THE PULMONARY ARTERY

Malignant Fibrous Histiocytoma (Sarcoma)

Sarcoma of the pulmonary artery includes a heterogeneous group of neoplasms showing variable degrees of differentiation along several mesenchymal lines.[166, 167] More than 100 have been reported, mostly as single case reports. Few of these cases were subject to either immunocytochemistry or electron microscopy. Most sarcomas of the pulmonary artery have been previously classified as undifferentiated, and those given a more specific categorization (e.g., chondrosarcoma, osteosarcoma, angiosarcoma, liposarcoma, rhabdomyosarcoma) were often diagnosed at postmortem examination in the absence of ancillary studies. The largest review of such cases from a single institution, which included immunohistochemistry and electron microscopy, was a series of six endarterectomy cases of pulmonary artery sarcomas reported by Boue and colleagues.[168] The authors concluded, from a review of the immunocytochemistry findings in their material and 15 previous similarly examined cases in the literature, that pulmonary artery sarcoma was not a grossly homogeneous neoplasm, because background stromal elements varied from myxoid, gelatinous, and polypoid to firm, fibrous, and concentric, including a combination of forms in the same tumor. The tumors were invasive and often embolized to the lungs, but distant metastases were rare. Most pulmonary artery sarcomas were best classified as malignant fibrous histiocytoma (five of their six cases). Immunohistochemical staining tended to be positive for vimentin, α_1-antichymotrypsin, α_1-antitrypsin, neuron-specific enolase, and muscle-specific actin, and negative for cytokeratin, lysozyme, Ulex europaeus, factor VIII–related antigen, chromogranin, S100, and neurofilament antigen. Electron microscopy is helpful in excluding specific differentiation. A pulmonary artery sarcoma may present as benign thromboembolic disease and can be an unanticipated finding in endarterectomy specimens.

ANGIOCENTRIC LUNG TUMORS

Inflammatory Pseudotumor

Inflammatory pseudotumor (IPT), or plasma cell granuloma, is a well-recognized entity both in the lung and other organs. It tends to occur in young people less than 30 years of age and may mimic a lung tumor clinically.[169] Some pulmonary pseudotumors exhibit angioinfiltrative behavior,[170] and four of the seven cases reported by Nonomura and associates[169] showed vascular invasion of medium-sized blood vessels at the periphery of the lesions. Those authors stated that an angioinvasive growth

pattern might not be infrequent. A case of IPT affecting major epicardial coronary arteries has also been reported.[171] Immunostaining with p53 has been used to distinguish IPT from sarcoma involving the lung.[172] Although IPT is widely believed to be an inflammatory/reactive lesion rather than a neoplasm, a first report of clonal cytogenetic changes in a pulmonary IPT suggested it might be a true neoplasm.[173]

Lymphomatoid Granulomatosis

Lymphomatoid granulomatosis[174] is an angiocentric, necrotizing (coagulative necrosis) lymphoproliferative disorder, which is now regarded as a form of T-cell lymphoma. Partially necrotic, tumor-like masses in the lung measuring from a few millimeters to 10 cm in diameter (Fig. 7-35) are centered on pulmonary arterial or venous branches, which are often characterized by preservation of the outline of the infiltrated blood vessels and intact elastic laminae on elastic van Gieson stain. The necrotic lesions may cavitate. Histologically, the pleomorphic lymphoid infiltrate has a mildly granulomatous appearance in some areas.

Epithelioid or Histiocytoid Hemangioendothelioma

This condition, previously termed intravascular bronchioloalveolar tumor or IVBAT, is a rare tumor derived from vasoformative cells.[175] It affects women approximately 30 years of age who develop multiple pulmonary nodules. Tumor cells (Fig. 7-36) grow intravascularly and also fill alveoli and bronchioles.

CONDITIONS AFFECTING PULMONARY VEINS

Anomalous Pulmonary Venous Connection

The term anomalous pulmonary venous connection indicates the anatomic condition in which a pulmonary vein fails to join the left atrium, but, instead, joins the right atrium or a systemic vein. Total anomalous pulmonary venous connection (TAPVC) is a serious condition in which none of the pulmonary veins join the left atrium. A partial anomalous venous connection is more likely to be encountered in later life than TAPVC.

Age-Related Changes in Pulmonary Venules

In the peripheral pulmonary veins (i.e., medium-sized veins, small veins, and postcapillary venules), the severity of intimal thickening is age dependent.[176] Collagenous venular intimal thickening is common after 20 years of age. The pathogenesis and clinical significance of age-related intimal thickening of pulmonary veins awaits elucidation. For example, it is not known whether these changes influence the respiratory function of normal individuals.

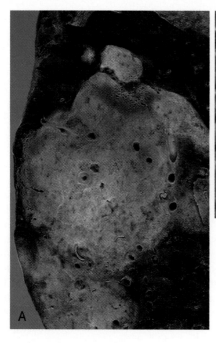

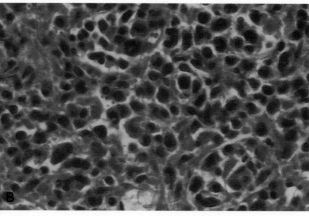

Figure 7-35 • Lymphomatoid granulomatosis. *A,* Solid pulmonary tumor mass showing clear outlines of preexisting blood vessels within the lesion. *B,* Lymphomatous infiltrate of atypical-looking lymphocytes (H&E stain).

Pulmonary Venoocclusive Disease

Pulmonary venoocclusive disease (PVOD), has been referred to earlier. It is a primary pulmonary venular thrombotic process leading to luminal obstruction by intimal fibrosis (see Fig. 7-22). Findings consistent with organized thrombi include fibrous webs and septa with multiple smaller lumens between them in pulmonary venules (a colander-like appearance). Secondary changes in the pulmonary arteries are of a lesser order and are overshadowed by prominent venous changes. Computerized tomography may yield findings suggestive of PVOD, but definitive diagnosis requires lung biopsy.[177] PVOD may have a multifactorial etiology. About one third of cases occur in childhood with an equal sex distribution; in adults, there is a slight male preponderence; occasionally, the condition is familial. Many patients have no antecedent symptoms or associated conditions, whereas some may have ingested bush tea containing *Crotalaria* alkaloids.[178] Patients may also have had a pulmonary viral infection; no agents may have been cultured; or the patient might be affected by drug toxicity (e.g., bleomycin therapy for lymphoma,[179, 180] mitomycin, treatment with the nitrosourea BCNU[181]). It is claimed that PVOD may be associated with lymphoma per se.[182] Alkylating agents used to treat patients with cancer may damage parenchymal veins throughout the body, and the general venous system should be carefully examined in such patients.[183] PVOD occuring in a patient with SLE has been reported.[184] The condition has also complicated both bone marrow transplantation[185] and use of oral contraceptives.[186] An association between PVOD and hypertrophic cardiomyopathy has been noted.[187, 188] The coexistence of these two rare conditions appears to be more than a chance association. Genetic studies of patients with PVOD are indicated to explore the possibility of a common genetic context for their coexistence in a single patient.

Pyemic Abscesses of the Lung

Any systemic suppurative process (e.g., right-sided infective endocarditis [RIE], liver abscess, renal infection, otitis media) may lead to pyemic abscesses in the lung caused by embolism of infected material. Apart from RIE, the other processes involve venous thrombosis with secondary infection of the thrombus and thrombolysis in the pathogenesis of the pyemic lung abscesses (see the infectious causes of arteritis, discussed earlier).

Lung Inflammation as a Source of Systemic Embolism

Inflammatory lesions within the lung, such as a lung abscess or multiple pyemic abscesses; a septic, infected infarct; or bronchiectasis, which may sometimes be asso-

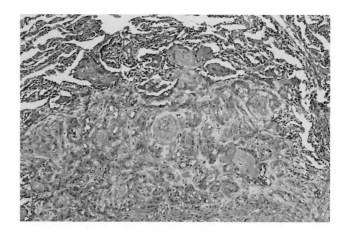

Figure 7-36 • Epithelioid or histiocytoid hemangioendothelioma (previously named intravascular bronchioloalveolar tumor [IVBAT]). Multiple hyalinized nodules with tumor cells at their margins fill alveoli, bronchioles, and small blood vessels (H&E stain).

ciated with mucoviscidosis and tuberculosis, may lead to secondary thrombosis of a pulmonary vein or venule. This thrombus may be either bland or infected. Its detachment leads to systemic thromboembolism because the pulmonary veins connect directly with the left atrium. This easily overlooked source of systemic thromboembolism exists in some cases of a suspected paradoxical embolism in which there is no other apparent source for systemic emboli.

Kubo and colleagues[189] angioscopically examined the peripheral pulmonary arteries in 14 patients with chronic lung diseases. Abnormal findings were more frequent in chronic bronchitis and pulmonary tuberculosis than in chronic emphysema. "Vasculitis" and thrombus exist in the peripheral pulmonary arteries of chronic lung diseases, and angioscopy may provide more details about the vascular wall and lumen compared with those of pulmonary angiography.

CONDITIONS AFFECTING BRONCHIAL ARTERIES

There are two major groups of bronchial arteries: (1) the posterior arteries arise from intercostal vessels or directly from the aorta, and (2) accessory bronchial arteries, including those passing to the trachea and carina, arise from the innominate artery proximal to its bifurcation. Bronchial arteries, which supply the lamina propria of large bronchi, characteristically have a predominance of longitudinal smooth muscle in their wall and possess only an inner elastic lamina. In the lung periphery, it may be difficult to distinguish bronchial arteries from diseased pulmonary vessels without injection studies.

Bronchial arteries may achieve major significance[190] in two circumstances: (1) in diseases of the bronchial tree including bronchiectasis, in which there is evidence of new vessel formation; (2) in certain forms of congenital heart disease, such as right-sided ventricular outflow tract obstruction of pulmonary atresia, which produces pulmonary oligemia unless the ductus arteriosus remains patent. In such situations, some bronchial arteries become greatly enlarged and tortuous (Fig. 7-37). In severe pulmonary hypertension, the bronchial circulation may act as a collateral system for the pulmonary arterial tree, because there is usually a precapillary bronchopulmonary arterial linkup, both within the lung and via pleural adhesions.

PULMONARY EDEMA

Pulmonary edema may have a hemodynamic cause or result from microvascular injury, negative pressure, or idiopathic mechanisms.

Hemodynamic Edema

Pulmonary edema is a common occurrence in patients with congestive cardiac failure, no matter what its cause, and is a result of pulmonary congestion leading to hydrostatic force in the pulmonary capillary bed exceeding the

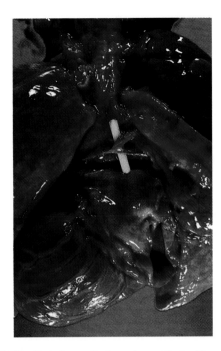

Figure 7-37 • Posterior mediastinum in a patient with severe tetralogy of Fallot. An enlarged bronchial collateral artery, defined by marker, arises from the descending thoracic aorta and bifurcates to supply both lungs.

colloid oncotic pressure. Decreased oncotic pressure resulting from hypoalbuminemia (i.e., caused by protein-losing enteropathy, nephrotic syndrome, liver disease, or lymphatic obstruction) may also induce pulmonary edema.

Edema Caused by Microvascular Injury

A wide variety of stimuli, including infectious agents such as viruses or *Mycoplasma;* inhaled gases (e.g., ammonia nitrogen dioxide in silo fillers disease, smoke, sulfur dioxide); aspirated liquids (e.g., gastric juice, paraffin); drugs/chemicals (e.g., bleomycin, amphotericin B, paraquat); and miscellaneous causes, including shock, uremia, acute pancreatitis, radiation, and extracorporeal circulation, may all induce microvascular injury and promote an outpouring of edema fluid.

Negative Pressure Pulmonary Edema

Acute pulmonary edema caused by upper airway obstruction has been rarely reported in adults[191] but may be underdiagnosed. Upper airway obstruction caused by obstructed endotracheal tubes may at times be an unrecognized cause of pulmonary edema in intensive care units.[192] Factors contributing to this type of pulmonary edema include: (1) the main mechanism, which is negative intrathoracic and transpulmonary pressure; (2) an acquired permeability defect in alveolar capillary membranes secondary to vigorous inspiration; (3) hypoxia; (4) inflammation; and (5) reflex vasoconstriction induced by hypoxia.

Idiopathic Pulmonary Edema

High-Altitude Pulmonary Edema

Persons living at lower altitudes who suddenly travel to very high altitudes (e.g., mountaineers who ascend rapidly to heights greater than 2500 m), may develop pulmonary edema through a mechanism that is not well understood. Vigorous young men are most susceptible to high-altitude pulmonary edema (HAPE). The pathophysiology of HAPE is unknown, but hypoxia-induced pulmonary artery hypertension is a cardinal feature.[193] The edema fluid has a high protein content and resembles that encountered in so-called neurogenic pulmonary edema, in pulmonary edema following relief of airway obstruction, in pulmonary edema that occurs after surgery to augment pulmonary blood flow in congenital heart disease,[194] or in pulmonary edema resulting from heroin overdose.[195] Scherrer and associates[196] reported that inhalation of nitric oxide improves arterial oxygenation in HAPE because of its favorable action on blood flow distribution in the lungs. The authors postulated two sites where nitric oxide may exert its beneficial effect: (1) the muscular pulmonary arteries in which persons prone to HAPE may have defects in nitric-oxide-mediated vasodilatation, and (2) the capillary bed, where defective synthesis of nitric oxide may increase leakage of water, protein, and cells. Jerome and Severinghaus[194] suggested a unifying hypothesis whereby HAPE results from the stress failure of overdistended, relatively thin-walled pulmonary arteries, rather than from capillary rupture. A role for sympathetic nervous system overactivity, such as occurs in neurogenic, postobstructive and heroin–overdose-induced pulmonary edema, cannot be excluded in HAPE.

"Neurogenic" Pulmonary Edema

Raised intracranial, pressure may lead to pulmonary edema, which is thought to be caused by a neurogenic mechanism. However, the experimental work of Novitzky and colleagues[197] with regard to the effects of brain death on the cardiac transplant donor patient has shown that so-called neurogenic edema (Fig. 7-38) is really caused by a hemodynamic mechanism. During the initial phase of

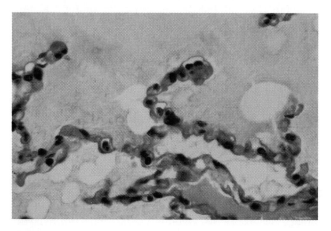

Figure 7-38 • Experimentally induced and erroneously so-called "neurogenic" pulmonary edema produced by elevating intracranial pressure in an anesthetized baboon (H&E stain).

intracranial hypertension, Cushing reflex—the release of endogenous catecholamines at cardiac and vascular levels—induces a massive increase of the systemic vascular resistance and the mean arterial pressure.[198] These hemodynamic changes acutely increase myocardial wall stress, resulting in acute subendocardial coronary insufficiency. When systemic vascular resistance is maximally elevated, cardiac output decreases and left atrial pressure increases above the mean pulmonary artery pressure, occasionally exceeding 90 mm Hg. This is caused by mitral insufficiency from papillary muscle dysfunction induced by subendocardial ischemia. A transient increase in left atrial pressure may result in pulmonary edema. When systemic vascular resistance decreases, the left atrial pressure returns to levels before brain death.

LUNG TRANSPLANTATION

The pulmonary microcirculation is affected in both acute and chronic rejection. However, perivascular lymphoid infiltration is not specific for acute rejection, because it may be a feature of certain viral infections (e.g., cytomegalovirus inclusion body disease[199]).

Acute Rejection

Acute rejection occurs most commonly within the first 3 months after transplantation. Many centers perform unilateral lung transplants. The grading system shown in Table 7-4 is used.[200] Inflammation of the venules (Figs. 7-39 and 7-40) within interlobular septa may also be noted in acute rejection, but thrombosis of the lymphocyte infiltrated vessels is rare.

Chronic Rejection

Bronchiolitis obliterans is the major feature of chronic rejection. In addition, graft arteriopathy is concomitant with similar changes in donor coronary arteries, if a combined heart-lung transplantation was done. Most long-term survivors of lung transplantation have severe bronchiectasis. The effect of the latter on the bronchial circulation has been alluded to earlier.

TABLE 7-4 • **Grading System Used in Acute Rejection of the Lung**

Grade 1:	Minimal rejection	Perivascular lymphoid infiltrate only affects occasional small vessels in transbronchial lung biopsies (see Fig. 7–38)
Grade 2:	Mild rejection	Plentiful and larger perivascular, mononuclear cell infiltrates easily seen at low power; frequent subendothelial infiltration and endothelialitis
Grade 3:	Moderate rejection	Perivascular infiltrates extend into adjacent alveolar septae and alveolar sacs
Grade 4:	Severe rejection	Changes as in grade 3, but with extensive alveolar septal involvement and diffuse alveolar damage

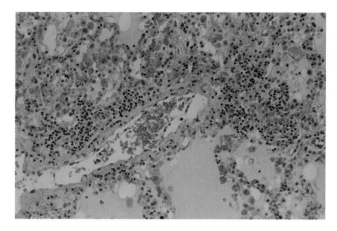

Figure 7-39 • Mild acute venulitis caused by mild acute grade 2 rejection of donor lung (H&E).

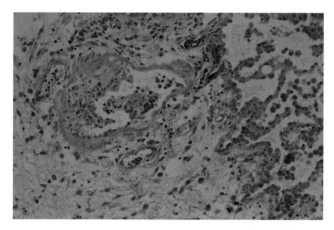

Figure 7-40 • Lung rejection. Mild acute grade 2 rejection is characterized by a modest perivascular infiltration of lymphocytes. Some edema is also evident (H&E stain).

REFERENCES

1. Rich S, Braunwald E, Grossman W: Pulmonary hypertension. In: Braunwald E (ed): Heart Disease. A Textbook of Cardiovascular Medicine. 5th ed. Philadelphia, WB Saunders, 1997, p 780
2. Gravanis MB, Fransh RH, Pine JR: Pulmonary hypertension and cor pulmonale. In: Gravanis MB (ed): Cardiovascular Pathophysiology. New York, McGraw-Hill, 1987, p 115
3. Friedman WF, Molony DA, Kirkpatrick SE: Prostaglandins: Physiological and clinical correlations. Adv Pediatr 25:151, 1978
4. Roberts JD, Fineman JR, Morin FC III, et al: Inhaled nitrous oxide and persistent pulmonary hypertension of the newborn. N Engl J Med 336:605, 1997
5. Davidson WR Jr, Fee EC: Influence of aging on pulmonary hemodynamics in a population free of coronary artery disease. Am J Cardiol 65:1454, 1990
6. Heath D: Structural changes in the pulmonary vasculature associated with aging. In: Carder L, Moyer JH (eds): Aging of the Lung. New York, Grune & Stratton, 1964, p 70
7. Konstantinides S, Geibel A, Olschewski M, et al: A comparison of surgical and medical therapy for atrial septal defects in adults. N Engl J Med 333:469, 1995
8. Saha A, Balakrishnan KG, Jaiswal PK, et al: Prognosis for patients with Eisenmenger's syndrome of various etiology. Int J Cardiol 45:199, 1994
9. Warnes CA: The adult with congenital heart disease: Problems for the patient, cardiologist, and pathologist. Paper presented at the Society of Cardiovascular Pathology Meeting, Orlando, Florida, Companion Meeting to the 86th Annual Meeting of the US-CAP, March 2, 1997
10. Edwards JE: Anomalous coronary arteries with special reference to arteriovenous-like communications (editorial). Circulation 17:1001, 1958
11. Cowie MR, Mahmood S, Ell PJ: The diagnosis and assessment of an adult with anomalous origin of the left coronary artery from the pulmonary artery. Eur J Nucl Med 21:1017, 1994
12. Angelini P: Normal and anomalous coronary arteries: Definitions and classification. Am Heart J 117:418, 1989
13. Wilson CL, Dlabal PW, Holeyfield RW, et al.: Anomalous origin of left coronary artery from pulmonary artery: Case reports and review of literature concerning teenagers and adults. J Thorac Cardiovasc Surg 73:887, 1977
14. Likar I, Criley JM, Lewis KB: Anomalous left coronary artery arising from the pulmonary artery in an adult. A review of the therapeutic problem. Circulation 33:727, 1966
15. Suzuki Y, Murakami T, Kawai C: Detection of anomalous origin of left coronary artery from pulmonary artery by real-time Doppler color flow mapping in a 53-year-old asymptomatic female. Int J Cardiol 34:339, 1992
16. Taylor AJ, Virmani R, Rogan KM: Congenital coronary artery anomalies in the young: Risk for sudden death. J Am Coll Cardiol 19(suppl A):288A, 1992
17. Barth CW, Roberts WC: Left main coronary artery originating from the right sinus of Valsalva and coursing between the aorta and pulmonary trunk. J Am Coll Cardiol 7:366, 1986
18. Levin SE, Kemp DH: Sudden cardiac death of a child caused by aberrant origin of left coronary artery from the right sinus of Valsalva. Cardiovasc J S Afr 5:62, 1994
19. Gentles TL, Lock JE, Perry SB: High pressure balloon angioplasty for branch pulmonary artery stenosis: Early experience. J Am Coll Cardiol 22:867, 1993
20. Ing FF, Grifka RG, Nihill MR, Mullins CE: Repeat dilation of intravascular stents in congenital heart defects. Circulation 92:893, 1995
21. Hwang B, Lu JH, Meng CC: Percutaneous balloon valvuloplasty for congenital critical pulmonary stenosis in neonates. Chin Med J 53:228, 1994
22. Pool PE, Vogel JHK, Blount SG: Congenital unilateral absence of a pulmonary artery. Am J Cardiol 10:706, 1962
23. Wagenvoort CA, Wagenvoort N: Pathology of Pulmonary Hypertension. New York, John Wiley & Sons, 1977
24. Wagenvoort CA, Wagenvoort N: Diseases of the pulmonary circulation. In: Silver MD (ed): Cardiovascular Pathology. 2nd ed. New York, Churchill Livingstone, 1991.
25. Rose AG: Etiology of valvular heart disease. Curr Opin Cardiol 11:98, 1996
26. Udwadia AD, Khambadkone S, Bharucha BA, et al: Familial congenital valvar pulmonary stenosis: Autosomal dominant inheritance. Pediatr Cardiol 17:407, 1996
27. Grant SC, Scarffe JH, Brooks NH: Failure of balloon dilatation of the pulmonary valve in carcinoid pulmonary stenosis. Br Heart J 67:450, 1992
28. Yurdakul Y, Atasoy S, Sariosmanoglu N, et al: Congenital absence of the pulmonary valve associated with pulmonary stenosis, large duct arteriosus and intact ventricular septum. Turk J Pediatr 36:163, 1994
29. Abuhamad AZ, Bass T, Katz ME, Heyl PS: Familial recurrence of pulmonary sequestration. Obstet Gynecol 87:843, 1996
30. Oshika H, Morishita M, Yoshikawa K, et al: Successful embolization of bronchial artery in racemose hemangioma. Jpn J Thorac Dis 31:257, 1993
31. Haimoto H, Tsutsumi Y, Nagura H, et al: Immunohistochemical study of so-called sclerosing haemangioma of the lung. Virchows Arch A Pathol Anat 407:419, 1985
32. Tonner PH, Scholz J: Possible lung embolism following embolization of a hemangioma with fibrin glue. [German]. Anaesthetist 43:614, 1994
33. Srivastava D, Preminger T, Locke JE, et al: Hepatic venous blood and the development of pulmonary arteriovenous malformations in congenital heart disease. Circulation 92:1217, 1995
34. Rich S, Chomka E, Hasara L, et al. The prevalence of pulmonary hypertension in the United States. Chest 96:236, 1989

35. Rose AG: Pathology of natural heart valves and indications for heart valve replacement. In: Pathology of Heart Valve Replacement. Lancaster, United Kingdom, MTP Press Limited (Kluwer Academic Publishers Group), 1987

36. Colman NC: Pathophysiology of pulmonary embolism. In: Leclerc JR (ed): Venous Thromboembolic Disorders. Philadelphia, Lea & Febiger, 1991

37. Leu HJ, Leu AJ: Phlebosclerosis, phlebothrombosis, and thrombophlebitis: A current perspective. Cardiovasc Pathol 5:183, 1996

38. Simioni P, Prandoni P, Leusing AWA, et al: The risk of recurrent venous thromboembolism in patients with an Arg^{506} to Gln mutation in the gene for factor V (factor V Leiden). N Engl J Med 336:399, 1977

39. Greaves M: Thrombophilia—investigation and management. Bull R Coll Pathol 97:6, 1997 (Recent College Symposia: Abstracts and References October–November 1996)

40. Den Heijer M, Koster T, Blom HJ, et al: Hyperhomocysteinemia as a risk factor for deep-vein thrombosis. N Engl J Med 334:759, 1996

41. Mandel H, Brenner B, Berant M, et al: Coexistence of hereditary homocystinuria and factor V Leiden—effect on thrombosis. N Engl J Med 334:763, 1996

42. Rivero MA, Marcial MA, Reyes A: Pathology of pulmonary hypertension and schistosomiasis mansoni. Puerto Rico Health Sci J 12:43, 1993

43. Vuong PN, Bayssade-Dufour C, Albaret JL, Farhati K: Histopathological observations in new and classic models of experimental *Schistosoma haematobium* infections. Trop Med Int Health 1:348, 1996

44. Shields DJ, Edwards WD: Pulmonary hypertension attributable to neoplastic emboli: An autopsy study of 20 cases and a review of literature. Cardiovasc Pathol 1:279, 1992

45. Roberts LR, Kamath PS: Pathophysiology and treatment of variceal hemorrhage. Mayo Clin Proc 71:973, 1996

46. Coard K, Silver MD, Perkins G, et al: Isobutyl-2-cyanoacrylate pulmonary emboli associated with occlusive embolotherapy of cerebral arteriovenous malformations. Histopathology 8:917, 1984

47. Walley VM: The morphologic appearance of Vasoseal (letter to the editor). Cardiovasc Pathol 3:137, 1994

48. Kottke-Marchant K: Extracardiac thrombotic, embolic, and hemorrhagic causes of sudden death. Cardiovasc Pathol 3:129, 1994

49. Kay JM: Hypoxia, obstructive sleep apnea syndrome, and pulmonary hypertension (editorial). Hum Pathol 28:261, 1997

50. Heath D: Longitudinal muscle in pulmonary arteries. J Pathol Bacteriol 85:407, 1963

51. Nattie EE, Dobble EA: Threshold of intermittent hypoxia-induced right ventricular hypertrophy in the rat. Respir Physiol 56:253, 1984

52. Kay JM, Suyama KL, Keane PM: Effect of intermittent normoxia on muscularization of pulmonary arterioles induced by chronic hypoxia in rats. Am Rev Respir Dis 121:993, 1980

53. Kay JM: Vascular disease. In: Thurlbeck WM, Churg AM (eds): Pathology of the Lung. 2nd ed. New York, Thieme, 1995, p 931

54. Wagenvoort CA, Wagenvoort N: Pulmonary venous changes in chronic hypoxia. Virchows Arch A Pathol Anat Histol 372:51, 1976

55. Ahmed Q, Chung-Park M, Tomashefski JF: Cardiopulmonary pathology in patients with sleep apnea/obesity hypoventilation syndrome. Hum Pathol 28:264, 1977

56. Douglas NJ: Respiratory dreams and nightmares. Thorax 51:882, 1996

57. Chaouat A, Weitzenblum E, Krieger J, et al: Pulmonary hemodynamics in the obstructive sleep apnea syndrome. Results in 220 consecutive patients. Chest 109:380, 1996

58. Fleetham JA: A wake up call for sleep disordered breathing. Evidence of ill effects is conflicting and inconclusive (editorial). Br Med J 314:839, 1997

59. Wright J, Johns R, Watt I, et al: Health effects of obstructive sleep apnea and the effectiveness of continuous positive airways pressure: A systematic review of the research evidence. Br Med J 314:851, 1997

60. Schrand JR: Is sleep apnea a predisposing factor for tobacco use? Med Hypotheses 47:443, 1996

61. Heath D, Edwards JE: The pathology of hypertensive pulmonary vascular disease. A description of six grades of structural changes in the pulmonary arteries with special reference to congenital cardiac septal defects. Circulation 18:533, 1958

62. Pietra GG, Edwards WD, Kay JM, et al: Histopathology of primary pulmonary hypertension. A qualitative and quantitative study of pulmonary blood vessels from 58 patients in the National Heart, Lung, and Blood Institute, Primary Pulmonary Hypertension Registry. Circulation 80:1198, 1989

63. Kanjuh VI, Sellers RD, Edwards JE: Pulmonary vascular plexiform lesion. Arch Pathol 78:513, 1964

64. Katzenstein AA: Pulmonary hypertension and other vascular disorders. In: Katzenstein and Askin's Surgical Pathology of Non-Neoplastic Lung Disease. 3rd ed. Philadelphia, WB Saunders Company, 1997

65. Defaria JL: Cor pulmonale in Manson's schistosomiasis. I. Frequency in necropsy material; pulmonary vascular changes caused by schistosome ova. Am J Pathol 30:167, 1954

66. Rabinovitch M, Haworth SG, Castaneda AR, et al: Lung biopsy in congenital heart disease: A morphometric approach to pulmonary vascular disease. Circulation 58:1107, 1978

67. Rabinovitch M, Haworth SG, Vance Z, et al: Early pulmonary vascular changes in congenital heart disease studied in biopsy tissue. Hum Pathol 11(suppl): 499, 1980

68. Winkler J. Primary pulmonary hypertension (review, German). Z Gesamte Inn Med 48:555, 1993

69. Hatano S, Strasser T (eds): Primary pulmonary hypertension: Report on a WHO meeting. World Health Organization. Geneva, 1975, p 7

70. Higgenbottam T, Stenmark K, Simonneau G: Treatments for severe pulmonary hypertension (commentary). Lancet 353:338 1999

71. Barst RJ, Rubin LJ, McGoon MD, et al: Survival in primary pulmonary hypertension with long-term continuous intravenous prostacyclin. Ann Intern Med 121:409, 1994

72. Fuster V, Steele PM, Edwards WD, et al: Primary pulmonary hypertension: Natural history and the importance of thrombosis. Circulation 70:580, 1984

73. Petitpretz P, Brenot F, Azarian R, et al: Pulmonary hypertension in patients with human immunodeficiency virus infection. Comparison with primary pulmonary hypertension. Circulation 89:2722, 1994

74. Michaels AD, Lederman RJ, MacGregor JS, Cheitlin MD: Cardiovascular involvement in AIDS. Curr Probl Cardiol, 22:115, 1997

75. Gurtner HP, Gertsch M, Salzmann C, et al: Haufen sich die primar vaskularen formens des chronischen cor pulmonale? Schweiz Med Wochenschr 98:1579, 1968

76. Brenot F, Herve P, Petitpretz F, et al: Primary pulmonary hypertension and fenfluramine use. Br Heart J 70: 537, 1993

77. Naeije R, Maggiorini M, Delcroix M, et al: Effects of chronic dexfenfluramine treatment on pulmonary hemodynamics in dogs. Am J Respir Crit Care Med 154:1347, 1996

78. Weir EK, Reeve HL, Huang JM, et al: Anorexic agents aminorex, fenfluramine, and dexfenfluramine inhibit potassium current in rat pulmonary vascular smooth muscle and cause pulmonary vasoconstriction. Circulation 94:2216, 1996

79. McGoon MD, Vanhoutte PM: Aggregating platelets contract isolated canine pulmonary arteries by releasing 5-hydroxytryptamine. J Clin Invest 74:828, 1984

80. Nemecek GM, Coughlin SR, Handley DA, Moskowitz MA: Stimulation of aortic smooth muscle mitogenesis by serotonin. Proc Natl Acad Sci U S A 83:674, 1986

81. Connolly HM, Crary JL, McGoon MD, et al: Valvular heart disease associated with fenfluramine-phentermine. N Engl J Med 337:581, 1997

82. Devereux RB: Appetite suppressants and valvular heart disease (editorial). N Engl J Med 339:765, 1998

83. Khan MA, Herzog CA, St Peter JV, et al: The prevalence of cardiac valvular insufficiency assessed by transthoracic echocardiography in obese patients treated with appetite-suppressant drugs. N Engl J Med 339:713, 1998

84. Edwards WD, Edwards JE: Clinical primary hypertension—three pathological types. Circulation 56:884, 1977

85. Tron V, Magee F, Wright JL, et al: Pulmonary capillary hemangiomatosis. Hum Pathol 17:1144, 1986

86. Wagenvoort CA, Beetstra A, Spijker J: Capillary hemangiomatosis of the lungs. Histopathology 2:401, 1978

87. Faber CN, Yousem SA, Dauber JH, et al: Pulmonary capillary hemangiomatosis. A report of three cases and a review of the literature. Am Rev Respir Dis 140:808, 1989

88. Wagenvoort CA: Misalignment of lung vessels: A syndrome causing persistent neonatal pulmonary hypertension. Hum Pathol 17:727, 1986

89. Oldenburgh J, Van der Pal HJH, Schrevel LS, et al: Malalignment of lung vessels and alveolar capillary dysplasia. Histopathology 27:192, 1995

90. Clausen KP, Geer JC: Hypertensive pulmonary arteritis. Am J Dis Child 118:718, 1969

91. Shiue ST, McNally DP: Pulmonary hypertension from prominent vascular involvement in diffuse amyloidosis. Arch Intern Med 148:687, 1988

92. Veinot JP, Edwards WD, Kyle RA: Pulmonary vascular amyloid causing pulmonary hypertension: Report of a case and review of literature. Cardiovasc Pathol 2:231, 1993

93. Roertgen KE, Lund EM, O'Brien TD, et al: Apolipoprotein AI-derived pulmonary vascular amyloid in aged dogs. Am J Pathol 147:1311, 1995

94. Matsuki Y, Suzuki K, Tanaka N, et al: Amyloidosis secondary to rheumatoid arthritis associated with plexiform change in bilateral temporal lobes. Intern Med 33:764, 1994

95. Lie JT, Price DD: Plexogenic pulmonary hypertension associated with intravenous cocaine abuse. Cardiovasc Pathol 4:235, 1995

96. Levin PJ, Klaff LJ, Rose AG, Ferguson AD: Pulmonary effects of contact exposure to paraquat: A clinical and experimental study. Thorax 34:150, 1979

97. Walley VM, Virmani R, Silver MD: Pulmonary arterial dissections and ruptures: To be considered in patients with pulmonary arterial hypertension presenting with cardiogenic shock or sudden death. Pathology 22:1, 1990

98. Heath D, Kay JM, Flenley DC: Respiratory system. In: MacSween RNM, Whaley K (eds): Muir's Textbook of Pathology. 13th ed. Edward Arnold, London, 1992

99. Report of an Expert Committee: Chronic cor pulmonale. WHO Techn Rep 213:1, 1961

99a. Woodard JP, Gulbahce E, Shreve M, et al: Pulmonary cytolytic thrombi: A newly recognized complication of stem cell transplantation. Bone Marrow Transplant 25:293, 2000.

99b. Gulbahce HE, Manivel JC, Jesserun J: Pulmonary cytolytic thrombi. A previously unrecognized complication of bone marrow transplantation. Am J Surg Path (in press).

100. Parums DV: The arteritides. Histopathology 25:1, 1994

101. Robles M, Reyes PA: Takayasu's arteritis in Mexico: A clinical review of 44 consecutive cases. Clin Exp Rheum 12:381, 1994

102. Ishikawa K: Natural history and classification of occlusive thromboaortopathy (Takayasu's disease). Circulation 57:27, 1978

103. Castellote E, Romero R, Bonet J, et al: Takayasu's arteritis as a cause of renovascular hypertension in a non-Asian population. J Hum Hypertens 9:841, 1995

104. Virmani R, Burke A: Pathologic features of aortitis. Cardiovasc Pathol 3:205, 1994

105. Pantanowitz D, Immelman EJ, Rose AG, et al: Arteritis: Part II. Takayasu disease. Cardiovasc J S Afr 4:74, 1993

106. Lie JT. Occidental (temporal) and oriental (Takayasu) giant cell arteritis. Cardiovasc Pathol 3:227, 1994

107. Lupi-Herrera E, Sanchez-Torres G, Marcushamer J, et al: Takayasu's arteritis: Clinical study of 107 cases. Am Heart J 93:94, 1977

108. Arend WP, Michel BA, Bloch DA, et al: The American College of Rheumatology 1990 criteria for the classification of Takayasu arteritis. Arthritis Rheum 33:1129, 1990

109. Rangel-Abundis A, Fraga A, Badui E, et al: Takaysu's arteritis associated with heart valve disease (pulmonary and aortic) and arteritis (coronary and renal). [Spanish]. Arch Inst Cardiol Mex 62:33, 1992

110. Sharma S, Talwar KK, Rajani M: Coronary artery to pulmonary collaterals in nonspecific aortoarteritis involving the pulmonary valves. Cardiovasc Intervent Radiol 16:111, 1993

111. Koyabu S, Isaka N, Yada T, et al: Severe respiratory failure caused by recurrent pulmonary hemorrhage in Takayasu's arteritis. Chest 104:1905, 1993

112. Caver MA, Maicas C, Silva L, et al: Takayasu's disease causing pulmonary hypertension and right heart failure. Am Heart J 127:450, 1994

113. Gur H, Ehrenfeld M, Izsak E: Pleural effusion as a presenting manifestation of giant cell arteritis. Clin Rheumatol 15:200, 1996

114. Ladanyi M, Fraser RS: Pulmonary involvement in giant cell arteritis. Arch Pathol Lab Med 111:1178, 1987

115. Chassagne P, Gligorov J, Dominique S: Pulmonary artery obstruction and giant cell arteritis (letter). Ann Intern Med 122:732, 1995

116. de Heide LJ, Pieterman H, Henneman G: Pulmonary infarction caused by giant-cell arteritis of the pulmonary artery. Neth J Med 46:36, 1995

117. Wagenaar SSC, van den Bosch JMM, Westermann CJ, et al: Isolated granulomatous giant cell vasculitis of the pulmonary elastic arteries. Arch Pathol Lab Med 110:962, 1986

118. Erkan F, Cavdar T: Pulmonary vasculitis in Behçet's disease. Am Rev Respir Dis 146:232, 1992

119. Lakhanpal S, Tani K, Lie JT, et al: Pathologic features of Behçet's syndrome: A review of Japanese autopsy registry data. Hum Pathol 16:790, 1985

120. Gamble CN, Wiesner KB, Shapiro RF, Boyer WJ: The immune complex pathogenesis of glomerulonephritis and pulmonary vasculitis in Behçet's disease. Am J Med 66:1031, 1979

121. Matsumoto T, Uekusa T, Fukuda Y: Vasculo-Behçet disease: A pathologic study of eight cases. Hum Pathol 22:45, 1991

122. Rose AG, Halper J, Factor SM: Pulmonary arteriopathy in Takayasu's disease. Arch Pathol Lab Med 108:644, 1984

123. Turiaf J, Battesti P, Marland P, et al: Sarcoidosis involving large pulmonary arteries. In: Williams JW, Davies BH (eds): Eighth International Conference on Sarcoidosis and Other Granulomatous Diseases. Cardiff, Wales, Alpha Omega, 1980, p 3

124. Rosen Y: Sarcoidosis. In: Dail DH, Hammar SP (eds): Pulmonary Pathology. New York, Springer-Verlag, 1988, p 427

125. Rosen Y, Moon S, Huang CT, et al: Granulomatous pulmonary angiitis in sarcoidosis. Arch Pathol Lab Med 101:170, 1977

126. Salazar A, Mana J, Sala J, et al: Combined portal and pulmonary hypertension in sarcoidosis. Respiration 61:117, 1994

127. Heatly T, Sekela M, Berger R: Single lung transplantation involving a donor with documented pulmonary sarcoidosis. J Heart Lung Transplant 13:720, 1994

128. Liebow AA: The J Burns Amberson Lecture. Pulmonary angiitis and granulomatosis. Am Rev Respir Dis 108:1, 1973

129. Sadoun D, Kambouchner M, Tazi A, et al: Necrotizing sarcoid granulomatosis. Apropos of 4 cases (review). Ann Med Int 145:230, 1994

130. Tsukamato K, Honda A, Kotani I, et al: A case of necrotizing sarcoid granulomatosis. Jpn J Thorac Dis 33:181, 1995

131. Wegener F: Uber eine eigenartige rhinogene granulomatose mit besonderer beteiligung des arteriensystems und der nieren. Beitr Pathol Anat 102:36, 1939

132. Travis WD: Common and uncommon manifestations of Wegener's granulomatosis. Cardiovasc Pathol 3:217, 1994

133. Kallenberg CG: Overlapping syndromes, undifferentiated connective tissue disease, and other fibrosing conditions (review). Curr Opin Rheumatol 7:568, 1995

134. Watanabe R, Tatsumi K, Uchimaya T, et al: Puerperal secondary pulmonary hypertension in a patient with mixed connective disease. Jpn J Thorac Dis 33:883, 1995

135. Okawa-Takatsuji M, Aotsuka S, Uwatoko S, et al: Enhanced synthesis of cytokines by peripheral blood monocytes cultured in the presence of autoantibodies against U1-ribonucleoprotein and/or negatively charged molecules: Implication in the pathogenesis of pulmonary hypertension in mixed connective tissue disease (MCTD). Clin Exp Immunol 98:427, 1994

136. Mikami Y, Sawai T: Pulmonary hypertension in autopsy cases of mixed connective tissue disease. Ryumachi 33:117, 1993

137. Friedman DM, Mitnick HJ, Danilowicz D: Recovery from pulmonary hypertension in an adolescent with mixed connective tissue disease. Ann Rheumatol Dis 51:1001, 1992

138. Rose AG: Hypertension and diseases of medium-sized arteries. In: Silver MD (ed): Cardiovascular Pathology. 2nd ed. New York, Churchill Livingstone, 1991, p 385

139. Matsumoto T, Homma S, Okada M, et al: The lung in polyarteritis nodosa: A pathologic study of 10 cases. Hum Pathol 24:717, 1993

140. Koss MN, Antonovych T, Hochholzer L: Allergic granulomatosis

(Churg-Strauss syndrome). Pulmonary and renal morphologic findings. Am J Surg Pathol 5:21, 1981

141. Churg J: Systemic necrotizing vasculitis. Cardiovasc Pathol 3:197, 1994

142. Jennette JC, Falk RJ, Andrassy K, et al: Nomenclature of systemic vasculitides: Proposal of an international consensus conference. Arthritis Rheum 37:187, 1994

143. Akikusa B, Sato T, Ogawa M, et al: Necrotizing alveolar capillaritis in autopsy cases of microscopic polyangiitis. Incidence, histopathogenesis, and relationship with systemic vasculitis. Arch Pathol Lab Med 121:144, 1997

144. Travis WD, Koss MN: Vasculitis. In: Dail DH, Hammar SP (eds): Pulmonary Pathology. New York, Springer-Verlag, 1994, p 1027

145. Mulherin D, Bresnihan B: Systemic lupus erythematosus (review). Baillieres Clin Rheumatol 7:31, 1993

146. Ford SE, Ford PM: The cardiovascular pathology of phospholipid antibodies: An illustrative case and review of the literature. Cardiovasc Pathol 4:111, 1995

147. Simonson JS, Schiller NB, Petri M, Hellmann DB: Pulmonary hypertension in systemic lupus erythematosus. J Rheumatol 16:918, 1989

148. Goldman J, Edwards WD: Plexogenic pulmonary hypertension in systemic lupus erythematosus: Report of two cases and review of the literature. Cardiovasc Pathol 3:65, 1994

149. Grateau G, Roux ME, Franck N, et al: Pulmonary hypertension in a case of dermatomyositis (letter). J Rheumatol 20:1452, 1993

150. Stupi AM, Steen VD, Owens GR, et al: Pulmonary hypertension in the CREST syndrome variant of systemic sclerosis. Arthritis Rheum 29:515, 1986

151. Young ID, Ford SE, Ford PM: The association of pulmonary hypertension with rheumatoid arthritis. J Rheumatol 16:1266, 1989

152. Slavin RE, Gonzalez-Vitale JC: Segmental mediolytic arteritis: A clinical pathologic study. Lab Invest 35:23, 1976

153. Lie JT: Systemic, cerebral, and pulmonary segmental mediolytic arteriopathy: Villainous masqueraders of vasculitis. Cardiovasc Pathol 5:305, 1996

154. Slavin RE, Cafferty L, Cartwright L, Cartwright J Jr: Segmental mediolytic arteritis: A clinicopathologic and ultrastructural study of two cases. Am J Surg Pathol 13:588, 1989

155. Ahn JM, Im JG, Ryoo JW et al: Thoracic manifestations of Behçet syndrome: Radiographic and CT findings in nine patients. Radiology 194:199, 1995

156. Bartter T, Irwin RS, Nash G: Aneurysms of the pulmonary arteries. Chest 94:1065, 1988

157. Plokker HWM, Wagenaar SS, Bruschke AVG, Wagenvoort CA: Aneurysm of a pulmonary artery branch: An uncommon cause of a coin lesion. Chest 68:258, 1975

158. D'Aunoy R, Von Haam E: Aneurysm of the pulmonary artery with patent ductus arteriosus (Botallo's duct): Report of two cases and review of the literature. J Pathol Bacteriol 38:39, 1934

159. Ross RS, Feder FP, Spencer FP: Aneurysms of the previously ligated patent ductus arteriosus. Circulation 23:350, 1961

160. Selzer A, Lewis AE: The occurrence of chronic cyanosis in cases of atrial septal defect. Am J Med Sci 218:516, 1949

161. Walley VM, Virmani R, Silver MD: Pulmonary arterial dissections and ruptures: To be considered in patients with pulmonary artery hypertension presenting with cardiogenic shock or sudden death. Pathology 22:1, 1990

162. Green NJ, Rollason TP: Pulmonary artery rupture in pregnancy complicating patent ductus arteriosus. Br Heart J 68:616, 1992

163. Rau AN, Glass MN, Waller BF et al: Right pulmonary artery occlusion secondary to a dissecting aortic aneurysm. Clin Cardiol 18:178, 1995

164. Plenat F, Vert P, Didier F, Andre M: Pulmonary interstitial emphysema. Clin Perinatol 5:351, 1978

165. Rudd PT, Wigglesworth JS: Oxygen embolism during mechanical ventilation with disappearance of signs after death. Arch Dis Child 57:237, 1982

166. Burke AP, Virmani R: Sarcomas of the great vessels: A clinicopathologic study. Cancer 71:1761, 1993

167. Kruger I, Borowski A, Horst M, et al: Symptoms, diagnosis, and therapy of primary sarcomas of the pulmonary artery. Thorac Cardiovasc Surg 38:91, 1990

168. Boue DR, Frank JG, Haghighi P, Russack V: Pulmonary artery sarcoma in endarterectomy specimens: Clinicopathologic study of 6 cases. Cardiovasc Pathbiol 1:48, 1996

169. Nonomura A, Mizukami Y, Matsubara F, et al: Seven patients with plasma cell granuloma (inflammatory pseudotumor) of the lung, including two with intrabronchial growth: An immunohistochemical and electron microscopic study. Intern Med 31:756, 1992

170. Warter A, Stage D, Roeslin N: Angioinvasive plasma cell granuloma of the lung. Cancer 59:435, 1987

171. Rose AG, McCormick S, Cooper K, Titus JL: Inflammatory pseudotumor (plasma cell granuloma) of the heart. Report of two cases and literature review. Arch Pathol Lab Med 120:549, 1996

172. Ledet SC, Brown RW, Cagle PT: P53 immunostaining in the differentiation of inflammatory pseudotumor from sarcoma involving the lung. Mod Pathol 8:282, 1995

173. Snyders CS, Dell'Aquila M, Haghighi P, et al: Clonal changes in inflammatory pseudotumor of the lung: A case report. Cancer 76: 1545, 1995

174. Gibbs AR, Whimster WF: Tumors of the lung and pleura. In: Fletcher CDM (ed): Diagnostic Histopathology of Tumors. New York, Churchill Livingstone, 1995, p 127

175. Corrin B, Manners B, Millard M, et al: Histogenesis of the so-called "intravascular bronchiolo-alveolar tumor." J Pathol 128:163, 1979

176. Sageshima M, Masuda H, Kawamura K, Shozawa T: Intimal thickening of peripheral pulmonary vein: Analysis of 139 consecutive autopsy cases. Cardiovasc Pathol 1:169, 1992

177. Swensen SJ, Tashjian JH, Myers JL et al: Pulmonary veno-occlusive disease: CT findings in eight patients. Am J Roentgenol 167: 937, 1996

178. Bras G, Berry DM, Gyorgy P: Plants as aetiological factors in veno-occlusive disease of the liver. Lancet 1:960, 1957

179. Rose AG: Pulmonary veno-occlusive disease due to bleomycin therapy for lymphoma. Case reports. S Afr Med J 64:636, 1983

180. Knight BK, Rose AG: Pulmonary veno-occlusive disease after chemotherapy. Thorax 40:874, 1985

181. Lombard CM, Churg A, Winokur S: Pulmonary venoocclusive disease following therapy for malignant neoplasms. Chest 92:871, 1987

182. Capewell SJ, Wright AJ, Ellis DA: Pulmonary veno-occlusive disease in association with Hodgkin's disease. Thorax 39:554, 1984

183. Rose AG: Pulmonary veno-occlusive disease after chemotherapy with bleomycin (letter). Hum Pathol 15:199, 1984

184. Kishida Y, Kanai Y, Kuramochi S, Hosoda Y: Pulmonary veno-occlusive disease in a patient with systemic lupus erythematosus. J Rheumatol 20:2161, 1963

185. Troussard X, Bernaudin JF, Cordonnier C, et al: Pulmonary veno-occlusive disease after bone marrow transplantation. Thorax 39: 763, 1984

186. Townsend JN, Roberts DH, Jones EL, Davies MK: Fatal pulmonary venoocclusive disease after use of oral contraceptives. Am Heart J 124:1643, 1992

187. Rose AG, Learmonth GM, Benatar SR: Pulmonary veno-occlusive disease associated with hypertrophic cardiomyopathy (letter). Arch Pathol Lab Med 108:267, 1984

188. Chetty R, Rose AG, Commerford PJ, Taylor DA: Pulmonary veno-occlusive disease associated with hypertrophic cardiomyopathy. Cardiovasc Pathol 289:289, 1992

189. Kubo S, Fujita K, Nakatomi M: Angioscopic findings of the peripheral pulmonary arteries in patients with chronic pulmonary diseases. Jpn J Thorac Dis 30:2018, 1992

190. Skidmore FD: Part II. The development of the pulmonary circulation. In: Goor DA, Lillehei CW (eds): Congenital Malformations of the Heart. New York, Grune & Stratton, 1975, p 89

191. Lang SA, Duncan PG, Shephard DA, Ha HC: Pulmonary edema associated with airway obstruction. Can J Anaesth 37:210, 1990

192. Eid AA, Agabani M, Grady K: Negative-pressure pulmonary edema: A cautionary tale. Cleve Clin J Med 64:151, 1997

193. Jerome EH, Severinghaus JW: High-altitude pulmonary edema (editorial). N Engl J Med 334:662, 1996

194. Okita Y, Miki S, Kusuhara K, et al: Acute pulmonary edema after Blalock-Taussig anastomosis. Ann Thorac Surg 53:684, 1992

195. Wetli CV, Davis JH, Blackbourne BD: Narcotic addiction in Dade County, Florida: An analysis of 100 consecutive autopsies. Arch Pathol 93:330, 1972

196. Scherrer U, Vollenweider L, Delabays A, et al: Inhaled nitric

oxide for high-altitude pulmonary edema. N Engl J Med 334:624, 1996
197. Novitzky D, Wicomb WN, Rose AG, Reichart B: Pathophysiology of pulmonary edema following experimental brain death in the Chacma baboon. Ann Thorac Surg 43:288, 1987
198. Novitzky D: Selection and management of cardiac allograft donors. Curr Opin Cardiol 11:174, 1996
199. Nakhleh RE, Bolman RM III, Henke CA, Hertz MI: Lung transplant pathology: A comparative study of pulmonary acute rejection and cytomegalovirus infection. Am J Surg Pathol 15:1197, 1991
200. Yousem SA, Berry GJ, Brunt EM, et al: A working formulation for the standardization of nomenclature in the diagnosis of heart and lung rejection: Lung study group. J Heart Transplant 9:593, 1990

Chapter 8

Myocardial Cell Death, Including Ischemic Heart Disease and Its Complications

·····

Giorgio Baroldi

In defining the injury or death of a cell, a pathologist should consider its structure and function in relation to anabolic and catabolic turnover and to extracellular and intracellular exchange as well as the morphologic signs that establish both the point of no return (at which damage becomes irreversible) and the cause-and-effect relationships involved, so as to distinguish whether dysfunction precedes demonstrable cell lesions or vice versa. This is particularly true for myocardial cells, or myocells.

Impairment of the complex interaction of ions and molecules within specialized cell structures is the obvious yet morphologically undetectable pathogenic mechanism of dysfunction. However, the function of a healthy organ in a dead person may return to normal if, within a critical period, its metabolic turnover is reestablished, as is shown in the transplantation of donor organs. Similarly, after acute coronary artery occlusion, the subtending myocardium immediately loses its function but returns to normal, without evidence of morphologic ischemic damage, if blood flow is reestablished within 20 minutes.[1] In comparison, infectious agents of any type, toxic cells, interstitial and intracellular storage of many substances, and so forth may damage cell structure first and subsequently damage its function. The need, therefore, is to demonstrate or discover the earliest morphologic signs, including mobile ions and molecular structures, to prove irreversibility—that is, cell death. This task is not easy but will be achieved by improved, reliable, biomolecular techniques that enable the examiner to discriminate different and specific disorders in each type of injury.

Several forms of morphologically distinct myocardial cell injury and death are currently recognizable (Table 8-1) and will be discussed, but before doing so, I want to briefly recall myocell architecture in relation to its rhythmic cycle of contraction and relaxation, which starts at the end of the third fetal week and ends when a person dies. (Cardiac arrest is the major cause of death in Western societies.)

THE FUNCTIONAL ANATOMY OF THE MYOCARDIAL CELL

Myocardial cells form a functional but not anatomic syncytium (their anatomy is fully reported in Chapter 2). In fact, they are joined at their extremities by intercalated disks and have lateral connections with adjacent myocells and a fibrillar collagen matrix forming a network that connects neighboring myocells, their cytoskeleton, and vascular walls.[2] The contractile apparatus consists of my-

ofibrils subdivided into sarcomeres separated by dark, subtle Z lines and constituted by thin actin and thick L-meromyosin filaments. Thick filaments have lateral (H-meromyosin) digitations that correspond to the tropomyosin and troponin digitations of the thin filaments. These digitations are the active sites of the biochemical "hinge" that regulates the contraction-relaxation cycle, the sarcomere being the true morphofunctional unit. According to the "sliding theory" of myocardial contraction, the cycle is achieved by a back-and-forth movement of thin filaments that penetrate the other half of the sarcomere by sliding on thick filaments. In diastole, the tropomyosin/troponin complex inhibits contraction. The binding of Ca^{++} to troponin removes inhibition and permits systolic contraction. This means a rhythmic pumping of Ca^{++} from where it is stored in the sarcoplasmic reticulum to the myofibrils and back again. The systolic length of sarcomeres ranges from 1.86 to 1.95 μm and the diastolic length from 2.05 to 2.15 μm. The length that gives maximal active tension in relationship to the Starling phenomenon is between 2.20 and 2.35 μm (end-diastolic reserve.)[3]

All myofibrils have a registered order that gives the myocell its characteristic regular cross-striation pattern and bands, which vary according to cell function (Fig. 8-1 and see Fig. 2-15). Alterations in this functional morphology may present various aspects.

MYOCARDIAL CELL INJURY AND DEATH IN RELATION TO THE MYOCARDIAL CONTRACTION CYCLE

Three distinct structural types of myocardial cell injury and death are distinguished in relation to the contraction-relaxation cycle.[4, 5] Thus, the myocell may arrest in relaxation or in contraction or may progressively lose its contractile compliance.

Myocell Injury and Death in Irreversible Relaxation: Infarct Necrosis

In infarct necrosis, or atonic death, a myocardial cell loses its ability to contract and becomes a passive, extensible element. Within a few seconds of experimental coronary occlusion, ischemic myocardium loses contractility,[1] becomes cyanosed, and bulges (systolic paradoxical bulging) because of intraventricular pressure. An expression of this flaccid paralysis is thinning and attenuation of mildly eosinophilic myocells and the elongation of nuclei

TABLE 8-1 • **Morphologic Forms of Myocardial Cell Injury and Death**

Infarct or coagulation necrosis
Coagulative myocytolysis or contraction band necrosis
Paradiscal band or zonal lesion
Reflow or reperfusion
Cutting-edge band lesion
Colliquative myocytolysis or myofibrillar loss
Myocellular vacuolization
Coagulative myocyte necrosis
Apoptosis
Infectious/immune/parasitic/storage necrosis

and sarcomeres. Prominent I-bands[6] are the first structural changes seen and are obvious within 1 hour of the coronary occlusion (Fig. 8-2).[7, 8] Classically, the irreversibility of this lesion is established histologically only after 6 to 8 hours, when polymorphonuclear leukocytes first marginate within vessels at the periphery of the affected area and then penetrate centripetally into the necrotic tissue. This infiltration, which is usually not associated with a marked exudate of fibrin and red cells, disappears in approximately 1 week, without evidence of dissolution or lysis of necrotic myocells. (Apoptosis as an earlier sign of myocardial infarction is discussed later.)

A myocardial infarct is a nonhemorrhagic, monofocal lesion that exists in the absence of wall rupture and fibrinolytic therapy.[9] Only in large infarcts does a palisade, crowded with polymorphonuclear leukocytes, appear at the edge of the infarct, giving it an abscess-like image by light microscopy (Fig. 8-3). This seems to occur because leukocyte penetration is blocked, possibly by maximal stretching of the dead tissue. Postmortem injection fails to fill intramural arterial vessels in an infarcted zone in the acute phase (the avascular area). Thinning of the cardiac wall is always associated with an acute infarct affecting more than 30% of the left ventricular mass. Stretching of the infarcted wall with cohesion of the paralyzed myocells may be an important compressive factor in limiting or abolishing blood flow to infarcted myocardium and its sequestration from pharmacologic penetration. To control the role of this factor, I examined from the files of the

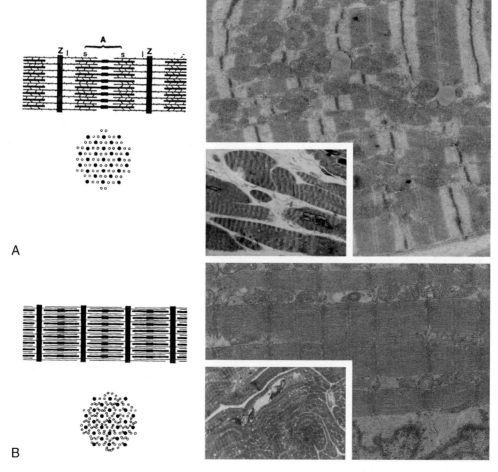

Figure 8-1 • Normal contraction-relaxation cycle of the myocardial cell, illustrated photographically and diagramatically with fibers in longitudinal and cross section. *A*, Relaxation phase showing different bands (EM; inset, toluidine blue). *B*, Contraction phase with disappearance of I-bands. Z lines show normal thickness. By light microscopy, they become more distinct in hypercontraction. At low magnification, the clear cross-striations in the relaxed cells correspond to two adjacent I-bands without clear-cut evidence of the limiting Z line. The dark band is formed by the A-band. (EM; inset, toluidine blue.)

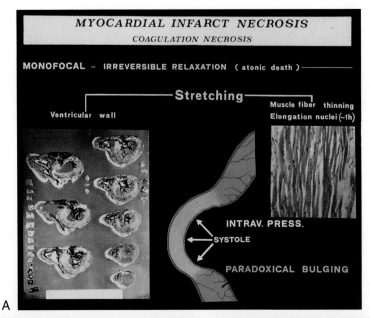

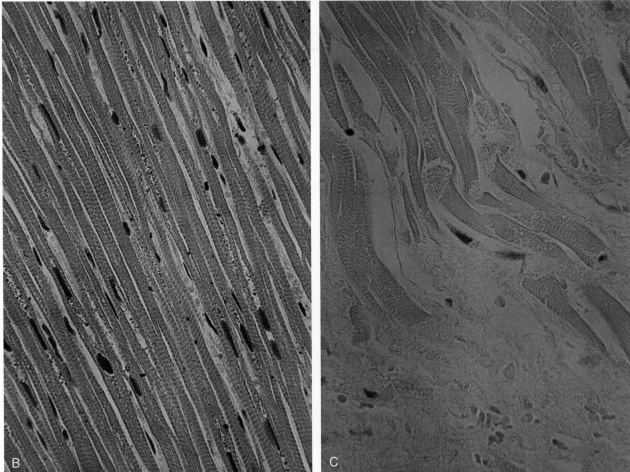

Figure 8-2 • Infarct necrosis with loss of contraction. *A*, Macroscopic view of a posterior acute infarct and peripheral histologic views of hyperdistended dead myocardial fibers with nuclei elongated by intraventricular pressure. *B*, Early stage (H&E stain). *C*, Late stage. The regular order of sarcomeres is maintained in the pale remnant myocells of the 25-day-old infarct in its late stage of healing (H&E stain).

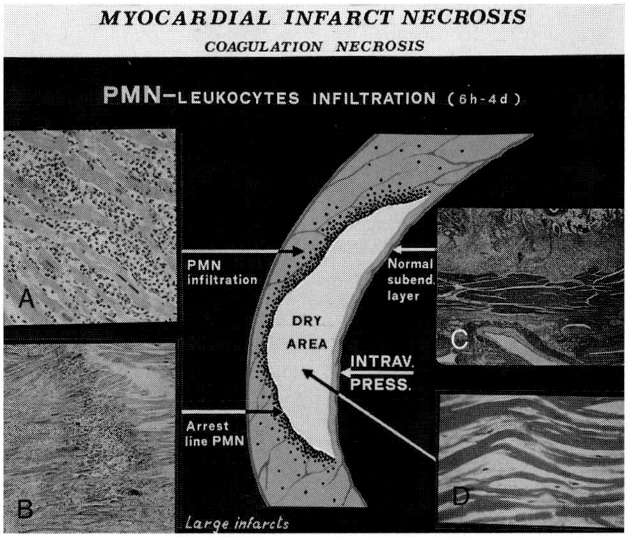

MYOCARDIAL INFARCT NECROSIS
COAGULATION NECROSIS

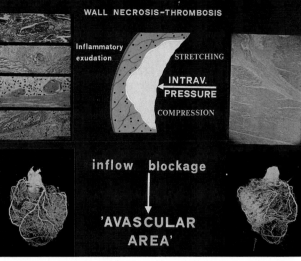

Figure 8-3 • Infarct necrosis showing in counterclockwise inserts. *A,* Polymorphonuclear leukocyte (PMN) infiltration (H&E stain). *B,* Extensive PMN infiltration with abscess-like formation and myocell destruction along a clear-cut line within the necrotic myocardium. The centripetal infiltration is blocked around a central "dry" area (H&E stain). *C,* Stretching of dead myocells (H&E stain). *D,* Note preservation of subendocardial myocardium (Movat stain). Intrav pressure, Intraventricular pressure.

Armed Forces Institute of Pathology 13 cases of severe constrictive pericarditis because I considered that this condition would limit or abolish ventricular wall expansion associated with severe and multiple, obstructive coronary atherosclerosis. Not one case had extensive myocardial fibrosis and a history of myocardial infarction. A Marlex mesh that was positioned before infarct induction by coronary artery ligature in sheep prevented a massive scar with aneurysm of the cardiac wall and both hemodynamic and cardiac dysfunction.[9a] In the necrotic zone, secondary thrombosis of intramural vessels is always present and is likely, in part, caused by these dynamic changes (Fig. 8-4).

Another peculiar alteration is an intimal obliterative proliferation in small arteries at the periphery of an infarct; it is already noticeable when healing begins (Fig. 8-5). Some authors consider repair a process of granulation tissue formation and fibrosis. In our opinion, healing is not accomplished by granulation tissue but by digestion of necrotic structures within the sarcolemmal sheaths by macrophages.[10] The result is an alveolar pattern of tubes within which macrophages laden with lipofuscin are found, followed by collagenization (Fig. 8-6). An important observation is that the myofibrillar apparatus always maintains a registered order of sarcomeres—that is, cross-striations do not disappear. They can be recognized in the last remnants of necrotic tissue in infarcts even where healing is almost complete (Fig. 8-2).

This form of myocardial injury is generally called *coagulation necrosis* despite the absence of any true coagulative process. The term *myocardial infarct necrosis* appears to be more appropriate and explicit. It must be stressed that extensive hemorrhage is not part of the natural history of this form of necrosis. It can be seen after

MYOCARDIAL INFARCT NECROSIS
COAGULATION NECROSIS

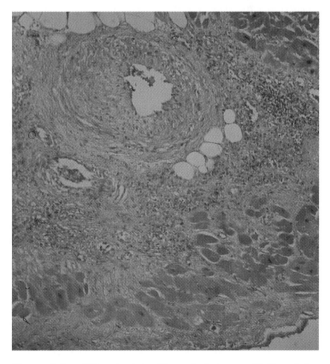

Figure 8-4 • Degeneration of the wall and thrombosis of intramural arterial vessels (upper left of photograph) secondary to infarct necrosis (lower left of photograph). An avascular area at the site of an acute infarct is shown in left anterior (to left of photograph) and right posterior cast views. The infarct is in the territory of an almost normal left anterior descending branch. There is right coronary occlusion. Its territory is vascularized by many intra- and intercoronary collaterals. There was no infarct in the right coronary territory (All H&E stain). Intrav pressure, Intraventricular pressure (From Baroldi G, Scomazzoni G: Coronary Circulation in the Normal and Pathologic Heart. In: American Registry of Pathology, A.F.I.P. [ed]: Washington, DC, U.S. Government Printing Office, 1967.)

Figure 8-5 • Obliterative intimal hyperplasia (upper mid edge of photograph) in an arteriole surviving at the edge of an infarct (H&E stain).

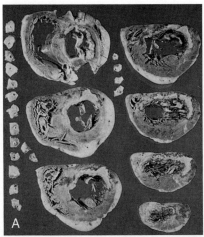

Figure 8-6 • Repair of infarct necrosis *A*, Gross view of a sliced heart with an inferolateral 10-day-old infarct in the left ventricle. The lesion shows yellow, necrotic, myocardium surrounded by red rim. *B*, Centripetal macrophagic digestion of necrotic tissue within sarcolemmal sheaths starting from the periphery of the infarct. No evidence of granulation tissue (H&E stain). *C*, For comparison, highly vascularized granulation tissue organizing an intracavitary thrombus at the site of a healing infarct. In the latter, there is no evidence of neovascularization. Postmortem coronary injection of radiopaque material (Movat pentachrome stain).

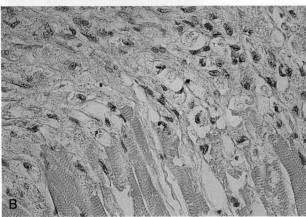

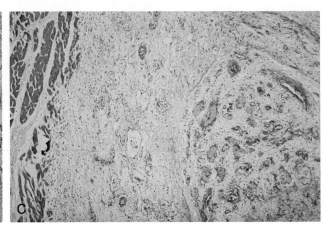

cardiac wall rupture and fibrinolytic therapy. (For more details, see the later section discussing acute myocardial infarction.)

Myocell Injury and Death in Irreversible Hypercontraction

In tetanic death, the structural and functional pattern is opposite that seen in infarct necrosis. Here, the myocardial cell stops activity in contraction. More precisely, we should speak of hypercontraction, because sarcomere length is significantly less than that calculated for physiologic maximal contraction. Several different structural aspects of this type of injury can be distinguished.

Coagulative Myocytolysis, or Contraction Band Necrosis

The lesion that characterizes catecholamine cardiotoxicity is a nonhemorrhagic coagulative myocytolysis that includes pancellular and paradiscal forms.

Pancellular Lesion

Pancellular lesions manifest, experimentally, within 15 minutes of the intravenous infusion of norpinephrine or isoproterenol. Markedly eosinophilic myocells become hypercontracted and then fragment into irregular, transverse, total, or partial acidophilic bands, or both, or some

develop a diffuse, granular aspect (myofibrillar degeneration). By electron microscopy, the bands appear as small groups of hypercontracted, extremely short sarcomeres with highly thickened Z lines or as amorphous dark material suggesting the coagulation of contractile proteins. The clear spaces between bands are partially filled with normal or slightly swollen mitochondria with dense, fine granules and occasional rupture of their cristae. The sarcotubular system is completely destroyed, whereas the basement membrane is practically intact, with only an occasional disruption. The folding of the sarcolemma is a characteristic feature at the site of hypercontracted sarcomeres. Glycogen deposits disappear without evidence of intracellular or interstitial edema or damage to vessels or platelet aggregates. Fragmentation or total disintegration of these rigid, inextensible myocells in irreversible hypercontraction may be due to the mechanical action of surrounding normal, contracting myocardium. Pancellular destruction (Fig. 8-7) is a clear sign of cell death, but it is still not clear whether the hypercontraction of intact eosinophilic myocells with thickened Z lines (Fig. 8-8) is reversible or irreversible. Apparently, the Z-line thickening reflects an agglomeration of contractile proteins. If it reverts to normal, we should include in the sliding theory the concept of a reversible rolling-up of filaments at the Z-line level.

The pancellular lesion may involve one single myocell among thousands of normal ones, foci of the few myo-

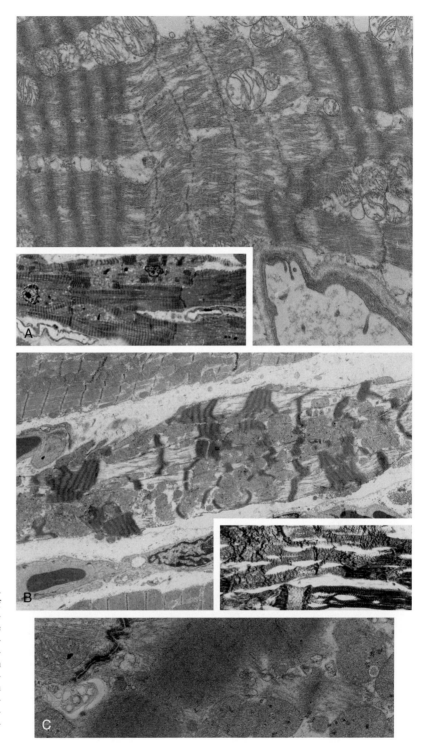

Figure 8-7 • Coagulative myocytolysis (contraction band necrosis). Different stages of disruption of hypercontracted myocells. *A,* Heart excised from ischemic heart disease patient at transplantation. Note markedly thickened Z lines and very short sarcomeres alternated with stretched sarcomeres (EM; inset, toluidine blue). *B,* Destruction of myocells with band of hypercontracted sarcomeres, granular appearance, and rhexis. (EM; intravenous norepinephrine in dog; inset PTHA is from the myocardium surrounding an acute infarct in human.) *C,* Coagulated sarcomeres with faint Z lines still visible (EM; intravenous norepinephrine in dog).

cells, or a large area of myocardial fibers. In the experimental catecholamine infusion model, extension of cellular damage is directly related to the dose administered. The higher the dose, the greater the number of necrotic foci and damaged myocells per focus. The early acute lesion does not provoke an inflammatory cell exudate or infiltrate of any type. Its repair is similar to that previously described for infarct necrosis; that is, macrophagic digestion followed by an alveolar pattern and collagenization of the sarcolemmal tubes. Even in healing, there is

no evidence of vessel changes.[11, 12] Mineralization, or increased intramyocellular Ca^{++}, has been reported experimentally,[13] a finding in line with the pathogenic theory of Ca^{++} influx. The frequent finding of calcified myocells in conditions with increased Ca^{++} metabolism may be an extreme pattern of this lesion.

This type of myonecrosis and injury has been described in many pathologic conditions in humans (e.g., pheochromocytoma, intracranial lesions, transplanted heart, thrombotic thrombocytopenic purpura, "stone heart," scle-

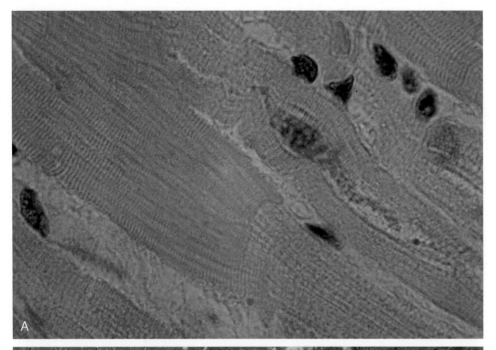

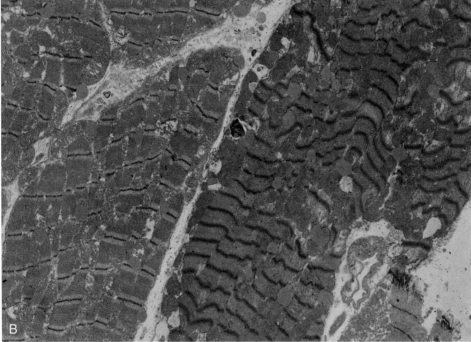

Figure 8-8 • Hypercontraction of the myocell. This is the first change in experimental catecholamine cardiotoxicity; it is frequently observed in the hearts of human subjects under a variety of conditions in the absence of hemorrhage *A*, Chronic ischemic heart disease (H&E stain). *B*, Electron micrograph showing experimental norepinephrine intravenous infusion in dog. Note thickening of the Z lines (×4,765). (From Todd GL, Baroldi G, Pieper GM, et al: Experimental catecholamine-induced myocardial necrosis. I. Morphology, quantification and regional distribution of acute contraction band lesions. J Mol Cell Cardiol 17:317, 1985.)

roderma, malignant hyperthermia, ischemic heart disease) and in experimental models, (e.g., catecholamine infusion, stellate ganglion stimulation, electric shock, magnesium deficit, psychological stress).[5, 13–15] In a series of cardiac diseases we studied, coagulative myocytolysis was always found to have varying ranges of frequency and extent (Table 8-2). Such ubiquity raises doubts about the significance of this finding. Among healthy subjects who died of head trauma, those who died instantaneously had no such lesions, whereas in those who survived for at least 1 hour, their frequency was 47%.[16] This suggests that adrenergic overstimulation may induce catecholamine myotox-

icity in the agonal period. We urge that any time the role of coagulative myocytolysis, or contraction band necrosis, has to be evaluated, the frequency, number of foci and affected myocells per square millimeter, and their ages all be considered.

The profusion of synonyms used for this type of myocardial damage (e.g., microinfarct, focal myocytolysis, focal myocarditis, infarct-like necrosis, hyaline degeneration, myocytolysis with major contraction bands, myofibrillar degeneration and contraction band necrosis) causes confusion and does not help to determine its precise frequency in human or experimental pathology. To

TABLE 8-2 • **Frequency of Coagulative Myocytolysis in Various Pathologic Conditions and Healthy Controls**

| | | | Coagulative Myocytolysis† | | | | | |
| | | | Semiquantitation | | | Morphologic Form | | |
Source	Number of Cases	Total Showing Change	+	++	+++	Cross Band	Alveolar	Healing
Accidental death in normals	97	19	16	1	2	14	4	1
Sudden/unexpected coronary death	208	149	88	38	23	95	28	26
Acute myocardial infarct	200	196	—	—	196	70	74	56
Pheochromocytoma	65	56	25	17	14	30	13	13
AIDS	38	25	9	8	8	19	6	—
Sudden/unexpected death in Chagas disease	34	17	4	3	10	8	5	4
Intracranial hemorrhage	27	24	3	2	19	13	9	2
Ischemic heart disease*	63	59	14	14	31	27	12	20
Dilated cardiomyopathy*	63	53	12	19	22	35	6	12
Valvulopathy*	18	14	—	4	10	3	7	4
Transplanted hearts	38	33	4	13	16	8	18	7
Survival <6 months	23	23	3	8	12	5	14	4
≥6 months	15	10	1	5	4	3	4	3

+, ≤5 foci; ++, 6–20 foci; +++, >20 foci.
* Hearts excised at transplantation.
† Coagulative myocytolysis includes pancellular and paradiscal lesions.

maintain a terminology already established in the literature, I have adopted the term *myocytolysis*,[17] adding the adjective *coagulative* to better characterize this myofibrillar damage with coagulation of contractile proteins, or use the old German term *Zenker necrosis*.[5]

Paradiscal Contraction Band

A paradiscal contraction band, usually associated with a pancellular lesion, is observed in human pathology and, experimentally, as a single contraction band adjacent to an intercalated disk. The band is formed by fewer than 15

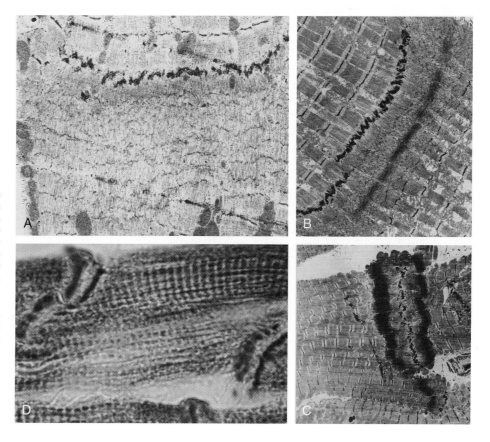

Figure 8-9 • Paradiscal contraction bands. Different aspects of contraction bands confined to the extremity of an otherwise normal myocell, close to the intercalated disc and induced by intravenous infusion of norpinephrine in the dog. These bands are formed by 10 to 15 hypercontracted sarcomeres with ill defined, thin Z lines. *A*, Clear appearance (EM). *B*, Increased electron density along a line (EM). *C*, Very dark aspect (EM). *D*, Histologic equivalent of dark paradiscal bands (toluidine blue). (From Todd GL, Baroldi G, Pieper GM, et al: Experimental catecholamine-induced myocardial necrosis. I. Morphology, quantification and regional distribution of acute contraction band lesions. J Mol Cell Cardiol 17:317, 1985.)

hypercontracted sarcomeres; the remaining part of the myocell is normal. In contrast to the pancellular lesion, its ultrastructure reveals extremely short sarcomeres, closely packed together with thinner Z lines that are often fragmented or ill-defined. Myofilaments are visible and are without evidence of rhexis. Only an increased electron density of different degrees may cross the whole band. However, all transitional patterns, from clear to deeply dark bands, are seen, often on both sides of the same intercalated disk (Fig. 8-9). In cross section, myocells are larger and may assume a spoked-wheel aspect, especially with phosphotungstic acid–hematoxylin stain. Hypercontraction of this band, as with other bands found in the pancellular lesion, is demonstrated by an increased myocell diameter, concomitant scalloped sarcolemma, displacement or squeezing of mitochondria, and waviness of contiguous normal myocells (Fig. 8-10).[11]

The paradiscal lesion may be observed within 5 minutes of a catecholamine intravenous infusion; it is similar to the zonal lesion described in hemorrhagic shock.[18, 19] Both are prevented by β-blocking agents.[7, 20] Its subsequent evolution is not known. Its dark aspect could represent the usual hypercontraction phase with thickened Z lines, whereas clearing of these dark bands could indicate rebuilding to a normal structure, suggesting that the paradiscal lesion is reversible. One may speculate that segmental hypercontraction adjacent to a disk is "protected" from fragmentation by its position at the extremity of an otherwise normally functioning myocell. It should be noted that in acute catecholamine cardiotoxicity, no other form of myocardial necrosis was seen.[11, 12]

Contraction Bands at the Cut Edges of Living Myocardium

Coagulative myocytolysis must be distinguished from other contraction band patterns.[4, 5] In endomyocardial and other heart biopsy material and in hearts excised at transplantation, myocell retraction, formed by eosinophilic segments of hypercontracted sarcomeres with thickened Z lines in the absence of myofibrillar disruption, is visible along cut edges (Fig. 8-11). The depth of this lesion from the cut margin has been calculated to be 0.2 to 0.5 mm.[11] This type of band could easily be confused with coagulative myocytolysis or other changes, particularly in transverse sections of areas with alternated hypercontracted and stretched myocells, resulting in pseudovacuolization at the level of the stretched I-band. Practically and in biopsy material, the lesion is regarded as an artifact.

Reflow or Reperfusion Injury

Contraction bands with total disruption of myocells, as seen in coagulative myocytolysis, are observed with the experimental temporary occlusion of a coronary artery[21] and in patients who have had long-lasting resuscitative attempts or cardiac surgery.[22] However, in these circumstances, the myocardial damage is associated with extensive hemorrhage, vessel damage, platelet aggregates, and scanty polymorphonuclear leukocytes (Fig. 8-12). In general, this is an extensive focal or confluent lesion, but it may involve the whole inner part of the left ventricle and the interventricular septum (concentric hemorrhagic necrosis)[23] and produce a "stone heart" clinically. In experimental temporary coronary occlusion, reflow is often associated with malignant arrhythmias.[24] The latter and structural lesions can be prevented by β-blockers.[7, 25] Frequently interpreted as infarct or ischemic necrosis, reflow necrosis seems to be related to an increase of flow after ischemia or anoxia in which catecholamines[26] and Ca^{++} may play an important role in the Ca^{++} paradox phenomenon; after temporary hypocalcemia, normocalcemia induces contraction band lesions.[27]

Myocell Injury and Death Associated With Progressive Loss of Cardiac Function

In contrast to the two previous morphofunctional forms of myoinjury, a myocardial cell can perform with reduced function as is seen in congestive heart failure ("failing death"). The main structural change in this circumstance is the progressive loss of myofibrils observed in many heart muscle diseases (e.g., alcoholism, peripartum disorders, Keshan and dilated cardiomyopathies, ischemic heart disease) (see Chapter 10).

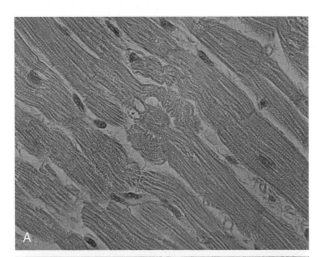

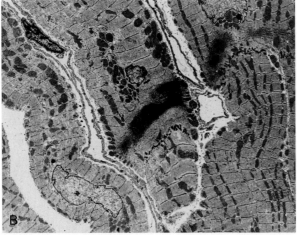

Figure 8-10 • Wavy fibers appear as undulating normal myocells surrounding a hypercontracted myocell. *A,* Excised human heart at transplantation (H&E stain). *B,* Experimental catecholamine infusion in dog (EM). (From Todd GL, Baroldi G, Pieper GM, et al: Experimental catecholamine-induced myocardial necrosis. I. Morphology, quantification and regional distribution of acute contraction band lesions. J Mol Cell Cardiol 17:317, 1985).

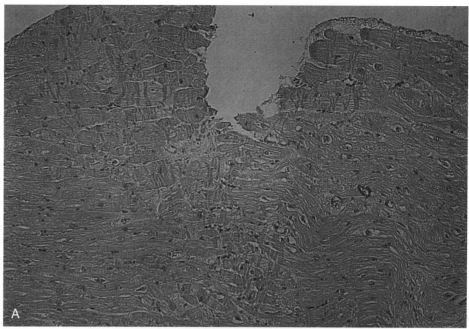

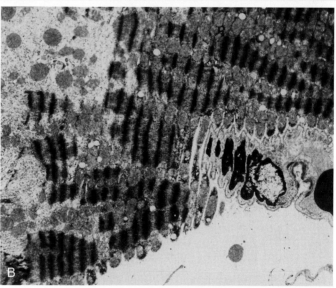

Figure 8-11 • Cutting-edge band lesion at edges of sections made in living myocardium. It is formed by very thickened Z lines and highly shortened sarcomeres without rhexis or fragmentation. *A*, Heart excised at transplantation (H&E stain). *B*, Specimen of cardiac biopsy (EM).

In 144 hearts excised consecutively from patients undergoing heart transplant to correct intractable end-stage heart failure resulting from various causes, we found all degrees of myofibrillar loss, from mild vacuolization that induced a moth-eaten pattern to total disappearance of myofibrils and an alveolar pattern often associated with an edematous aspect of the myocell (Fig. 8-13). The histologic difference from the alveolar aspect seen in coagulative myocytolysis is an absence of macrophages or other reactive cells. The impression is that there is colliquation of myofibrils rather than digestion by active monocytes—a kind of washout that leaves a "clean" alveolar appearance that is initially obvious around an apparently normal nucleus. The loss of myofibrils (colliquative myocytolysis) is a diffuse phenomenon that seems to begin preferentially in the subendocardium and the inner part of the cardiac wall. Often, by light microscopy, the space devoid of myofibrils has a homogeneous or fine granular appearance that, by electron microscopy, is attributable to edema, packed mitochondria, or both (Fig. 8-14).[28]

CAUSES AND PATHOGENESIS OF THE THREE FORMS OF DYSFUNCTIONAL MYONECROSIS

The clearly defined structures of the acute phases of the three types of myonecrosis and their relationship to various functional conditions indicate that each is a distinct entity rather than a different expression of a single pathologic process. That is, each has a dissimilar biochemical disorder, the nature of which is controversial and a matter for investigation.[5] It is assumed (1) that in irreversible relaxation, intracellular acidosis displaces Ca^{++}

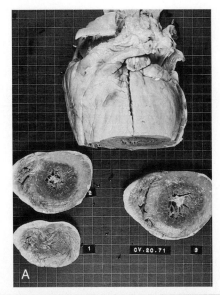

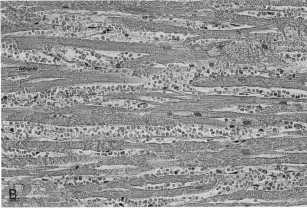

Figure 8-12 • Myocardial reflow or reperfusion necrosis. *A,* Concentric hemorrhagic necrosis. *B,* Histology presents diffuse contraction band necrosis associated with extensive hemorrhage. This pattern is not seen in human catecholamine cardiotoxicity or in that induced in the experimental setting (H&E stain).

from troponin, resulting in loss of contraction[29]; (2) that intracellular alkalosis induces a rapid loss of adenosine triphosphate (ATP) with a lack of energy to remove Ca^{++} from troponin[30] or a massive intracellular influx of Ca^{++} by means of increased membrane permeability that leads, through activation of myofibrillar adenosinetriphosphatase (ATPase), to (hyper)contraction and ATP consumption[31]; and (3) that there is reduced ability of the sarcotubular system and mitochondria to bind Ca^{++} in failing death.[32]

The rule on which we base this nosologic classification is that a pathogenic mechanism always produces the same type of morphologic lesion. Infarct necrosis is the result of a critical sudden reduction of nutrient flow. Coagulative myocytolysis (or contraction band necrosis) and hypercontraction damage are probably caused by adrenergic stimulation or any factor acting through free-radical–mediated lipid peroxidation,[33] whereas colliquative myocytolysis is possibly linked with catecholamine depletion, reduced intracellular Ca^{++}, loss of K^+, and increased intracellular Na^+. Myofibrillar lysis follows prolonged β-blocking therapy,[34] hypokalemia,[35] and hypocalcemia.[36]

ASSOCIATION BETWEEN THE VARIOUS FORMS OF MYOCARDIAL INJURY AND ISCHEMIC HEART DISEASE

The previous sections stress that irreversible relaxation injury is pathognomonic of a myocardial infarction, irreversible hypercontraction is induced experimentally by catecholamines and is found in many ischemic and nonischemic conditions, and colliquative myocytolysis is an indication of congestive heart failure, independent of its cause. It is important, however, to emphasize the association, between these three forms of myocardial injury and ischemic heart disease. Thus, in all acute myocardial infarcts, a rim of coagulative myocytolysis of varying widths is observed at the periphery and in continuity with the infarct. In 85% of acute myocardial infarcts, isolated or confluent foci of coagulative myocytolysis not associated with hemorrhage are found in nonischemic myocardium surrounding the infarct zone or in other regions of the heart (Fig. 8-15),[37, 38] a finding also observed in experimental myocardial infarction.[7] An experiment conducted in a dog that demonstrated a temporary coronary occlusion lasting 18, 20, 40 and 60 minutes or a 10-minute occlusion followed by 5-minute reflow repeated four times (conditioning), induced a progressive increase in the number of foci and myocells × 100 mm² showing coagulative myocytolysis in parallel with the duration of occlusion and maximal after conditioning. The extent of the lesion, often associated with ventricular fibrillation, was similar in both ischemic and nonischemic myocardium. This form of necrosis was not blood flow-dependent as shown by the injection of radioactive microspheres. In these studies, both pathologic contraction bands and ventricular fibrillation were prevented by a β-blocker (presented for publication). In humans, coagulative myocytolysis is unrelated to infarct size, heart weight, or severity of coronary atherosclerosis and is related only to adventitial lymphoplasmacellular infiltrates in atherosclerotic plaque. Because the centripetal infiltration of polymorphonuclear leukocytes begins at an infarct's periphery, where blood flow is present and increased, only in this myocardial layer is coagulative myocytolysis related to these leukocytes.

In 38% of acute infarcts, particularly in patients with chronic ischemia, colliquative myocytolysis has been demonstrated in subendocardial and perivascular myocardial layers; it is usually free of infarct necrosis and observed around myocardial fibrosis (Fig. 8-16).

In sudden and unexpected coronary deaths, coagulative myocytolysis was the only acute myocardial lesion found in 72% of hearts, and it was associated with a documented infarct in 14% of cases. Only in 8% of cases was colliquative myocytolysis observed, generally at the site of extensive myocardial fibrosis.[39] The association of these three forms of injury has to be considered in relation to an early diagnosis and the size of the acute myocardial infarct.

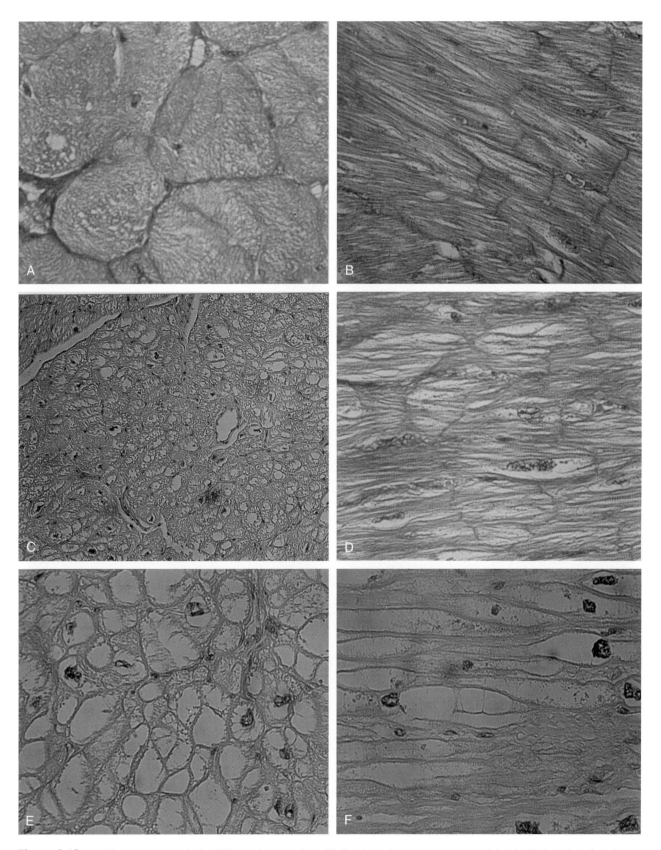

Figure 8-13 • Colliquative myocytolysis. Different degrees of myofibrillar loss, shown in transverse and longitudinal sections from human hearts excised at transplantation for congestive heart failure. *A* and *B*, Minimal patterns (*A*, Mallory; *B*, (H&E stain). *C* and *D*, Median patterns (*C*, (H&E stain); *D*, Mallory). *E* and *F*, Severe pattern with almost total loss of myofibrillar apparatus (both H&E stain).

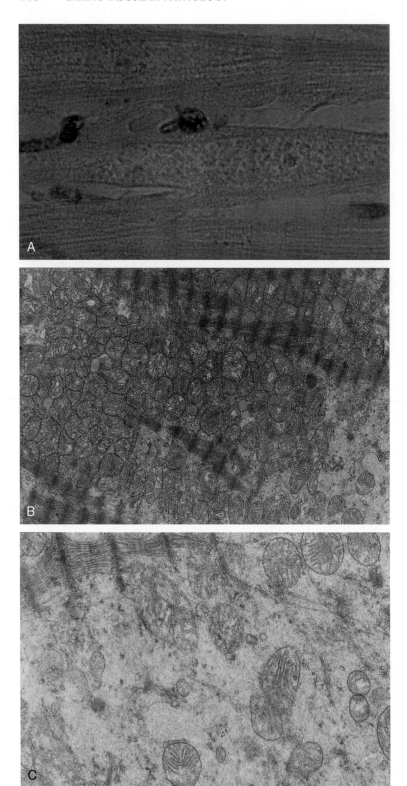

Figure 8-14 • Colliquative myocytolysis in human hearts excised at transplantation *A,* Severe loss of myofibrils with granular appearance (H&E stain). *B,* By electron microscopy, the myocell is filled by mitochondria. (EM, ×3000). *C,* It may also show edema (EM).

REVERSIBLE AND IRREVERSIBLE MYOCARDIAL INJURY IN RELATION TO MYOCARDIAL DYSFUNCTION IN VIVO

In describing the morphologic changes in these three forms of functional myocardial injury, the possible histologic signs of irreversibility, polymorphonuclear infiltrates, disruption of myofibrils, and subtotal loss of myofibrils have been mentioned, and the approximate period from functional arrest to myocellular death has been reported. Only for colliquative myocytolysis do we lack information on both timing and repair.

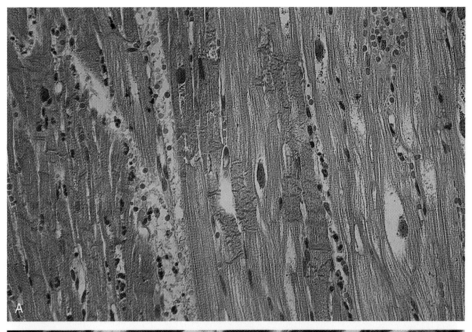

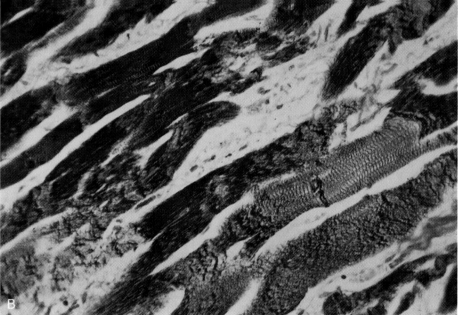

Figure 8-15 • Coagulative myocytolysis associated with acute infarct necrosis. *A*, Lesion close to the edge of an infarct (H&E stain). *B*, Lesion in myocardium of noninfarcted zone (PTAH). Note the absence of hemorrhage.

We are still unable to document histologically the point of no return of any myocardial injury or to correlate regional or global dysfunction shown by radionuclide angiography or echocardiography with its morphologic substratum. Dysfunction, or asynergy, is divided into three main patterns: (1) hypokinesis, or reduced contractility; (2) akinesis, or loss of contraction; and (3) dyskinesis, or paradoxical systolic bulging of noncontracting myocardium. The functional recovery of asynergic myocardium has been reported for some time; more recently, however, the concept of a viable but nonfunctioning myocardium has produced correct diagnosis and therapy in relation to permanent and temporary asynergic areas.[40] Dobutamine infusion predicted improvement in 198 of 205 segments that recovered function after surgery.[41]

At present, two patterns of viable but nonfunctioning myocardium are distinguishable. One, a chronic ischemic state, is a *hibernating myocardium,* defined as "a state of persistently impaired myocardial and left ventricular function at rest due to reduced coronary blood flow that can be partially or completely restored to normal if the myocardial oxygen supply/demand relationship is favorably altered either by improving blood flow and/or reducing demand."[42] This is a situation in which a "smart" heart stops contracting to save its structures but is ready to function again as soon as flow is reestablished. Less clear is how a hibernating myocardium could reduce demand and resume contracting. The other type of nonfunctioning viable myocardium is the *stunned myocardium,* a circumstance that occurs following reflow after temporary exper-

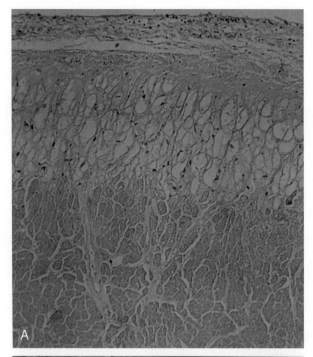

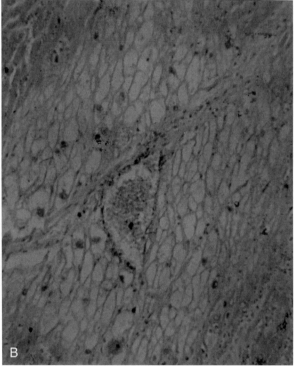

Figure 8-16 • Colliquative myocytolysis associated with acute infarct in *A*, subendocardial myocardium. *B*, Perivascular myocardium (H&E stain).

imental ischemia; hours or weeks are required for the myocardium to return to proper functioning.[43–45, 50a] These two apparently divergent patterns of viable myocardium—acute ischemia plus reflow in stunning and chronic ischemia in hibernation—do not have clear-cut histologic hallmarks. In a variety of experimental models, occlusions plus reflow did not show histologic findings in stunned myocardium in contrast to relaxation of myocells with wide I-bands, margination of nuclear chromatin, glycogen depletion, intracellular and extracellular edema,[46] and marked alterations of collagen matrix[47] occurring after an increasing number of brief coronary occlusions ("sensitization"). In chronic ischemic patients, transmural biopsies of dysfunctioning myocardium reveal cellular swelling, loss of myofibrils, and glycogen accumulation to be the main changes,[48] with time-dependent deterioration and fibrosis impairing recovery after revascularization[50b] and considered an incomplete progressive degenerative adaptation to ischemia.[50c] The structural changes are similar to those we define as colliquative myocytolysis. They were related to repeated episodes of ischemia rather than to chronic hypoperfusion[49] and were interpreted as reversible "dedifferentiation," the delayed functional recovery being due to slow resynthesis of myofibrils.[50] The relationship between blood flow and viable but nonfunctioning myocardium is still unclear. The examination of 102 dyssynergic segments recovered from 21 patients, 1 month after they had received thrombolytic treatment associated with an acute anterior infarction, revealed 36 were necrotic and 66 viable. Perfusion defects were recorded in 30 of the latter (hibernation) whereas the other 36 had preserved resting perfusion (stunning). Flow response to dobutamine was markedly reduced in necrotic segments but not in hibernated or stunned ones, with an improved function in 55% of stunned versus 16% of hibernated and 11% of necrotic myocardium. The lack of functional response was unrelated to an abolished vasodilating capacity.[50d] This was not confirmed by others.[50e] In patients with end-stage cardiac failure who underwent heart transplantation, myocardial blood flow was reduced equally in viable and fibrotic areas, suggesting that mechanisms other than coronary lesions and myocardial fibrosis caused the blood flow reduction.[51] At present, a histologic definition of hibernating or stunned myocardium is lacking; false-positive findings (asynergy with normal, contracting myocardium) and false-negative findings (myocardial damage without asynergy) are common.[52]

In this uncertainty, we are confined to hypotheses. If we consider the functional myocardial injuries and their basic morphologic changes, the working postulate could be that stunning following reflow is an impairment of the contraction-relaxation cycle with prevailing contraction (reduced capability of the Ca^{++} pump to remove this ion from actin/myosin interdigitation) and reduced relaxation; the reverse could be so for hibernation, that is, prevailing relaxation with reduced contraction.

A final comment about the concept of myocell death: In a recent review,[53] two main patterns of cell death were proposed—apoptosis (see later section) and oncosis. The term *oncosis* is derived from the Greek word *onkos*, swelling. It has the structural hallmarks of swelling, vacuolization, and blebbing (increased permeability) and ends in coagulation necrosis with karyolysis followed by a phagocytic and inflammatory reaction. This is typical ischemic cell death. The previous concepts may be valid for other tissues, but they appear to be inadequate for myocell death. In fact, infarct necrosis of the myocell is not an oncotic phenomenon and never shows, at any

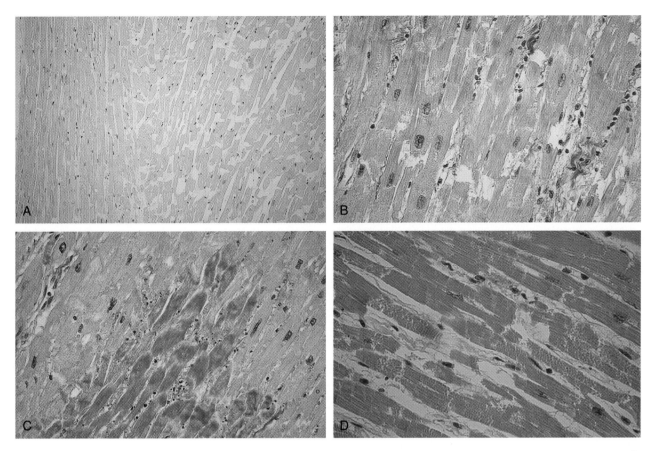

Figure 8-17 • Ventricular fibrillation damage. *A,* Area of distended myocells (left) adjacent to an area of contracted and segmented myocells (H&E stain). *B,* Contracted and segmented myocells without affinity for stain. *C,* Myocells with coagulative myocytolysis (Afog). *D,* Contracted myocells plus stretched disks alternating with distended myocells showing granular aspect (H&E stain). This pattern may be confused with coagulative myocytolysis.

stage of its evolution, the changes typical of oncosis. Only in colliquative myocytolysis with intracellular edema may the term *swelling* be appropriate. However, this lesion cannot be defined as an ischemic lesion, does not show coagulation necrosis, and is typical of end-stage heart failure as a consequence, not as a cause, of the latter.[28] In this discussion, the myocardial changes possibly linked with malignant arrhythmia and ventricular fibrillation (Fig. 8-17) must be considered (see the later section on cardiac arrest).

OTHER MYOCARDIAL CELL INJURIES

In other pathologic conditions, different patterns of myocardial cell injury not secondary to dysfunction are seen. They include myocarditis (see Chapter 9), tropical and parasitic diseases, metabolic and familial diseases (see Chapter 16), and so forth. Also, many descriptive terms, such as hydropic degeneration, cloudy swelling, hyaline and fatty degeneration, vacuolization, and zonal lesion, are used to describe changes. The impression is that many pertain to one of the functional injuries previously described. Allowing for conditions in which we can demonstrate infectious or parasitic agents or storage substances (glycogen, for example) within myocells, the visible histologic changes are quite nonspecific. In parasitic

disease we may see parasites without evidence of any reaction, whereas in myocarditis, bacterial or mycotic agents may be seen in necrotic foci of myocardium. In virus or autoimmune myocarditis, myotoxic lymphocytes may destroy myocells. In this section, morphologic changes that may affect diagnosis and interpretation are emphasized.

Myocarditis

According to the Dallas criteria,[54] a diagnosis is made when myocytotoxic elements affect and destroy myocells (see Chapter 9). We note that the appearance of necrotic, "cross-banded" myocells surrounded by reactive oligodendritic monocytes may simulate myocarditis (Fig. 8-18). This fact must be kept in mind because of the high frequency of this myocardial injury in human pathology.

Vacuolization

Vacuolization of the myocell is a very common nonspecific finding in a variety of injuries. Empty vacuoles in myocells can be seen in any storage disease, in fat degeneration, or as a possible artifact, particularly in histologic transverse sections (e.g., perinuclear halo, stretched myocells sectioned at I-bands). However, the pattern most commonly associated with vacuolization is the previously

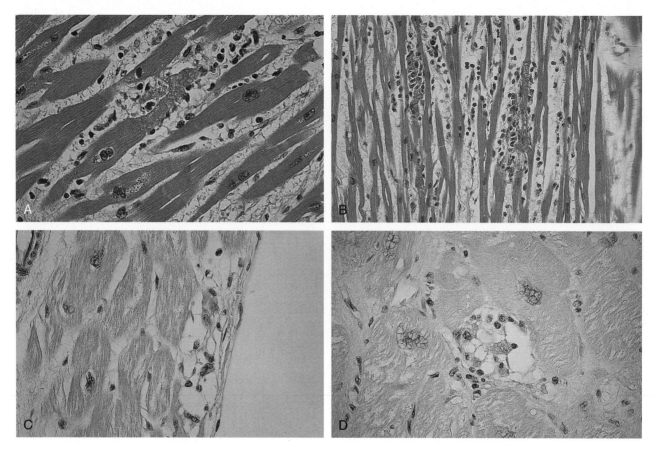

Figure 8-18 • *A* and *B*, Coagulative myocytolysis associated with monocyte reaction in a patient with AIDS. This is "pseudomyocarditis," a pattern shown in all conditions with coagulative myocytolysis. *C*, Two dead myocells with monocytes at the interstitial margin in a case with chronic valvulopathy. *D*, One dead myocell with monocytes within the myocardium in a case of dilated cardiomyopathy of unknown origin (All H&E stain).

described colliquative myocytolysis extensively present in all hearts with end-stage failure due to various causes[28] and found in 38% of fatal acute myocardial infarcts.[5] It is interpreted as a marker of ischemia in post-transplant biopsies[55] and in cases of sudden death.[56] However, vacuolization is not seen in the early phases of infarct necrosis.

Coagulative Myocyte Necrosis

This recent definition describes an ischemic necrosis that includes "myocyte hypereosinophilia, loss of nuclei, smudging, and loss of cytoplasmic detail and scattered polymorphonuclear leukocytes" in endomyocardial biopsies removed from transplanted hearts.[57] This lesion, which is similar if not identical to coagulative myocytolysis, can be interpreted as an expression of catecholamine cardiotoxicity in denervated hearts sensitized to catecholamines.[58, 58a] The frequency and extent of this lesion in transplanted hearts (see Table 8-2) has been previously mentioned.

Apoptosis

This term defines an old concept in embryology and pathology that indicates a "physiologic, genetically con-

trolled, cellular death" that maintains homeostasis in a tissue; that is, a balance between cellular birth and death. An error in this balance may induce pathology. The morphology of this type of cellular death is well established: early nuclear and cellular shrinkage, nuclear pyknosis ("half-moon" or "sickle" nuclei), followed by budding and karyorhexis with breakup into a cluster of apoptotic bodies phagocyted by macrophages or nearby cells. The term *apoptosis* is from the Greek *apo* (from) and *ptosis* (fall) and suggests leaves dropping here and there from a tree as opposed to the massive and simultaneous cell death of an infarct.[53] An increasing number of papers have demonstrated a high frequency of myocardial and coronary apoptosis by means of the immunostaining of exposed nuclear molecular endings of DNA fragments. Apoptosis has been recognized in smooth muscle cells and macrophages of human atherosclerotic plaques,[58b] in experimental vascular injury,[59, 60] in the myocardium after reperfusion,[61] in acute infarction,[62] in dilated cardiomyopathy,[63] in end-stage heart failure,[64] in arrhythmogenic right ventricular dysplasia,[65] and after myocardial stretching in hibernating myocardium.[58c, 66] Apoptosis, therefore, needs to be considered in the natural history of most, if not all, cardiovascular diseases. Its ubiquity, however, engenders some doubts about its significance. In our histologic studies, we were unable to show any morphologic evidence of apoptotic changes (nuclear shrinkage, apoptotic bodies, etc.) in the three forms of morphofunctional injury. Neither in amitosis of myocell nuclei[66a] nor in hibernating myocardium by electron microscopy and immunohistochemistry[66b, 66c] were nuclear changes typical for apoptosis documented. TUNEL (in situ nick end-labeling) detects not only DNA fragmentation but also single-stranded DNA breaks with free 3'-OH terminals.[66c] The nature of apoptosis in myocardial pathology is a matter for continuing investigation.[67–68a, 69]

REPAIR OF MYOCARDIAL INJURIES

With the exception of apoptosis, in which dead cells simply disappear, and colliquative myocytolysis, which does not seem to induce any cellular reaction or repair, the other two forms of myocardial repair show the same mechanism of collagenization based on macrophagic phagocytosis within sarcolemmal tubes followed by collagen fiber deposition as was described earlier. The resulting infarct scar is variable in size and is formed by dense fibrous tissue with straight collagen fibers. Coagulative myocytolysis heals in plurifocal, often confluent, fibrous foci with marked waviness of collagen fibers (Fig. 8-19). A common finding in myocardial scars is obliterative

hyperplasia and hypertrophy of the smooth muscle cells of the tunica media of small vessels (Fig. 8-20). The medial hyperplasia may transform to fibrous tissue.[5] The question is whether, in cardiac hypertrophy, the increased interstitial/perivascular or intermyocellular connective tissue is caused by the proliferation of collagen fibers and collagen matrix related to increased myocardial mass[2] or to a substitutive, ongoing process of necrosis, particularly coagulative myocytolysis (see Fig. 8-18), affecting a few cells, or to both (see the subsequent discussion of remodeling).

CARDIAC ARREST

The heart may arrest its function in several ways.[70] It may stop in ventricular fibrillation whether or not preceded by a malignant arrhythmia possibly linked with adrenergic stimulation[71]; or in asystole occurring after neural bradycardia/hypotension[72]; or in electromechanical dissociation[73] in which a normal electrocardiogram is associated with a loss of mechanical function (pulse, blood pressure, heart sounds, and consciousness) not always explained at autopsy (e.g., pulmonary embolism, heart rupture with tamponade).[74]

The structural counterpart of each pattern of cardiac

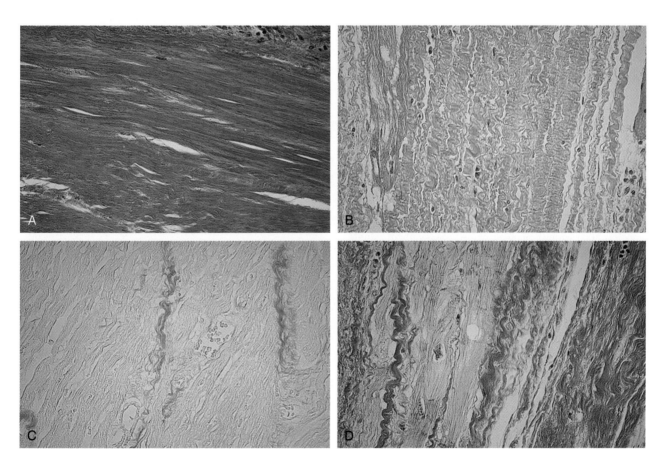

Figure 8-19 • Different types of myocardial scar. *A*, Dense, compact fibrous tissue with straight fibers in healed infarct (Gomori). *B*, Wavy collagen fibers in an extensive scar associated with contracting myocells in a sudden and unexpected death case (H&E stain). *C*, Waviness of interstitial collagen fibers in a hypertrophied, chronic ischemic heart with minimal interstitial fibrosis (Picrosirius red). *D*, Dense infarct scar (right) and wavy interstitial fibrosis in surrounding normal myocardium (Gomori stain).

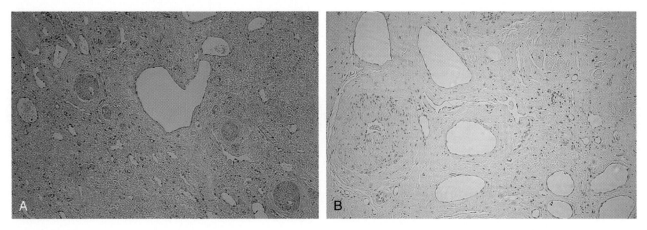

Figure 8-20 • *A* and *B*, Marked obliterative hyperplasia of smooth muscle cells of the tunica media of arterioles in myocardial scar. This is a secondary phenomenon (H&E stain).

arrest is unknown. The type of cardiac arrest could be important in relation to the pathophysiology of death and its implication in forensic pathology. At present, we know that ventricular fibrillation prevails in ischemic heart disease as is shown by successful defibrillation[75] and by patients who die suddenly during Holter monitoring.[76] Defined as "chaotic, random, asynchronous electrical activity of the ventricles due to repetitive re-entrant excitation and/or rapid focal discharge,"[77] ventricular fibrillation may have a morphologic hallmark that is now generally interpreted as an artifact.

As early as 1907, segmentation of myocardial fibers was related to a severe myocell contraction and proposed as a change possibly linked with ventricular fibrillation (quoted in Staemmler[78]). In many conditions we observed the following histologic, often associated, changes: bundles of hyperdistended myocardial cells with occasional focal disruption alternating with bundles of hypercontracted myocells with thickened Z lines, and the widening or segmentation of the intercalated disks. Hypercontraction was associated with prevailing "square" nuclei in contrast to the rectangular appearance of hyperdistended myocells. The same changes were observed in single myocells or groups of myocells in alternating hypercontracted and hyperdistended states. Often a hyperdistended myocell assumed a focal or diffuse granular aspect with fragmentation. These changes did not show the affinity for eosin or any other stain seen in coagulative myocytolysis (see Fig. 8-17), being distinct from the latter and seen in most (80%) sudden and unexpected coronary deaths, in 52% of brain hemorrhage cases without ischemic heart disease, in 24% of cases involving acquired immunodeficiency syndrome, in 95% of normal subjects who died following electrocution, and in 91% of cases following head trauma.[5] The criticism that this damage is an artifact of histologic procedures seems contradicted by the negative findings in more than 150 hearts excised at transplantation.[28] Furthermore, rigor mortis[79, 80] and ventricular fibrillation in dogs (electrical stimulus or intracoronary infusion of potassium chloride) maintained for 30 minutes and in calves maintained for 1 to 40 hours[81] did not induce this morphology. The variability in the extent of this change may distinguish successful (small myocardial areas triggering electrical instability with disruption of syncytial function) from unsuccessful defibrillation.

NATURAL HISTORY OF ISCHEMIC HEART DISEASE

Ischemic heart disease (IHD) is caused by a critical regional reduction of nutrient blood flow to the myocardium secondary to obstructive atherosclerosis of the extramural coronary arteries and their branches. Six main clinical patterns result. They are defined in Table 8-3. Each may transform to another, as the disease is characterized by great variability in course and complications. A major effort is under way to correlate clinical and morphologic findings obtained at autopsy or from surgical specimens. Morphology found in fatal cases helps to define the natural history of coronary atherosclerosis and its related clinical course.

TABLE 8-3 • **Clinical Patterns of Ischemic Heart Disease**

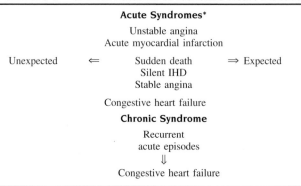

	Acute Syndromes*	
	Unstable angina	
	Acute myocardial infarction	
Unexpected ⇐	Sudden death	⇒ Expected
	Silent IHD	
	Stable angina	
	Congestive heart failure	
	Chronic Syndrome	
	Recurrent	
	acute episodes	
	⇓	
	Congestive heart failure	

*Each acute syndrome may occur in a normal individual or a patient with a previous episode of IHD (See text).

Natural History of the Coronary Atherosclerotic Plaque

The epidemiology, pathogenesis, and morphology of atherosclerosis are discussed in Chapter 4. Here, only a few points peculiar to coronary atherosclerosis are made so as to allow a better understanding of the relationship between morphologic changes and clinical disorders.

Hemodynamics

Epicardial coronary arteries and their branches are muscular arteries and so are prone to atherosclerosis. Hemodynamics influence the latter as is shown by rare adult cases in which the right coronary artery arises anomalously from the pulmonary artery. The left vessel arising from the aorta is severely atherosclerotic but not the one originating from the low-pressure pulmonary artery,[82, 83] an impressive example that stresses the role of hemodynamics, as compared with other factors.

Fibromuscular Intimal Thickening

On the other hand, the extramural coronary arteries and their branches show physiologic thickening at birth. It is progressive and affects the whole intima diffusely by the second decade. This process starts with smooth muscle cell hyperplasia with hyperelastosis and is followed by fibrous transformation with age[84] (see Chapter 3 also). It is interpreted as a response of the coronary wall to various dynamic forces enhanced by the peculiar coronary blood flow that fills the extramural vessels in systole without discharge into intramural vessels compressed by myocardial contraction; only in diastole is flow free to penetrate intramurally. However, the finding of a non-thickened coronary intima in animals (e.g., dogs) with cardiac morphophysiology identical to that of humans invites consideration of whether humans have the proper neuroadrenergic component to control wall tone in these vessels running free on the surface of the heart; they are, therefore, more subject to the effects of hemodynamic forces because of the absence of a surrounding support. This physiologic intimal thickening, sometimes erroneously interpreted as an early sign of atherosclerosis, is, at maximum, a predisposing factor. Intramural arterial vessels and "mural" tracts of extramural coronary arteries[85] do not show physiologic intimal thickening and myohyperplastic atherosclerotic plaques, possibly because of the protective effect of a lower blood pulse and support from surrounding myocardium.

Types of Atherosclerotic Plaque

A second point is that the atherosclerotic plaques in IHD patients without familial hyperlipidemia seem to have a natural history different from those observed in hyperlipidemic subjects and those induced experimentally by hypercholesterol diets.[5] The hypercholesterol plaque is characterized by early lipoprotein transendothelial infiltration followed by a macrophagic reaction.[5] In contrast, the plaque seen in nonhyperlipidemic IHD patients begins with a nodular, possibly "monoclonal,"[86] smooth muscle

TABLE 8-4 • **Progression of Myohyperplastic Atherosclerotic Plaque in Relation to Increasing Intimal Thickness and Lumen Reduction**

Intimal Thickness/μm	Morphologic Variables	Lumen-diameter Reduction (%)
>300	Nodular smooth myocellular hyperplasia $\Downarrow$ Fibrosis	<50
>600	Fibrosis + basophilia Early adventitial/intimal inflammatory reaction	50–69
>1000	Basophilia Calcification Inflammatory reaction Vascularization Hemorrhage Rupture Thrombosis	>70

cell and elastic intimal hyperplasia, defined as a smooth myocell hyperplastic plaque or a myohyperplastic plaque, followed by muscle cell degeneration and fibrosis. From this early nodular lesion, the plaque[5] progresses by means of various changes, with increasing intimal thickening and lumen reduction (Table 8-4).

Progression and Complications of the Myohyperplastic Atherosclerotic Plaque

Fissuring or rupture of an atherosclerotic plaque evokes coronary thrombosis or embolization or both, which in turn cause acute coronary syndromes.[87, 88] Fissuring combined with mural thrombi occurs even in the absence of clinical symptoms that explain plaque progression and increasing lumen reduction.[89] The molecular bases of plaque rupture are of paramount importance in understanding both the natural history of atherosclerotic plaque and IHD and their etiopathogenesis. Briefly, the thin fibrous cap that covers the lipid core of a "vulnerable" plaque, often undetected angiographically, breaks down by means of a complex interaction of factors, derived from T lymphocytes, macrophage-foam cells, and activated smooth muscle cells. The smooth muscle cells synthesize the extracellular matrix protein, collagen, and elastin from amino acids. In an unstable plaque, interferon-γ (IFN-γ) secreted by activated T cells may inhibit collagen synthesis and activated macrophages secrete metalloproteinase that can break down both collagen and elastin peptides and, eventually, aminoacids, leading to plaque rupture and coronary syndromes.[90]

Our histologic studies of selected coronary myohyperplastic plaques[91] revealed, deep to the fibrous cap of the early fibrotic plaque and near the media, a proteoglycan accumulation in which lipoprotein and cholesterol or calcium salts or both accumulate because of their affinity with proteoglycans[92] (Fig. 8-21). Recurrence of these phenomena gives rise to the tridimensional (longitudinal, circumferential, radial) progression of a plaque and leads to lumen reduction. This continuous, and pathologic reshap-

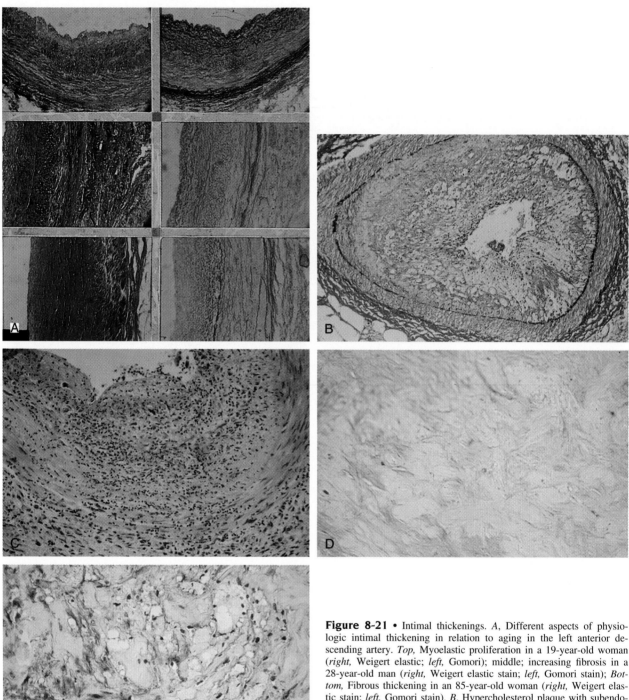

Figure 8-21 • Intimal thickenings. *A,* Different aspects of physiologic intimal thickening in relation to aging in the left anterior descending artery. *Top,* Myoelastic proliferation in a 19-year-old woman (*right,* Weigert elastic; *left,* Gomori); middle; increasing fibrosis in a 28-year-old man (*right,* Weigert elastic stain; *left,* Gomori stain); *Bottom,* Fibrous thickening in an 85-year-old woman (*right,* Weigert elastic stain; *left,* Gomori stain). *B,* Hypercholesterol plaque with subendothelial lipoprotein infiltration and foam cells from a hyperlipidemic patient (Movat stain). *C,* Myohyperplastic plaque with nodular smooth muscle cell and elastic tissue hyperplasia as first stage of the lesion (H&E stain). *D,* Proteoglycan accumulation. *E,* Interstitial and macrophage (foam cells) lipoprotein storage in the proteoglycan pool (*D, E,* Movat stain).

ing of the intima explains the varying histology among plaques (Fig. 8-22) and along the course of any one plaque, in which atheroma or fibrosis may prevail (Fig. 8-23). On this morphologic background, other subsequent changes or complications of atherosclerosis are grafted. They are, respectively, adventitial and intimal lympho-plasmacellular infiltrates that have a peculiar tropism for

nerves adjacent to the media (Fig. 8-24); vascularization; intimal hemorrhage; rupture of the plaque at the atheroma site; and mural, or occlusive, thrombosis. It must be stressed that in a large series of coronary sections from patients with various patterns of IHD and from 97 normal subjects who died by accident, platelet aggregates, fibrinomural thrombi, and subendothelial lipoprotein/choles-

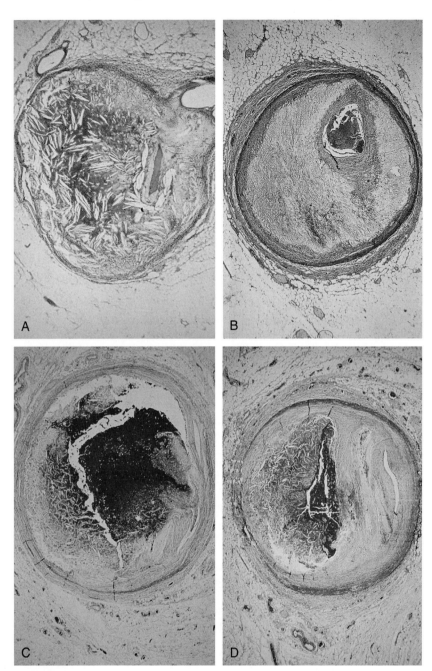

Figure 8-22 • Different aspects of the atherosclerotic plaque. *A*, Atheromatous hemorrhagic plaque with very small residual lumen at right. *B*, Fibrous plaque with small eccentrically placed lumen obstructed by an acute thrombus. *C*, Hemorrhagic rupture of a plaque proximal to *D*. *D* Severe stenosis occluded by a small thrombus (All Movat stain).

terol deposition were not seen in 1519 coronary sections with normal lumen and physiologic intimal thickening (≤ 300 μm) or in 1319 sections with less than 70% lumen reduction, or in 743 sections with intimal thickening less than 1000 μm. Quantified plaque variables had a significantly different incidence among patients with various patterns of IHD when plaques causing identical lumen reduction were compared.[5, 91] (For a discussion of atherosclerotic coronary aneurysms, see a later section.)

Lumen Reduction. In coronary angiographic studies,[93–97] the reduction or disappearance of luminal stenosis has been reported. This change is attributed to recanalization of a thrombus or lysis of an embolus[98] or to resolution of vasoconstriction or spasm. The likelihood of plaque regression arose from observations that ad-

vanced plaques are rare in adult cachectic people and that an experimental hypercholesterol plaque regresses after suspension of an atherogenic diet,[99] a concept essential to controlling atherosclerosis by this method. However, images are not always comparable in follow-up cineangiographic studies, and the frequency of regression was observed in only 4% of 1063 coronary angiographic segments.[100] In discussing plaque regression, the previous distinction between hypercholesterol and myohyperplastic plaques may explain the divergencies. Intensive lipid-lowering therapy resulting in angiographic regression associated with clinical improvement in patients with hyperapolipoprotein, IHD, and a family history of vascular disease[101] could be explained by resorption of lipids. It remains to be proved whether the

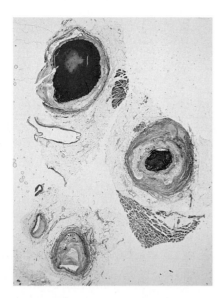

Figure 8-23 • Different histological levels of the same plaque. *Top,* an "occlusive" luminal coagulum with an almost normal vessel wall (with minor proteoglycan accumulation); *Middle,* occlusive thrombosis in severe stenosis with two areas of proteoglycan accumulation; *Lower,* subocclusive stenosis without thrombotic occlusion. (All Movat stain).

myohyperplastic plaque, found most often in IHD patients, resorbs.

Collaterals. The anastomotic, or collateral, coronary system, which may bypass a stenosis is another, often disregarded, variable in the natural history of coronary atherosclerotic plaques. These vessels exist at birth, are present everywhere in normal hearts, and may join branches of the same coronary artery, *homocoronary collaterals,* or branches of two or more coronary arteries, *intercoronary collaterals* (Figs. 8-25 and 8-26). In humans they are intramyocardial, and all increase in length and diameter in cardiac hypertrophy and chronic hypoxia such as anemia. In the case of a severe luminal stenosis, the collaterals in its direct topographic area enlarge (Fig. 8-27). Here we may speak of a *satellite collateral system* that may show two different patterns despite an identical coronary obstructive lesion. One apparently compensates by relatively few, highly enlarged collaterals that are easy to detect by angiography, and the other compensates by innumerable smaller collaterals not seen angiographically (Fig. 8-28). The differing architectures of satellite collaterals can be explained by subsequent atherosclerotic involvement of coronary arteries and by the loss of vessels in the infarcted zone (the avascular area; see Fig. 8-4), with further enlargement of surviving collaterals (Fig. 8-29). The increased anastomotic network connecting adventitial and intimal vessels with the residual lumen can be included in this satellite system.[102]

In our opinion, collateral development is not angiogenesis[103] but angiohyperplasia,[5] that is, hyperplasia of all wall components of preexisting vessels, which leads to increased diameter and length and to the remodeling of the normal wall structure in relation to enhanced flow[104] or to endothelial cell growth factors or both.[105] A similar remodeling occurs in cardiac hypertrophy.[100, 102] The role of ischemia in collateral development[106] is contradicted by

the fact that on occasion, only one collateral dramatically enlarges whereas most in the same zone do not (Fig. 8-30).

From an anatomic viewpoint, coronary vessels are not end arteries. Rather, they have innumerable collateral connections at every level of the intramural coronary system.[102] In contrast to those of the dog, vascular connections on the surface of the heart between extramural arteries and their branches are exceptional in humans.

From the clinical standpoint, findings on collaterals that are shown by coronary cineangiography support the mistaken belief that they do not protect in cases of IHD.[107] This argument will be discussed further. Here, it is sufficient to recall that human collaterals have a structure similar to that of capillaries.[102]

Postmortem and Clinical Imaging of Coronary Atherosclerotic Plaques

Lumen reduction is considered an index of ischemia. The degree of stenosis and number of coronary vessels with severe stenoses show great variability in different groups of IHD patients, noncardiac patients, and normal subjects (Table 8-5). Other modifications of a plaque, such as rupture or fissure of its surface leading to intimal hemorrhage, thrombosis, and embolization, cause unstable angina, myocardial infarction, sudden death, or all three. The rationale, therefore, is to demonstrate all of these variations in vivo for diagnostic, prognostic, and therapeutic purposes.

Coronary Cineangiography

This is a major source of clinical information, and terms such as "luminal irregularities," "haziness with ill-defined margins," "intraluminal lucencies," "menstruum persistence," and so forth are used to describe plaque alterations. The latter may be minor or may extend to angiographic cutoff, suggesting vessel occlusion. These cineangiographic images occur in persons who are ill; we

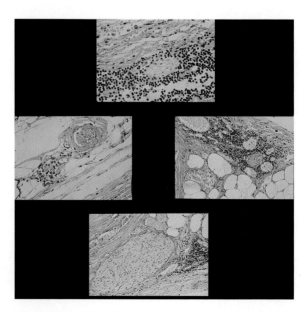

Figure 8-24 • Adventitial lymphoplasmacellular infiltrates. Various, aspects of pericoronary nerve involvement near the media (H&E stain).

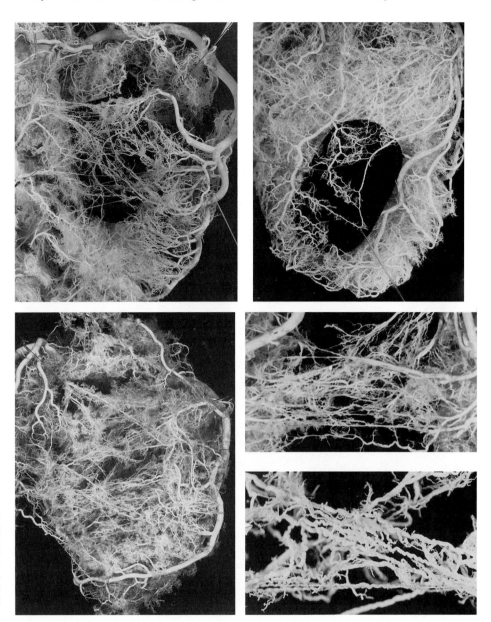

Figure 8-25 • Homo-intercoronary anastomoses (or collaterals) showing their characteristic corkscrew appearance. (From Baroldi G, Scomazzoni G: Coronary Circulation in the Normal and Pathologic Heart. American Registry of Pathology, A.F.I.P. [ed]: Washington, D.C., U.S. Government Printing Office, 1967.)

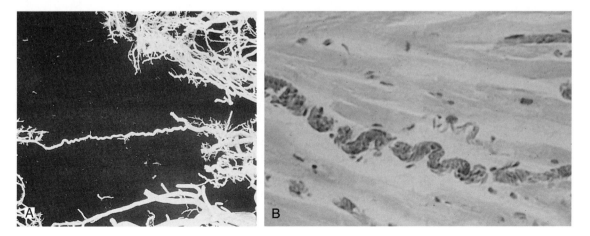

Figure 8-26 • *A*, Cast of isolated normal homocoronary collateral with characteristic corkscrew aspect. *B*, Equivalent histologic image (H&E stain). (From Baroldi G, Scomazzoni G: Coronary Circulation in the Normal and Pathologic Heart. American Registry of Pathology, A.F.I.P. [ed]: Washington, D.C., U.S. Government Printing Office, 1967.)

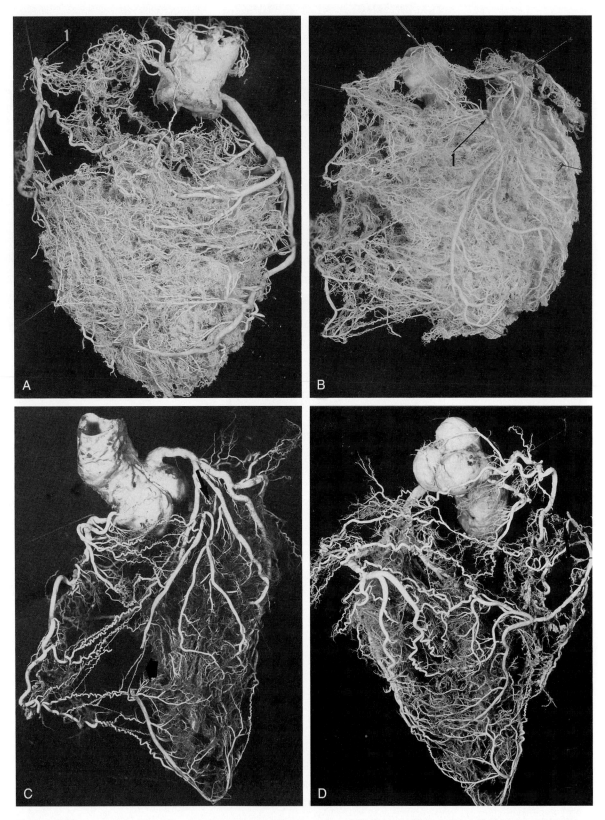

Figure 8-27 • Coronary plastic casts with dramatic collateral enlargement. *A*, A 71-year-old man with occlusion of the RCA but no IHD; microfocal myocardial fibrosis; death due to brain hemorrhage. *B*, A 39-year-old man with occlusion of the LAD and the first segment of RCA (not shown). Acute infarct of the inferior left ventricle. *C, D*, Anterior view showing double occlusion of LAD (*C*), and posterior view showing occlusion of RCA. *D*, A 66-year-old man dying of a brain hemorrhage without IHD or myocardial damage. (RCA, right coronary artery; LAD, left anterior descending artery.) (From Baroldi G, Scomazzoni G: Coronary Circulation in the Normal and Pathologic Heart. American Registry of Pathology, A.F.I.P. [ed]: Washington, D.C., U.S. Government Printing Office, 1967.)

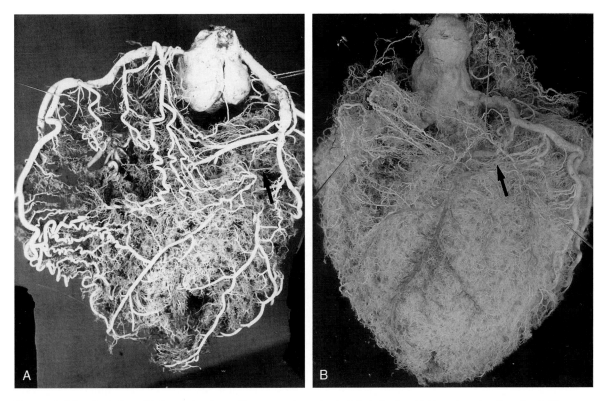

Figure 8-28 • Occlusion of left anterior descending artery (arrows). *A*, Relatively few highly enlarged collaterals. *B*, Numerous relatively small collaterals. (From Baroldi G, Scomazzoni G: Coronary Circulation in the Normal and Pathologic Heart. American Registry of Pathology, A.F.I.P. [ed]: Washington, D.C., U.S. Government Printing Office, 1967.)

do not know how commonly similar images occur in the healthy population. Nevertheless, healthy subjects who have died by accident and without a history of IHD have, at postmortem examination, coronary atherosclerotic plaques with various degrees of lumen reduction (see Table 8-5).[5, 39]

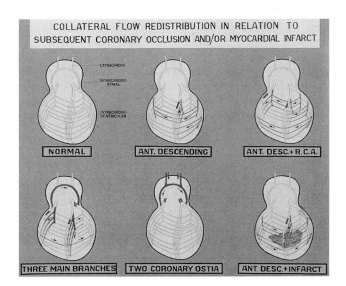

Figure 8-29 • Collateral flow redistribution in relationship to subsequent coronary occlusions or myocardial infarction or both. (From Baroldi G, Scomazzoni G: Coronary Circulation in the Normal and Pathologic Heart. American Registry of Pathology, A.F.I.P. [ed]: Washington, D.C., U.S. Government Printing Office, 1967.)

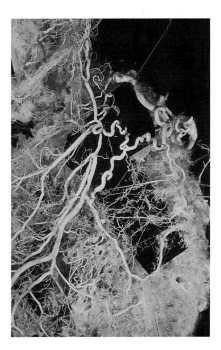

Figure 8-30 • One large "satellite" collateral from the left circumflex branch bypassing occlusion of the left anterior descending branch. Note numerous normal collaterals. Not all collaterals in an ischemic area increase in diameter and length. (From Baroldi G, Scomazzoni G: Coronary Circulation in the Normal and Pathologic Heart. American Registry of Pathology, A.F.I.P. [ed]: Washington, D.C., U.S. Government Printing Office, 1967.)

TABLE 8-5 • **Maximal Lumen Reduction and Number of Main
Extramural Coronary Arteries with Severe (≥70% Lumen Diameter) Stenosis**

Source	Number of Cases	Maximal Lumen Reduction (%)						Severe Stenosis (Vessels)		
		0	< 50	50–69	70–79	80–89	≥ 90	1	2	3
AMI 1st	145	3	8	6	29	45	54	61	48	19
AMI chr	55	1	1	—	8	11	35	16	22	16
Total	200	9	9	6	37	56	89	77	71	35
SUCD 1st	133	18	18	18	21	39	27	40	34	13
SUCD chr	75	—	—	5	8	14	48	13	26	31
Total	208	18	18	23	29	53	75	53	60	44
NCA	100	10	10	17	11	24	31	26	18	22
AD	97	20	20	31	19	13	6	22	13	3

Abbreviations: AD, normal subjects dying from accident; AMI, acute myocardial infarct; NCA, noncardiac atherosclerotic patients; SUCD, sudden/unexpected coronary death; 1st, first episode of ischemic heart disease (IHD); chr, chronic IHD.

Angioscopy

Angioscopy is another method that is believed to allow a distinction to be made between white thrombi, in unstable angina, and red, in stable angina,[108] and to allow greater precision than angiography provides in defining atherosclerotic lesions.[109] In reality, the angioscopic image is limited to the surface of the vessel intima, in a very unnatural condition, the presence of underlying lesions cannot be established correctly. Angioscopic images of white or red thrombi need histologic confirmation before any diagnosis is established.

Intravascular Ultrasound Imaging

Intravascular ultrasound imaging is, perhaps, the most promising of all diagnostic techniques.[110–115] It provides more precise information about the shape of the stenosis, which can be categorized as sagittal, cylindrical, or lumen cast.[114] Nevertheless, *ultrasonic histology* is too ambitious a term to use for the procedure. At present, every histologic change found in the natural history of an atherosclerotic plaque cannot be recognized by this investigative method. Among the many variables of atherosclerotic plaque, calcification is easily detected by various methods in vivo. However, its presence does not correlate with lumen reduction,[115a] and its demonstration by electron beam computed tomography does not predict the outcome in high-risk IHD patients.[115b] One point needs discussion—the relationship between the caliber of a catheter and the coronary lumen any time a catheter is introduced. The mean diameters of the lumens of the three main coronary arteries, or branches, calculated on the basis of plastic casts of normal hearts, are 3600 μm for the left anterior descending branch, 3000 μm for the left circumflex, and 3200 μm for the right coronary artery.[102] A 70%, 80%, and 90% lumen reduction, respectively, means a reduction to 1080 μm, 720 μm, and 360 μm for the first vessel, 900 μm, 600 μm, and 300 μm for the second vessel, and 960 μm, 640 μm, and 320 μm for the third vessel. The distribution of a maximal stenosis in each of 408 IHD cases was 70% stenosis in 16%, 80% stenosis in 27%, and 90% stenosis in 40% of individuals. These data raise doubts about catheterization because of the discrepancy between the diameter of a catheter (about 1500 μm) and the lumen it crosses (see Fig. 8-21). It must be noted that this traumatic intervention may induce iatrogenic morphofunctional changes that must be considered when dynamic measurements and diagnostic evaluations are made, particularly during angioplasty.

A last comment concerns differences between pathologists and angiographers when estimating the degree of coronary stenosis. The claim is that the former may overcall a stenosis because in vivo the filling pressure distends the vessel wall (see Chapter 1). In general, agreement exists when a correct quantification of angiographic and histologic imagings of severe, concentric stenoses is made. There is disagreement with regard to small concentric and semilunar plaques. It is to be noted that quantification of stenoses with any degree of lumen reduction gave similar results in 100 acute infarct cases with and without postmortem coronary injection under pressure.[5]

Vessel wall architecture is modified according to variations in flow dynamics and related stresses.[115c] Progression of the atherosclerotic process interacts with both. Vascular enlargement that is either post- or prestenotic or at the plaque level was recognized long ago.[115d] Pre- and poststenotic dilation must be considered when angiographic quantification of a stenosis is calculated. Enlargement at the plaque level makes unreliable any lumen measurement expressed as a percentage of a cross-sectional area. A normal or mild lumen stenosis may appear severe in a highly enlarged plaque. This prompted me, from the beginning of my studies, to evaluate a stenosis by calculating the average diameter of the residual lumen on a histologic section and to consider its percent of dilation in relation to the normal diameter of the corresponding vessel estimated on the plastic cast. I doubt that when plaque enlargement occurs, it can be teleologically defined as a compensatory phenomenon.[115e] The fact remains that most patients at their first episode of IHD had one or more severe lumen reductions, and the only demonstrable compensatory phenomenon was enlarged collaterals.[101]

Magnetic Resonance Imaging

Fayad and colleagues described in vivo, high-resolution magnetic resonance imaging of atherosclerotic lesions in genetically engineered mice, suggesting that this technique is a powerful tool for investigating serially and noninvasively the progression and regression of atherosclerotic lesions in an intact animal.[116]

Acute Coronary Syndromes

Acute coronary events include three main syndromes (see Table 8-3). Angina pectoris may exist by itself or be the first symptom of an infarct or a sudden death; an infarct may rapidly convert to sudden death; or an infarct and sudden death may arise without angina or other subjective symptoms. Each clinical pattern may occur in an apparently normal subject who is without a cardiac history and is enjoying life, or develop in a patient who has had previous episodes of IHD. This distinction between the first episode and the acute coronary syndrome that occurs in chronic IHD helps to define the natural history of each syndrome. In the absence of clinical information and in cases of silent IHD, this distinction can be made by a pathologist when a large focus of myocardial fibrosis that is more than 10% of the left ventricular mass is present or absent at autopsy.[5]

From the etiopathogenic viewpoint, a further distinction can be made because acute coronary syndromes occur in the presence of atherosclerotic and nonatherosclerotic coronary disease, such as dissecting aneurysm, emboli, ostial malformation, coronary arteritis, and with normal coronary arteries. The rare forms of nonatherosclerotic coronary diseases causing IHD (see later section) have a different history and pathophysiologic background even if they share the symptoms, signs, and pathogenetic mechanisms linked to complications with coronary atherosclerotic disease. The last group includes acute coronary syndromes occurring in the presence of coronary arteries with normal or minor lumen reduction; acute infarcts[37, 38, 117] or sudden or unexpected death[39] in the absence of significant coronary atherosclerosis. Cases have been reported at autopsy (see Table 8-5) and in most coronary angiographic studies.[5] In the latter situation, the pathogenetic hypotheses are that platelet or fibrin thromboemboli[118, 119] or coronary spasm of the main extramural arteries or branches[120] or intramural vessels[121–123] are responsible for the acute ischemia.

Coronary spasm was postulated long ago[124] and was demonstrated cineangiographically in angina pectoris with coronary atherosclerosis[120, 125] and in acute myocardial infarction.[126–129] At present, we do not know its exact causes, although several hypotheses have been formulated,[130] including release of a vasoactive substance by pericoronary mast cells[131] and endothelial cells.[132] Apart from some questionable histologic findings—smooth muscle cell contraction in the coronary media[122] or constriction of intramyocardial vessels in an experimental model[121]—a pathologist has no satisfactory way of demonstrating spasm postmortem. By quantitative measurement of medial thickness, it is possible to say that, despite medial reduction at plaque level, the structure of the remaining media is sufficient for functional vasoconstriction.[91] In an instance in which a serial section was performed on a coronary artery that showed angiographic spasm shortly before death, the spasm occurred in a severely stenosed atherosclerotic vessel.[128] In patients who had focal spasm induced by ergonovine maleate, small atherosclerotic plaques, undetected angiographically, were demonstrated by intravascular ultrasonography.[133] Spasm in a morphologically normal coronary artery (an artery without any pathologic change) has to be proved. In fact, the finding that isolated coronary artery spasm was the cause of arrhythmogenic cardiac arrest in seven resuscitated people with normal coronary arteries who subsequently demonstrated a positive reaction to the ergonovine test[133a] cannot be trusted. A normal coronary angiogram does not exclude the presence of an undetected "active" plaque (see later section).

The concept of spasm of the intramural vessels is an unsupported hypothesis. It is a conclusion that applies to many other conditions in which spasm is considered the cause of an acute coronary syndrome; for example, ischemia in chronic cocaine abusers. A review of the literature demonstrates that angiographic documentation of spasm has never been reported in cocaine abusers. Furthermore, the unique myocardial lesion found is acute contraction band necrosis, that is, coagulative myocytolysis. Its frequency is similar to that found in normal controls; no acute or old ischemic myocardial lesions were seen in 26 chronic cocaine abusers.[16]

Another condition reported in some cases of sudden coronary death[134] is the presence of extramural vessels covered by myocardial bridges,[85] which are considered a possible cause of vasoconstriction.[135] Surgical debridging is successful in preventing such deaths.[136]

Angina Pectoris

Cardiogenic chest pain can be confused with pain originating from noncardiac sources. Nevertheless, the main patterns of angina pectoris or its equivalents are listed in Table 8-6. Exact morphoclinical correlation is difficult in these conditions because a pathologist may examine only cases of angina followed by sudden death or fatal infarcts. However, cineangiographic studies have contributed to our understanding of stenoses of the main extramural coronary vessels and of plaque findings in such patients. "Complex and acute thrombotic" changes consisting of the "presence of luminal irregularity or haziness with ill-defined margins, a smudged appearance, inhomogeneous opacification within the lumen, or changes suggesting ulceration or plaque rupture"[137] are described. About

TABLE 8-6 • **Main Patterns of Angina Pectoris or Equivalents**

Stable angina (physical effort, cold, etc.)
Unstable angina (at rest)
Mixed when stable and unstable angina coexistent
Variant or Prinzmetal angina (coronary spasm)[312]
Cardiac syndrome X angina (women + positive exercise test and normal angiogram)[313]
Postinfarction angina
Angina equivalents: abrupt dyspnea, exhaustion, fatigue, fainting, arrhythmias

58% of patients with unstable angina showed angiographic evidence of a coronary thrombus[137, 138] in contrast to 5% of patients with stable angina. More precisely, angiographic stenoses were classified into four categories: *concentric,* symmetric with smooth margin; *eccentric,* asymmetric and further subdivided; *type I,* smooth border and a broad neck; and *type II,* convex obstruction and irregular or scalloped borders and multiple irregularities formed by closely spaced, severe obstructions. Type II coronary stenosis is interpreted as a disrupted atherosclerotic plaque or a partially occlusive or lysed thrombus expressing plaque evolution and a signal of impending infarction. Such plaques were found in 71% of patients with unstable angina, in 16% of those with stable angina, and in 66% of those with acute (within 12 hours) or recent (within 1–2 weeks) or healing (within 2–10 weeks) myocardial infarctions.[139, 140] These angiographic findings are supported by a morphologic study that showed a complicated plaque, rupture, hemorrhage, thrombus, and so forth in only 11% of angiographic type I stenoses in contrast to 79% in angiographic type II stenoses.[141] Despite the limitation of intimal scanning, discussed previously, directional coronary atherectomy revealed mural thrombosis in 35% of patients with unstable angina and in 17% of patients with stable angina.[142] Of patients with unstable angina or a recent (2-week-old) myocardial infarction, 44% had a fresh, large, "thrombus" of 3000 μm^2 or larger that was characterized by layered platelet aggregates, fibrin, and erythrocytes.[143]

An increasing number of angiographic reports claim the frequent occurrence of a thrombotic occlusion at the site of a noncritical atherosclerotic lesion. This opinion was derived from the angiographic finding that occlusion had occurred in an infarct-related artery that, in a previous coronary angiogram, had shown an obstructive stenosis of <50%.[144, 145] At restudy, progression of the small atherosclerotic plaques was uncommon in non–infarct-related vessels, so the conclusion was that small atherosclerotic plaques not detectable angiographically may rupture and cause occlusive thrombosis.[146]

The relationship between clinical and histologic imaging will be commented on later. Here, it is important to note a general agreement when the angiographic and histologic degree of severity of stenoses and their number in coronary arteries and branches are compared.[5] The concordant finding is that at their first episode of acute coronary syndrome, most patients show one or all main vessels with severe stenosis ranging from 70% to more than 90%. When a distinction is made between a first-episode and a chronic case, the latter showed a higher frequency of 90% stenosis and three-vessel disease (see Table 8-5).

Acute Myocardial Infarction

More frequent in men (the male/female ratio is 2:1), an infarct may occur in the fourth decade or even earlier if associated with hyperlipidemia, but maximal frequency occurs in the seventh decade. Uncommon in women younger than 60 years old, infarcts in this gender reach maximal frequency in the eighth decade.[37, 38] Future changes in these figures may be expected because of the increasing mean age and changing lifestyles of women.

Clinical Diagnosis

The diagnosis of a typical myocardial infarction is made when an individual has chest pain, electrocardiographic abnormalities, and an elevation of cardiac-specific serum enzymes. The substernal chest pain is severe and is described as a weight or tightness in the chest, with radiation to the neck or left arm. However, sometimes myocardial infarction may occur without symptoms, particularly in elderly or diabetic patients (a so-called silent myocardial infarction; see a later section). Shortness of breath and signs of adrenergic hyperstimulation such as sweating and tachycardia are also common, particulary when left ventricular dysfunction complicates myocardial infarction. Conversely, bradycardia is common in inferior myocardial infarction because of stimulation of vagal afferent nerve endings.

The typical electrocardiographic changes in the acute stage include ST segment elevation (equal to or greater than 1 mV) in contiguous leads or new-onset left bundle branch block; T-wave inversion and abnormal Q waves develop later during the subacute phase but may be absent (non–Q-wave myocardial infarction).

Myocardial necrosis is associated with the release into the plasma of cardiac enzymes and proteins. Many have been tested as markers of acute myocardial infarction. The serial evaluation of creatine-kinase (CK and its cardiac-specific isoenzyme MB [muscle-brain]) is a sensitive and specific marker of myocardial damage. Serum MB-CK starts rising 6 to 10 hours after symptom onset. It peaks at 14 to 36 hours, and returns to normal at 48 to 72 hours after an acute myocardial infarction. Normal CK and CK-MB serum levels rule out a myocardial infarction in 95% of cases. Frequent assessments are required to avoid false-negative results; false-positive results may be due to associated extensive skeletal muscle damage, which can usually be recognized in appropriate clinical conditions. Measurements of myoglobin and troponin are evolving as sensitive and specific early markers of myocardial injury.[147–149b]

Other nonspecific findings include fever, leukocytosis and, in the acute phase, erythrocyte sedimentation rate and C-reactive protein increase. Noninvasive imaging techniques, including echocardiography and radionuclide studies, allow quantification of myocardial infarct extension and residual left ventricular function and are useful for risk stratification.

By coronary cineangiography, a total or subtotal coronary occlusion was present in 87% and 10%, respectively, of patients examined within 4 hours of the onset of symptoms related to an acute Q-wave or transmural infarction. The frequency was lower—17 and 16%, respectively, when similar patients were observed after 6 hours.[150] In non–Q-wave or subendocardial infarcts, patients investigated within 24 hours, within 24 to 72 hours, and within 72 hours to 7 days after peak symptoms a total occlusion was seen in 26, 37, and 42%, and a subtotal occlusion was seen in 34, 25, and 18%, respectively.[151] Of patients with the definite angiographic features of an occlusive thrombus who had emergency surgical revascularization, 88% had a "thrombus" that was recovered by a Fogarty catheter.[150] From the earliest pathologic reports,[152-154] the frequency of an occlusive "white" thrombus, usually found related to a severe atherosclerotic stenosis, ranged from 38 to 91% and was more common in large transmural infarcts.[37, 38, 155-157] Thrombus formation correlates with many variables. In contrast with sudden and unexpected death, thrombus frequency is similar in both first-episode and chronic acute infarcts.[5]

Histologic and Ultrastructural Changes

The main histologic changes that occur in a myocardial infarct have been described, their time course reported, and the difficulty of early histologic diagnosis stressed. Grossly, an infarct 6 to 8 hours old can be outlined by incubating heart slices in a solution of nitroblue tetrazolium. It is reduced to a dark blue formazan by dehydrogenase enzymes contained in normal myocardium. Depletion of these enzymes following necrosis results in an unstained area.[158] Scarred areas of myocardium do not take up the stain either. A variant of this technique is the postmortem coronary perfusion of nitroblue tetrazolium.[159] The results of many other histochemical and immunohistochemical methods used to show the loss of various substances (glycogen, myoglobin, intracellular diffusion of IgG,[160] fibrinogen complement C5b-9,[161, 162] caeruloplasmin, C-reactive protein,[163] cytoskeletal proteins vinculin, desmin, α-actinin,[164] etc.) led to the conclusion that all markers were nonspecific and possibly were linked to agonal changes.[163]

Diagnosis by standard histologic techniques is still limited to the observation, at 6 to 8 hours, of polymorphonuclear leukocyte margination in vessels, and their early infiltration at the periphery of dead tissue. "Wavy fibers"—that is, undulating myocardial fibers[165]—and foci of coagulative myocytolysis or myocell stretching are early signs of an acute myocardial infarct but are not specific per se. The claim that the detection of apoptosis may demonstrate myocardial ischemic cell death as early as 2 to 4 hours[62] needs further investigation.

The close topographic association between infarct necrosis and coagulative myocytolysis defines a need to discriminate between these two forms of injury any time a technique is used to detect an early infarct. For instance, the hematoxylin–basic fuchsin–picric acid stain,[166] positive within 30 minutes of damage, beautifully stains contraction band necrosis which, besides having an association with infarcts, is found in many different ischemic and nonischemic conditions. The same criticism applies in the clinical setting when serum levels of CK-MB enzymes or other types of molecules released from necrotic tissue are measured to indirectly determine infarct size and stratification of risk in acute coronary syndromes.[167] The material measured reflects all forms of myocardial injury and necrosis that occur in association with an infarct, whereas, for clarity, their individual and possibly different contributions should be considered. Positive technetium Tc 99m stannous pyrophosphate myocardial scintigrams from patients with complicated postinfarct courses showed "myocytolytic" degeneration.[168] Recently, serum tumor necrosis factor alpha[169] and cardiac I troponins[170] and T troponins[171] were considered effective in determining infarct size and establishing the risk of death. However, the levels of troponin I were similar, independent of the number of vessels with severe stenoses and the presence of "angiographic" thrombi,[168] suggesting that other nonischemic damage may be present (see earlier discussion).

The association of the three different forms of myocardial injury and necrosis, mentioned previously, questions the timetables for healing defined by the histologic appearance or disappearance of involved cells (Table 8-7).[172, 173] It is to be noted that these timetables were developed in the past and do not take into consideration modern knowledge about the onset of clinical symptoms and infarction or the varying morphology of myocardial necrosis. As mentioned earlier, the healing of an infarct and contraction band necrosis is not accomplished by granulation tissue formation, and the evolution of colliquative myocytolysis is unknown. It is to be noted that the various stages of coagulative myocytolysis were incompletely defined in an experimental model of "myofibrillar degeneration," or coagulative myocytolysis, obtained by electrical current discharge on the surface of canine hearts.[13]

Our understanding of early ultrastructural changes and their time course in acute myocardial infarction is limited to experimental acute coronary occlusion and has no application to autopsy material. They are similar to changes observed in anoxia or following autolysis. In acute ischemia, glycogen depletion begins in the first minute of coronary occlusion and is almost complete after 40 minutes; mitochondrial swelling begins within 10 to 12 minutes and the organelles show diffuse disintegration of cristae and vacuolization after 30 minutes and rupture of their membranes at 5 hours; nuclei show chromatin clumping at 15 minutes and rupture of their membranes after 3 to 4 hours; sarcotubular system swelling is established by 30 minutes; myofibrils are relatively resistant and the sarcolemma may rupture within 5 hours. It must

TABLE 8-7 • **Chronology of Histologic Changes in Acute Myocardial Infarction**

Histologic Changes	Mallory et al[172]* 1939 Start/End	Lodge-Patch[173] 1951 Start/End
Edema	—	2/3
Myocell nuclei	—	4/11
Myocell necrosis	20/180†	6/28
Phagocyte remotion†	5/180	6/28
Polymorphonuclear leukocyte infiltration	6–24/180	6/10
Basophilic ground substance	—	20/14
Pigmented macrophages	6/365	3/>365
Lymphocytes-plasma cells	6/60	5/180
Eosinophilic leukocytes	6/28	10/30
Fibroblasts	4/90	4/60
Collagen	14/>365	10/>365
Angiogenesis	5/90	4/90

* Mallory, White, and Salcedo-Salgar described nonhemorrhagic contraction band necrosis at the periphery of acute infarcts.
† See original text for definition of "remotion."
Boldface italic = hours; lightface = days.

TABLE 8-8 • **Location of Myocardial Infarcts in 200 Consecutive Cases**

Ventricular Wall	%
Left anterior	7
Lateral	7
Inferior	10
Interventricular septum	3
Anteroseptal	48
Inferoseptal	14
Anterolateral	2
Inferolateral	9

be noted that even within 15 to 30 minutes, the stretching of myocells and pronounced I-bands are visible.[6]

Location, Wall Extension, and Size of Acute Myocardial Infarcts

The main location of an acute infarct is the left ventricle. Despite the frequent occlusion of the right coronary artery, an isolated infarct of that ventricle is rare, because the thin wall of the latter is nourished by intracavitary blood.[174, 175] However, in 40% of inferior wall infarcts of the left ventricle, the adjacent right ventricular wall is also involved. Isolated right ventricular infarction is a potentially reversible cause of cardiogenic shock, and its clinical recognition is based on right-sided heart failure with no left-sided signs, a right ventricular third or fourth heart sound, elevated jugular venous pressure, arterial hypotension, ventricular dilation, decreased right ventricular ejection fraction, and specific electrocardiographic findings.[176] In our study we did not demonstrate any ischemic lesion of the right ventricle in 18 cases with cor pulmonale, of whom one had right coronary occlusion and three had severe right coronary obstruction.[102] Atria are rarely affected by isolated infarcts. The relatively high frequency—8.5%[177, 178]—of atrial involvement, especially of the right atrium in left ventricular infarcts, needs further study.

The distribution of acute infarcts in the 200 consecutive cases we studied[5] is indicated in Table 8-8. In 11.5% of cases, the infarct involved the inner one third of the ventricular wall, in 31% it involved the inner two thirds, and in 57.5% it was transmural. The infarcted zone had a very irregular, tridimensional shape and its planimetrically measured size ranged from less than 10% of the left ventricular mass to more than 50% (Table 8-9). No correlation was found between infarct size and the number of severe stenoses in the coronary system.[37, 38]

TABLE 8-10 • **Complications of Myocardial Infarction**

Acute (2 wk)	Long-term
Arrhythmias	Arrhythmias
Sudden death	Sudden death
Denervation of noninfarcted myocardium	
Cardiogenic shock	
Pericarditis	Dressler syndrome

Rupture
  Free wall
  Interventricular septum
  Papillary muscle	

Mitral insufficiency due to:
  Papillary muscle
  Rupture
  Infarct
  Dyssynchronous impulse
	Mitral insufficiency due to:
	  Papillary muscle
	  Dysfunction/atrophy
	  Spatial separation by aneurysm
	  Annular dilation

Congestive heart failure	Congestive heart failure
Aneurysm	Aneurysm
Mural thrombosis	Mural thrombosis
Thromboembolism	Thromboembolism

Cardiac Remodeling

After a patient has a myocardial infarct, the collagenous network in the infarcted area is first degraded. This may induce myocardial wall thinning and cardiac dilation. Patients who have echocardiographic evidence of such infarct expansion are at risk for cardiac rupture. Long-term complications of infarct expansion include congestive heart failure, aneurysm formation, additional ischemic events, and premature cardiac mortality. Subsequently, new collagen is synthesized and a scar is formed that prevents further dilation and cardiac rupture. Nevertheless, these changes may induce myocardial stiffness and conducting system disturbances. Remaining viable myocytes in the infarcted region reattach to this now dense collagen matrix. This process is called remodeling.[180] Cleutjens and colleagues[180] studied collagen changes following myocardial infarction in the rat heart. Interstitial cells, not cardiomyocytes, produced the new collagens from myofibroblasts in the infarcted zone and fibroblast in noninfarcted myocardium.

Complications

The main morphologic complications of a myocardial infarct are listed in Table 8-10 and are discussed here.

TABLE 8-9 • **Percentage Distribution of Infarct Size (% Left Ventricular Mass) in 200 Consecutive Acute Infarct Cases Without (AMI First-Episode) and With (AMI Chronic) Extensive Myocardial Fibrosis**

Source	Number of Cases	Infarct Size (%)					
		≤10	11–20	21–30	31–40	41–50	>50
AMI first	145	22	21	22	16	10	9
AMI chronic	55	51	13	22	5	7	2
Total	200	30	19	22	13	9	7

AMI, acute myocardial infarct; first, first episode of IHD; chronic, acute myocardial infarct in chronic patients.

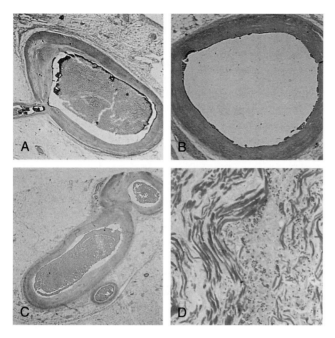

Figure 8-31 • Rupture of a left anterior infarcted wall with massive hemorrhage, absence of contraction bands, and normal coronary lumen with small, nonstenosing, atherosclerotic plaques without thrombosis. *A,* Anterior descending; *B,* left circumflex; *C,* right coronary; *D,* massive hemorrhage (all H&E stain). *A, B,* and *C* are seen after postmortem coronary injection of barium sulfate.

Fibrinous Pericarditis

An acute pericardial inflammatory reaction may extend into the immediately adjacent subepicardial myocardium. It has been reported in 7 to 16% of clinical cases[181] and in 13 to 45% of postmortem examinations.[182] It is associ-

ated primarily with a transmural infarct. Fibrous adhesions follow in healing and may obliterate the pericardial cavity, but constriction is uncommon. This fibrinous pericarditis must be distinguished from the Dressler syndrome which becomes manifest 10 days to 2 years after infarction.[183] These lesions are discussed in Chapter 12.

Cardiac Rupture

Cardiac rupture at the site of an acute infarct occurred in 17% of our cases.

Location. In our series of 200 acute infarcts, 27 patients died of cardiac tamponade secondary to rupture of the left ventricular free wall at the site of a transmural infarction. In 2 other cases there was perforation of the interventricular septum and in 5 the left anterior (2 cases) or posterior (3 cases) papillary muscle had ruptured. Of these 34 cases with rupture, 31 (93%) were first-episode IHD cases with the infarct involving 11 to 20% of left ventricular mass. In that series, no relationship was found with the presence or absence of an occlusive thrombus (Fig. 8-31). In free-wall rupture, the main site is the distal third of the anterior left ventricle (Fig. 8-32A). This complication may be the presenting manifestation of a myocardial infarction with the associated hemopericardium of between 250 and 350 ml of fluid and clotted blood causing cardiac tamponade and sudden death. It may develop less than 24 hours after infarction (rapid rupture) or 3 to 5 or 7 to 10 days after infarction (slow rupture).[184] In the latter instance, rupture may be associated with early aneurysm formation.[185] Rupture of the inferior free wall may follow an extended pathway. It may pass to the posterior interventricular septum either in myocardium or in epicardial fat and rupture into the pericardial cavity on the posterior surface of the right ventricle or into the right ventricular cavity. In the latter instance, the total lesion

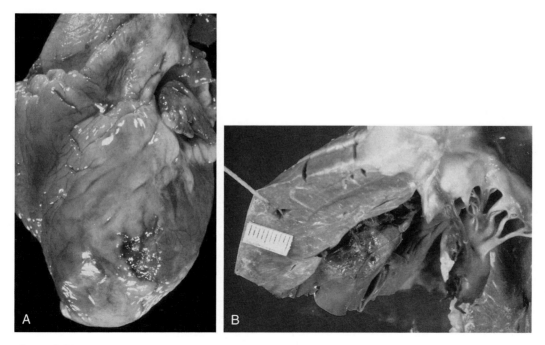

Figure 8-32 • *A,* Free wall rupture of lower third of the anterior left ventricle. *B,* Rupture of the anterior papillary muscle at an infarct site. (Courtesy of M.D. Silver, MD.)

clinically simulates a ruptured interventricular septum.[185] Rupture of the right ventricle, its papillary muscles, and of the atria have been reported but all are rare.[186]

Pathogenesis. Free-wall, interventricular septal, and some papillary muscle ruptures (Fig. 8-32B) following myocardial infarction are associated with an endocardial tear and subsequent dissection of blood through the infarcted myocardium. Final pathology depends upon the speed and direction of the dissection and whether the endocardial tear gapes.[185] Usually, in a free-wall rupture, the dissection rapidly follows a serpiginous path to the epicardial surface. In a very rare pattern, the dissection is limited to the internal part of the wall, which produces a partial rupture, or diverticulum, that can be obliterated by thrombus. Such diverticuli may reach the epicardial surface, causing it to bulge and rupture subsequently. In one case observed personally, the left ventricle showed two equally sized chambers communicating through a 2-cm hole. The "external" chamber was practically filled with thrombus. That this finding was not a pseudoaneurysm— that is, a total cardiac wall rupture with a hematoma circumscribed by adherent pericardium—was established by coronary injection with plastic material, which showed a normal disposition of extramural arteries and branches on the surface of the dissected heart.[187]

Many factors are thought to predispose to cardiac rupture. They include the destruction of the cardiac skeleton, massive polymorphonuclear infiltrate with dissolution of necrotic myocardium by release of proteolytic enzymes, and exertion or hypertension after infarction. An old observation of an excess of heart ruptures—73% among 22 mental patients with acute myocardial infarction[188]— raises the hypothesis that the brain-heart interrelationship may induce this complication via adrenergic overstimulation (see later section).[5]

Cardiac Tamponade. When cardiac tamponade follows cardiac wall rupture, it is easily recognized clinically by electromechanical dissociation, echocardiography, and other tests. Pathologically, it presents with a bluish, bulging pericardium. Rupture of an interventricular septum and of a papillary muscle may be treated surgically and, in very special circumstances, a rupture of the free wall has been occluded successfully (see Chapter 12 also).

Aneurysm

An aneurysm may be an early or late complication of myocardial infarction. The first functional sign of an infarct is the loss of contraction of dead myocells in the affected area and passive stretching by means of interventricular pressure. Bulging (acute aneurysm) of the functionless muscle is related to large transmural infarcts; those of the anterior left ventricle are particularly prone to this complication. Subsequently, an aneurysm wall can thin and, in extreme form, be only a few millimeters thick, whereas the lesion bulges markedly from the heart's surface. Calcium may deposit in the wall (Fig. 8-33A). At this stage, mural thrombus may fill most of the aneurysm lumen, but this is not a universal finding. Endocardium not covered with thrombus is white, thickened, and lacks the trabeculation usually formed by trabeculae carneae. The endocardium shows fibroelastotic thickening and may have fresh, organizing, or organized mural thrombus attached to it. Depending upon the length of time after the infarct, the aneurysm wall shows histologic variability related to the repair process and presents dense scar containing a variable number of stretched but viable hypertrophied myocells (Fig. 8-33B). Lipomatous metaplasia (see later section) is found in the scars of 55% of aneurysms removed surgically. The overlying pericardial cavity becomes obliterated by fibrous adhesions and small epicardial coronary arteries show obliterative intimal thickening. Some surgical pathology specimens contain little scar, quite unlike the classic aneurysm wall at autopsy. Nevertheless, that excised area, when imaged, would have bulged during systole, fulfilling the definition of an aneurysm.

Extension of an infarct, contractility of surrounding normal myocardium, and speed of repair are the three main factors that determine aneurysm wall structure. The aneurysm is rarely saccular, and rupture of a healed aneurysm is infrequent. Intracavitary thrombosis with associated thromboembolism (for example, see Chapter 15) and worsening ventricular function may have fatal results. A marked decrease of tissue norepinephrine and denervation paralleled by an increase of β1-adrenoceptors have been demonstrated in myocardium bordering an aneurysm scar

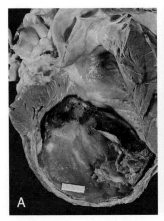
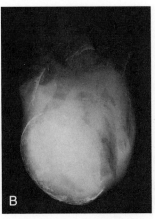
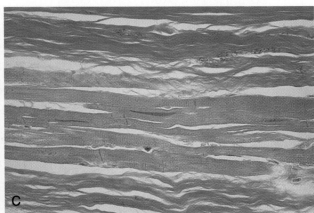

Figure 8-33 • *A,* Gross view of a postinfarct aneurysm of the anterior left ventricle. Its lumen is filled with thrombus (scale indicates 2 cm). *B,* Postmortem radiograph shows calcification of aneurysm wall. (*B,* Courtesy of M.D. Silver, MD.) *C,* Stretched but viable myocells in dense scar in a left ventricular aneurysm wall excised at surgery (Gomori stain).

removed surgically. This profound impairment of the adrenergic system in perianeurysmal myocardium may play a role in the recurrent sustained ventricular tachycardia that develops in some patients with postinfarction aneurysm,[189] prompting surgical ablation or electrocautery. A question is whether myocardial catecholamine toxicity may progressively expand the area of necrosis, and thus cause a continuous risk of arrhythmias and ventricular fibrillation. The other complication of left ventricular aneurysm is congestive heart failure (see later section). The excellent results achieved by surgical excision emphasize the life-threatening risk of this dysfunctional lesion.

Mitral Valve Regurgitation

Mitral valve regurgitation, a complication that is more common in the absence of papillary muscle rupture,[186] may occur within the first week of a transmural or subendocardial acute infarct involving either the left ventricular free wall or the interventricular septum or both, or it may develop long after an infarct has healed (see Chapter 14 also). Acute severe mitral insufficiency following myocardial infarction is usually caused by papillary muscle rupture. It develops within the first week and is associated more often with rupture of the posteromedial papillary muscle than the anterolateral muscle at a 4:1 ratio. Clinical effects depend on the site of rupture. Thus, a rupture occurring at mid-belly releases chordae attached to adjacent sides of both leaflets and is likely to induce severe valvular regurgitation. On the other hand, rupture of the tip or avulsion of chordae from the tip, the latter erroneously called chordal rupture, has less severe effects. The complication is amenable to valve replacement.[185] Right ventricular papillary muscle rupture occurs but is rare. Mitral regurgitation is rarely a severe acute event, as it is mainly a chronic process with varying degrees of dysfunction that is recognized in the postinfarction period.

Papillary Muscle Dysfunction

Papillary muscle dysfunction, which leads to mitral regurgitation, is a consequence of (1) infarct scarring involving the subendocardium and papillary muscle; (2) postinfarct atrophy of the papillary muscle; (3) a dyssynchronous conducting system impulse activating the papillary muscles; or (4) mechanical separation of papillary muscles, for example, by an aneurysm. Congestive heart failure may aggravate a preexisting papillary muscle dysfunction by causing annular dilation and mitral regurgitation.[185] The latter mechanism also explains functional tricuspid incompetence, another common accompaniment of myocardial infarction.

Denervation

In experimental transmural infarction in the dog, heterogeneous sympathetic denervation in noninfarcted myocardium distal to the area of necrosis is documented[190] by measuring endocardial and epicardial effective refractory period changes during left and right stellate stimulation[184] or by scintigraphy in canine transmural and non-transmural infarction[190a] and in sheep in which sympathetic denervation occurred in presence of a normal blood flow and blood flow reserve.[190b] By scintigraphy, abnormalities were shown in sympathetic innervation related to ventricular arrhythmia ("denervation supersensitivity") in ischemic heart disease[191] and in the absence of coronary disease[192]

as well as in stunned myocardium[193] in vasospastic angina,[193a-c] in arrhythmogenic right ventricular cardiomyopathy,[193d] and in Chagas disease,[193e, 193f] the role of intramural nerves is worth investigation to determine: (1) all cardiac conditions in which sympathetic denervation occurs; (2) its etiopathogenetic mechanisms; and (3) its relationship with cardiac complications and death.[193g] As already mentioned, myocardial denervation may result in myocellular supersensitivity linked with contraction band necrosis and malignant arrhythmia/ventricular fibrillation. We do not know whether and when reinnervation is reestablished.[193h, 193i] In human orthotopic transplanted hearts, it requires 15 years.[193j]

Endocardial Thrombosis and Thromboembolism

Mural thrombi may develop any time after an infarct, and vary greatly in thickness and diameter (Fig. 8-34). Histology may show a continuum of thrombus deposition, reparative processes, and calcification. Several methods— for example, angiocardiography, indium-III platelet scanning, magnetic resonance imaging, and echocardiography—enable a clinician to both recognize and follow the fate of laminar thrombi or those projecting into the lumen. Echocardiography is the most reliable (and a relatively inexpensive) noninvasive technique used in detecting intracardiac masses, including those in the atria by means of transesophageal echocardiography. It has a 90% sensitivity and specificity compared with data from aneurysmectomy or autopsy.[194] Endocardial thrombi occurring after acute infarcts are most often found on the anterior left ventricular wall (39%) and are least often associated with inferior infarcts (1%).[190] An endocardial thrombus was found in 31% of 124 patients with anterior infarction immediately preceding discharge from hospital, and none was found in 74 patients with inferior infarction ($p < .001$), without relation to early thrombolytic therapy but rather with relation to location, a low ejection fraction of less than 35%, and apical dyskinesia or aneurysm but not akinesia. Follow-up showed disappearance of the thrombus in 48% of cases; it was related to predischarge apical akinesia or warfarin therapy. Systemic thromboembolism occurred in six patients, each of whom had a predischarge mobile thrombus,[195] which is a severe risk factor,

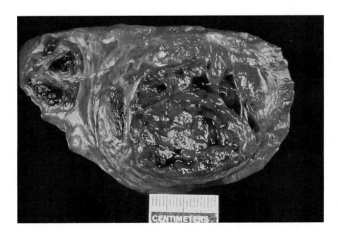

Figure 8-34 • Intracavitary endocardial thrombosis associated with an acute infarct. (Courtesy of M.D. Silver, MD.)

particularly for brain damage. Rarely, peripheral thromboembolism is the first sign of a myocardial infarct (see Chapter 15 also).

Cardiac Arrhythmias and Conduction System Defects

A patient with an acute myocardial infarction is prone to life-threatening arrhythmias at any time, particularly in the early phase. However, malignant arrhythmias resulting in fatal ventricular fibrillation have been reduced by modern therapy, β-blockers, antiarrhythmic drugs, and so forth (see the section on cardiac arrest). Serial section study of the conduction system in cases of acute myocardial infarct shows that it is rarely infarcted.[196] Of 556 patients with acute infarction, various types of conduction block were found in 186: (1) complete left bundle branch block in 23; (2) complete right bundle branch block in 8; (3) lone left anterior hemiblock in 72; (4) lone left posterior hemiblock in 32; and (5) complete atrioventricular block in 51. There was a maximal mortality rate of 60 to 70% in the first group and in patients with combined right bundle branch block and left anterior hemiblock.[197] Conduction disturbances may be transient and are probably due to reversible injuries accompanying an infarct (see Chapter 20 also).

Cardiogenic Shock

Cardiogenic shock used to be a relatively frequent, often fatal complication of an infarct that exceeded 40% of the left ventricular myocardial mass.[198] Now its frequency has been greatly reduced. A question is whether this reduction is the result of decreased infarct size. In 100 consecutive cases of acute myocardial infarct examined in 1974,[37] 26 died in cardiogenic shock. The sizes of the infarcts in these 26 cases were less than 40% in 92% and between 41 and 50% in 15%; none of the infarcts was greater than 50%. Among 58 cases without cardiogenic shock, the percentage of distribution was 86, 9, and 5%, respectively. A similar distribution of infarct size was observed in a 1980 series.[38] These data open to question the relationship between infarct size and cardiogenic shock, suggesting that other neurohormonal mechanisms may explain cardiogenic shock.

Acute Congestive Failure

Acute congestive failure of the left ventricle is also a common complication of acute infarct and is responsible for other disorders, such as pulmonary hypertension, deep vein thrombosis, right ventricular dysfunction, and so forth.

Sudden Coronary Death

Most definitions of sudden death are more or less satisfactory in that among the selective criteria, a survival time, which ranges from 1 to 24 hours, is included. Sudden death implies (1) a mystery from the clinical standpoint; (2) occurrence in an apparently healthy subject; or (3) occurrence during an inactive phase of a recognized disease. We prefer a definition that considers (1) rapid onset without any specific chronologic limit; (2) unexpectedness, both subjectively and objectively; and (3) occurrence without any clinical evaluation and in an apparently healthy person (*primary, or unexpected, sudden*

death) or in a patient during an apparently benign phase in the course of a disease (*secondary, or expected, sudden death*).[5]

A comparison of studies of sudden death reported in the literature is difficult, if not impossible, because of different selection criteria, dissimilar methods of examination, and divergent definitions. For instance, in some studies only ischemic cases with coronary stenosis greater than 75% of luminal area were selected, creating an obvious bias in the findings and conclusions. Furthermore, in several studies, lumen reduction at plaque level was calculated as a percentage of the cross-sectional area (see previous discussion); a distinction between different forms of myocardial damage was not made; infarct size was never calculated nor related to coronary alterations; the collaterals were never investigated and their role in ischemic heart disease was ignored[198a-d]; and a distinction between cases with and without cardiopulmonary resuscitation was never considered. Similarly, cases involving survival of 1 to 24 hours may include agonal changes unrelated to death, and a lack of discrimination between unexpected and expected deaths can lead to misinterpretation. This is a fundamental distinction because sudden coronary death is a unique entity with its own causes and pathogenetic mechanisms. It is not synonymous with acute myocardial infarction. Most patients resuscitated by defibrillation[199, 200] and the majority of patients who die suddenly while being monitored by a Holter device[76, 201] do not show electrocardiographic signs of acute Q-wave infarction. Therefore, the inability to demonstrate an acute infarct in unexpected sudden death is not a result of technical problems but occurs because most cases do not involve an infarct. For instance, most cases of sudden death in unstable angina[87, 88] are sudden *expected* deaths following documented acute myocardial infarction.

In a 1995 review, we pooled data from previous studies,[5] and the following observations about sudden coronary death emerged: (1) It occurred prevalently in men, with a man/woman ratio ranging from 1 to 16, mean 6 ± 4, with the mean age of occurrence in women being 63 ± 6 years, higher than the men's mean of 58 ± 4 years; (2) A functional reduction in lumen diameter (70% or more) due to coronary atherosclerotic stenosis was present in 84% of cases. This stenosis involved only one main artery in 13%, two arteries in 21%, and three arteries in 58%; (3) In contrast to the opinions of some,[202] collaterals followed the rules found in IHD in general; (4) A coronary occlusive thrombus was present in 29% of cases. In first-episode cases, the frequency of white occlusive thrombi was 8%; in chronic cases, it was 28%. Coronary mural thrombi were mentioned in only a few of the pooled reports, occurring with a frequency of 22%, an incidence twice that found for white mural thrombi in our cases. The frequency of plaque rupture ranged from 5 to 31%. Plaque fissuring was observed in 103 of 115 vessels showing either mural or occlusive red or white thrombi.[86] Disrupted plaque associated with acute thrombus was reported in 30% of 90 cases of sudden coronary death, acute thrombus alone in 23%, and disrupted plaque without thrombus in 3%. No distinction was made between occlusive and mural thrombi;[198a] (5) The acute myocardial injury was reported as an infarct in 21 studies. The frequency ranged from 22 to 68%, with a mean of 43%. In contrast, among 72% of our cases, coagulative myocytolysis was the unique acute myocardial necrosis found and colliquative myocytolysis was present in only 8%, mainly around extensive myocardial fibrosis. Apparently, this finding differs from an observation of 6 sudden coronary deaths showing as the main myocardial lesion an extensive colliquative myocytolysis in areas unstained by triphenyl tetrazolium chloride and related to a severely obstructed vessel. The authors' conclusion was that colliquative myocytolysis is a pathologic marker of myocardial ischemia.[56] However, all 6 cases underwent aggressive resuscitation; (6) Heart weight was pathological (≥ 500 g)[203] in 46% of 1279 cases reported in the literature. In our 133 first-episode cases of coronary sudden and unexpected death, the frequency was 43%, whereas in 75 chronic cases it was 76%; (7) Platelet aggregates or fibrin-platelet thrombi and emboli of the intramural vessels were found in coronary sudden death[118, 204] and were considered responsible for focal or coalescent myocardial necrosis defined as "myocytolysis or myofibrillar lesions"[205] or "microfocal necrotic deeply eosinophilic hypercontracted muscle cells or fine connective stroma after resolution of dead myocells"[87] or "recent microinfarcts."[88] In our sudden and unexpected cases fibrin-platelet thrombi were never found, and the frequency and number of vessels containing platelet aggregates did not differ from those observed in controls who died by accident; (8) no evidence surfaced which indicated that sudden and unexpected death in IHD is due to changes in the conduction system, despite intimal thickening of pertinent arteries[206] and degenerative changes in neural structure.[207, 208]

The relationship between strenuous exercise and IHD is controversial.[209] Among 2324 pooled sudden death cases in which physical effort at demise was investigated, deaths occurred mainly at rest (69%). Sudden death among young athletes was not often due to the IHD. Of 78 cases reported in the literature, only 3 presented an acute event possibly linked with death. They included rupture of the aorta in 2 cases and pulmonary thromboembolism in 1 case. The other lesions found had been present a long time (e.g., anomalous origin of the coronary arteries; hypoplasia of a right coronary artery; "mural" left anterior descending branch; hypertrophic cardiomyopathy; floppy mitral valve; heart tumor; right ventricular dysplasia; and coronary atherosclerosis). The last was the estimated cause of death in 3% of subjects younger than 20 years of age, in 40% of those between 20 and 29, in 7% of those between 30 and 39, and in 100% of those older than 40 years of age. Similarly, coronary atherosclerosis was the leading cause in 91% of 36 joggers. I had the opportunity to examine the hearts of a few cases of marathon runners who died suddenly.[210] They showed foci of coagulative myocytolysis and pericoronary nerve lymphoplasmacellular inflammation, which was associated with severe obstructive coronary atherosclerosis and extensive myocardial fibrosis that had been unrecognized clinically. In 25 cases of sudden coronary death associated with physical or emotional stress, rupture of an atherosclerotic plaque was observed in 68%, in contrast to 23% of 116 patients who died suddenly at rest. A hemorrhage into the plaque had a frequency of 72 and 41%, respectively.[198d] On this subject, we examined a

case of sudden and unexpected death of a 32-year-old body buider while weight-lifting at a gymnasium. He was an androgenic-anabolic steroids user. The unique autopsy finding was a 20% myocardial infarction of the anterolateral cardiac wall, with a histologic age of approximately 15 to 20 days. The infarct necrosis was surrounded by young connective tissue and many macrophages. External to the fibrous tissue was early extensive coagulative myocytolysis without evidence of macrophagic repair. The coronary arteries cross-sectioned at a 3-mm interval were normal, without histologic evidence of atherosclerosis, hemorrhage, or any other pathologic change (presented for publication). It is notable that hemorrhage is found mainly in advanced atherosclerotic plaque in infarct-related vessels[5, 91] (see Chapter 11 for further discussion).

Silent Acute Ischemic Heart Disease

A patient without or with minor nonspecific symptoms but with typical signs of IHD is defined as a case of *silent ischemic heart disease.*[211] The morphologic demonstration of this event is an infarct with a histologic age of more than 6 to 12 hours, found in an apparently healthy subject who was living a normal life and who died suddenly and unexpectedly without evidence of subjective symptoms.[39] Silent myocardial infarction occurs in diabetic patients in whom it is possibly linked with neuropathy of the afferent nerves that conduct pain[212] and with an increased sympathetic tone, which could explain the high percentage of sudden deaths.[213] In the Framingham study, 39% of diabetic patients had had a silent myocardial infarction as compared to a rate of 22% in nondiabetic individuals.[214]

Chronic Ischemic Heart Disease

The prevention of acute coronary syndromes and a reduction in the rate of mortality resulting from them in some Western countries has increased the number of patients with chronic ischemia. As a result, the natural history of IHD shows a trend toward congestive heart failure. This pattern, often defined as *ischemic cardiomyopathy* (see Chapter 10), is attributed mainly to a progressive expansion of ischemic myocardial fibrosis, including the thickening of the collagen matrix. Our studies showed that myocardial fibrosis is more extensive in IHD than in other conditions with identical congestive heart failure. However, even in congestive heart failure secondary to IHD, there exists the structural paradox of normal or reduced myocardial wall thickness and myocell size despite increased myocardial mass. The current explanations for this weight/size paradox are the stretching of myocells, the longitudinal cleavage of hypertrophied myocells when heart weight exceeds 500 g,[203] myocellular slippage,[2, 203, 215] and apoptosis.[63, 64] However, myocell stretching has not been confirmed,[203] and amitosis without myocell cleavage is the only type of nuclear division of myocells found in normal, atrophic, or hypertrophied hearts.[67] In reality, myocell slippage is difficult to establish because the myocardium is a network of cellular units connected by short myofibrillar bridges and a fibrillar collagen network. If slippage was the cause of cardiac wall thickness reduction (from 3 to 1.5 cm) all the essential interstitial structures (blood vessels, lymphatics, and nerves) should undergo massive destruction consequent to such a widespread myocellular interpenetration.[28] Finally, the role of apoptosis is still under investigation but the process, by definition, should be associated with normal or reduced heart weight.

In discussing the role of myocardial fibrosis in the genesis of congestive heart failure, the structure and extent of fibrous tissue must be considered. In a comparative morphometric and histologic study of 63 ischemic hearts, 63 hearts with dilated cardiomyopathy of unknown nature, and 18 hearts with chronic valvulopathy, all excised at transplantation because of irreversible congestive failure, the following main findings were observed.[28]

First: Three different aspects of myocardial fibrosis were found: (1) a dense, monofocal scar formed by straight and compact collagen fibers as an end result of infarct necrosis (see Fig. 8-19); (2) plurifocal or focal/confluent fibrosis with marked waviness of the collagen fibers marking repair of coagulative myocytolysis at the periphery of an infarct or in nonischemic myocardium; and (3) increased interstitial/perivascular or intermyocellular fibrosis, again formed by wavy collagen fibers and found in zones of histologically viable myocardium (see Fig. 8-19). The undulate structure of the fibrous tissue in the last two conditions indicates that collagen protein synthesis occurs in a beating myocardium and adapts these fibers to contraction. It appears unlikely that these two types of fibrosis reduce contractility.

Second: Myocardial fibrosis of any type was absent or minimal in 77% of histologic sections in dilated cardiomyopathy, in 68% of sections in valvulopathy, and in 43% of sections in IHD. However, even in this last group the "fibrous index," expressed as a ratio between the total area of fibrosis and the total histologic area in square millimeters $\times$ 100 as assessed at 16 examined sites per heart, showed that the histologic area of viable myocardium greatly exceeded the area of fibrosis. This finding was supported by the presence of thallium uptake in large zones of these hearts in vivo despite depressed flow.[216] These two observations undermine the belief that congestive heart failure is caused by myocardial fibrosis and suggests a distorted, longitudinal sarcomerogenesis following biochemically reduced relaxation that results in an "abortive" hypertrophy.[28] This hypothesis is supported by increased myocyte length and maladaptive rearrangement of myocyte shape, that is, increased myocyte length-to-width ratio, which is found in ischemic hearts excised at transplantation.[217]

Third: The more common occurrence of varying phases of coagulative myocytolysis was found in most hearts, especially in the ischemic group, indicating that this form of myocell injury is an ongoing phenomenon even in the absence of acute myocardial infarction. Thus, in our view, the mild progression of myocardial fibrosis seems to be a consequence of repetitive episodes of catecholamine myotoxicity more than of ischemia, a concept that agrees with the lack of correlation between infarct

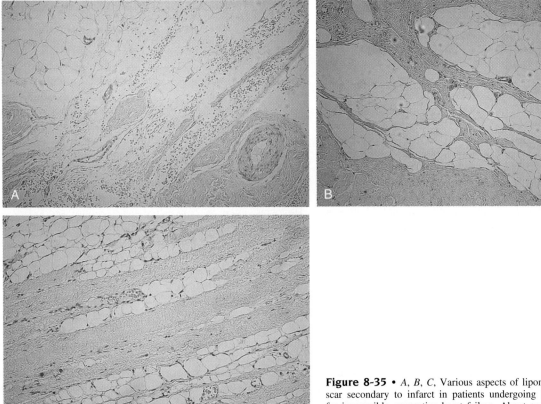

Figure 8-35 • *A, B, C,* Various aspects of lipomatous metaplasia in scar secondary to infarct in patients undergoing heart transplantation for irreversible congestive heart failure. About one half of the scar in *C* was replaced by fat. (All H&E stain).

size (measured by technetium Tc 99m sestamibi, end-systolic and end-diastolic volumes, or ejection fraction) at hospital discharge and the observation 1 year later of a significant left ventricular dilation, particularly in patients who had large infarcts.[218] These facts support the concept that congestive heart failure is linked to biochemical myocellular disorders of unknown cause that are likely to be related to neurohormonal disorders.[28]

Fourth: There was extensive transformation of compact scar into adipose tissue (Fig. 8-35). This lipomatous metaplasia[219] was present in 68% of cases of ischemic hearts, in 37% of cases of chronic valvulopathy, and in 26% of cases of dilated cardiomyopathy. It is a phenomenon to be considered (1) in the functional evaluation of a scar, as adipose tissue is more compressible and "sliding"; (2) in cardiac imaging so as to avoid nuclear markers captured by fat cells' being misinterpreted as viable myocardium; (3) in quantitative morphology in which the extent of adipose tissue may not be calculated in the total scar size; and (4) in qualitative and quantitative biochemical analysis of myocardial tissue.

Among these cases of congestive heart failure of varying natures, we observed endocardial thickening caused by organized thrombus and, more frequently, another form of myoelastofibrous endocardial thickening that consists of smooth muscle hyperplasia with bundle formation. Elastic tissue hyperplasia, smooth myocell degeneration, and fibrous replacement are evolutionary phases of this lesion.[28] This finding, which had a similar frequency and extent in ischemic and dilated cardiomyopathy and in valvulopathy, and was absent in normal control hearts, indicates that a possible common denominator acts in these three conditions of congestive heart failure and other pathologic conditions.[28]

NONATHEROSCLEROTIC CAUSES OF ACUTE CORONARY SYNDROMES

Obliterative Intimal Thickening

Nonatherosclerotic obliterative intimal thickening of the coronary arteries is a pathologic process found in a variety of human conditions, such as coarctation of the aorta,[220] the transplanted human[221–223] (and dog[224]) heart, aortocoronary saphenous vein grafts,[225, 226] infectious immune processes such as tuberculosis,[227] polyarteritis nodosa,[228] Kawasaki disease,[228] giant cell arteritis,[229] rheumatic fever,[230] and systemic lupus erythematosus,[231] and in experimental hypertension[232, 233] as well as in cases of variation of flow volume[234, 235] and of trauma.[235] Histologically, this process presents a diffuse proliferation of smooth muscle cells with absent or minimal elastic hyperplasia, increased proteoglycans, and interstitial fibrosis. The internal elastic membrane is intact and none of the typical changes seen in the atherosclerotic plaque, even in the subocclusive phase, are present (Fig. 8-36). This intimal thickening has been improperly defined as accelerated atherosclerosis.[236] I object to this term because the word *accelerated* suggests that it evolves with the same sequence of changes but in a shorter period. This is not

the case, even if in some chronic conditions such as transplanted human hearts with long survival, atherosclerosis is superimposed. Today, in transplanted hearts this coronary arteriopathy is considered a major problem that limits their effectiveness (see Chapter 23).

Coronary Ostial Stenosis

This group of conditions includes nonatherosclerotic coronary ostial diseases consequent to inflammatory or degenerative processes involving the ascending aorta, such as syphilis, Takayasu disease, spondylitis, aortic dissecting aneurysm, supravalvular stenosis due to severe intimal thickening, adhesion of the free edge of aortic cusps to the aortic intima above the coronary ostia, and occlusion by embolus[237] or papillary fibroelastoma of an aortic cusp.[238]

Coronary Artery Anomalies

Sudden death has been reported in 27% of subjects, all young males, with ostial dislocation of the left coronary artery or its circumflex branch from the right aortic sinus. A slit-like opening and sharp angulation with compression of the segment running between the aorta and the pulmonary arteries are used to explain subsequent ischemia and sudden death[239] (see Chapter 11 also). In most reports on major coronary artery anomalies with left-to-right shunts (fistulas[240] or anomalous origin from the pulmonary artery[241]), there is no clinical evidence of angina and cardiac insufficiency despite myocardial damage in childhood, whereas in adults, cardiac failure, ischemia, bacterial endocarditis, or rupture of the fistula may be present.[240] Coronary anomalies, if recognized, can be successfully treated surgically.

Coronary Aneurysm, Dissection, and Embolism

An aneurysm is a circumscribed dilation of the artery wall that is not to be confused with ectasia, which refers to dilation of the whole vessel as occurs, for instance, in old age secondary to loss of elasticity. The genesis of a vascular aneurysm is any condition that destroys a circumscribed portion of the vessel wall, such as atherosclerosis, arteritis, polyarteritis nodosa, Kawasaki syndrome, septic embolus, trauma, or focal congenital myoelastic defects. In a review of 89 adult patients, 66 men and 23 women, the total number of coronary artery aneurysms was 127, of which 35 were in the left main trunk, 15 in the left anterior descending branch, 15 in the left circumflex branch, 1 in the left posterior descending branch, and 61 in the right coronary artery. Of the 127 aneurysms, 17% were congenital, 52% atherosclerotic, 11% mycotic, 4% syphilitic, 11% dissecting, and 5% unclassified.[242] The main complications were rupture with hemorrhage, thrombosis with embolism, and compression.

Other pathologic conditions in which myocardial infarction and sudden death are observed are the rare instances of a primary dissecting aneurysm in a coronary artery (see Chapter 16 also) or a coronary embolism.

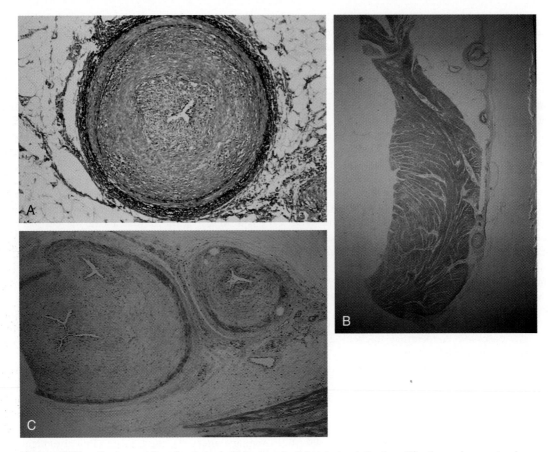

Figure 8-36 • Coronary obliterative intimal thickening. *A,* Subocclusive intimal proliferation, minor proteoglycan deposition, and normal internal elastic lamina in a transplanted heart in situ 8 months (Weigert elastic). *B* and *C,* Transplanted heart in a patient with a survival of 19 months (H&E stain). Note that many subepicardial arterial vessels are severely stenosed.

Both conditions imply an abrupt coronary occlusion. Of 25 cases involving a dissecting aneurysm, 21 were female, 8 in the postpartum state, and 18 died suddenly and unexpectedly. At autopsy, it was found that 6 had had an acute myocardial infarction that preceded their sudden demise by days. The dissection occurred most commonly—in 18 cases—in the outer media of the left anterior descending branch, causing luminal occlusion by lifting the superficial media and intima into the lumina. The cause and pathogenesis of the dissections are still matters of investigation. Cystic medial necrosis was described in three cases; in others, nonspecific changes included foci of granulation tissue, scar, degeneration of the internal elastic lamina and, often, a more or less diffuse adventitial and periadventitial inflammatory reaction formed by eosinophils, lymphocytes, plasmacells, and histiocytes, and rare polymorphonuclear leukocytes were reported.[243, 244] Coronary artery dissection is also induced by trauma (see the following section).

In 74 cases of coronary artery embolism, sudden death occurred in 60%. The associated pathologic conditions were infective endocarditis, 64%, intracavitary endocardial thrombus, 11%, syphilitic aortitis, 5%, ulcerated aortic atherosclerotic plaque, 4%, paradoxic embolus through a patent foramen ovale, 4%, aortic thrombus, 3%, proximal coronary thrombus, 3%, pulmonary thrombus, caseous tuberculous material, neoplastic tissue, or calcific valve, 1%, not established, 1%.[245] Coronary embolism occurs as a result of ulcerated calcium nodules on natural heart valves. Also, thrombi or fragments of prosthetic valves may be released during diagnostic or surgical procedures (see Chapter 21). Cholesterol emboli, frequently found in spleen, kidney, and brain, are rare in the myocardium and are an infrequent finding in cases of sudden death occurring during unstable angina: 4 cases in 25[88] and 2 cases in 90.[87] In the two latter studies, postmortem injection could be the cause of a relative higher frequency. Embolism of myocardium has occurred after surgical treatment of hypertrophic cardiomyopathy.[245a]

Trauma

Finally, we must consider blunt or nonpenetrating trauma of the chest as a possible cause of myocardial infarction due to vascular contusion[246] as well as iatrogenic coronary disease secondary to therapeutic interventions such as the occlusion by suture of the left circumflex coronary branch during mitral valve replacement, with a subsequent posterior/superior left ventricular wall myocardial infarction, or the tying or compression of a coronary artery with high take-off during aortotomy, peri-aortic dissection, or low cross-clamping of the aorta.[83]

Coronary dissection is a very rare event during coronary angiography.[247] It occurs focally at the site of the aortocoronary bypass graft insertion. On the other hand a "therapeutic" dissection produced by percutaneous transluminal coronary angioplasty is required to establish an improved luminal diameter (see Chapter 22). Nevertheless, this is a safe procedure with a mortality rate of 0.9%.[248] Obliterative intimal thickening of coronary ostia following high-pressure coronary perfusion[249] may develop, and chest radiation for malignant neoplasms can result in bizarre fibroblasts, adventitial and medial fibrosis, and obliterative intimal thickening.[250] Oral contraceptives are suspected of causing acute coronary syndromes in young women, apparently when associated with hyperlipidemia, hypertension, and excessive cigarette smoking.[251] (See Chapter 17 also.)

UNANSWERED QUESTIONS

It is difficult to establish a cause-and-effect relationship between the morphology and the clinical events found in IHD. The prevailing concept is that clinical patterns are caused by coronary atherosclerosis and its complications. From that viewpoint, at a critical degree a coronary artery stenosis causes ischemia, collaterals are absent or unable to compensate for flow reduction, and acute clinical patterns have a common pathogenetic background. This leads to such statements as "Evidence from serial coronary arteriography and that obtained after reperfusion by thrombolysis, at operation during acute coronary syndromes, and from postmortem arteriography have also confirmed the importance of plaque disruption and thrombosis. Indeed, these acute or subacute changes in coronary arterial anatomy appear to be the most frequent cause of all the acute coronary syndromes, including unstable angina, myocardial infarction, and ischemic sudden death. If we accept the premise that all three acute coronary syndromes may evolve from acute plaque disruption followed by thrombosis or spasm or both, we can construct an unifying theory."[252] The point is whether or not we can accept this premise. The last part of this chapter is devoted to a review of the functional meaning of the main morphologic aspects of IHD so as to better understand its natural history and review current pathogenetic concepts. Unfortunately, all postmortem and in vivo studies are done after the onset of a clinical event. So far, there has been little opportunity to follow the changes that precede an event. Therefore, we deal with hypotheses.

Coronary Atherosclerotic Lumen Reduction

No doubt exists that most patients, at the time of their first clinical episode, usually show severe atherosclerotic damage of extramural coronary arteries and their branches. More precisely, the frequency of one or more stenoses causing more than a 70% reduction in lumen diameter, which is equivalent to 90% lumen area, was 88% in first-episode acute infarct cases, 98% in acute infarct in chronic patients, 66% in first-episode sudden coronary death, and 93% in chronic cases, that is, those with extensive myocardial fibrosis. The question is whether atherosclerotic stenosis determines ischemia. If one thinks like a plumber when looking at the stenosis, the answer is obvious. Nevertheless, flow reduction depends on many variables, as it is directly proportional to the fourth power of luminal radius and inversely proportional to fluid viscosity and the length of the tube. In particular, the pressure difference across a constricted segment is determined by pressure on the upstream side, the resistance to flow through the segment, and the peripheral resistance of the vascular bed distal to the constriction.[253] The responsivity of a complex atherosclerotic plaque to many variables (such as spasm, collateral flow, increased peripheral resistance by vascular compression in asynergic zones, inflammatory nerve irritation at the outer media, increased coagulability following tissue necrosis, etc.) makes unreliable any measurement of flow by catheterization in patients. Several facts place in doubt the ideas that flow reduction is caused by coronary atherosclerotic plaque and that an atherosclerotic plaque may determine a chronic blood flow reduction or ischemia:

1. Of normal people who die accidentally, 92% have stenosing atherosclerotic plaques, and that number increases to 96% in those over 50 years of age. Severe stenoses were observed in 39% (46% in those over 50 years of age), with those stenoses affecting two vessels in 13% and three vessels in 3%. In noncardiac patients, the rate of severe stenosis is 66%, with a distribution close to that found in ischemic groups. No extensive myocardial fibrosis was found in any of these subjects.[5, 39]

2. Severe stenoses exist months or years before onset of the first symptoms in people enjoying normal, often stressful lives. This means that collateral flow has been adequate, at least until the first episode.

3. There is no relationship between the degree of coronary damage and the onset, course, complications, and mortality associated with acute coronary syndromes. In other words, an individual may experience a first infarct or may die suddenly without severe stenosis or occlusion, 8% and 21.5%, respectively, or may have 70 to 90% stenosis or more than 90% stenosis in all main vessels. There is no critical point of coronary obstructive atherosclerosis at which the disease invariably starts.

4. Infarct size does not relate to the number of severe stenoses in the coronary system. This is a contradictory point because it might be expected that a patient with a greater number of severe stenoses would have greater ischemia and thus larger infarcts. This is not the case.[5, 37, 38]

5. Infarct size and survival are nonrelated variables, as they should be.[5, 37, 38]

6. Old thrombotic occlusions are found without a related healed infarct,[5, 156] and on angiographic restudy, new occlusions are seen without clinical evidence of an infarct.[146]

7. A patient can have bilateral coronary ostial occlusion or subocclusion but no myocardial infarct (see later section).[5]

It must be stressed that atherosclerosis progresses slowly and there is plenty of time for collateral enlargement.[254] This means we are dealing with an enlarged collateral system when the disease becomes manifest clinically. The postmortem anatomic demonstration by tridimensional plastic casts of enlarged satellite collaterals, always present and proportional to an increased number of severe coronary stenoses and independent of the presence or absence of a history of IHD, is proof that a pressure gradient is capable of promoting a compensatory flow.[5, 102] The adequacy of the latter is shown by means of experimental occlusion of a previous severe coronary stenosis that does not produce any change in cardiac function or in myocardial morphology but is associated with a dramatic increase in enlarged collaterals.[255, 256] The intramural system, including collaterals, is poorly visualized by cineangiography; this technique selectively injects one coronary artery, allowing limited vision of anastomotic channels because of competing nonradiopaque blood flowing from noninjected arteries. The compensatory function of normal collaterals in humans is demonstrated by cases in which there has been surgical occlusion of a damaged coronary artery after a chest wound but an infarct has not followed.[257-262] Nevertheless, some angiographic data speak in favor of collateral function; for example, prevention of postinfarct aneurysm formation, reduction in infarct size, improved ventricular function, and so forth[5] and, in particular, the fact that repetitive coronary occlusion at the site of a stenosis caused by angioplastic inflation recruits collaterals,[263, 264] a result also obtained experimentally in the absence of coronary stenosis,[265] even in the absence of collaterals investigated by contrast echocardiography with decreasing ischemia from the first to the third occlusion;[264a] the myocardial tolerance to repeated occlusions in a human is owed to collateral recruitment and not to intracoronary adenosine infusion.[264b] A recovery of myocardial contractility does not depend on increased collateral flow.[264c] Thus, collaterals develop within a few days,[256] disappear as soon as a stenosis is removed, and reappear immediately when the latter is reestablished.[266] Possibly, this is caused by spasm of the parent vessels or by regional myocardial asynergy following this highly traumatic, invasive technique. Nevertheless, despite repetitive occlusions, function returns to normal, with rapid electrocardiographic normalization and the disappearance of chest pain.

The factors that trigger myohyperplasia as a starting point of the *myohyperplastic* atherosclerotic plaque (see previous section) are unknown. There is no evidence that platelet growth factor[267] acts in promoting the *hypercholesterolemic plaque* (see previous discussion). Gotlieb and Silver also discuss atherogenesis and platelet growth factor in Chapter 4. The roles of catecholamines,[268] endothelial factors,[132] and other multifunctional cell factors capable of transforming wall structures in relation to hemodynamic functions[269] are matters for investigation. The lymphoplasmacellular inflammation around the media

is not a promoting factor as it appears only at the proteoglycan stage of plaque evolution. However, it seems to intensify radial progression. In fact, this inflammation in acute infarct cases correlates significantly with short but severe stenoses.[91] Finally, the high variability in location of atherosclerotic coronary plaques in various subjects is still unexplained.

Coronary Thrombosis and Occlusion

Is a thrombus the cause of an acute coronary syndrome? The hypothesis is based on postmortem findings of an occlusive thrombus associated with plaque rupture as well as platelet embolization in the vascular bed supplying the affected myocardium,[87, 88] on cineangiographic demonstration of coronary occlusion in most patients with acute myocardial infarction, and on recovery of a thrombus proximal to a stenosis in most patients undergoing emergency bypass surgery.[150] In these patients, the cineangiographic image was positive for coronary thrombosis, showing persistent staining of intraluminal material by contrast agent, which is most commonly detectable in patients with total or subtotal occlusion. However, coronary angiography fails to visualize all coronary lesions found at autopsy.[270] Serial-section study of plaques subject to postmortem coronary injection of radiopaque menstruum showed arterioles and a well-formed tunica media within the thickened intima. They connected with an intimal angiomatous plexus, the residual lumen, and large adventitial vessels[5] (Figs. 8-37, 8-38). Is persistent staining of intraluminal material an expression of this type of plaque vascularization? Angiographically, "irregular lesions," or plaque ruptures, persist for many years,[97] and there is no correlation between histologic stability or instability and stable or unstable angina.[271]

Thrombus

In this discussion, several points must be considered. The first is the differentiation between a thrombus and a coagulum,[272] the latter often referred to as a "red" thrombus. Each has a different, although often related, pathogenic mechanism. A thrombus is initiated by platelet adhesion at a site of damaged endothelium; this is followed by their aggregation and the subsequent deposition of layers of fibrin and platelets (Zahn lines). It heals by means of granulation tissue, and the resultant fibrosis fills the lumen. It may contain vessels that recanalize the lumen. The chronological sequence of thrombus organization varies among vessels and among those of differing luminal diameter. In major coronary arteries, the main changes after 3 days are (1) early endothelial sprouting and capillary growth (3 to 8 days); (2) presence of capillaries, fibroblasts, and hemosiderin and early deposition of collagen fibrils (9 to 19 days); (3) presence of fibrocytes and connective tissue and recanalization (after 20 days).[273] Recanalizing vessels may or may not contribute to distal coronary flow because of competing preexisting collaterals. Recanalizing capillary-like vessels may discharge flow into the plaque's vascular network without

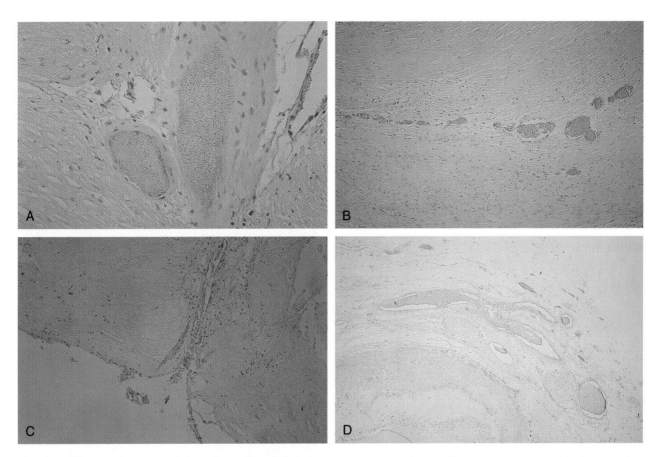

Figure 8-37 • Vascularization of atherosclerotic intimal thickening (serial section in hearts with postmortem coronary injection of barium sulfate). *A*, Arteriole with well-developed tunica media. *B*, The latter connected with a capillary-like plexus. *C*, Residual lumen. *D*, Large adventitial vessels (All H&E stain).

making a major contribution to flow redistribution. In contrast, recanalizing vessels with a well-developed tunica media may indicate a consistent flow that is able to remodel the vessel wall and allow increased function. Experimentally, recanalization of an occlusive thrombus takes more than 15 days to begin.[274]

Red Coagulum

A coagulum, or clot, is formed by elements in the same proportion in which they exist in flowing blood — that is, mainly red cells, with leukocytes entangled in a fine network of fibrin. Its fate is unknown but organization per se has never been proven. In our experience, an old vein graft inserted years before may show a nonatherosclerotic wall and a lumen filled with atheromatous, toothpaste-like material that is easily squeezed from the lumen; this finding suggests that a coagulum, instead of organizing, breaks down and changes into atheromatous material.[5] In an atheromatous plaque, the pultaceous content may result from repeated hemorrhage.[275] Finally, a coagulum cannot be the cause of ischemia because it develops secondary to the cessation of or a great reduction in blood flow; in the latter condition, layering of the various elements occurs. The coagulum is easily lysed when flow is restored. The layered "thrombus" recovered

from a patient with an acute infarction[150] and found in atherectomy material[143] seems to be more a coagulum than a thrombus. In our studies, a coagulum was differentiated from a thrombus,[5, 155] and the overall frequency of an occlusive thrombus was 41% in cases of acute infarct and 15% in cases of sudden death. The frequency of mural thrombi, which included the so-called intraintimal thrombi, was 18% and 11%, respectively. They were found mainly in severe, long, and concentric stenoses.[5, 155] This means that the occlusion is ineffective probably because the thrombus formed in a stenosis already bypassed by collaterals. Their compensatory function is supported both by the absence of disease before the acute event and by experiment.[250] Does the occlusion of a small residual lumen, per se, abolish flow in the presence of an already functioning collateral flow (Fig. 8-39)? The question is moot.

Other arguments have been offered concerning the significance of the occlusive thrombus.[5] Based on the correlations we have made, its development appears to be a multivariant phenomenon (Fig. 8-40), and what is important is not its frequency but its significance in the natural history of IHD. Much new data about events occurring in the plaque[5, 91] suggest that the thrombus is an epiphenomenon — an important one by today's understanding, perhaps, but an epiphenomenon nonetheless (Figs. 8-41, 8-

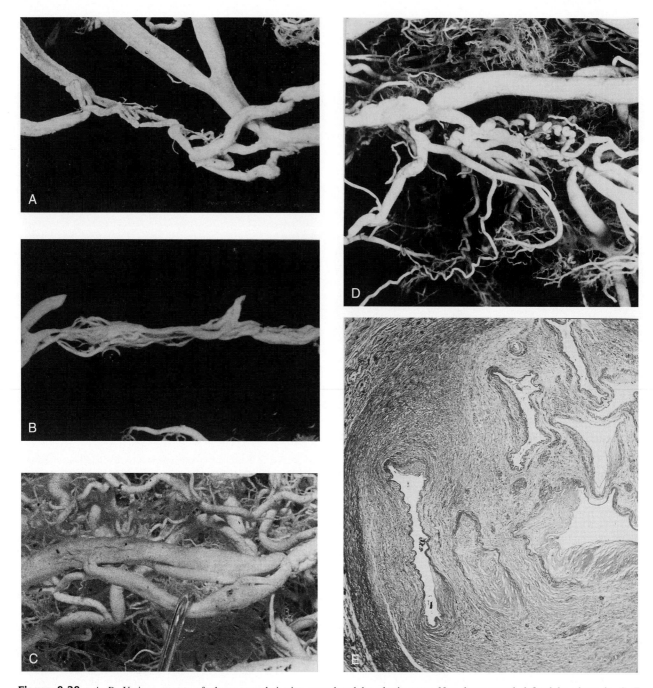

Figure 8-38 • *A–D,* Various aspects of plaque vascularization reproduced by plastic casts. Note large vessel defined by clamp in *C. E,* Histologic section at site of recanalized occlusion. Note large vessels in arterial wall (H&E stain).

42). In that eventuality, it is useful to question why billions of dollars are spent dissolving or bypassing occlusive coronary thrombi when all efforts should be invested in understanding the phenomena associated with a plaque so as to prevent its formation and complications.

Illustrative Case Report

At the beginning of this chapter, emphasis was placed on the need to observe a phenomenon before and after its occurrence. At our institute, we had the opportunity to witness the beginning and follow the establishment of an infarct during cineangiography[276] and to study the heart excised at transplantation 1 year later.

The case documented some facts and suggested some considerations. First, if we believe that the first ischemic change on electrocardiogram (ECG) was the beginning of the infarct, the case indicates that an infarct may start in the absence of a coronary occlusion, which occurs as a secondary event. In contrast, if we consider the first imaging of occlusion as a starting point, it must be noted that there were no ECG or hemodynamic changes or

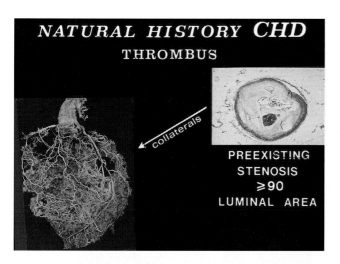

Figure 8-39 • *Left,* Cast showing an enlarged collateral system in a case of severe stenosis *Right,* Occlusion of the small residual lumen by thrombus or any other occlusive cause seems to have no significance in reducing the blood flow. (Movat stain). (From Baroldi G, Scomazzoni G: Coronary Circulation in the Normal and Pathologic Heart. American Registry of Pathology, A.F.I.P. [ed]: Washington, D.C., U.S. Government Printing Office, 1967.)

subjective symptoms after coronary occlusion. Only 70 minutes after the first occlusion—and despite an intracoronary vasodilator, a Ca^{++} antagonist, urokinase, and successful angioplasty—were there ECG changes and chest pain without evidence, during temporary recanalization by urokinase, of images suggesting plaque rupture, thrombosis, or distal embolization.

Second, this case shows that cineangiographic occlusion can be an apparent occlusion caused by stoppage of flow because of intramural flow blockage, with clotting, not thrombosis, of blood at the origin of the vessel where the left circumflex branch, with unrestricted flow, is located (retrograde progressive pseudo-occlusion) (Fig. 8-43). Spontaneous permanent and intermittent coronary occlusion have been attributed to a combination of thrombosis and vasoconstriction.[277] Neither was demonstrated in this case.

Third, the case indicates how rapidly—in 20 to 70 minutes—a large transmural infarct can develop despite

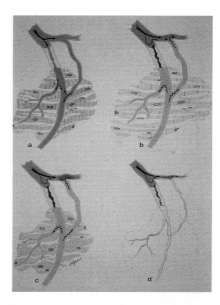

Figure 8-41 • Changes in contractility in the related myocardial region as a cause of increased peripheral resistance. a, Severe coronary stenosis in the presence of a functioning collateral system and normally contracting myocardium. b, Atonic stretched myocardium. c, Tetanic hypercontracted myocardium. d, Coronary spasm. These are all causes of increased peripheral resistance and of secondary hemorrhage and rupture within the plaque.

all the therapeutic approaches available today, and that chest pain is an unreliable sign for timing the event.

Fourth, the case demonstrates that occlusion by thrombus may occur without infarction, as shown by the right occlusive thrombus.

Finally, it confirms that myocardial dysfunction precedes electrocardiographic ischemic change and pain[278, 279] and may aggravate coronary atherosclerosis—90% stenosis along the whole course of the left anterior descending artery—in the relatively short period of 12 months. This suggests that diffuse and severe coronary

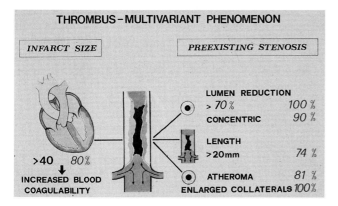

Figure 8-40 • Illustration that coronary thrombosis is a multivariant phenomenon.

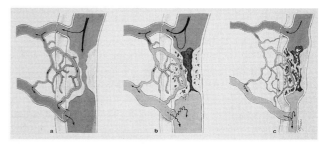

Figure 8-42 • Effects of retrograde collateral flow or spasm on the atherosclerotic plaque. a, Intimal vascularization of an atherosclerotic plaque through the vasa vasorum network originating from secondary branches both proximal and distal to a stenosis. Proximal flow reduction is counterbalanced by distal retrograde collateral flow (left). b, Stagnation and change in flow distribution consequent to stasis distal to stenosis and secondary thrombus formation in lumen (middle). c, Spasm at the level of or distal to stenosis, again with thrombi forming in lumen (right). Mechanisms depicted in the middle and right illustrations may be responsible for secondary intimal hemorrhage or rupture of atheroma as epiphenomena of increased peripheral resistance or of mechanical effects (spasm, wall motion secondary to exerted contractility) on the atherosclerotic plaque.

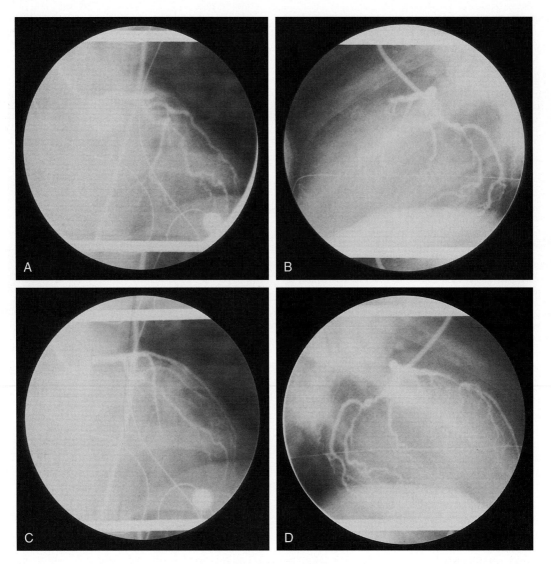

Figure 8-43 • Series of cineangiographic images. *A*, Severe stenoses of the left anterior descending artery. *B*, Occlusion after 20 minutes resulting from ischemic changes as seen on ECG. *C* and *D*, During the short period of recanalization, the "occlusion" progressively ascends to the origin of the branch. This angiographic pseudo-occlusion was a unique case in whom it was possible to follow events. (From Baroldi G, Marzilli M, L'Abbate A, et al: Coronary occlusion: Cause or consequence of acute myocardial infarction. A case report. Clin Cardiol 13:49, 1990.)

atherosclerosis in patients with chronic disease is secondary to myocardial asynergy rather than being a progression of myohyperplastic atherosclerosis. It also raises questions concerning the previously reported opinion of some angiographers on rupture plus thrombosis of small atherosclerotic plaques. They did not consider (1) the differing dynamics in vessels that were or were not related to asynergic regions, (2) pseudo-occlusion, and (3) the lack of any documentation[5, 277a] of occlusive thrombi in small plaques at autopsy despite an extremely high frequency of small plaques in the general population (see Table 8-5).

Obviously, we do not know how many infarcts have the pathogenesis illustrated in this case, and we do not know the exact cause of intramural flow blockage even if there is no support for spasm of intramural arteries and no reflow phenomenon. Data suggest that extravascular compression of a noncontracting wall by an infarct that developed in a previously demonstrated hypokinetic zone is a possible cause. However, the basic question is, how many of the angiographic occlusions seen in 87% of cases within 1 to 4 hours after the onset of symptoms are "apparent" occlusions? This is a very important point in relation to present aggressive therapy during which a positive reaction may be caused by mechanisms different from those we believe are active. For instance, it has been shown, in isolated rat hearts with global ischemia and, therefore, in the absence of thrombus and platelet aggregates, that streptokinase improves myocardial contraction following reoxygenation and reperfusion[280]; or fibrinolysis may be active in that it reduces hypercoagulability secondary to infarct necrosis by improving contractility rather than by dissolving nonexistent thrombus. These divergent opinions demonstrate the need for new clinical approaches that routinely monitor the sequence of all events and the need for an experimental model capable of mimicking human IHD.

Finally, this patient with unstable angina who survived a large infarct did not show coronary spasm, plaque rupture, or embolization and its histologic sequelae in small vessels. The case permits commentary (1) on the fissuring of a plaque as a possible artifact. Such fissuring was defined as "a connection between an intraintimal platelet/fibrin thrombus and the lumen that is demonstrable by the presence of injection media within the plaque,"[87] forgetting plaque vascularization as a carrier of injection media; (2) on sudden death within 6 hours in patients with unstable angina in whom emboli have been demonstrated histologically.[87, 88] Most of the latter cases had documented infarct necrosis, which usually shows secondary thrombosis of intramural vessels. Even though these cases were selected as examples of sudden death within 6 hours and even within 1 hour, many events may occur in that period, and final morphologic findings cannot predict their exact sequence. It is known that 38% of patients with unstable angina are hypersensitive to spasmogenic stimuli, in contrast to 20% of patients with acute infarct, 6% with old infarct, and 4% with stable angina.[281] Patients with unstable angina who die suddenly are a subset of the IHD population in whom the pathologic findings, interpreted as a cause of the event, could be considered secondary phenomena. In particular, the "microinfarcts" described in these cases correspond to various stages of coagulative myocytolysis always present around an acute infarct; and, as was noted, most patients experienced acute infarct.

Other Mechanisms of Coronary Ischemia

Several attractive hypotheses were formulated to explain acute and chronic IHD. A brief discussion may be useful to review their roles in the natural history of this disease.

Infarct at a Distance[174]

This is thought to occur when there is occlusion in the parent main branch from which collaterals supplying another vascular territory originate and when there exists a steal syndrome[282] in which collaterals steal blood flow from the territory of the parent vessels. Both these hypotheses are difficult to substantiate in a network system like that of the coronary arteries.

Mural Coronary Arteries

The dipping of coronary arteries or branches into the myocardium for a variable distance is a relatively common phenomenon that occurs in 25% of cases.[85] The rhythmic coronary occlusion in systole and its "milking" effect[135] may result in ischemia in limited and still unclear circumstances during which tachycardia may occur.

Coronary Ostial Obstruction

In our studies, atherosclerotic severe stenosis or occlusion of a coronary ostium was found in only 0.9 and 0.5% of cases, respectively.[102] In inflammatory diseases of the aorta, syphilis, Takayasu disease, and so on, a severe stenosis or occlusion may occur and may be considered the cause of ischemia. However, in the files of the Armed Forces Institute of Pathology, there were 11 cases—5 men and 6 women—with occlusion or severe stenosis of all coronary ostia due to aortitis. The ages ranged from 10 to 63 years and the heart weighed from 200 to 700 g. Only 1 patient died suddenly. Microfocal subendocardial fibrosis, recent in 2 and old in 4, were the histologic findings. None had a history of IHD. These cases support the concept of adequate compensatory function of extracardiac coronary anastomoses, particularly from bronchial arteries.[283]

Small Vessel Diseases

These include a variety of conditions. We indicated previously that in our studies, platelet aggregates had a similar frequency in cases of sudden and unexpected death and in healthy controls, the number of vessels with aggregates being proportional to the duration of the terminal episode, with progressive reduction of blood flow velocity and a layering effect of blood elements having differing masses.[284] On the other hand, in human pathology, diseases exist that are "experiments" of nature. One is thrombotic thrombocytopenic purpura (TTP) in which, despite a diffuse occlusive microangiopathy of intramural arterioles and occlusive platelet aggregates in most normal intramural vessels (Fig. 8-44 and see Fig. 16-18B&C), plus extremely severe hemolytic anemia, hemorrhages, and neurologic disorders, not 1 patient of 39 cases examined had clinical symptoms or signs of IHD or histologic evidence of an infarct, and not 1 died suddenly.[285] Another experiment is sickle cell anemia in which, despite the plugging of small vessels and of the terminal bed by sickled erythrocytes during acute episodes, not one patient of 53 cases examined had a history or histologic evidence of an acute or chronic coronary syndrome.[286] Contraction abnormalities, electrocardiographic changes, and MB isoenzymes were not observed during sickle cell crises.[287] (TTP and the chronic effects of sickle cell anemia are also discussed in Chapter 16.) It should be noted that in all our studies, "cholesterol" emboli were exceptions (Fig. 8-45).

Perivascular Fibrosis

This fibrosis in the intramural system has been proposed as a factor that limits vasodilation and produces ischemia and infarction without coronary disease.[288] This hypothesis is apparently contradicted by the absence of ischemic events in rheumatic heart disease when intramural perivascular fibrosis predominates.

No-reflow Phenomenon

This consists of interstitial exudation or hemorrhage and swelling of parenchymal cells, with vascular compression described in the kidney, brain, and heart[289–291] but not proven in the natural history of ischemic heart disease. If this term is applied to extravascular compres-

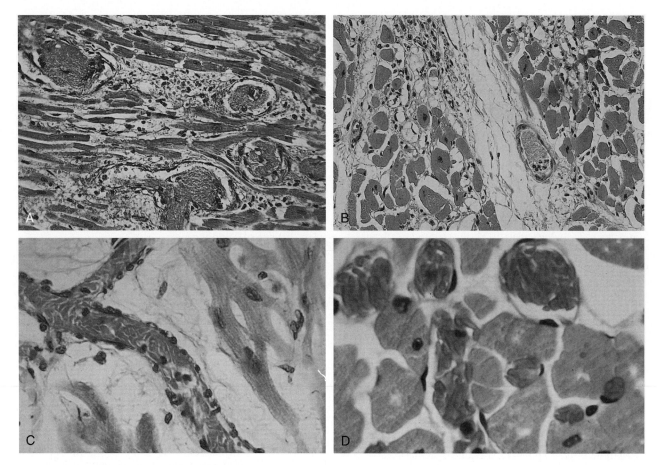

Figure 8-44 • Small vessel disease without ischemic effects. Thrombotic thrombocytopenic purpura with *A*, severe occlusive microangiopathy and *B*, platelet aggregates in most normal arteriolar vessels (Both Movat stain); *C* and *D*, sickle cell anemia with vascular "plugging" in acute phase of disease (Both H&E stain).

sion by an asynergic, stretched, or hypercontracted myocardium with blockage of flow, the no-reflow phenomenon becomes a fundamental mechanism of infarction and is the first signal of ischemia, occurring before electrocardiographic changes and pain.[278, 279]

Relative Coronary Insufficiency

Any time there is an increasing metabolic demand, nutrient blood flow may become insufficient. This is claimed to explain acute coronary syndromes in the absence of other main factors. Apart from the absence of any relationship between sudden death or acute infarction and increased physical exercise, the concept of relative coronary insufficiency pertains particularly to cardiac hypertrophy. The belief is that there is no rebuilding of the vasculature proportional to the increased mass of the myocardium and that the increased myocell diameter reduces the metabolic exchange with capillaries. First, extramural coronary arteries remodel in terms of length to the increased heart mass and they enlarge their diameters as well.[102] Second, using the usual count of one capillary to one myocell to calculate metabolic exchange does not take into account the fact that the terminal bed includes a myriad of collaterals with capillary-like structures so that any myocell is included in a capillary network more extensive than one capillary per myocell. Finally, most heavy hearts show only microfocal subendocardial fibrosis which, often interpreted as ischemic in nature, is the re-

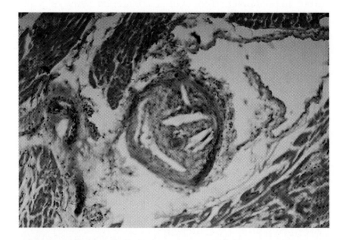

Figure 8-45 • Cholesterol embolus in normal myocardium in a case of sudden and unexpected coronary death (H&E stain). This was the only cholesterol embolus found in all cases we studied.[5]

sult of coagulative myocytolysis as seen in experimental hypertrophy.[30]

Coronary Spasm

The difficulty in establishing the role of spasm of subepicardial arteries or branches in the natural history of IHD has been mentioned. However, the possibility that spasm may induce ventricular fibrillation and sudden death is a theoretical possibility supported by experimental acute coronary occlusion. Such experiments induce ventricular fibrillation and death within the first hour in the dog. Foci of coagulative myocytolysis are visible and β-blockers prevent both the latter and the former.[7] (See previous section.) Sudden permanent or transitory ischemia may induce hypoakinesis, which activates compensatory adrenergic stimulation via nerve reflexes.

Activity of Atherosclerotic Myohyperplastic Plaque

The term *active*, in this sense, defines a dynamic rather than a static, inactive system. The myohyperplastic plaque is a structure in which two main morphofunctional dynamics act. One is the continuous blood flow through connections between adventitia, intima, and residual lumen, which can be altered by local or peripheral increased resistance. The other dynamic is an inflammatory process that has two aspects: (1) inflammatory macrophages that act not only as antigen-presenting cells for T lymphocytes but also as scavenger cells to remove noxious material and as a source of growth-regulatory molecules and cytokines[292] and of metalloproteinase, which dissolves connective tissue and leads to plaque rupture.[90] (See Chapter 4.) This pattern is more pertinent to the hypercholesterol plaque in which "inflammation" seems a reparative rather than an inflammatory process that follows lipoprotein infiltration; (2) T lymphocytes and plasma cells found in the intima and in the adventitia close to the media. Described long ago,[153, 268, 275, 293, 294] they were considered a minor complication[294] and interpreted as an autoimmune process.[295, 296] The importance of this inflammatory process is its significant presence in and extension around periaortic and pericoronary nerves adjacent to the media in ischemic patients in contrast to healthy people with an equal degree of coronary stenosis and intimal thickening.[5, 91] This process suggests that plaque activity is linked with this inflammatory process. It may act by means of nerve irritation or degeneration or coronary constriction or by means of regional myocardial contractility and injury. As with any chronic process, it may present periods of activity alternating with periods of inactivity, thus explaining the clinical variability in IHD. Several clinical studies indicate that an inflammatory index, measured as C-reactive protein, predicts an increased mortality in unstable angina and in non-Q infarcts.[296a–c] C-reactive protein and serum amyloid A protein are markers of hypersensitivity of the inflammatory system, even to small stimuli, rather than of plaque rupture.[296b] The nature, type, and localization of both of these agents in the atherosclerotic process and in the natural history of IHD has to be determined (see previous section).

Infarct Size, Complications, and Death in Ischemic Heart Disease

It is a generally accepted concept that complications and death in IHD are related to ischemia. In the past 20 years all effort has been aimed at abolishing borderline ischemia and reducing or limiting infarct size by restoring blood flow abolished by thrombosis, or spasm, or both. With this point of view, it becomes essential to establish the length of the interval between the onset of an infarct and its complete evolution in order to therapeutically arrest its progression. With permanent coronary occlusion in dogs, an infarct is fully formed in 1 hour. If blood flow is restored within 20 minutes the infarct does not evolve.[1] The question is whether we may accept this experiment as a model of the natural history of coronary occlusion in human IHD. First, the experimental occlusion is performed on a normal dog heart, not in a severely obstructed atherosclerotic coronary artery as in IHD; and second, the dog heart is not comparable to the human heart because the former has collaterals joining extramural arteries and branches on the surface of the heart whereas in the human heart, collaterals are intramural. This means that in the dog, superficial collaterals may rapidly function to redistribute flow, as they are not restricted or occluded by systolic contraction or loss of contractility plus stretching by intraventricular pressure; these phenomena occur within a few seconds of experimental occlusion. The function of extramural collaterals explains the small size of the infarct, which is limited to the posterior papillary muscle and the adjacent subendocardium despite occlusion of the left circumflex branch, which predominates in this animal and gives origin to the posterior descending branch.

In the clinical setting, the onset of a transmural infarct can be referred only to the onset of typical chest pain and the time interval calculated accordingly. In the case mentioned earlier, chest pain began 90 minutes after the first electrocardiographic sign of ischemia, and all clinical data indicate that the infarct probably had fully evolved at that time. However, the general belief is that this time interval ranges from 3 to 6 hours, as was deduced from another experimental model in the dog. Temporary occlusion for 40 minutes followed by 2 to 4 days of reperfusion as well as reperfusion after reocclusion for 3 to 4 hours produced a wave-front phenomenon[21] with progressive transmural expansion of the lesion. Defined as reperfusion injury (see an earlier section), characteristic contraction bands are its morphologic marker.[297] However, this lesion also shows massive interstitial hemorrhage and is commonly associated with malignant arrhythmia and ventricular fibrillation. The impression is that an overlapping of experimental findings and human conditions exists, and there is a need to distinguish coagulative myocytolysis from reperfusion injury as two different entities.

The first question is, how many times can reperfusion injury be documented in the natural history of IHD? We have not demonstrated histologic evidence that an infarct may expand, that is, that a central area of infarction of one age is encircled by infarcted myocardium of younger age, nor have we demonstrated, in 200 consecutive myocardial infarcts not treated with fibrinolytic therapy, that a hemorrhage was present in the myocardium. Hemorrhage is seen only following heart rupture[5] or is reported in patients treated by fibrinolytic agents.[9] Similarly, we have not seen lesions described as the wavefront phenomenon in reflow necrosis.[21] We have mentioned that reperfusion injury is occasionally seen after cardiac surgery. However, it is to be noted that despite innumerable reperfusion and vascularization procedures done on millions of patients by means of thrombolysis, angioplasty, or coronary bypass, reperfusion injury has never been proven. Therefore, any discussion of the advantage or disadvantage of reperfusion procedures,[297] although theoretically useful, is meaningless in human IHD. The size of a fatal infarct necrosis was small (less than 20%) in half of our first-episode cases and in 64% of chronic patients (see Table 8-9), and only 11% of these infarcts were subendocardial. In our experience, the pathophysiologic distinction between subendocardial and transmural infarcts[291] is still unclear. We believe that complications and death are related more to nonischemic disorders linked with catecholamine myotoxicity or congestive failure than to infarct size or reperfusion. Nonhemorrhagic coagulative myocytolysis of various extents is always seen at the periphery of all infarcts. This suggests that catecholamine or catecholamine-like myotoxicity is linked with malignant arrhythmia. This lesion needs blood flow to develop and to allow Ca^{++} influx, and blood flow is increased around an infarct as has been shown experimentally[298] and deduced histologically by the polymorphonuclear infiltration that starts in the border zone. An increased contractility,[299] probably stimulated by mechanoreceptors,[300] follows loss of contraction in the infarcted zone. These conditions may explain increased adrenergic activity around the infarct, a concept that is further supported by the prevention of contraction band necrosis and ventricular fibrillation by β-blockers in experimental infarction[7] and in transient ischemia,[264] and by denervation in permanent coronary occlusion[301] and use of lidocaine,[302] lipid peroxidation,[303] superoxide dismutase,[304] or regional pre-conditioning.[305] A similar increase of adrenergic activity can be suspected for the myocardial necrosis documented by creatine kinase-MB elevation in 19% of patients who underwent coronary intervention—as PTCA, rotational atherectomy, and so forth—without complication, and would be more frequent in those with diffuse atherosclerosis[305a] (adventitial perinerve inflammation?), with enzyme level being important for prognostic and therapeutic approaches.[305b] It should be noted that abrupt angioplastic occlusion impairs baroreflex modulation of vagal and sympathetic outflow.[305c]

Coagulative myocytolysis, or contraction band necrosis, is generally considered an ischemic lesion because it is found associated with infarct necrosis. However, all data indicate the two lesions should be separated in terms of cause and pathogenesis. All aspects of IHD present a composite syndrome with several concurrent pathogenic mechanisms in which colliquative myocytolysis, as a signal of congestive heart failure, must be included. On the subject, it should be realized that *chronic ischemia* is still difficult to define. The likelihood that a chronic reduction of regional blood flow explains hibernation has already been questioned. On the other hand, and more precisely, by *chronic ischemic heart disease* we mean its continuance through several acute episodes without any possibility of arresting its course. When an individual becomes a patient, he or she is likely to remain a patient and to receive uninterrupted therapy. In this chronic course, neuromediated factors may play an important role. In this context and for unknown reasons, the myocardium may fail and a new complication, congestive heart failure, may ensue. Blood flow reduction in poorly beating but viable myocardium[216] may be due simply to reduced myocell function, a concept supported by the lack of histologic documentation of ischemic injury and by the absence of energy deficiency as shown by lactate production, oxygen and pH reduction in coronary sinus blood, and symptoms of ischemia in patients with congestive heart failure of various origins.[306] In reality, the ischemia per se and the ischemic factors are ill defined and their relationship with

TABLE 8-11 • **Cardiac Pump Adaptation in Ischemic Heart Disease—Sequence of Events**

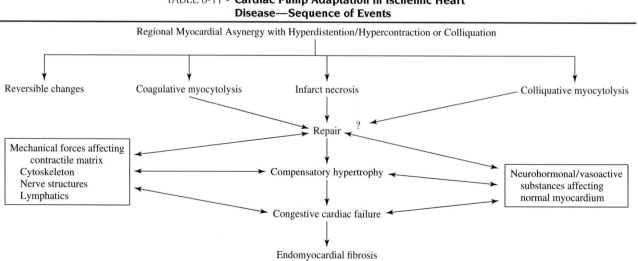

adrenergic stress still cloudy. At present, more attention is paid to resistance vessels and endothelial vasoactive substances. An increased metabolic demand by atrial pacing in IHD patients determines vasoconstriction rather than a maximal vasodilation as shown by intracoronary adenosine infusion[306a]; and in acute myocardial infarct patients, there is a global flow reduction, which is 45% lower than normal at 90 minutes in both nonculprit and reopened culprit coronary arteries.[306b] More aggressive therapy in the United States versus that of Canada does not change the outcome at 1 year[306c]; no differences were found in treating an acute infarct by angioplasty or by intravenous thrombolysis[306d]; β-blocker therapy was effective[306e]; and the major risk factors for IHD, namely, cigarette smoking[306f] and psychological factors,[306g] act via excessive sympathetic nervous system activation.

Structural Readaptive Changes in Ischemic Heart Disease

The natural history of IHD is characterized by an interaction of various interdependent pathogenic mechanisms that act on a complex contracting structure (Table 8-11). We have emphasized that different forms of myocardial injury and death may depend on (1) the mechanical forces of normal contraction on asynergic myocardium; (2) myotoxicity caused primarily by adrenergic stimulation via nervous reflexes; and (3) other ion and molecular disorders. However, in the cardiac pump addi-

tional morphologic parameters exist, such as collagen matrix, myocell cytoskeleton, intramyocardial nerve axons and their terminal ends, and lymphatics. We do not have information on lymphatics and we have only indirect evidence of possible destruction of intramyocardial nerve structures (see the section concerning denervation in infarct complications). There are additional data concerning changes to the collagen matrix and cytoskeleton,[2, 307–309] although their meanings are still unclear, as is whether the finding is an epiphenomenon. In conclusion, the need is to reasses the cause of death not only clinically[309a] but also pathologically, giving to any changes their real functional meaning, and when they are not known, to say so pending further study. What is often defined as a remodeling of a pump is an alternating sequence of destructive and repair processes with hypertrophy of surviving myocardium and possible other undetermined factors leading to congestive heart failure and its own structural changes. On this subject, endocardial myoelastofibrosis found in failing hearts (Fig. 8-46) must be considered.[28]

Pathologic Diagnosis of Sudden Coronary Death

The diagnosis of sudden coronary death is one of the more difficult diagnoses for a pathologist. The high frequency of occurrence of (1) coronary atherosclerotic plaques not associated with extensive myocardial fibrosis in apparently normal people dying from accident and (2)

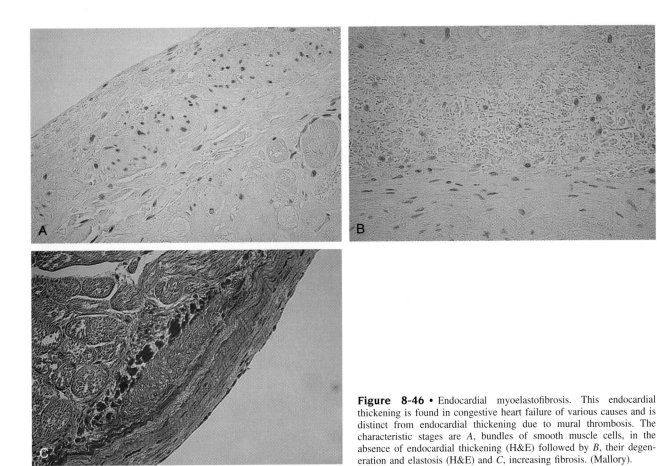

Figure 8-46 • Endocardial myoelastofibrosis. This endocardial thickening is found in congestive heart failure of various causes and is distinct from endocardial thickening due to mural thrombosis. The characteristic stages are *A*, bundles of smooth muscle cells, in the absence of endocardial thickening (H&E) followed by *B*, their degeneration and elastosis (H&E) and *C*, increasing fibrosis. (Mallory).

TABLE 8-12 • **Histologic Diagnosis of Sudden Coronary Death**

Criteria		
Coronary Atherosclerotic Plaque	Myocardium	Diagnosis
Absent	Normal	Not likely
Uncomplicated*	Normal	Not likely
	Extensive fibrosis	Possible†
	Coagulative myocytolysis at varying histologic stages	Absolute
Complicated	Normal	Possible
	Coagulative myocytolysis at varying histologic stages and/or infarct necrosis	Absolute

* For definitions of uncomplicated versus complicated atherosclerotic plaque, see text.

† If clinical circumstances are suggestive.

acute foci of coagulative myocytolysis found in the latter with a longer survival time render both these pathologic parameters, per se, nonspecific. In terms of a diagnosis, we need to define a variety of stages of coagulative myocytolysis, from acute cross-band foci to alveolar, healing, and healed foci or microfoci. This indicates an ongoing adrenergic myotoxic phenomenon that may be linked to malignant arrhythmia and ventricular fibrillation. From the coronary side, we should distinguish between complicated (with hemorrhage, fissuring embolization, thrombosis, and adventitial lymphoplasma cellular inflammatory reaction) and uncomplicated atherosclerotic plaques. A variety of possible combinations in a subject who dies suddenly can be proposed (Table 8-12) to help in making practical diagnoses in this condition. It should be noted that spasm of a normal coronary artery has been never documented and we lack reliable histologic hallmarks of coronary artery spasm.

CONCLUSION

Despite many preventive and therapeutical approaches, IHD remains the primary medical problem in advanced societies in terms of cost of hospitalization, diagnostic procedures, and therapy, and is the main cause of death, disability, and early retirement. In the United States, the National Health International Review indicates that in 1989, the incidence of IHD was 2.9% of the total population; 86/1000 of patients were males between 45 and 64 years of age, and 169/1000 were males between 65 and 74 years of age, whereas among females, the figures were 26/1000 and 113/1000, respectively. In women, a dramatic increase in occurrence is seen after menopause, whether natural or surgical. There are 800,000 new acute IHD episodes per year and 450,000 recurrent attacks. Following an infarct, morbidity and mortality are between two and nine times more likely than in the normal population, and there is a higher frequency of (1) reinfarction within 6 years in 23% of men and 31% of women; (2) angina pectoris in 41% of men and 34% of women; (3) congestive heart failure in 20%; (4) brain infarction in 9% of men and 18% of women; (5) sudden death in 13%

of men and 6% of women. In two thirds of patients there is no complete recovery even if 88% return to their usual activities. In 1989, 498,000 deaths due to IHD were registered, and they were commonly sudden and unexpected, particularly in men.[310] A similar incidence of this disease is seen in Italy, where until 1945 IHD in general and acute myocardial infarct in particular were rarely found in those seen in the autopsy room. After that time, a dramatic increase in industrialization combined with a higher consumer standard of living took place, and in a few years, an incidence of IHD similar to that in the United States and other Western countries was seen, a fact that should stimulate a review of the roles of many risk factors and their possible association.

All data indicate how poorly we have succeeded in controlling this disease and how unsatisfactory is the current interpretation of its pathophysiology.[297]

The merit of the "unifying" theory[252] mentioned previously is that it promotes discussion. However, its oversimplification contrasts with the complexity of this disease, which is aggravated by the lack of an adequate experimental model; coronary occlusion in animals imitates the pattern of nonatherosclerotic acute coronary syndromes only. The alternative points of view expressed here are an attempt to answer three main questions: why we develop IHD, why it takes a variable clinical course and does not have a definite recovery, and why individuals with IHD die. Despite many postulates and consequent preventive and therapeutic measures taken during the past 50 years, IHD remains the number one killer in this society. In some countries, for undetermined reasons, the related mortality has been reduced. However, no figures indicate that morbidity has changed.[310] The result is an increasing number of chronic patients treated variously with multiple, often uncontrolled approaches and with incomplete knowledge of their real therapeutic values and excessive social cost. A critical revision of the meaning of any technologic approach is needed, particularly when the approach is à la mode as is, for instance, the current enthusiasm for apoptosis in heart disease, including ischemic disease, when the sensitivity and specificity of the immunohistochemical methods used to diagnose the condition must be established.[311]

REFERENCES

1. Jennings RB: Early phase of myocardial ischemic injury and infarction. Am J Cardiol 24:753, 1969
2. Weber KT: Cardiac interstitium in health and disease: The fibrillar collagen network. J Am Coll Cardiol 13:1637, 1989
3. Spiro D, Spotnitz H, Sonnenblick EH: The relation of cardiac fine structure to function. In: Gould SE (ed): Pathology of the Heart and Blood Vessels. Springfield, CC Thomas, 1968, p 131
4. Baroldi G: Different types of myocardial necrosis in coronary heart disease: a pathophysiological review of their functional significance. Am Heart J 89:742, 1975
5. Baroldi G, Silver MD: Sudden death in ischemic heart disease: an alternative view on the significance of morphologic findings. RG Landes Austin, TX, Springer-Verlag, New York, 1995
6. Korb G, Totovic V: Electron microscopical studies on experimental ischemic lesions of the heart. Ann NY Acad Sci 105:135, 1969
7. Baroldi G, Silver MD, Lixfield W, et al: Irreversible myocardial damage resembling catecholamine necrosis secondary to acute cor-

onary occlusion in dogs: its prevention by propranolol. J Molec Cell Cardiol 9:687, 1977

8. Hort W: Mikroskopische Beobachtung an menschlichen Infarktherzen. Virchows Arch 345:61, 1968

9. Fujiwara H, Onodera T, Tanaka M, et al: A clinicopathologic study of patients with hemorrhagic myocardial infarction treated with selective thrombolysis with urokinase. Circulation 73:749, 1986

9a. Kelley ST, Malekan R, Gorman JH, et al: Restraining infarct expansion preserves left ventricular geometry and function after acute anterolateral infarction. Circulation 99:135, 1999

10. Baroldi G, Silver MD: The healing of myocardial infarcts in man. G Ital Cardiol 5:465, 1975

11. Todd GL, Baroldi G, Pieper GM, et al: Experimental catecholamine-induced myocardial necrosis. I. Morphology, quantification and regional distribution of acute contraction band lesions. J Mol Cell Cardiol 17:317, 1985

12. Todd GL, Baroldi G, Pieper GM, et al: Experimental catecholamine-induced myocardial necrosis. II. Temporal development of isoproterenol-induced contraction band lesions correlated with ECG, hemodynamic and biochemical changes. J Mol Cell Cardiol 17:647, 1985

13. Reichenbach D, Benditt EP: Myofibrillar degeneration: a common form of cardiac muscle injury. Ann NY Acad Sci 156:164, 1969

14. Reichenbach DD, Benditt EP: Catecholamine and cardiomyopathy: the pathogenesis and potential importance of myofibrillar degeneration. Hum Pathol 1:125, 1970

15. Rona G, Chappel CI, Balazs T, et al: An infarct-like myocardial lesion and other toxic manifestations produced by isoproterenol in rat. Arch Pathol 67:443, 1959

16. Fineschi V, Welti EV, Di Paolo M, Baroldi G: Myocardial necrosis and cocaine: A quantitative morphologic study in 26 cocaine-associated deaths. Int J Leg Med 3:164, 1997

17. Schlesinger MJ, Reiner L: Focal myocytolysis of the heart: Am J Pathol 31:443, 1955

18. Martin AM, Hackel DB: The myocardium of the dog in hemorrhagic shock. An histochemical study. Lab Invest 12:77, 1963

19. Martin AM, Hackel DB: An electron microscopic study of the progression of myocardial lesions in the dog after hemorrhagic shock. Lab Invest 15:243, 1966

20. Entman ML, Hackel DB, Martin AM, et al: Prevention of myocardial lesions during hemorrhagic shock in dogs by pronethalol. Arch Pathol 83:392, 1965

21. Reimer KA, Lowe JE, Rasmussen MM, et al: The wavefront phenomenon of ischemic cell death. I. Myocardial infarct size vs duration of coronary occlusion in dogs. Circulation 56:786, 1977

22. Lie JT, Lawrie GM, Morris GC, et al: Hemorrhagic myocardial infarction associated with aortocoronary bypass revascularization. Am Heart J 96:295, 1978

23. Gottlieb A, Masse S, Allard J, et al: Concentric hemorrhagic necrosis of the myocardium: A morphological and clinical study. Hum Pathol 8:27, 1977

24. Reimer KA, Jennings RB: The changing anatomic reference base of evolving myocardial infarction. Underestimation of myocardial collateral blood flow and overestimation of experimental anatomic infarct size due to edema, hemorrhage and acute inflammation. Circulation 60:866, 1979

25. Reimer KA, Rasmussen MM, Jennings RB: On the nature of protection by propranolol against myocardial necrosis after temporary coronary occlusion in dogs. Am J Cardiol 37:520, 1976

26. Raab W: Preventive myocardiology, fundamentals and targets. In: Kugelmass NI (ed): Bannerstone Division of American Lectures in Living Chemistry. Springfield, IL, CC Thomas, 1970, pp 57

27. Zimmermann ANE, Daems W, Hulsmann WC, et al: Morphopathological changes of heart muscle caused by successive perfusion with calcium-free and calcium-containing solutions (calcium paradox). Cardiovasc Res 1:201, 1967

28. Baroldi G, Silver MD, De Maria R, Pellegrini A: Pathology and pathogenesis of congestive heart failure: A quantitative morphologic study of 144 hearts excised at transplantation. Pathogenesis 3:33, 1998

29. Katz AM: Cellular mechanisms in congestive heart failure. Am J Cardiol 62:3A, 1988

30. Meerson FZ: The myocardium in hyperfunction, hypertophy and heart failure. Circ Res 25(suppl 2):1, 1969

31. Fleckenstein A, Janke J, Doring HJ, et al: Myocardial fiber necrosis due to intracellular Ca^{++} overload. A new principle in cardiac pathophysiology. In: Dhallas NS (ed): Recent Advances in Studies on Cardiac Structure and Metabolism. Vol 4. Baltimore, University Park Press, 1975, p 563

32. Bing RJ, Tillmanns H, Fauvel JM, et al: Effect of prolonged alcohol administration on calcium transport in heart muscle of the dog. Circ Res 35:33, 1974

33. Mak T, Weiglicki WB: Protection by beta-blocking agents against free radical-mediated sarcolemmal lipid peroxidation. Circ Res 63:262, 1988

34. Sun SC, Burch GE, De Pasquale NP: Histochemical and electron microscopy study of heart muscle after beta-adrenergic blockade. Am Heart J 74:340, 1967

35. Emberson JW, Muir AR: Changes in ultrastructure of rat myocardium induced by hypokalaemia. J Exp Physiol 54:36, 1969

36. Weiss DL, Subswicz B, Rubenstein I: Myocardial lesions of calcium deficiency causing irreversible myocardial failure. Am J Pathol 48:653, 1966

37. Baroldi G, Radice F, Schmid C, et al: Morphology of acute myocardial infarction in relation to coronary thrombosis. Am Heart J 87:65, 1974

38. Silver MD, Baroldi G, Mariani F: The relationship between acute occlusive coronary thrombi and myocardial infarction studies in 100 consecutive patients. Circulation 61:219, 1980

39. Baroldi G, Falzi G, Mariani F: Sudden coronary death. A postmortem study in 208 selected cases compared to 97 "control" subjects. Am Heart J 98:20, 1979

40. Pierard LA, De Landsheere CM, Berthe C, et al: Identification of viable myocardium by echocardiography during dobutamine infusion in patients with myocardial infarction after thrombolytic therapy: Comparison with positron emission tomography. J Am Coll Cardiol 15:1021, 1990

41. La Canna G, Alfieri O, Giubbini R, et al: Echocardiography during infusion of dobutamine for identification of reversible dysfunction in patients with chronic coronary artery disease. J Am Coll Cardiol 23:617, 1994

42. Rahimtoola SH: The hibernating myocardium. Am Heart J 117:21, 1989

43. Kloner RA, Allen J, Zheng Y, et al: Myocardial stunning following exercise treadmill testing in man. J Am Coll Cardiol 15:203A, 1990

44. Kloner RA, Przyklenk K, Patel B: Altered myocardial states. The stunned and hibernating myocardium. Am J Med 86(supp 1A):14, 1989

45. Taylor AL, Murphree S, Buja ML, et al: Segmental systolic response to brief ischemia and reperfusion in the hypertrophied canine left ventricle. J Am Coll Cardiol 20:994, 1992

46. Schroder ES, Sirna SJ, Kieso RA, et al: Sensitization of reperfused myocardium to subsequent coronary flow reductions: An extension of the concept of myocardial stunning. Circulation 78:717, 1988

47. Zhao M, Zhang H, Robinson TF, et al: Profound structural alterations of the extracellular collagen matrix in postischemic dysfunctional ("stunned") but viable myocardium. J Am Coll Cardiol 10:1322, 1987

48. Flameng W, Van Belle H, Vanhaecke J, et al: Relation between coronary artery stenosis and myocardial purine metabolism, histology and regional function in humans. J Am Coll Cardiol 9:1235, 1987

49. Vanoverschelde J, Wijns W, Depré C, et al: Mechanisms of chronic regional postischemic dysfunction in humans. New insights from the study of noninfarcted collateral-dependent myocardium. Circulation 87:1513, 1993

50. Borgers M, Thoné F, Wouters L, et al: Structural correlates of regional myocardial dysfunction in patients with critical coronary stenosis: Chronic hibernation? Cardiovasc Pathol 2:237, 1993

50a. Kloner RA, Bolli R, Marban E, et al: Medical and cellular implications of stunning, hibernating and preconditioning. Circulation 97:1848, 1998

50b. Schwartz ER, Schoendube FA, Kostin S, et al: Prolonged myocardial hibernation exacerbates cardiomyocyte degeneration and impairs recovery of function after revascularization. J Am Coll Cardiol 31:118, 1998

50c. Elsasser A, Schlepper M, Klovekorn WP et al: Hibernating myocardium. An incomplete adaptation to ischemia. Circulation 96:2920, 1997

50d. Sambuceti G, Giorgetti A, Corsiglia L, et al: Perfusion-contraction mismatch during inotropic stimulation in hibernating myocardium. J Nucl Med 39:396, 1998

50e. Camici P, Wijn W, Borgers M, et al: Pathophysiologic mechanism of chronic reversible left ventricular dysfunction due to coronary artery disease (hibernating myocardium). Circulation 96:3205, 1997

51. Parodi O, De Maria R, Oltrona L, et al: Myocardial blood flow distribution in patients with ischemic heart disease or dilated cardiomyopathy undergoing heart transplantation. Circulation 88:509, 1993

52. Cabin HS, Clubb KS, Vita N, et al: Regional dysfunction by equilibrium radionuclide angiocardiography: A clinicopathologic study evaluating the relation of degree of dysfunction to the presence and extent of myocardial infarction. J Am Coll Cardiol 4: 743, 1987

53. Majno G, Joris I: Apoptosis, oncosis and necrosis. An overview of cell death. Am J Pathol 146:3, 1995

54. Aretz HT: Myocarditis: The Dallas criteria. Hum Pathol 18:619, 1987

55. Clausell N, Butany J, Gladstone P, et al: Myocardial vacuolization, a marker of ischemic injury, in surveillance of cardiac biopsies post transplant: Correlations with morphologic vascular disease and endothelial dysfunction. Cardiovasc Pathol 5:29, 1996

56. Adegboyega PA, Haque AK, Boor PJ: Extensive myocytolysis as a marker of sudden cardiac death. Cardiovasc Pathol 5:315, 1996

57. Fyfe B, Loth E, Winters GI, et al: Heart transplantation. Associated perioperative ischemic myocardial injury. Morphologic features and clinical significance. Circulation 93:1133, 1996

58. Donald DE: Myocardial performance after excision of the extrinsic nerves in the dog. Circ Res 34:317, 1974

58a. Inoue H, Zipes DP: Results of sympathetic denervation in the canine heart: supersensitivity that may be arrhythmogenic. Circulation 78:877, 1987

58b. Isner JM, Kearney M, Bortman S, Passeri J: Apoptosis in human atherosclerosis and restenosis. Circulation 91:2703, 1995

58c. Chen C, Ma L, Linfert DR, et al: Myocardial cell death and apoptosis in hibernating myocardium. J Am Coll Cardiol 30:1407, 1997

59. Hand DKM, Haudenshild CC, Hong MK, et al: Evidence for apoptosis in human atherogenesis and in rat vascular injury model. Am J Pathol 147:267, 1995

60. Geng YJ, Libby P: Evidence for apoptosis in advanced human atheroma: Colocalization with interleukin-1b-converting enzyme. Am J Pathol 147:251, 1995

61. Gottlieb R, Burleson KO, Kloner RA, et al: Reperfusion injury induces apoptosis in rabbit cardiomyocytes. J Clin Invest 94:1621, 1994

62. Bardales RH, Hailey SL, Su Su X, et al: In situ apoptosis assay for detection of early acute infarction. Am J Pathol 149:821, 1996

63. Katz AM: The cardiomyopathy of overload: An unnatural growth response. Eur Heart J 16(suppl 0):110, 1995

64. Narula J, Heider N, Virmani N, et al: Apoptosis in myocytes in end-stage heart failure. N Engl J Med 335:1182, 1996

65. Mallat Z, Tedgni A, Fontaliran F, et al: Evidence of apoptosis in arrhythmogenic right ventricular dysplasia. N Engl J Med 335: 1190, 1996

66. Cheng W, Li B, Kajstura L, et al: Stretch-induced programmed myocyte cell death. J Clin Invest 96:2247, 1995

66a. Baroldi G, Falzi G, Lampertico P: The nuclear patterns of cardiac muscle fibers. Cardiologica 51:109, 1967

66b. Dispersyn GD, Ausma J, Thone F, et al: Cardiomyocyte remodelling during myocardial hibernation and atrial fibrillation: Prelude to apoptosis. Cardiovasc Res 43:947, 1999

66c. Kanoh M, Takemura G, Misao J, et al: Significance of myocytes with positive DNA in situ nick end-labeling (TUNEL) in hearts with dilated cardiomyopathy: Not apoptosis but DNA repair. Circulation 99:2757, 1999

67. Martin SJ: Apoptosis: Suicide, execution or murder? Trends Cell Biol 3:141, 1993

68. Ohno M, Takemura G, Ohno A, et al: "Apoptotic" myocytes in infarcted area of rabbit hearts may be oncotic myocytes with DNA fragmentation. Circulation 98:1422, 1998

68a. William SR: Apoptosis and heart failure. N Engl J Med 341:759, 1999

69. Buja LM, Entman ML: Modes of myocardial cell injury and cell death in ischemic heart disease. Circulation 98:1355, 1998

70. Fisch C, Armstrong WP, Bigger TJ, et al: Sudden cardiac death. Clinical electrophysiology and electrocardiography: Summary. J Am Coll Cardiol 5(suppl 6):27B, 1985

71. Surawicz B: Ventricular fibrillation. J Am Coll Cardiol 5(suppl 6): 42B, 1985

72. Milstein S, Buetikofer J, Lesser J, et al: Cardiac asystole: A manifestation of neurally mediated hypotension-bradycardia. J Am Coll Cardiol 14:1626, 1989

73. Fozzard HA: Electromechanical dissociation and its possible role in sudden cardiac death. J Am Coll Cardiol 5(suppl 6):31B, 1985

74. Hackel DB, Reimer KA: Sudden Death: Cardiac and Other Causes. Durham, NC, Carolina Academic Press, 1993

75. Cobb LA, Werner JA, Trobaugh GB: Sudden cardiac death. I. A decade's experience with out-of-hospital resuscitation. Mod Concepts Cardiovasc Dis 6:31, 1980

76. Bayés de Luna A, Coumel P, Leclercq JF: Ambulatory sudden cardiac death: Mechanisms of production of fatal arrhythmia on the basis of data from 157 cases. Am Heart J 117:15, 1989

77. Zipes DP: Electrophysiological mechanism involved in ventricular fibrillation. Circulation 51–52(suppl 3):3, 1975

78. Staemmler M: Herzt. In: Kaufmann E (ed): Lehrbuch der speziellen pathologischen Anatomie. Berlin, Georg Riemer, 1911, p 3

79. Vanderwer MA, Humphrey SM, Gavin JB, et al: Changes in the contractile state: Fine structure and metabolism of cardiac muscle cells during the development of rigor mortis. Virchows Arch 35: 159, 1981

80. Lowe JE, Cummings RG, Adams DH, et al: Evidence that ischemic cell death begins in the subendocardium independent of variations in collateral flow or wall tension. Circulation 68:190, 1983

81. Ghidoni JJ, Liotta D, Thomas H: Massive subendocardial damage accompanying prolonged ventricular fibrillation. Am J Path 56:15, 1969

82. Burch GE, De Pasquale NP: Arteriosclerosis in high pressure and low pressure coronary arteries. Am Heart J 63:720, 1962

83. Blake HA, Manion WC, Mattingly TW, et al: Coronary artery anomalies. Circulation 30:927, 1964

84. Wolkoff K: Ueber die Atherosklerose der Coronarterien des Herzens. Beitr Path Anat 82:555, 1929

85. Geiringer E: The mural coronary. Am Heart J 41:359, 1951

86. Benditt EP: Evidence for a monoclonal origin of human atherosclerotic plaques and some implications. Circulation 50:650, 1974

87. Davies MJ, Thomas A: Thrombosis and acute coronary artery lesions in sudden cardiac ischemic death. N Engl J Med 310:1137, 1984

88. Falk E: Unstable angina with fatal outcome: Dynamic coronary thrombosis leading to infarction and/or sudden death. Autopsy evidence of recurrent mural thrombosis with peripheral embolization culminating in total vascular occlusion. Circulation 71:699, 1985

89. Davies MJ: A macro and micro view of coronary vascular insult in ischemic heart disease. Circulation 82(suppl II):32, 1990

90. Libby P: Molecular bases of the acute coronary syndromes. Circulation 91:2844, 1995

91. Baroldi G, Silver MD, Mariani F, et al: Correlation of morphological variables in the coronary atherosclerotic plaque with clinical patterns of ischemic heart disease. Am J Cardiovasc Pathol 2:159, 1988

92. Wight TN, Curwen KD, Litrenta MM, et al: Effect of endothelium on glycosaminoglycan accumulation in injured rabbit aorta. Am J Pathol 113:156, 1983

93. Bemis CE, Gorlin R, Kemp HC, et al: Progression of coronary artery disease: A clinical arteriographic study. Circulation 47:455, 1973

94. Gensini GG, Kelly AE: Incidence and progression of coronary artery disease: An angiographic correlation in 1263 patients. Arch Intern Med 129:814, 1972

95. Laks H, Kaiser GC, Mudd JG, et al: Revascularization of the right coronary artery. Am J Cardiol 43:1109, 1979

96. Rafflenbeul W, Smith LR, Rogers WL, et al: Quantitative coronary arteriography. Coronary anatomy of patients with unstable angina pectoris reexamined 1 year after optimal medical therapy. Am J Cardiol 43:699, 1979

97. Haft JI, Al-Zarka AM: Comparison of the natural history of irregular and smooth coronary lesions: Insights into the pathogenesis, progression and prognosis of coronary atherosclerosis. Am Heart J 126:551, 1993

98. O'Reilly RJ, Spellberg RD: Rapid resolution of coronary arterial emboli. Myocardial infarction and subsequent normal coronary arteriograms. Ann Intern Med 81:348, 1974

99. Wissler RW: Current status of regression studies. In: Paoletti R, Gotto AM Jr (eds): Atherosclerosis Review. Vol 3. New York, Raven, 1978, p 213

100. Jost S, Deckers JW, Nikutta P, et al: Progression of coronary artery disease is dependent on anatomic location and diameter. J Am Coll Cardiol 2:1339, 1993

101. Brown G, Albers JJ, Fisher LD, et al: Regression of coronary artery disease as a result of intensive lipid-lowering therapy in men with high levels of apolipoprotein B. N Engl J Med 323:1289, 1990

102. Baroldi G, Scomazzoni G: Coronary Circulation in the Normal and Pathologic Heart. In: American Registry of Pathology, A.F.I.P. (ed): Washington, DC, U.S. Government Printing Office, 1967

103. Unger EF, Sheffield CD, Epstein SE: Creation of anastomoses between an extracardiac artery and the coronary circulation. Circulation 82:1449, 1990

104. Flynn MS, Kern MJ, Donohue TJ, et al: Alterations of coronary collateral blood flow velocity during intraaortic balloon pumping. Am J Cardiol 71:1451, 1993

105. D'Amore PA, Thompson RW: Mechanisms of angiogenesis. Ann Rev Physiol 49:453, 1987

106. Chilian WM, Mass HJ, Williams SM, et al: Microvascular occlusions promote coronary collateral growth. Am J Physiol 258(Heart Circ Physiol 27): H1103, 1990

107. Helfant RH, Kemp HG, Gorlin R: The interrelation between extent of coronary artery disease, presence of collaterals, ventriculographic abnormalities and hemodynamics. Am J Cardiol 25:102, 1970

108. Mizuno K, Satomura K, Miyamoto A, et al: Angioscopic evaluation of coronary artery thrombi in acute coronary syndrome. N Engl J Med 326:287, 1992

109. Feyter de PJ, Ozaki Y, Baptista J, et al: Ischemia-related lesion characteristics in patients with stable or unstable angina: A study with intracoronary angioscopy and ultrasound. Circulation 92:1408, 1995

110. Coy KM, Park JC, Fishbein MC, et al: In vitro validation of three-dimensional intravascular ultrasound for the evaluation of arterial injury after balloon angioplasty. J Am Coll Cardiol 20:692, 1992

111. Hodgson JM, Reddy KG, Suneja R, et al: Intracoronary ultrasound imaging: Correlation of plaque morphology with angiography, clinical syndrome and procedural results in patients undergoing coronary angioplasty. J Am Coll Cardiol 21:35, 1993

112. Mints GS, Painter JA, Pichard AD, et al: Atherosclerosis in angiographically "normal" coronary artery reference segments: An intravascular ultrasound study with clinical correlation. J Am Coll Cardiol 25:1479, 1995

113. Potkin BN, Bartorelli AL, Gessert BS, et al: Coronary artery imaging with intravascular high-frequency ultrasound. Circulation 81:1575, 1990

114. Roelandt JRTC, Di Mario C, Pandian NG, et al: Three-dimensional reconstruction of intracoronary ultrasound images. Rationale, approaches, problems and directions. Circulation 90:1044, 1994

115. Tobis JM, Mallery J, Mahon D, et al: Intravascular ultrasound assessment of lumen size and wall morphology in normal subjects and patients with coronary artery disease. Circulation 84:1087, 1991

115a. Sangiorgi G, Rumberger JA, Severson A, et al: Arterial calcification and not lumen stenosis is highly correlated with atherosclerotic plaque burden in human: A histologic study of 723 coronary artery segments using nondecalcifying method. J Am Coll Cardiol 31:126, 1998

115b. Detrano RC, Wong ND, Doherty JM, et al: Coronary calcium does not accurately predict near-term future coronary events in high-risk adults. Circulation 99:2633, 1999

115c. Rodbard S: Vascular modification induced by flow. Am Heart J 51:926, 1956

115d. Rodbard S: Physical factors in arterial sclerosis and stenosis. Angiology 22:267, 1971

115e. Glagov S, Weisemberg E, Zarnes CK, et al: Compensatory enlargement of human atherosclerotic coronary arteries. N Engl J Med 316:1371, 1987

116. Fayad ZA, Fallon JT, Shinnar M, et al. Noninvasive in vivo high-resolution magnetic resonance imaging of atherosclerotic lesions in genetically engineered mice. Circulation 98:1541, 1998

117. Eliot RS, Baroldi G, Leone A: Necropsy studies in myocardial infarction with minimal or no coronary luminal reduction due to atherosclerosis. Circulation 49:1127, 1974

118. Haerem JW: Platelet aggregates in intramyocardial vessels of patients dying suddenly and unexpectedly of coronary artery disease. Atherosclerosis 15:199, 1972

119. Davies MJ, Thomas AC, Knapman PA, et al: Intramyocardial platelet aggregation in patients with unstable angina suffering sudden ischemic cardiac death. Circulation 73:418, 1986

120. Oliva PB, Breckinridge JC: Arteriographic evidence of coronary arterial spasm in acute myocardial infarction. Circulation 56:366, 1977

121. Factor SM, Minase T, Cho S, et al: Microvascular spasm in the cardiomyopathic Syrian hamster: A preventable cause of focal myocardial necrosis. Circulation 66:342, 1982

122. Factor SM: Smooth muscle contraction bands in the media of coronary arteries: A postmortem marker of antemortem coronary spasm. J Am Coll Cardiol 6:1326, 1985

123. Hellstrom HR: The injury-spasm (ischemia-induced hemostatic vasoconstrictive) and vascular autoregulatory hypothesis of ischemic disease. Resistance vessel-spasm hypothesis of ischemic disease. Am J Cardiol 49:802, 1982

124. Leary T: Coronary spasm as a possible factor in producing sudden death. Am Heart J 10:338, 1935

125. Dhurandhar RW, Watt DL, Silver MD, et al: Printzmetal's variant form of angina with arteriographic evidence of coronary arterial spasm. Am J Cardiol 30:902, 1972

126. Cheng TO, Bashour T, Shing BK, et al: Myocardial infarction in the absence of coronary arteriosclerosis. Am J Cardiol 30:680, 1972

127. Oliva PB, Hammill SC, Edwards WD: Cardiac rupture, a clinically predictable complication of acute myocardial infarction: Report of 70 cases with clinicopathologic correlations. J Am Coll Cardiol 22:720, 1993

128. Maseri A, L'Abbate A, Baroldi G, et al: Coronary vasospasm as a possible cause of myocardial infarction: A conclusion derived from the study of "preinfarction" angina. N Engl J Med 299:1271, 1978

129. Vincent MG, Anderson JL, Marshall HW: Coronary spasm producing coronary thrombosis and myocardial infarction. N Engl J Med 309:220, 1983

130. Shepherd JT, Vanhoutte PM: Mechanism responsible for coronary vasospasm. J Am Coll Cardiol 8:5A, 1986.

131. Laine P, Keartiness M, Pentilla A, et al: Association between myocardial infarction and the mastcells in the adventitia of the infarct related coronary artery. Circulation 99:361, 1999

132. Ware JA, Heistad DD: Platelet-endothelium interactions. N Engl J Med 328:628, 1993

133. Yamagashi M, Miyatake K, Tamai J, et al: Intravascular ultrasound detection of atherosclerosis at the site of focal vasospasm in angiographically normal or minimally narrowed coronary segments. J Am Coll Cardiol 23:352, 1994

133a. Chevalier P, Dacosta A, Defaye P, et al: Arrhythmic cardiac arrest due to isolated coronary artery spasm: Long term outcome of seven resuscitated patients. J Am Coll Cardiol 31:57, 1998

134. Morales AR, Romanelli R, Boucek RJ: The mural left anterior descending coronary artery, strenuous exercise and sudden death. Circulation 62:230, 1980

135. Noble J, Bourassa MG, Peticlerc R, et al: Myocardial bridging and milking effect of the left anterior descending coronary artery: Normal variant or obstruction? Am J Cardiol 37:993, 1976

136. Faruqui AMA, Maloy WC, Felner JM, et al: Symptomatic myocardial bridging of coronary artery. Am J Cardiol 41:1305, 1978

137. Cowley MJ, Disciascio G, Rehr RB, et al: Angiographic observations and clinical relevance of coronary thrombus in unstable angina pectoris. Am J Cardiol 63:108E, 1989

138. Gotoh K, Minamino T, Katoh O, et al: The role of intracoronary thrombus in unstable angina: Angiographic assessment and thrombolytic therapy during ongoing anginal attacks. Circulation 77:526, 1988

139. Ambrose JA, Winters SL, Arora RR, et al: Coronary angiographic morphology in myocardial infarction: A link between the pathogenesis of unstable angina and myocardial infarction. J Am Coll Cardiol 6:1233, 1985

140. Ambrose JA, Winters SL, Stern A, et al: Angiographic morphology and pathogenesis of unstable angina pectoris. J Am Coll Cardiol 5:609, 1985

141. Levin DC, Fallon JT: Significance of the angiographic morphology of localized coronary stenoses: Histopathologic correlations. Circulation 66:316, 1982

142. Arbustini E, De Servi S, Bramucci E, et al: Comparison of coro-

nary lesions obtained by directional coronary atherectomy in unstable angina, stable angina, and restenosis after either atherectomy or angioplasty. Am J Cardiol 75:675, 1995

143. Rosenschein U, Ellis SG, Handenschild CC, et al: Comparison of histopathologic coronary artery lesions obtained from directional atherectomy in stable angina versus acute coronary syndromes. Am J Cardiol 73:508, 1994

144. Hackett D, Verwilghen J, Davies G, et al: Coronary stenoses before and after acute myocardial infarction. Am J Cardiol 63:1517, 1989

145. Little WC, Constantinescu M, Applegate RJ, et al: Can coronary angiography predict the site of a subsequent myocardial infarction in patients with mild-to-moderate coronary artery disease? Circulation 78:1157, 1988

146. Ambrose JA, Tannenbaum MA, Alexopoulos D, et al: Angiographic progression of coronary artery disease and the development of myocardial infarction. J Am Coll Cardiol 12:56, 1988

147. Mair J, Morandell D, Genser N, et al: Equivalent early sensitivities of myoglobin, creatine kinase MB mass, creatine kinase isoform ratios and cardiac troponins I and T for acute myocardial infarction. Clin Chem 41:1266, 1995

148. Hamm CW, Goldman BU, Heeschen C, et al: Emergency room triage of patients with acute chest pain by means of rapid testing for cardiac troponin T or troponin I. N Engl J Med 337:1648, 1997

149. Hlatky MA: Evaluation of chest pain in the emergency department (editorial). N Engl J Med 337:1687, 1997

149a. Newby LK, Christenson RH, Ohman EM, et al: Value of serial troponin T measures for early and late risk stratification in patients with acute coronary syndromes. Circulation 98:1853, 1998

149b. Roberts R, Fromm RE: Management of acute coronary syndromes based on risk stratification by biochemical markers: An idea whose time has come (editorial). Circulation 98:1831, 1998

150. DeWood MA, Spores J, Notske R, et al: Prevalence of total coronary occlusion during the early hours of transmural myocardial infarction. N Engl J Med 303:897, 1980

151. DeWood MA, Stifter WF, Simpson CS, et al: Coronary arteriographic findings soon after non–Q-wave myocardial infarction. N Engl J Med 315:417, 1986

152. Hammer A: Ein Fall von trombotischen Verschlusse einer der Kranzarterien des Herzens. Wiener Medizinische Wochenschrift 5:83, 1878

153. Herrick JB: Clinical features of sudden obstruction of the coronary arteries. JAMA 59:87, 1912

154. Herrick JB: Thrombosis of the coronary arteries. JAMA 72:93, 1919

155. Baroldi G: Acute coronary occlusion as a cause of myocardial infarct and sudden coronary heart death. Am J Cardiol 16:859, 1965

156. Chandler AB, Chapman I, Erhardt LR, et al: Coronary thrombosis in myocardial infarction. Report of a workshop on the role of coronary thrombosis in the pathogenesis of acute myocardial infarction. Am J Cardiol 34:823, 1974

157. Freifeld AG, Schuster EH, Bulkley BH: Nontransmural versus transmural myocardial infarction. A morphological study. Am J Med 75:423, 1983

158. Nachlas MM, Shnitka TK: Macroscopic identification of early myocardial infarcts by alterations in dehydrogenase activity. Am J Pathol 42:379, 1963

159. Feldman S, Glagov S, Wissler RW, Hughes RH: Postmortem delineation of infarcted myocardium. Coronary perfusion with nitro-blue tetrazolium. Arch Pathol Lab Med 100:55, 1976

160. Kent SP: Diffusion of myoglobin in the diagnosis of early myocardial ischemia. Lab Invest 46:270, 1982

161. Brinkman B, Sepulchre MA, Fechner G: The application of selected histochemical and immunohistochemical markers and procedures to the diagnosis of early myocardial damage. Int J Leg Med 106:135, 1993

162. Thomsen H, Held H: Immunohistochemical detection of C5b-9 in myocardium: An aid in distinguishing infarction-induced ischemic heart muscle necrosis from other forms of lethal myocardium injury. Forensic Sci Int 71:87, 1995

163. Leadbeatter S, Nawman HM, Jasani B: Further evaluation of immunocytochemical staining in the diagnosis of early ischaemic/hypoxic damage. Forensic Sci Int 45:135, 1990

164. Zhang JM, Riddlck L: Cytosckeleton immunohistochemical study of early ischemic myocardium. Forensic Sci Int 80:229, 1996

165. Bouchardy B, Majno G: A new approach to the histologic diagnosis of early myocardial infarcts. Cardiology 56:327, 1971–72

166. Lie JT, Holley KE, Kampa WR, Titus JL: New histochemical method for morphologic diagnosis of early stages of myocardial ischemia. Mayo Clin Proc 46:316, 1971

167. Erhardt L: Biochemical markers in acute myocardial infarction: The beginning of a new era. Eur Heart J 17:1781, 1996

168. Buja ML, Poliner LR, Parkey RW, et al: Clinicopathologic study of persistently positive technetium-99 stannous pyrophosphate myocardial scintigrams and myocytolytic degeneration after myocardial infarction. Circulation 56:1016, 1977

169. Hirschl MM, Gwechenberger M, Binder T, et al: Assessment of myocardial injury by serum tumour necrosis factor alpha measurements in acute myocardial infarction. Eur Heart J 17:1852, 1996

170. Antman EM, Tanasijevic MJ, Thompson B, et al: Cardiac-specific troponin I levels to predict the risk of mortality in patients with acute coronary syndromes. N Engl J Med 335:1342, 1996

171. Ohman ME, Armstrong PW, Christenson RH, et al: Cardiac troponin T levels for risk stratification in acute myocardial ischemia. N Engl J Med 335:1333, 1966

172. Mallory GK, White PD, Salcedo-Salgar G: The speed of healing of myocardial infarct. A study of the pathologic anatomy in 72 cases. Am Heart J 18:647, 1939

173. Lodge-Patch I: The aging of cardiac infarcts and its influence on cardiac rupture. Br Heart J 13:37, 1951

174. Blumgart HL, Schlesinger MJ, Davis D: Studies on the relation of the clinical manifestations of angina pectoris, coronary thrombosis and myocardial infarction to the pathologic findings with particular reference to the significance of the collateral circulation. Am Heart J 19:1, 1940

175. Wade WB: The pathogenesis of infarction of the right ventricle. Br Heart J 21:545, 1959

176. Hurst JW, King SB, Friesinger GB, et al: Atherosclerotic coronary heart disease: Recognition, prognosis and treatment. In: Hurst WS, Logue RB, Rackley CE, et al (eds): The Heart. 6th ed. New York, McGraw-Hill, 1986, p 981

177. McCain FH, Kline EM, Gilson JS: A clinical study of 281 autopsy reports on patients with myocardial infarction. Am Heart J 39:263, 1950

178. Wartman WB, Souders JC: Localization of myocardial infarcts with respect to the muscle bundles of the heart. Arch Pathol 50:329, 1950

179. Antman EM, Braunwald E: Acute myocardial infarction in heart disease. In: Braunwald E (ed): Heart Disease, 5th ed. Philadelphia, WB Saunders, 1997, pp 1195–1196

180. Cleutjens JPM, Verluyten MJA, Smits JFM, Daemen MJAP. Collagen remodeling after myocardial infarction in the rat heart. Am J Pathol 147:325, 1995

181. Kahn AH: Pericarditis of myocardial infarction. Review of the literature with case presentation. Am Heart J 90:788, 1975

182. Toole JC, Silverman ME: Pericarditis of acute myocardial infarction. Chest 67:647, 1975

183. Kennedy HL, Das SK: Postmyocardial infarction (Dressler's) syndrome: Report of a case with immunologic and viral studies. Am Heart J 91:233, 1976

184. Becker AE, Mantgem JP: Cardiac tamponade: A study of 50 hearts. Eur J Cardiol 3:349, 1975

185. Silver MD, Butany J, Chiasson DA: The pathology of myocardial infarction and its mechanical complications. In: David TE (ed): Mechanical complications of myocardial infarction. RG Landes, 1993, p 4

186. Vlodaver Z, Edwards JE: Rupture of ventricular septum or papillary muscle complicating myocardial infarction. Circulation 55:815, 1977

187. Scomazzoni G, Baroldi G, Mantero O: Studio anatomo-clinico su di un singolare caso di aneurisma dissecante del miocardio. Ospedale Maggiore 45:1, 1957

188. Jetter WW, White PD: Rupture of the heart in patients in mental institutions. Ann Intern Med 21:783, 1944

189. Bevilacqua M, Norbiato G, Vago T, et al: Alterations in norepinephrine content and beta adrenoceptor regulation in myocardium bordering aneurysm in human heart: Their possible role in the genesis of ventricular tachycardia. Eur J Clin Invest 16:163, 1986

190. Barber MJ, Mueller TM, Henry DP, et al: Transmural myocardial infarction in the dog produces sympathectomy in noninfarcted myocardium. Circulation 67:787, 1983

190a. Dae MW, Herre JM, O'Connel WJ, et al: Scintigraphic assessment of sympathetic innervation after transmural versus nontransmural myocardial infarction. J Am Coll Cardiol 17:1416, 1991

190b. Kramer CM, Nicol PD, Rogers WJ, et al: Reduced sympathetic innervation underlies adjacent noninfarcted region dysfunction during left ventricular remodeling. J Am Coll Cardiol 30:1079, 1997

191. Calkins H, Allman K, Bolling S, et al: Correlation between scintigraphic evidence of regional sympathetic neuronal dysfunction and ventricular refractoriness in human heart. Circulation 89:172, 1993

192. Mitrani RD, Klein SL, Miles WH, et al: Regional sympathetic denervation in patients with ventricular tachycardia in absence of coronary artery disease. J Am Coll Cardiol 22:1344, 1993

193. Ciuffo AA, Ouyang P, Becker LC, et al: Reduction of sympathetic inotropic response after ischemia in dog. Contributor to stunned myocardium. J Clin Invest 75:1504, 1985

193a. Sakata K, Shirotani M, Yoshida H, Kurata C: Iodine-123 metaiodobenzylguanidine cardiac imaging to identify and localize vasospastic angina without significant coronary artery narrowing. Am J Coll Cardiol 30:370, 1997

193b. Sakata K, Miura F, Sugino H, et al: Assessment of regional sympathetic nerve activity in vasospastic angina: Analysis of iodine-123-labeled metaiodobenzylguanidine scintigraphy. Am Heart J 133:484, 1997

193c. Takano H, Nakamura T, Satou T et al: Regional myocardial sympathetic dysinnervation in patients with coronary vasospasm. Am J Cardiol 75:324, 1997

193d. Wichert T, Hindriks G, Lerch H, et al: Regional myocardial sympathetic dysinnervation in arrhythmogenic right ventricular cardiomyopathy. Circulation 89:667, 1994

193e. Emdin M, Marin Neto A, Carpeggiani C, et al: Heart rate variability and cardiac denervation in Chagas' disease. J Ambul Monit 5:251, 1992

193f. Baroldi G, Oliveira SJM, Silver MD: Sudden and unexpected death in clinically "silent" Chagas disease. A hypothesis. Int J Cardiol 58:263, 1997

193g. Nakata T, Miyamoto K, Doi A, et al: Cardiac death prediction and impaired cardiac sympathetic innervation assessed by MIBG in patients with failing and nonfailing hearts. J Nucl Cardiol 5: 579, 1998

193h. De Marco T, Dae M, Yuen-Green MSF, et al: Iodine-123 metaiodobenzylguanidine scintigraphic assessment of the transplanted human heart: evidence for late innervation. J Am Coll Cardiol 25: 927, 1995

193i. Wilson RF, Laxson DD, Christensen BV, McGinn AL, et al: Regional differences in sympathetic reinnervation after human orthotopic cardiac transplantation. Circulation 88:165, 1993

193j. Bengel FM, Neberfuhr P, Ziegler SI, et al: Serial assessment of sympathetic reinnervation after orthotopic heart transplantation. A longitudinal study using PET and C-11 hydroxyephedrine. Circulation 99:1866, 1999

194. Dantzig JM, Delemarre BJ, Bot H, Visser A: Left ventricular thrombus in acute myocardial infarction. Eur Heart J 17:1640, 1996

195. Keren A, Goldberg S, Gottlieb S, et al: Natural history of left ventricular thrombi: their appearance and resolution in the hospitalization period of acute myocardial infarction. J Am Coll Cardiol 15:790, 1990

196. Ekelund LG, Morberg A, Olsson AG, Oro L: Recent myocardial infarction and the conduction system: A clinicopathological correlation. Br Heart J 34:744, 1972

197. Jones ME, Terry G, Kenmure ACF: Frequency and significance of conduction defects in acute myocardial infarction. Am Heart J 94: 163, 1977

198. Page DL, Caulfield JB, Kastor JA, et al: Myocardial changes associated with cardiogenic shock. N Engl J Med 285:133, 1971

198a. Roberts WC, Jones AA: Quantitation of coronary arterial narrowing at necropsy in sudden coronary death. Am J Cardiol 44:39, 1979

198b. Farb A, Tang AL, Burke AP, et al: Sudden coronary death. Frequency of active coronary lesions, inactive coronary lesions and myocardial infarction. Circulation 92:1701, 1995

198c. Burke AP, Farb A, Malcolm GT, et al: Coronary risk factors and plaque morphology in men with coronary disease who died suddenly. N Engl J Med 336:1276, 1997

198d. Burke AP, Farb A, Malcolm GT, et al: Plaque rupture and sudden death related to exertion in men with coronary artery disease. JAMA 281:921, 1999

199. Cobb LA, Baum RS, Schaffer WA: Resuscitation from out-of-

hospital ventricular fibrillation: 4 years' follow-up. Circulation 51–52(suppl 3):223, 1975

200. Goldstein S, Landis JR, Leighton R, et al: Characteristics of the resuscitated out-of-hospital cardiac arrest victim with coronary heart disease. Circulation 64:977, 1981

201. Bayés de Luna A, J Guindo: Sudden death in ischemic heart disease. Rev Port Cardiol 9:473, 1990

202. Spain DM, Bradess VA, Iral P, et al: Intercoronary anastomotic channels and sudden unexpected death from advanced coronary atherosclerosis. Circulation 27:12, 1963

203. Linzbach AJ: Heart failure from the point of view of quantitative anatomy. Am J Cardiol 5:370, 1960

204. Jorgensen L, Haerem JW, Chandler BA, et al: The pathology of acute coronary death. Acta Anesth Scand 29:193, 1968

205. El-Maraghi N, Genton E: The relevance of platelet and fibrin thromboembolism of the coronary microcirculation, with special reference to sudden cardiac death. Circulation 62:936, 1980

206. Burke AP, Subramanian R, Smialek J, et al: Nonatherosclerotic narrowing of the atrioventricular node artery and sudden death. J Am Coll Cardiol 21:117, 1993

207. James TN: Degenerative lesions of a coronary chemoreceptor and nearby neural elements in the heart of victims of sudden death. J Am Coll Cardiol 8:12A, 1986

208. Shvalev VN, Virkhert AM, Stropus RA, et al: Changes in neural and humoral mechanisms of the heart in sudden death due to myocardial abnormalities. J Am Coll Cardiol 8:55A, 1986

209. Gibbons LW, Copper KH, Meyer BM, et al: The acute cardiac risk of strenuous exercise. JAMA 244:1799, 1980

210. Noakes TD, LH Opie, Rose AG: Autopsy-proved coronary atherosclerosis in marathon runners. N Engl J Med 301:86, 1979

211. Cohn PF: Silent myocardial ischemia and infarction. 2nd ed. New York, Marcel Dekker, 1989

212. Faerman I, Faccio E, Mile J, et al: Autonomic neuropathy and painless myocardial infarction in diabetic patients. Diabetes 26: 1147, 1977

213. Jacoby RM, Nesto RW: Acute myocardial infarction in the diabetic patient: Pathophysiology, clinical course and prognosis. J Am Coll Cardiol 20:736, 1992

214. Kannel WB, McGhee DL: Diabetes and cardiovascular risk factors: The Framingham study. Circulation 59:8, 1979

215. Beltrami CA, Finato N, Rocco M, et al: Structural basis of end-stage failure in ischemic cardiomyopathy in humans. Circulation 89:151, 1994

216. De Maria R, Parodi O, Baroldi G, et al: Morphological bases for thallium-201 uptake in cardiac imaging and correlates with myocardial blood flow distribution. Eur Heart J 17:951, 1996

217. Gerdes MA, Kellerman SE, Moore AJ, et al: Structural remodeling of cardiac myocytes in patients with ischemic cardiomyopathy. Circulation 86:426, 1992

218. Chareconthaitawee P, Christian TF, Hirose K, et al: Relation of initial infarct size to extent of left ventricular remodeling in the year after acute myocardial infarction. J Am Coll Cardiol 25:567, 1995

219. Baroldi G, Silver MD, De Maria R, et al: Lipomatous metaplasia in left ventricular scar. Can J Cardiol 13:65, 1997

220. Vlodaver Z, Neufeld HN: The coronary arteries in coarctation of the aorta. Circulation 37:449, 1968

221. Cooley DA, Bloodwell RD, Hallman GL, et al: Human cardiac transplantation. Circulation (suppl I):1, 1969

222. Thomson JG: Production of severe atheroma in a transplanted human heart. Lancet 2:1088, 1969

223. Billingham ME: The postsurgical heart. The pathology of cardiac transplantation. Am J Cardiovasc Path 1:319, 1988

224. Kosek JC, Chartrand C, Hurley EJ, et al: Arteries in canine cardiac homografts. Ultrastructure during acute rejection. Lab Invest 21:328, 1969

225. Johnson DW, Flemma RJ, Lepley D: Direct reconstruction of flow to small distal coronary arteries. Am J Cardiol 25:105, 1970

226. Kern WH, Dermer GB, Lindesmith GG: The intimal proliferation in aortic-coronary saphenous vein grafts. Light and electron microscopic studies. Am Heart J 84:771, 1972

227. Gouley BA, Bellet S, McMillan TM: Tuberculosis of the myocardium. Report of six cases with observations on involvement of the coronary arteries. Arch Intern Med 51:244, 1933

228. Holsinger DR, Ormundson PJ, Edwards JE: The heart in periarteritis nodosa. Circulation 25:610, 1962

229. Harrison CV: Giant-cell or temporal arteritis: A review. Am J Clin Pathol 1:197, 1948

230. Gross L, Kugel MA, Epstein EZ: Lesions of the coronary arteries and their branches in rheumatic fever. Am J Pathol 11:253, 1935

231. Bonfiglio TA, Botti RE, Hagstrom JWC: Coronary arteritis, occlusion and myocardial infarction due to lupus erythematosus. Am Heart J 83: 153, 1972

232. Spiro D, Lattes RG, Wiener J: The cellular pathology of experimental hypertension. I. Hyperplastic arteriosclerosis. Am J Pathol 47:19, 1965

233. Wolinsky H: Effects of estrogen and progestogen treatment on the response of the aorta of male rats to hypertension. Morphological studies. Circ Res 30:341, 1972

234. Rodbard S: Vascular modifications induced by flow. Am Heart J 51:926, 1956

235. Hassler O: The origin of the cell constituting arterial intima thickening. An experimental autoradiographic study with the use of H^3-thymidine. Lab Invest 2:286, 1970

236. Bulkley BH, Hutchins GM: Accelerated "atherosclerosis": A morphologic study of 97 saphenous vein coronary artery bypass grafts. Circulation 55:163, 1977

237. Vlodaver Z, Neufeld HN, Edwards JE: Pathology of angina pectoris. Circulation 46:1048, 1972

238. Cheitlin MD, McAllister HA, De Castro CM: Myocardial infarction without atherosclerosis. JAMA 231:951, 1975

239. Cheitlin MD, De Castro CM, McAllister HA: Sudden death as a complication of anomalous left coronary origin from the anterior sinus of Valsalva: A not-so-minor congenital anomaly. Circulation 50:780, 1974

240. Neufeld NH, Lester RG, Adams P, et al: Congenital communications of a coronary artery with a cardiac chamber or the pulmonary trunk (coronary artery fistula). Circulation 24:171, 1961

241. McClellan JT, Jokle E: Congenital anomalies of coronary arteries as cause of sudden death associated with physical exertion. Am J Clin Pathol 50:229, 1968

242. Daoud AS, Pankin D, Tulgan H, et al: Aneurysm of the coronary artery. Report of ten cases and review of the literature. Am J Cardiol 11:228, 1963

243. Claudon DG, Claudon DB, Edwards JE: Primary dissecting aneurysm of coronary artery. A cause of acute myocardial ischemia. Circulation 45:259, 1972

244. Silver MD: Medial hemorrhage and dissection in a coronary artery: An unusual cause of coronary occlusion. CMAJ 32:99, 1968

245. Wenger NK, Bauer S: Coronary embolism. Review of the literature and presentation of fifteen cases. Am J Med 25:549, 1958

245a. Chan S, Silver MD: Fatal myocardial embolus after myectomy. Can J Cardiol 16:207, 2000

246. Vlay SC, Blumenthal DS, Shoback D, et al: Delayed acute myocardial infarction after blunt chest trauma in a young women. Am Heart J 100:907, 1980

247. Virmani R, Forman MB, Rabinowitz M, McAllister HA: Coronary artery dissections. Cardiol Clin 2:633, 1984

248. Dorros G, Cowley MI, Janke L, et al: In-hospital mortality rate in the National Heart, Lung and Blood Institutes percutaneous transluminal coronary angioplasty registry. Am J Cardiol 53:7C, 1984

249. Silver MD, Wigle ED, Trimble AS et al: Iatrogenic coronary ostial stenosis. Arch Pathol 88:73, 1969

250. Applefeld MM, Wiernik PH: Cardiac disease after radiation therapy for Hodgkin's disease: Analysis of 48 patients. Am J Cardiol 51:1679, 1983

251. Oliver MF: Oral contraceptives and myocardial infarction. Br Med J 2:210, 1970

252. Gorlin R, Fuster V, Ambrose JA: Anatomic-physiologic links between acute coronary syndromes. Circulation 74:6, 1986

253. Gregg DE: Coronary Circulation in Health and Disease. Philadelphia, Lea & Febiger, 1950

254. Gregg DE: The natural history of collateral development. Circ Res 35:335, 1974

255. Gregg DE, Patterson RE: Functional importance of the coronary collaterals. New Engl J Med 303:1404, 1980

256. Khouri EM, Gregg DE, Lowesohn HS: Flow in the major branches of the left coronary artery during experimental coronary insufficiency in the unanesthetized dog. Circ Res 23:99, 1968

257. Bean WB: Bullet wound of the heart with coronary artery ligation. Am Heart J 21:375, 1944

258. Bradbury S: Thirty years after ligation of the anterior descending branch of the left coronary artery. Am Heart J 24:562, 1942

259. Carleton RA, Boyd T: Traumatic laceration of the anterior coronary artery treated by ligation without myocardial infarction: Report of a case with a review of the literature. Am Heart J 56:136, 1958

260. Pagenstecher: Weiterer Beitrag zur Herzchirurgie. Die Unterbindung der verletzen Arteria Coronaria. Dtsch Med Wochenschr 4: 56, 1901

261. Parmley WW: Factors causing arrhythmias in chronic congestive heart failure. Am Heart J 114:1267, 1987

262. Zerbini EJ: Coronary ligation in wounds of the heart. Report of a case in which ligation of the anterior descending branch of the left coronary artery was followed by complete recovery. J Thorac Surg 12:642, 1943

263. Cribier A, Korsatz L, Koning R, et al: Improved myocardial ischemic response and enhanced collateral circulation with long repetitive coronary occlusion during angioplasty: A prospective study. J Am Coll Cardiol 20:578, 1992

264. Deutsch E, Berger M, Kussmaul WG, et al: Adaptation to ischemia during percutaneous transluminal coronary angioplasty: Clinical, hemodynamic and metabolic features. Circulation 82:2044, 1990

264a. Sakata Y, Kodama K, Kitanaza M, et al: Different mechanism of ischemic adaptation to repeated coronary occlusions in patients with and without recruitable collateral circulation. J Am Coll Cardiol 30:1679, 1997

264b. Billinger M, Fleish M, Eberli FR, et al: Is the development of myocardial tolerance to repeated ischemia in humans due to preconditioning or to collateral recruitment? J Am Coll Cardiol 33: 1027, 1999

264c. Barilli F, De Vincentis G, Maugieri E, et al: Recovery of contractility of viable myocardium during inotropic stimulation is not dependent on an increase of myocardial blood flow in the absence of collateral filling. J Am Coll Cardiol 33:697, 1999

265. Yamamoto H, Tomoike H, Shimokawa H, et al: Development of collateral function with repetitive coronary occlusion in a canine model reduces myocardial reactive hyperemia in the absence of significant coronary stenosis. Circ Res 55:623, 1984

266. Khouri EM, Gregg DE, McGranahan GM: Regression and reappearance of coronary collaterals. Am J Physiol 220:655, 1971

267. Ross R: The arterial wall and atherosclerosis. Ann Rev Med 30:1, 1979

268. Velican C, Velican D: Natural history of coronary atherosclerosis. Boca Raton, FL, CRC, 1989

269. Wissler RW: The arterial medial cell: Smooth muscle of multifunctional mesenchyme? Circulation 36:1, 1967

270. Dietz WA, Tobis JM, Isner JM: Failure of angiography to accurately depict the extent of coronary artery narrowing in three fatal cases of percutaneous transluminal coronary angioplasty. J Am Coll Cardiol 19:1261, 1992

271. van der Wal AC, Becker AE, Koch KT, et al: Clinically stable angina pectoris is not necessarily associated with histologically stable atherosclerotic plaques. Heart 76:312, 1996

272. Boyd W: A Textbook of Pathology: Structure and Function in Disease. 7th ed. Philadelphia, Lea & Febiger, p 196

273. Irniger W: Histologische Alterbestimmung von Thrombosen und Embolien. Virchows Arch 336:220, 1963

274. Weisse AB, Lehan PH, Ettinger PO, et al: The fate of experimentally induced coronary thrombosis. Am J Cardiol 23:229, 1969

275. Morgan AD: The Pathogenesis of Coronary Occlusion. Oxford, UK, Blackwell Scientific, 1956

276. Baroldi G, Marzilli M, L'Abbate A, et al: Coronary occlusion: Cause or consequence of acute myocardial infarction? A case report. Clin Cardiol 13:49, 1990

277. Hackett D, Davies G, Chierchia S, Maseri A: Intermittent coronary occlusion in acute myocardial infarction: Value of combined thrombolytic and vasodilator therapy. N Engl J Med 317:1055, 1987

277a. Fishbein MC, Siegel RJ: How big are coronary atherosclerotic plaques that rupture? Circulation 94:2662, 1996

278. Nesto R, Kowalchuk G: The ischemic cascade: Temporal sequence

of hemodynamic, electrocardiographic and symptomatic expression of ischemia. Am J Cardiol 59:23C, 1987

279. Taki J, Yasuda T, Gold HK, et al: Characteristic of transient left ventricular dysfunction detected by ambulatory left ventricular function monitoring device in patients with coronary artery disease (abstract). Circulation 76(suppl 4):366, 1987

280. Fung AY, Rabkin SW: Beneficial effects of streptokinase on left ventricular function after myocardial reoxygenation and reperfusion following global ischemia in the isolated rabbit heart. J Cardiovasc Pharmacol 6:429, 1984

281. Bertrand ME, LaBlanche JM, Tilmant P, et al: Frequency of provoked coronary arterial spasm in 1089 consecutive patients undergoing coronary arteriography. Circulation 65:1299, 1982

282. Leachman RD, Cokkinos DV, Zamalloa O, Del Rio C: Intercoronary artery steal. Cardiovasc Res Cent Bull 10:71, 1972

283. Moberg A: Anastomoses between extracardiac vessels and coronary arteries. Acta Med Scand 485(suppl):1, 1968

284. Baroldi G, Falzi G. Mariani F, et al: Morphology, frequency and significance of intramural arterial lesions in sudden coronary death. G Ital Cardiol 10:644, 1980

285. Baroldi G, Manion WC: Microcirculatory disturbances and human myocardial infarction. Am Heart J 74:171, 1967

286. Baroldi G: High resistance of the human myocardium to shock and red blood cell aggregation (sludge). Cardiologia 54:271, 1969

287. Val-Mejias J, Lee WK, Weisse AB, et al: Left ventricular performance during and after sickle cell crisis. Am Heart J 97:585, 1974

288. Reagan TJ, Wu CF, Weisse AB, et al: Acute myocardial infarction in toxic cadiomyopathy without coronary obstruction. Circulation 51:453, 1975

289. Sommers HM, Jennings RB: Ventricular fibrillation and myocardial necrosis after transient ischemia. Effect of treatment with oxygen, procainamide, reserpine and propranolol. Arch Int Med 129:780, 1972

290. Majno G, Ames A, Chaing J, et al: No-reflow after cerebral ischemia. Lancet 2:569, 1967

291. Kloner RA, Ganote CE, Jennings RB: The "no-reflow" phenomenon after temporary coronary occlusion in the dog. J Clin Invest 54:1496, 1974

292. Ross R: The pathogenesis of atherosclerosis: A perspective for the 1990s. Nature 362:801, 1993

293. Kochi K, Takebayashi S, Hikori T, et al: Significance of adventitial inflammation of the coronary artery in patients with unstable angina: Results at autopsy. Circulation 71:709, 1985

294. Schwartz CJ, Mitchell JRA: Cellular infiltration of the human arterial adventitia associated with atheromatous plaque. Circulation 26:73, 1962

295. Parums D, Mitchinson MJ: Demonstration of immunoglobulin in the neighbourhood of advanced atherosclerotic plaques. Atherosclerosis 38:211, 1981

296. van der Wal AC, Das PK, van der Berg DB, et al: Atherosclerotic lesions in humans. In situ immunophenotypic analysis suggesting an immune-mediated response. Lab Invest 61:166, 1989

296a. Morrow DA, Rifai N, Antman EM, et al: C-reactive protein is a potent predictor of mortality independently of and in combination with troponin T in acute coronary syndromes. A TIMI 11A substudy. J Am Coll Cardiol 31:1460, 1998

296b. Liuzzo G, Buffon A, Biasucci LM, et al: Enhanced inflammatory response to coronary angioplasty in patients with severe unstable angina. Circulation 98:2370, 1998

296c. Vakeva AP, Azah A, Rollins SA, et al: Myocardial infarction and apoptosis after myocardial ischemia and reperfusion. Role of the terminal complements and inhibition by anti-C5 therapy. Circulation 97:2259, 1998

297. Factor SM, Bache RJ: Pathophysiology of myocardial ischemia. In: Hurst JW (ed): The Heart. New York, McGraw-Hill, 1994, p 1119

298. Hood WB: Experimental myocardial infarction. III. Recovery of left ventricular function in the healing phase. Contribution of increased fiber shortening in noninfarcted myocardium. Am Heart J 79:531, 1970

299. Goldstein RE, Borer JS, Epstein SE: Augmentation of contractility

following ischemia in the isolated supported heart. Am J Cardiol 29:265, 1972

300. Malliani A, Schwartz PJ, Zanchetti A: A sympathetic reflex elicited by experimental coronary occlusion. Am J Physiol 217:703, 1979

301. Jones CE, Devous MD, Thomas JX, et al: The effect of chronic cardiac denervation on infarct size following acute coronary occlusion. Am Heart J 95:738, 1978

302. Nasser FN, Walls JT, Edwards WD, et al: Lidocaine-induced reduction in size of experimental myocardial infarction. Am J Cardiol 46:967, 1980

303. Meerson FZ, Kagan VE, Kozlov YP, et al: The role of lipid peroxidation in pathogenesis of ischemic damage and the antioxidant protection of the heart. Basic Res Cardiol 77:465, 1982

304. Przyklenk K, Kloner RA: Superoxide dismutase plus catalase improve contractile function in the canine model of the stunned myocardium. Circ Res 58:148, 1986

305. Przyklenk K, Bauer B, Ovize M, et al: Regional ischemic "preconditioning" protects remote virgin myocardium from subsequent sustained coronary occlusion. Circulation 87:893, 1993

305a. Kini A, Marmur JD, Kini S, et al: Creatine kinase-MB elevation after coronary intervention correlates with diffuse atherosclerosis and low-to-medium level elevation has a benign clinical course. J Am Coll Cardiol 34:663, 1999

305b. Calif RM, Abdelmeguid AE, Kuntz RE, et al: Myonecrosis after revascularization procedures. J Am Coll Cardiol 31:241, 1998

305c. Airaksinen KEJ, Tahvanain KUD, Ecberg DE, et al: Arterial baroreflex impairment in patients during acute coronary occlusion. J Am Coll Cardiol 32:1641, 1998

306. Pool-Wilson PA: Relation of pathophysiologic mechanisms to outcome in heart failure. J Am Coll Cardiol 22(supp A):A22, 1993

306a. Sambuceti G, Marzilli M, Maraccini P, et al: Coronary vasoconstriction during myocardial ischemia induced by rises in metabolic demand in patients with coronary artery disease. Circulation 95:2652, 1997

306b. Gibson MC, Ryan KA, Murphy SA, et al: Impaired coronary blood flow in nonculprit arteries in the setting of acute myocardial infarction. J Am Coll Cardiol 34:974, 1999

306c. Mark DB, Naylor DC, Heatki MA, et al: Use of medical resource and quality of life after acute myocardial infarction in Canada and United States. N Engl J Med 331:1130, 1994

306d. Dauchin N, Vaur L, Genes N, et al. Treatment of acute myocardial infarction by primary coronary angioplasty or intravenous thrombolysis in the "real world." One-year results from a nationwide French survey. Circulation 99:2639, 1999

306e. Leicht JW, McElduff P, Dolson A, Heller R: Outcome with calcium channel antagonist after myocardial infarction: A community-based study. J Am Coll Cardiol 31:11, 1998

306f. Narkiewiez K, De Borne van PJH, Hausberg M, et al: Cigarette smoking increases sympathetic outflow in humans. Circulation 98:528, 1998

306g. Rozanski A, Blumenthal JA, Kaplan J: Impact of psychological factors on the pathogenesis of cardiovascular diseases and implication for therapy. Circulation 99:2196, 1999

307. Ganote C, Armstrong S: Ischemia and the myocyte cytoskeleton: Review and speculations. Cardiovasc Res 27:1387, 1993

308. Hein S, Sheffold T, Schaper J: Ischemia induces early changes to cytoskeletal and contractile proteins in diseases human myocardium. J Thorac Cardiovasc Surg 110:89, 1995

309. Hein S, Schaper J: The cytoskeleton of cardiomyocytes is altered in the failing human heart. Heart Failure 12:128, 1996

309a. Laner MS, Blackstone EH, Young JB, Topol EJ: Cause of death in clinical research. Time for a reassessment? J Am Coll Cardiol 34:618, 1999

310. Kannel WB, Thom TJ: Incidence, prevalence and mortality of cardiovascular disease. In: Hurst JW (ed): The Heart. New York, McGraw-Hill, 1994, p 200

311. Colucci WS: Apoptosis in the heart. N Engl J Med 335:1224, 1996

312. Lanza GA, Pedrotti P, Pasceri V, et al: Autonomic changes associated with spontaneous coronary spasm in patients with variant angina. J Am Coll Cardiol 28:1249, 1996

313. Kaski JC, Rosano GMC, Collins P, et al: Cardiac syndrome X: Clinical characteristic and left ventricular function. J Am Coll Cardiol 25:807, 1995

Chapter 9

Myocarditis

· · · · ·

Gayle L. Winters • Bruce M. McManus

Myocarditis is nonischemic myocardial inflammation of known or unknown causes. It most often results from infectious agents, hypersensitivity responses, or immune-related injury. Viruses are the most common infectious causes of myocarditis acquired in the community. The major causes of myocarditis are listed in Table 9-1.[1–5]

Although myocarditis is clearly less common than other forms of heart disease, such as coronary artery atherosclerosis, hypertension, and valvular heart disease, the true incidence is difficult to ascertain. Clinical presentations, which range from subclinical to fulminant cardiac failure, are frequently nonspecific, and, as such, myocarditis does not have reliable clinical diagnostic criteria. The incidence of myocarditis in autopsy series varies from less than 1 to 10%,[6–9] and the frequency with which myocarditis is diagnosed on endomyocardial biopsy has been reported in various studies as 0 to 63%.[10–13] These data, however, are not based on standardized diagnostic criteria and include a heterogeneous group of patients. In numerous studies, investigators incorporate patients with idiopathic dilated cardiomyopathy, a condition that may be a long-term sequela of myocarditis. A more realistic estimate of incidence is a rate of 1 to 5%[14, 15] at autopsy, depending on the extent of histologic sectioning, and 4 to 10%[16–18] in biopsy specimens from patients presenting with acute heart failure and ventricular dilation.

Historically, myocarditis has been the source of much clinical and pathologic confusion and controversy. Although the term *myocarditis* dates to the 1800s, it was not until 1941 that Saphir was able to separate histologic myocarditis from ischemic heart disease.[19] From that time until the introduction of the endomyocardial bioptome in 1962,[20] myocarditis was a presumptive (and frequently incorrect) clinical diagnosis, often in young patients manifesting heart failure preceded by a febrile illness, or, alternatively, the diagnosis of myocarditis was first made at autopsy. The endomyocardial biopsy (EMB) allowed tissue to be obtained from living patients for histologic diagnosis. The confusion was further enhanced by lack of agreement among clinicians regarding indications for EMB as well as treatment of biopsy findings[21] and among pathologists as to what constitutes the histologic criteria for myocarditis.[22] It has become increasingly apparent that histologic descriptors alone may not be sufficient to characterize this disease fully, and consideration must be given to serologic, molecular, immunologic, and immunogenetic factors.

The clinical outcome of patients with myocarditis is extremely variable and somewhat dependent on the extent of myocardial involvement. Subclinical cases of focal myocarditis appear as an incidental finding at autopsy in patients who clearly died of unrelated causes. More extensive myocardial involvement may result in fulminant cardiac failure, leading to death or cardiac transplantation. Myocarditis accounts for a small percentage of sudden cardiac deaths: 5% of cases, excluding those with severe coronary atherosclerotic heart disease.[23] If a patient survives the acute phase of myocarditis, inflammatory lesions may either resolve or heal by progressive fibrosis. A certain number of these cases may progress to idiopathic dilated cardiomyopathy (see later and Chapter 10).

CLASSIFICATION

Myocarditis has been classified on the basis of etiology, chronology, and histology. Etiologic classification includes *primary myocarditis,* an idiopathic process, and *secondary myocarditis,* which has an identifiable apparent cause. However, because the inflammatory responses are often nonspecific, attempting to assign an etiology on the basis of histologic findings is often futile. In addition, although most cases of myocarditis in the West are believed to be caused by viruses, it has been difficult to prove viral etiology. Thus, many cases that may have this cause are called *idiopathic myocarditis.*

Chronologic classification schemes attempt to correlate clinical course with pathologic features and divide myocarditis into *acute* and *chronic,*[24–27] with some classifications also using *fulminant,*[27] *recurrent,*[25] or *rapidly progressive,*[26] and some subdividing *chronic* into *active* and *persistent.*[27] In these systems, there is no reference to etiology or pathogenesis. Proponents of these temporal-based systems state their advantage as that of being able to provide suggestions about the probable course of the disease and the likelihood of response to immunosuppressive therapy. However, it is difficult to know the natural history of the disease and the specific point in its evolution at which tissue was obtained for examination. A source of great confusion stems from use of the term *chronic myocarditis* interchangeably with idiopathic dilated cardiomyopathy. There is reasonable clinical and experimental evidence that myocarditis may lead to dilated cardiomyopathy and that the two entities may very well represent two stages of the same disease (see later); however, dilated cardiomyopathy represents the end stage of a number of insults to the myocardium, which include but are not limited to inflammation. The use of the term chronic myocarditis, therefore, is discouraged.

In 1995, the World Health Organization/International Society and Federation of Cardiology Task Force on the Definition and Classification of Cardiomyopathies included *inflammatory cardiomyopathy* (defined as myocarditis in association with cardiac dysfunction) as a subtype

TABLE 9-1 • **Major Causes of Myocarditis**

Infections	Immune Reactions	Cardiotoxic Drugs	Unknown
Viruses	**Drug hypersensitivity**	Cocaine	Sarcoidosis
Coxsackieviruses A and B	Antibiotics	Catecholamines	Kawasaki disease
Echoviruses	Diuretics		
Influenza viruses	Antihypertensive agents		
Adenoviruses			
Herpesviruses (CMV, EBV)	**Poststreptococcal (rheumatic fever)**		
HIV			
	Systemic lupus erythematosus		
Bacteria			
Diphtheria	**Giant cell myocarditis**		
Tuberculosis			
Borrelia (Lyme disease)	**Transplant rejection**		
Fungi			
Candida			
Aspergillus			
Protozoa			
Trypanosoma (Chagas disease)			
Toxoplasma			
Helminths			
Trichinella			
Taenia (cysticercosis)			
Echinococcus (hydatid disease)			
Schistosoma			

CMV, cytomegalovirus; EBV, Epstein-Barr virus; HIV, human immunodeficiency virus.

of specific cardiomyopathies,[28] heart muscle diseases that are associated with specific cardiac or systemic disorders. The Dallas criteria for diagnosis and classification of myocarditis on EMB specimens are discussed in detail below.

The approach to myocarditis taken in this chapter is from the standpoint of a pathologist faced with a particular histologic picture. The focus is on the more common forms of the disease and on problems encountered in daily practice. Cardiac transplant rejection, which may be considered a form of myocarditis, is discussed in Chapter 23.

ENDOMYOCARDIAL BIOPSY DIAGNOSIS OF MYOCARDITIS

The development of the EMB technique allowed direct examination of myocardial tissue during life as well as the opportunity to obtain insights into the etiology, pathogenesis, and natural history of myocarditis.[29] Right ventricular EMB is most often employed, and, because most

TABLE 9-2 • **Common Challenges in the Diagnosis of Myocarditis on Endomyocardial Biopsy**

1. Timing of biopsy in relation to acute symptoms
2. Sampling error
3. Bias from clinical diagnosis
4. Variation in diagnostic criteria among pathologists
5. Presence of inflammatory cells in normal myocardium; how much is normal?
6. Inflammatory infiltrates in cardiomyopathy
7. Lack of specificity of myocardial infiltrates (e.g., confusion with ischemic injury, catecholamine effect)
8. Drug-induced toxicity/hypersensitivity

diseases under consideration are widespread in heart muscle, it is assumed that the right side of the ventricular septum contains representative pathology.[30, 31] It should be noted, however, that sampling error can occur in disease processes that are potentially focal, such as myocarditis.[32, 33] The role of the biopsy is to (1) establish a morphologic diagnosis of myocarditis, (2) exclude other causes of myocardial disease that have similar clinical manifestations, and (3) monitor the effect of therapy. Historically, difficulties in diagnostic interpretation of EMB findings[22, 34, 35] (Table 9-2) resulted in widely divergent reports of the incidence of myocarditis and the inability to compare natural history, clinical outcome, or effectiveness of therapy for patients diagnosed at different centers.

The Dallas Criteria

Definition

In order to develop uniform, reproducible morphologic criteria for the diagnosis of myocarditis based on EMB specimens in support of a multicenter international myocarditis treatment trial, a group of eight cardiac pathologists met in 1984. They devised what have become known as the Dallas criteria.[36-38] The Dallas criteria define idiopathic myocarditis as *"an inflammatory infiltrate of the myocardium with necrosis and/or degeneration of adjacent myocytes not typical of the ischemic damage associated with coronary artery disease."*

Histopathology

The intensity and distribution of the inflammatory infiltrate are highly variable, ranging from a solitary small focus to multifocal aggregates to diffuse myocardial involvement. The inflammatory infiltrate is usually apparent

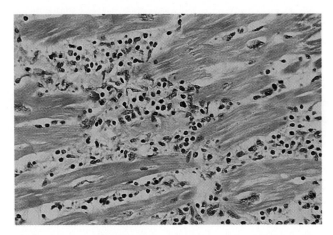

Figure 9-1 • Lymphocytic myocarditis that fulfills the Dallas criteria. There is an interstitial lymphocytic infiltrate with associated myocyte damage (H&E stain).

TABLE 9-3 • Inflammatory Infiltrates and the Differential Diagnosis of Myocarditis

Lymphocytes	Neutrophils
Idiopathic	Idiopathic (early)
Viral infections (including AIDS)	Viral infections (early)
Immune response	Pressor effect
Collagen vascular disease	Ischemic injury/infarction
Drug toxicity	Bacterial infections
Sarcoidosis	Drug toxicity
Kawasaki disease	
Lyme disease	
Lymphoma (atypical)	

Eosinophils	Giant Cells
Hypersensitivity	Idiopathic
Parasitic infestation	Sarcoidosis
Hypereosinophilic syndromes/restrictive cardiomyopathy	Granulomatous infections
Idiopathic	Hypersensitivity
Asthmatic bronchitis	Rheumatoid diseases
Mycoplasma pneumoniae	Rheumatic fever

AIDS, acquired immunodeficiency syndrome.

at low power in biopsy specimens with diagnostic features of myocarditis. A high-power search for an occasional lymphocyte is generally not necessary and may lead to a false-positive diagnosis. Many interstitial cells may be difficult to characterize on routine hematoxylin eosin (H&E)–stained sections, and normal myocardial components such as mast cells, fibroblast nuclei cut in cross section, pericytes, histiocytes, and endothelial cells may resemble lymphocytes.[13] In addition, a small number of inflammatory cells, including lymphocytes, may be found in normal myocardium. On examination of 20 high-power (×400) microscope fields on H&E sections of normal myocardium, Edwards and colleagues found the mean number of interstitial lymphocytes to be <5/high-power field.[39] Linder[40] and Schnitt[41] and their associates, using immunoperoxidase stain for leukocyte common antigen, found an average of 13 immunoreactive cells/mm² in "uninflamed" biopsy specimens. Tazelaar and Billingham found foci of inflammatory cells (>5 inflammatory cells/focus) in 9.3% of 86 cardiac transplant donor hearts.[42] Interstitial fibrosis is a common but nonspecific finding in hypertrophied, nonischemic hearts. It may be perivascular or patchy, replacing individual or clusters of myocytes. Lymphocytes within fibrous tissue are not considered diagnostic of active myocarditis.

The difficulty that then arises is differentiation of low-grade lymphocytic myocarditis from "normal" myocardium. Strict adherence to the Dallas criteria, which require the presence of myocyte damage (Fig. 9-1) in addition to the inflammatory infiltrate, appears to have eliminated the need to quantify lymphocytes. It should be noted that giant cells, granulomas, or clusters of eosinophils in the heart are abnormal and may be sufficient to warrant a diagnosis of myocarditis. The composition of the cellular infiltrate helps to distinguish the etiology of the myocarditis,[13, 37, 38] and some of the more common differential diagnoses suggested by the predominant cellular components are summarized in Table 9-3.

Myocyte damage may be characterized by necrosis or degenerative changes such as myocyte dropout, myocyte vacuolization, irregular myocyte contours, or cellular dis-

ruption with lymphocytes closely applied to the sarcolemma. The myocardium away from the inflammatory infiltrate frequently shows few pathologic changes and may appear entirely normal. Interstitial edema and myocyte necrosis with contraction bands are not reliable diagnostic criteria, as biopsy artifacts may simulate both processes.[43, 44]

Classification

Two separate classifications are used for the first biopsy and subsequent biopsies (Table 9-4), because healing or healed myocarditis cannot be reliably diagnosed on first EMB and such terms should be used only in instances when unequivocal myocarditis has been diagnosed previously. The use of terms with a temporal inference (i.e., acute, subacute, chronic) should be avoided.

Borderline myocarditis (Fig. 9-2) implies that the degree of inflammation is too sparse or that myocyte damage is not demonstrated. An unequivocal diagnosis of myocarditis cannot be rendered. In such cases, additional

TABLE 9-4 • Endomyocardial Biopsy Diagnosis of Myocarditis: The Dallas Criteria

Classification

First biopsy
Myocarditis with or without fibrosis
Borderline myocarditis (second biopsy may be indicated)
No myocarditis

Subsequent biopsies
Ongoing (persistent) myocarditis with or without fibrosis
Resolving (healing) myocarditis with or without fibrosis
Resolved (healed) myocarditis with or without fibrosis

Descriptors

	Inflammatory Infiltrate	Fibrosis
Distribution	Focal, confluent, diffuse	Endocardial, interstitial
Extent	Mild, moderate, severe	Mild, moderate, severe
Type	Lymphocytic, eosinophilic, granulomatous, giant cell, neutrophilic, mixed	Perivascular, replacement

tissue levels should be obtained from the paraffin block. If clinical suspicion is strong, the clinician may elect to repeat the biopsy.

Ongoing (persistent) myocarditis indicates that the inflammatory infiltrate is as extensive as in the previous biopsy, and *resolving (healing) myocarditis* implies that the inflammation is less extensive. *Resolved (healed) myocarditis* indicates that the inflammatory infiltrate is no longer present. Lymphocytes may be associated with an area of fibrosis or scarring after total resolution of active myocarditis and do not necessarily imply ongoing myocarditis (Fig. 9-3). Myocarditis may recur after complete histologic resolution. The biopsy in which recurrence is diagnosed should be considered a "first" biopsy and serve as the reference point for subsequent biopsies.

Technical Considerations

Because myocarditis may be focal, sampling error is the single most common cause of false-negative diagnoses. The most important factor in sampling is the number of pieces obtained by EMB. It is recommended that a minimum of three but preferably at least five individual tissue pieces be examined when myocarditis is strongly suspected.[36] Because the goal is to sample different areas of the myocardium, myocardial samples should not be divided once obtained by the bioptome in order to provide the required number of pieces. When a small-jawed bioptome or femoral approach is used, obtaining more tissue samples increases sensitivity. In two studies that compared the sensitivity of myocardial biopsy samples with multiple sections of myocardium from hearts with known myocarditis obtained at autopsy, the likelihood of a false-negative diagnosis on EMB was nearly 40%, even when as many as 10 biopsy samples were obtained.[32, 33] Therefore, only positive biopsy findings are considered diagnostic; a negative biopsy finding does not exclude the diagnosis of myocarditis. Some clinicians, however, consider exclusionary information obtained on biopsy material to be valuable in patient management.

It is essential that sufficient EMB samples be obtained and examined by light microscopy. Special studies, in-

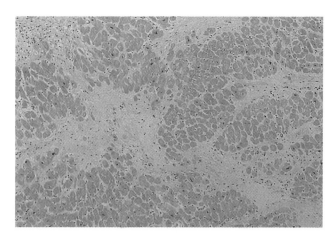

Figure 9-3 • Healed myocarditis. An irregular pattern of myocardial fibrosis in an explanted heart from a patient with previously biopsy-proven myocarditis. Other areas of this heart contained active and healing myocarditis (H&E stain).

cluding immunohistochemistry for viral antigens, electron microscopy, in situ hybridization (ISH), and gene amplification, may provide additional information even in cases with negative histology (see below). If such studies are desired, sections from the pieces so used should also be examined by light microscopy, or additional pieces should be obtained at biopsy to meet the minimum number of pieces required.

After fixation and processing, ribbons of tissue from at least three different levels should be cut from the paraffin block. Serial sectioning may enhance the yield of a positive diagnosis, particularly in cases of focal myocarditis.[45] Additional unstained slides for special stains are cut at this time to avoid wasting tissue in the paraffin block. In addition to H&E stain, a connective tissue stain (i.e., Masson trichrome) is helpful for assessing the amount and distribution of interstitial fibrosis and aids in the detection of myocyte damage.

Because one of the most common causes of false-positive diagnoses is that of the pathologist being swayed by strong clinical bias, it is often recommended that the biopsy specimen be assessed initially without knowledge of clinical history. However, a final diagnosis should not be rendered without knowing clinical details that may help elucidate the cause of inflammatory changes detected histologically. Clinical information of potential pertinence to the biopsy includes age, sex, duration of illness, status of coronary arteries (determined by angiography), history of myocardial infarction, viral illness or recent pregnancy, ejection fraction, arrhythmias, assessment of ventricular size and function, drug history (i.e., alcohol, pressors, controlled substances, hypersensitivity-related or known cardiotoxic drugs, immunosuppressive and chemotherapeutic agents), and other systemic illnesses (i.e., infectious, autoimmune).[12, 36]

LYMPHOCYTIC MYOCARDITIS

Lymphocytic myocarditis is the most common form of the disease. Most cases of such histologic subtype are

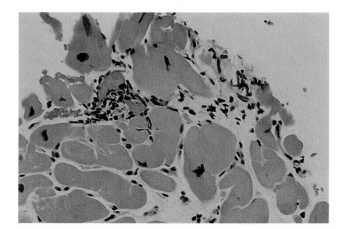

Figure 9-2 • Borderline myocarditis. An interstitial lymphocytic infiltrate is present without associated myocyte degeneration or necrosis (H&E stain).

documented or presumed to be of viral origin. The most frequently implicated agents are coxsackievirus groups A and B and other enteroviruses (polioviruses, echoviruses), adenoviruses, and influenza viruses. Less common etiologic agents, which are especially important in immunosuppressed individuals, include herpesviruses, such as cytomegalovirus (CMV), and human immunodeficiency virus (HIV-1) (see later).

Gross Pathology

During the active phase of myocarditis, the gross appearance of the heart may be quite variable, as involvement of the myocardium may be focal, patchy, or diffuse. The heart may appear entirely normal, particularly when the extent of disease is limited. With more extensive disease, the heart often appears enlarged, with dilation of either ventricle or all cardiac chambers. The myocardium is often mottled, with pale foci and hyperemic-hemorrhagic areas (Fig. 9-4). Mural thrombi may be present, particularly in dilated hearts. An associated fibrinous pericarditis results in a dull, shaggy appearance of the epicardial-pericardial surface. Healed myocarditis may reflect few residual changes arising from the active episode. However, focal or geographic scarring may be present, a feature indistinguishable from that seen in idiopathic dilated cardiomyopathy (see later). The pattern of fibrosis is usually distinct from that of healed myocardial infarction, which occurs in the distribution of a specific coronary artery and which reflects the watershed zones of perfusion. However, differentiation of healed myocarditis from foci of ischemic replacement fibrosis may not always be possible.

Histopathology

Myocarditis is most frequently characterized by an interstitial mononuclear inflammatory infiltrate, predominantly lymphocytic, with damage to adjacent myocytes. The interstitium containing the inflammatory cells is often widened and edematous. The inflammatory infiltrates may be focal, multifocal, or diffuse (Fig. 9-5A–C). Myocyte damage, which may take the form of myocytolysis (vacuolization), irregular myocyte contours, or frank necrosis-apoptosis, also varies in extent and is only roughly proportional to the amount of inflammation. Rarely, the histologic picture mirrors that of an acute myocardial infarction or a myocardial abscess. Myocyte damage is generally not seen away from areas of inflammation. Myocyte hypertrophy and fibrosis may reflect underlying disease or healing and compensatory processes. However, the diagnosis of myocarditis should be made with extreme caution in the setting of minimal inflammation and extensive chronic myocardial changes that may explain the patient's cardiac failure.

Detection of Viral Etiology

The diagnostic approach to myocarditis at the beginning of the 21st century rests on an evolving set of

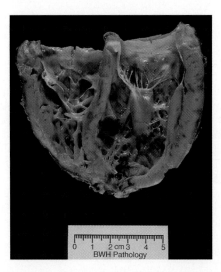

Figure 9-4 • Explanted heart with lymphocytic myocarditis diagnosed on endomyocardial biopsy 2 weeks previously. There is biventricular dilation. The myocardium appears mottled and focally hemorrhagic. A left ventricular assist device had been inserted into the left ventricular apex.

concepts. Clinical findings in patients with myocarditis have long been known to be fickle and misleading. Serologic diagnoses of viral myocarditis are also notoriously difficult, primarily because of the polyclonal immune response to viruses in the same antigenic group. Similarly, the histopathologic diagnosis, although based on standardized criteria (i.e., Dallas criteria), is not without deficiencies or difficulties in application. As noted previously, sensitivity of detection of classic histopathologic features of myocarditis in endomyocardial biopsy specimens is also limited. Fortunately, new tools are now available, and a multifaceted approach to establishing the nature of, and potential treatment for, myocarditis can include immunohistochemical and molecular observations. The latter strategies are based largely on evidence and suspicion that cardiotropic viruses are a common cause of community-acquired myocarditis and associated systemic infectious syndromes.[46–49] Thus, the identification of a causative agent or the unearthing of a pathogenetic process for myocarditis in humans has become a challenging, broad-based, exercise reliant on molecular acumen as well as traditional structural and virologic information.

Studies in the 1950s and early 1960s convinced pathologists and clinicians of the major role enteroviruses have in frequently fatal cases of neonatal and infantile myocarditis.[50, 51] In that early era, the detection of viruses was achieved on the basis of classic agar overlay plaque assays,[52] revealing the presence of live virus in various bodily materials, including stool and nasopharyngeal secretions, during life and in portions of solid organs such as heart, liver, pancreas, brain, and spleen at autopsy.

Through the 1960s, efforts to secure a microbiologic diagnosis were advanced by application of immunofluorescent techniques.[53] The immunofluorescence tools were considered unreliable by many observers, partly because of the lack of high-quality antibody reagents. Similarly, it was recognized that the ultrastructural features of the

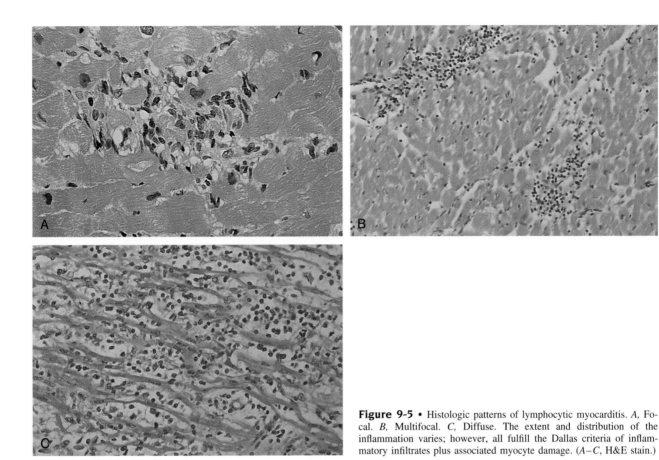

Figure 9-5 • Histologic patterns of lymphocytic myocarditis. *A,* Focal. *B,* Multifocal. *C,* Diffuse. The extent and distribution of the inflammation varies; however, all fulfill the Dallas criteria of inflammatory infiltrates plus associated myocyte damage. (*A–C,* H&E stain.)

most commonly suspected pathogens, coxsackieviruses, included a diameter (~28 μm) and electron density consistent with ribosomes.[54, 55] Despite extensive pathogenetic work on murine models of myocarditis over more than three decades, it was not until 1986 that Bowles and others[56] initiated a new era of understanding regarding viral heart disease in humans, especially for patients in whom clinical myocarditis or inflammatory cardiomyopathy had no apparent etiologic basis. Their molecular application for diagnostic purposes represented a conceptual breakthrough that would be followed rapidly by other efforts to identify and localize viral genomes in presumably infected hearts. Enteroviral genome was the most vigorously sought of all viruses because of the serologic impression garnered by the World Health Organization in its 1975–85 surveillance data.[57, 58] Such data indicated that the most common serogroup associated with clinical cardiovascular disease or dysfunction was coxsackievirus group B (30 to 35 cardiovascular disorders per 1000 serologic infections). Conventional wisdom evolved that coxsackievirus B3 was the most common viral cause of human heart muscle disease, and this serotype remains the leading virus of interest.

Importantly, enteroviral genome detected in tissue or cells may not only reflect a current, active, or recent infection, but can also serve as a "flag" for remote, prior, or ongoing (persistent) infections. Accumulated worldwide data on enteroviral genome in heart muscle have

verified that regardless of whether an idiopathic cardiomyopathy is acute or chronic, inflammatory or noninflammatory, and regardless of the exact molecular tools used to detect the genome—dot blots, slot blots, ISH, or various forms of gene amplification (i.e., polymerase chain reaction [PCR])—a significant frequency of myocardial positivity for enteroviral genome should be expected.[59-67] The range of molecular positivity extends from 0% in certain series[68] to >50% in selected patient populations.[69, 70] In general, adult patients with histopathologic myocarditis have a 25 to 35% chance of having enteroviral genome in their myocardium. This compares with a frequency of about 5% in control patients without acute cardiomyopathy. It also compares with an even lower likelihood of isolating virus from the same hearts by classic virologic techniques.

In Situ Hybridization

Since the pioneering work of Kandolf and colleagues,[71] ISH has become recognized as an excellent tool in the assessment of enteroviruses or other viruses as potential causes of myocarditis or cardiomyopathy.[48, 65] ISH has several virtues diagnostically. First, it is very sensitive, and, in an optimized reference version of the technique, as few as 50 copies of positive-strand viral genome can be detected in paraffin-embedded tissue sections (unpublished observations, Dr. R. Kandolf). Second, and perhaps most importantly, ISH allows localization of the genome in particular cells. Because of the latter attribute, ISH and in situ gene amplification[72] have clearly demonstrated that infection of heart muscle involves endothelium, whether on vessel walls or on cardiac cavitary surfaces. The patterns of viral genome distribution in infected hearts have been established in experimental models,[73] and ISH for the viral genome allows one to observe the co-localization of cell injury and death, elements of the immune response, and other histopathologic features.[74] Thus, ISH has helped validate the histopathologic evidence that most myocyte cell death in myocarditis occurs in concert with direct viral infection of these cells,[75, 76] preceding the tissue-based immune cell invasion. In addition, through the use of serial tissue sections, it is readily possible to show not only whether a particular myocyte is infected, but also whether it is apoptotic (by DNA nick end-labeling techniques) or necrotic (by altered tinctorial properties on trichrome stains or with immunohistochemical staining for myofilament proteins like actin). Third, ISH can be used effectively to demonstrate the presence of an actively replicating enterovirus. This is possible because enteroviruses replicate through a negative-strand intermediate, and, by using both sense- and antisense probes, both negative- and positive-strand viral RNA, respectively, can be detected on serial sections of the same cells.[77] Not all viral species have an intermediate strand of reverse polarity; thus, the use of ISH to demonstrate active replication is most pertinent to cardiotropic agents like coxsackieviruses and echoviruses. The unequivocal presence of positive-strand genome in the absence of negative-strand genome suggests quiescent or persistent enteroviral infection, with downregulated viral transcription.

ISH as a diagnostic tool for viral infections of the heart depends on the quality of the tissue, the probes, and the actual version of the technique applied. Although RNases and DNases may eliminate the RNA and DNA of particular viruses during a postmortem period, efforts to schedule an early autopsy, rapid triage of explanted hearts at transplantation, and timely handling of EMB fragments from the catheterization suite are helpful. Disagreement exists regarding whether it is best to freeze or fix tissue rapidly for molecular virologic purposes. To preserve RNA and DNA, it is best to fix tissue as soon as possible, but pieces of tissue should also be flash frozen in order to obtain the best chance of successful gene amplification.

Sensitivity of ISH is known to be highly related to the length of probe used. The molecular cloning and characterization of the single, positive-strand genomic RNA of a cardiotropic coxsackievirus B3 allowed the generation of probes several hundred bases long, covering the length of the genome. These probes are not only sensitive, but also allow detection of a broad range of cardiotropic enteroviral genomes in tissue sections. In other words, given the genomic similarity of enteroviruses, the full-length probes may pick up in a single assay any number of coxsackieviruses or echoviruses potentially resident in infected heart muscle cells. In consideration of the apparent similarity of clinical course and the lack of a virus-specific therapy for the cardiotropic viruses, such reliable "broad-spectrum"

detection of genome is sufficient for clinical management. The complementary use of enterovirus group–specific and capsid protein–specific antisera[78, 79] allows the detection of enteroviral proteins in serial tissue sections by immunohistochemistry. Both monoclonal and polyclonal antibodies are available for such purposes. Although double labeling by ISH for genome and by immunohistochemistry for capsid proteins has long been possible,[80, 81] it is perhaps more revealing and convenient if serial sections cut 3 μm thick are used.

Molecular Probes

The use of cDNA probes labeled with ^{35}S to detect enteroviral genomes in tissue sections of human hearts has been replaced in many laboratories by nonradioactive, biotinylated riboprobes, both having similar sensitivity and the latter being less expensive and safer. Also, if the RNase step is omitted from the latter protocol, many additional signals may be detected emanating from the "loose" ends of biotinylated probes hybridized to target viral genome. Biotinylated enterovirus-specific complementary DNA probes have also been used to visualize colloidal gold–conjugated antibodies at the ultrastructural level.[82] Such an approach is normally reserved for investigative studies, as the standard ISH approach on paraffin sections should detect a clinically relevant infectious agent.

Polymerase Chain Reaction

The use of gene amplification strategies based on polymerase chain reaction (PCR) is another way of assessing biopsy tissue, explants, and hearts obtained at autopsy for the presence of enteroviruses or other potential pathogens causing heart muscle damage and failure.[60, 62] Although many efforts have been made to use PCR diagnostically in this setting, the results are variable and conflicting. A number of technical considerations may be pertinent to discuss in this context. Central to any diagnostic technique, and perhaps most critical with PCR, is optimization of each step and reaction in the procedure. Expression of sensitivity for detecting viral genomes in clinical samples is largely lacking. Variable approaches have been published, including the number of infected cells per ten thousand or per million, number of plaque-forming units (without any knowledge of the number of genomes present), or absence of evaluation at all. None have actually provided sensitivity for detection of a given number of genomes in tissue sections. We made an attempt to acquire this kind of data, and the optimized protocol is presented in Figure 9-6. This protocol attends to annealing temperature, magnesium concentration, and number of amplification cycles. The latter two considerations affect both the reverse transcriptase step and the PCR step. Through this approach, we improved our sensitivity of detection of enteroviral positive-strand genome to between 1.5 and 15 viral genomic copies in a background of 5 ng of nonspecific RNA. This sensitivity must be tempered by the impact of "real-life" conditions of RNA evaluation in heart tissue in the clinical setting. Additional strategies, such as a PCR mimic or the introduction

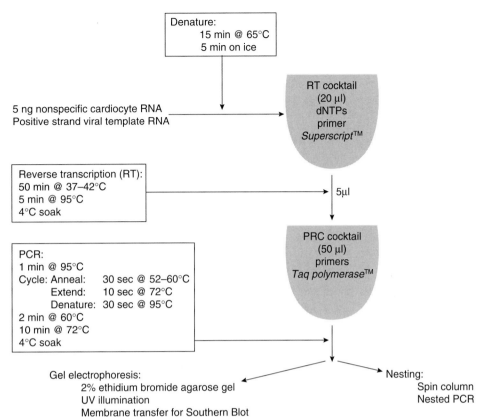

Figure 9-6 • Protocol for reverse transcriptase–polymerase chain reaction for RNA of positive-strand viruses such as coxsackieviruses.

of a restriction site in a known quantity of standard "competitor," have also been used by us and reported by others.[83]

Immunophenotyping

Despite uncertainty regarding etiologic agents in idiopathic myocarditis, the immunohistochemical phenotype of infiltrating immune cells[84, 85] suggests a stereotypic immunologic response. Thus, the predominance of T cells and macrophages in the infiltrates, regardless of the diversity of infiltrative patterns or the amount of tissue necrosis, in fatal and nonfatal human case material (unpublished data) implies a uniform host response to viral infection. Efforts to identify predominant T-cell subsets in the infiltrate—for example, CD4+ or CD8+ T cells or other cells such as natural killer (NK) cells—have not been particularly helpful, even though experiments in immunodeficient models clearly show that these cells are important in the host response to viral infection of target organs such as the heart.[86] An admixture of cells is present and can be grown out of infected tissue under the influence of cytokines such as interleukin-2 (IL-2).[87, 88] Liu and colleagues[88a] have illustrated the complexity of immune phenomena within the heart in viral myocarditis.

Many observations on the phenotype of cells circulating in the peripheral blood of myocarditis patients have been made.[89, 90] These suggested a reduction in NK cell cytotoxicity of peripheral blood mononuclear cells in myocarditis patients.[18, 91] A stronger immune response, including elevated NK cell counts, appears to correlate with less severe myocardial disease,[18] but the clinicopathologic value of this information is uncertain. Higher peripheral blood CD2+ T-cell counts have been associated with a greater risk of death.[18]

Histocompatibility

In related immunogenetic observations, there is discrepancy and controversy as to the relative importance of major histocompatibility types underlying patient susceptibility to idiopathic dilated cardiomyopathy or myocarditis. Although an excess of DR4 antigens had been suggested for patients with idiopathic dilated cardiomyopathy by previous serologic studies,[92] more recent work at the molecular level does not support this viewpoint.[93] Indeed, the molecular histocompatibility data implicate DR12 and DQB1*0503, DQB1*0301 and/or *0304 in idiopathic dilated cardiomyopathy susceptibility and DQ5 and DQB1*0501 in myocarditis susceptibility.[93] Upregulated expression of class I and II major histocompatibility antigens on myocardial cells in myocarditis has been suggested as a useful albeit nonspecific marker of the inflammatory process.[94–96]

Autoimmunity

Autoimmunity induced by an episode of viral myocarditis has been invoked as pathogenetic for heart muscle injury or failure.[18, 97–99] A long list of candidate autoantibodies is available, including those that are cardiac specific, ranging from antibodies against major structural

TABLE 9-5 • **Basic Diagnostic Approach to Patients with Possible Myocarditis**

Signs/symptoms
 Flulike illness, shortness of breath, +/− chest pain, +/− palpitations, other syndromes

Laboratory tests
 Endomyocardial biopsy, fecal virus isolation, WBC count, chest film, electrocardiogram, echocardiogram, serum enzymes (creatine phosphokinase/troponin I), viral serology

Evaluation of endomyocardial biopsy tissue
 Histopathologic
  Negative for myocarditis
  Positive for myocarditis
   Immunohistochemistry for leukocyte subsets
 Molecular
  In situ hybridization
  In situ PCR
  Immunohistochemistry for viral capsid proteins

WBC, white blood cell; PCR, polymerase chain reaction.

proteins to those involved in cellular metabolism. A specific relationship between these antibodies and cardiac injury or dysfunction in humans has not been shown. Immunofluorescence studies of immunoglobulin and complement deposits in such hearts[100] has not led to routinely useful diagnostic information.

Diagnostic Approach

The availability of ISH and other techniques to detect viral genomes, along with immunohistochemistry to detect viral capsid proteins, has changed the overall approach to the pathologic diagnosis of myocarditis (Table 9-5). Employing histopathologic, ISH, and immunohistochemical information, PCR results, viral culture, and yet other approaches may be necessary in certain cases. A comparative approach to the molecular or classic virologic detection of such pathogens as coxsackieviruses may depend on the relative virtues of given tools and the clinical question being asked (Table 9-6). Indeed, a composite of tests and assays may be necessary. A certain constellation of laboratory findings may suggest a differ-

ent therapeutic approach for one group of patients versus another. EMB results may be histopathologically negative but molecularly positive for virus. On the other hand, biopsy results may be strikingly abnormal histopathologically but negative for viruses sought by molecular means. Just what probes, primers, and antibodies to use remains a matter of arbitrary choice, economics, and technical expertise at many centers. Many inflamed heart biopsy specimens no doubt have an as yet undetected pathogen present. The detection of myocardial enzymes released from injured myocardium into the blood may provide adjunctive information,[101] but they are neither specific for viral injury nor predictive of outcome. If the heart muscle is actively infected, antiviral or immune-enhancing therapies may be considered.[67, 102, 103] If the myocardium is without viral genome or has evidence only of persistent infection, a supportive or perhaps immunosuppressive approach may be warranted.[104, 105] Currently, the best diagnostic approach to any type of viral heart muscle disease remains obscure. At the very least, molecular tools combined with other data offer the chance of a firm diagnosis, something not possible in the past. Still at issue is the standardization of an inclusive histopathologic-virologic-molecular phenotypic approach for use in certain reference laboratories.

Despite strong evidence of enteroviral infection of the heart muscle, as well as other organs, in humans and in murine models, we are still not certain of the viral etiology of many clinical cases of pediatric and adult myocarditis. Enteroviruses are not the whole story in "idiopathic" myocarditis. In fact, apart from neonatal cases and those acquired in the nursery,[106] it is likely now that although enteroviruses account for the most cardiac infections of all virus genuses, they may still cause a minority of all idiopathic myocarditis seen. Similarly, although molecular epidemiologic data suggest that coxsackieviruses are the commonest enteroviruses to infect the heart,[70, 107–109] other data suggest that adenoviruses, herpes simplex virus, and CMV also play a significant role in the pathogenesis of human cardiomyopathy.[110] There is a need to study a large series of failed hearts with more than one molecular tool, searching for more than one set of viruses, in order to resolve current questions and confusion about the etiology of viral heart disease in humans.

TABLE 9-6 • **Comparative Value of Different Methods in Detection of Enterovirus in Fluids, Cells, and Tissues**

	RT PCR	Nested PCR	ISH	Plaque Assay
Sensitivity	++	++++	+++	+
Specificity	+++	++++	++++	+++
Reproducibility	+++	++	+++	+++
Economy (financial)	+++	++	++	++
Economy (time)	++++	+++	+++	++
Quantitation	+	+	+++	+++
Localization	+	+	++++	++
Suggested "ideal" application and value	Detection of acute viral infection	Detection of persistent viral genome	Localization of viral genome and replication in tissues and cells	Determination of virulence

RT, reverse transcription; PCR, polymerase chain reaction; ISH, in situ hybridization.

Pathobiology

Mechanisms of Myocyte Damage

When viruses cause myocarditis, the process of injury evolves through quite well-defined stages.[74, 75] Most of our knowledge regarding the behavior of cardiotropic viruses in vivo and the response of the host has been garnered from studies of coxsackievirus variants in various murine hosts.[46] Although there are at least three "competing" hypotheses regarding pathogenesis in vivo— direct injury, autoimmunity, and molecular mimicry[48]— the features of myocarditis are, in part, a reflection of linked temporal events measurable by virologic, immunologic, and pathologic assays. Initially, the infection is a systemic primary viremia; however, it soon localizes to lymphatic and nonlymphatic tissues, whereupon secondary viremia is fostered and the next series of viral and host events unfold. The engagement of lymphatic tissues such as lymph nodes, thymus, and spleen[81, 111] triggers both innate and antigen-specific immune responses, whereas elsewhere the virus is already infecting "target-organ" cells and beginning to cause cell death.

The infective preference of coxsackieviruses for certain cells rests with several host and viral factors. These include not only the innate immune responses as vital components of early host efforts to contain the invading virus, but also the presence and activity of cell-surface viral receptors, the intracellular replicative environment, and the capacity of the cell to package and export virions.[112]

The molecular mechanisms underlying innate immunity are now partly understood.[112] The initiation of phosphorylation events, partly through the action of interferon, and the activation of interferon-inducible protein kinase contribute to the relative balance of viral and host protein synthesis and cytokine responses.[113] Induction of inducible nitric oxide synthase (iNOS) reflects another host mechanism by which control of viral replication may be achieved[114] although, on the other hand, iNOS can induce tissue injury.[115] Nitric oxide derived through iNOS activity may be induced in a range of parenchymal and inflammatory cells. Both NK cells and γ-δ T cells contribute to host defense, the latter being activated by heat-shock proteins and likely contributing to apoptotic and necrotic mechanisms of host cell death.[112] Antigen-specific T- and B-cell responses are also important in the course of disease. The Th1 CD4+ responses correlate with strong inflammatory responses in murine coxsackievirus infections, as in other viral and parasitic conditions, whereas Th2 responses may limit such target-organ inflammatory sequelae.[112] Another important factor is the nature, frequency, and timing of heterotypic enterovirus infections, wherein exposure of the host immune system to viral group-specific antigens markedly alters the outcome of subsequent infections.[116] In addition to the immune recognition phenomena that underlie a successful host response to viruses, there is a complex cytokine response that may contribute to ventricular dysfunction, especially through TNF-α.[117] The roles of autoimmunity and molecular mimicry in the actual pathogenetic process of myocardial injury in the postinfectious period remain interesting but speculative.[112]

Although a functional receptor for coxsackieviruses was partly characterized in the 1980s,[118, 119] it was not until the late 1990s that definitive identification and molecular evaluation of the coxsackievirus-adenovirus receptor (CAR) were achieved,[120, 121] with high homology demonstrated for the receptor in humans and mice. The particular roles of decay-accelerating factor,[122] putative nucleolin receptor,[123] and antibody-mediated endocytosis[124] in viral pathogenesis in vivo remain to be established. It is intriguing that mRNA expression patterns of murine CAR do not necessarily correspond to the patterns or extent of viral RNA detection by ISH. Thus, the role of replicative determinants may be very important in the cellular pathogenesis of coxsackievirus, including the interaction of host cell proteins with the 5′ and 3′ nontranslated regulatory regions.[125, 126] Several proteins that interact with the positive-strand viral RNA or the negative-strand replicative intermediate have been identified.[127] Differences in the host protein constituency of different cell types may prove to be crucial in the likelihood of replication to high titers and cellular signaling and injury and in determining immune responses.

The sequence of events during an infectious episode provides important clues to the pathogenesis of tissue injury and ventricular failure. By careful light microscopic evaluation and according to molecular and virologic data, the majority of target-organ injury and cell death occurs prior to visible immune cell accumulation in such sites as cardiac muscle.[75, 76] Thus, destructive lesions associated with ISH positivity are evident by day 2 after infection, and these foci progress to peak replication of virus between days 3 and 5 following infection. It is only at this point that an inflammatory infiltrate is detectable. The peak influx of immune cells between days 6 and 10 is associated with destruction of infected myocytes and stromal collapse. Variable early calcification of dying myocytes is a reflection of the variable rapidity of cell death and is primarily a consequence of direct viral injury and loss of normal calcium homeostasis.[128] Viral proteases such as 2B are known to affect cellular calcium homeostasis significantly. By day 14 following infection, healing is advancing, although positive-strand viral genome is still present in many hearts. Downregulation of replication in the weeks following infection, reflected by the lack of negative-strand genome, is associated with the development of persistence, a condition that can be maintained for weeks even in immunocompetent animals. The role of persistent virus in the conversion of the acutely inflamed heart to one that is cardiomyopathic remains to be understood.

Host and viral genetics are important determinants of disease in murine models and undoubtedly in humans. Host genetic factors relate to well-known factors such as sex hormones and immunogenetic background; however, the genetics of the immune response, stress-signaling proteins,[113] factors that determine life or death of an infected cell,[129] other regulatory proteins involved in cell activation and in structural gene expression are also important determinants of disease expression. The regulation of phosphorylation events and of proteins that interact with regulatory regions of the viral genome are just now being elucidated.

In summary, a dynamic "struggle" between virus and host is played out in the collision of host and viral genetic determinants and environmental modulators of molecular and cellular processes. Further insights into the modes of viral traffic, viral sequestration, viral killing, viral persistence, and viral modulation of cell signaling will allow future molecular manipulation of infective episodes in favor of the host.

Can "Focal Myocarditis" Cause Death?

Among the many enigmas associated with human myocarditis, the extent of myocarditis needed to cause clinical events remains uncertain. The following appears to be generally true: Most patients with unexplained heart failure, on EMB, are found not to have myocarditis but the morphologic characteristics of idiopathic dilated cardiomyopathy. The latter hearts may have widely distributed mononuclear cells,[130, 131] the significance of which is uncertain. A second truism is that when biopsy-proven myocarditis[36] is found in patients with unexplained, often recent-onset heart failure, the nature of the disease (as defined by biopsy) is most frequently focal. Indeed, numerous patients have so-called borderline myocarditis,[18] wherein a small infiltrate cannot be closely associated with tissue injury. Only a minority have extensive inflammatory infiltrates and prominent myocyte injury or death. In the larger subset of patients with focal myocarditis on biopsy, it should be remembered that if there is even one small focus in a randomly acquired biopsy specimen, there is a good likelihood that other foci are present throughout the heart or regionally in the heart.

When the issue of focal myocarditis is extended to a whole explanted heart or one obtained at autopsy, the perspective may be somewhat different. A single focus of myocarditis found in 5 to 10 sections representative of the left and right ventricular myocardium and the atria assumes a diminishing significance. Furthermore, two or three widely separated foci may not be compelling. However, it should be remembered that even patients with idiopathic dilated cardiomyopathy may die suddenly 25% of the time;[132] and excluding the possibility that a small focus or two of myocarditis could be the cause of a rapid cardiac demise becomes more difficult. The latter comparisons do not acknowledge that the hearts with idiopathic dilated cardiomyopathy have markedly increased muscle mass (in adults the average heart weight of this subset is >600 g), whereas the acutely myocarditic heart, however inflamed, may be dilated and edematous but may not have increased muscle mass. Because increased heart weight is a risk factor for sudden death, it may not be surprising that patients with idiopathic dilated cardiomyopathy often die suddenly. The basis of sudden death in the setting of focal myocarditis may be related to electrical microreentry or through other mechanisms of ectopic automaticity. Involvement of the conduction system itself can occur, but this is generally not considered specific or uniquely important (also see Chapter 20). Further, the occurrence of clinically mild myocarditis, the most common expression of enteroviral heart disease, may be associated with aberrant release of cytokines in the cardiac microenvironment. Cytokines such as TNF-α are known to contribute to depressed ventricular function[133] and could be related to aberrant automaticity. Finally, in our experience, whereas most patients in the community who die suddenly of natural and unexpected causes, and who have myocarditis, have large and often confluent areas of active disease, there is still a subset for whom no better answer can be derived than that implied from tiny, isolated foci of inflammation and injury. This area of ignorance invites further examination.

In the face of uncertainty painted in the foregoing discussion, we recommend that for hearts of sudden-death victims, for whom no immediate cause can be found, at least two representative transmural tissue blocks be taken from each of the left and right ventricular free walls and from the ventricular septum. Only after these sections have been perused histologically would we take the conduction system or other heart tissue to search for inflammatory foci. The finding of rare inflammatory foci in these settings, even in an unexplained motor vehicle accident, should be regarded conservatively but considered a plausible factor in the death.

Clinicopathologic Correlations

Clinical Manifestations

The clinical diagnosis of myocarditis is confounded by the lack of a distinct clinical syndrome. The clinical manifestations are broad and frequently nonspecific, ranging from asymptomatic to acute or late-onset congestive heart failure to sudden cardiac death (Fig. 9-7). Fever, chest pain, and arrhythmia may be present. The clinical presentation may be similar to other cardiac disorders (i.e., acute myocardial infarction,[134–136] idiopathic dilated cardiomyopathy[137, 138]), resulting in false-positive and false-negative clinical diagnoses.

The prototypical clinical presentation is a previously asymptomatic young adult who experiences rapid-onset congestive heart failure with or without arrhythmias in the setting of a recent viral-type illness. Although an EMB is most often performed in this setting, the presence or absence of these and other clinical characteristics are not reliably predictive of a histologic diagnosis.

In addition to a history of viral-type illness, other historical information may be helpful, including a drug history (i.e., hypersensitivity reactions, use of vasopressors, immunosuppressive agents, and controlled substances), history of alcohol use, and family history of heart disease (i.e., idiopathic dilated cardiomyopathy). Laboratory tests including leukocyte count, erythrocyte sedimentation rate, serum creatinine phosphokinase, cardiac troponins, and viral serology may provide supportive information but are rarely diagnostic. Electrocardiographic changes are nonspecific and may include sinus tachycardia, diffuse ST-T wave abnormalities, premature atrial and ventricular beats, and interventricular conduction delays. Occasionally, Q waves and ST-T changes may mimic an acute myocardial infarction. The cardiac silhouette on chest radiograph may be normal to massively enlarged. Echocardiographic findings are also nonspecific but may show a dilated left

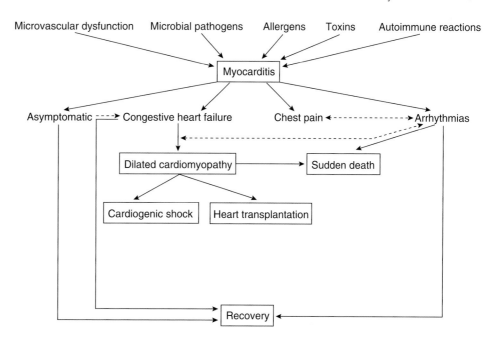

Figure 9-7 • Myocarditis: etiologies, clinical manifestations, and possible outcomes.

ventricle with global or regional left ventricular wall motion abnormalities. Pericardial effusion, ventricular thrombi, and restrictive ventricular filling patterns may be present.[2, 139, 140]

The clinical outcome of patients who survive one or more episodes of myocarditis is also highly variable and may be related to different offending agents or differing genetic susceptibility, or both. In general, patients can be divided into three categories: (1) those whose disease is self-limited and resolves completely, (2) those who have a visibly progressive deterioration with heart failure or intractable arrhythmias leading to death or cardiac transplantation, and (3) those who progress to dilated cardiomyopathy after a long latency period (see later).

Radionuclide Imaging

A definitive diagnosis of myocarditis requires EMB. Despite its specificity, EMB lacks sensitivity due to sampling error if the inflammation is patchy or focal. Desire for a noninvasive method of screening patients with clinically suspected myocarditis prior to biopsy led to investigation of radionuclide scans that detect inflammation or necrotic changes in the myocardium.

Gallium 67 has an affinity for inflammatory cells, and scans have been used clinically to localize abscesses. Although highly sensitive, these scans are not specific enough to be a practical screening tool.[141, 142] Indium 111 imaging of monoclonal antibodies to cardiac myosin can be used to detect myocardial necrosis. When compared with right ventricular EMB to detect myocarditis, antimyosin antibody imaging had a sensitivity of 100% but a specificity of only 58%.[143] More recently, magnetic resonance imaging with gadolinium-induced signal enhancement as a marker of inflammation has shown promise as a noninvasive diagnostic tool in acute myocarditis.[144] Imaging of 44 patients with clinical symptoms of acute myocarditis demonstrated evolution from a focal to a dis-

seminated process during the first 2 weeks after onset of symptoms. If the reliability of this technique is confirmed, it would allow repeated studies over the course of the disease without application of radiation, radioactive material, or invasive procedures.

Treatment of Myocarditis

Definitive therapies for lymphocytic (viral, idiopathic) myocarditis are not available. Because many patients spontaneously recover, it is unclear whether any form of treatment influences the ultimate outcome of the disease. The mainstay of medical management has been supportive cardiovascular therapy. Because hypoxia and exercise intensify the damage from myocarditis, adequate oxygenation and bed rest are indicated. Congestive heart failure and arrhythmias are treated with standard medical management.

The introduction of the EMB allowed the identification of a subset of patients presenting with clinical manifestations of myocarditis who have histologic evidence of the disease. Because the histology of myocarditis resembles that of acute allograft rejection, it was thought that immunosuppression might produce histologic and perhaps clinical improvement. A number of small, uncontrolled studies reported improvement when immunosuppressive agents such as prednisone and azathioprine were administered to patients with biopsy-proven myocarditis.[26, 142, 145, 146] Favorable results, however, were not universal.

The Myocarditis Treatment Trial, a large multicenter study in which patients were prospectively randomized to receive either immunosuppressive therapy or conventional therapy alone, was conducted in the mid-1980s.[18] The results revealed no significant difference in outcomes of patients treated or not treated with immunosuppressive agents and, therefore, do not support the routine use of immunosuppression in treatment. However, pathologic criteria for inclusion in the trial were based solely on the results of light microscopy and excluded cases of giant cell myocarditis, hypersensitivity myocarditis, and cardiac sarcoidosis. The immunosuppressive therapy used, including the drugs, dosages, and duration of administration, do not represent all possible immunosuppressive strategies.

Recent data support the concept that antiviral and immunologically augmentative therapy along with cardiologic support of ventricular dysfunction may be beneficial in certain patients. On the other hand, gamma globulin has been evaluated in children with myocarditis. In one study, children so treated were more likely than controls to have normal ventricular function at 1 year, suggesting a role for immune therapy.[147] It is likely that management of patients with histopathologic myocarditis will require multiple approaches, depending on the stage of disease at detection, the nature of the infiltrate, and the age of the patient.

The diagnosis of active lymphocytic myocarditis may be considered an indication for cardiac transplantation when congestive heart failure is refractory to medical management. The Registry of the International Society for Heart and Lung Transplantation reports that <1% of patients undergoing heart transplantation have active myocarditis.[148] However, patients with active myocarditis who undergo heart transplantation reject the allograft earlier, with higher frequency, and with increased severity compared with heart transplant recipients with other preoperative diagnoses.[149] Detection of recurrent lymphocytic myocarditis in the allograft is precluded by the identical histologic appearance of this process and acute cellular rejection. Recurrence of forms of myocarditis with other distinguishing histologic characteristics, such as giant cell myocarditis or sarcoidosis, has been reported (see also Chapter 23.)

Relationship Between Myocarditis and Idiopathic Dilated Cardiomyopathy

Dilated cardiomyopathy is considered an idiopathic disorder that represents the end stage of a number of possible insults to the myocardium (see Chapter 10). An association between viral myocarditis and dilated cardiomyopathy initially arose when a number of patients with coxsackievirus B infection subsequently developed dilated cardiomyopathy.[150-152]

Although abnormal electrocardiograms suggestive of myocarditis have been documented during influenza epidemics, it has not been possible to analyze the pathogenetic events from initiation of viral infection to the development of dilated cardiomyopathy in humans. However, in a murine model infected with coxsackievirus B3, a self-limited acute infection of the myocardium was followed by cell-mediated immune responses after the virus was cleared, culminating in a histologic picture similar to human dilated cardiomyopathy.[142, 153]

Evidence in humans supporting the development of dilated cardiomyopathy from viral myocarditis is circumstantial. (1) A high incidence of cardiac abnormalities follow recovery from a documented coxsackievirus group B infection.[154] Based on clinical evidence, in up to 30% of patients diagnosed with active viral myocarditis, chronic cardiac disease with clinical manifestations indistinguishable from those of idiopathic dilated cardiomyopathy developed.[155, 156] However, caution is warranted in interpreting these data because, in the absence of tissue confirmation, overdiagnosis may have resulted. (2) Many patients with dilated cardiomyopathy have elevated antibody titers to cardiotropic viruses.[157, 158] (3) Enteroviral genomes have been identified in EMB specimens obtained from patients with dilated cardiomyopathy. However, because enteroviruses are very common pathogens, the presence of viral genome does not establish an enteroviral etiology for the myocarditis.[56] (4) Myocarditis has been diagnosed in EMB specimens obtained from patients with a clinical diagnosis of dilated cardiomyopathy.[152, 159] However, neither the histologic characteristics nor the clinical features at presentation necessarily correlated with patient outcome, regardless of whether treatment with immunosuppressive drugs was administered.

It remains unknown as to why some, but not all, individuals actively infected with cardiotropic viruses ultimately may develop a dilated cardiomyopathy. Hereditary immunoregulatory defects may explain a predisposition. Proof of such mechanisms will solidify the theory that viral myocarditis and dilated cardiomyopathy are opposite ends of the spectrum of the same disease.

GIANT CELL MYOCARDITIS

Giant cell myocarditis is a rare, morphologically distinct form of myocarditis with a clinical course that is usually more fulminant than that of lymphocytic myocarditis and is frequently fatal.[160-162] First described by Salykow in 1905,[163] giant cell myocarditis was frequently classified with granulomatous lesions and by a variety of other names, including granulomatous myocarditis and Fiedler myocarditis, which were used interchangeably. Characterization of giant cell myocarditis histologically and clinically has been aided by data collected on cases diagnosed by EMB as well as on explanted and autopsy hearts. Idiopathic giant cell myocarditis, which lacks granuloma formation, is now considered to be a separate entity from granulomatous myocarditis[164, 165] (see later).

Gross Pathology

Because myocardial involvement by giant cell myocarditis is usually extensive, hearts of patients with acute clinical presentations are typically dilated with flaccid ventricular walls (Fig. 9-8A, B). The cut surface of the myocardium contains serpiginous pale areas, which correspond to areas of intense inflammation. Scarring is not characteristic of the acute disease but may appear in hearts of patients with longer survival.

Histopathology

Three histologic phases of giant cell myocarditis (acute, healing, and healed) have been described and may coincide within a single heart[165] (Fig. 9-9A–C). Histologic findings in the acute phase consist of a widespread

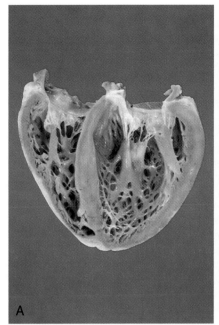

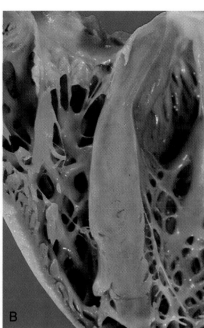

Figure 9-8 • Giant cell myocarditis. *A,* Explanted heart with biventricular dilation. *B,* High-power view of the interventricular septum shows mottled myocardium with focal pale areas.

mixed inflammatory infiltrate composed of lymphocytes, histiocytes, plasma cells, and eosinophils. Numerous multinucleated macrophagic giant cells are admixed with the other cells in the inflammatory infiltrate, particularly at the margin of necrotic zones of myocardium, but true granulomas are absent. Organisms (mycobacteria, fungi, spirochetes, viral inclusions) and foreign bodies cannot be demonstrated. There is typically multifocal or widespread geographic necrosis. The uninvolved myocardium, endocardium, and pericardium are usually normal. The healing

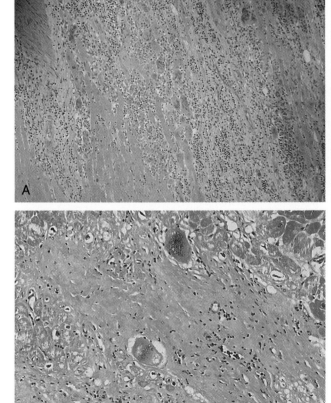

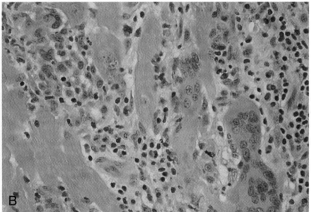

Figure 9-9 • Giant cell myocarditis. *A,* Low-power histology of the interventricular septum of the heart depicted in Figure 9-8. An extensive inflammatory infiltrate with multinucleated giant cells is evident. *B,* Higher power shows a mixed inflammatory infiltrate, multinucleated giant cells, and extensive myocyte damage. *C,* Healing giant cell myocarditis presents areas of fibrosis with occasional giant cells and inflammatory cells. Healed giant cell myocarditis may consist of areas of fibrosis similar to those in Figure 9-3. (*A–C,* H&E stain.)

phase consists of granulation tissue and collagen with macrophagic and myogenic giant cells and occasional lymphocytes. Myocyte necrosis is far less evident than in the acute phase. The healed phase consists of fibrosis, which may contain a sparse lymphocytic infiltrate, but giant cells are not present.

Pathobiology

The histogenesis of the giant cells has long been debated. Early observations of the contiguous arrangement of giant cells with myocytes and electron microscopic analysis showing fragments of myofibrils within the cytoplasm of giant cells suggested a myogenic origin.[164, 166] Other studies, however, demonstrated well-developed endoplasmic reticulum and lysosomal granules supporting the macrophage-histiocytic origin of giant cells.[161] Other histochemical and immunohistochemical studies support two lineages of giant cells, both macrophage[160, 165, 167–171] and myocyte[172, 173] in origin. The derivation of giant cells is possibly related to the type or phase of injury or the nature of the response evoked, or both.

Although the etiology of giant cell myocarditis may be unclear, in some patients there appears to be an association with immunologic abnormalities such as active rheumatic disease, thymoma with or without myasthenia gravis,[174–177] lymphoma,[178] systemic lupus erythematosus, dermatomyositis, thyroiditis, orbital myositis,[179, 180] pernicious anemia,[181] and ulcerative colitis.[182–184] It is postulated that giant cell myocarditis may be either a de novo autoimmune disease or may arise after an infective myocarditis, likely viral, in a patient with altered immunity. However, numerous attempts to identify an infective agent have not been successful.

Experimental giant cell myocarditis can be produced in Lewis rats by autoimmunization with myosin.[185, 186] Human and experimental giant cell myocarditis is characterized by an infiltrate of T lymphocytes and histiocytes and both have a similar clinical course, suggesting that a similar pathogenesis may underlie both diseases. In experimental models, therapy with cyclosporine and anti–T lymphocytes can prevent giant cell myocarditis.[187, 188] The presence of circulating antiheart antibodies and a favorable response to immunosuppressive therapy have been reported in some patients (see later).

Clinicopathologic Correlations

Because giant cell myocarditis is a rare condition, little was known about the natural history or response to therapy. The largest series consists of 63 cases from multiple centers worldwide (reported by Cooper and others[162]). The authors found giant cell myocarditis to be a disease of relatively young (mean age 43 years), previously healthy adults with no gender predilection. Most patients manifested congestive heart failure (75%), and 19% had associated autoimmune disorders. Sustained, refractory ventricular tachycardia developed in almost half the patients during the course of their illness. The rate of death or cardiac transplantation was 89%. Median survival of 5.5 months was much worse than for lympho-

cytic myocarditis. Others, however, have reported longer survival, up to 10 years.[189] Patients treated with corticosteroids and cyclosporine, azathioprine, or both therapies survived longer (average 12 months) as compared with those who received no immunosuppressive therapy (average 3 months). In view of the poor prognosis, cardiac transplantation remains the only possibility for long-term survival. Giant cell myocarditis is known to recur in the transplanted heart[190–192] and was identified by post-transplant EMB in 26% of 34 patients reported by Cooper and others. However, the outcome among such transplant recipients has been better than that of patients who do not undergo transplantation.

GRANULOMATOUS MYOCARDITIS

The designation *granulomatous myocarditis* should be reserved for the forms in which there are well-defined granulomas. It should be distinguished from giant cell myocarditis (see earlier), as the etiology and pathogenesis may be markedly different. Granulomatous myocarditis may be due to one of several known etiologies (i.e., infections, hypersensitivity, foreign bodies) or of unknown etiology (i.e., sarcoidosis). Necrotizing granulomas suggest an infectious (fungal or mycobacterial) etiology. Poorly formed granulomas may occur in hypersensitivity myocarditis (see later) and are typically associated with a prominent eosinophilic infiltrate.

Sarcoidosis

Cardiac involvement by sarcoidosis has been reported in 20 to 30% of patients with sarcoidosis at autopsy. However, less than 5% of patients with sarcoidosis have cardiac symptoms, and only 40 to 50% of patients with cardiac sarcoidosis at autopsy were diagnosed during life.[193, 194]

Gross Pathology

Sarcoid may involve a small portion of the myocardium, may be patchy, or affect large confluent areas (Fig. 9-10A). Although any area may be involved, areas of predilection include the left ventricular free wall (including papillary muscle), basal portion of the ventricular septum, conduction system, and atrial walls.[195] This distribution of granulomas may explain the conduction system disturbances that occur in up to half of the patients. The involved areas are sharply demarcated from uninvolved myocardium. Healed sarcoid results in patchy or serpiginous fibrosis, which, when extensive and transmural, often results in aneurysm formation.

Histopathology

Histologic features are similar to those of extracardiac sarcoid and consist of well-formed non-necrotizing granulomas replacing the myocardium (Fig. 9-10B). Giant cells are usually present, but, unlike giant cell myocarditis, myocyte necrosis is typically absent and eosinophils are rare (Table 9-7). Areas with lymphocytic infiltrates may

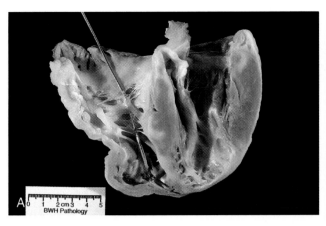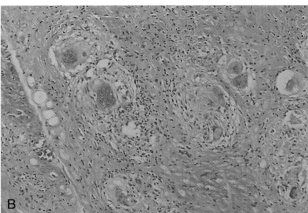

Figure 9-10 • Sarcoidosis. *A*, Explanted heart with patchy myocardial fibrosis, focally transmural, involving the right and left ventricles and the tricuspid valve. *B*, Histology showing well-formed noncaseating granulomas. Results of stains for fungal organisms and acid-fast bacilli were negative (H&E stain).

occur close to the granulomas, and, if these areas alone are captured on EMB, confusion with lymphocytic myocarditis may result. Sarcoid granulomas frequently surround the intramural coronary arteries and may extend into the adventitia and media of these vessels.[196] The arterial lumina may be narrowed by intimal proliferation. Lymph nodes and lungs are frequently involved. The diagnosis of sarcoidosis is by exclusion, and special stains are needed to rule out other causes of granulomatous myocarditis, especially mycobacterial and fungal infections. Healed sarcoidosis reflects the replacement of granulomatous areas by dense fibrosis.

Clinicopathologic Correlations

Myocardial sarcoidosis is a disease of young or middle-aged adults of either sex and may appear with or without evidence of disease elsewhere. Generalized cutaneous anergy and increased serum antiogensin-converting enzyme levels are helpful diagnostic adjuvants. In the absence of extracardiac signs, the disease may be difficult to diagnose. Clinical presentations of myocardial sarcoidosis are protean, including restrictive or dilated cardiomyopathy, congestive heart failure, ventricular arrhythmias, heart block, and pericarditis. Sudden death is the initial presentation in approximately 20% of patients.[195, 196] EMB is positive in up to 50% of patients with presumed myo-

cardial involvement by sarcoid[197]; however, because of the patchy nature of the disease, a negative biopsy result does not exclude the diagnosis.

Treatment of ventricular arrhythmias, conduction disturbances, and congestive heart failure is important to consider clinically.[198, 199] In addition to standard antiarrhythmic pharmacologic agents, implantation of pacemakers and automatic implantable cardioverter-defibrillators, as well as radiofrequency ablation of arrhythmogenic foci, may be necessary. Long-term corticosteroid therapy may result in improvement of symptoms, reversal of electrocardiographic disturbances, complete or partial resolution of thallium perfusion defects, and improvement in prognosis. Cardiac transplantation may benefit some patients with myocardial sarcoidosis but remains controversial because of the potential for recurrence in the allograft.[200, 201]

Tuberculosis

Tuberculous involvement of the myocardium, apart from direct extension of tuberculous pericarditis, is extremely rare. Myocardial tuberculosis is most often clinically silent and diagnosed only at autopsy.[202, 203] Myocardial tuberculosis may occur as localized necrotizing granulomas with giant cells, miliary granulomatous lesions with or without necrosis, or diffuse infiltration. Identification of mycobacterial organisms by histochemical stains or culture, or both, is necessary to confirm the diagnosis. Clinical symptoms of myocardial tuberculosis include arrhythmias and complete heart block, congestive heart failure, left ventricular aneurysms, and sudden death.

EOSINOPHILIC MYOCARDITIS

Eosinophilic infiltrates in the endomyocardium may be divided into three general categories: (1) hypersensitivity myocarditis, (2) hypereosinophilic syndrome, and (3) parasitic infections. In addition, peripheral eosinophilia

TABLE 9-7 • **Pathologic Features of Giant Cell Myocarditis Versus Sarcoidosis**

	Giant Cell Myocarditis	Sarcoidosis
T lymphocytes	+++	+++
B lymphocytes	+	+
Macrophages	+++	+++
Eosinophils	+++	0 (+/−)
Plasma cells	++	+
Macrophage giant cells	+++	++
Myogenic giant cells	+	0
Granulomas	0	+++
Myocyte necrosis	+++	0
Extracardiac granulomas/ giant cells	0	+++

with myocardial involvement may occur in association with other underlying disorders such as malignancy (leukemia, lymphoma, Hodgkin disease, lung carcinoma, malignant melanoma), or vasculitis (polyarteritis nodosa, Churg-Strauss syndrome).[204]

Hypersensitivity Myocarditis

Hypersensitivity to a variety of pharmacologic agents may result in inflammatory reactions that involve the myocardium and resolve without sequelae upon withdrawal of the offending agent. Hypersensitivity myocarditis is not dose dependent and may arise at any time during or after use of the offending agent. More than 30 drugs have been implicated as possible etiologic agents[205]; however, the specific agent is often difficult to identify because patients may be exposed to many agents and there is often an uncertain temporal relationship between therapy and myocarditis. Although methyldopa, sulfonamides, and penicillin traditionally accounted for more than 75% of reported cases,[206] an expanding list of causative drugs includes antibiotics, antihypertensive agents, diuretics, and antiepileptic drugs (see also Chapter 17). The incidence of this disease is difficult to establish because it is frequently not suspected clinically and may go unnoticed. Occasionally, the condition has been documented on EMB. In an unselected autopsy series, the incidence was 0.5%.[207] In explanted hearts from cardiac transplant recipients, who are typically on a variety of medications, the incidence in some series exceeds 20% (see also Chapter 23).[208–210]

Gross Pathology and Histopathology

The gross findings in hearts with hypersensitivity myocarditis varies from normal to a mottled, flaccid appearance with biventricular dilation similar to that seen in lymphocytic myocarditis. Hypersensitivity myocarditis is characterized histologically by a patchy inflammatory infiltrate consisting of lymphocytes (some atypical), plasma cells, histiocytes, and an increased proportion of eosinophils (Fig. 9-11). The infiltrate usually involves all cardiac chambers and is predominantly along tissue planes in interstitial or perivascular locations, or both, often with associated edema.[205] Myocyte necrosis is not a prominent feature, but occasional degenerating myocytes may be seen at the edge of the infiltrate. The severity of the infiltrate is clearly disproportionate to the amount of myocyte damage. Occasional giant cells and poorly formed granulomas may be present. All inflammatory lesions are at approximately the same stage; fibrosis and granulation tissue are typically absent. A non-necrotizing vasculitis may be present.

Pathobiology

The time from initial drug exposure to the development of hypersensitivity myocarditis varies from hours to months. Hypersensitivity drug reactions are not mediated directly against the drug but develop to chemically reactive drug metabolites that act as haptens and generate a

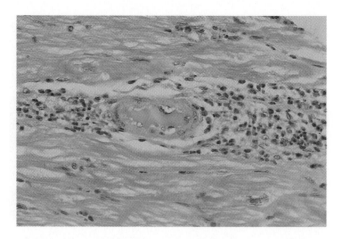

Figure 9-11 • Hypersensitivity myocarditis. Perivascular inflammatory infiltrate with predominance of eosinophils. The infiltrate is confined to the interstitium with no associated myocyte damage (H&E stain).

delayed-type hypersensitivity response.[211, 212] Long-lived haptens or breakdown of peripheral tolerance to normal self-antigens can lead to ongoing immune responses even after therapy with the drug is discontinued. Local and persistent T-lymphocyte activation then yields a host of cytokines that mediate the local vascular and tissue changes. The prominent accumulation of eosinophils is most likely related to the specific cytokines (i.e., IL-5), elaborated by the T cells involved.

Clinicopathologic Correlations

The typical patient is often middle-aged to elderly, is taking multiple medications, and may have known allergies. Peripheral eosinophilia is common, and symptoms may include rash, fever, the appearance of new electrocardiographic changes, mildly elevated cardiac enzymes, mild cardiomegaly, or unexplained tachycardia. Most patients who have hypersensitivity myocarditis are not seriously ill, but occasional patients die suddenly, presumably from an arrhythmia.

Hypersensitivity myocarditis can occasionally follow a more fulminant course, persisting even after drug cessation and resulting in the patient's death. This condition most likely represents the more severe end of the spectrum of hypersensitivity myocarditis and has been termed *acute eosinophilic necrotizing myocarditis*.[213–215] The latter cases are characterized by a more severe and extensive eosinophil-rich mononuclear infiltrate with marked edema and myocyte necrosis (Fig. 9-12). No extracardiac pathology is evident. Although usually diagnosed at autopsy, an occasional premortem diagnosis has been made and successfully treated with high-dose corticosteroids.[214]

Hypereosinophilic Syndrome

Hypereosinophilic syndrome represents a spectrum of diseases, including Loeffler endocarditis and endomyocardial fibrosis, which are discussed in detail in Chapter 10. The following features help differentiate hypereosinophilic syndrome from hypersensitivity myocarditis (see

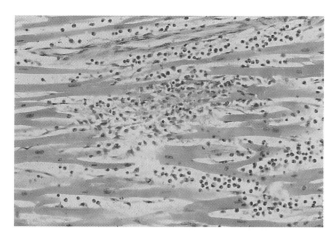

Figure 9-12 • Acute eosinophilic necrotizing myocarditis. Eosinophil-rich inflammatory infiltrate with associated interstitial edema and myocyte necrosis (H&E stain).

above): (1) eosinophils make up a large proportion of the inflammatory cells, and degranulation is often evident; (2) myocyte necrosis is prominent; (3) eosinophilic microabscesses and granulomas may be present; (4) the endocardium is extensively infiltrated by eosinophils, and mural thrombi with eosinophils are characteristic; (5) endocardial scarring results in a restrictive cardiomyopathy; (6) peripheral eosinophilia is uniformly present during the necrotic phase but tends to diminish as the disease progresses; and (7) multiorgan infiltration by eosinophils is common.

Parasitic Infections

Parasitic disease involving the heart may elicit a hypersensitivity-type reaction with prominent eosinophils. The major parasites that infect the myocardium include *Taenia solium* (cysticercosis), *Echinococcus granulosus* (hydatid disease), *Schistosoma, Trichinella spiralis,* and visceral larva migrans.[216] Toxoplasmosis and trypanosomiasis (Chagas disease) are discussed below. Cardiac involvement by parasitic diseases may be the primary manifestation resulting in specifically or predominantly cardiac disorders (i.e., trichinosis, schistosomiasis) or may involve the heart as part of systemic disease (i.e., hydatid disease, cysticercosis).

Parasitic infections that elicit an eosinophilic response are usually limited to helminthic parasites and are more pronounced if tissues are invaded (i.e., trichinosis) than if encystment occurs (i.e., cysticercosis). Eosinophils participate in the immune response against these multicellular parasites by releasing unique toxic inflammatory mediators.

NEUTROPHILIC MYOCARDITIS

Myocyte necrosis with a neutrophilic infiltrate is common in bacterial and some fungal infections. Infection of the myocardium may be acquired through generalized sepsis or spread by continuity from infective endocarditis. Special stains for bacteria and fungi are necessary to establish the causative organisms. Multiple microabscesses containing the offending organisms are frequently present.

OTHER SPECIFIC FORMS OF MYOCARDITIS

HIV-Associated Myocarditis

Cardiac involvement in acquired immunodeficiency syndrome (AIDS) may be divided into pericardial, myocardial, and endocardial processes[217]; myocardial disease may be further subdivided into dilated cardiomyopathy (see Chapter 10) and myocarditis, as well as involvement by neoplasia (i.e., Kaposi sarcoma, lymphoma) and drug toxicity.[218–222] Cardiac involvement occurs in one quarter to one half of patients with AIDS, although clinically significant disease is present in less than 10%.

As in other immunosuppressed individuals, AIDS patients are at increased risk for opportunistic infections (see below) that may involve the myocardium. More typical, however, is focal lymphocytic myocarditis with associated myocyte necrosis or "borderline" myocarditis, in which myocyte necrosis is not evident (Fig. 9-13). In most cases, a pathogenic agent cannot be identified. The pathogenesis of HIV-associated myocarditis is probably multifactorial.[219] A viral etiology is likely, at least for some cases. Evidence suggests that the idiopathic myocarditis is due to HIV itself.[223] With a variety of techniques, including ISH and PCR, the HIV genome has been detected in cardiac myocytes and dendritic cells of patients with AIDS.[224–227] However, no conclusive evidence exists that this is a direct cause of myocarditis, and the presence of detectable HIV genome does not always correlate with histologic myocarditis. Myocardial cell abnormalities have been observed in the absence of inflammation, suggesting that HIV may exert either a direct toxic effect on myo-

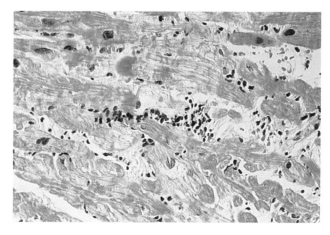

Figure 9-13 • Human immunodeficiency virus associated–myocarditis. Focal lymphocytic infiltrate without obvious myocyte damage resembling other forms of viral "borderline" myocarditis (H&E stain).

TABLE 9-8 • **Opportunistic Myocardial Infections in Immunosuppressed Patients**

Bacterial	Viral
Mycobacterium avium–intracellulare	Cytomegalovirus
Mycobacterium tuberculosis	Herpes simplex virus
Fungal	**Protozoan**
Aspergillus fumigatus	*Pneumocystis carinii*
Candida albicans	*Toxoplasma gondii*
Coccidioides immitis	
Cryptococcus neoformans	
Histoplasma capsulatum	

cytes or an indirect effect by inducing cytokine production such as TNF. The HIV-related myocarditis may result in dilated cardiomyopathy.

Myocarditis in Immunosuppressed Patients (Opportunistic Infections)

Immunosuppressed patients, including organ transplant recipients (see also Chapter 23), patients with AIDS, and patients undergoing chemotherapy for neoplasia are at increased risk of opportunistic infections that may involve the myocardium. The more common bacterial, fungal, viral, and protozoan organisms are listed in Table 9-8. Illustrative cases of common fungal (*Aspergillus*), viral (CMV), and protozoan (*Toxoplasma*) organisms are presented in Figure 9-14A–F.

The gross appearance of a heart involved by opportunistic infection ranges from an incidental finding that is not grossly apparent to multiple foci of necrosis and large abscesses. Microscopic examination may show the inflammatory response characterisitic of the various organisms (i.e., granulomatous for *Mycobacterium* and *Histoplasma;* hemorrhagic necrosis for *Aspergillus*). However, the inflammatory response may be severely blunted in the immune-compromised patient such that inflammation is not present. Special studies such as histochemical stains (i.e., Grocott-Gomori methenamine–silver nitrate and periodic acid–Schiff [PAS]), immunohistochemistry (i.e., CMV), ISH, and PCR (i.e., CMV) can be used to establish the diagnosis. Infection by multiple pathogens is common.

The myocardium is often an incidental site of infection when there is systemic blood-borne infection. Patients may be asymptomatic from a cardiac standpoint or may manifest contractile dysfunction and conduction system abnormalities.

Lyme Disease Myocarditis

Lyme disease is caused by the spirochetal organism *Borrelia burgdorferi* and is passed to humans by several species of ticks of the genus *Ixodes* (deer tick).[228, 229] *B. burgdorferi* is endemic to most of North America, Europe, the former Soviet Union, China, Japan, and Australia. Most Northern Hemisphere human infections occur during the months of May through August, when the vector larval stage activity and human outdoor activity

are at their peak. In recent years, more than 10,000 new cases have been reported each year to the Centers for Disease Control and Prevention in Atlanta.[230, 231]

Cardiac involvement occurs in about 10% of patients during the first 3 months of infection,[232, 233] most commonly manifested by variable degrees of A-V block associated with a myocarditis consisting of a myocardial infiltrate of lymphocytes as well as plasma cells and macrophages resembling a viral myocarditis (Fig. 9-15A and C). A band-like collection of lymphocytes in the endocardium is characteristic and may be detected on EMB. Involvement of the conduction system, particularly the A-V node, may be prominent and correlates with the clinical presentation of A-V heart block.

Lymphoplasmacytic infiltrates may extend into the visceral pericardium and pericardial fat. Rare extracellular *B. burgdorferi* organisms can be demonstrated in the myocardium using modified silver stains (Fig. 9-15B and D), and the organism has been isolated from the myocardium.[234] The demonstration of spirochetes in myocardial tissue suggests that the myocarditis is due to a direct toxic effect, although there is speculation that immune-mediated mechanisms also play a role. The organism may persist in the myocardium despite antibiotic therapy.[235] Isolation of *B. burgdorferi* from the myocardium of a patient with long-standing cardiomyopathy has also been described.

Lyme disease is characterized by three stages.[229] The first, or acute, stage consists of a characteristic skin rash, erythema migrans, which begins at the site of the tick bite. Fever, minor constitutional symptoms, or regional lymphadenopathy may also be present. The second, or disseminated, stage is marked by neurologic, cardiac, or musculoskeletal symptoms, which appear within weeks to months of the bite. The third stage, persistent infection, is characterized by prolonged arthritis of large joints, typically the knee. Treatment consists of antibiotic therapy, although the optimal regimen remains controversial. In general, the sooner the disease is recognized and the sooner antibiotics are started, the better the chance for eradication of the organism. A vaccine effective in preventing the disease in humans has been developed.[236, 237]

Chagas Disease

Chagas disease (American trypanosomiasis), caused by the protozoan *Trypanosoma cruzi,* is the most important cause of heart disease in Latin America, where it is estimated that 16 million people are infected by the parasite and another 90 million are at risk.[238] The heaviest concentration of Chagas disease is in rural Brazil. Although the prevalence in the United States in unknown, it is estimated that 50,000 to 100,000 immigrants have *T. cruzi* infection.[239]

T. cruzi is present in mammalian hosts such as armadillos, rodents, and opossums and is transmitted to humans by reduviid bugs via fecal contamination while they are feeding.[238, 240] Two distinct forms of the parasite develop in the infected human: amastigotes (aflagellate forms), which are intracellular, and trypomastigotes (flagellate forms), which circulate in the blood. Muscle, in-

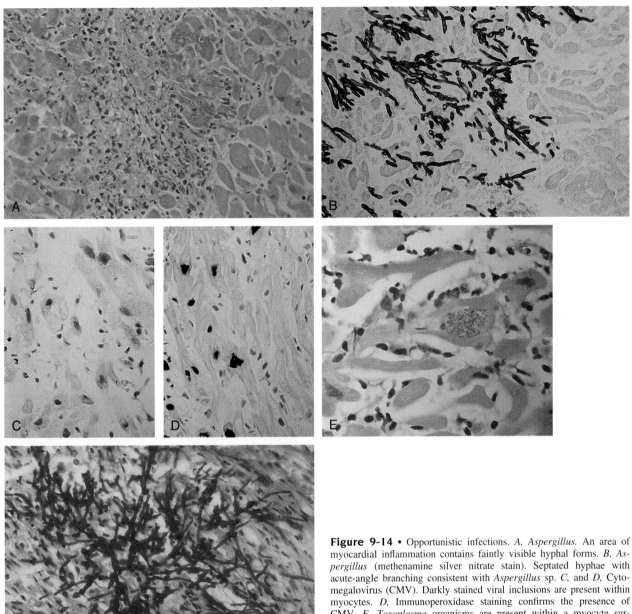

Figure 9-14 • Opportunistic infections. *A, Aspergillus.* An area of myocardial inflammation contains faintly visible hyphal forms. *B, Aspergillus* (methenamine silver nitrate stain). Septated hyphae with acute-angle branching consistent with *Aspergillus* sp. *C,* and *D,* Cytomegalovirus (CMV). Darkly stained viral inclusions are present within myocytes. *D,* Immunoperoxidase staining confirms the presence of CMV. *E, Toxoplasma* organisms are present within a myocyte surrounded by a mononuclear cell infiltrate. *F, Candida* (periodic acid–Schiff stain). Cluster of pseudohyphae in the myocardium of a child with disseminated candidiasis. (All H&E stain.)

cluding the heart, may be parasitized, and intracellular replication of the parasite may lead to cell rupture. The parasite can also invade the nervous system.

The diagnosis of Chagas disease is based on the triad of positive epidemiology, positive serology, and a combination of clinical findings, which include prominent cardiovascular manifestations. Chagas disease may be divided into acute and chronic forms.

Acute Chagas Disease

Acute chagasic myocarditis is characterized by an inflammatory infiltrate of lymphocytes and plasma cells, interstitial edema, and extensive myocyte necrosis. Amastigote forms of *T. cruzi* may be identified within myo-

cytes (Fig. 9-16), which may rupture, leading to abscess formation. Organisms may also be present in noninflamed myocardium. The amastigotes are 2- to 3-μm spheric organisms with rod-shaped kinetoplasts and spheric nuclei. *T. cruzi* organisms may be distinguished from *Toxoplasma* organisms by PAS staining, which is positive for *Toxoplasma* and negative for *Trypanosoma*.

Cardiac damage induced by *T. cruzi* results from direct mechanical damage to the myocyte by the penetrating organism, which may lead to myofibrillar rupture.[238] An intense inflammatory response ensues, including cytotoxic T lymphocytes, which are sensitized by *T. cruzi* antigens. Antibodies are produced that might cross-react with tissue. Infection of endothelial cells may lead to microvascular thrombosis, spasm, or both, with resultant focal ische-

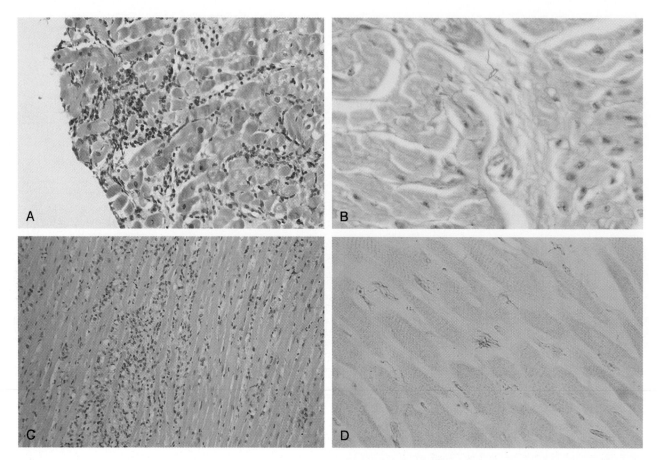

Figure 9-15 • Lyme disease myocarditis. *A,* Endomyocardial biopsy with mononuclear cell infiltrate from a young adult who was successfully treated with intravenous ceftriaxone (H&E stain). *B,* Modified Steiner stain demonstrates extracellular *Borrelia burgdorferi* organism within the myocardium. *C,* Mouse model of Lyme disease with intense mononuclear cell infiltrate in the myocardium (H&E stain). *D,* Numerous *B. burgdorferi* organisms are present on modified Steiner stain. (*A* to *D,* courtesy of P. Duray, MD.)

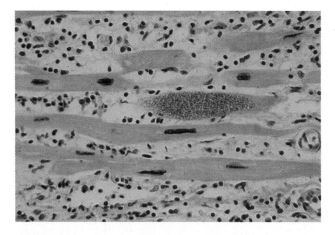

Figure 9-16 • Acute chagasic myocarditis showing *Trypanosoma cruzi*–packed cyst, interstitial lymphocytic infiltrate, and myocyte degeneration (H&E stain). (From von Lichtenberg F: Infectious disease. In: Cotran RS, Kumar V, Robbins SL [eds]: Pathologic Basis of Disease. Philadelphia, WB Saunders, 1989, p 408).

mic injury. In addition, *Trypanosoma* contains enzymes such as collagenases and proteases, which may degrade the extracellular matrix, resulting in aneurysmal thinning of the apex, a characteristic of the chronic form of the disease.

Most infected individuals, often children, lack evidence of clinical disease. The infection goes unnoticed but may become evident later in life. When symptomatic, acute Chagas disease is manifested by fever and malaise. The Romaña sign—unilateral bipalpebral edema, conjunctivitis, and swelling of satellite lymph nodes—is useful clinically. The presence of arryhthmias, heart block, or congestive heart failure during the acute phase foretells a poor prognosis. The fatality rate during the acute phase is 5 to 10%.

Chronic Chagas Disease

In approximately 10 to 30% of infected individuals, chronic Chagas disease develops years after the initial infection.[239] The heart is typically enlarged, with four-chamber dilation. A left ventricular apical aneurysm, which may contain mural thrombus, is present in approximately 50% of patients.[241] Right ventricular apical aneurysms have been found at autopsy in 10 to 20% of patients. The myocardium may contain an inflammatory infiltrate comprised of lymphocytes, plasma cells, and occasional eosinophils. Amastigotes may be difficult or impossible to identify. Marked interstitial fibrosis is often a prominent myocardial finding, separating atrophic myofibers, particularly near the ventricular apices.

The pathogenesis of chronic Chagas disease is incompletely understood, and several mechanisms have been proposed[242]: (1) continued invasion of the myocardium by *T. cruzi,* (2) destruction of the parasympathetic ganglion cells in the heart, resulting in neurogenic heart disease, (3) autoimmune mechanisms, supported by a negative correlation between the severity of disease and the level of parasitemia, and (4) microvascular changes, resulting in focal myocyte necrosis with associated interstitial fibrosis and inflammatory mononuclear cells.

Clinically, patients may present with congestive heart failure, arrhythmias, thromboembolic events, or sudden death. In the United States, Chagas disease may mimic coronary artery disease or idiopathic dilated cardiomyopathy and, therefore, be underdiagnosed.[243] Positive serologic tests for *T. cruzi* antibodies help confirm the diagnosis. Cardiac transplantation has been done for advanced chronic Chagas disease but is associated with a high rate of *Trypanosoma* infection of the allograft despite preoperative parasiticidal treatment.[244, 245]

Toxic Myocarditis

Myocardial degeneration and necrosis with resultant inflammation may be caused by a variety of chemical or biologic toxins. For a discussion of the cardiac effects of drugs (including chemotherapeutic agents), chemicals, and substances of abuse (including cocaine), see Chapter 17.

Diphtheria

Although rarely seen today, diphtheria may result in myocardial involvement, which occurs in approximately one quarter of cases and is the most common cause of death in affected individuals.[246] Cardiac damage is caused by exotoxin liberated by the bacterium *Corynebacterium diphtheriae* rather than by direct invasion by the microorganism. The toxin inhibits protein synthesis by interfering with amino acid transfer from RNA to polypeptide chains under construction.

Involved hearts appear flabby and dilated with pale areas of myocardium. The early stages of myocardial involvement are characterized by extensive hyaline degeneration, myocytolysis, and intracellular fat accumulation. A mononuclear cell response occurs but is disproportionately mild compared to the extent of myocyte damage. Later stages are characterized by interstitial myocardial fibrosis. There is a propensity for the disease to involve the conduction system, resulting in partial or complete heart block. Treatment includes antitoxin, antibiotics, and pacemaker placement.

Myocarditis Associated with Systemic Diseases

Myocarditis associated with rheumatoid arthritis; collagen vascular diseases, including systemic lupus erythematosus, scleroderma, and polymyositis-dermatomyositis; and Whipple disease is discussed in Chapter 16. Acute rheumatic carditis is discussed in Chapter 13.

CONDITIONS THAT MIMIC MYOCARDITIS

Not all myocardial inflammation constitutes myocarditis. The presence of inflammatory cells in the myocardium alone is insufficient to warrant a diagnosis of myocarditis, and small infiltrates may be found in a number of other conditions. Although obtaining a more detailed clinical history may be helpful, a number of these conditions may have clinical presentations that mimic myocarditis. Furthermore, in rare instances, two conditions may coexist.

Idiopathic Dilated Cardiomyopathy

The diagnosis of idiopathic dilated cardiomyopathy is based primarily on exclusion of other known or established causes of heart failure. Histologic findings such as myocyte hypertrophy and degeneration and varying degrees of one or more of interstitial, replacement, or endocardial fibrosis are characteristic but nonspecific. Whether one accepts the premise that idiopathic dilated cardiomyopathy is the same entity as end-stage "chronic" myocarditis, sufficient sampling of these hearts reveals a high proportion of inflammatory infiltrates. One study that examined the explanted hearts of patients with idiopathic dilated cardiomyopathy undergoing cardiac transplantation found at least one focus of inflammatory infiltrates in 87% of 108 cases.[130] The infiltrates are predominantly lymphocytic and are frequently associated with areas of fibrosis (Fig. 9-17). Distinguishing features are extensive, chronic changes in the myocardium (hypertrophy, atrophy, myofibrillar loss, fibrosis, endocardial thickening), which, along with clinical history and duration of illness, should help differentiate idiopathic dilated cardiomyopathy from active myocarditis.

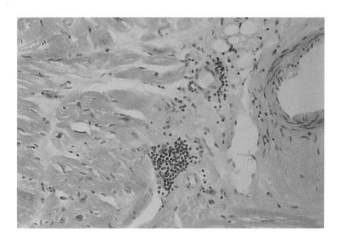

Figure 9-17 • Idiopathic dilated cardiomyopathy. Focal lymphocytic infiltrate associated with an area of perivascular fibrosis (H&E stain).

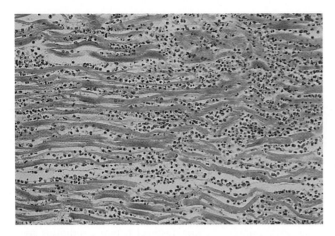

Figure 9-18 • Acute myocardial infarction. Extensive neutrophilic infiltrate associated with myocardial coagulative necrosis (H&E stain).

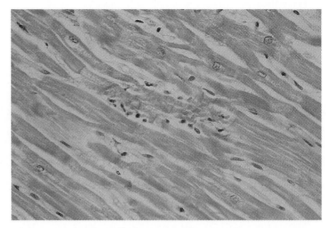

Figure 9-20 • Catecholamine effect. Necrosis with contraction bands in the myocardium of a patient with bilateral pheochromocytomas (H&E stain).

Ischemic Injury

Myocardial Infarction

In contrast to multiple small areas of myocyte injury due to myocarditis, myocardial infarction is characterized by bandlike zones of coagulative necrosis in the distribution of a coronary artery. Hearts with myocardial injury due to myocarditis lack such concordance. Neutrophils are recruited to an infarcted area acutely (Fig. 9-18), followed by a mixed inflammatory infiltrate, including lymphocytes, plasma cells, and pigment-laden macrophages, during the healing phase. A myocardial infarction typically spares the few cell layers of myocardium immediately deep to the endocardium, as these layers are perfused by blood from within the ventricular cavity. Myocarditis often involves the endocardium and immediately adjacent myocardium. Clinical history, including angiographic status of the coronary arteries, should be known prior to rendering a final pathologic diagnosis. With a history of myocardial infarction, documented coronary artery disease, or evidence of ischemic myocardial damage,

the diagnosis of myocarditis should be rendered only with great skepticism, if at all.

Hypotension and Ischemic Reperfusion

Patients who experience an episode of hypotension or who are resuscitated from a cardiac arrest may have ischemic myocardial injury that may be confused with myocarditis. Myocyte necrosis results from ischemia, and these irreversibly injured myocytes respond to reperfusion by developing prominent contraction bands (Fig. 9-19). Ischemic injury to capillaries often results in hemorrhage when blood flow is restored. Neutrophils may be present in areas of contraction band necrosis, but often this type of injury fails to elicit the typical generalized early neutrophilic response.[247, 248]

Pressor Effect

Exogenous

In patients who have received high-dose pressor agents, such as dopamine, focal or multifocal aggregates

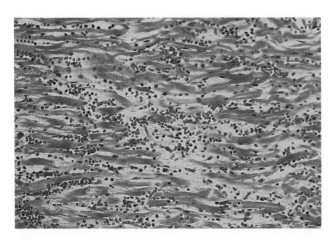

Figure 9-19 • Ischemic reperfusion. Reperfused ischemic myocardium with hemorrhage, contraction bands, and focal neutrophilic infiltrate (H&E stain).

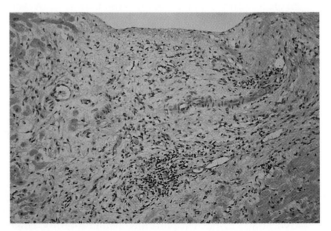

Figure 9-21 • Biopsy site. Subendocardial area of granulation tissue containing a focally dense collection of lymphocytes (H&E stain).

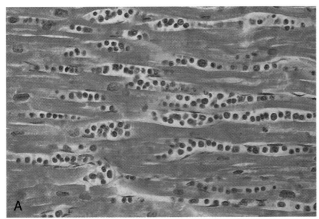 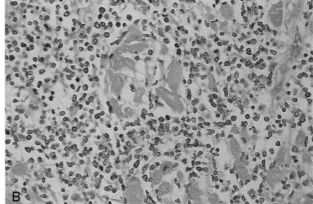

Figure 9-22 • Atypical lymphoid infiltrates. *A,* Acute myeloblastic leukemia involving the myocardium. *B,* Myocardial involvement by large cell lymphoma (H&E stain).

of mononuclear cells (predominantly macrophages) and occasional neutrophils associated with a small number of necrotic myocytes (often < 10 cells) may develop. Contraction bands are prominent early, after which the myocyte nuclei become pyknotic and disappear.[249] A basophilic, granular material may be present with the myocytes, which presumably represents mitochondrial calcification. These changes, known as "catecholamine effect," must be differentiated from myocarditis, particularly in patients with congestive heart failure who have been treated aggressively with pressor agents.

Endogenous

Endogenous catecholamines usually result from catecholamine-producing neoplasms such as pheochromocytoma. Similar to the effect of exogenous catecholamines, the characteristic histologic feature is contraction band necrosis (Fig. 9-20).[250] As in myocarditis, an excess of catecholamines may result in acute heart failure with cardiac dilation or even sudden death.

Biopsy Site

Patients who have undergone previous EMBs may have tissue obtained from healing biopsy sites during subsequent biopsy procedures. Because myocyte injury and an inflammatory infiltrate may be present (Fig. 9-21), misinterpretation as myocarditis can occur. Differentiating features include the following: (1) lesions that are endocardially based with focal endocardial disruption and, often, overlying fibrin thrombus; (2) the presence of granulation tissue with pigmented macrophages; and (3) myocyte disarray at the base of the lesion. Of course, the clinical history of a previous biopsy procedure is helpful.

Atypical Lymphoid Infiltrates (Hematologic Malignancies)

Leukemias, lymphomas, and Epstein-Barr virus–related lymphoproliferative disorders may involve the myocardium. The neoplastic infiltrates are usually monomor-

phic and have malignant cytologic characteristics (Fig. 9-22*A* and *B*). Unlike myocarditis, myocyte damage is often limited unless the infiltrate is extensive.

Cardiac Transplant Rejection

Acute rejection after cardiac transplantation (see also Chapter 23) is indistinguishable from lymphocytic myocarditis. Therefore, history is of paramount importance. Only the presence of other distinguishing characteristics for specific forms of myocarditis such as parasites (*Toxoplasma*), viral inclusions (CMV), and giant cells (giant cell myocarditis) allow for differentiation between transplant rejection and myocarditis.

REFERENCES

1. Herskowitz A, Baughman KL: Myocarditis. In: Gravanis MB (ed): Cardiovascular Disorders: Pathogenesis and Pathophysiology. St. Louis, Mosby, 1993, p 178
2. Wynne J, Braunwald E: The cardiomyopathies and myocarditides. In: Braunwald E (ed): Heart Disease. Philadelphia, WB Saunders, 1997, p 1404
3. Aretz HT: Diseases of the myocardium. In: Bloom S (ed): Diagnostic Criteria for Cardiovascular Pathology: Acquired Diseases. Philadelphia, Lippincott-Raven, 1997, p 1
4. Schoen FJ: The heart. In: Cotran RS, Kumar V, Collins T (eds): Pathologic Basis of Disease. Philadelphia, WB Saunders, 1999, p 543
5. McManus BM, Kandolf R: Myocarditis. In: McManus BM, Braunwald E (eds): Atlas of Cardiovascular Pathology. Philadelphia, Current Medicine, in press
6. Gore I, Saphir O: Myocarditis: A classification of 1402 cases. Am Heart J 34:827, 1947
7. Kline IK, Kline TS, Saphir O: Myocarditis in senescence. Am Heart J 65:446, 1963
8. Abelmann WH: Myocarditis. N Engl J Med 275:832, 1966
9. Okada R, Wakafuji S: Myocarditis in autopsy. In: Sekiguchi M, Olsen EGJ, Goodwin JF (eds): Proceedings of the International Symposium on Cardiomyopathy and Myocarditis. New York, Springer-Verlag, 1985
10. Zee-Chang CS, Tsai CC, Palmer DC, et al: High incidence of myocarditis by endomyocardial biopsy in patients with idiopathic congestive cardiomyopathy. J Am Coll Cardiol 3:63, 1984
11. Kereiakes DJ, Parmley WW: Myocarditis and cardiomyopathy. Am Heart J 108:1318, 1984

12. Marboe CC, Fenoglio JJ: Biopsy diagnosis of myocarditis. In: Waller BF (ed): Contemporary Issues in Cardiovascular Pathology. Philadelphia, FA Davis, 1988, p 137

13. Hauck AJ, Edwards ED: Histopathologic examination of tissues obtained by endomyocardial biopsy. In: Fowles RE (ed): Cardiac Biopsy. Mount Kisco, NY, Futura, 1992, p 95

14. Gravanis MB, Sternby NH: Incidence of myocarditis. Arch Pathol Lab Med 115:390, 1991

15. Passarino G, Burlo P, Ciccone G, et al: Prevalence of myocarditis at autopsy in Turin, Italy. Arch Pathol Lab Med 121:619, 1997

16. Chow LC, Dittrich HC, Shabetai R: Endomyocardial biopsy in patients with unexplained congestive heart failure. Ann Intern Med 109:535, 1988

17. Aretz HT, Billingham ME, Edwards WD, et al: The utility of the Dallas criteria for the histopathological diagnosis of myocarditis in endomyocardial biopsy specimens (abstract). Circulation 88 (suppl):I-552, 1993

18. Mason JW, O'Connell JB, Herskowitz A, et al: A clinical trial of immunosuppressive therapy for myocarditis. N Engl J Med 333: 269, 1995

19. Saphir O: Myocarditis, a general review with an analysis of 240 cases. Arch Pathol 32:1000, 1941

20. Sakakibara S, Konno S: Endomyocardial biopsy. Jpn Heart J 3: 537, 1962

21. Hrobon P, Kuntz KM, Hare JM: Should endomyocardial biopsy be performed for detection of myocarditis? A decision analytic approach. J Heart Lung Transplant 17:479, 1998

22. Shanes JG, Ghali J, Billingham ME, et al: Interobserver variability in the pathologic interpretation of endomyocardial biopsy results. Circulation 75:401, 1987

23. Virmani R, Burke AP, Farb A, Smialek J: Problems in forensic cardiovascular pathology. In: Schoen FJ, Gimbrone MA Jr (eds): Cardiovascular Pathology: Clinicopathologic Correlations and Pathogenetic Mechanisms. Baltimore, Williams & Wilkins, 1995, p 173

24. Burch GE, Ray CT: Myocarditis and myocardial degeneration. Bull Tulane Medical Faculty 8:1, 1948

25. Lustock MJ, Chase J, Lubitz JM: Myocarditis: A clinical and pathologic study of forty-five cases. Dis Chest 28:243, 1955

26. Fenoglio JJ Jr, Ursell PC, Kellogg CF, et al: Diagnosis and classification of myocarditis by endomyocardial biopsy. N Engl J Med 308:12, 1983

27. Lieberman EB, Hutchins GM, Herskowitz A, et al: Clinicopathologic description of myocarditis. J Am Coll Cardiol 18:1617, 1991

28. Richardson P, McKenna W, Bristow M, et al: Report of the 1995 World Health Organization/International Society and Federation of Cardiology Task Force on the Definition and Classification of Cardiomyopathies. Circulation 93:841, 1996

29. Mason JW, O'Connell JB: Clinical merit of endomyocardial biopsy. Circulation 79:971, 1989

30. Baandrup U, Florio RA, Olsen EG: Do endomyocardial biopsies represent the morphology of the rest of the myocardium? A quantitative light microscopic study of single v. multiple biopsies with the King's bioptome. Eur Heart J 3:171, 1982

31. Fowles RE, Anderson JL: Instruments and techniques for cardiac biopsy. In: Fowles RE (ed): Cardiac Biopsy. Mount Kisco, NY, Futura, 1992, p 43

32. Chow LH, Radio SJ, Sears TD, McManus BM: Insensitivity of right ventricular endomyocardial biopsy in the diagnosis of myocarditis. J Am Coll Cardiol 14:915, 1989

33. Hauck AJ, Kearney DL, Edwards WD: Evaluation of postmortem endomyocardial biopsy specimens from 38 patients with lymphocytic myocarditis: Implications for role of sampling error. Mayo Clin Proc 64:1235, 1989

34. Billingham ME: The diagnostic criteria of myocarditis by endomyocardial biopsy. Heart Vessels 1(suppl):133, 1985

35. Schoen FJ: Myocardial, pericardial, and endocardial heart disease. In: Interventional and Surgical Cardiovascular Pathology. Philadelphia, WB Saunders, 1989, p 173

36. Aretz HT, Billingham ME, Edwards WD, et al: Myocarditis: A histopathologic definition and classification. Am J Cardiovasc Pathol 1:3, 1987

37. Aretz HT: Myocarditis: The Dallas criteria. Hum Pathol 18:619, 1987

38. Aretz HT: Myocarditis: The Dallas classification. In: Virmani R, Atkinson JB, Fenoglio JJ (eds): Cardiovascular Pathology. Philadelphia, WB Saunders, 1991, p 246

39. Edwards WD, Holmes DR, Reeder GS: Diagnosis of active lymphocytic myocarditis by endomyocardial biopsy: Quantitative criteria for light microscopy. Mayo Clin Proc 57:419, 1982

40. Linder J, Cassling RS, Rogler WC, et al: Immunohistochemical characterization of lymphocytes in uninflamed ventricular myocardium. Arch Pathol Lab Med 109:917, 1985

41. Schnitt SJ, Ciano PS, Schoen FJ: Quantitation of lymphocytes in endomyocardial biopsies: Use and limitations of antibodies to leukocyte common antigen. Hum Pathol 18:796, 1987

42. Tazelaar HD, Billingham ME: Myocardial lymphocytes: Fact, fancy, or myocarditis? Am J Cardiovasc Pathol 1:47, 1986

43. Billingham ME: The role of endomyocardial biopsy in the diagnosis and treatment of heart disease. In: Silver MD (ed): Cardiovascular Pathology. Vol 2. New York, Churchill Livingstone, 1983, p 1205

44. Karch SB, Billingham ME: Myocardial contraction bands revisited. Hum Pathol 17:9, 1986

45. Burke AP, Farb A, Robinowitz M, Virmani R: Serial sectioning and multiple level examination of endomyocardial biopsies for the diagnosis of myocarditis. Mod Pathol 4:690, 1991

46. McManus BM, Kandolf R: Myocarditis: Evolving concepts of cause, consequences, and control. Curr Opin Cardiol 6:418, 1991

47. Martino TA, Liu P, Sole MJ: Viral infection and the pathogenesis of dilated cardiomyopathy. Circ Res 74:182, 1994

48. Carthy CM, Yang D, Anderson DR, et al: Myocarditis as systemic disease: New perspectives on pathogenesis. Clin Exp Pharmacol Physiol 24:997, 1997

49. Kandolf R: Enteroviral myocarditis and dilated cardiomyopathy. Med Klin 93:215, 1998

50. Rabin ER, Melnick JL: Viral myocarditis. Cardiovasc Res Center Bull 4:2, 1965

51. Artenstein MS, Cadigan FC Jr, Buescher EL: Clinical and epidemiological features of coxsackie group B virus infections. Ann Intern Med 63:597, 1965

52. Godman GC: The cytopathology of enteroviral infection. Int Rev Exp Pathol 5:67, 1966

53. Burch GE, Sun SC, Chu KC, et al: Interstitial and coxsackievirus B myocarditis in infants and children: A comparative histologic and immunofluorescent study of 50 autopsied hearts. JAMA 203:1, 1968

54. Burch GE, Harb J: Coxsackie B4 virus crystal formation in mouse pancreas. Proc Soc Exp Biol Med 149:893, 1975

55. Kandolf R, Canu A, Hofschneider PH: Coxsackie B3 virus can replicate in cultured human foetal heart cells and is inhibited by interferon. J Mol Cell Cardiol 17:167, 1985

56. Bowles NE, Richardson PJ, Olsen EG, Archard LC: Detection of coxsackie-B-virus–specific RNA sequences in myocardial biopsy samples from patients with myocarditis and dilated cardiomyopathy. Lancet 1:1120, 1986

57. Grist NR, Bell EJ, Reid D: The epidemiology of enteroviruses. Scott Med J 20:27, 1975

58. Grist NR, Reid D: General pathogenicity and epidemiology. In: Bendinelli M, Friedman H (eds): Coxsackieviruses: A General Update. New York, Plenum Press, 1988, p 221

59. Easton AJ, Eglin RP: The detection of coxsackievirus RNA in cardiac tissue by in situ hybridization. J Gen Virol 69:285, 1988

60. Weiss LM, Movahed LA, Billingham ME, Cleary ML: Detection of coxsackievirus B3 RNA in myocardial tissues by the polymerase chain reaction. Am J Pathol 138:497, 1991

61. Bowles NE, Rose ML, Taylor P, et al: End-stage dilated cardiomyopathy: Persistence of enterovirus RNA in myocardium at cardiac transplantation and lack of immune response. Circulation 80: 1128, 1989

62. Kandolf R, Canu A, Klingel K, et al: Molecular studies on enteroviral heart disease. In: Brinton MA, Heinz FX (eds): New Aspects of Positive-Strand RNA Viruses. Washington, DC, American Society of Microbiology, 1990, p 340

63. Tracy SM, Wiegard V, McManus BM, et al: Enteroviruses in the myocarditic and myopathic heart: Roles and dilemmas. J Am Coll Cardiol 15:1688, 1990

64. Ou J, Sole M, Butany J, et al: Detection of enterovirus RNA in

myocardial biopsies from patients with myocarditis and cardiomyopathy using gene amplification by polymerase chain reaction. Circulation 82:8, 1990

65. Tracy SM, Chapman NM, McManus BM, et al: A molecular and serologic evaluation of enterovirus involvement in human myocarditis. J Mol Cell Cardiol 22:403, 1990
66. Ueno H, Yokota Y, Shiotani H, et al: Significance of detection of enterovirus RNA in myocardial tissues by reverse transcription–polymerase chain reaction. Int J Cardiol 51:157, 1995
67. Figulla HR, Stille-Siegener M, Mall G, et al: Myocardial enterovirus infection with left ventricular dysfunction: A benign disease compared with idiopathic dilated cardiomyopathy. J Am Coll Cardiol 25:1170, 1995
68. Grasso M, Arbustini E, Silini E, et al: Search for coxsackievirus B3 RNA in idiopathic dilated cardiomyopathy using gene amplification by polymerase chain reaction. Am J Cardiol 69:658, 1992
69. Kandolf R: The molecular pathogenesis of enterovirus myocarditis: Virus persistence and chronic inflammation. Internist 36:430, 1995
70. Muir P, Micholson F, Illavia SJ, et al: Serological and molecular evidence of enterovirus infection in patients with end-stage dilated cardiomyopathy. Heart 76:243, 1996
71. Kandolf R, Ameis D, Kirschner P: In situ detection of enteroviral genomes in myocardial cells by nucleic acid hybridization: An approach to the diagnosis of viral heart disease. Proc Natl Acad Sci U S A 84:6272, 1987
72. Berger MM, Redl B, Aymard M, Bruno L: Direct in situ transcriptase polymerase chain reaction for the detection of enterovirus genome in liver tissues. J Virol Methods 65:55, 1997
73. Klingel K, Hohenadl C, Canu A, et al: Ongoing enterovirus-induced myocarditis is associated with persistent heart muscle infection: Quantitative analysis of virus replication, tissue damage, and inflammation. Proc Natl Acad Sci U S A 89:314, 1992
74. Chow LH, Gauntt CJ, McManus BM: Differential effects of myocarditic variants of coxsackievirus B3 in inbred mice: A pathologic characterization of heart tissue damage. Lab Invest 64:55, 1991
75. McManus BM, Chow LH, Wilson JE, et al: Direct myocardial injury by enterovirus: A central role in the evolution of murine myocarditis. Clin Immunol Immunopathol 68:159, 1993
76. McManus BM, Chow LH, Wilson JE, et al: Direct damage of myocardium by enterovirus: Old and new evidence for a preeminent injurious role in murine myocarditis. In: Figulla HR, Kandolf R, McManus BM: Idiopathic Dilated Cardiomyopathy: Cellular and Molecular Mechanisms, Clinical Consequences. Berlin, Springer Verlag, 1993, p 284
77. Hohenadl C, Klingel K, Mertsching J, et al: Strand-specific detection of enteroviral RNA in myocardial tissue by in situ hybridization. Mol Cell Probes 5:11, 1991
78. Hohenadl C, Klingel K, Rieger P, et al: Investigation of the coxsackievirus B3 nonstructural proteins 2B, 2C, and 3AB: Generation of specific polyclonal antisera and detection of replicating virus in infected tissue. J Virol Methods 47:279, 1994
79. Klingel K, McManus BM, Kandolf R: Enterovirus-infected immune cells of spleen and lymph nodes in the murine model of chronic myocarditis: A role in pathogenesis? Eur Heart J 16(suppl O):42, 1995
80. Brahic M, Stowring L, Ventura P, Haase AT: Gene expression in visna virus infection in sheep. Nature 292:240, 1981
81. Klingel K, Stephan S, Sauter M, et al: Pathogenesis of murine enterovirus myocarditis: Virus dissemination and immune cell targets. J Virol 70:8888, 1996
82. Klingel K, Rieger P, Mall G, et al: Visualization of enteroviral replication in myocardial tissue by ultrastructural in situ hybridization: Identification of target cells and cytopathic effects. Lab Invest 78:1227, 1998
83. Martino TA, Sole MJ, Penn LZ, et al: Quantitation of enteroviral RNA by competitive polymerase chain reaction. J Clin Microbiol 31:2634, 1993
84. Chow LH, Ye YL, Gauntt CJ, McManus BM: Early cellular infiltrates in coxsackievirus B3 murine myocarditis. In: Schultheiss HP (ed): New Concepts in Viral Heart Disease. Berlin, Springer Verlag, 1988, p 205
85. Chow LH, Ye YL, Linder J, McManus BM: Phenotypic analysis of infiltrating cells in human myocarditis: An immunohistochemi-

cal study in paraffin-embedded tissue. Arch Pathol Lab Med 113:1357, 1989
86. Chow LH, Beisel KW, McManus BM: Enteroviral infection of mice with severe combined immunodeficiency: Evidence for direct viral pathogenesis of myocardial injury. Lab Invest 66:24, 1992
87. Kishimoto C, Kurnick JT, Fallon JT, et al: Characteristics of lymphocytes cultured from murine viral myocarditis specimens: A preliminary and technical report. J Am Coll Cardiol 14:799, 1989
88. Chow LH, Switzer BL, McManus BM, Johnson DR: In vitro culture of cells infiltrating infected mouse hearts: Correlative studies with tissue histology. Lab Invest 60:18A, 1989
88a. Liu P, Aitlin K, Kong YY, et al: The tyrosine kinase p561ck is essential in coxsackievirus B3-mediated heart disease. Nat Med 6:429, 2000
89. Kanda T, Yokoyama T, Ohshima S, et al: T-lymphocyte subsets as noninvasive markers of cardiomyopathy. Clin Cardiol 13:617, 1990
90. Herzum M, Maisch B: Humoral and cellular immune reactions to the myocardium in myocarditis. Herz 17:91, 1992
91. McManus BM, Chow LH, Radio SJ, et al: Progress and challenges in the pathologic diagnosis of myocarditis. Eur Heart J 12:18, 1991
92. Anderson JL, Carlquist JF, Hammond EH: Deficient natural killer cell activity in patients with idiopathic dilated cardiomyopathy. Lancet 2:1124, 1982
93. Lozano MD, Rubocki RJ, Wilson JE, et al: Human leukocyte antigen class II associations in patients with idiopathic dilated cardiomyopathy. J Cardiac Failure 3:97, 1997
94. Herskowitz A, Ahmed-Ansari A, Neumann DA: Induction of major histocompatibility complex antigens within the myocardium of patients with active myocarditis: A nonhistologic marker of myocarditis. J Am Coll Cardiol 15:624, 1990
95. Hufnagel G, Maisch B: Expression of MHC class I and II antigens and the Il-2 receptor in rejection, myocarditis and dilated cardiomyopathy. Eur Heart J 12(suppl D):137, 1991
96. Hammond EH, Menlove RL, Yowell RL, Anderson JL: Vascular HLA-DR expression correlates with pathologic changes suggestive of ischemia in idiopathic dilated cardiomyopathy. Clin Immunol Immunopathol 68:197, 1993
97. Schultheiss HP, Schwimmbeck P, Bolte HD, Klingenberg M: The antigenic characteristics and the significance of the adenine nucleotide translocator as a major autoantigen to antimitochondrial antibodies in dilated cardiomyopathy. Adv Myocardiol 6:311, 1985
98. Caforio AL, Grazzini M, Mann JM, et al: Identification of alpha- and beta-cardiac myosin heavy chain isoforms as major autoantigens in dilated cardiomyopathy. Circulation 85:1734, 1992
99. Maisch B, Bauer E, Cirsi M, Kochsiek K: Cytolytic cross-reactive antibodies directed against the cardiac membrane and viral proteins in coxsackievirus B3 and B4 myocarditis: Characterization and pathogenetic relevance. Circulation 87 (suppl 5):IV-49, 1993
100. Hammond EH, Menlove RL, Anderson JL: Predictive value of immunofluorescence and electron microscopic evaluation of endomyocardial biopsies in the diagnosis and prognosis of myocarditis and idiopathic dilated cardiomyopathy. Am Heart J 114:1055, 1987
101. Smith SC, Ladenson JH, Mason JW, Jaffe AS: Elevations of cardiac troponin I associated with myocarditis: Experimental and clinical correlates. Circulation 95:163, 1997
102. Drucker NA, Colan SD, Lewis AB, et al: Gamma-globulin treatment of acute myocarditis in the pediatric population. Circulation 89:252, 1994
103. Heim A, Brehm C, Stille-Siegener M, et al: Cultured human myocardial fibroblasts of pediatric origin: Natural human interferon-alpha is more effective than recombinant interferon-alpha 2a in carrier-state coxsackievirus B3 replication. J Mol Cell Cardiol 27:2199, 1995
104. Kleinert S, Weintraub RG, Wilkinson JL, Chow CW: Myocarditis in children with dilated cardiomyopathy: Incidence and outcome after dual therapy immunosuppression. J Heart Lung Transplant 16:1248, 1997
105. Parillo JE: Myocarditis: How should we treat in 1998? J Heart Lung Transplant 17:941, 1998
106. Kaplan MH: Coxsackievirus infection in children under three

months of age. In: Bendinelli M, Friedman H (eds): Coxsackieviruses: A General Update. New York, Plenum Press, 1988, p 241

107. Nicholson F, Ajetunmobi JF, Li M, et al: Molecular detection and serotypic analysis of enterovirus RNA in archival specimens from patients with acute myocarditis. Br Heart J 74:522, 1995

108. Chiang FT, Lin LI, Tseng YZ, et al: Detection of enterovirus RNA in patients with idiopathic dilated cardiomyopathy by polymerase chain reaction. J Formos Med Assoc 91:569, 1992

109. Koide H, Kitaura Y, Deguchi H, et al: Genomic detection of enteroviruses in the myocardium—studies on animal hearts with coxsackievirus B3 myocarditis and endomyocardial biopsies from patients with myocarditis and dilated cardiomyopathy. Jpn Circ J 56:1081, 1992

110. Martin AB, Webber S, Fricker FJ, et al: Acute myocarditis: Rapid diagnosis by PCR in children. Circulation 90:330, 1994

111. Anderson DR, Wilson JE, Carthy CM, et al: Direct interactions of coxsackievirus B3 with immune cells in the splenic compartment of mice susceptible or resistant to myocarditis. J Virol 70:4632, 1996

112. Huber SA, Gauntt CJ, Sakkinen P: Enteroviruses and myocarditis: Viral pathogenesis through replication, cytokine induction, and immunopathogenicity. In: Advances in Virus Research. Vol 51. Maramorosch K: New York, Academic Press, 1999, p 35

113. Huber M, Watson KA, Selinka HC, et al: Cleavage of RasGAP and activation of mitogen-activated protein kinase in the course of coxsackievirus B3 replication. J Virol 73:3587, 1999

114. Zaragoza C, Ocampo C, Saura M, et al: The role of inducible nitric oxide synthase in the host response to coxsackievirus myocarditis. Proc Natl Acad Sci U S A 95:2469, 1998

115. Koglin J, Granville DJ, Glysing-Jensen T, et al: Attenuated acute cardiac rejection in NOS2-/- recipients correlates with reduced apoptosis. Circulation 99:836, 1999

116. Yu JZ, Wilson JE, Wood SM, et al: Secondary heterotypic versus homotypic infection by coxsackie B group viruses: Impact on early and late histopathological lesions and virus genome prominence. Cardiovasc Pathol 8:93, 1999

117. Kapadia S, Dibbs Z, Kurrelmeyer K: The role of cytokines in the failing human heart. Cardiol Clin 16:645, 1998

118. Mapoles JE, Krah DL, Crowell RL: Purification of a HeLa cell receptor protein for group B coxsackieviurses. J Virol 55:560, 1985

119. Hsu KH, Lonberg-Holm K, Alstein B, et al: A monoclonal antibody specific for the cellular receptor for the group B coxsackieviruses. J Virol 62:1647, 1988

120. Tomko RP, Xu R, Philipson L: HCAR and MCAR: The human and mouse cellular receptors for subgroup C adenoviruses and group B coxsackieviruses. Proc Natl Acad Sci U S A 94:3352, 1998

121. Bergelson JM, Krithivas A, Celi L, et al: The murine CAR homolog is a receptor for coxsackie B viruses and adenoviruses. J Virol 72:415, 1998

122. Martino TA, Petric M, Brown M, et al: Cardiovirulent coxsackieviruses and the decay-accelerating factor (CD55) receptor. Virology 244:302, 1998

123. Kramer B, Huber M, Kern C, et al: Chinese hamster ovary cells are non-permissive towards infection with coxsackie B3 despite functional virus-receptor interactions. Virus Res 48:149, 1997

124. Gauntt CJ: Specific and non-specific heart defenses in enteroviral infections. In: Figulla HR, Kandolf R, McManus BM (eds): Idiopathic Dilated Cardiomyopathy: Cellular and Molecular Mechanisms, Clinical Consequences. Berlin, Springer Verlag, 1993, p 310

125. Yang DC, Wilson JE, Anderson DR, et al: *In vitro* mutational and inhibitory analysis of the *cis*-acting translational elements within the 5′ untranslated region of coxsackievirus B3: Potential targets for antiviral action of antisense oligomer. Virology 228:63, 1997

126. Liu Z, Carthy CM, Cheung P, et al: Structural and functional analysis of the 5′ untranslated region of coxsackievirus B3 RNA: *In vivo* translational and infectivity studies of full-length mutants. Virology 265:206, 1999

127. Cheung PKM, Carthy CM, Watson K, et al: Specific interactions of HeLa cell proteins with the 5′ and 3′ untranslated regions of coxsackievirus B3 RNA. Under review

128. Van Kuppeveld FJ, Hoenderop JG, Smeets RL, et al: Coxsackievirus protein 2B modifies endoplasmic reticulum membrane and plasma membrane permeability and facilitates virus release. EMBO J 16:3519, 1997

129. Carthy CM, Granville D, Watson KA, et al: Caspase activation and cleavage of substrates following coxsackievirus B3−induced cytopathic effect in HeLa cells. J Virol 72:7669, 1998

130. Tazelaar HD, Billingham ME: Leukocyte infiltrates in idiopathic dilated cardiomopathy. A source of confusion with active myocarditis. Am J Surg Pathol 10:405, 1986

131. Kuhl U, Noutsias M, Seeberg B, Schultheiss HP: Immunohistological evidence for a chronic intramyocardial inflammatory process in dilated cardiomopathy. Heart 75:295, 1996

132. Roberts WC, Siegel RJ, McManus BM: Idiopathic dilated cardiomyopathy: Analysis of 152 necropsy patients. Am J Cardiol 60: 1340, 1987

133. Torre-Amione G, Kapadia S, Lee J, et al: Expression and functional significance of tumor necrosis factor receptors in human myocardium. Circulation 92:1487, 1995

134. Nemickas R, Fishman D, Killip T, et al: Massive myocardial necrosis in a young woman. Am Heart J 95:766, 1978

135. Miklozek CL, Crumpacker CS, Royal HD, et al: Myocarditis presenting as acute myocardial infarction. Am Heart J 115:768, 1988

136. Narula J, Khaw BA, Dec GW, et al: Brief report: Recognition of acute myocarditis masquerading as acute myocardial infarction. N Engl J Med 328:100, 1993

137. Kopecky SL, Gersh BJ: Dilated cardiomyopathy and myocarditis: Natural history, etiology, clinical manifestations, and management. Curr Probl Cardiol 12:569, 1987

138. Abelmann WH, Lorell BH: The challenge of cardiomyopathy. J Am Coll Cardiol 13:1219, 1989

139. Marboe CC, Fenoglio JJ Jr: Pathology and natural history of human myocarditis. Pathol Immunopathol Res 7:226, 1988

140. Herskowitz A, Ansari AA: Myocarditis. In: Braunwald E (ed): Atlas of Heart Disease. Philadelphia, Current Medicine, 1995, p 9.1

141. O'Connell JB, Henkin RE, Robinson JA, et al: Gallium-67 imaging in patients with dilated cardiomyopathy and biopsy-proven myocarditis. Circulation 70:58, 1984

142. O'Connell JB: Endomyocardial biopsy in the diagnosis and treatment of myocarditis. In: Fowles RE (ed): Cardiac Biopsy. Mount Kisco, NY, Futura, 1992, p 165

143. Yasuda T, Palacios IF, Dec GW, et al: Indium-111 monoclonal antimyosin imaging in the diagnosis of acute myocarditis. Circulation 76:306, 1987

144. Friedrich MG, Strohm O, Schulz-Menger J, et al: Contrast media−enhanced magnetic resonance imaging visualizes myocardial changes in the course of viral myocarditis. Circulation 97:1802, 1998

145. Mason JW, Billingham ME, Ricci DR: Treatment of acute inflammatory myocarditis assisted by endomyocardial biopsy. Am J Cardiol 45:1037, 1980

146. Mortensen SA, Baandrup U, Buch J, et al: Immunosuppressive therapy of biopsy-proven myocarditis: Experiences with corticosteroids and cyclosporine. Int J Immunother 1:35, 1985

147. McNamara DM, Rosenblum WD, Janosko KM, et al: Intravenous immune globulin in the therapy of myocarditis and acute cardiomyopathy. Circulation 95:2476, 1997

148. Hosenpud JD, Bennett LE, Keck BM, et al: The registry of the International Society for Heart and Lung Transplantation: Fifteenth official report—1998. J Heart Lung Transplant 17:656, 1998

149. O'Connell JR, Dec GW, Goldenberg IF, et al: Results of heart transplantation for active lymphocytic myocarditis. J Heart Lung Transplant 9:351, 1990

150. Abelmann WH: Myocarditis. N Engl J Med 275:994, 1966

151. Johnson RA, Palacios I: Dilated cardiomyopathies of the adult. N Engl J Med 307:1119, 1982

152. Fallon JT: Myocarditis and dilated cardiomyopathy: Different stages of the same disease? In: Waller BF (ed): Contemporary Issues in Cardiovascular Pathology. Philadelphia, FA Davis, 1988, p 155

153. O'Connell JB, Robinson JA: Coxsackie viral myocarditis. Postgrad Med J 61:1127, 1985

154. Orinius E: The late cardiac prognosis after Coxsackie-B infection. Acta Med Scand 183:235, 1968

155. Smith WG: Coxsackie B myopericarditis in adults. Am Heart J 80: 34, 1970

156. Gerzen P, Granath A, Holmgren B, Zetterquist S: Acute myocarditis: A follow-up study. Br Heart J 34:575, 1972

157. Cambridge G, MacArthur CGC, Waterson AP, et al: Antibodies to coxsackie B viruses in congestive cardiomyopathy. Br Heart J 41: 692, 1979

158. Kitura Y: Virological study of idiopathic cardiomyopathy: Serological study of virus antibodies and immunofluorescent study of myocardial biopsies. Jpn Circ J 41:279, 1981

159. Dec GW, Palacios IF, Fallon JT, et al: Active myocarditis in the spectrum of acute dilated cardiomyopathies: Clinical features, histologic correlates, and clinical outcome. N Engl J Med 312:885, 1985

160. Wilson MS, Barth RF, Baker PB, et al: Giant cell myocarditis. Am J Med 79:647, 1985

161. Cooper LT, Berry GJ, Rizeq M, Schroeder JS: Giant cell myocarditis. J Heart Lung Transplant 14:394, 1995

162. Cooper LT, Berry GJ, Shabetai R: Idiopathic giant cell myocarditis—natural history and treatment. N Engl J Med 336:1860, 1997

163. Saltykow S: Über diffuse myokarditis. Arch Pathol Lab Med Anat 182:1, 1905

164. Davies MJ, Pomerance A, Teare RD: Idiopathic giant cell myocarditis—a distinctive clinico-pathological entity. Br Heart J 37:192, 1975

165. Litovsky SH, Burke AP, Virmani R: Giant cell myocarditis: An entity distinct from sarcoidosis characterized by multiphasic myocyte destruction by cytotoxic T cells and histiocytic giant cells. Mod Pathol 9:1126, 1996

166. Pyun KS, Kim YH, Kalzenstein RE, Kikkawa Y: Giant cell myocarditis: Light and electron microscopic study. Arch Pathol 90:181, 1970

167. Rabson AB, Schoen FJ, Warhol MJ, et al: Giant cell myocarditis after mitral valve replacement: Case report and studies of the nature of giant cells. Hum Pathol 15:585, 1984

168. Theaker JM, Gatter KC, Brown DC, et al: An investigation into the nature of giant cells in cardiac and skeletal muscle. Hum Pathol 19:974, 1988

169. Kodama M, Matsumoto Y, Fujiwara M, et al: Characteristics of giant cells and factors related to the formation of giant cells in myocarditis. Circ Res 69:1042, 1991

170. Avellini C, Alampi G, Cocchi V, et al: Acute idiopathic interstitial giant cell myocarditis: A histological and immunohistological study of a case. Pathologica 83:229, 1991

171. Takeda A, Takeda N, Sakata A, et al: What is the nature of multinucleated giant cells in giant cell myocarditis? Cardiovasc Pathobiol 2:119, 1997

172. Tubbs RR, Sheibani K, Hawk WA: Giant cell myocarditis. Arch Pathol Lab Med 104:245, 1980

173. Tanaka M, Ichinohasama R, Kawahara Y, et al: Acute idiopathic interstitial myocarditis: A case report with special reference to morphological characteristics of the giant cells. J Clin Pathol 39: 1209, 1986

174. Langston JD, Wagman GF, Dickenman RC: Granulomatous myocarditis and myositis associated with thymoma. Arch Pathol 68: 367, 1959

175. Burke JS, Medline NM, Katz A: Giant cell myocarditis and myositis, associated with thymoma and myesthenia gravis. Arch Pathol 88:359, 1969

176. de Jongste MJ, Oosterhuis HJ, Lie KI: Intractable ventricular tachycardia in a patient with giant cell myocarditis, thymoma and myasthenia gravis. Int J Cardiol 13:374, 1986

177. Butany JW, McAuley P, Bergeron C, MacLaughlin P: Giant cell myocarditis and myositis associated with thymoma and leprosy. Can J Cardiol 7:141, 1991

178. Hales SA, Theaker JM, Gatter KC: Giant cell myocarditis associated with lymphoma: An immunocytochemical study. J Clin Pathol 40:1310, 1987

179. Klein BR, Hedges TR III, Dayal Y, Adelman LS: Orbital myositis and giant cell myocarditis. Neurology 39:988, 1989

180. Leib ML, Odel JG, Cooney MJ: Orbital polymyositis and giant cell myocarditis. Ophthalmology 101:950, 1994

181. Kloin JE: Pernicious anemia and giant cell myocarditis. Am J Med 78:355, 1985

182. McKeon J, Haagsma B, Bett JH, Boyle CM: Fatal giant cell myocarditis after colectomy for ulcerative colitis. Am Heart J 111: 1208, 1986

183. Ariza A, Lopez D, Mate JL, et al: Giant cell myocarditis: Monocytic immunophenotype of giant cells in a case associated with ulcerative colitis. Hum Pathol 126:121, 1995

184. Humbert P, Faivre R, Fellman D, et al: Giant cell myocarditis: An autoimmune disease? Am Heart J 115:485, 1988

185. Kodama M, Matsumoto Y, Fujiwara M, et al: A novel experimental model of giant cell myocarditis induced in rats by immunization with cardiac myosin fraction. Clin Immunol Immunopathol 57:250, 1990

186. Kodama M, Hanawa J, Sacki M, et al: Rat dilated cardiomyopathy after autoimmune giant cell myocarditis. Circ Res 75:278, 1994

187. Zhang S, Kodama M, Hanawa H, et al: Effects of cyclosporine, prednisolone and aspirin on rat autoimmune giant cell myocarditis. J Am Coll Cardiol 21:1254, 1993

188. Hanawa H, Kodama M, Inomata T, et al: Anti-alpha beta T cell receptor antibody prevents the progression of experimental autoimmune myocarditis. Clin Exp Immunol 96:470, 1994

189. Ren H, Poston RS, Hruban RH, et al: Long survival with giant cell myocarditis. Mod Pathol 6:402, 1993

190. Kong G, Madden B, Spyrou N, et al: Response of recurrent giant cell myocarditis in a transplanted heart to intensive immunosuppression. Eur Heart J 12:554, 1991

191. Gries W, Farkas D, Winters GL, Costanzo-Nordin MR: Giant cell myocarditis: First report of disease recurrence in the transplanted heart. J Heart Lung Transplant 11:370, 1992

192. Grant SCD: Recurrent giant cell myocarditis after transplantation. J Heart Lung Transplant 12:155, 1993

193. Silverman KJ, Hutchins GM, Bulkley BM: Cardiac sarcoid: A clinicopathologic evaluation of 84 unselected patients with systemic sarcoidosis. Circulation 58:1204, 1978

194. Glazier JJ: Specific heart muscle disease. In: Braunwald E (ed): Atlas of Heart Diseases: Cardiomyopathies, Myocarditis, and Pericardial Diseases. Philadelphia, Current Medicine, 1995, p 4.8

195. Roberts WC, McAllister HA, Ferrans VJ: Sarcoidosis of the heart: A clinicopathologic study of 35 necropsy patients (group I) and review of 78 previously described necropsy patients (group II). Am J Med 63:86, 1977

196. Virmani R, Bures JC, Roberts WC: Cardiac sarcoidosis: A major cause of sudden death in young individuals. Chest 77:423, 1980

197. Ratner SJ, Fenoglio JJ Jr, Ursell PC: Utility of endomyocardial biopsy in the diagnosis of cardiac sarcoidosis. Chest 90:528, 1986

198. Sekiguchi M, Yazaki Y, Isobe M, Hiroe M: Cardiac sarcoidosis: Diagnostic, prognostic, and therapeutic considerations. Cardiovasc Drugs Ther 10:495, 1996

199. Sharma OP: Cardiac and neurologic dysfunction in sarcoidosis. Clin Chest Med 18:813, 1997

200. Valantine HA, Tazelaar HD, Macoviak J, et al: Cardiac sarcoidosis: Response to steroids and transplantation. J Heart Lung Transplant 6:244, 1987

201. Oni AA, Hershberger RE, Norman DJ, et al: Recurrence of sarcoidosis in a cardiac allograft: Control with augmented corticosteroids. J Heart Lung Transplant 11:367, 1992

202. Bali HK, Wahi S, Sharma BK, et al: Myocardial tuberculosis presenting as restrictive cardiomyopathy. Am Heart J 120:703, 1990

203. Chan AC, Dickens P: Tuberculous myocarditis presenting as sudden cardiac death. Forensic Sci Int 57:45, 1992

204. Rothenberg ME: Eosinophilia. N Engl J Med 338:1592, 1998

205. Burke AP, Saenger J, Mullick F, Virmani R: Hypersensitivity myocarditis. Arch Pathol Lab Med 115:764, 1991

206. Kounis NG, Zavras GM, Soufras GD, Kitrou MP: Hypersensitivity myocarditis. Ann Allergy 62:71, 1989

207. Seeverens H, deBruin C, Jordan J: Myocarditis and methyldopa. Acta Med Scand 211:233, 1982

208. Gravanis MB, Hertzler GL, Franch RH, et al: Hypersensitivity myocarditis in heart transplant candidates. J Heart Lung Transplant 10:688, 1991

209. Lewin D, d'Amati G, Lewis W: Hypersensitivity myocarditis: Findings in native and transplanted hearts. Cardiovasc Pathol 1: 225, 1992

210. de Alava E, Panizo-Santos A, Fernandez-Gonzalez AL, Pardo-

Mindan FJ: Eosinophilic myocarditis in patients waiting for heart transplantation. Cardiovasc Pathol 4:43, 1995

211. Kendall KR, Day JD, Hruban RH, et al: Intimate association of eosinophils to collagen bundles in eosinophilic myocarditis and ranitidine-induced hypersensitivity myocarditis. Arch Pathol Lab Med 119:1154, 1995

212. McManus BM, Wood SM: Inflammatory mechanisms of toxic and allergic injury of the heart and blood vessels. In: Sipes IG, McQueen CA, Gandolfi AJ (eds): Comprehensive Toxicology. Vol 6. Cardiovascular Toxicology. New York, Elsevier, 1997, p 411

213. Herzog CA, Snover DC, Staley NA: Acute necrotising eosinophilic myocarditis. Br Heart J 52:343, 1984

214. Getz MA, Subramanian R, Logemann T, Ballantyne F: Acute necrotizing eosinophilic myocarditis as a manifestation of severe hypersensitivity myocarditis: Antemortem diagnosis and successful treatment. Ann Intern Med 115:201, 1991

215. Parrillo JE: Heart disease and the eosinophil. N Engl J Med 323:1560, 1990

216. Baily GG: Parasitic infections of the heart. J Infect 37:2, 1998

217. Cammarosano C, Lewis W: Cardiac lesions in acquired immune deficiency syndrome (AIDS). J Am Coll Cardiol 5:703, 1985

218. Roldan EO, Moskowitz L, Hensley GT: Pathology of the heart in acquired immunodeficiency syndrome. Arch Pathol Lab Med 111:943, 1987

219. Anderson DW, Virmani R: Emerging patterns of heart disease in human immunodeficiency virus infection. Hum Pathol 21:253, 1990

220. Patel RC, Frishman WH: AIDS and the heart: Clinicopathologic assessment. Cardiovasc Pathol 4:173, 1995

221. Harrity PJ, Subramanian R: Human immunodeficiency virus infection cardiac lesions. In: Connor DH, Chandler FW, Schwartz DA, et al (eds): Pathology of Infectious Diseases. Vol 1. Stamford CT, Appleton & Lange, 1997, p 153

222. Barbaro G, Di Lorenzo G, Grisorio B, Barbarini G: Incidence of dilated cardiomyopathy and detection of HIV in myocardial cells of HIV-positive patients. N Engl J Med 339:1093, 1998

223. Ho DD, Pomerantz RJ, Kaplan JC: Pathogenesis of infection with human immunodeficiency virus. N Engl J Med 317:278, 1987

224. Grody WW, Cheng L, Lewis W: Infection of the heart by the human immunodeficiency virus. Am J Cardiol 66:203, 1990

225. Lipshultz SE, Fox CH, Perez-Atayde AT, et al: Identification of human immunodeficiency virus-1 RNA and DNA in the heart of a child with cardiovascular abnormalities and congenital acquired immune deficiency syndrome. Am J Cardiol 66:246, 1990

226. Cenacchi G, Re MC, Furlini G, et al: Human immunodeficiency virus type 1 antigen detection in endomyocardial biopsy: An immunomorphological study. Microbiologica 13:145, 1990

227. Rodriguez ER, Nasim S, Hsia J, et al: Cardiac myocytes and dendritic cells harbor human immunodeficiency virus in infected patients with and without cardiac dysfunction: Detection by multiplex, nested, polymerase chain reaction in individually microdissected cells from right ventricular endomyocardial biopsy tissue. Am J Cardiol 68:1511, 1991

228. Burgdorfer W, Barbour AG, Hayes SF, et al: Lyme disease—a tick-borne spirochetosis? Science 216:1317, 1982

229. Steere AC: Lyme disease. N Engl J Med 321:586, 1989

230. Spach DH, Liles WC, Campbell GL, et al: Tick-borne diseases in the United States. N Engl J Med 329:936, 1993

231. Lyme disease—United States, 1995. MMWR Morb Mortal Wkly Rep 45:481, 1996

232. Steere AC, Batsford WP, Weinberg M, et al: Lyme carditis: Cardiac abnormalities of Lyme disease. Ann Intern Med 93:8, 1980

233. Duray PH, Chandler FW: Lyme disease. In: Connor DH, Chandler FW, Schwartz DA, et al (eds): Pathology of Infectious Diseases. Vol 1. Appleton & Lange, Stamford, 1997, p 635

234. Stanek G, Klein J, Bittner R, Glogar D: Isolation of Borrelia burgdorferi from the myocardium of a patient with longstanding cardiomyopathy. N Engl J Med 322:249, 1990

235. Preacmur V, Weber K, Pfister HW, et al: Survival of Borrelia burgdorferi in antibiotically treated patients with Lyme borreliosis. Infection 17:355, 1989

236. Steere AC, Sikand VK, Meurice F, et al: Vaccination against Lyme disease with recombinant Borrelia burgdorferi outer-surface lipoprotein A with adjuvant. N Engl J Med 339:209, 1998

237. Sigal LH, Zahradnik JM, Lavin P, et al: A vaccine consisting of recombinant Borrelia burgdorferi outer-surface protein A to prevent Lyme disease. N Engl J Med 339:216, 1998

238. Acquatella H: Chagas' disease. In: Braunwald E (ed): Atlas of Heart Diseases: Cardiomyopathies, Myocarditis, and Pericardial Disease. Philadelphia, Current Medicine, 1995, p 8.1

239. Kirchhoff LV: American trypanosomiasis (Chagas' disease)—a tropical disease now in the United States. N Engl J Med 329:639, 1993

240. Lack EE, Filie A: American trypanosomiasis. In: Connor DH, Chandler FW, Schwartz DA, et al (eds): Pathology of Infectious Diseases. Vol 2. Stamford, CT Appleton & Lange, 1997, p 1297

241. Oliveira JS, Mello De Olivera JA, Frederigue U Jr, Lima Filho EC: Apical aneurysm of Chagas' heart disease. Br Heart J 46:432, 1981

242. Rossi MA, Ramos SG: Pathogenesis of chronic Chagas' myocarditis: An overview. Cardiovasc Pathol 5:197, 1996

243. Hagar JM, Rahimtoola SH: Chagas' heart disease in the United States. N Engl J Med 325:763, 1991

244. Bocchi EA, Bellotti G, Uip D, et al: Long-term follow-up after heart transplantation in Chagas' disease. Transplant Proc 25:1329, 1993

245. Almeida DR, Carvalho AC, Branco JN, et al: Chagas' disease reactivation after heart transplantation: Efficacy of allopurinol treatment. J Heart Lung Transplant 15:988, 1996

246. Stockins BA, Lanas FT, Saavedra JG, Opazo JA: Prognosis in patients with diphtheric myocarditis and bradyarrhythmias: Assessment of results of ventricular pacing. Br Heart J 72:190, 1994

247. Cowan MJ, Reichenbach D, Turner P, Thostenson C: Cellular response of the evolving myocardial infarction after therapeutic coronary artery reperfusion. Hum Pathol 22:154, 1991

248. Reichenbach D, Cowan MJ: Healing of myocardial infarction with and without reperfusion. In: Virmani R, Atkinson JB, Fenoglio JJ (eds): Cardiovascular Pathology. Philadelphia, WB Saunders, 1991, p 86

249. Todd GL, Baroldi G, Pieper GM, et al: Experimental catecholamine-induced myocardial necrosis. I. Morphology, quantification and regional distribution of acute contraction band lesions. J Mol Cell Cardiol 17:317, 1985

250. Case records of the Massachusetts General Hospital (Case 15-1988). N Engl J Med 318:970, 1988

Chapter 10

Cardiomyopathies

. . . . .

Pietro Gallo • Giulia d'Amati

DEFINITION OF CARDIOMYOPATHY

Until recently, the unifying feature of cardiomyopathies was an ignorance of their etiology; indeed, they were defined by the World Health Organization/International Society and Federation of Cardiology (WHO/ISFC) as "heart muscle diseases of unknown cause."[1] Cardiomyopathies have also been called "primary" diseases because of their unknown cause and because they are limited to the myocardium. In fact, a "specific heart muscle disease," as distinct from cardiomyopathy, was defined by the WHO/ISFC as "heart muscle disease of known cause or associated with disorders of other systems." The 1980 classification defined three groups: dilated, hypertrophic, and restrictive cardiomyopathy. The last was restricted to Loeffler endocarditis and endomyocardial fibrosis.

In the early 1990s, a revision of the WHO/ISFC classification was considered necessary to encompass two newly described entities: "primary" restrictive cardiomyopathy and arrhythmogenic "right ventricular" cardiomyopathy.[2] Moreover, a genetic predisposition, in terms of either etiology or pathogenesis, has been identified in patients with many cardiomyopathies, and a genetic background was considered a unifying and common trait. However, sporadic forms of each cardiomyopathy share the same clinical, functional, and pathologic features as familial ones, and even within the same family, among patients having the same genetic defect, there is much phenotypic variability. Therefore, genetic information demonstrated that cardiomyopathies are not always of unknown cause, but it did not produce common pathogenetic mechanisms. As a consequence, a new WHO/ISFC task force[3] defined cardiomyopathies as "diseases of the myocardium associated with clinical dysfunction," disregarding their primary nature. However, even if genetic defects are increasingly accepted as etiologic factors, the pathogenetic triggers are still largely obscure, and we accordingly prefer to maintain the primary nature of cardiomyopathies as a defining trait.

The individual cardiomyopathies are defined according to their functional characteristics (e.g., dilated, restrictive, or arrhythmogenic) instead of their etiologic or pathologic traits. This is justified by continuing uncertainty about etiology, with complex links between proved genetic background, marked phenotypic variability, and intervening acquired factors; and by the presence of common functional patterns between different forms: hypertrophic cardiomyopathies with either a dilated or restrictive physiology; arrhythmogenic cardiomyopathies with adipose replacement of the right ventricular myocardium and dilation of the left ventricle; genetic mimics, such as mitochondrial cardiomyopathies, which may manifest with either a hypertrophic or a dilated pattern; or Noonan syndrome, which can produce either a hypertrophic or a restrictive pattern.

In conclusion, we define cardiomyopathies as myocardial diseases characterized by obscure etiologies, often with a mixture of genetic and acquired factors; by the coexistence of distinctive pathologic traits and nonspecific features; and by overlapping natural histories and functional patterns.

CLASSIFICATION OF CARDIOMYOPATHIES

There is at present no way of providing a proper classification of cardiomyopathies; they can only be itemized. This chapter describes four major classes of cardiomyopathies—dilated, hypertrophic, restrictive, and arrhythmogenic forms (Table 10-1)—as well as a group of "specific" cardiomyopathies, such as the ones occurring in muscular dystrophies, neuromuscular disorders, and myopathies. The 1995 WHO/ISFC classification[3] also includes a group of "unclassified cardiomyopathies," such as endocardial fibroelastosis, mildly dilated cardiomyopathy, and mitochondrial cardiomyopathies; these are covered here under separate headings.

DILATED CARDIOMYOPATHY

Definition

Dilated cardiomyopathy is a primary myocardial disease "characterized by dilatation and impaired contraction of the left ventricle or both ventricles."[3] Valvular, hypertensive, congenital, or ischemic conditions may cause a similar dysfunction, and must be excluded. A chance finding of coronary atherosclerosis does not rule out a diagnosis of dilated cardiomyopathy, provided "the degree of myocardial dysfunction is not explained by the extent of ischemic damage."[3] Even though genetic, viral, toxic, metabolic, or immunologic causes have been described, they apply to only a minority of cases and seemingly have a nonspecific predisposing or triggering role. The reference standard accordingly remains the idiopathic disease, and in this chapter the term dilated cardiomyopathy refers to the idiopathic form if not otherwise stated. An account of what is known of etiology and pathogenesis is given under the appropriate headings.

TABLE 10-1 • **Comparison of Pathologic, Etiologic, and Natural History Features in the Four Major Classes of Cardiomyopathy**

Cardiomyopathy	Major Pathologic Features	Possible Causes	Natural History
Dilated	LV (usually biventricular) eccentric hypertrophy Myocyte hypertrophy with myofibril loss	Autosomal dominant heredity (candidate genes on Ch 1, 3, 9, 10) Autosomal recessive heredity X-linked heredity (dystrophin gene) Viral infections Autoimmunity Myocardial toxicity	Biventricular pump failure Sudden death Steady course or improvement
Hypertrophic	LV/biventricular asymmetric (less frequently symmetric) hypertrophy Myocardial disarrangement at gross, microscopic, ultrastructural, and cytoarchitectural levels	Autosomal dominant heredity (genes on Ch 14q, 1q, 15q, 11p, 7q) Genetic mimics: Noonan and Costello syndromes, lentiginosis, mitochondrial cardiomyopathies	Sudden death Subaortic obstruction LV pump failure Impaired ventricular compliance
Restrictive	Ventricular stiffness (e.g., myocardial fibrosis, amyloidosis) and/or endocardial fibro(elasto)sis Enlarged atria	Unknown cause Genetic Infiltrative disease Acquired factors (virus, toxic, ion deficiency) Congenital	Impaired ventricular compliance Reduced diastolic LV or biventricular volume
Arrhythmogenic	RV (frequently biventricular) adipose or fibroadipose replacement RV aneurysms LV dilation	Autosomal dominant heredity (candidate genes on Ch 14, 1, 2, 3) Autosomal recessive heredity (candidate gene on Ch 17) Myocarditis	Concealed form (sudden death) Overt electrical disorder (threatening arrhythmias) RV failure (maintained LV function) Biventricular pump failure

Ch, chromosome; LV, left ventricular; RV, right ventricular.

Pathology

Gross Anatomy

Hearts with dilated cardiomyopathy have a striking gross appearance. There is a huge increase in mass (Fig. 10-1A), and heart weight exceeds 500 g (cor bovinum) in more than half of the cases.[4–6] On average, long-term survivors have significantly heavier hearts than those who die in the short term,[4, 7] whereas the inverse is true for the isolated weight of the right ventricle.[4] Also, because of ventricular dilation and apical rounding, the heart shape is modified. When dilation affects mainly the left ven-

tricular cavity, the right ventricle may appear displaced, but the usual configuration is of four-chamber dilation (see Fig. 10-1A), the heart appearing almost spherical, and a proper apex is not obvious. The epicardium is usually normal and coronary arteries appear straight, even stretched (see Fig. 10-5C). The myocardium is rather flabby, and the ventricular wall usually collapses when sectioned.

For clinical pathologic correlation, the most appropriate way of opening the heart is along an echocardiographic plane, either an apical four-chamber view or a short-axis section. On cut surface, the ventricles show an

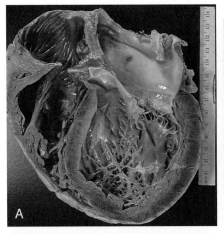 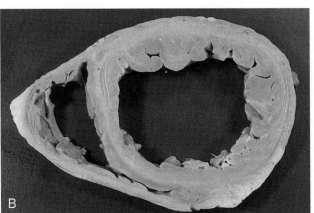

Figure 10-1 • Dilated cardiomyopathy. *A,* Four-chamber section of the heart of a 58-year-old man. All chambers are dilated, and the left ventricle has a globoid appearance, with rightward deviation of the ventricular septum. *B,* Native heart of a 55-year-old man, transplanted for dilated cardiomyopathy. The specimen was cut along a short-axis echocardiographic plane. Both ventricles show eccentric hypertrophy, with walls of normal thickness and prominent dilation of cavities, leading to marked reduction of the parietal thickness/cavity diameter ratio (left ventricle is to the right in photograph).

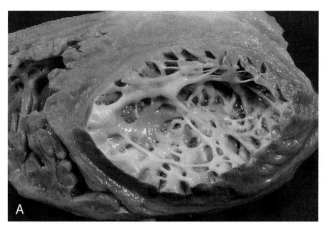
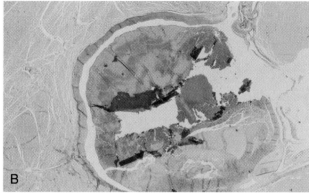

Figure 10-2 • *A,* Native heart of a 52-year-old man, transplanted for dilated cardiomyopathy. The specimen was cut along a short-axis plane passing near the apex and shows an irregularly thickened endocardium. *B,* Native heart of a 40-year-old man, transplanted for dilated cardiomyopathy. A trabecular recess of the left ventricle is filled with thrombotic material (Mallory trichrome stain).

eccentric hypertrophy (Fig. 10-1*B*) (i.e., a mass increase with chamber volume enlargement).[8] Although hypertrophy is demonstrated by cardiac weight increase, this is not always grossly evident because of dilation: the free wall width may be normal,[9] or thinned, as happens in short-term survivors.[4, 7] Because of the striking dilation of the cavity, there is a marked reduction in the ratio of parietal thickness to cavity diameter (see Fig. 10-1*B*), dropping from 0.48 (normal subjects) to 0.21 or even 0.17 (dilated cardiomyopathy with, respectively, long-term and short-term survival).[7] Fibrosis is frequent, and larger areas of replacement scarring are possible, raising a differential diagnosis with ischemic heart disease or some inflammatory disease, such as sarcoidosis.

Endocardial fibrosis is a common finding, especially at the apex (Fig. 10-2*A*). Albeit occasionally diffuse, it is usually focal, sometimes with the appearance of raised patches, which supposedly derive from the organization of mural thrombi. These thrombi occur frequently, especially in short-term survivors[7]; they are located mainly at the apex and may be in various stages of organization. Thrombus formation is fostered by the reduced ejection fraction, which converts the apex into a sort of caput mortuum. Thrombosis begins in small recesses within the trabecular myocardium (Fig. 10-2*B*). These endocardial thrombi may be the source of distant emboli. Kidneys, spleen, brain, and limbs are the most common sites of systemic embolization, but thrombosis of right-sided chambers and pulmonary embolism are not rare.[4]

Short-axis sections done by a pathologist demonstrate the dilation of ventricles well. When left ventricular distention prevails, its cavity gains a circular outline, and herniation of the ventricular septum causes a reduction in right ventricular cavity size. In biventricular dilation, the ventricular septum assumes an almost straight configuration, and the ventricles look like two adjoined letter Ds (Fig. 10-3*A*). Atrial dilation is usually prominent although less impressive than in other conditions such as atrioventricular valve stenosis or restrictive cardiomyopathy, and is thought to be the result of atrial involvement in the myopathic process.[10]

A primary valve disease must be excluded by definition. The semilunar valves are usually normal, whereas atrioventricular valves, and particularly the mitral valve, often display secondary insufficiency caused by the dilation of the valvular ring, with rolling of leaflet edges (Fig. 10-3*B*).

Histopathology

The histologic picture of dilated cardiomyopathy could be defined as a peculiar complex of nonspecific features. Although a cardiomyopathic pattern is recognizable at a glance, it consists of a list of features common to most end-stage cardiac conditions (Fig. 10-4*A*), which seem to be the consequence of a rise in parietal stress rather than its cause.

No myocardial component is spared by the disease: myocytes, interstitium, small vessels, and endocardium are all affected, but, as expected, myocytes show the most prominent changes. Histologic features are in keeping with the gross appearance of eccentric hypertrophy. Hypertrophy is usually associated with a marked increase in the area of a large population of myocytes (see later discussion) and is defined by a generalized enlargement of hyperchromatic, often bizarrely shaped nuclei (see Fig. 10-4*A*); dilation is marked by thinning and occasional "waving" of variable numbers of myocytes, caused by their lengthening[11–13] and by their side-to-side slippage[14] within muscular bundles. Attenuated myocytes (Fig. 10-4*B*) are easily recognizable not only in longitudinal sections but also in transverse slices passing through the nucleus. The enlarged nucleus tends to occupy the entire cross-sectional area, its rounded outline being remodeled to a rectangular one by sarcoplasmic stretching. The simultaneous presence of large hypertrophied cells and small attenuated elements in the same endomyocardial specimen characteristically produces an increased variability in the myocellular area.[15]

Another histopathologic equivalent to contractility failure is the typical finding of myofibril loss, which causes hydropic changes within the myocyte that range from a

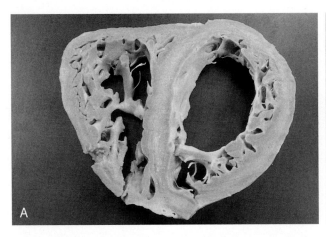
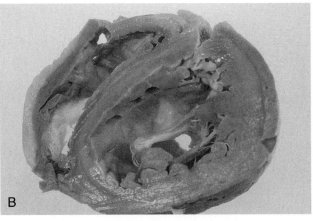

Figure 10-3 • *A,* Native heart of a 57-year-old man, transplanted for dilated cardiomyopathy. The specimen was cut along a midventricular short-axis plane. The ventricles show comparable eccentric hypertrophy, with a straight ventricular septum and biventricular endocardial fibrosis. *B,* The same heart as in Figure 10-2*A.* The valvular plane is viewed from below. Mitral valve leaflets have rolled edges as a result of secondary valvular incompetence.

perinuclear halo to a pattern of colliquative myocytolysis (see Chapter 8). These diffuse but nonspecific features are often present in the subendocardial layer. Myocellular derangement is also documented by immunohistochemistry, which shows a nonspecific increase and disorderly arrangement of desmin intermediate filaments,[16] and by electron microscopy (see later discussion).

An increase in intramyocardial fibrillar collagen (see Fig. 10-4*A*), and especially in the type I/type III ratio,[17] is a constant feature in this cardiomyopathy. Classically, fibrosis has been subdivided microscopically into replacement, interfiber, perivascular, and plexiform types.[18] Interfiber and perivascular fibroses usually prevail, especially in the left ventricle, but replacement sclerosis may be evident focally. Endocardial fibrosis may be characterized by a proliferation of smooth muscle cells, transformed into secreting cells.

The myocardium may be infiltrated by some inflammatory cells.[19] Usually, there are only a few lymphocytes, mainly adjacent to areas of replacement fibrosis. Their paucity and peculiar topographic distribution do not allow

a diagnosis of myocarditis.[20, 21] However, a differential diagnosis may be difficult, especially given the limited sampling offered by an endomyocardial biopsy.

The coronary arteries show, by definition, only mild lesions, proportional to the patient's age. Intramyocardial branches sometimes display a nonspecific proliferation of medial smooth muscle cells, with a luminal narrowing said to correlate with the ultrastructural finding of small vessels disease occasionally observed in these patients.[22]

Ultrastructure

Electron microscopy, like histology, fails to reveal any specific changes in dilated cardiomyopathy but may provide additional information, mainly about the nature of hypertrophy and myofibril loss.[4, 16]

Nuclei are enlarged and have irregular shape, with deep infoldings of the nuclear membrane that may mimic nuclear duplication.[23] Multiple nucleoli, inclusions of sarcoplasmic components,[24] and true double nuclei are not exceptional. Other changes consistent with myocellular

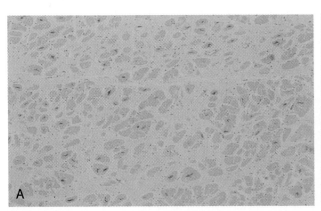
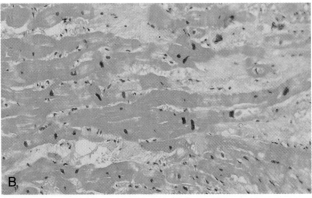

Figure 10-4 • *A,* Left ventricular specimen from a patient who died of dilated cardiomyopathy. Cardiomyopathic change is evident: hypertrophied myocytes, often with bizarrely shaped hyperchromatic nuclei, lie on a fibrous background, intermingled with small myocytes. *B,* Left ventricular endomyocardial biopsy from a 59-year-old male patient who had a dilated cardiomyopathy. Myocytes are attenuated and display transversely arranged hyperchromatic nuclei. Two months after the biopsy procedure, the patient underwent cardiac transplantation (H&E stain).

hypertrophy are the dilation and proliferation of T tubules, the occurrence of rough endoplasmic reticulum, and increased numbers of sarcomeres and mitochondria.[25] Rough endoplasmic reticulum is common in atrial cells and is associated with the secretion of natriuretic peptide. The frequent presence of this structure in ventricular myocytes[26] is supposedly related to the ventricular production of this peptide.[23] So-called mitochondriosis is by itself a nonspecific feature, although it is frequently encountered in mitochondrial cardiomyopathies (see later discussion).

Myofibril loss ranges from rarefaction to complete absence of sarcomeres.[16] Other degenerative changes include mitochondrial abnormalities,[27] deposits reminiscent of the "rod bodies" of nemaline myopathy,[23] myelin figures, and increased glycogen, lipid droplets, and phagolysosomes.

Electron microscopy may detect a series of lesions affecting capillaries and arterioles (up to 100 or sometimes to 200 μm in diameter) encompassed by the term small vessels disease. These pathologic changes may include a manifold thickening of the vascular basement membrane,[22] hyperplasia of smooth muscle cells of the arteriolar media,[28] and some changes affecting endothelial cells, ranging from regressive phenomena to cytoplasmic swelling.

Morphometry

Morphometry has long been employed to study dilated cardiomyopathy, reviewing both gross specimens and endomyocardial biopsies examined by light or electron microscopy. Its purposes have been several: to compare morphometric data with clinical and hemodynamic parameters,[29, 30] especially to understand the functional meaning of myocellular enlargement[30-32]; to predict a patient's prognosis[29, 31, 33-36]; to determine responsiveness to long-term β-blocker treatment[37-38]; and to compare atrial and ventricular pathologic features.[39]

Morphometry has given a quantitative basis to the finding of eccentric hypertrophy, demonstrating a volume increase of ventricular myocytes[9] accompanied by nuclear enlargement[30, 40] and signs of decompensation, such as myofibril loss[30, 41] and myocellular lengthening.[9] Degenerative phenomena culminate in a myocellular loss, documented by a reduced myocellular volume fraction in the myocardium[9] and by the occurrence of replacement fibrosis. Despite this widespread myocellular loss, the preservation of total myocyte number suggests that some myocellular proliferation must take place in the ventricular myocardium.[9]

As to the relationship between morphometric variables and functional status and outcome, the most consistent results were achieved with two morphometric variables: nuclear area and myofibril volume fraction (i.e., the ratio of the sarcoplasmic volume occupied by myofibrils). A nuclear enlargement is associated with both a worse functional status[30] and poorer prognosis[36]; the same is true of a reduced myofibril volume fraction (myofibril loss), in terms of both clinicopathologic correlation[30, 42, 43] and outcome.[31, 36] Conversely, conflicting results are obtained by evaluating the total area of myocytes: a myocellular enlargement has been associated with either a worse functional status[29, 32, 43] and poorer prognosis[29, 35, 44] or with no significant hemodynamic change,[30, 45, 46] or even with a

better outcome.[31] However, myocellular enlargement cannot properly be considered equivalent to myocellular hypertrophy because it is also caused by degenerative phenomena.

Indications for Endomyocardial Biopsy

In the first years of endomyocardial biopsy use, its effectiveness as a diagnostic tool in patients with dilated cardiomyopathy was controversial.[47-49] A biopsy was not considered diagnostic because dilated cardiomyopathy does not display a specific histopathologic picture, and it seemed to give additional information in only a limited number of cases, from as few as 10 to 15%[47, 50] up to 26%.[51] In a more recent series, however, a biopsy was found to modify the original diagnosis of dilated cardiomyopathy in as many as 50% of cases,[25] confirming its diagnostic value.

The indications for endomyocardial biopsy remain controversial in terms of risk and effectiveness. Nevertheless, it is reasonable to affirm that because an endomyocardial biopsy adds minimal risk to a cardiac catheterization,[25, 52-54] even though it is not strictly necessary for diagnostic purposes, it should be considered a useful complement to any invasive procedure. Another controversial point is whether cardiac catheterization should be restricted to a selected group of patients[55] or whether its use should be extended. The noninvasive assessment of dilated cardiomyopathy has shown a predictive value and diagnostic sensitivity of only 66 and 59%, respectively.[56] In the particular instance of ischemic cardiomyopathy, coronary angiography is not only necessary[57] but sometimes not even sufficient[58] for correct diagnosis.

But why is a biopsy useful? Histologic assessment allows an observer to exclude a specific cardiomyopathy[46, 48] or a myocarditis,[25, 47, 59, 60] or to suspect a mitochondrial cardiomyopathy.[25] Biopsy also permits clinical-hemodynamic correlations and prognostic inferences by means of morphometric (described earlier) or biochemical[47] analysis and provides material for research, such as studies of the correlation of dilated cardiomyopathy with immunologic markers,[61] the release of atrial natriuretic peptide,[62] or the effect of growth hormone.[63]

Etiology and Pathogenesis

The etiology and pathogenesis of idiopathic dilated cardiomyopathy are said to be unknown, because ischemic, valvular, and inflammatory causes are excluded from this diagnosis, but a series of putative causative agents have been identified, and dilated cardiomyopathy could be their nonspecific end point. Here, the causative roles of genetics, viral infections, and autoimmunity are discussed briefly, whereas the relationships of dilated cardiomyopathy to pregnancy, metabolic disorders, and cardiotoxicity are dealt with under separate headings.

Genetics

A familial inheritance has been detected in 20 to 30% of patients with dilated cardiomyopathy, with a prevalent autosomal dominant trait and variable penetrance.[64] Other familiar dilated cardiomyopathies are X-linked (X-linked cardiomyopathy, and neuromuscular disorders; see later discussions) or they manifest a pattern of maternal inheritance resulting from mitochondrial DNA mutations (mitochondrial cardiomyopathies; see later discussion). Rare recessive forms of dilated cardiomyopathy[65] characterized by worse prognosis[65a] have also been described. Homozygosis (DD) for the angiotensin-converting enzyme (ACE) gene correlates with the development of not only ischemic heart disease but also dilated cardiomyopathy.[66] (Chapter 16 describes cardiomyopathies associated with some other systemic diseases and conditions.)

Autosomal Dominant Dilated Cardiomyopathy

Despite the relatively high prevalence of autosomal dominant dilated cardiomyopathy, the molecular basis of myocardial dysfunction in these patients is still not known. Five associated loci have been mapped: two occur on chromosome 1[67, 68] and one each on chromosomes 3,[69] 9,[70] and 10.[71] The clinical phenotypes described vary from "pure" dilated cardiomyopathy[70] to an association of dilated cardiomyopathy with mitral valve prolapse[71] to a clinical picture dominated by conduction abnormalities.[67, 69] Pathologic findings are not dissimilar in familial and nonfamilial cardiomyopathies, and they cannot be distinguished morphologically.[72] In contrast to other cardiomyopathies (e.g., familial hypertrophic cardiomyopathy and long QT syndrome) the genetic defect or defects underlying autosomal dominant dilated cardiomyopathy are not known. Possible candidate genes could be those involved in immune regulation,[73] according to the autoimmune hypothesis of dilated cardiomyopathy, or they could be the ones responsible for normal heart function (i.e., encoding for contractile or muscle membrane proteins). An altered myosin light chain gene expression has been excluded as a cause of dilated cardiomyopathy.[74] However, a protease-mediated cleavage of the myosin regulatory light chain, with a significant impact on myocardial function, has been described.[75]

X-Linked Dilated Cardiomyopathy

X-linked dilated cardiomyopathy[76] is a familial heart disease inherited with the X chromosome in a dominant fashion. It affects young men in their late teens to early twenties with rapidly progressive congestive heart failure. Dilated cardiomyopathy may also affect female carriers, but with a later onset and slower progression. Clinical signs of skeletal myopathy are not observed in these patients; however, an increased serum creatine kinase (MM-CK) concentration is common. The dystrophin gene[77] is responsible, as it is for both Duchenne and Becker X-linked muscular dystrophies. Further analyses of several families revealed deletions encompassing both the dystrophin muscle promoter and first muscle exon.[78] More recently, a point mutation was detected in a large population of kindred[79] which abolished expression of the major dystrophin messenger RNA isoforms (muscle, brain, and Purkinje cell isoforms) in the myocardium. Skeletal muscle of cardiomyopathic patients was functionally normal but showed overexpression of brain and Purkinje cell dystrophin isoforms, whereas the muscle isoform was absent. These findings indicate that myocardial function is strictly dependent on the expression of muscle dystrophin isoform. Unlike skeletal muscle, the myocar-

dium of patients with X-linked cardiomyopathy is unable to express dystrophin from alternate promoters in a compensatory mechanism.

Exhaustive reports on gross and microscopic cardiac pathology in X-linked dilated cardiomyopathy are not available. Nevertheless, because of similarities in their pathogenetic mechanism, one can infer that the morphologic features would be similar to those of cardiomyopathy found in Duchenne and Becker dystrophies (see later discussion).

Viral Infections and Myocarditis

In animal models, especially in mice,[80] a persistent viral infection of myocardial cells causes myocarditis and leads to dilated cardiomyopathy. Also, cases of progression from a biopsy-proven viral myocarditis to a pathologically documented dilated cardiomyopathy have been reported in humans.[81, 82] Through the use of in situ hybridization and polymerase chain reaction, viral RNA sequences are demonstrable in a subset of dilated cardiomyopathy patients.[83] The frequency of enteroviral genome varies from 10%, when the search is restricted to coxsackieviruses to 25 to 30%,[84–86] when it is expanded to all enteroviruses. Patients with enteroviral RNA persistence are said to represent a clinically distinct subset of dilated cardiomyopathy cases. In one series, they exhibited greater mortality than their enterovirus-negative counterparts,[86] whereas in another they showed better functional status and outcome.[84]

Proposed explanations for the role of viral infection in the pathogenesis of dilated cardiomyopathy are direct viral cytotoxicity, immunologic response, and persistence of viral RNA.[87] An explanation of the direct myocardial toxicity of coxsackieviruses, and possibly of the sequence from viral infection to cardiomyopathy, has been given: Enteroviral protease 2A was shown to cleave dystrophin, thereby impairing both structure and function of the myocyte cytoskeleton.[87a]

Autoimmunity

That a chronic autoimmune process may be active in a significant number of patients is suggested by both the T nature of occasional lymphocytes found in the myocardium[88] and by the frequent activation of endothelial and myocardial interstitial cells, that express major histocompatibility antigens and adhesion molecules.[89] Several autoantibodies in the sera of cardiomyopathic patients have an ability to bind to myocellular proteins such as myosin light chain, tropomyosin, actin, and heat shock protein-60 (HSP-60),[90] to the second extracellular loop of the β_1-adrenoceptor,[91] and to the adenosine diphosphate–adenosine triphosphate carrier.[92] Although they are present in a limited subset, from one third to almost one half of patients,[73, 90, 93] autoantibodies do not seem to be a secondary phenomenon but may actually have an etiologic role, because they demonstrably impair myocardial function in vivo.[92] The presence of autoantibodies can be (1) genetically mediated (e.g., anti-β-adrenoceptor antibodies were found in 59% of affected members of a family with a hereditary cardiomyopathy),[73] (2) triggered by a viral infection, or (3) a result of currently unknown factors. What limits consideration of autoantibodies in the etiology of dilated cardiomyopathy is their high incidence in control patients: anti–HSP-60 autoantibodies were found in 42% of those with ischemic heart disease,[90] and anti-β-adrenoceptor antibodies in 22% of nonaffected members of the previously mentioned cardiomyopathic family.[73] Further support for autoimmune pathogenesis derives from reports of a significant association between dilated cardiomyopathy and celiac disease.[93a, 93b]

Pathogenesis

The existence of the etiologic factors mentioned previously has been demonstrated in only limited subsets of patients, and that favors a hypothesis of etiologic heterogeneity. However, these causative agents are not necessarily mutually exclusive: for example, one could inherit a predisposition to autoimmunity and hence to a cardiomyopathy triggered by viral infection. Even though the causes of dilated cardiomyopathy may differ, its pathogenesis could have a common mechanism, that is, inability to cope with functional derangement and destruction of myocytes by apoptosis[94] and inability to develop an effective compensatory hypertrophy. Despite the myocardial mass increase, myocytes characteristically exhibit myofibril loss that probably makes the enlarged myocytes less effective functionally. The physiopathologic importance of myofibril loss is stressed by the unique observation of a woman with postpartum hypopituitarism (Sheehan syndrome), who had a dilated cardiomyopathy caused by chronic growth hormone deficiency.[63] On endomyocardial biopsy, myocytes demonstrated marked myofibril loss, but after administration of recombinant human growth hormone, the patient showed a dramatic improvement both in cardiac function and myocyte myofibrillar content. The potential therapeutic role of growth hormone, however, was not confirmed in patients with the idiopathic form of dilated cardiomyopathy.[95, 96]

Functional impairment of myocytes could also derive from a dysfunction of contractile proteins, as suggested by the finding of mutations in the gene for α-cardiac actin in familial dilated cardiomyopathy.[96a] A pathogenetic role for myocyte cytoskeleton impairment has already been postulated for dilated cardiomyopathy associated with dystrophinopathies. This hypothesis has been confirmed by the discovery of mutations in the genes coding for other cytoskeletal proteins, such as desmin,[96b] metavinculin,[96c] and lamin A/C[96d] in patients with familial dilated cardiomyopathy.

Clinical Pathologic Correlation

Clinical Features and Diagnosis

From a clinical standpoint, dilated cardiomyopathy is characterized by left ventricular dilation, impaired systolic function, and symptoms of congestive heart failure.

The importance of ventricular enlargement was questioned by Keren and coworkers[97] who described patients with clinical and hemodynamic features of idiopathic pump failure but little or no ventricular dilation. In this condition, named "mildly dilated congestive cardiomyopathy," there were neither pathologic findings typical of other cardiomyopathies nor biopsy features of myocarditis. The histologic picture was nonspecific but, at variance with classic cases of dilated cardiomyopathy, it did not include significant myofibril loss. This observation suggests that myofibril loss is more related to ventricular dilation than to pump failure.[98] A subset of cases show that this condition can be considered an early stage of dilated cardiomyopathy because patients undergo progressive ventricular dilation during the follow-up period. However, in a substantial number of patients clinical status deteriorates without significant increase in ventricular diameter.[98, 99] This favors the existence of mildly dilated cardiomyopathy as a distinct entity.

Symptoms of dilated cardiomyopathy include fatigue, exercise intolerance, and, in one third of patients, chest pain. The diagnosis is made by a sequence of examinations whose invasiveness is directly related to their accuracy.[100] Physical examination demonstrates a variable degree of cardiomegaly and features of congestive pump failure; systolic murmurs resulting from mitral regurgitation are common. Chest radiography confirms cardiac enlargement and shows pulmonary vascular redistribution. Electrocardiography usually displays atrial or ventricular tachyarrhythmias. Complex ventricular arrhythmias are common, and their relationship to the degree of left ventricular functional impairment has been both suggested[101, 102] and questioned.[103, 104] In our experience,[105] they are associated with right-sided heart impairment rather than left ventricular dysfunction, and with extensive interstitial fibrosis. Regardless of their origin, frequent or complex ventricular arrhythmias predict mortality if not necessarily sudden death.[105, 106] In the pediatric setting, recurrent or incessant supraventricular tachycardias may be the cause, and not the effect, of ventricular dysfunction, because therapeutic control of arrhythmias may induce improvement, or even regression, of cardiomyopathic changes.[107] Echocardiography has the best accuracy/invasiveness ratio and offers a comprehensive anatomic and functional appraisal of this heart condition (Fig. 10-5A). Furthermore, it helps to exclude secondary forms of left ventricular dilation and detects both primary valvular incompetence and segmental, or inducible, wall motion abnormalities. Radionuclide ventriculography adds little information to results of echocardiography unless the latter are affected by technical problems. Echocardiographic imaging is so pervasive nowadays that pathologists must be accustomed to cutting dilated cardiomyopathy hearts for clinicopathologic correlation according to short-axis or four-chamber views. The usefulness of cardiac catheterization, angiocardiography, coronary angiography, and endomyocardial biopsy depends mainly on pragmatism in the approach to these patients. On one side are those with end-stage ventricular dysfunction, who could benefit only from cardiac transplantation and who could be labeled as having a presumptive idiopathic dilated cardiomyopathy without undergoing invasive assessment; on the other are potentially treatable patients, who might have either a myocarditis or a specific cardiomyopathy and those who could be successfully revascularized. Once an invasive assessment is completed, one gains information through left ventriculography (Fig. 10-5B),

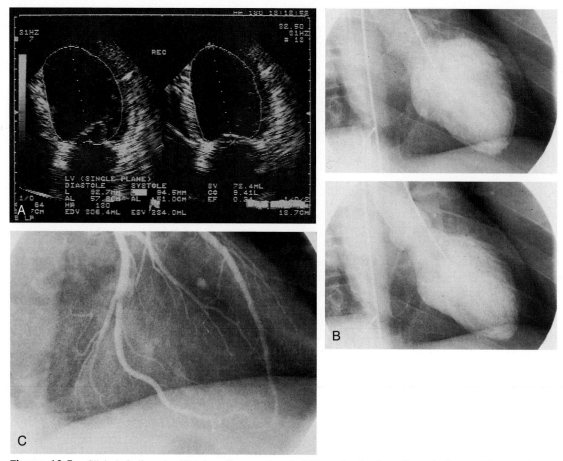

Figure 10-5 • Clinical findings in dilated cardiomyopathy. *A,* Bidimensional echocardiograph from a 51-year-old man. Dilation and global hypokinesia of left ventricle (ejection fraction, 18%) are evident; there is little difference between the left ventricular profile in systole *(right)* and diastole *(left).* *B,* Left ventriculogram from a 41-year-old man. The telesystolic volume *(below)* is quite similar to the telediastolic one *(above).* No endoventricular thrombi are apparent. *C,* Coronary arteriogram from a 54-year-old man. The left ventricle is dilated, the telediastolic diameter being 62 mm. Coronary arteries appear stretched and thread-like. *(A, B,* and *C* courtesy of F. Fedele, MD, Rome.)

which allows study of segmental wall motion abnormalities, assessment of many hemodynamic variables, identification of intraventricular thrombi, and evaluation of the degree and nature of mitral regurgitation. Primary valve pathology must be ruled out to make a diagnosis of dilated cardiomyopathy, but mitral regurgitation secondary to left ventricular dilation is a frequent occurrence. Coronary arteriography (Fig. 10-5*C*) allows study of coronary artery anatomy and function, and endomyocardial biopsy provides further information.

Natural History and Complications

Determining the expected length of survival of patients with dilated cardiomyopathy is hampered by three sets of problems: the source of data, the effects of early diagnosis and therapy, and heterogeneity in the study population. The classic notion is that one fourth of patients die within the first year of follow-up, and half within the fifth year,[100] but the origin of data influences the survival estimation. Most studies come from patient populations referred to major clinical centers, whereas the long-term fate of a population-based cohort proved much better than that of a referred one.[108] In the 1980s, patients with di-

lated cardiomyopathy had a median survival period after diagnosis of about 2 years.[109, 110] More recently, a marked improvement in survival has been observed. In a large study population subdivided into three study groups according to the period of enrollment (1978–1982, 1983–1987, and 1988–1992), the 2-year cumulative survival rates during those periods were 73.8%, 87.7%, and 90.3%, respectively, and the 4-year survival rates were 53.8%, 72.3%, and 82.9%.[111] Such dramatic improvement is commonly attributed to the combined effect of earlier diagnosis and new therapies, mainly ACE inhibitors and β-blockers. The third major source of variability is a heterogeneity in evolution of dilated cardiomyopathy. Three main types of natural history and mode of death have emerged: progressive deterioration, sudden and unexpected death, and a steady course, if with no improvement.

In the past, patients with dilated cardiomyopathy manifested heart failure and rapid deterioration. Death was the result of untreatable congestive failure or of complications such as systemic or pulmonary embolism.[4] Predictors of reduced survival were studied extensively, and independent determinants of poor prognosis were identified among clinical, hemodynamic, and histomorphometric variables. The major clinical or hemodynamic factors of bad prognosis[7, 35, 99, 109, 111, 112] proved to be older age; longer duration of heart failure symptoms; higher cardiothoracic index, mean right atrial pressure, left ventricular end-diastolic and systolic pressures, and left ventricular end-systolic volume; and lower cardiac index and ejection fraction. The significance of histomorphometric variables has already been discussed. Sudden death is infrequent in patients with dilated cardiomyopathy, and it does not depend on the degree of ventricular dilation, because this mode of death has the same frequency in both dilated and mildly dilated cardiomyopathy (7.0% versus 6.7%).[99]

A variable but substantial percentage of dilated cardiomyopathy patients, ranging from 23[109] to 39%[31] and even to 47% in pediatric cases,[107] showed a steady course or even some improvement of their condition. Regression of symptoms has been attributed to an earlier diagnosis and more effective treatment,[111] or to a missed diagnosis of myocarditis,[60] but it could also be a result of specific treatment in exceptional cases of endocrine disorders that lead to dilated cardiomyopathy, such as growth hormone deficiency[63] or thyrotoxicosis.[113]

Patients affected by dilated cardiomyopathy are the most suitable candidates for cardiac transplantation for several reasons: their disease is limited to the heart; they are not likely to have had previous cardiac surgery when transplanted; and they have a progressive, incurable disease but remain in steady state long enough to be enrolled on a waiting list. Cardiomyopathic patients account for 51.1% of recipients of heart transplant.[114]

Alternative surgical procedures are currently used in nontransplant eligible patients. They include partial left ventriculectomy as proposed by Batista and coworkers,[115] left ventriculoplasty to exclude the anteroseptal wall, and isolated mitral valve reconstruction to correct secondary mitral regurgitation. In selected groups, these procedures give encouraging results.[115a, 115b]

Peripartum Cardiomyopathy

This is a rare cardiac disorder of unknown cause, in which unexplained left ventricular dysfunction develops during late pregnancy or the early puerperium.[116] It is uncommon before the last month of pregnancy and much more common up to 5 months after delivery.[117] Its reported incidence varies in different geographic regions.[117] The diagnosis is considered only when other conditions associated with perinatal heart failure have been excluded. Risk factors include advanced maternal age, multiparity, African descent, and twinning. Familial occurrence has been described.[118] Although several attempts have been made to uncover the origin of this condition, no study has identified a distinct cause. This may be a result of the coexistence of multiple etiologic factors or of differences in inclusion criteria of the patients in published series.

The most frequent clinical symptoms are dyspnea, cough, orthopnea, and chest pain; hemoptysis may be the initial feature of pulmonary embolism, to which these patients are particularly predisposed.[119] Electrocardiography may reveal sinus tachycardia, and on echocardiography, left ventricular dilation and impaired performance are observed.[117] Pathologic findings are no different from those observed in other cases of dilated cardiomyopathy. Gross examination generally demonstrates biventricular dilation with occasional endocardial thickening and mural thrombi. Histologic findings include variable degrees of myocyte hypertrophy and degeneration, interstitial fibrosis, and, occasionally, lymphocytic infiltrates. A number of studies have demonstrated evidence of myocarditis in endomyocardial biopsies from affected women, but the frequency of this finding among series is highly variable.[120–122] Prognosis is related to the recovery of left ventricular function within 6 months of diagnosis.[119] Reported mortality rates range from 25 to 50%.[116]

Endocardial Fibroelastosis, Dilated Form

Endocardial fibroelastosis (EFE) is a condition with homogeneous pathologic features, thought to be the nonspecific reaction of a growing heart to a number of endocardial insults. A distinction is made between a secondary form, associated with congenital heart disease, and a primary form, in which no other anatomic cardiac abnormalities are found. The former may show a restrictive pattern and is discussed in the section on restrictive cardiomyopathy; the latter generally causes marked left ventricular dilation (Fig. 10-6A), with a combined dilated and restrictive functional pattern. Rarely, the left ventricle can be of normal size or hypoplastic, with enlargement of both atria and the right ventricle ("contracted" type).

Primary EFE is a rare disease; in the last few decades, its incidence has declined to less than 1 in 5000 live births.[123] Its prevalence has a reverse correlation with patient age, being rare after infancy.

Clinical features of EFE include congestive heart failure or, in the so-called contracted form, a clinical picture of left-sided obstructive disease. Left atrial and pulmonary artery pressure are elevated. Sudden death can be the initial feature.

On gross examination, the left ventricular chamber is usually dilated, although in the contracted form of the disease a small left ventricular cavity can be observed infrequently. The ventricular endocardium is extremely thickened, usually obscuring trabeculae (see Fig. 10-6A) and openings of thebesian veins. The process is diffuse within the left (or both) ventricles and must not be confused macroscopically with focal fibrous endocardial thickening, as is seen in jet lesions, endomyocardial fibrosis, or dilated cardiomyopathy (see Fig. 10-2A). Papillary muscles and chordae tendineae may be involved, causing mitral regurgitation. Aortic regurgitation resulting from encroachment of the fibroelastotic process to the aortic cusps is also observed. The left ventricular wall is hypertrophied.

Microscopically, coarse elastic lamellas are prominent within the fibrotic endocardium (Fig. 10-6B), extending into the subendocardium and arranged tangentially to the ventricular lumen. Elastin fibrils are much thicker in endocardial fibroelastosis than in similar conditions acquired in adult life, such as on the mural aspect of healed transmural myocardial infarcts.[124] The latter condition indicates a reaction to abnormal pressure and/or wall resistance.

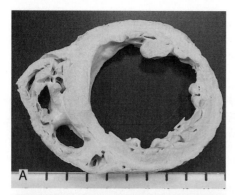

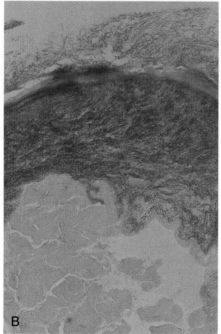

Figure 10-6 • *A,* Native heart of an 8-year-old girl, transplanted for endocardial fibroelastosis, dilated type. The specimen was cut along a midventricular short-axis plane. The left ventricular endocardium is extremely thickened, whitish, and china-like, with obliteration of the trabecular pattern. The left ventricle is dilated. (The scale is in centimeters). *B,* Left ventricular endomyocardial biopsy from a 14-year-old female patient affected by endocardial fibroelastosis, dilated type. The endocardium is thickened, with layered coarse elastic fibers (van Gieson-elastic stain).

A number of pathogenetic mechanisms have been proposed. The primary form of endocardial fibroelastosis could be the result of inadequate subendocardial blood flow or of increased endocardial mural tension and overstretching resulting from myocarditis with left ventricular dilation.[125] Presumably, the younger the patient, the more intimal fibroblasts and vascular smooth muscle cells can react to injury by producing elastin in greater amounts relative to collagen production. Data have been published supporting the hypothesis that endocardial fibroelastosis is a sequel of viral myocarditis in the newborn or infant, in particular mumps virus infection.[126] The introduction of mumps vaccine may explain the decline in incidence of EFE in the United States during the last few decades.[123] Finally, genetic forms of the disease with a wide range of inheritance patterns have been described.[127]

HYPERTROPHIC CARDIOMYOPATHY

Definition

Heterogeneity in pathology, hemodynamic pattern, and natural history are the hallmarks of hypertrophic cardiomyopathy. In 1980, the WHO[1] gave a detailed description of this condition and provided a unifying term to such confusing names as asymmetric (septal) hypertrophy, hypertrophic (muscular) subaortic stenosis, and obstructive cardiomyopathy. More recently,[3] the WHO/ISFC defined hypertrophic cardiomyopathy as being "characterized by left and/or right ventricular hypertrophy, which is usually asymmetric and involves the interventricular septum."

Pathology

Classic Form

The classic form of hypertrophic cardiomyopathy is that described by Teare in 1958.[128] Its gross, microscopic, and ultrastructural features are dominated by two hallmarks: myocardial hypertrophy and structural derangement (Table 10-2).

Gross Anatomy

Myocardial hypertrophy is strikingly variable in distribution and extent. In archetypal cases, it is distinctively asymmetric (Fig. 10-7*A*; see Fig. 11–25 also), whereas the frequency of symmetric hypertrophy (a diffuse concentric hypertrophy of the left ventricle) varies from 1[130]

TABLE 10-2 • **Myocardial Hypertrophy and Structural Derangement in Hypertrophic Cardiomyopathy**

Pathology	Gross Anatomy	Histopathology	Ultrastructure
Myocardial hypertrophy	Mostly asymmetric thickening of the ventricular septum and/or wall (prevalent localization: left ventricle, anteroseptal segment)	Irregular enlargement of both myocytes and nuclei, sometimes with a clear perinuclear halo	Commensurate increase in sarcomeres, mitochondria, and energy stores (glycogen, lipid)
Structural derangement	Irregular distribution of muscular bundles in the hypertrophic segment, reminiscent of the cut surface of a myometrial leiomyoma	Disarray of bundles, myocytes, myofibrils, desmin intermediate filaments, and specialized intercellular junctions	Disarray of myofibrils, myofilaments, and Z bands

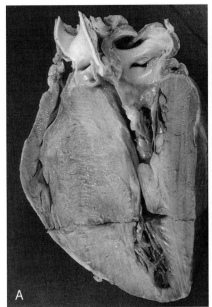

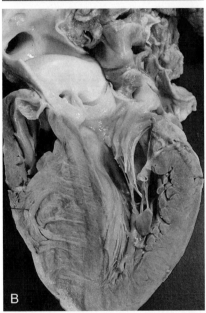

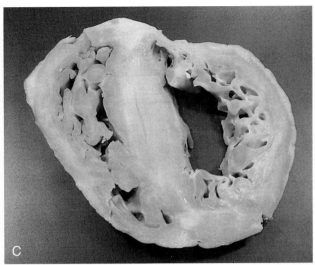

Figure 10-7 • Gross morphology of hypertrophic cardiomyopathy. *A,* Heart of a 17-year-old male patient who died after a cerebellar septic embolism. The specimen was cut in a long-axis plane. Septal hypertrophy is distinctively asymmetric: the ventricular septum and left ventricular inferior free wall, respectively, are 44 and 15 mm thick. The anteromedial leaflet of the mitral valve is thickened, with a corresponding area of fibrosis in the septal endocardium. (From Gallo P: Cuore e Pericardio. In: Ascenzi A, Mottura G (eds): Trattato di Anatomia Patulogica per il Medico Pratico, 5th ed. Turin, UTET, 1997, p 304). *B,* The heart of a 14-year-old male patient with asymmetric midseptal hypertrophic cardiomyopathy who died suddenly. The specimen was cut along a long-axis plane. The ventricular septum shows an irregular distribution of muscular bundles, mimicking the cut surface of a myometrial lieomyoma. Slight fibrosis of the septal endocardium is also present. *C,* Native heart of a 49-year-old man, transplanted for hypertrophic cardiomyopathy, dilated form. The specimen was cut along a midventricular short-axis plane. The ventricular septum and right ventricular lateral wall are thickened. The ventricular septum and anteroseptal region also show areas of replacement fibrosis.

to 34%[131] in different series. Diagnosis of symmetric hypertrophic cardiomyopathy implies a strict exclusion of any primary cause of left ventricular hypertrophy—from an exaggerated response to physiologic stimuli, to hypertension, to any type of left ventricular outflow obstruction—and a differential diagnosis from clinical mimics. Asymmetric hypertrophy may involve any ventricular segment, although the anterior portion of the ventricular septum, alone or in association with other segments, is the most commonly affected (see Fig. 10-7A): 96% in the large echocardiographic series of Klues and associates.[130] In the comprehensive pathologic study by Davies and McKenna,[131] left ventricular hypertrophy was distributed as follows: anteroseptal in 23 of 43 asymmetric cases (53%); anteroseptal plus lateral in 8; anterior, septal, or posteroseptal in 2 cases each; anterolateral or posterolateral in 1 case each (see Fig. 10-10A). Posterior or "in-

verted" hypertrophy seems to have specific clinical implications, in that patients are younger than the average patient with hypertrophic cardiomyopathy, are severely symptomatic, and have an obstructive hemodynamic pattern.[132] Asymmetric apical involvement, which is common in a distinct set of Japanese patients,[133] is rare in Europe and America, affecting 1% in the series of Klues and associates.[130] Right ventricular involvement is not uncommon, 18% in the series of Davies and McKenna,[131] and may give rise to a distinctive right ventricular outflow obstruction[134] because of the encroachment of septal hypertrophy on, and distortion of, the infundibulum. Even if no obstructive changes exist, a widening of the crista supraventricularis is a peculiar finding that may draw the pathologist's attention to the diagnosis of right or left ventricular involvement. Also, the extent of asymmetric hypertrophy is variable. In a comprehensive survey,[130] hypertrophy affected only one echocardiographic segment in 28% of cases, two segments in 38%, and three or more in 34%. Myocardial disarrangement is evident on macroscopic inspection (Fig. 10-7B; see Table 10-2). Fibrosis is often macroscopically evident, too, especially in areas of hypertrophy, and may present either a diffuse interstitial pattern, contributing to the structurally deranged appearance of the cut surface, or a pattern of substitution (Fig. 10-7C).

Interest in mitral valve morphology relates to its systolic anterior motion. However, pathologic and echocardiographic investigations demonstrate frequent structural derangement of this structure, as well. The valve is often congenitally dysplastic[135] or floppy,[136] with dysplastic features of both leaflets, which may be wide or elongated,[137] and of the tensor apparatus; sometimes direct insertion of papillary muscles into leaflets is seen.[138] Also, anterior displacement of the ventricular insertion of papillary muscles may play a role in determining irregular valve mobility.[139] In its systolic anterior motion, a rather frequent occurrence in these patients, the anteroseptal leaflet hits the ventricular septum, leading to fibrosis of both the valvular free edge and the septal endocardium (see Fig.

10-7A). This was seen in 32% of Davies and McKenna's cases.[131] The area of contact (and zone of fibrosis) varies in extent,[137] but damage to valvular tissue may be responsible for complications such as chordal rupture[131] or the development of infective endocarditis (see Fig. 10-12) with subsequent pyemic embolism.

Subepicardial coronary arteries are usually normal, but an intramyocardial tunneling of the left anterior descending branch has been described,[140] and it may be part of a general structural derangement in these hearts. A systematic study of recipient hearts removed in our Cardiac Transplantation Unit demonstrated myocardial bridging in 40% of the hearts with hypertrophic cardiomyopathy (see Fig. 10-11), compared with 6% of specimens with dilated cardiomyopathy and 5% of those with ischemic heart disease.

Histopathology

Myocardial hypertrophy and derangement are appreciable at light microscopy (see Table 10-2). For descriptive purposes, myocardial disarray has been classified in various ways.[141, 142] It presents a complex structural disorder that can be appreciated at different levels and includes (1)

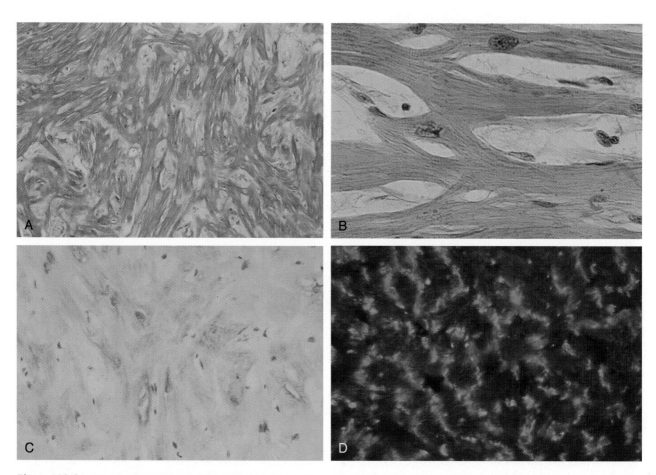

Figure 10-8 • Microscopy in hypertrophic cardiomyopathy. *A,* Myocardial disarray at the myocellular level. Myocytes intersect at various angles and show somewhat whorled appearance (trichrome stain). *B,* Disarray at the myofibrillar level (same case as in Fig. 10-7C). When the condenser is lowered, myofibrils can be seen running in different directions (H&E stain). *C,* Myocardial disarray at the level of intermediate filaments. Intercalated disks have not been stained, and Z bands are labeled only focally; a myocyte (*bottom, middle*) shows longitudinal arrangement of desmin intermediate filaments (Immunohistochemical staining for desmin). *D,* Myocardial disarray at the level of specialized intercellular junctions. There is an uneven labeling of connexin43, the main protein of cardiac gap junctions, suggesting an irregular distribution and an abnormally folded and convoluted shape of these intercellular junctions (Immunofluorescence staining for connexin43).

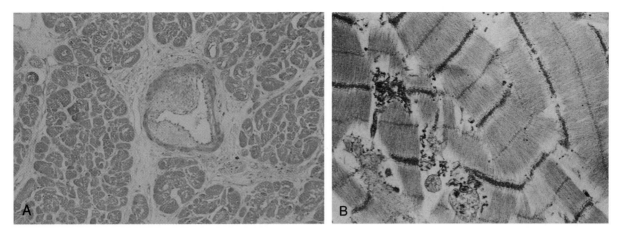

Figure 10-9 • Microscopy in hypertrophic cardiomyopathy. *A,* Stenosis of intramural coronary artery. The lumen is narrowed by intimal hyperplasia caused by smooth muscle cell proliferation (Trichrome stain). *B,* Electron microscopy showing myocardial disarray at the myofilament level. Myofibrils have a disorderly arrangement.

bundles of myocytes that cross with a herringbone pattern; (2) myocytes that display bizarre forms (Fig. 10-8*A*) with increased Y-shaped branching, frequent side-to-side junctions, or even a characteristic whorled appearance, usually around a central fibrous core; (3) myofibrils that insert not only on intercalated disks but also on the lateral sarcolemmal membrane (Fig. 10-8*B*); (4) desmin intermediate filaments (which contribute to the maintenance of myocyte shape) that show, in areas of myocyte disarray, a decrease or loss of labeling of intercalated disks and Z bands (Fig. 10-8*C*) and that may exhibit a longitudinal arrangement (see Fig. 10-8*C*) or a granular patchy distribution,[143] specific for disarray of hypertrophic cardiomyopathy[144]; and (5) specialized intercellular junctions that are demonstrably affected, in areas of disarray, by an irregular distribution of connexin43 immunolabeling (Fig. 10-8*D*) and an increased number of antidesmosomal protein–positive dots.[145] A relationship between these structural abnormalities and both contractile and arrhythmic peculiarities of hypertrophic cardiomyopathy is easy to hypothesize. Although it is a hallmark of hypertrophic cardiomyopathy, myocardial disarray is not limited to that condition. In fact, a nonspecific disarray of myocytes may affect the right ventricular outflow tract in tetralogy of Fallot, pulmonary atresia, or cor pulmonale; may affect the left ventricle in aortic atresia or hypertensive heart disease; may be related to areas of myocardial scarring, including those in endomyocardial biopsies; and may occur in normal hearts where cells converge at acute angles (e.g., at the junction of the ventricular free wall with the septum). Myocardial disarray is said to be characteristic of hypertrophic cardiomyopathy when it occupies at least 20% of one or more tissue blocks.[131]

Microscopic examination also confirms the presence of both interstitial and replacement fibrosis.[146] Interstitial fibrosis is said to be a primary morphologic abnormality in the disease spectrum,[146a] whereas the areas of myocardial scarring are currently interpreted as an ischemic effect resulting from stenosis of intramural coronary arteries.[147] Thickened arteries are a frequent finding, being observed in 40[131] to 83%[147] of cases in areas of hypertrophy.

Thickening is caused by smooth muscle cell proliferation in both medial and intimal layers (Fig. 10-9*A*). It is not clear whether these vascular lesions are primary or secondary to myocardial hypertrophy and hypercontractility. Electron microscopy provides little additional information in the study of hypertrophic cardiomyopathy (Fig. 10-9*B*; see Table 10-2).

Endomyocardial Biopsy in Hypertrophic Cardiomyopathy

Endomyocardial biopsy is not useful in hypertrophic cardiomyopathy because myocardial disarray is usually deep in the ventricular wall and beyond the bioptome's reach. Nevertheless, in the pediatric series of Laetherbury and coworkers,[25] a biopsy was made in two patients with a clinical diagnosis of hypertrophic cardiomyopathy. In the first, the histologic picture was normal and a septal fibroma was subsequently demonstrated; in the second, electron microscopic observation suggested a mitochondrial cardiomyopathy.

Restrictive Form

Idiopathic restrictive cardiomyopathy (see later discussion) is characterized by atrial dilation, small nonhypertrophic ventricles, and the histologic feature of widespread interstitial fibrosis. McKenna and colleagues[148] described a group of patients who not only showed a ventricular filling pattern typical of restrictive cardiomyopathy (Fig. 10-10*A*) and diffuse interstitial fibrosis (Fig. 10-10*B*) but also exhibited extensive myocardial disarray (see Fig. 10-10*B*). They usually inherit their disease as an autosomal dominant trait but do not necessarily present with myocardial hypertrophy. Whether these cases should be considered as an expression of the phenotypic variability of hypertrophic cardiomyopathy (hypertrophic cardiomyopathy, restrictive pattern) or as an extension of the spectrum of restrictive cardiomyopathy (restrictive cardiomyopathy with myocardial disarray) is essentially a problem of semantics. In our experience, these hearts show a typical and extensive myocardial disarray, including an altered desmin pattern,[144] and a diffuse interstitial fibrosis

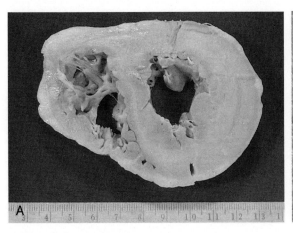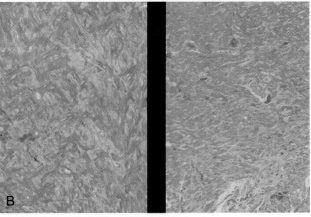

Figure 10-10 • Native heart of a 17-year-old male patient, transplanted for hypertrophic cardiomyopathy, restrictive form. *A,* The specimen was cut along a midventricular short-axis plane. The left ventricular cavity is slightly reduced and there is asymmetric hypertrophy of its lateral free wall. (The scale is in centimeters.) *B,* Histologic section showing *(left)* myocardial disarray and interstitial fibrosis, and *(right)* diffuse interstitial fibrosis, often surrounding individual myocytes (*A* and *B,* Mallory's azan stain.)

that is more widespread than the one commonly encountered in hypertrophic cardiomyopathy and less diffuse than that observed in idiopathic restrictive cardiomyopathy. They could represent an intermediate form in a continuous spectrum of pathology ranging from hypertrophic to restrictive cardiomyopathy.

Dilated Form

In the experience of Hina and associates,[149] 16% of patients diagnosed with "classic" hypertrophic cardiomyopathy underwent progressive left ventricular dilation during the follow-up period. At pathologic examination, segments of the left ventricle or septum known to be hypertrophic appeared to be converted into thin scars (Fig. 10-11), leading to ventricular dilation. Histology revealed extensive replacement fibrosis and more than average

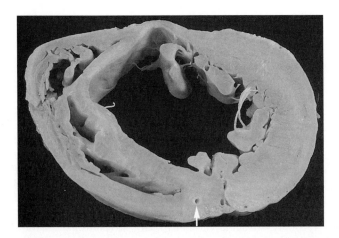

Figure 10-11 • Native heart of a 44-year-old male patient, transplanted for hypertrophic cardiomyopathy, dilated form. The specimen was cut along a midventricular short-axis plane. The left ventricular cavity is remarkably dilated; the inferior left ventricular wall and ventricular septum are thinned and display large areas of substitution fibrosis. Myocardial tunneling of the left anterior descending coronary branch is visible *(arrow).*

narrowing of intramyocardial coronary artery branches.[150] Also, myocardial disarray was more extensive and more diffusely distributed. Were it not for the clinical history, a differential pathologic diagnosis from dilated cardiomyopathy or ischemic heart disease could be difficult. Residual areas of asymmetric hypertrophy and the histologic features of extensive myocardial disarray and small vessel disease aided the diagnosis.

Genetics

The growing evidence of a familial distribution of the disease and subsequent identification of some responsible genes mapping for contractile proteins suggest that the familial form is the archetype and is accompanied by a series of pathologic, genetic, and clinical mimics.[151] Actually, the disease's heterogeneity is such that there may be a wide variation in both pathology[131] and evolution,[152] even within the same family with a shared mutation of the same gene. Accordingly, this section provides a unifying genetic basis for this cardiomyopathy and subsequently deals with its phenotypic variability in terms of pathology, hemodynamics, and evolution.

Since 1989, when the first gene associated with the disease was mapped on chromosome 14q1,[153] familial hypertrophic cardiomyopathy has become the paradigm for inherited cardiac disorders. Linkage studies and candidate-gene approaches demonstrated that about half of the patients with hypertrophic cardiomyopathy have mutations in one of eight disease genes: β-heavy chain cardiac myosin (β-MHC)[154] on chromosome 14q; troponin T[155] on chromosome 1q;[156] α-tropomyosin[155] on chromosome 15q;[157] cardiac myosin-binding protein C[158] on chromosome 11p;[159] essential and regulatory light chains of ventricular myosin;[160] troponin and alpha-cardiac actin.[161a] All of these are sarcomeric proteins or parts of the intrasarcomeric cytoskeleton (myosin binding protein C) involved in myocyte contraction. Gene mutations altering their structure may also adversely affect their function and, consequently, both myocyte shape and contractile activity. The hypothesis is supported by results of functional transfection studies in which cells expressing mutant forms of β-MHC show disruption of sarcomeric assembly.[162, 163] Cardiac hypertrophy, which is almost invariably observed in hypertrophic cardiomyopathy, could then be interpreted as a compensatory phenomenon for myocyte abnormalities induced by mutant proteins. In addition, a distinct form of hypertrophic cardiomyopathy associated with Wolff-Parkinson-White syndrome has been described in a large family in which a close linkage to DNA markers on chromosome 7q3 was found.[164]

A significant proportion of cases (20 to 30%) are caused by mutations in the β-MHC gene on chromosome 14.[165] More than 40 such mutations and one deletion have been identified so far, and their number is still increasing. Genotype-phenotype studies show that some mutations (e.g., Gly256Glu[166] and Leu908Val[167]) bear a favorable prognosis, whereas others (e.g., Arg719Trp, Arg403Gln, Arg453Cys) are associated with a high frequency of cardiac sudden death.[166–169] Mutations in the gene for cardiac myosin-binding protein C account for approximately 15% of cases of familial hypertrophic cardiomyopathy. The clinical expression of these mutations is often delayed until middle or old age, with a favorable clinical course.[169a] These findings underline the importance of genetic counseling for affected patients and their relatives, because it has both diagnostic purposes and prognostic implications.

At present, a familial distribution has been assessed in about half of cases. However, a more rigorous exclusion of clinical mimics, the extension of familial screening to genetic rather than phenotypic analysis,[170] and increased knowledge of genetics applied to cardiomyopathies will probably lead to detection of a genetic defect in most patients with hypertrophic cardiomyopathy. (See further discussion in Chapter 24.)

Differential Diagnosis

Other Genetic Disorders

Cardiomyopathic changes resembling those observed in familial hypertrophic cardiomyopathy have been described in several other genetic disorders.

Noonan syndrome is a pleiotropic pathologic condition[171] transmitted as an autosomal dominant trait. Its clinical features are highly variable and include short stature, cubitus valgus, lymphedema, cryptorchidism, mental dullness, ptosis, and facial dysmorphism.[172] Cardiovascular symptoms are common and affect as many as 70% of cases.[173] The most common are pulmonary valve stenosis and hypertrophic cardiomyopathy,[174] the latter characterized by symmetric or asymmetric left ventricular hypertrophy. Histologic studies often reveal myofiber disarray. However, it is never as extensive as in familial hypertrophic cardiomyopathy.[175] Less frequent cardiac findings include atrial septal defect (often associated with pulmonary stenosis), ventricular septal defect, and patent ductus arteriosus. Little is known about the etiology and pathogenesis of Noonan syndrome. A gene for the disease has been mapped on the long arm of chromosome 12[176] but has yet to be identified.

Lentiginosis is a rare disorder of skin pigmentation of neural crest origin that causes multiple skin macules affecting trunk, limbs, and face. It is often associated with left ventricular hypertrophy with an obstructive pattern; in about 30% of cases, right ventricular outflow tract obstruction is also present. Lentiginosis usually manifests in children and can be associated with sensorineural deafness, psychic and somatic infantilism, genital hypoplasia, and an autosomal dominant mode of transmission (LEOPARD syndrome)[177]; however, sporadic cases of adult onset and an absence of findings have been described.[178] The disease should be suspected in patients having multiple cutaneous macules, electrocardiographic abnormalities, and a systolic murmur.

Costello syndrome, a rare genetic disease, has an autosomal recessive pattern of inheritance. Cases are characterized by the association of cardiomyopathy with a hypertrophic pattern and rhythm disturbances, nasal papillomas, mental retardation, and craniofacial abnormalities.

Mitochondrial cardiomyopathies may also manifest with a hypertrophic pattern.

Exaggerated Hypertrophies

Various conditions that share a morphologic resemblance to archetypal hypertrophic cardiomyopathy can be grouped under this heading.

Hypertensive Left Ventricular Hypertrophy

A subset of hypertensive patients develop left ventricular hypertrophy that is disproportionate for the degree of hypertension. Subjects are characteristically older than the average hypertensive patient (old age hypertrophy), most commonly female and black (Afro-Caribbean hypertensive cardiomegaly), and their disease does not have any familial distribution. From a pathologic standpoint, they show marked left ventricular hypertrophy with cardiac weight frequently exceeding 550 g. Myocardial hypertrophy may be either symmetric, with reduced cavity size and restrictive filling pattern, or asymmetric, with septal involvement, but histologic examination does not reveal significant myocardial disarray. These patients are not prone to sudden death. In the past, this subset was tentatively described as a variant of hypertrophic cardiomyopathy,[179] but more recent studies allow discrimination on both hemodynamic and histopathologic terms.[180]

Athlete's Heart

Young competitive athletes may develop a slight symmetric left ventricular hypertrophy and diastolic cavity dimension increase (athlete's heart),[181] which can prompt a problem in diagnosis. Distinction from hypertrophic cardiomyopathy is important, because the latter is the most common cause of sudden unexpected death in young athletes,[182] and a tentative diagnosis of the condition could lead to an athlete's unnecessary disqualification from competition. The classic athlete's heart and hypertrophic cardiomyopathy share no relation, but some competitive athletes, especially those participating in sports such as distance running, swimming, cycling, rowing, or canoeing and those using enhancing steroids may develop a slight (13- to 16-mm), symmetric left ventricular hypertrophy that creates a "gray zone" in differential diagnosis with milder symmetric forms of hypertrophic cardiomyopathy.[183] Detection of a familial distribution provides definitive evidence for hypertrophic cardiomyopathy, whereas an enlarged left ventricular cavity contradicts such a diagnosis. In extreme cases, it may be necessary to interrupt the athlete's training and watch for a decrease in cardiac mass with athletic deconditioning.[184] (See discussion in Chapter 11 also.)

Neonatal Cardiomegaly

Neonatal and fetal echocardiography sometimes reveals a picture of severe cardiomegaly reminiscent of the pattern of hypertrophic cardiomyopathy. Such a diagnosis should not be made at this age. At postmortem examination, a range of cardiovascular defects, from aortic coarctation to malformation of coronary arteries, is detected. There remains a small subset of patients who show only left ventricular hypertrophy: in these cases, cardiomegaly may be the result of chronic renal failure or maternal diabetes. In infants who survive, myocardial hypertrophy may regress.

Clinical Mimics

Exaggerated hypertrophies may be difficult to distinguish from hypertrophic cardiomyopathy. Other pathologic conditions mimic hypertrophic cardiomyopathy at echocardiography but are easily discriminated on pathologic grounds at postmortem examination or if endomyocardial biopsy is available. Among such conditions, the most common are amyloidosis, glycogen storage disease, and Fabry disease.

Clinical Pathologic Correlation

Physiopathologic Correlation

The three pathologic phenotypes of hypertrophic cardiomyopathy are associated with three physiopathologic patterns: obstructive, restrictive, and dilated.

Obstructive Pattern

The dynamic subaortic pressure gradient, which characterizes the classic, "obstructive" form of the disease, has anatomic as well as functional causes. Anatomically, the left ventricular outflow tract is frequently narrowed by a bulging septal myocardium covered by patchy endocardial fibrous thickening (see Fig. 10-7A), and by an anterior displacement of the papillary muscles.[139] Functionally, the outlet is further narrowed by systolic anterior motion of the mitral valve. In midsystole, the anteromedial mitral leaflet crosses and restricts the outflow tract. Moreover, its distal portion hits against the septal endocardium, producing endocardial thickening. This systolic anterior motion has been related to increased ejection velocities that create a Venturi effect and attract the mitral leaflets anteriorly. However, systolic anterior motion often begins in protosystole, when ejection velocity is still low and also occurs in the absence of septal hypertrophy. Therefore, an alternate theory has arisen.[185] It attributes systolic motion to anterior displacement of the papillary muscles and the following succession of events: the vortex normally created throughout diastole is reversed, and it positions the systolic outflow stream close to the posterior wall, where it strikes the posterior side of the mitral leaflets, creating drag forces that initiate anterior displacement of the closing mitral leaflets. Figure 11–26C presents the echocardiographic morphology from a case with both asymmetric septal hypertrophy and systolic anterior movement of the anterior mitral valve.

Restrictive Pattern

A diastolic dysfunction, leading to a left ventricular filling defect, is present in most hypertrophic cardiomyopathy patients. It is related to an impaired left ventricular relaxation and distensibility, which are independent of the degree and distribution of myocardial hypertrophy and probably depend on myocardial disarray and interstitial fibrosis. When prominent, this diastolic dysfunction produces a restrictive cardiomyopathic pattern.

Dilated Pattern

Left ventricular dilation in hypertrophic cardiomyopathy is largely caused by myocardial ischemia, a combined result of narrowing of intramyocardial coronary branches, increased oxygen requirements, raised filling pressures (which mainly affect the subendocardial myocardium), and, in older patients, obstructive epicardial coronary artery atherosclerosis.[186]

Clinical Features and Diagnosis

Most patients are only mildly symptomatic or even asymptomatic. In these cases, the diagnosis of hypertrophic cardiomyopathy is often made either during screening of relatives of a recognized patient or at postmortem examination in cases of unexpected, and usually sudden, death. When symptoms occur, clinical diagnosis is usually made without difficulty. The most frequent symptoms are dyspnea, which is mainly related to the diastolic dysfunction common to all patients, angina pectoris, fatigue, and syncope. All are exacerbated by exertion; syncope and presyncope are particularly ominous, because they are associated with an increased risk of sudden death. The severity of symptoms is usually related to the extent of hypertrophy. The relative prevalence of left ventricular outflow pressure gradient, diastolic stiffness, and myocardial ischemia accounts for the resulting physiopathologic pattern.

Diagnosis may be made by a succession of steps. Physical examination may be noncontributory in asymptomatic patients. When an outflow gradient is present, a crescendo-decrescendo systolic murmur is typical. It must be differentiated from the one elicited by fixed aortic stenosis. In dynamic obstruction, initial ejection from the left ventricle is enhanced, whereas in fixed aortic stenosis, left ventricular emptying is obstructed from the beginning of systole. Accordingly, the two murmurs have different characteristics, and these differences can be enhanced by maneuvers that modify the gradient intensity.[187] With the exclusion of a limited set of patients who have localized nonobstructive left ventricular hypertrophy, the electrocardiogram is usually abnormal, with the most common changes being ST-segment and T-wave abnormalities; tall QRS complexes, a sign of left ventricular hypertrophy; and, less frequently, prominent Q waves. Giant negative

T waves in midprecordial leads are considered characteristic of segmental, mainly apical, left ventricular involvement. Accessory atrioventricular pathways are uncommon,[188] albeit not so rare as to represent a chance association. Rhythm disturbances are frequent and can be exposed by treadmill testing. They comprise ventricular arrhythmias, supraventricular tachycardia, and atrial fibrillation. The predictive role of spontaneous nonsustained or inducible sustained ventricular tachycardia in identifying patients at increased risk of sudden death is controversial.[189, 190] Echocardiography is extremely useful both in studying patients with hypertrophic cardiomyopathy and in screening their relatives. It allows the detection and quantification of morphologic features, in terms of both diagnosis and evolution of the disease, as well as functional and hemodynamic findings. Moreover, the echocardiogram has value not only in determining the degree of hypertrophy but also the architecture of myocardium (quantitative texture analysis); the features of subaortic obstruction and of mitral systolic anterior motion and prolapse; the diameter of cavities; the type of motion, thickening, and thinning of the septal and parietal walls; and many other variables. If the reliability of echocardiography is limited by technical restraints, thallium scanning is helpful. Gated radionuclide ventriculography allows evaluation of septal and ventricular wall motion. Magnetic resonance imaging is used to carefully assess the distribution and severity of myocardial hypertrophy[191] and three-dimensional left ventricular motion and deformation in vivo.[192] Invasive procedures allow evaluation of the systolic gradient, the diastolic filling defect, mitral valve motion and regurgitation, and the coronary tree. They are particularly useful to study the right ventricle and pulmonary circulation. The value of endomyocardial biopsy has been discussed.

Natural History and Complications

The clinical course of hypertrophic cardiomyopathy is variable, even within the same family[152] (i.e., among patients sharing the same mutation). The majority of adults remain stable for decades. They have an annual mortality rate of 1.7 to 3%,[193, 194] but children have a death rate twice as high.[195] Only rarely is death caused by complications, such as infective endocarditis[196] (Fig. 10-12) or myocardial infarction.[197] The majority of patients die suddenly and unexpectedly, with death often being the first manifestation of disease in young members of affected families who have no time to develop either symptoms or echocardiographic features of the disease.[198] Predictive factors of sudden death have been investigated intensively. The typical profile of a candidate for sudden death[194] is a young, asymptomatic patient with substantial left ventricular hypertrophy who dies during sedentary or modest physical activities; only a minority die during exertion, including competitive athletics. The most consistent risk factors include young age at diagnosis, a "malignant" family history of sudden death, a particularly marked and diffuse left ventricular hypertrophy,[199] nonsustained ventricular tachycardia during Holter monitoring, inducibility of sustained supraventricular or ventricu-

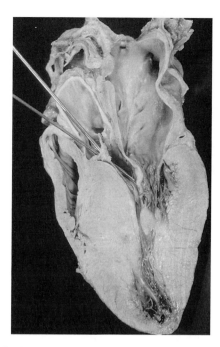

Figure 10-12 • The heart of an adult man, affected by hypertrophic cardiomyopathy, who died from infective endocarditis of aortic and mitral valves and septic embolism. The specimen was cut along a long-axis plane. Asymmetric septal hypertrophy, fibrous thickening of the anteroseptal leaflet of the mitral valve, and aortic cusp perforations *(probes)* are seen.

lar tachycardia, bradyarrhythmias, prior occurrence of syncope or cardiac arrest, and some particular β-MHC gene mutations (see earlier discussion). The sudden death is presumed to be arrhythmic: ventricular tachyarrhythmias, bradyarrhythmias, and atrial arrhythmias associated with hypotension are suspected. (See discussion in Chapter 11 also.) A minority of patients, as many as 16% in the series of Hina and colleagues,[149] deteriorated progressively[200] and either died of congestive heart failure or underwent cardiac transplantation. They show a functional and pathologic dilated pattern.

Patients who are symptomatic and have a subaortic gradient higher than 50 mm Hg could benefit from surgical excision of the subaortic obstruction, a procedure commonly performed in North America. A myotomy-myectomy of the hypertrophied septum is done, most often through a transaortic approach. The operation usually relieves obstruction and alleviates mitral regurgitation associated with systolic anterior movement of the mitral leaflet. Several grams of myocardium, in pieces, are received in surgical pathology, and some may show endocardial thickening. If fragments are small, it is important to sample them by both longitudinal and transverse sections if myocardial disarray is to be recognized, usually in deeper parts of the fragments. Connective tissue stains may help in this examination. However, in some instances, the pathologist may not be able to substantiate histologically a clinical diagnosis of hypertrophic cardiomyopathy.

In healing and with time, the operative site appears as a shallow, saucer-like depression in the septal wall, with overlying endocardial thickening and fibrosis extending

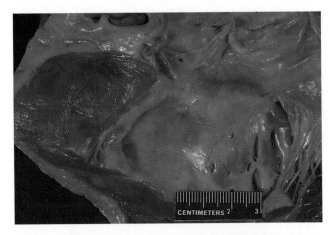

Figure 10-13 • Healed myotomy-myectomy wound appearing as a saucer-shaped depression lined by thickened endocardium. Note asymmetric hypertrophy in the basal septum. The patient was a 34-year-old man who died of noncardiac causes 6 years after surgery. Scale indicates 3 cm. (Courtesy of M.D. Silver, MD, Toronto.)

into the immediately adjacent septal muscle (Fig. 10-13). The surgical procedure usually produces a left bundle branch block.

Rarely, the septum is perforated by this procedure and a postoperative, fatal myocardial infarct may result from embolization of a fragment of disarrayed myocardium to the left anterior descending coronary artery after a myotomy-myectomy.[200a]

RESTRICTIVE CARDIOMYOPATHY

Definition

Among cardiomyopathies, the restrictive form is the least common in Western countries. Its hallmark is a reduced diastolic relaxation of either the left or both ventricles, with impeded diastolic filling and increased ventricular filling pressure. Systolic function is generally normal or nearly so. A variety of specific pathologic processes can cause restrictive cardiomyopathy. They may be divided into two distinct groups: conditions with predominant endocardial involvement, and others with predominant myocardial involvement.

Conditions with Predominant Endocardial Involvement

Endomyocardial Fibrosis

Worldwide, endomyocardial fibrosis (EMF) is the most common cause of restrictive cardiomyopathy. Two distinct clinicopathologic entities produce EMF: Loeffler endocarditis and tropical endomyocardial fibrosis. Despite the similarities of pathologic findings in end-stage disease (see later discussion), these two entities differ in geographic, age, and gender distribution; clinical presentation; and evolution.

Loeffler Endocarditis

This is a rare disease that generally affects men living in temperate zones who are in their fourth decade of life. It is typically associated with systemic eosinophilia (hypereosinophilic syndrome), often of unknown cause, although in some cases it may be secondary to hematologic or allergic disorders or parasitic infestation.[201]

Clinically, the disease tends to be rapidly progressive. It may manifest in the acute phase, with hypereosinophilia, systemic embolism, and congestive heart failure. Echocardiography commonly shows thickening of the posterobasal left ventricular wall, with limited motion of the posterior mitral leaflet.[202, 203] Systolic function is often well preserved. At a later stage, as a result of dense endocardial scarring, there is a reduction in ventricular cavity size (Fig. 10-14A), with abnormal diastolic filling caused by increased ventricular wall stiffness; the atria are usually dilated.

At gross examination, there is a diffuse deposition of mural thrombus over the ventricular endocardium, with a predilection for the inflow tract and apex of both ventricles. Mural thrombus generally surrounds papillary muscles and may spread onto heart valves; it often causes distal embolization. The endocardium is subsequently converted into a whitish fibrous plaque (up to 1 cm thick), incorporating the thrombotic material (Fig. 10-14B). On histologic examination,[203, 204] the disease process begins with an eosinophilic necrotizing myocarditis,[205] extending to the overlying endocardium. Endocardial damage is likely to cause thrombotic deposition, which is in turn infiltrated by eosinophils. Intramural coronary arteritis can be found. In the end, one can observe a stratification of thrombotic material over a dense myocardial fibrous scar, with the interposition of a layer of granulation tissue (Fig. 10-14C). Fibrous scarring, in which calcification or even ossification can be found, extends irregularly through the superficial myocardium to about a third of its depth. Loeffler endocarditis is caused by myocardial and endocardial tissue damage produced by major basic and cationic proteins derived from activated eosinophils. Thrombus deposition is secondary to endocardial damage.

Tropical Endomyocardial Fibrosis

This condition is restricted to the tropical areas of Africa, India, and South America, where it is a relatively frequent cause of congestive heart failure. In contrast to Loeffler endocarditis, the disease is equally common in both men and women and is more common in children and young adults, although individuals of any age can be affected.[202, 206] Eosinophilia is infrequent; when present, it may reflect a parasitic infection.

Clinical manifestations depend on which ventricle is affected: left-sided involvement is associated with pulmonary congestion, whereas predominantly right-sided disease may result in clinical symptoms suggestive of a constrictive pericarditis, such as raised jugular venous pressure, liver enlargement, and ascites. However, biventricular involvement is most frequent and shows the additional finding of low cardiac output. The atrioventricular valves are often involved, resulting in regurgitation.[207, 208]

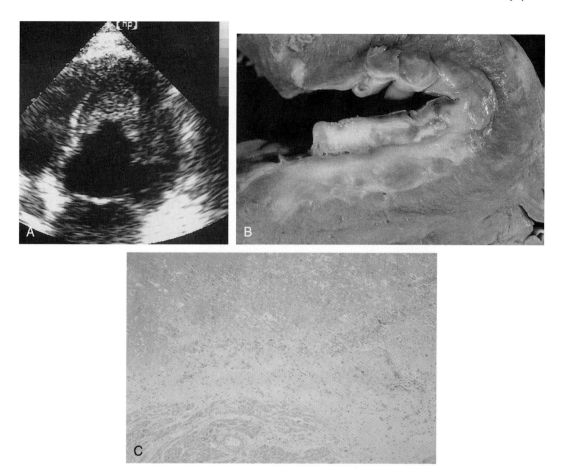

Figure 10-14 • Loeffler endocarditis. *A,* Bidimensional echocardiographic assessment of an adult man admitted with hypereosinophilic syndrome. The left ventricular cavity apex is obliterated by thrombotic material. *B,* The heart of a 44-year-old man who died from eosinophilic leukemia. The specimen was cut along a midventricular short-axis plane. Marked fibrosis of both endocardium and subendocardial myocardium is apparent. The endocardium is covered by thick, heterogeneous, thrombotic material. *C,* Histologic section of the left ventricle of a 36-year-old woman who died of crescentic glomerulonephritis. Eosinophilic infiltration within myocardium *(bottom),* endocardial fibrosis *(middle),* and thrombotic material *(top)* are seen (H&E stain). (*A,* Courtesy of V. Greco, MD, Rome).

The disease has an insidious onset and a relentless course. Death is caused either by congestive heart failure or malignant arrythmias. Endocardial surgical excision with atrioventricular valve replacement leads to substantial symptomatic improvement, especially in patients with predominant left ventricular involvement.[209]

Hearts have biatrial enlargement and normal ventricular chamber size; ventricular wall thickness is normal or slightly increased. The left ventricular endocardium shows dense fibrous thickening that is generally localized to the inflow tract and apex and surrounds the papillary muscles; in about half of the cases, the right ventricle is also involved.

Histologically, the affected endocardium shows a thick layer of hyaline collagen separated from the underlying myocardium by more loosely arranged fibrous connective tissue.[210] Collagenous septa extend into the myocardium. Eosinophils and surface thrombotic material are absent, even in the early stages of the disease.

There are several hypotheses regarding the pathogenesis of tropical endomyocardial fibrosis; it has been postu-

lated that cerium toxicity in conjunction with magnesium deficiency may cause the disease.[211] Cerium, a lanthanide, is present in leafy vegetables and root tubers, such as cassava, which constitute the main dietary intake of low socioeconomic classes in the tropics.[212]

Endocardial Fibroelastosis, Restrictive Form

EFE is commonly encountered in association with congenital heart disease involving the left ventricle, including congenital aortic or mitral valve stenosis, aortic coarctation, anomalous origin of the left coronary artery from the pulmonary trunk, and hypoplastic left heart syndrome (Fig. 10-15). These forms are collectively referred to as *secondary,* as opposed to *primary* forms, in which no other cardiac abnormalities can be found. The clinicopathologic pattern is that of a small, hypoplastic left ventricle with decreased diastolic compliance, but a dilated form can also be observed.

Pathologic features are similar to those observed in primary EFE. Focal areas of valvular or mural endocar-

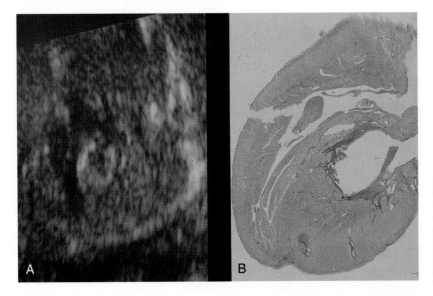

Figure 10-15 • Endocardial fibroelastosis, restrictive form, in a 28-week fetus with aortic atresia. *A,* The in utero echocardiogram shows a reduced left ventricular cavity, with hyperechogenic boundaries. *B,* Postmortem examination confirmed the hypoplasia of the left ventricle and showed endocardial fibroelastosis as well as subendocardial calcific deposits, visible as empty clefts. (*A,* Courtesy of E. Maggi, MD, Rome; *B,* Trichrome stain.)

dial thickening are observed in association with cardiac malformations. The left ventricle may be either small and hypoplastic or enlarged. As in the primary form, the pathogenetic mechanism underlying secondary EFE could be an endocardial reaction to high intracameral pressure or decreased wall resistance, or both, which in turn could be related to the observed cardiac malformations.

Conditions with Predominant Myocardial Involvement

Idiopathic Restrictive Cardiomyopathy

This is a rare entity that is sometimes familial and can be associated with a distal skeletal myopathy. Autosomal dominant restrictive cardiomyopathy with variable penetrance has been described in association with complete heart block and/or skeletal myopathy.[213, 214, 214a] A familial, nonhypertrophic form of cardiomyopathy with echo-

cardiographic and hemodynamic features of restrictive type is found associated with Noonan syndrome.[215] Restrictive cardiomyopathy occurring as the sole clinical finding has also been described in a family setting.[216]

Pathologic features include biatrial enlargement with normal ventricular cavity size and wall thickness. Patchy endocardial fibrosis can be observed. Histologic examination may reveal variable degrees of myofiber hypertrophy in the absence of myocellular disarrangement. The exclusion of myofiber disarray in these patients is important in the differential diagnosis from a variant of hypertrophic cardiomyopathy with restrictive physiology and normal ventricular wall thickness. The most characteristic feature is the presence of interstitial fibrosis surrounding both groups of myofibers and single myocytes (Fig. 10-16). Interstitial fibrosis acts as a straightjacket for cardiac myocytes, affecting ventricular diastolic relaxation. There may be fibrosis of the sinoatrial and atrioventricular nodes, accounting for conduction disturbances observed in a subset of patients with idiopathic restrictive cardiomyopathy.

Infiltrative Heart Disease

Amyloid Heart Disease

Cardiac amyloidosis is usually part of a systemic deposition of twisted β-pleated sheet fibrils (see Chapter 16). In addition to these nonbranching fibrils, a minor second component of globular structure, the so-called *P component,* is always present.

There are several types of amyloidosis in humans, but cardiac involvement is more commonly encountered in the so-called *primary,* or immunoglobulin-type, amyloidosis (amyloid AL), which is caused by production of an amyloid protein derived from immunoglobulin light chains. Amyloid AL is associated with B-cell dyscrasias.[217]

Secondary amyloidosis (AA), is caused by the deposition of a nonimmunoglobulin protein associated with chronic inflammatory conditions.[218] Rheumatoid arthritis

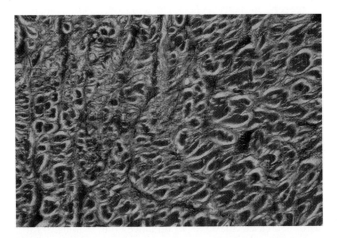

Figure 10-16 • Necropsy specimen of a 23-year-old woman who died from idiopathic restrictive cardiomyopathy. Diffuse plexiform fibrosis surrounds individual myocytes (Mallory's azan stain).

and chronic inflammatory bowel disease are the major causes in Western countries.

Familial amyloidosis is induced by the deposition of mutant forms of transthyretin and apolipoprotein A-1.[219, 220, 220a, 220b] This is a plasma protein that transports retinol-binding protein and thyroxine. Familial amyloidosis is a late-onset disease transmitted with an autosomal dominant pattern of inheritance. More than 50 amyloidogenic transthyretin mutations have been reported.[221] One of these (isoleucine 122) is prevalent in persons of African descent and seems to play a role in the increased prevalence of "isolated" cardiac amyloidosis in elderly blacks.[222] Although familial amyloidosis is usually a systemic disease, the most frequent clinical manifestations are cardiomyopathy and/or polyneuropathy[217]; the former is clinically similar to senile amyloidosis.

Senile amyloidosis, caused by the deposition of non-mutant forms of transthyretin or of an atrial natriuretic-like protein,[218–223] is becoming increasingly frequent as the population ages. It is uncommon in persons younger than 70 years of age. The cause of amyloid formation in these patients is unknown. In senile amyloidosis, the deposits are most commonly found in the vessel walls and myocardium. The disease is usually asymptomatic, except in patients with massive myocardial infiltration, which causes cardiac insufficiency or conduction disturbances (see Chapter 20 also).

Clinically, cardiac involvement is quite frequent in systemic amyloidosis. It is the main cause of death in patients with AL amyloid. Cardiac signs do not usually manifest before the fourth decade. The most frequent presentation is that of a restrictive cardiomyopathy, but congestive heart failure due to systolic dysfunction can also be a feature.[220] Orthostatic hypotension, probably caused by amyloid infiltration of the autonomic nervous system, and arrhythmias have also been described.[224]

On gross examination, myocardium infiltrated by amyloid is tan, firm, and rubbery. The ventricular cavities can be normal, small, or slightly enlarged. The ventricular wall may show a considerable thickness, which sometimes mainly involves the septum, mimicking hypertrophic cardiomyopathy on echocardiographic examination. The atria are mildly enlarged and, particularly in senile forms, may show small, translucent endocardial nodules, more evident after formalin fixation (Fig. 10-17). Amyloid deposits often result in focal or marked thickening of valve cusps and leaflets. On microscopic examination, interstitial deposits of amyloid appear as hyaline, eosinophilic material surrounding cardiac myofibers, which often appear atrophic. The deposits are also found in endocardium and valve leaflets and, as medial and adventitial deposits, in the intramural coronary arteries and veins. Amyloid deposits are best identified by their characteristic staining qualities and ultrastructural morphology.[225] Immunohistochemical stain is required for accurate classification of amyloidosis on tissue.[226] Interstitial deposits of eosinophilic, hyaline material resembling but distinct from amyloid have been described in cyclosporin-treated cardiac transplantation patients[227] and in a recently described type of infiltrative heart disease, microfibrillar cardiomyopathy. The latter is characterized by interstitial,

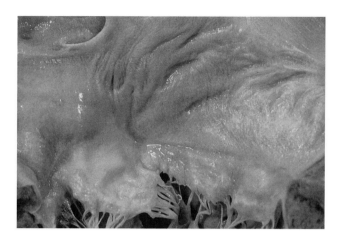

Figure 10-17 • Postmortem specimen from a 69-year-old man who died from restrictive cardiomyopathy. The left atrial endocardium and mitral valve leaflets show scattered small yellowish nodules, caused by amyloid deposits.

subendocardial, and perivascular deposits that do not stain with Congo red, have ultrastructural features distinct from amyloid, and, on immunohistochemistry, are identified as fibrillin microfibrils.[228]

Endomyocardial biopsy is useful in the diagnosis of cardiac amyloidosis. It is recommended in the differential diagnosis of constrictive pericarditis in patients who exhibit a restrictive hemodynamic pattern.

Other Infiltrative Heart Diseases

A number of other infiltrative conditions and storage diseases, often familiar, can result in restrictive cardiomyopathy (see Chapter 16).

Cardiac Sarcoidosis

This affects 20 to 30% of patients with the generalized disease; however, only a small proportion of cases are symptomatic.[229] It typically affects young adults of either gender who have clinical signs of systemic sarcoidosis. The disease has a variable course: in some patients it progresses rapidly to congestive heart failure; others present with sudden death or heart block, presumably caused by involvement of the conduction system by the inflammatory process[230] (see Chapters 9 and 20). The myocardial inflammatory infiltrate usually impairs diastolic function; the presence of fibrosis may also influence systolic contractile function. The gross appearance of the heart varies with the extent and activity of the granulomas, but grossly visible scars are common. They are often transmural and thin, with the right ventricular wall allowing transillumination and requiring differential diagnosis from arrhythmogenic cardiomyopathy; sometimes aneurysms form. Microscopically, the characteristic non-caseating granulomas, or scars resulting from them, replace cardiac muscle. Endomyocardial biopsy may be useful in diagnosis but, because the granulomas are focal, a negative biopsy does not exclude the disease.[231]

Iron Storage Disease

It may occur as an autosomal recessive hereditary disease, as a primary or idiopathic hemochromatosis, or as a

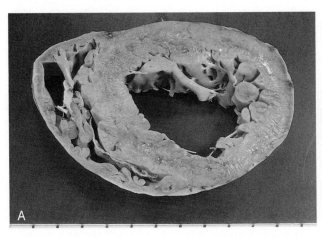
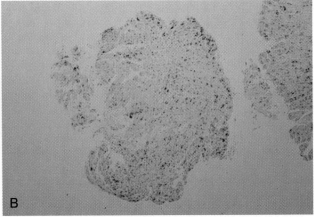

Figure 10-18 • Iron storage disease of myocardium. *A,* Heart of a boy affected by thalassemia who died from dilated cardiomyopathy secondary to hemosiderosis. The specimen was cut along a midventricular short-axis plane. The left ventricular myocardium is hypertrophied and is a typical rusty-brown. (Scale in centimeters.) *B,* Left ventricular endomyocardial biopsy from a 51-year-old man affected by hemochromatosis. Myocyte iron deposits appear blue with Perl stain.

consequence of secondary iron overload due to excessive iron intake, ineffective erythropoiesis, liver disease, or hemolytic anemia. Iron deposition occurs in a variety of parenchymal tissues, including the heart; the severity of myocardial involvement varies from patient to patient and can lead to an association of restrictive and dilated pattern, often with arrhythmias; some patients remain asymptomatic despite echocardiographic evidence of myocardial involvement. Myocardial damage is thought to be the result of direct iron toxicity to myocytes.[232] The affected heart has a rusty-brown, hypertrophied left ventricle (Fig. 10-18*A*). Microscopically, the marked accumulation of hemosiderin in cardiac myocytes (Fig. 10-18*B*), particularly in the perinuclear region, is associated with varying degrees of cellular degeneration and replacement fibrosis. In primary hemochromatosis, iron deposits are more evident in the subepicardium, followed by the subendocardium and midwall region[233]; there is a direct correlation between the amount of iron deposited and the degree of cardiac dysfunction.[234] Ultrastructurally, cardiac myocytes contain abundant siderosomes, mainly in the perinuclear region. Endomyocardial biopsy is important to confirm the clinical diagnosis and grade the disease.[235] In all iron storage conditions, the cardiomyopathy may resolve if iron is leached from tissues.

Inborn Errors of Metabolism

Several inborn metabolic diseases affect the myocardium, because of the accumulation of abnormal metabolites in cardiac myocytes (see Chapter 16). Typically they produce a restrictive pattern with impaired diastolic ventricular filling, but systolic function may also be affected.

Fabry disease (angiokeratoma corporis diffusum universale) is an X-linked disease that results from deficiency of the lysosomal enzyme α-galactosidase A. It is characterized by intracellular accumulation of ceramide trihexoside, with preferential localization in kidneys, skin, and myocardium. Histologic findings in the heart include prominent vacuolization of both working and conduction myocytes (Fig. 10-19*A*) and endothelial cells. On frozen section, the vacuoles are sudanophilic, periodic acid–

Schiff (PAS)–positive, and strongly birefringent. At the ultrastructural level, ceramide trihexoside deposits form concentric or parallel lamellas. From a clinical standpoint, the disease is characterized by angina resulting from endothelial lipid deposits with intramural coronary artery stenosis, increased left ventricular thickness, and impaired ventricular compliance and systolic function.

Gaucher disease is a recessive disorder resulting from mutations at the glucocerebrosidase locus on chromosome lq21. Histologically, it is marked by accumulation of cerebrosides in the brain and in phagocytes of various parenchymal organs and myocardium. The last appears to be infiltrated by macrophages laden with cerebrosides.

Glycogen storage diseases result from defects in enzymes involved in glycogen synthesis or catabolism. Cardiac involvement is prominent in deficiency of acid maltase, which leads to lysosomal storage of glycogen (type II glycogenosis, Pompe disease). The heart shows an apparent left ventricular hypertrophy, often mimicking hypertrophic cardiomyopathy. On microscopic examination, myocytes show prominent vacuolization due to the presence of intracellular glycogen deposits (Fig. 10-19*B*). These can be demonstrated with routine histochemical methods and by electron microscopy.

Clinical Features and Diagnosis

Restrictive cardiomyopathy is similar to constrictive pericarditis, which may also manifest with "restrictive physiology" but, in comparison to the former, is often cured surgically. Accordingly, a diagnosis of restrictive cardiomyopathy must both discriminate this entity from constrictive pericarditis and define therapeutic options. The feature of restrictive cardiomyopathy is abnormal diastolic ventricular filling in the presence of normal or almost normal systolic function.[100, 236] Clinical symptoms include weakness, dyspnea, exercise intolerance, and, in severe cases, peripheral edema, ascites, and anasarca resulting from the elevated central venous pressure. Conduction disturbances are common in both amyloidosis and

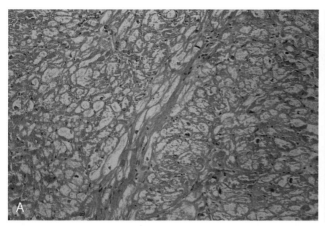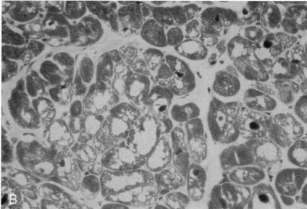

Figure 10-19 • Inborn metabolic diseases of myocardium. *A,* Fabry disease. Necropsy specimen. Myocyte vacuolization is prominent (H&E stain). *B,* Glycogenosis. Left ventricular endomyocardial biopsy from a patient with type II glycogenosis (Pompe disease). Intracellular glycogen deposits are evident on periodic acid–Schiff stain.

sarcoidosis. Angina may be a feature of Fabry disease and amyloidosis.

Physical examination may reveal jugular vein distention and a jugular venous pulse that fails to fall during inspiration and may actually rise (Kussmaul sign). Chest radiography shows ventricular chambers of normal size, usually with enlarged atria and vascular pulmonary congestion, as well as interstitial edema. Electrocardiography shows nonspecific S-T and T-wave abnormalities; conduction defects may be seen in specific conditions (see earlier discussion). Echocardiography usually demonstrates normal-sized ventricular cavities with enlarged atria.[237] An increase in ventricular wall thickening may be observed in patients with infiltrative heart disease.[202] Restrictive cardiomyopathy has a typical pattern of mitral-inflow velocity, marked by increased early diastolic filling velocity and decreased atrial filling velocity, deceleration time, and isovolumetric relaxation time.[236] Other noninvasive tests, such as computed tomographic scanning and magnetic resonance imaging, give the same information as echocardiography but may also be useful in excluding pericardial pathology. On cardiac catheterization, a characteristic feature is the presence of the dip-and-plateau diastolic filling curve (square root sign). Endomyocardial biopsy may aid in differentiating restrictive cardiomyopathy from constrictive pericarditis, which has normal myocardial features, and in demonstrating specific causes of restrictive cardiomyopathy (see earlier discussion).

The prognosis is variable but often dismal, with steady progression and high mortality.

ARRHYTHMOGENIC CARDIOMYOPATHY

Definition

Arrhythmogenic cardiomyopathy is a primary disease characterized by progressive adipose or fibroadipose replacement of the ventricular myocardium. It was formerly described as "right ventricular arrhythmogenic dysplasia,"[238] a term that focuses on its arrhythmogenic poten-

tial but implies a congenital anomaly as the cause. This pathologic entity has been differentiated from Uhl's anomaly, and its progressive postnatal development has been definitively assessed.[239] The inclusion of such an entity in the WHO classification of cardiomyopathies was long proposed,[2] in view of its primary nature, postnatal development, and frequent genetic background, and has now been achieved.[3] Although there is unanimous consensus on the progressive involvement of the left ventricle, and in spite of our proposal[240] for naming this condition "arrhythmogenic cardiomyopathy," the term "right ventricular arrhythmogenic cardiomyopathy" is still widely used. Consistent with our proposal, the former term is adopted in this chapter. This condition is also discussed in Chapter 11 with emphasis on sudden death. Figures 11–27 to 11–29 present mophologic findings also.

Pathology

Gross Anatomy

A striking feature in arrhythmogenic cardiomyopathy is a fibroadipose replacement of the ventricular myocardium. This process is more evident, and probably occurs earlier, in the right ventricle, where it may become transmural.

Right Ventricular Involvement

External inspection is often noncontributory, because the right ventricular myocardium is not generally discernible through the subepicardial fat, but palpation may disclose areas of reduced consistency or even of indentation, corresponding to the dome-shaped aneurysms detected in vivo (Fig. 10-20*A*). A generalized volume or mass increase is often present,[241] and the average heart weight is above normal limits.[242]

On cut surface, the striking feature is the fatty replacement of the ventricular myocardium. The adipose tissue appears to be an extension of the subepicardial layer, replacing the myocardium to a variable degree (see Fig. 10-20*A*, right-hand photograph). Effacement of the external two thirds of the parietal myocardium is frequent, and

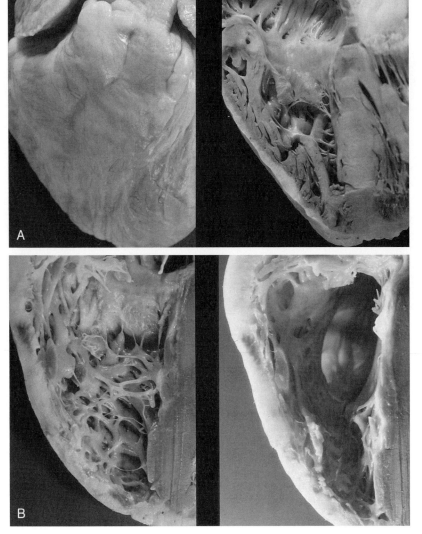

Figure 10-20 • Arrhythmogenic cardiomyopathy. *A*, Heart of a 12-year-old boy affected by familial arrhythmogenic cardiomyopathy who died suddenly. The external aspect of the right ventricle shows two areas of introflection of the anterior infundibular wall *(left)*. On a four-chamber section, the myocardium of the right ventricular wall appears replaced by adipose tissue. Right trabecular myocardium and the ventricular septum are spared *(right)*. *B*, The heart of a 32-year-old man who also died suddenly. The specimen was cut along a four-chamber plane and the section is viewed from behind. Transmural adipose replacement of the right ventricular wall, with an occasional area of persisting myocardium *(left)*. The ventricular septum is only focally affected. On transillumination, the pulmonary infundibulum and the right ventricular apex, two corners of the "triangle of dysplasia," are transparent *(right)*.

myocardial replacement may be transmural, with occasional islands of persisting muscular tissue (Fig. 10-20*B*). Even in advanced cases, the trabecular myocardium and a thin rim of subendocardial myocardium are usually spared, but trabeculae may appear shrunken, with fibroadipose replacement. Transillumination (see Fig. 10-20*B*, right-hand photograph) may prove particularly helpful in detecting the areas of adipose replacement.[242] Adipose replacement may be either diffuse or regional.[241] When focal, it is most frequently located at the angles of the "triangle of displasia"[243]: the pulmonary infundibulum (see Fig. 10-20*A*), the right ventricular apex, and the inferior wall of the right ventricle (Fig. 10-21, *A* and *C*). In spite of myocardial replacement, the parietal width is not noticeably reduced or is even increased. This contrasts with the hypothesis of a congenital absence of ventricular myocardium—as was suggested by the term "dysplasia"—and allows this condition to be distinguished from "parchment heart"[244] and from Uhl's anomaly.[245] In these latter malformations the parietal right ventricular wall is parchment thin, the myocardium being focally absent, and there is direct continuity of endocar-

dial and epicardial layers. Other differential features from arrhythmogenic cardiomyopathy include the absence of male preponderance and familial distribution, a younger age at clinical presentation, and the rarity of arrhythmias.[246] Parietal thinning, as well as endocardial thickening, may be evident in arrhythmogenic cardiomyopathy, too, in areas of aneurysmal dilation.[241] Aside from these zones, endocardial fibrous thickening is not a common feature, whereas fibrous replacement of the subendocardial myocardium is frequent. Myxoid change and prolapse of the atrioventricular valves have been described.[242] Coronary arteries are usually normal, considering the relatively young age of patients coming to observation, but critical stenoses have been reported.[242]

Biventricular Involvement

Some left ventricular involvement in "right ventricular" arrhythmogenic cardiomyopathy had been reported sporadically, but the biventricular nature of this cardiomyopathy was thoroughly assessed in contemporary and independent work of the Rome[240] and Trieste[247] groups, respectively based on pathologic and echocardiographic

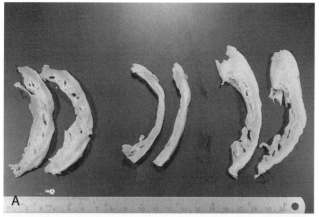

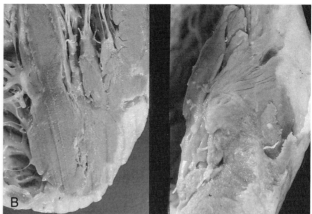

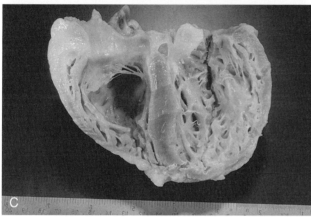

Figure 10-21 • Arrhythmogenic cardiomyopathy. *A,* Ventricular slices from the native heart of a 40-year-old woman who received a heart transplant. The slices were taken from the left ventricle *(left)* and from the anterior *(middle)* and inferior *(right)* walls of the right ventricle. The patient had left ventricular fibroadipose replacement and inferior right ventricular adipose substitution. *B,* Same case as *A.* Both pictures show parts of the left ventricle and illustrate a case of biventricular arrhythmogenic cardiomyopathy, adipose type. There is mild adipose replacement of the apical zone *(left)* and a much more extensive adipose substitution of the basal ventricular wall *(right). C,* Same case as in *A.* The native heart, devoid of its atrial caps, was cut along a four-chamber plane. The picture illustrates biventricular arrhythmogenic cardiomyopathy, with adipose replacement of the right ventricle and fibroadipose replacement of the left ventricle. The ventricular septum is spared.

grounds. Because of the greater left ventricular thickness, the fibroadipose replacement only exceptionally becomes transmural on the left side.[248] As a consequence, parietal thinning and focal aneurysms[249] have rarely been described, whereas a generalized ventricular dilation may ensue, sometimes with apical thrombus formation. The presence of left ventricular fatty replacement cannot be easily guessed from the exterior, but on cut surface a considerable subepicardial substitution may be obvious (Fig. 10-21*B*). Along with adipose infiltration, some fibrous scarring is commonly seen (Fig. 10-21, *A* and *C*). At variance with the right ventricle, preferential sites of involvement have not been identified, even if a basal-to-apical gradient has been reported.[250] The ventricular septum is usually spared or only superficially affected (see Fig. 10-20*B*), but massive septal involvement has been described occasionally.[251] Apart from unique cases,[252] left ventricular involvement in arrhythmogenic cardiomyopathy is constantly accompanied by a more extensive right ventricular change. It is noteworthy that in comparison to patients with monoventricular right disease, the ones with biventricular involvement are slightly older, have heavier hearts, and have a significantly higher frequency of right ventricular aneurysms.[241]

Histopathology

Microscopically, two main patterns have been defined[239]: a fatty or adipose type and a fibrofatty or fibroadipose one. We favor a distinction based on histologic evaluation of both the nature of the replacing tissue

and the myocellular features. Accordingly, we define an infiltrative and a cardiomyopathic pattern.

Infiltrative Pattern

The infiltrative pattern shows normal—or slightly atrophic—myocytes being replaced by mature adipocytes in a lacelike way. The fatty cells are contiguous to, and indistinguishable from, subepicardial adipose tissue, and that suggests an infiltration from the outside; in some cases, a thin edge of myocardial cells persists as a reminder of the effaced boundary between epicardial fat and myocardium (Fig. 10–22*A*). The subendocardial layer is usually normal. At the boundary with the adipose front, persisting myocytes appear as thin interlacing strands, giving full reason for the electric instability of the parietal myocardium. Small muscular islands, or even isolated disperse myocytes, are often seen within the adipose tissue. The infiltrative pattern of arrhythmogenic cardiomyopathy is predominantly associated with a right ventricular localization, with infrequent involvement of all the sites of the triangle of dysplasia. An adipose pattern is maintained and is usually limited to the outer ventricular layers.[240] Hearts with the infiltrative pattern are slightly heavier than normal, show only infrequently aneurysmal dilations and foci of active myocarditis, and often exhibit mitral valve prolapse.[240a]

Cardiomyopathic Pattern

In this pattern, there is massive myocardial replacement by fibrofatty tissue. Residual myocytes, often arranged in nests encircled by fibrous tissue (Fig. 10–22*B*),

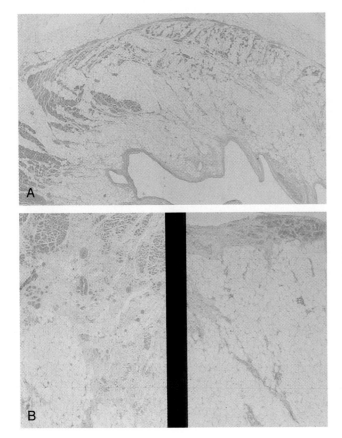

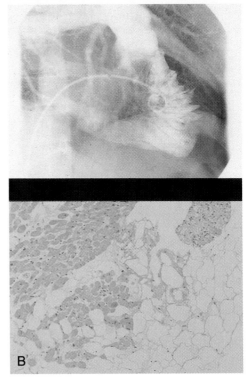

Figure 10-22 • Histology of arrhythmogenic cardiomyopathy. *A,* Right ventricular wall. The adipose replacement is transmural, extending to the endocardium *(bottom)*. A thin edge of myocardial cells marks the boundary between the former subepicardial adipose tissue *(top)* and the replaced myocardium. *B,* Left ventricular wall of an adult man who suddenly died of biventricular arrhythmogenic cardiomyopathy, cardiomyopathic pattern. Myocardium is largely replaced by adipose and fibrous tissues *(left)*. The residual subendocardial myocardium is embedded within fibrous tissue. Scattered lymphocytic infiltrates are apparent within the adipose tissue underneath *(right)*. (All H&E stain.)

are enlarged and show myofibril loss. The cardiomyopathic pattern is associated with extensive right ventricular involvement and an almost constant extension to the left ventricle, where myocardial replacement can be nearly transmural and is usually more fibrous than in the right ventricle. Myocardial fibroadipose replacement, characteristic of the cardiomyopathic pattern, has been statistically associated with older age of patients, thinner right ventricular wall, and higher occurrence of both right ventricular aneurysms and microscopic features of focal myocarditis.[241, 241a] In the cardiomyopathic pattern we also observed features suggestive of transdifferentiation from myocytes to adipose cells.[241b]

Ultrastructure

Electron microscopic examination adds little further information. Ultrastructural changes of myocytes ("flattening" of intercalated discs) have been reported,[253, 254] but more recently they have been either considered nonspecific[242] or not confirmed.[241]

Indications for Endomyocardial Biopsy

Of all cardiomyopathies, the arrhythmogenic one is the easiest to identify by endomyocardial biopsy.[255, 256] Provided the biopsy is taken at an affected area, adipose or fibroadipose replacement is easy to recognize (Fig. 10-23). The problem is that fatty infiltration is very common in endomyocardial biopsy specimens taken for widely different reasons,[257] so that a diagnosis of arrhythmogenic cardiomyopathy can be suspected only if the percentage

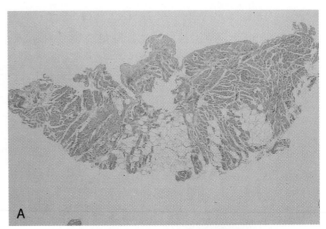

Figure 10-23 • Right ventricular endomyocardial biopsy from a 52-year-old woman affected by arrhythmogenic cardiomyopathy. *A,* Adipose replacement is evident, covering 13.8% of the total specimen area. *B,* Right ventriculogram showing the typical "pile of plates" pattern of the right ventricular apical region *(top)*. Endomyocardial biopsy specimen of the same patient, showing extensive adipose replacement *(bottom)*. (*A,* From Gallo P: La biopsia endomiocardia nella patologia cardiovascolare pediatrica. G Ital Cardiol 25:1499, 1995. *B,* Top, courtesy of P. Loschiavo, MD, Rome; bottom, (H&E stain).

of adipose replacement exceeds a given threshold. The mean percentage area covered by adipose tissue in arrhythmogenic cardiomyopathy biopsy samples ranges from 13.3[258] to 19.8%,[257] but in the Padua experience[258] adipose replacement involving more than 3.2% of the total biopsy area is said to allow a diagnosis of arrhythmogenic cardiomyopathy with a 67% sensitivity and a 91.5% specificity.

Etiology and Pathogenesis

In spite of much research, and because of conflicting evidence, the etiology and pathogenesis of arrhythmogenic cardiomyopathy are still unknown. Several causes have been tentatively suggested.

Congenital Defect

The first hypothesis was that of a congenital aplasia of ventricular myocardium, as implied by adoption of the term "dysplasia." Actually, arrhythmogenic cardiomyopathy is not usually detected in infancy, it has been differentiated from Uhl's anomaly (see earlier discussion), and its progressive development in adult life has been documented.[247] The hypothesis of a congenital basis has been retained on genetic grounds.

Genetics

At present, the cause of the disease is still unknown. However, in about 30% of cases, familial transmission with an autosomal dominant pattern of inheritance[259-261] and variable penetrance has been documented. Arrhythmogenic cardiomyopathy variability, both in clinical expression and penetrance, suggests that defects in various genes could underlie the disease phenotype. Linkage studies performed on several large kindreds identified three distinct loci on the long arm of chromosome 14 (ARVD1, ARVD3), whose mutation can give rise to arrhythmogenic cardiomyopathy.[262, 263, 263a] In additional families, the disease was mapped respectively to the long arm of chromosome 1 (ARVD2)[264] and chromosome 2 (ARVD4),[264a] and on the short arm of chromosome 10 (ARVD6).[264b] In addition, the gene for Naxos disease (arrhythmogenic right ventricular cardiomyopathy, palmoplantar keratoderma, woolly hair, and recessive inheritance) has been mapped to 17q21.[264c] The finding of genetic defects in arrhythmogenic cardiomyopathy favors the hypothesis of a genetically induced myocardial atrophy; alternatively, genetic factors could play a role in the susceptibility to myocardial inflammation, with consequent myocyte loss and adipose replacement.

Acquired Factors

Arrhythmogenic cardiomyopathy has been supposed to be a result of a chronic myocarditis.[265-267] A lymphocytic infiltrate is often present, at least in the cardiomyopathic pattern, and the disappearance of the ventricular myocytes—with the consequent fibroadipose replacement—could be the result of a myocarditis (Fig. 10-24). In chronic Chagas heart disease, a condition believed to be the result of an immunomediated myocarditis, classic ar-

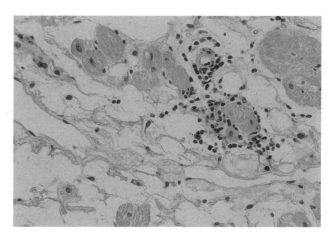

Figure 10-24 • Right ventricular specimen from the native heart of a 21-year-old man, transplanted for familial myocarditis and arrhythmogenic cardiomyopathy. Residual myocytes are surrounded by lymphocytes and lipoblasts (H&E stain).

rhythmogenic cardiomyopathy may ensue.[268] Actually, the genetic and inflammatory pathogenetic hypotheses are not necessarily mutually exclusive. There could be a genetic predisposition either to viral infections with preferential right ventricular involvement[269, 270] or to autoimmune myocarditis.[271] We have recently observed[272] two siblings with a family history of dilated cardiomyopathy and myocarditis, who underwent heart transplantation with a clinical diagnosis of mildly dilated cardiomyopathy and subsequently were found to have arrhythmogenic cardiomyopathy associated with myocarditis. At least in these siblings, the association between arrhythmogenic cardiomyopathy and myocarditis appeared to be of genetic origin. The myocellular damage, whatever the trigger, could be apoptoic in nature.[273]

Clinical Pathologic Correlation

Arrhythmogenic cardiomyopathy is usually diagnosed in young adults. As to gender distribution, a strong male predominance is reported in the United States[240a] and Canada,[241a] whereas a lower male to female ratio is described in Europe[241, 273a] (1.4 : 1 in our series). In the United States, the disease is said to cause fewer than 1% of adult sudden cardiac deaths[274, 275] and 3% of sports-related deaths.[274] In Italy, in the Veneto region, a substantially higher prevalence was reported in a series of young adults dying suddenly (see Chapter 11). Such a geographical distribution has been attributed to either genetic factors or a selection bias. This cardiomyopathy is still poorly known and, because one detects what one knows, unless the unopened heart is sent to a referral center (as in the Veneto program), the diagnosis of arrhythmogenic cardiomyopathy may be missed. A heart featuring this cardiomyopathy may even escape the close scrutiny of an expert cardiac surgeon. Among a series of 1068 cardiac transplants, three such hearts escaped notice: two were used as grafts, causing death of the recipients, and the third was discarded in time because it suddenly arrested during harvesting.[276]

Natural History

There is a wide spectrum of clinical presentation, mainly depending on the stage of the natural history. Four patterns have been traced, which probably correspond to as many subsequent steps in the natural history of the disease.[241, 276a]

Concealed Form

In this phase, the patient experiences only minor arrhythmias,[277] which usually go unnoticed, and the diagnosis is made either at postmortem examination in cases of unexpected sudden death or during screening of relatives of a recognized patient.

Overt Electrical Heart Disorder

This is the typical clinical presentation, with severe, usually symptomatic, ventricular arrhythmias (see later discussion) and impending cardiac arrest. This pattern, and especially the occurrence of syncope and ventricular couplets, is more common in young patients than in adults.[278]

Right Ventricular Failure

There is right ventricular pump failure because of extensive myocardial replacement, whereas the left ventricular function is relatively preserved.

Biventricular Pump Failure

It develops late in the natural history of the disease and is characterized by a progressive dilation of right[279] and left[247] ventricles—with an exceptional finding of right[280] or left[281] ventricular rupture—that causes pump failure and death or requires heart transplantation. The decompensation is mainly ascribed to the biventricular evolution of the disease[282] and is more common in familial cases and in those with the cardiomyopathic pattern.[283]

Associated Conditions

The association of arrhythmogenic cardiomyopathy with mitral valve prolapse is described with increasing frequency.[240a, 241a, 284, 285] In our experience, the correlation extends to tricuspid valve prolapse and patent foramen ovale, and is peculiar to the infiltrative pattern.

Clinical Features and Diagnosis

As stated previously, a patient with arrhythmogenic cardiomyopathy may seek medical advice because of overt arrhythmias or cardiomyopathic features of pump failure, or in the setting of a family screening. Physical examination is usually noncontributory. In a minority of patients, there are findings such as asymmetry of the precordium, because of right ventricular enlargement, and third and fourth heart sounds. On chest radiography, the heart may be globular and enlarged; 73% of patients in the series of Marcus and Fontaine[286] had a cardiothoracic ratio of 50% or more. The resting electrocardiogram offers several diagnostic clues: (1) a QRS prolongation (more than 110 msec), which is a highly specific but scarcely sensitive sign[287]; (2) an epsilon wave—a small upright deflection just after the QRS complex—that is particularly evident in lead V_1 and may be observed in one third of patients[286]; (3) inversion of T waves in the right precordial leads, which is present in half of these patients; and (4) premature ventricular complexes with a left bundle branch block configuration. These are commonly observed, especially during spontaneous ventricular tachycardia.[243] The signal-averaged electrocardiogram is usually abnormal in patients with ventricular arrhythmias,[288] in the frequency domain rather than in time. Electrophysiologic studies show only few, and nonspecific, conduction abnormalities. Ventricular tachycardia induced by either electrophysiologic studies or exercise stress testing is usually like that occurring spontaneously. Holter electrocardiography monitoring may help register not only the ventricular tachycardia but also ventricular extrasystoles, which may be particularly frequent. Echocardiography gives useful information,[289] provided the study is performed in multiple planes and focuses on both chamber dimensions and an analytical appraisal of wall motion pattern. The most prominent findings are dilation of the right ventricle, with increased end-diastolic and end-systolic diameters, and a raised right ventricular/left ventricular end-diastolic diameter ratio; localized bulging and dyskinesia of a ventricular segment; and highly reflective and irregularly shaped ventricular tracts. Radionuclide angiography allows both quantification of contractile abnormalities and assessment of a wall-motion score.[290] Electron-beam computed tomography[291] and magnetic resonance imaging[292] not only permit examination of right ventricular dimensions and contractility but also direct visualization of subepicardial adipose replacement. On a magnetic resonance scan, both adipose and fibroadipose replacement tissues[241] give a bright signal and are accordingly readily detectable. For diagnostic purposes, magnetic resonance imaging has proved highly specific but scarcely sensitive.[293, 294] In spite of the abundant information given by noninvasive techniques, right ventricular angiography remains the reference method for evaluating these patients[286] and allows an endomyocardial biopsy to be taken. The most frequent angiographic feature is the "pile of plates" pattern (see Fig. 10-23B), observed in the right ventricular apical region and caused by transversely arranged hypertrophic trabeculae separated by deep fissures.[295] This pattern, together with a ventricular aneurysm in the "triangle of dysplasia," has high specificity and sensitivity.

Criteria for Diagnosis

A consensus on standardized diagnostic principles has been reached,[261] based on the identification of major and minor criteria for diagnosis (Table 10-3). A diagnosis of arrhythmogenic cardiomyopathy is permissible in the presence of either two major criteria, or one major plus two minor criteria, or four minor criteria taken from different groups.

TABLE 10-3 • **Criteria for Diagnosis of Arrhythmogenic Cardiomyopathy**

Group	Major Criteria	Minor Criteria
Global and/or regional dysfunction and structural alterations detected in vivo	Severe dilation and reduction of RV ejection fraction with no (or only mild) LV impairment Localized RV aneurysms (akinetic or dyskinetic areas with diastolic bulging) Severe segmental dilation of the RV	Mild global RV dilation and/or ejection fraction reduction with normal LV Mild segmental dilation of the RV Regional RV hypokinesia
Tissue characterization of walls	(Fibro)adipose replacement of myocardium on endomyocardial biopsy	
Repolarization abnormalities		Inverted T waves in right precordial leads (V2 and V3) (people aged >12 yr, in absence of right bundle branch block)
Depolarization/conduction abnormalities	Epsilon waves or localized prolongation (>110 msec) of the QRS complex in right precordial leads (V1–V3)	Late potentials (signal-averaged ECG)
Arrhythmias		Left bundle branch block type ventricular tachycardia (sustained and nonsustained) (ECG, Holter, exercise testing) Frequent ventricular extrasystoles (>1000/24 h) (Holter)
Familial history	Familial disease confirmed at necropsy or surgery	Familial history of premature sudden death (<35 yr) due to suspected arrhythmogenic cardiomyopathy Familial history (clinical diagnosis based on present criteria)

ECG, electrocardiography; LV, left ventricle; RV, right ventricle.
Modified from McKenna WJ, Thiene G, Nava A, et al: Diagnosis of arrhythmogenic right ventricular dysplasia/cardiomyopathy. Br Heart J 71:215, 1994.

SPECIFIC CARDIOMYOPATHIES

According to the 1995 WHO classification, the term "specific cardiomyopathy" defines heart muscle disease associated with specific cardiac or systemic disorders. These were previously described as specific heart muscle diseases. Specific cardiomyopathies include several well-known systemic, metabolic, and neuromuscular disorders affecting the heart. Some of these conditions, with emphasis on other specifics, are also discussed in Chapters 6, 11, 16, and 20.

Muscular Dystrophies

Duchenne and Becker Muscular Dystrophies

Duchenne muscular dystrophy is a lethal neuromuscular disorder with an incidence of 1 in 3500 male births.[296] Clinically, it is characterized by progressive muscular weakness. Symptoms begin in the second year of life, although an elevated serum creatine kinase concentration is present at birth. Heart involvement is observed in more than 80% of patients and takes the form of dilated cardiomyopathy.[297] Yet, despite the frequency of cardiomyopathy, heart failure is responsible for only 10% of deaths in the condition.[297] Disturbances of cardiac rhythm and conduction have also been reported.[298] The typical autopsy finding is epimyocardial fibrosis, especially involving the posterobasal left ventricular wall.[299] In our experience, histologic features of arrhythmogenic right ventricular cardiomyopathy with biventricular involvement can be observed in Duchenne muscular dystrophy. Histology reveals degenerative changes and marked variability in myofiber shape and size, associated with areas of replacement fibrosis. Dilated cardiomyopathy also complicates Becker muscular dystrophy but appears to be unrelated to the severity of the muscoloskeletal involvement.[300]

Both Duchenne and Becker muscular dystrophies are caused by defects of the dystrophin gene on chromosome Xp21.[301, 302] Dystrophin is a large membrane cytoskeletal protein, closely associated with a number of sarcolemmal proteins.[303] Its putative role is to stabilize muscle cell membranes during contraction (for an excellent review on dystrophin structure and function see Ohlendieck[303]). Myopathy and cardiomyopathy in Duchenne muscular dystrophy are caused by an absence of dystrophin from sarcolemmal membranes. This is easily recognized on histologic sections treated with antidystrophin antibodies. In the milder allelic variant of Becker, the protein is partially conserved.[304] The hypothetic functional role of dystrophin may explain the posterobasal fibrosis observed in these hearts.[305] In comparison with the anterior left ventricular wall, where myocyte bundles are "mesh-like," those in the inferior wall have a parallel longitudinal arrangement; therefore, during contraction, forces acting on them are directed axially. If the role of dystrophin is to reinforce sarcolemma against axial forces, its absence would cause specific myocellular damage, followed by replacement fibrosis, in this area.

Myotonic Dystrophy

Inherited as an autosomal dominant trait, myotonic muscular dystrophy has a genetic abnormality in that an increased number of cytosine-thymine-guanine (CTG) repeats occur in the untranslated region of a protein kinase gene on chromosome 19q13.3.[306] Clinically, there is progressive muscle weakness (dystrophy) and delayed relaxation after contraction (myotonia), associated with systemic features such as cataracts, premature baldness, testicular atrophy, and mental deterioration.[307] Cardiac involvement is frequent, manifesting chiefly as conduction disturbances, whereas working myocardial dysfunction is seldom clinically evident.[308] Histologic changes in the conduction system consist of fibrosis and adipose infiltration of both sinus and atrioventricular nodes.[309, 310] Nonspecific myocardial changes such as increased interstitial fibrosis and myofibrillar degeneration are also found.

Miscellaneous Conditions

Other conditions associated with cardiomyopathy, generally of dilated pattern, are Emery-Dreifuss muscular dystrophy, limb-girdle muscular dystrophy, and autosomal recessive muscular dystrophy. The last is attributed to a deficiency of the 50-kd dystrophin-associated glycoprotein adhalin.[311]

Neuromuscular Disorders and Myopathies

Dilated or hypertrophic cardiomyopathies develop in several neuromuscular disorders and myopathies. From a cardiologic standpoint, the most important types are mitochondrial (cardio)myopathies, Friedreich ataxia, and desmin-related myopathies. Also the juvenile form of spinal muscular atrophy (Kugelberg-Welander disease) may be associated with congestive heart failure.[312]

Mitochondrial Cardiomyopathy

Etiology and Pathogenesis

Mitochondria are cytoplasmic organelles responsible for energy production from carbohydrates, fats, and proteins via oxidative phosphorylation. They possess their own genetic material, which is a 16,569–base-pair, double-stranded circular molecule of DNA.[313] The molecule contains tightly compacted genes for 22 transfer RNAs, two ribosomal RNAs, and 13 polypeptides, the latter all subunits of oxidative phosphorylation enzyme complexes. All other mitochondrial polypeptides are encoded by nuclear DNA and transported into mitochondria.[314] A mitochondrial cardiomyopathy is defined as one caused by mitochondrial DNA (mtDNA) mutation. The first reports on the pathogenetic role of point mutations and deletions of mtDNA in human disease date from 1988.[315, 316] Since then, at least 50 mtDNA point mutations have been associated with a variety of clinical disorders that preferentially affect the tissues most dependent on oxidative metabolism (skeletal muscle, brain, and myocardium). Because mtDNA is carried only by the oocyte, these disorders are transmitted through maternal inheritance. Moreover, because each cell possesses hundreds of mitochondria, mutations may result in the coexistence of mutated and wild-type mtDNA (so-called heteroplasmy). The phenotypic expression of a mutation depends on the relative proportion of mutated mtDNA within the cells (threshold effect).[317] Cardiac disorders in affected patients can be part of a multisystem disease or present as the sole, or predominant, clinical feature. In either case, cardiac involvement consists of cardiomyopathy and/or arrhythmias (mainly conduction block or pre-excitation syndrome).

Genetic classification includes sporadic, mendelian-inherited, and maternally inherited forms.

Sporadic cardiomyopathy is observed in the Kearns-Sayre/chronic external ophthalmoplegia syndrome. The disease is the result of mtDNA deletions or duplication[318, 319] and is characterized by early-onset (before 20 years) of ophthalmoplegia, atypical retinitis pigmentosa, myopathy, and one of the following: cardiac conduction defects, which can be associated with impaired myocardial contractility; cerebellar dysfunction; or elevated cerebrospinal fluid proteins.

Mitochondrial cardiomyopathies with mendelian inheritance are exceedingly rare. They are caused either by mutations in nuclear DNA encoding for mitochondrial polypeptides or by defects of intergenomic communication. An example of the latter is autosomal recessive progressive external ophthalmoplegia and cardiomyopathy.[320]

Maternally inherited mitochondrial cardiomyopathies are the most frequent and likely represent a large proportion of all familial cardiomyopathies. They are the consequence of mtDNA point mutations.[321] Cardiomyopathy can be associated with other signs of oxidative phosphorylation disease, such as encephalomyopathy or lactic acidemia, or can be the sole clinical feature. Examples of maternally inherited encephalomyopathy with cardiomyopathy include the MELAS syndrome (mitochondrial encephalomyopathy with lactic acidosis and stroke-like episodes), associated with cardiomyopathy in 20% of cases and usually with a hypertrophic pattern[322]; the MERRF syndrome[323] (myoclonic epilepsy and ragged red fiber disease), in which dilated cardiomyopathy and ventricular arrhythmias develop; and maternally inherited myopathy and cardiomyopathy, in which systemic signs of oxidative phosphorylation derangements are associated with myocardial hypertrophy or dilatation.[324]

There are increasing reports describing cardiomyopathy as the sole or prevalent manifestation of mtDNA point mutations.[325–328] In contrast to neuromuscular diseases like MELAS and MERRF, there is no predominant point mutation among these patients, although transfer RNA is generally affected.

Pathology

Despite an expanding literature on mitochondrial cardiomyopathies, information about the clinicopathologic pattern of the disease is still scarce. This is largely because reported cases have been studied mainly from neurologic and genetic standpoints. However, information available from reported cases suggests that left ventricular concentric hypertrophy is the prevalent pattern[329, 330]; a dilated form of mitochondrial cardiomyopathy has also been reported.[331] In our experience,[332] mitochondrial cardiomyopathy may manifest in a hypertrophic form, with diffuse concentric hypertrophy progressing toward a dilated pattern. Histologic findings generally include myocyte hypertrophy with perinuclear vacuolation (Fig. 10-25A).[327, 333] Myofiber disarray can be observed, but it is never so extensive as to suggest familial hypertrophic cardiomyopathy. Ragged red fibers (Fig. 10-25B), com-

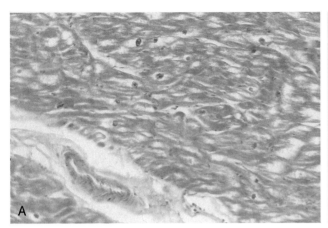 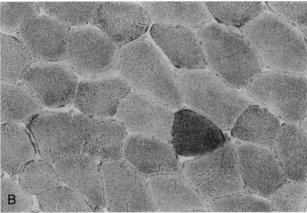

Figure 10-25 • Maternally inherited mitochondrial cardiomyopathy. *A,* Left ventricular specimen taken, after transplantation, from the native heart of a 33-year-old man, with features of concentric hypertrophic cardiomyopathy. Myocytes show perinuclear vacuolization, the light microscopic equivalent to mitochondriosis (H&E stain). *B,* Skeletal muscle biopsy from this case, showing a "ragged red fiber." These muscular fibers, which are actually red with the modified Gomori stain, are replete with mitochondria. In this section, stained to reveal the nuclear-coded mitochondrial enzyme succinic dehydrogenase, the pathologic fiber was a deep blue.

monly found in skeletal muscle in mitochondrial disease, are infrequently detected in the myocardium. Variable amounts of interstitial fibrosis are seen. Histochemical stain for cytochrome C oxidase may help diagnosis, revealing either a decrease or total loss of enzymatic activity within single cells or aggregates of cardiomyocytes.[330, 333] However, this finding is not constant and does not exclude the diagnosis. A defective pattern in myocellular enzymatic activity can also be revealed with the use of antibodies to cytochrome C oxidase subunits.[330] Myocyte ultrastructural findings include an increased number of mitochondria (mitochondriosis), which are often abnormally shaped and may show concentric or parallel lamellar arrangement of cristae and/or crystalline inclusions. Intracytoplasmatic lipid droplets have been described occasionally.

Clinical Pathologic Correlation

Increased awareness among cardiologists and neurologists of disorders affecting both heart and skeletal muscle has led to the more frequent diagnosis of heart involvement in patients with mitochondrial disease. However, the occurence of cardiomyopathy as the sole clinical manifestation can raise a problem in differential diagnosis with other inherited forms of cardiomyopathy, mainly familial hypertrophic cardiomyopathy. In our opinion, maternal inheritance should strongly suggest an underlying mitochondrial etiology. Noncardiac signs of mitochondrial disease must be carefully sought in these patients, and blood tests such as creatine kinase, lactic acid dehydrogenase, lactic acid, and carnitine dosages must be performed. Endomyocardial biopsy can be useful in patients presenting with a cardiomyopathy as the sole clinical manifestation of mitochondrial disease. However, genetic analysis on blood or on muscular or myocardial tissue is required to make a definite diagnosis.

Friedreich Ataxia

This is the most common inherited ataxia. It is transmitted as an autosomal recessive trait and is clinically

characterized by ataxia of all four limbs and the trunk, absence of tendon reflexes in the lower limbs, sensory loss, and pyramidal signs.[334] Usually the disease has its onset before 20 years of age and symptoms progress without remission. Cardiac involvement is extremely common and is often the cause of death.[335] The most common finding on echocardiography is symmetric or, less frequently, asymmetric left ventricular hypertrophy. At variance with familial hypertrophic cardiomyopathy, both systolic and diastolic left ventricular functions are normal[336] and patients do not show an increased risk of malignant ventricular arrhythmias. Less commonly, patients present with clinical and echocardiographic features of dilated cardiomyopathy, which almost invariably progresses to congestive heart failure, giving this latter form a much worse prognosis.[335, 337] Atrial and ventricular arrhythmias are not infrequent in these patients.[335]

Congestive heart failure associated with neurologic lesions mimicking those of Friedreich ataxia may be caused by abetalipoproteinemia (Bassen-Kornzweig disease), a lipid disorder featuring myocardial fibrosis.[338]

Whatever the clinical presentation, hearts generally show ventricular hypertrophy, as assessed by an increased weight, associated with biventricular dilation[339, 340] on pathologic examination. Histology reveals nonspecific myocardial changes: myocellular hypertrophy with large, hyperchromatic nuclei; focal degenerative changes; and increased interstitial fibrosis (Fig. 10-26). Small areas of myofiber disarray can also be found, but they are not more extensive than those seen in nonspecific myocardial hypertrophy. Disease of small intramural coronary arteries (see Fig. 10-26), with a wide range of vessel changes (such as medial degeneration and fibrosis, intimal proliferation, and either subintimal or medial deposition of PAS-positive material) has been reported by several authors.[339, 341, 342] It is unclear, however, whether small vessel stenosis contributes to the pathogenesis of myocardial dysfunction, at least in a subset of these patients. Finally, conduction system abnormalities, such as sinus node fibrosis, are occasionally described in patients with atrial arrhythmias.[342]

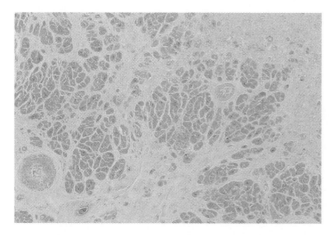

Figure 10-26 • Left ventricular specimen from the heart of a 28-year-old patient who died from Friedreich ataxia. The gross features were those of a dilated cardiomyopathy. Microscopically, hypertrophy of myocytes, extensive substitution fibrosis, and stenosis of intramural coronary arteries are observed (H&E stain).

The genetic defect underlying Friedreich ataxia has been identified as the presence of unstable expansions of a GAA repeat in the frataxin gene on chromosome 9.[343, 344] The function of the protein encoded by this gene is still unknown, as are possible pathogenetic mechanisms underlying neurologic and cardiac symptoms. However, there is a correlation between the size of the GAA expansions and the frequency of cardiomyopathy and loss of upper limb reflexes.[345]

Desmin-Related Myopathies

Desmin is an intermediate filament found exclusively in muscle cells. It plays a crucial role in maintaining normal cellular architecture, by linking neighboring Z bands to each other and to the sarcoplasmic membrane[346]; a role in the functional, and possibly spatial, relationship between nucleus and plasma membrane has also been attributed to this type of intermediate filament.[347] Desmin accumulation may be a secondary finding in congenital myotonic dystrophy or in regenerating muscle fibers of infantile spinal muscular atrophy.[348] Moreover, rare congenital myopathies, such as multicore myopathy and nemaline rod myopathy, characterized respectively by granular/filamentous cellular desmin inclusions and rod bodies, have been described. These are either sporadic or familial, and they can be associated with cardiomyopathy.[349-351]

Multicore myopathy is a skeletal muscle disorder with proximal skeletal muscle weakness, frequent occurrence of respiratory insufficiency, and the presence of many pink, hyaline myocellular inclusions on skeletal muscle biopsy. Its association with cardiomyopathy is reported.[352-354] Cardiac pathologic features vary from a dilated pattern, with myocardial hypertrophy and biventricular enlargement, to a restrictive one; histology may also reveal cytoplasmic eosinophilic inclusions,[355] but this is not a constant finding. Both skeletal and cardiac muscle inclusions show a positive reaction with antidesmin antibodies. Electron microscopy is required for the diagnosis of desmin cardiomyopathy.[214a] Ultrastructural findings include the presence of electron-dense granular and filamentous material between myofibrils or in the subsarcolemmal space.[351, 354, 355]

Nemaline myopathy, a term coined by Shy and associates,[356] is a congenital nonprogressive myopathy of either autosomal dominant or recessive inheritance. Occasional sporadic cases occur. Cardiac involvement is not frequent, but may be fatal, and is described in the sporadic form. It generally manifests as dilated cardiomyopathy. The histologic hallmark of nemaline myopathy is the presence of rod bodies within muscle fibers; these are found only sporadically within cardiac myocytes.[357] On immunohistochemistry, rod bodies are positive for desmin and α-actinin; electron microscopy shows the filamentous nature of the rods, which tend to be arranged parallel to the long axis of myocytes.

Histiocytoid Cardiomyopathy

Histiocytoid cardiomyopathy is a rare cardiac disorder of children. It characteristically affects female infants younger than 2 years of age. Clinically, the disease manifests as tachycardia or other dysrhythmias, refractory to treatment; less commonly, the presenting feature is sudden unexpected death.[358]

On gross examination, hearts fail to show major abnormalities, except for an increased weight. The characteristic feature of the disease is evident at the histologic level: it consists of large, polygonal cells with vacuolated or granular cytoplasm and round, central nuclei ("histiocytoid" cells) located within the myocardium. These abnormal cells may occur in a diffuse or focal pattern at any myocardial site, but they frequently follow a distribution reminiscent of the conduction system[359] (Fig. 10-27). Transitional cells, intermediate in morphologic abnormality between histiocytoid cells and normal myocytes, are sometimes observed. At the ultrastructural level, cells show a marked decrease of myofibrils. They lack a T-tubule system, contain desmosomes rather than side-to-side junctions, and are rich in mitochondria.[360-363] Immunohistochemistry reveals a patchy, perimembranous positivity for muscle-specific actin, while histiocytic markers are negative.[363]

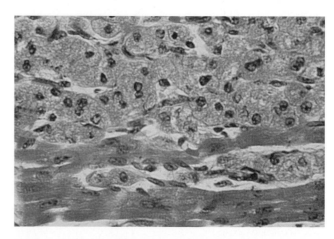

Figure 10-27 • Subendocardial oncocytic cells in right ventricular myocardium from a female infant who died with cardiac rhythm irregularities (Hematoxylin-phloxin-saffron [HPS] staining). (Courtesy of M.M. Silver, MB, BS, Toronto.)

The origin and pathogenesis of the disease are unclear. The view that it is a disorder of the atrioventricular conduction system is supported by some of the morphologic features of the cells and by their preferential left ventricular subendocardial distribution. However, the extensive increase in mitochondria, which is not a feature of Purkinje cells, has led to the consideration that these cells are oncocytes, like those described in a variety of other organs. This view is supported by the finding of oncocytosis in various glandular tissues of some patients with histiocytoid cardiomyopathy.[364] Therefore, the disease could be considered the result of hamartoma-like aggregates of cardiac myocytes with oncocytic changes.

Ischemic Cardiomyopathy

The term "ischemic cardiomyopathy" was first coined by Burch and coworkers in 1970[365] to describe a severe myocardial dysfunction associated with coronary artery disease, and it is used in that fashion by clinicians. Its clinical features are often indistinguishable from those of dilated cardiomyopathy. The development of a dilated pattern in ischemic heart disease can result from either chronic ischemia, leading to a failed heart with multifocal small areas of replacement fibrosis, or ventricular remodeling after acute myocardial infarction. The latter term describes complex alterations in left ventricular architecture involving both infarcted and noninfarcted areas and leading to ventricular enlargement.[366]

The 1995 WHO classification[3] defines ischemic cardiomyopathy as a "dilated cardiomyopathy with impaired contractile performance not explained by the extent of coronary artery disease or ischemic damage." Such a definition has a completely different meaning to that widely used by clinicians and is intended to delineate a cardiomyopathic subset in the population of patients with ischemic heart disease. We do not quite agree with this definition because it lacks a quantitative basis to establish the extent of coronary artery disease or ischemic myocardial damage. Moreover, severe atherosclerotic lesions have been described in normal hearts (70% or more).[367] In our experience, severe stenosis of a single coronary branch is found in a subset of hearts with gross and histologic features indistinguishable from those of "idiopathic" dilated cardiomyopathy, suggesting that isolated atherosclerotic lesions may be a superimposed phenomenon. According to these observations, the term ischemic cardiomyopathy—as proposed by WHO—could be of little use and is potentially misleading for clinicians.

REFERENCES

1. Brandenburg RO, Chazov E, Cherian G, et al: Report of the WHO/ISFC task force on the definition and classification of cardiomyopathies. Br Heart J 44:672, 1980
2. Boffa GM, Thiene G, Nava A, Dalla Volta S: Cardiomyopathy: A necessary revision of the WHO classification. Int J Cardiol 30:1, 1991
3. Richardson P, McKenna W, Bristow M, et al: Report of the 1995 World Health Organization/International Society and Federation of Cardiology task force on the definition and classification of cardiomyopathies. Circulation 93:841, 1996
4. Rose AG, Beck W: Dilated (congestive) cardiomyopathy: A syndrome of severe cardiac dysfunction with remarkably few morphological features of myocardial damage. Histopathology 9:367, 1985
5. Higginson J, Isaacson C, Simson I: The pathology of cryptogenic heart disease. A study of the pathological pattern in 80 cases of obscure heart failure in the South African Bantu Negro. Arch Pathol 70:497, 1960
6. Kallichurum S: The heart in cardiomyopathy. A postmortem study. S Afr Med J 50:1585, 1976
7. Benjamin IJ, Schuster EH, Bulkley BH: Cardiac hypertrophy in idiopathic dilated congestive cardiomyopathy: A clinicopathologic study. Circulation 64:442, 1981
8. Rossi MA, Carillo SV: Cardiac hypertrophy due to pressure and volume overload: Distinctly different biological phenomena? Int J Cardiol 31:133, 1991
9. Beltrami CA, Finato N, Rocco M, et al: The cellular basis of dilated cardiomyopathy in humans. J Mol Cell Cardiol 27:291, 1995
10. Triposkiadis F, Pitsavos C, Boudoulas H, et al: Left atrial myopathy in idiopathic dilated cardiomyopathy. Am Heart J 128:308, 1994
11. Linzbach AJ: Heart failure from the point of view of quantitative anatomy. Am J Cardiol 5:370, 1960
12. Astorri E, Bolognesi R, Colla B, et al: Left ventricular hypertrophy: A cytometric study on 42 human hearts. J Mol Cell Cardiol 9:763, 1977
13. Gerdes AM, Kellerman SE, Moore JA, et al: Structural remodeling of cardiac myocytes in patients with ischemic cardiomyopathy. Circulation 86:426, 1992
14. Anversa P, Capasso JM: Cardiac hypertrophy and ventricular remodeling. Lab Invest 64:441, 1991
15. Gallo P, Grillo LR, Pelliccia F, Baroldi G: Cardiomiopatia dilatativa. In: Baroldi G, Thiene G (eds): Biopsia Endomiocardica. Testo Atlante. Padua, Piccin, 1996, p 59
16. Schaper J, Froede R, Hein S, et al: Impairment of the myocardial ultrastructure and changes of the cytoskeleton in dilated cardiomyopathy. Circulation 83:504, 1991
17. Marijianowski MM, Teeling P, Mann J, Becker AE: Dilated cardiomyopathy is associated with an increase in the type I/type III collagen ratio: A quantitative assessment. J Am Coll Cardiol 25:1263, 1995
18. Anderson KR, Sutton MG St. J, Lie JT: Histopathological types of cardiac fibrosis in myocardial disease. J Pathol 128:79, 1979
19. Tazelaar HD, Billingham ME: Leukocyte infiltrates in idiopathic dilated cardiomyopathy. A source of confusion with active myocarditis. Am J Surg Pathol 10:405, 1986
20. Hammond EH, Menlove RL, Anderson JL: Predictive value of immunofluorescence and electron microscopic evaluation of endomyocardial biopsies in the diagnosis and prognosis of myocarditis and idiopathic dilated cardiomyopathy. Am Heart J 114:1055, 1987
21. Aretz HT, Billingham ME, Edwards WD, et al: Myocarditis. A histopathologic definition and classification. Am J Cardiovasc Pathol 1:3, 1986
22. Tanganelli P, Pierli C, Bravi A, et al: Small vessel disease (SVD) in patients with unexplained ventricular arrhythmia and dilated congestive cardiomyopathy. Am J Cardiovasc Pathol 3:13, 1990
23. Valente M, Danieli D, Calabrese F: Ultrastruttura del miocardio nelle cardiomiopatie. In: Baroldi G, Thiene G (eds): Biopsia Endomiocardica. Testo Atlante. Piccin, Padua, 1996, p 277
24. Knieriem H-J: Electron-microscopic findings in congestive cardiomyopathy. In: Kaltenbach M, Loogen F, Olsen EGJ (eds): Cardiomyopathy and Myocardial Biopsy. Berlin, Springer-Verlag, 1978, p 71
25. Leatherbury L, Chandra RS, Shapiro SR, Perry LW: Value of endomyocardial biopsy in infants, children and adolescents with dilated or hypertrophic cardiomyopathy and myocarditis. J Am Coll Cardiol 12:1547, 1988
26. Tanaka M, Hiroe M, Nishikawa T, et al: Cellular localization and structural characterization of natriuretic peptide-expressing ventricular myocytes from patients with dilated cardiomyopathy. J Histochem Cytochem 42:1207, 1994
27. Urie PM, Billingham ME: Ultrastructural features of familial cardiomyopathy. Am J Cardiol 62:325, 1988
28. Mosseri M, Yarom R, Gotsman MS, Hasin Y: Histologic evidence for small-vessel coronary artery disease in patients with angina pectoris and patent large coronary arteries. Circulation 74:964, 1986

29. Tanganelli P, Di Lenarda A, Bianciardi G, et al: Correlation between histomorphometric findings on endomyocardial biopsy and clinical findings in idiopathic dilated cardiomyopathy. Am J Cardiol 64:504, 1989

30. Gallo P, Bernucci P, d'Amati G, et al: Functional significance of myocellular hypertrophy in dilated cardiomyopathy: Histomorphometric analysis on 40 endomyocardial biopsies. Am J Cardiovasc Pathol 5:11, 1994

31. Figulla HR, Rahlf G, Nieger M, et al: Spontaneous hemodynamic improvement or stabilization and associated biopsy findings in patients with congestive cardiomyopathy. Circulation 71:1095, 1985

32. Nakayama Y, Shimizu G, Hirota Y, et al: Functional and histopathologic correlation in patients with dilated cardiomyopathy: An integrated evaluation by multivariate analysis. J Am Coll Cardiol 10:186, 1987

33. Breithardt G, Kuhn H, Knierem HJ: Prognostic significance of endomyocardial biopsy in patients with congestive heart failure. In: Kaltenbach M, Loogen F, Olsen EGJ (eds): Cardiomyopathy and Myocardial Biopsy. New York, Springer, 1978, p 258

34. Shirey EK, Proudfit WL, Hawk WA: Primary myocardial disease: Correlation with clinical findings, angiographic and biopsy diagnosis. Am Heart J 99:198, 1980

35. Schwarz F, Mall G, Zebe H, et al: Determinants of survival in patients with congestive cardiomyopathy: Quantitative morphologic findings and left ventricular hemodynamics. Circulation 70:923, 1984

36. Pelliccia F, d'Amati G, Cianfrocca C, et al: Histomorphometric features predict 1-year outcome of patients with idiopathic dilated cardiomyopathy considered to be at low priority for cardiac transplantation. Am Heart J 128:316, 1994

37. Yamada T, Fukunami M, Ohmori M, et al: Which subgroup of patients with dilated cardiomyopathy would benefit from long-term β-blocker therapy? A histologic viewpoint. J Am Coll Cardiol 21:628, 1993

38. Sinagra G, Rakar S, Zecchin M, et al: Nonpredictive value of fibrosis in dilated cardiomyopathy treated with metoprolol. Cardiovasc Pathol 5:21, 1996

39. Ohtani K, Yutani C, Nagata S, et al: High prevalence of atrial fibrosis in patients with dilated cardiomyopathy. J Am Coll Cardiol 25:1162, 1995

40. Scholz D, Diener W, Schaper J: Altered nucleus/cytoplasm relationship and degenerative structural changes in human dilated cardiomyopathy. Cardioscience 5:127, 1994

41. Tashiro A, Masuda T, Segawa I: Morphometric comparison of mitochondria and myofibrils between hypertrophic and dilated cardiomyopathies. Virchows Arch [Pathol Anat] 416:473, 1990

42. Mall G, Schwarz F, Derks H: Clinicopathologic correlations in congestive cardiomyopathy: A study on endomyocardial biopsies. Virchows Arch [Pathol Anat] 397:67, 1982

43. Zimmer G, Zimmermann R, Hess OM, et al: Decreased concentration of myofibrils and myofiber hypertrophy are structural determinants of impaired left ventricular function in patients with chronic heart diseases: A multiple logistic regression analysis. J Am Coll Cardiol 20:1135, 1992

44. Unverferth DV, Magorien RD, Moeschberger ML, et al: Factors influencing the one-year mortality of dilated cardiomyopathy. Am J Cardiol 54:147, 1984

45. Baandrup U, Olsen EGJ: Critical analysis of endomyocardial biopsies from patients suspected as having cardiomyopathy: Morphological and morphometric aspects. Br Heart J 45:475, 1981

46. Yonesaka S, Becker AE: Dilated cardiomyopathy: Diagnostic accuracy of endomyocardial biopsy. Br Heart J 58:156, 1987

47. O'Connell JB, Robinson JA, Buramanian R, Scanlon PJ: Endomyocardial biopsy: Techniques and applications in heart disease of unknown cause. Heart Transpl 3:132, 1984

48. Mason JW: Indications for endomyocardial biopsy. In: Fenoglio JJ (ed): Endomyocardial Biopsy: Techniques and Applications. Boca Raton, CRC Press, 1982, p 48

49. Fowles RE: Current uses and indications for cardiac biopsy. In: Fowles RE (ed): Cardiac Biopsy. Mount Kisco, NY, Futura, 1992, p 19

50. MacKay EH, Littler WA, Sleight P: Critical assessment of diagnostic value of endomyocardial biopsy. Br Heart J 40:69, 1978

51. Olsen EGJ: Special investigations of COCM (congestive cardiomyopathy): Endomyocardial biopsies (morphological analysis). Postgrad Med J 54:486, 1978

52. Sekiguchi M, Hiroe M, Ogasawara S, Nishikawa T: Practical aspects of endomyocardial biopsy. Ann Acad Med Singapore 10: S115, 1981

53. Laser JA, Fowles RE, Mason JW: Endomyocardial biopsy. Cardiovasc Clin 15:141, 1985

54. Craven CM, Allred T, Garry SL, et al: Three cases of fatal cardiac tamponade following ventricular endocardial biopsy. Arch Pathol Lab Med 114:836, 1990

55. Dec GW, Fuster V: Medical progress: Idiopathic dilated cardiomyopathy. N Engl J Med 331:1564, 1994

56. Figulla HR, Kellermann AB, Stille Siegener M, et al: Significance of coronary angiography, left heart catheterization, and endomyocardial biopsy for the diagnosis of idiopathic dilated cardiomyopathy. Am Heart J 124:1251, 1992

57. Hare JM, Walford GD, Hruban RH, et al: Ischemic cardiomyopathy: Endomyocardial biopsy and ventriculographic evaluation of patients with congestive heart failure, dilated cardiomyopathy and coronary artery disease. J Am Coll Cardiol 20:1318, 1992

58. Bortman G, Sellanes M, Odell DS, et al: Discrepancy between pre- and post-transplant diagnosis of end-stage dilated cardiomyopathy. Am J Cardiol 74:921, 1994

59. Zee-Cheng C-S, Tsai CC, Palmer DC, et al: High incidence of myocarditis by endomyocardial biopsy in patients with idiopathic congestive cardiomyopathy. J Am Coll Cardiol 3:63, 1984

60. Grogan M, Redfield, MM, Bailey KR, et al: Long-term outcome of patients with biopsy-proved myocarditis: Comparison with idiopathic dilated cardiomyopathy. J Am Coll Cardiol 26:80, 1995

61. Kuhl U, Daun B, Seeberg B, et al: Dilatative kardiomyopathie—Eine chronische myokarditis? Immunohistologische charakterisierung lymphozytarer infiltrate. Herz 17:97, 1992

62. Jougasaki M, Yasue H, Okumura K, et al: Atrial natriuretic peptide in the ventricles of patients with dilated cardiomyopathy and human foetuses. Histochem J 21:715, 1989

63. Frustaci A, Perrone GA, Gentiloni N, Russo MA: Reversible dilated cardiomyopathy due to growth hormone deficiency. Am J Clin Pathol 97:503, 1992

64. Mestroni L, Krajinovic M, Severini GM, et al: Molecular genetics of dilated cardiomyopathy. Herz 19:97, 1994

65. Goldblatt J, Melmed J, Rose AG: Autosomal recessive inheritance of idiopathic dilated cardiomyopathy in a Madeira Portuguese kindred. Clin Genet 31:249, 1987

65a. Mestroni L, Rocco C, Gregori D, et al: Familial dilated cardiomyopathy: evidence for genetic and phenotypic heterogeneity. Heart Muscle Disease Group. J Am Coll Cardiol 34:181, 1999.

66. Raynolds MV, Bristow MR, Bush EW, et al: Angiotensin-converting enzyme DD genotype in patients with ischemic or idiopathic dilated cardiomyopathy. Lancet 342:1073, 1993

67. Kass S, MacRae C, Graber HL, et al: A genetic defect that causes conduction system disease and dilated cardiomyopathy maps to 1p1-1q1. Nat Genet 7:546, 1994.

68. Durand JB, Bachinski LL, Bieling LC, et al: Localization of a gene responsible for familial hypertrophic cardiomyopathy to chromosome 1q32. Circulation 92:3387, 1995

69. Olson TM, Keating MT: Mapping a cardiomyopathy locus to chromosome 3p22-p25. J Clin Invest 97:528, 1996

70. Krajinovic M, Pinamonti B, Sinagra G, et al: Linkage of familial dilated cardiomyopathy to chromosome 9. Am J Hum Genet 57: 846, 1995

71. Bowles KR, Gajarski R, Porter P, et al: Gene mapping of familial autosomal dominant dilated cardiomyopathy to chromosome 10q21-23. J Clin Invest 98:1355, 1996

72. Michels VV, Tazelaar HD, Driscoll DJ, et al: Histopathology of familial versus nonfamilial dilated cardiomyopathy. Cardiovasc Pathol 2:219, 1993

73. Limas C, Limas CJ, Boudoulas H, et al: Anti-β-receptor antibodies in familial cardiomyopathy: Correlation with HLA-DR and HLA-DQ gene polymorphisms. Am Heart J 127:382, 1994

74. Holt JC, Caulfield JB, Norton P, et al: Human cardiac myosin light chains: Sequence comparisons between myosin LC1 and LC2 from normal and idiopathic dilated cardiomyopathic hearts. Mol Cell Biochem 145:89, 1995

75. Margossian SS, White H, Caulfield JB, et al: Light chain 2 profile and activity of human ventricular myosin during dilated cardiomy-

opathy: Identification of a causal agent for impaired myocardial function. Circulation 85:1720, 1992

76. Berko BA, Swift M: X-linked dilated cardiomyopathy. N Engl J Med 316:1186, 1987

77. Towbin JA, Hejtmancik F, Brink P, et al: X-linked dilated cardiomyopathy: Genetic evidence of linkage to the Duchenne muscular dystrophy gene at the Xp21 locus. Circulation 87:1854, 1993

78. Muntoni F, Cau M, Ganau A, et al: Brief report: Deletion of the dystrophin muscle-promoter region associated with X-linked dilated cardiomyopathy. N Engl J Med 329:921, 1993

79. Milasin J, Muntoni F, Severini GM, et al: A point mutation in the 5′ splice site of the dystrophin gene first intron responsible for X-linked dilated cardiomyopathy. Hum Mol Genet 5:73, 1996

80. Schnitt SJ, Stillman IE, Owings DV, et al: Myocardial fibrin deposition in experimental viral myocarditis that progresses to dilated cardiomyopathy. Circ Res 72:914, 1993

81. Tazelaar HD, Billingham ME: Leukocytic infiltrates in idiopathic dilated cardiomyopathy: A source of confusion with active myocarditis. Am J Surg Parthol 10:405, 1986

82. Matoba Y, Matsumori A, Ohtani H, et al: A case of biopsy-proven myocarditis progressing to autopsy-proven dilated cardiomyopathy. Clin Cardiol 13:732, 1990

83. Jin O, Sole MJ, Butany JW, et al: Detection of enterovirus RNA in myocardial biopsies from patients with myocarditis and cardiomyopathy using gene amplification by polymerase chain reaction. Circulation 82:8, 1990

84. Figulla HR, Stille-Siegener M, Mall G, et al: Myocardial enterovirus infection with left ventricular dysfunction: A benign disease compared with idiopathic dilated cardiomyopathy. J Am Coll Cardiol 25:1170, 1995

85. Schwaiger A, Umlauft F, Weyrer K, et al: Detection of enteroviral ribonucleic acid in myocardial biopsies from patients with idiopathic dilated cardiomyopathy by polymerase chain reaction. Am Heart J 126:406, 1993

86. Why HJ, Meany BT, Richardson PJ, et al: Clinical and prognostic significance of detection of enteroviral RNA in the myocardium of patients with myocarditis or dilated cardiomyopathy. Circulation 89:2582, 1994

87. Martino TA, Liu P, Sole MJ: Viral infection and the pathogenesis of dilated cardiomyopathy. Circ Res 74:182, 1994

87a. Badorff C, Lee G-H, Lamphear BJ, et al: Enteroviral protease 2A cleaves dystrophin: Evidence of cytoskeletal disruption in an acquired cardiomyopathy. Nat Med 5:320, 1999.

88. Holzinger C, Schollhammer A, Imhof M, et al: Phenotypic patterns of mononuclear cells in dilated cardiomyopathy. Circulation 92:2876, 1995

89. Kuhl U, Noutsias M, Seeberg B, Schultheiss HP: Immunohistological evidence for a chronic intramyocardial process in dilated cardiomyopathy. Heart 75:295, 1996

90. Latif N, Baker CS, Dunn MJ, et al: Frequency and specificity of antiheart antibodies in patients with dilated cardiomyopathy detected using SDS-PAGE and western blotting. J Am Coll Cardiol 22:1378, 1993

91. Magnusson Y, Wallukat G, Waagstein F, et al: Autoimmunity in idiopathic dilated cardiomyopathy: Characterization of antibodies against the β1-adrenoceptor with positive chronotropic effect. Circulation 89:2760, 1994

92. Schulze K, Becker BF, Schauer R, Schultheiss HP: Antibodies to ADP-ATP carrier—an autoantigen in myocarditis and dilated cardiomyopathy—impair cardiac function. Circulation 81:959, 1990

93. Magnusson Y, Marullo S, Hoyer S, et al: Mapping of a functional autoimmune epitope on the β1-adrenergic receptor in patients with idiopathic dilated cardiomyopathy. J Clin Invest 86:1658, 1990

93a. Curione M, Barbato M, De Biase L, et al: Prevalence of coeliac disease in idiopathic dilated cardiomyopathy. Lancet 354:222, 1999

93b. Fonager K, Sørensen HT, Nørgård B, Thulstrup AM: Cardiomyopathy in Danish patients with coeliac disease. Lancet 354:1561, 1999.

94. Yao M, Keogh A, Spratt P, et al: Elevated DNase I levels in human idiopathic dilated cardiomyopathy: An indicator of apoptosis? J Mol Cell Cardiol 28:95, 1996

95. Fazio S, Sabatini D, Capaldo B, et al: A preliminary study of growth hormone in the treatment of dilated cardiomyopathy. N Engl J Med 334:810, 1996

96. Frustaci A, Gentiloni N, Russo MA: Growth hormone in the treatment of dilated cardiomyopathy. N Engl J Med 335:672, 1996

96a. Olson TM, Michels VV, Thibodeau SN, et al: Actin mutations in dilated cardiomyopathy, a heritable form of heart failure. Science 280:750, 1998

96b. Li D, Tapscoft T, Gonzalez O, et al: Desmin mutation responsible for idiopathic dilated cardiomyopathy. Circulation 100:461, 1999

96c. Maeda M, Holder E, Lowes B, et al: Dilated cardiomyopathy associated with deficiency of the cytoskeletal protein metavinculin. Circulation 95:17, 1997

96d. Brodsky GL, Muntoni F, Miocic S, et al: Lamin A/C mutation associated with dilated cardiomyopathy with variable skeletal muscle involvement. Circulation 101:473, 2000

97. Keren A, Billingham ME, Weintraub D, et al: Mildly dilated congestive cardiomyopathy. Circulation 72:302, 1985

98. Keren A, Gottlieb S, Tzivoni D, et al: Mildly dilated congestive cardiomyopathy: Use of prospective diagnostic criteria and description of the clinical course without heart transplantation. Circulation 81:506, 1990

99. Gavazzi A, De Maria R, Renosto G, et al: The spectrum of left ventricular size in dilated cardiomyopathy: Clinical correlates and prognostic implications. Am Heart J 125:410, 1993

100. Braunwald E: Heart Disease: A Textbook of Cardiovascular Medicine. Philadelphia, WB Saunders, 1997

101. Holmes J, Kubo SH, Cody RJ, Kligfield P: Arrhythmia in ischemic and nonischemic dilated cardiomyopathy: Prediction of mortality by ambulatory monitoring. Am J Cardiol 55:146, 1985

102. Neri, R, Mestroni L, Salvi A, Camerini F: Arrhythmias in dilated cardiomyopathy. Postgrad Med J 62:593, 1986

103. Huang SK, Messer JV, Denes P: Significance of ventricular tachycardia in idiopathic dilated cardiomyopathy: Observations in 35 patients. Am J Cardiol 51:507, 1983

104. Meinertz T, Hogmann T, Kasper W, et al: Significance of ventricular arrhythmias in idiopathic dilated cardiomyopathy. Am J Cardiol 53:902, 1984

105. Pelliccia F, Gallo P, Cianfrocca C, et al: Relation of complex ventricular arrhythmias to presenting features and prognosis in dilated cardiomyopathy. Int J Cardiol 29:47, 1990

106. De Maria R, Gavazzi A, Caroli A, et al: Ventricular arrhythmias in dilated cardiomyopathy as an independent prognostic marker. Italian Multicenter Cardiomyopathy Study (SPIC) Group. Am J Cardiol 69:1451, 1992

107. Ciszewski A, Bilinska ZT, Lubiszewska B, et al: Dilated cardiomyopathy in children: Clinical course and prognosis. Pediatr Cardiol 15:121, 1994

108. Sugrue DD, Rodeheffer RJ, Codd MB, et al: The clinical course of idiopathic dilated cardiomyopathy: A population-based study. Ann Intern Med 117:117, 1992

109. Fuster V, Gersh BJ, Giuliani ER, et al: The natural history of idiopathic dilated cardiomyopathy. Am J Cardiol 47:525, 1981

110. Franciosa JA, Wilen M, Ziesche S, Cohn JN: Survival in men with severe chronic left ventricular failure due to either coronary heart disease or idiopathic dilated cardiomyopathy. Am J Cardiol 51:831, 1983

111. Di Lenarda A, Secoli G, Perkan A, et al: Changing mortality in dilated cardiomyopathy. Br Heart J 72:S46, 1994

112. Romeo F, Pelliccia F, Cianfrocca C, et al: Determinants of end-stage idiopathic dilated cardiomyopathy: A multivariate analysis of 104 patients. Clin Cardiol 12:387, 1989

113. Kantharia BK, Richards HB, Battaglia J: Reversible dilated cardiomyopathy: An unusual case of thyrotoxicosis. Am Heart J 129:1030, 1995

114. Hosenpud JD, Bennett LE, Keck BM, et al: The registry of the International Society for Heart and Lung Transplantation: Fourteenth official report—1997. J Heart Lung Transpl 16:691, 1997

115. Batista RJ, Santos JL, Takeshita N, et al: Partial left ventriculectomy to improve left ventricular function in end-stage heart disease. J Card Surg 11:96, 1996.

115a. Calafiore AM, Gallina S, Contini M, et al: Surgical treatment of dilated cardiomyopathy with conventional techniques. Eur J Cardiothorac Surg 16:S73, 1999

115b. Isomura T, Suma H, Horii T, et al: Partial left ventriculectomy, ventriculoplasty or valvular surgery for idiopathic dilated cardiomyopathy. The role of intra-operative echocardiography. Eur J Cardiothorac Surg 17:239, 2000

116. Lampert MB, Lang R: Peripartum cardiomyopathy. Am Heart J 130:860, 1995

117. Homans DC: Peripartum cardiomyopathy. N Engl J Med 312:1432, 1985

118. Pearl W: Familial occurrence of peripartum cardiomyopathy. Am Heart J 129:421, 1995

119. Demakis JG, Rahimtoola SH, Sutton GC, et al: Natural course of peripartum cardiomyopathy. Circulation 44:1053, 1971

120. Sanderson JE, Olsen EGJ, Gratei D: Peripartum heart disease: An endomyocardial biopsy study. Br Heart J 56:285, 1986

121. Midei MG, DeMent SH, Feldman AM, et al: Peripartum myocarditis and cardiomyopathy. Circulation 81:922, 1990

122. Rizeq MN, Rickenbacher PR, Fowler MB, Billingham ME: Incidence of myocarditis in peripartum cardiomyopathy. Am J Cardiol 74:474, 1994

123. Opitz JM: Genetic aspects of endocardial fibroelastosis. Am J Med Genet 11:92, 1992

124. Hutchins GM, Bannayan GA: Development of endocardial fibroelastosis following myocardial infarction. Arch Pathol 91:113, 1971

125. Hutchins GM, Vie SA: The progression of interstitial myocarditis to idiopathic endocardial fibroelastosis. Am J Pathol 66:483, 1972

126. Ni J, Bowles NE, Kim YH, et al: Viral infection of the myocardium in endocardial fibroelastosis: Molecular evidence for the role of mumps virus as an etiologic agent. Circulation 95:133, 1997

127. Hunter AS, Keay AJ: Primary endocardial fibroelastosis: An inherited condition. Arch Dis Child 48:66, 1973

128. Teare D: Asymmetrical hypertrophy of the heart in young adults. Br Heart J 20:1, 1958

129. Gallo P: Cuore e Pericardio. In: Ascenzi A, Mottura G (eds): Trattato di Anatomia Patologica per il Medico Pratico. 5th ed. Turin, UTET, 1997, p 304

130. Klues HG, Schiffers A, Maron BJ: Phenotypic spectrum and patterns of left ventricular hypertrophy in hypertrophic cardiomyopathy: Morphologic observations and significance as assessed by two-dimensional echocardiography in 600 patients. J Am Coll Cardiol 26:1699, 1995

131. Davies MJ, McKenna WJ: Hypertrophic cardiomyopathy: Pathology and pathogenesis. Histopathology 26:493, 1995

132. Lewis JF, Maron BJ: Hypertrophic cardiomyopathy characterized by marked hypertrophy of the posterior left ventricular free wall: Significance and clinical implications. J Am Coll Cardiol 18:421, 1991

133. Yamaguchi H, Ishimura T, Nishiyama S, et al: Hypertrophic non-obstructive cardiomyopathy with giant negative T waves (apical hypertrophy): Ventriculographic and echocardiographic features in 30 patients. Am J Cardiol 44:401, 1979

134. Maron BJ, McIntosh CL, Klues HG, et al: Morphological basis for obstruction to right ventricular outflow in hypertrophic cardiomyopathy. Am J Cardiol 71:1089, 1993

135. Formigari R, Francalanci P, Gallo P, et al: Pathology of atrioventricular valve dysplasia. Cardiovasc Pathol 2:137, 1993

136. Petrone RK, Klues HG, Panza JA, et al: Coexistence of mitral valve prolapse in a consecutive group of 528 patients with hypertrophic cardiomyopathy assessed with echocardiography. J Am Coll Cardiol 20:55, 1992

137. Klues HG, Roberts WC, Maron BJ: Morphological determinants of echocardiographic patterns of mitral valve systolic anterior motion in obstructive hypertrophic cardiomyopathy. Circulation 87:1570, 1993

138. Klues HG, Maron BJ, Dollar AL, Roberts WC: Diversity of structural mitral valve alterations in hypertrophic cardiomyopathy. Circulation 85:1651, 1992

139. Lefebvre XP, Yoganathan AP, Levine RA: Insights from in-vitro flow visualization into the mechanism of systolic anterior motion of the mitral valve in hypertrophic cardiomyopathy under steady flow conditions. J Biomech Eng 114:406, 1992

140. Achrafi H: Hypertrophic cardiomyopathy and myocardial bridging. Int J Cardiol 37:111, 1992

141. van der Bel-Kahn J: Muscle fiber disarray in common heart diseases. Am J Cardiol 40:355, 1977

142. Maron BJ, Roberts WC: Quantitative analysis of cardiac muscle

cell disorganization in the ventricular septum of patients with hypertrophic cardiomyopathy. Circulation 59:687, 1979

143. d'Amati G, Kahn HJ, Butany J, Silver MD: Altered distribution of desmin filaments in hypertrophic cardiomyopathy: An immunohistochemical study. Mod Pathol 5:165, 1992

144. Francalanci P, Gallo P, Bernucci P, et al: The pattern of desmin filaments in myocardial disarray. Hum Pathol 26:262, 1995

145. d'Amati G, Francalanci P, Bernucci P, Gallo P: Myofiber intercalated disks in cardiomyopathies: An immunofluorescence study. Mod Pathol 8:31A, 1995

146. Factor SM, Butany J, Sole MJ, et al: Pathologic fibrosis and matrix connective tissue in the subaortic myocardium of patients with hypertophic cardiomyopathy. J Am Coll Cardiol 17:1343, 1991

146a. Shirani J, Pick R, Roberts WC, Maron BJ: Morphology and significance of the left ventricular collagen network in young patients with hypertrophic cardiomyopathy and sudden cardiac death. J Am Coll Cardiol 35:36, 2000

147. Maron BJ, Wolfson JK, Epstein SE, Roberts WC: Intramural ("small vessel") coronary artery disease in hypertrophic cardiomyopathy. J Am Coll Cardiol 8:545, 1986

148. McKenna WJ, Stewart JT, Nihoyannopoulos P, et al: Hypertrophic cardiomyopathy without hypertrophy: Two families with myocardial disarray in the absence of increased myocardial mass. Br Heart J 63:287, 1990

149. Hina K, Kusachi S, Iwasaki K, et al: Progression of left ventricular enlargement in patients with hypertrophic cardiomyopathy: Incidence and prognostic value. Clin Cardiol 16:403, 1993

150. Kawashima T, Yokota Y, Yokoyama M, Itoh H: Pathological analysis of hypertrophic cardiomyopathy simulating dilated cardiomyopathy. Acta Pathol Jpn 43:304, 1993

151. Davies MJ, Mann JM: The cardiovascular system: Part B. Acquired diseases of the heart. In: Symmers WStC (ed): Systemic Pathology. Vol. 10. New York, Churchill Livingstone, 1995

152. Hecht G, Klues H, Roberts W, Maron B: Coexistence of sudden cardiac death and end-stage heart failure in familial hypertrophic cardiomyopathy. J Am Coll Cardiol 22:489, 1993

153. Jarcho JA, McKenna W, Peter Pare JA, et al: Mapping a gene for familial hypertrophic cardiomyopathy to chromosome 14q1. N Engl J Med 321: 1372, 1989

154. Geisterfer-Lowrance AA, Kass S, Tanigawa G, et al: A molecular basis for familial hypertrophic cardiomyopathy: A β-cardiac myosin heavy chain gene missense mutation. Cell 62:999, 1990

155. Thierfelder L, Watkins H, McRae C, et al: Alpha-tropomyosin and cardiac troponin T mutations cause familial hypertrophic cardiomyopathy: A disease of the sarcomere. Cell 77:701,1994

156. Watkins H, MacRae C, Thierfelder L, et al: A disease locus for familial hypertrophic cardiomyopathy maps to chromosome 1q3. Nat Genet 3:333, 1993

157. Thierfelder L, MacRae C, Watkins H, et al: A familial hypertrophic cardiomyopathy locus maps to chromosome 15q2. Proc Natl Acad Sci U S A 90:6270, 1993

158. Watkins H, Conner D, Thierfelder L, et al: Mutations in the cardiac myosin binding protein-C gene on chromosome 11 cause familial hypertrophic cardiomyopathy. Nat Genet 11:434, 1995

159. Carrier L, Hegstenberg C, Beckmann JS, et al: Mapping of a novel gene for familial hypertrophic cardiomyopathy to chromosome 11. Nat Genet 4:311, 1993

160. Poetter K, Jang H, Hassanzadeh S, et al: Mutations in either the essential and regulatory light chains of myosin are associated with a rare myopathy in human heart and skeletal muscle. Nat Genet 13:63, 1996

161. Kimura A, Harada H, Park JE, et al: Mutations in the cardiac troponin I gene associated with hypertrophic cardiomyopathy. Nat Genet 16:379, 1997

161a. Mogensen J, Klausen IC, Pedersen AK, et al: Alpha-cardiac actin is a novel disease gene in familial hypertrophic cardiomyopathy. J Clin Invest 103:R39, 1999

162. Marian AJ, Yu Q-T, Mann DL, et al: Expression of a mutation causing hypertrophic cardiomyopathy disrupts sarcomere assembly in adult feline cardiac myocytes. Circ Res 77:98, 1995

163. Stracesky AJ, Geisterfer-Lawrance AA, Seidman CE, et al: Functional analysis of myosin missense mutations in familial hypertrophic cardiomyopathy. Proc Natl Acad Sci U S A 91:589, 1994

164. MacRae CA, Ghaisas N, Donnelly S, et al: Familial hypertrophic

cardiomyopathy with Wolff-Parkinson-White syndrome maps to a locus on chromosome 7q3. J Clin Invest 96:1216, 1995

165. Marian AJ, Roberts R: Molecular genetics of hypertrophic cardiomyopathy. Ann Rev Med 46:213, 1995

166. Watkins H, Rosenzweig A, Hwang D, et al: Characteristics and prognostic implications of myosin missense mutations in familial hypertrophic cardiomyopathy. N Engl J Med 326:1108, 1992

167. Epstein ND, Cohn GM, Cyran F, Fananapazir L: Differences in clinical expression of hypertrophic cardiomyopathy associated with two distinct mutations in the β-myosin heavy chain gene: A 908 Leu-Val mutation and a 403 Arg-Gln mutation. Circulation 86:345, 1992

168. Anan R, Greve G, Thierfelder L, et al: Prognostic implications of novel β-myosin heavy chain gene mutations that cause familial hypertrophic cardiomyopathy. J Clin Invest 93:280, 1994

169. Marian AJ, Mares A Jr, Kelly DP, et al: Sudden cardiac death in hypertrophic cardiomyopathy: Variability in phenotypic expression of β-myosin heavy chain mutations. Eur Heart J 16:368, 1995

169a. Niimura H, Bachinski LL, Sangwatanaroj S, et al: Mutations in the gene for cardiac myosin-binding protein C and late-onset familial hypertrophic cardiomyopathy. New Engl J Med 338:1248, 1998

170. Rosenzweig A, Watkins H, Hwang D-S, et al: Preclinical diagnosis of familial hypertrophic cardiomyopathy by genetic analysis of blood lymphocytes. N Engl J Med 325:1753, 1991

171. Mendez HMM, Opitz JM: Noonan syndrome: A review. Am J Med Genet 21:493, 1985

172. Allanson JE: Noonan syndrome. J Med Genet 24:9, 1987

173. Pearl W: Cardiovascular anomalies in Noonan syndrome. Chest 71:677, 1977

174. Sharland M, Burch M, McKenna WM, Paton MA: A clinical study of Noonan syndrome. Arch Dis Child 67:178, 1992

175. Burch M, Mann JM, Sharland M, et al: Myocardial disarray in Noonan syndrome. Br Heart J 68:586,1992

176. Jamienson CR, van der Burgt I, Brady AF, et al: Mapping a gene for Noonan syndrome to the long arm of chromosome 12. Nat Genet 8:357, 1994

177. Moynahan EJ: Progressive cardiomyopathic lentiginosis: First report of autopsy findings in a recently recognized inheritable disorder (autosomal dominant). Proc R Soc Med 63:448, 1970

178. St. John Sutton MG, Tajik AJ, Giuliani ER, et al: Hypertrophic obstructive cardiomyopathy and lentiginosis: A little known neural ectodermal syndrome. Am J Cardiol 47:214, 1981

179. Topol EJ, Traill TA, Fortuin NJ: Hypertensive hypertrophic cardiomyopathy of the elderly. N Engl J Med 312:277, 1985

180. Shimizu M, Sugihara N, Shimizu K, et al: Asymmetrical septal hypertrophy in patients with hypertension: A type of hypertensive left ventricular hypertrophy or hypertrophic cardiomyopathy combined with hypertension? Clin Cardiol 16:41, 1993

181. Maron BJ: Structural features of the athlete heart as defined by echocardiography. J Am Coll Cardiol 7:190, 1986

182. Maron BJ, Epstein SE, Roberts WC: Causes of sudden death in the competitive athlete. J Am Coll Cardiol 7:204, 1986

183. Maron BJ, Pelliccia A, Spirito P: Cardiac disease in young trained athletes. Insights into methods for distinguishing athlete's heart from structural heart disease, with particular emphasis on hypertrophic cardiomyopathy. Circulation 91:1596, 1995

184. Maron BJ, Pelliccia A, Spataro A, Granata M: Reduction in left ventricular wall thickness after deconditioning in highly trained Olympic athletes. Br Heart J 69:125, 1993

185. Lefebvre XP, He S, Levine RA, Yoganathan AP: Systolic anterior motion of the mitral valve in hypertrophic cardiomyopathy: An in vivo pulsatile flow study. J Heart Valve Dis 4:422, 1995

186. Walston A 2nd, Behar VS: Spectrum of coronary artery disease in idiopathic hypertrophic subaortic stenosis. Am J Cardiol 38:12, 1976

187. Frank S, Braunwald E: Idiopathic hypertrophic subaortic stenosis. Clinical analysis of 126 patients with emphasis on the natural history. Circulation 37:759, 1968

188. Fananapazir L, Tracy CM, Leon MB, et al: Electrophysiologic abnormalities in patients with hypertrophic cardiomyopathy. A consecutive analysis in 155 patients. Circulation 80:1259, 1989

189. DeRose JJ Jr, Banas JS Jr, Winters SL: Current perspectives on sudden cardiac death in hypertrophic cardiomyopathy. Prog Cardiovasc Dis 36:475, 1994

190. Maron BJ, Cecchi F, McKenna WJ: Risk factors and stratification for sudden death in patients with hypertrophic cardiomyopathy. Br Heart J 72:S13, 1994

191. Park JH, Kim YM, Chung JW, et al: MR imaging of hypertrophic cardiomyopathy. Radiology 185:441, 1992

192. Young AA, Kramer CM, Ferrari VA, et al: Three-dimensional left ventricular deformation in hypertrophic cardiomyopathy. Circulation 90:854, 1994

193. Hecht GM, Panza JA, Maron BJ: Clinical course of middle-aged asymptomatic patients with hypertrophic cardiomyopathy. Am J Cardiol 69:935, 1992

194. Maron BJ, Fananapazir L: Sudden cardiac death in hypertrophic cardiomyopathy. Circulation 85:157, 1992

195. Clark AL, Coats AJ: Screening for hypertrophic cardiomyopathy. Br Med J 306:409, 1993

196. Roberts WC, Kishel JC, McIntosh CL, et al: Severe mitral or aortic valve regurgitation, or both, requiring valve replacement for infective endocarditis complicating hypertrophic cardiomyopathy. J Am Coll Cardiol 19:365, 1992

197. Maron BJ, Epstein SE, Roberts WC: Hypertrophic cardiomyopathy and transmural myocardial infarction without significant atherosclerosis of the extramural coronary arteries. Am J Cardiol 43:1086, 1979

198. Maron BJ, Kragel AH, Roberts WC: Sudden death in hypertrophic cardiomyopathy with normal left ventricular mass. Br Heart J 63: 308, 1990

199. Spirito P, Maron BJ: Relation between extent of left ventricular hypertrophy and occurrence of sudden cardiac death in hypertrophic cardiomyopathy. J Am Coll Cardiol 15:1521, 1990

200. Horita Y, Shimizu, M, Sugihara N, et al: An autopsy case of hypertrophic cardiomyopathy showing dilated cardiomyopathy-like features by serial ventriculography. Jpn J Med 29:448, 1990

200a. Chan S, Silver MD: Fatal myocardial embolus after myectomy. Can J Cardiol 16:207, 2000

201. Roberts WC, Ferrans BJ: Pathologic anatomy of the cardiomyopathies. Idiopathic dilated and hypertrophic types, infiltrative types and endomyocardial disease with and without eosinophilia. Hum Pathol 6:287, 1975

202. Child JS, Perloff JK: The restrictive cardiomyopathies. Cardiol Clin 6:289, 1988

203. Spyrou N, Foale R: Restrictive cardiomyopathies. Curr Opin Cardiol 9:344, 1994

204. Weller PF, Bubley GJ: The idiopathic hypereosinophilic syndrome. Blood 83:2759, 1994

205. Herzog CA, Snover DC, Staley NA: Acute necrotizing eosinophilic myocarditis. Br Heart J 52:343, 1984

206. Gupta PN, Valiathan MS, Balakrishan KG, et al: Clinical course of endomyocardial fibrosis. Br Heart J 62:450, 1989

207. Vijayaraghavan G, Balakrishnan M, Sadanandan S, Cherian G: Pattern of cardiac calcification in tropical endomyocardial fibrosis. Heart Vessels 5(suppl):4, 1990

208. Shaper AG: What's new in endomyocardial fibrosis? Lancet 342: 255, 1993

209. de Oliveira SA, Pereira-Barreto AC, Mady C, et al: Surgical treatment of endomyocardial fibrosis: A new approach. J Am Coll Cardiol 16:1246, 1990

210. Chopra P, Narula J, Talwar KK, et al: Histomorphologic characteristics of endomyocardial fibrosis: An endomyocardial biopsy study. Hum Pathol 21:613, 1990

211. Valiathan MS, Rathinam K, Khartha CC: A geochemical basis for endomyocardial fibrosis. Cardiovasc Res 23:647, 1989

212. Sezi CL: Effect of protein deficiency cassava diet on *Cercopithecus aethiops* hearts and its possible role in the aetiology and pathogenesis of endomyocardial fibrosis in man. East Afr Med J 73:S11, 1996

213. Fitzpatrick AP, Shapiro LM, Rickards AF, Poole-Wilson PA: Familial restrictive cardiomyopathy with atrioventricular block and skeletal myopathy. Br Heart J 63:114, 1990

214. Katritsis D, Wilmshurst PT, Wendon JA, et al: Primary restrictive cardiomyopathy: Clinical and pathologic characteristics. J Am Coll Cardiol 18:1230, 1991

214a. Arbustini E, Morbini P, Grasso M, et al: Restrictive cardiomyopathy, atrioventricular block and mild to subclinical myopathy in patients with desmin-immunoreactive material deposits. J Am Coll Cardiol 31:645, 1998

215. Cooke RA, Chambers JB, Curry PV: Noonan's cardiomyopathy: A non-hypertrophic variant. Br Heart J 71:561, 1994

216. Aroney C, Bett N, Radford D: Familial restrictive cardiomyopathy. Aust N Z J Med 18:877, 1988

217. Gertz MA, Kyle RA, Noel P: Primary systemic amyloidosis: A rare complication of immunoglobulin M monoclonal gammopathy and Waldenström's macroglobulinemia. J Clin Oncol 11:94, 1993

218. Hesse A, Atland K, Linke RP, et al: Cardiac amyloidosis: A review and report of a new transthyretin (prealbumin) variant. Br Heart J 70:111, 1993

219. Skinner M: Familial amyloidotic cardiomyopathy. J Lab Clin Med 117:171, 1991

220. Kyle RA: Amyloidosis. Circulation 91:1269, 1995

220a. Hamidi AL, Liepnieks JJ, Hamidi AK, et al: Hereditary amyloid cardiomyopathy caused by a variant apolipoprotein A1. Am J Pathol 154:221, 1999

220b. Obici L, Bellotti V, Mangione P, et al: The new apolipoprotein A-1 variant leu(174) → Ser causes hereditary cardiac amyloidosis, and the amyloid fibrils are constituted by the 93-residue N-terminal polypeptide. Am J Pathol 155:695, 1999

221. Benson MD, Uemichi T: Transthyretin amyloidosis. Amyloid 3:44, 1996

222. Jacobson DR, Pastore RD, Yaghoubian R: Variant-sequence transthyretin (isoleucine 122) in late-onset cardiac amyloidosis in black Americans. N Engl J Med 336:466, 1997

223. Nichols WC, Liepnieks JJ, Snyder EL, Benson MD: Senile cardiac amyloidosis associated with homozygosity for a transthyretin variant (ILE-122). J Lab Clin Med 117:175, 1991

224. Gertz MA, Kyle RA, Thibodeau SN: Familial amyloidosis: A study of 52 North-American born patients examined during a 30-year period. Mayo Clin Proc 67:428, 1992

225. Roberts WC, Waller BF: Cardiac amyloidosis causing cardiac dysfunction: Analysis of 54 necropsy patients. Am J Cardiol 52:137, 1983

226. Linke RP, Nathrath WBJ, Eulitz M: Classification of amyloid syndromes from tissue sections using antibodies against various amyloid fibril proteins: Report of 142 cases. In: Glenner GG, Osserman EF, Benditt EP, et al (eds): Amyloidosis, 1986. New York, Plenum Publishers, 1986, p 599

227. Miles JL, Ratliff NB, McMahon JT, et al: Cyclosporin-associated microfibrils in cardiac transplant patients. Am J Cardiovasc Pathol 2:127, 1988

228. Factor SM, Menegus MA, Kress Y: Microfibrillar cardiomyopathy: An infiltrative heart disease resembling but distinct from cardiac amyloidosis. Cardiovasc Pathol 4:307, 1992

229. Gibbons WJ, Levy RD, Nava S, et al: Subclinical cardiac dysfunction in sarcoidosis. Chest 100:44, 1991

230. Virmani R, Bures JC, Roberts WC: Cardiac sarcoidosis: A major cause of sudden death in young individuals. Chest 77:423, 1980

231. Ratner SJ, Fenoglio JJ Jr, Ursell PC: Utility of endomyocardial biopsy in the diagnosis of cardiac sarcoidosis. Chest 90:528, 1986

232. Liu P, Olivieri N: Iron overload cardiomyopathies: New insights into an old disease. Cardiovasc Drugs Ther 8:101, 1994

233. Olson LJ, Edwards WD, McCall JT, et al: Cardiac iron deposition from idiopathic hemochromatosis: Histologic and analytic assessment of 14 hearts from autopsy. J Am Coll Cardiol 10:1239, 1987

234. Cecchetti G, Binda A, Piperno A: Cardiac alterations in 36 consecutive patients with idiopathic hemochromatosis: Polygraphic and echocardiographic evaluation. Eur Heart J 12:224, 1991

235. Barosi G, Arbustini E, Gavazzi A, et al: Myocardial iron grading by endomyocardial biopsy: A clinico-pathologic study on iron overloaded patients. Eur J Haematol 92:382, 1989

236. Kushwaha SS, Fallon JT, Fuster V: Restrictive cardiomyopathy. N Engl J Med 336:267, 1997

237. Appleton CP, Hatle LK, Popp RL: Demonstration of restrictive ventricular physiology by Doppler echocardiography. J Am Coll Cardiol 11:757, 1988

238. Frank R, Fontaine G, Vedel J, et al: Electrocardiologie de quatre cas de dysplasie ventriculaire droite arythmogène. Arch Mal Coeur Vaiss 71:963, 1978

239. Thiene G, Nava A, Corrado D, et al: Right ventricular cardiomyopathy and sudden death in young people. N Engl J Med 318:129, 1988

240. Gallo P, d'Amati G, Pelliccia F: Pathologic evidence of extensive left ventricular involvement in arrhythmogenic right ventricular cardiomyopathy. Hum Pathol 23:948, 1992

240a. Burke AP, Farb A, Tashko G, Virmani R: Arrhythmogenic right ventricular cardiomyopathy and fatty replacement of the right ventricular myocardium. Are they different diseases? Circulation 97:1571, 1998

241. Basso C, Thiene G, Corrado D, et al: Arrhythmogenic right ventricular cardiomyopathy: Dysplasia, dystrophy, or myocarditis? Circulation 94:983, 1996

241a. Lobo FV, Silver MD, Butany J, Heggtveit HA: Left ventricular involvement in right ventricular dysplasia/cardiomyopathy. Can J Cardiol 15:1239, 1999

241b. d'Amati G, di Gioia CRT, Giordano C, Gallo P: Myocyte transdifferentiation. Possible pathogenetic mechanism for arrhythmogenic right ventricular cardiomyopathy. Arch Pathol Lab Med 124:287, 2000

242. Lobo FV, Heggtveit HA, Butany J, et al: Right ventricular dysplasia: Morphological findings in 13 cases. Can J Cardiol 8:261, 1992

243. Marcus FI, Fontaine GH, Guiraudon G, et al: Right ventricular dysplasia: A report of 24 adult cases. Circulation 65:384, 1982

244. Osler WLM: The Principles and Practice of Medicine. 6th ed. New York, Appleton, 1905

245. Uhl HSM: A previously undescribed congenital malformation of the heart: Almost total absence of the myocardium of the right ventricle. Bull Johns Hopkins Hosp 91:197, 1952

246. Gerlis LM, Schmidt-Ott SC, Ho SY, et al: Dysplastic conditions of the right ventricular myocardium: Uhl's anomaly versus arrhythmogenic right ventricular dysplasia. Br Heart J 69:142, 1993

247. Pinamonti B, Sinagra G, Salvi A, et al: Left ventricular involvement in right ventricular dysplasia. Am Heart J 123:711, 1992

248. Segall HN: Parchment heart (Osler). Am Heart J 40:948, 1950

249. Waller BF, Smith ER, Blackbourne BD, et al: Congenital hypoplasia of portions of both right and left ventricular myocardial walls: Clinical and necropsy observations in two patients with parchment heart syndrome. Am J Cardiol 46:885, 1980

250. Beltrami CA, Finato N, Della Mea V, et al: Right ventricular dysplasia: Right and left ventricular involvement morphometrically evaluated. Cardiovasc Pathol 4:47, 1995

251. Bharati S, Ciraulo DA, Bilitch M, et al: Inexcitable right ventricle and bilateral bundle branch block in Uhl's disease. Circulation 57:636, 1978

252. Okabe M, Fukuda K, Nakashima Y, et al: An isolated left ventricular lesion associated with left ventricular tachycardia: Arrhythmogenic "left" ventricular dysplasia? Jpn Circ J 59:49, 1995

253. Guiraudon CM: Histological diagnosis of right ventricular dysplasia: A role for electron microscopy? Eur Heart J 10(suppl D):95, 1989

254. Roncalli L, Nico B, Locuratolo N, et al: Right ventricular dysplasia: An ultrastructural study. Eur Heart J 10(suppl D):97, 1989

255. Hasumi M, Sekiguki M, Hiroe M, et al: Endocardial biopsy approach to patients with ventricular tachycadia with special reference to arrhythmogenic right ventricular dysplasia. Jpn Circ J 5:242, 1987

256. Gallo P: La biopsia endomiocardica nella patologia cardiovascolare pediatrica. G Ital Cardiol 25:1499, 1995

257. Dembinski AS, Dobson JR 3rd, Wilson JE, et al: Frequency, extent, and distribution of endomyocardial adipose tissue: Morphometric analysis of endomyocardial biopsy specimens from 241 patients. Cardiovasc Pathol 3:33, 1994

258. Angelini A, Thiene G, Boffa GM, et al: Endomyocardial biopsy in right ventricular cardiomyopathy. Int J Cardiol 40:273, 1993

259. Nava A, Thiene G, Canciani B, et al: Familial occurrence of right ventricular dysplasia: A study involving nine families. J Am Coll Cardiol 12:1222, 1988

260. Miani D, Pinamonti B, Bussani R, et al: Right ventricular dysplasia: A clinical and pathologic study of two families with left ventricular involvement. Br Heart J 69:151, 1993

261. McKenna WJ, Thiene G, Nava A, et al: Diagnosis of arrhythmogenic right ventricular dysplasia/cardiomyopathy. Br Heart J 71:215, 1994

262. Rampazzo A, Nava A, Eme P, et al: The gene for arrhythmogenic right ventricular cardiomyopathy maps to chromosome 14q23-q24. Hum Mol Genet 4:2151, 1994

263. Severini GM, Krajinovic M, Pinamonti B, et al: A new locus for

arrhythmogenic right ventricular dysplasia on the long arm of chromosome 14. Genomics 31:193, 1996

263a. Severini GM, Krajinovic M, Pinamonti B, et al: A new locus for arrhythmogenic right ventricular dysplasia on the long arm of chromosome 14. Genomics 31:193, 1996

264. Rampazzo A, Nava A, Erne P, et al: A new locus for arrhythmogenic right ventricular cardiomyopathy (ARVD) maps to chromosome 1q42-q43. Hum Mol Genet 4:2151, 1995

264a. Rampazzo A, Nava A, Miorin M, et al: ARVD4, a new locus for arrhythmogenic right ventricular cardiomyopathy, maps to chromosome 2 long arm. Genomics 45:259, 1997

264b. Li D, Ahmad F, Gardner MJ, et al: The locus of a novel gene responsible for arrhythmogenic right-ventricular dysplasia characterized by early onset and high penetrance maps to chromosome 10p12-p14. Am J Hum Genet 66:148, 2000

264c. Coonar AS, Protonotarios N, Tsatsopoulou A, et al: Gene for arrhythmogenic right ventricular cardiomyopathy with diffuse non-epidermolitic palmoplantar keratoderma and woolly hair (Naxos disease) maps to 17q21. Circulation 97:2049, 1998

265. Thiene G, Corrado A, Rossi L: Right ventricular cardiomyopathy: Is there evidence of an inflammatory aetiology? Eur Heart J 12:22, 1991

266. Fontaliran F, Fontaine G, Brestescher C, et al: Signification des infiltrats lymphoplasmocytaires dans la dysplasie ventriculaire droite arythmogène. Arch Mal Coer Vaiss 88:1021, 1995

267. Pinamonti B, Miani D, Sinagra G, et al: Familial right ventricular dysplasia with biventricular involvement and inflammatory infiltration. Heart 76:66, 1996

268. Rossi MA: Comparison of Chagas' heart disease to arrhythmogenic right ventricular cardiomyopathy. Am Heart J 129:626, 1995

269. Matsumori A, Kawai C: Coxackie virus B3 perimyocarditis in BALB/c mice: Experimental model of chronic perimyocarditis in the right ventricle. J Pathol 131:97, 1980

270. Zolezzi F, Filippi E, Rosso R, et al: Chronic myocarditis leading to a right ventricular cardiomyopathy. G Ital Cardiol 16:273, 1986.

271. O'Connell JB, Fowles RE, Robinson JA, et al: Clinical and pathological findings of myocarditis in two families with dilated cardiomyopathy. Am J Cardiol 107:127, 1984

272. d'Amati G, Fiore F, Giordano C, et al: Pathologic evidence of arrhythmogenic cardiomyopathy and myocarditis in two siblings. Cardiovasc Pathol 7:39, 1998

273. James TN: Normal and abnormal consequences of apoptosis in the human heart: From postnatal morphogenesis to paroxysmal arrhythmias. Circulation 90:556, 1994

273a. Corrado D, Basso C, Thiene G, et al: Spectrum of clinicopathologic manifestations of arrhythmogenic right ventricular cardiomyopathy/dysplasia: A multicenter study. J Am Coll Cardiol 30:1512, 1997

274. Burke AP, Farb A, Virmani R, et al: Sports-related and non-sports-related sudden cardiac death in young adults. Am Heart J 121:568, 1991

275. Goodin JC, Farb A, Smialek JE, et al: Right ventricular dysplasia associated with sudden death in young athletes. Mod Pathol 4:702, 1991

276. Gallo P, Baroldi G, Thiene G, et al: When and why do heart transplant recipients die? A 7 year experience of 1068 cardiac transplants. Virchows Arch [Pathol Anat] 422:453, 1993

276a. Corrado D, Fontaine G, Marcus FI, et al: Arrhythmogenic right ventricular dysplasia/cardiomyopathy: Need for an international registry. Circulation 101:e101, 2000

277. Nava A, Thiene G, Canciani B, et al: Clinical profile of concealed form of arrhythmogenic right ventricular cardiomyopathy presenting with apparently idiopathic ventricular arrhythmias. Int J Cardiol 35:195, 1992

278. Daliento L, Turrini P, Nava A, et al: Arrhythmogenic right ventricular cardiomyopathy in young versus adult patients: Similarities and differences. J Am Coll Cardiol 25:655, 1995

279. Peters S: Age related dilatation of the right ventricle in arrhythmogenic right ventricular dysplasia-cardiomyopathy. Int J Cardiol 56: 163, 1996

280. Kusano I, Shiraishi T, Marimoto R, et al: Cardiac rupture due to severe fatty infiltration in the right ventricular wall. J Forensic Sci 364:1246, 1991

281. Borkowski P, Cespedes E, Agatston AS, Robinson MJ: Left ventricular rupture through an area of fatty infiltration: Case report and review of the literature. Cardiovasc Pathol 5:85, 1996

282. Pinamonti B, Di Lenarda A, Sinagra G, et al: Long-term evolution of right ventricular dysplasia-cardiomyopathy. Am Heart J 129: 412, 1995

283. Fontaine G, Brestescher C, Fontaliran F, et al: Modalités évolutives de la dysplasie ventriculaire droite arythmogène: À propos de 4 observations. Arch Mal Cœur Vaiss 88:973, 1995

284. Loperfido F, Marino B, Schiavon G, et al: Uhl's disease associated with mitral valve prolapse. Int J Cardiol 3:330, 1982

285. Martini B, Basso C, Thiene G: Sudden death in mitral valve prolapse with Holter monitoring–documented ventricular fibrillation: Evidence of coexisting arrhythmogenic right ventricular cardiomyopathy. Int J Cardiol 49:274, 1995

286. Marcus FI, Fontaine G: Arrhythmogenic right ventricular dysplasia/cardiomyopathy: A review. Pacing Clin Electrophysiol 18:1298, 1995

287. Fontaine G, Umemura J, Di Donna P, et al: La durée des complexes QRS dans la dysplasie ventriculaire droite arythmogène: Un noveau marquer diagnostique non invasif. Ann Cardiol Angeiol (Paris) 42:399, 1993

288. Blomstrom-Lundqvist C, Hirsch I, Olsson SB: Quantitative analysis of the signal-averaged QRS in patients with arrhythmogenic right ventricular dysplasia. Eur Heart J 9:301, 1988

289. Scognamiglio R, Fasoli G, Nava A, et al: Relevance of subtle echocardiographic findings in early diagnosis of the concealed form of right ventricular dysplasia. Eur Heart J 10(suppl D):27, 1989

290. Manyari DE, Duff HJ, Kostuk WJ, et al: Usefulness of noninvasive studies for diagnosis of right ventricular dysplasia. Am J Cardiol 57:1147, 1986

291. Hamada S, Takamiya M, Ohe T, et al: Arrhythmogenic right ventricular dysplasia: Evaluation with electron-beam CT. Radiology 187:723, 1993

292. Ricci C, Longo R, Pagnan L, et al: Magnetic resonance imaging in right ventricular dysplasia. Am J Cardiol 70:1589, 1992

293. Auffermann W, Wichter T, Breithardt G, et al: Arrhythmogenic right ventricular disease: MR imaging vs. angiography. Am J Radiol 161:549, 1993

294. Blake LM, Sheinmann MM, Higgins CB: Magnetic resonance features of arrhythmogenic right ventricular dysplasia. Am J Radiol 162:809, 1994

295. Daliento L, Rizzoli G, Thiene G, et al: Diagnostic accuracy of right ventriculography in arrhythmogenic right ventricular cardiomyopathy. Am J Cardiol 60:741, 1990

296. Engel AG, Yamamoto M, Fischbeck KH: Dystrophinopathies. In: Engel AG, Yamamoto M, Fischbeck KH (eds): Myology. 2nd ed. New York, McGraw-Hill, 1994, p 1133

297. Perloff JK, de Leon AC Jr, O'Doherty D: The cardiomyopathy of progressive muscular dystrophy. Circulation 33:625, 1966

298. Perloff JK, Moise NS, Stevenson WG, Gilmour RF: Cardiac electrophysiology in Duchenne muscular distrophy: From basic science to clinical expression. J Cardiovasc Electrophysiol 3:394, 1992

299. Frankel KA, Rosser RJ: The pathology of the heart in progressive muscular dystrophy: Epimyocardial fibrosis. Hum Pathol 7:375, 1976

300. Nigro G, Comi LI, Politano L, et al: Evaluation of the cardiomyopathy in Becker's muscular dystrophy. Muscle Nerve 18:283, 1995

301. Hoffman EP, Brown RH Jr, Kunkel LM: Dystrophin: The protein product of the Duchenne muscular dystrophy locus. Cell 51:919, 1987

302. Anderson MS, Kunkel LM: The molecular and biochemical basis of Duchenne muscular dystrophy. Trends Biochem Sci 17:289, 1992

303. Ohlendieck K: Towards an understanding of the dystrophin-glycoprotein complex: Linkage between the extracellular matrix and the membrane cytoskeleton in muscle fibers. Eur J Cell Biol 69:1, 1996

304. Maeda M, Nakao S, Miyazato H, et al: Cardiac dystrophin abnormalities in Becker muscular dystrophy assessed by endomyocardial biopsy. Am Heart J 129:702, 1995

305. Cziner DG, Levin RI: The cardiomyopathy of Duchenne's muscular dystrophy and the function of dystrophin. Med Hypotheses 40: 169, 1993

306. Mahadevan M, Tsilfidis C, Sabourin L, et al. Myotonic muscular dystrophy mutation: An unstable CTG repeat in the 3′ untranslated region of the gene. Science 255:1253, 1992

307. Harper PS: Myotonic Dystrophy. 2nd ed. Philadelphia, WB Saunders, 1989.

308. Perloff JK, Stevenson WG, Roberts NK, et al: Cardiac involvement in myotonic muscular dystrophy (Steinert's disease): A prospective study of 25 patients. Am J Cardiol 54:1074, 1984

309. Kennel AJ, Titus JL, Merideth J: Pathologic findings in the atrioventricular conduction system in myotonic dystrophy. Mayo Clin Proc 49:838, 1974

310. Nguyen HH, Wolfe JT 3rd, Holmes DR Jr, Edwards WD: Pathology of the cardiac conduction system in myotonic dystrophy: A study of 12 cases. J Am Coll Cardiol 11:662, 1988

311. Fadic R, Sunada Y, Waclawik AJ, et al: Brief report: Deficiency of a dystrophin-associated glycoprotein (adhalin) in a patient with muscular dystrophy and cardiomyopathy. N Engl J Med 334:362, 1996

312. Tanaka H, Uemura N, Toyama Y, et al: Cardiac involvement in the Kugelberg-Welander syndrome. Am J Cardiol 38:528, 1976

313. Anderson S, Bankier A, Barrel BG, et al: Sequence and organization of the human mitochondrial genome. Nature 290:457, 1981

314. Attardi G, Schatz G: Biogenesis of mitochondrial diseases. Ann Rev Cell Biol 4:289, 1988

315. Wallace DC, Singh G, Lott MT, et al: Mitochondrial DNA mutation associated with Leber's hereditary optic neuropathy. Science 242:1427, 1988

316. Holt J, Harding AE, Morgan-Hughes JA: Deletions of mitochondrial DNA in patients with mitochondrial cardiomyopathies. Nature 331:717, 1988

317. Wallace DC: Diseases of mitochondrial DNA. Annu Rev Biochem 61:1175, 1992

318. Moraes CT, Di Mauro S, Zeviani M, et al: Mitochondrial DNA deletions in progressive external ophthalmoplegia and Kearns-Sayre syndrome. N Engl J Med 320:1293, 1989

319. Poulton J, Deadman ME, Gardner RM: Duplications of mitochondrial DNA in mitochondrial myopathy. Lancet 1:236, 1989

320. Bolhega S, Tanji K, Santorelli F, et al: Multiple mitochondrial deletions associated with autosomal recessive ophthalmoplegia and severe cardiomyopathy. Neurology 46:1329, 1996

321. Shoffner JM, Wallace DC: Heart disease and mitochondrial DNA mutations. Heart Dis Stroke 1:235, 1992

322. Hirano M, Pavlakis S: Mitochondrial myopathy, encephalopathy, lactic acidosis and strokelike episodes (MELAS): Current concepts. J Child Neurol 9:4, 1994

323. Shoffner JM, Lott MT, Lezza AM, et al: Myoclonic epilepsy and ragged-red fiber disease (MERRF) is associated with a mitochondrial DNA tRNA(Lys) mutation. Cell 61:931, 1990

324. Wallace DC: Mitochondrial genetics: A new paradigm for aging and degenerative disease. Science 256:628, 1992

325. Tanaka M, Ino H, Ohno K, et al: Mitochondrial mutation in fatal infantile cardiomyopathy. Lancet 2:1452, 1990

326. Merante F, Tein I, Benson L, Robinson B: Maternally-inherited hypertrophic cardiomyopathy due to a novel T-to-C transition at nucleotide 9997 in the mitochondrial tRNA^{glycine} gene. Am J Hum Genet 55:437, 1994

327. Casali C, Santorelli F, d'Amati G, et al: A novel mtDNA point mutation in maternally inherited cardiomyopathy. Biochem Biophys Res Commun 213:588, 1995

327a. Casali C, d'Amati G, Bernucci P, et al: Maternally inherited cardiomyopathy: Clinical and molecular characterization of a large kindred harboring the A4300G point mutation in mitochondrial deoxyribonucleic acid. J Am Coll Cardiol, 33:1584, 1999

328. Santorelli FM, Mak SC, El-Shahawi M, et al: Maternally-inherited cardiomyopathy and hearing loss associated with a mitochondrial DNA point mutation in the mitochondrial tRNA^{lys} gene (G8363A). Am J Hum Genet 58:933, 1996

329. Anan R, Nakagawa M, Myata M, et al: Cardiac involvement in mitochondrial diseases. A study on 17 patients with documented mitochondrial DNA defects. Circulation 91:955, 1995

330. Müller-Höcker J, Ibel H, Paetzke I: Fatal infantile mitochondrial cardiomyopathy and myopathy with heterogeneous tissue expression of combined respiratory chain deficiencies. Virchows Arch [Pathol Anat] 419:355, 1991

331. Taniike M, Fukushima H, Yanagihara I, et al: Mitochondrial tRNA^{Ile} mutation in fatal cardiomyopathy. Biochem Byophys Res Commun 186:47, 1992

332. Bernucci P, d'Amati G, Casali C, et al: Cardiomiopatia mitocondriale: Una nuova entità nel campo della ricerca e della diagnosi cardiologica. G Ital Cardiol 26:1031, 1996

333. Schwartzkopff B, Zierz S, Frenzel H, et al: Ultrastructural abnormalities of mitochondria and deficiency of myocardial cytochrome C oxidase in a patient with ventricular tachycardia. Virchows Arch [Pathol Anat] 419:63, 1991

334. Harding AE: Friedreich's ataxia: A clinical and genetic study of 90 families with analysis of early diagnostic criteria and intrafamilial clustering of clinical features. Brain 104:589, 1981.

335. Child JS, Perloff JK, Bach PM, et al: Cardiac involvement in Friedreich's ataxia. J Am Coll Cardiol 7:1370, 1986

336. Giunta A, Maione S, Biagini R, et al: Noninvasive assessment of systolic and diastolic function in 50 patients with Friedreich's ataxia. Cardiology 75:321, 1988

337. Alboliras ET, Shub C, Gomez MR, et al: Spectrum of cardiac involvement in Friedreich's ataxia: Clinical, electrocardiographic and echocardiographic observations. Am J Cardiol 58:518, 1986.

338. Dische MR, Porro RS: The cardiac lesions in Bassen-Kornsweig syndrome. Report of a case, with autopsy findings. Am J Med 49:568, 1970

339. James TN, Fisch C: Observations on the cardiovascular involvement in Friedreich's ataxia. Am Heart J 66:164, 1963

340. Brumback RA, Panner BJ, Kingston WJ. The heart in Friedreich's ataxia. Arch Neurol 43:189, 1986

341. Ivemark B, Thorén C: The pathology of the heart in Friedreich's ataxia. Changes in coronary arteries and myocardium. Acta Med Scand 175:227, 1964

342. James TN, Cobbs BW, Coghlan HC, et al: Coronary disease, cardioneuropathy, and conduction system abnormalities in the cardiomyopathy of Friedreich's ataxia. Br Heart J 57:446, 1986

343. Chamberlain S, Shaw J, Rowland A, et al: Mapping of mutation causing Friedreich's ataxia to human chromosome 9. Nature 334:248, 1988

344. Campuzano V, Montermini L, Molto MD, et al: Friedreich's ataxia: Autosomal recessive disease caused by an intronic GAA triplet repeat expansion. Science 271:1423, 1996

345. Durr A, Cossee M, Agid Y, et al: Clinical and genetic abnormalities in patients with Friedreich's ataxia. N Engl J Med 335:1169, 1996

346. Lazarides E: Intermediate filaments as mechanical integrators of intercellular space. Nature 238:249,1980

347. Georgatos SD, Blobel G: Lamin B constitutes an intermediate filament attachment site at the nuclear envelope. J Cell Biol 105:115, 1987

348. Sarnat HB: Vimentin and desmin in maturing skeletal muscle and developmental myopathies. Neurology 42:1616, 1992

349. Calderon A, Becker LE, Murphy EG: Subsarcolemmal vermiform deposits in skeletal muscle, associated with familial cardiomyopathy: Report of two cases of a new entity. Pediatr Neurosci 13:108, 1987

350. Pellissier JF, Pouget J, Charpin C, Figarella D: Myopathy associated with desmin type intermediate filaments. An immunoelectron microscopic study. J Neurol Sci 89:49, 1989

351. Cameron CHS, Mirakhur M, Allen IV: Desmin myopathy with cardiomyopathy. Acta Neuropathol 89:560, 1995

352. Fardeau M, Godet-Guillain J, Tomé FMS, et al: Une nouvelle affection musculaire familiale, définie par accumulation intra-sarco-plasmique d'un matériel granulo-filamentaire dense en microscopie électronique. Rev Neurol (Paris) 131:411, 1978

353. Magliocco AM, Mitchell LB, Brownell AKW, Lester WM: Dilated cardiomyopathy in multicore myopathy. Am J Cardiol 63:150, 1988

354. Bertini E, Bosman C, Bevilacqua M, et al: Cardiomyopathy and multicore myopathy with accumulation of intermediate filaments. Eur J Pediatr 149:856, 1990

355. Ariza A, Coll J, Fernàndez-Figueras T, et al: Desmin myopathy: A multisystem disorder involving skeletal, cardiac, and smooth muscle. Hum Pathol 26:1032, 1995

356. Shy GM, Engel WK, Somers JE, et al: Nemaline myopathy. A new congenital myopathy. Brain 86:793, 1963

357. Ishibashi-Ueda H, Imakita M, Yutani C, et al: Congenital nemaline myopathy with dilated cardiomyopathy: An autopsy study. Hum Pathol 21:77, 1990

358. Malhotra V, Ferrans VJ, Virmani R: Infantile histiocytoid cardiomyopathy: Three cases and literature review. Am Heart J 128: 1009, 1994

359. Koponen MA, Siegel RJ: Histiocytoid cardiomyopathy and sudden death. Hum Pathol 27:420, 1996

360. Ferrans VJ, McAllister HA, Hase WH: Infantile cardiomyopathy with histiocytoid change in cardiac muscle cells. Report of 6 patients. Circulation 53:708, 1976

361. Amini M, Bosman C, Marino B: Histiocytoid cardiomyopathy in infancy: A new hypothesis? Chest 77:556, 1980

362. Zimmerman A, Diem P, Cottier H: Congenital "histiocytoid" cardiomyopathy: Evidence suggesting a developmental disorder of the Purkinje cell system of the heart. Virchows Arch [Pathol Anat] 396:187, 1982

363. Gelb AB, Van Meter SH, Billingham ME, et al: Infantile histiocytoid cardiomyopathy—Myocardial or conduction system hamartoma: What is the cell type involved? Hum Pathol 24:1226, 1993

364. Silver MM, Burns JE, Sethi RK, Rowe RD: Oncocytic cardiomyopathy with oncocytosis in exocrine and endocrine glands. Hum Pathol 11:598, 1980

365. Burch GE, Giles TD, Colcolough HL: Ischemic cardiomyopathy. Am Heart J 83:340, 1970

366. Pfeffer MA, Braunwald E: Ventricular remodeling after myocardial infarction. Circulation 81:1161, 1990

367. Baroldi G, Silver MD, Mariani F, Giuliano G: Correlation of morphological variables in the coronary atherosclerotic plaque with clinical patterns of ischemic heart disease. Am J Cardiovasc Pathol 2:159, 1988

Chapter 11

Cardiovascular Causes of Sudden Death

Gaetano Thiene • Cristina Basso • Domenico Corrado

Sudden, unexpected death cuts short human life, and cardiac arrest is its usual pathogenetic mechanism. It has been proved that electrical instability of the heart often provides the final common pathway. Nevertheless, although cardiac arrest is usually ascribable to an abrupt fatal arrhythmia, the event is rarely a mere functional disorder. A large spectrum of both congenital and acquired cardiovascular diseases form the organic substrate of life-threatening electrical dysfunction. The underlying abnormality is frequently concealed and discovered with surprise at postmortem examination. Nonetheless, we will prove that most diseases, although asymptomatic, are potentially detectable in life with proper imaging or electrophysiologic techniques.

In this chapter, we deal not only with the causes and mechanisms of cardiovascular sudden death but also briefly with the in vivo diagnosis of hidden heart defects to predict risk of, and eventually prevent, sudden death. Sudden infant death syndrome is excluded from this review.

DEFINITION

We define sudden death as a natural, unexpected fatal event occurring within 6 hours of the beginning of symptoms, in an apparently healthy subject, or one whose disease was not so severe that it would predict such an abrupt outcome.

The definition includes some fundamental issues that need discussion:

1. Sudden death is a mode of dying; in other words, it is a symptom, not a disease. The clinical condition causing it is frequently missed, so postmortem examination is mandatory to unveil the concealed morbid substrate.
2. Sudden death occurs in the natural history of several human diseases. Other causes, such as occult trauma, drowning, choking, drug addiction (e.g., cocaine abuse), or iatrogenic disorders should be excluded. In this regard, previous definitions of sudden death included the term "witnessed" to reinforce the reliability of a natural occurrence. However, most sudden deaths occur during sleep and are not witnessed. Therefore, this strict definition would exclude many natural deaths. For this reason, we do not require that death be witnessed in our definition. However, we strongly recommend toxicologic tests in such cases, in addition to an autopsy.
3. In definition, the time elapsing between the onset of final symptoms and death has been controversial, varying from a few minutes (instantaneous death) to 24 hours. An interval of 24 hours is too long because the concept of sudden death would then include many noncardiovascular diseases (e.g., cerebral stroke, fulminant bronchopneumonia, pancreatitis, adrenal apoplexy), in which cardiac arrest is secondary and usually delayed. "Instantaneous death," representing most sudden cardiac deaths, should be confined only to cases of abrupt irreversible ventricular fibrillation with immediate interruption of cerebral blood flow and loss of consciousness. Thus, an interval of 6 hours seems a wise compromise. Nevertheless, many authors are inclined to adopt a time of 1 hour.[1]
4. Although in most cases the underlying defect is clinically covert or poorly defined, there are sudden deaths that occur during the natural course of patently evident cardiac disease. This is the case, for instance, in symptomatic ischemic heart disease (before or after myocardial infarction) or in cardiomyopathies. Although sudden death may occur unexpectedly in an individual, thus fitting the definition, it is predicted by a yearly rate in a population affected by these morbid conditions and according to defined parameters. Risk stratification of sudden death is a major challenge in cardiac medicine.
5. Cardiac arrest may be reversible in the setting of resuscitative maneuvers, which are becoming more prompt, sophisticated, and effective. The term "aborted sudden death" has been introduced to refer to this situation and to patients who suffer but survive cardiac arrest. In terms of pathophysiology, the condition is equivalent to sudden death, although the difference is obviously immense. Many patients whose cardiac arrests are subsequently aborted develop myocardial infarctions. Nevertheless, aborted sudden death may not be followed by an overt acute myocardial infarction. It should be stressed that sometimes a cardiac rescue is achieved but irreversible cerebral damage follows the circulatory arrest, leading thereafter to a delayed cerebral death. This death, in all respects, should be considered sudden.

EPIDEMIOLOGY

There is general agreement that sudden death is a major issue in industrialized countries, but variability of definition and diagnosis, as well as factors such as missing information, lack of autopsy investigation, and different classifications of causes make epidemiologic evaluation difficult.[2]

In the United States, Gillum[3] estimated that more than 350,000 people die suddenly each year of cardiovascular causes. The annual incidence of sudden death in people between 35 and 74 years of age from 40 states was 191/ 100,000 in men and 57/100,000 in women. Almost half of all sudden deaths occur in people with known coronary artery disease.

Other studies from selected regions of the United States[4–11] suggested similar rates of sudden cardiac death, despite different definitions, populations, and time periods. In all, the incidence of sudden death is two to three times higher in men than in women, mostly parallelling the male/female ratio in ischemic heart disease. The proportion of sudden ischemic heart disease deaths is always 50 to 60%, except in the Framingham study in which results were lower (23%), probably because of exclusion of people with known coronary artery disease.[4]

As far as sudden deaths occurring in countries other than the United States, data are less well documented.[12] However, these international reports show the same patterns, except in Finland,[13] where rates are considerably higher than in the United States, again parallelling an increased rate of coronary artery disease mortality in that country.

Sudden cardiac death is uncommon in children and adolescents. Several studies have estimated the rate in those between 1 and 20 years of age is from 1.3 to 8.5/ 100,000 patients per year.[14] This would amount to at least 600 such deaths annually in the United States.[15] The incidence and causes of sudden death in a young adult population has not been well defined. Shen and colleagues[16] published the results of a 30-year population-based study in 54 young adults (20 to 40 years of age) who died suddenly; all were residents of Olmsted County, Minnesota. The incidence of sudden death was estimated on the basis of the ratio of observed events to relative census data for the Olmsted County population during the last three decades. An overall cohort incidence rate of 6.2/100,000 annually was calculated. Of the 54 cases who died suddenly, 19 were women (4.1/100,000 population annually) and 35 were men (8.7/100,000 population annually).

The major issue in interpreting epidemiologic data on sudden death, besides a lack of standardization in death certificate coding, is the variability in its definition. This includes differences in the time interval between symptom onset and death, the location of death, inclusion or exclusion of unwitnessed deaths, and consideration of the unexpected nature of death.[2] Time intervals used to define sudden death vary from 1 to 24 hours between the time of collapse and the loss of vital signs[17, 18]; in fact, the onset of symptoms is often difficult to define because patients have been unwell for days or weeks before sudden death. Noteworthy is that studies using a shorter time period (1 hour or less) in definition report a lower incidence of sudden death than those using a wider definition (up to 24 hours) in which most deaths may be clinically classified as due to myocardial infarction or stroke.[19]

Most authors accept that sudden and unexpected deaths should exclude those occurring in hospital. More recently, the definition has been extended to include deaths that occur in emergency rooms because of an increasing number of emergency services and prolonged life-support efforts.[3] As indicated, many studies exclude unwitnessed death because the exact times of symptom onset and

death cannot be established.[17] The probability of unwitnessed sudden death is higher in the setting of a shorter survival from symptom onset, among people living alone, in deaths occurring at home or during sleep, and in those without a history of known heart disease. As a consequence, exclusion of unwitnessed sudden deaths seriously biases a study by under-representing these conditions. On the other hand, inclusion of such sudden deaths implies a need to obtain detailed postmortem examinations and to interview clinicians and relatives about previous illnesses and symptoms. In this particular subgroup, as stressed earlier, the study should include toxicologic examination to rule out deaths due to drug addiction, excess alcohol intake, homicide, or suicide.

Finally, because as many as 50% of people who die suddenly have a previous history of heart disease, physicians tend to ascribe sudden death to coronary artery disease without further investigation, recording that on death certificates.[17]

PATHOPHYSIOLOGIC MECHANISMS OF SUDDEN DEATH

The final mechanism of death is cardiac arrest, but by no means are all sudden deaths cardiac or cardiovascular in nature. The heart may stop beating as a result of acute cerebral or respiratory failure. Thus, when considered as a primary loss of vital function, sudden death may be defined as cerebral, respiratory, or cardiovascular.

Sudden Cerebral Death

This occurs in the setting of abrupt brain apoplexy, usually a consequence of a hypertensive hemorrhage with ventricular flooding, or a subarachnoid hemorrhage secondary to rupture of a congenital aneurysm on the circle of Willis, or to an extensive hemispheric infarction after embolic occlusion of a carotid or cerebral artery.[20–22] The acute cerebral edema that results involves the brain stem, where cardiorespiratory centers are located, leading to a sudden loss of autonomous central respiratory function. The heart then stops, usually with a progressive sinus bradycardia to asystole.

In cerebral embolism, with the rare exception of paradoxical embolism, the source is the left side of the heart or the aorta and the embolus may be thrombotic, septic, or neoplastic. Thus, although the primary morbid disease is cardiovascular, sudden death due to cerebral embolism is a cerebral and not a cardiac phenomenon, because sudden death is a symptom rather than a disease, and it is classified according to the primary loss of vital function.

Sudden death may occur during epileptic seizures associated with respiratory muscle paralysis. Clearly, the abrupt dysfunction is cerebral in origin, whereas respiratory failure is secondary.[23] In some instances, the occurrence of bradycardia in association with apnea suggests involvement of cardiorespiratory reflexes.[24] However, there are cases of witnessed sudden death in subjects with a history of epilepsy, in whom the final episode does not occur associated with a convulsive seizure and in whom postmortem examination excludes cardiovascular causes of death. These cases are intriguing and difficult to fit into any classification.

Sudden Respiratory Death

In this instance, an abrupt airway obstruction accounts for an acute failure of ventilation and alveolar gas exchange, producing hypoxia, cyanosis, and final heart standstill. Accidental events such as tracheal obstruction following inhalation of a foreign body account for most of these cases, which should not strictly be considered sudden deaths. The sudden obstruction may be spontaneous in the setting of a congenital anomaly (tracheal or bronchial stenosis) or result from acquired conditions such as glottal edema complicating grippe or allergic bronchial asthma.[25–27] In the latter condition, airway obstruction is peripheral and diffuse. Amine release by inflammatory infiltrates in the bronchial wall explains the associated bronchospasm. Histology discloses eosinophils, typical thickening of bronchial basal membrane, and plugs in the bronchial lumen caused by hypersecretion of the mucinous glands. The latter aggravates airway obstruction.[27]

In cardiovascular or cerebral sudden deaths, immediate loss of consciousness occurs, whereas in airway obstruction, only ventilatory function is jeopardized, but circulation, including brain perfusion, is preserved during the attack. This implies that consciousness is maintained for minutes during desperate inspiratory efforts, until severe deoxygenation and asystole occur. In other words, the victim is witness to his impending death.

Sudden Cardiovascular Death

By cardiovascular, we mean the heart and the great arteries. The causes of cardiocirculatory arrest may reside in the aorta or the pulmonary artery or in one of the major cardiac structures, the integrity of which are essential for regular heart function. Thus, coronary arteries ensure adequate myocardial blood perfusion; normal myocardium guarantees not only an ordered contractility but also homogenous electric impulse propagation; valves and endocardium allow blood transit with no reflux during cardiac cycles; and the conduction system maintains electrical stability through a regular pace-making function and impulse transmission, with delay at the specialized atrioventricular (AV) junction allowing the sequence of atrial and ventricular contractility. Of course, to cause instantaneous death, dysfunction of any of these structures must be fulminant. As far as pathophysiology is concerned, cardiac arrest has two mechanisms.

Mechanical Arrest

The heart and circulatory functions are suddenly impeded by mechanical factors. This is the case, for instance, with aortic or cardiac rupture into the pericardial cavity, which produces hemopericardium.[28] Death occurs because cardiac tamponade impairs diastolic ventricular filling rather than because of hypovolemia, which is, instead, the mechanism with aortic rupture into the pleural and peritoneal cavities or the retroperitoneal space. Rupture of a mitral papillary muscle in the setting of myocardial infarction, or of chordae tendinae in the setting of mitral valve prolapse, may induce acute severe mitral incompetence and pulmonary edema.

Sudden, spontaneous hemorrhage may occur elsewhere, such as in the gastrointestinal tract, and may be so quick and massive as to induce loss of consciousness, shock, and cardiac arrest.[29]

Shock, defined as a discrepancy between the capacity of the circulatory system and the blood content, may also develop without hemorrhage in the setting of septic (Waterhouse-Friderichsen syndrome)[30] or allergic (beesting)[31] conditions. The fall of blood pressure may be sufficiently extensive to account for fulminant multiorgan failure and death within minutes or hours.

Another cause of mechanical cardiovascular sudden death is a saddle pulmonary thromboembolism, which abruptly blocks blood transit.[32, 33] Apart from conditions like orthopedic trauma or constrained postoperative position, in which the risk of pulmonary embolism is well known, such catastrophic events may happen in young women taking combined estrogen/progesterone therapy because of ovarian dysfunction or for contraception and among passengers on long-distance flights.

It is noteworthy that cardiac rupture, sudden heart failure with pulmonary edema and cardiogenic shock with myocardial infarction, are now all considered major subjects that are separate from sudden death.

Arrhythmic Cardiac Arrest

This is by far the most common pathophysiologic mechanism of sudden cardiac death. Although cerebral and respiratory functions behave normally, heart rhythm is suddenly upset with severe impairment of ventricular filling and emptying. As a consequence, cardiac output decreases, cerebral blood flow drops, and irreversible brain damage and death result. Ischemic myocardial damage, whether recent (myocardial necrosis) or past (myocardial fibrosis), is the most frequent substrate for an abrupt electrical disorder. However, arrhythmias also occur in the absence of ischemia (e.g., cardiomyopathy, conduction system abnormalities).

Tracings from Holter-monitored sudden deaths or on electrocardiograms (ECGs) recorded at resuscitative maneuvers revealed the following patterns during cardiac arrest[34–42]:

Ventricular Fibrillation (Nearly 70%)

Ventricular electrical activity consists of as many as 400 to 500 nonsynchronized beats per minute (bpm). This high frequency does not leave enough time for diastolic filling and systolic emptying; ventricular contractility is transformed in a vermicular, ineffective motion (Fig. 11-1).

Ventricular Tachycardia (Nearly 10%)

The ventricular rhythm, despite its high frequency (up to 250 bpm), is regular and presents as monomorphic, large, wide, and aberrant QRS complexes. The high rate does not allow enough blood flow to enter and exit the ventricles, so blood pressure drops and collapse may oc-

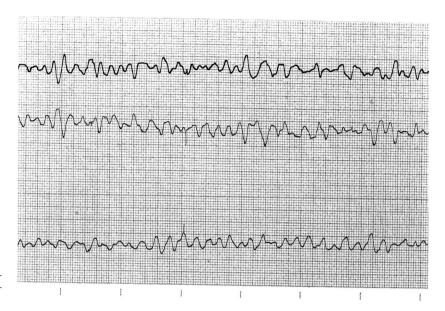

Figure 11-1 • Cardiac arrest in a case of sudden death; electrocardiographic tracing of recorded ventricular fibrillation.

cur, often in the presence of depressed left ventricular function. In this setting, ventricular tachycardia often degenerates into ventricular fibrillation.

Asystole (Nearly 15%)

There is a standstill of ventricular activity either because of sinus arrest or complete AV block. No QRS complexes are registered on the ECG, and that corresponds hemodynamically to absent ventricular systole.

Electromechanical Dissociation (Nearly 5%)

No pressure exists in the arterial system, although the ECG regularly registers QRS complexes. Electromechanical dissociation is usually secondary to cardiac tamponade or pulmonary embolism. However, conditions do exist, especially in the setting of acute and widespread myocardial ischemia, in which the phenomenon is primary because the myocardium becomes unexcitable.[34, 41] This is an odd phenomenon consisting of a split between myocardial excitation and contraction. Despite a regular onset and spread of electrical activity, no ventricular contraction follows.

Unexplained Sudden Death

Finally, there are cases in which a complete postmortem examination fails to identify a cause of sudden death. These cases should be considered separately. Nonetheless, if an extracardiac cause is excluded, these fatalities should be regarded as cardiac, considering that a cardiac arrest was the final mechanism of death.

PATHOPHYSIOLOGY OF VENTRICULAR TACHYARRHYTHMIAS

Excitation of the normal ventricular myocardium occurs via the His bundle branches–Purkinje network with final, rapid, fiber-to-fiber conduction. It is a wave-front phenomenon leading to quick, complete excitation, which corresponds to the QRS complex on the ECG (depolarization), so that the whole myocardium contracts almost simultaneously (systole). The muscle then becomes electrically refractory, which corresponds to the ST segment–T wave of the ECG (repolarization), and relaxation occurs (diastole). Ventricular arrhythmias may develop when electrical activity originates spontaneously from the ventricular myocardium and not from the regular excitation and conduction pathways. Clinical forms of ventricular arrhythmias include premature ventricular beats, nonsustained ventricular tachycardia (duration less than 30 seconds), sustained ventricular tachycardia (duration more than 30 seconds), or ventricular fibrillation.

Premature ventricular beats or ventricular tachycardia may arise from the right or left ventricle or from the ventricular septum. The source may be constant, giving rise to uniform QRS complexes; or variable, producing polymorphic QRS complexes.

The following three main mechanisms explain the onset of ventricular arrhythmias[43] and influence the ventricular fibrillation threshold:

1. *Automaticity:* Foci of ventricular myocardium spontaneously depolarize faster than the physiologic pacemaker. This mechanism may explain the arrhythmogenesis of acute focal myocarditis.
2. *Reentry:* The wave-front phenomenon of ventricular depolarization is disturbed by an interposition of necrotic tissue, fibrosis, or fat, which delays or blocks the conduction undirectionally within surviving scattered myocytes. The delayed impulse propagation reaches adjacent ventricular myocardium at the end of its phase of depolarization-repolarization when it is excitable. Therefore, intraventricular reentry occurs between the two pathways, with different electrophysiologic properties. This mechanism has been proved in conditions such as acute myocardial infarction or chronic ischemic heart disease and in cardiomyo-

pathies such as arrhythmogenic right ventricular cardiomyopathy.

3. *Triggered activity:* Because of the proarrhythmic effect of some drugs or a congenital abnormality of repolarization with ionic pump defects, myocytes may be triggered after depolarization. This manifests as ventricular arrhythmias, mainly torsade de points.

PREVALENCE OF MECHANISMS OF SUDDEN DEATH

Cardiovascular sudden death is by far the most frequent occurrence, followed by deaths induced by respiratory or cerebral causes. In our experience (the Veneto region study project of Juvenile Sudden Death), cardiovascular sudden death accounted for 81.5% of the collected cases, followed by cerebral (7.5%) and respiratory (5%) cases (Table 11-1)[44]; 6% of cases were unexplained. This by no means implies that fatal, acute cerebrovascular accidents are rare, but most of those fatalities are not sudden because their clinical courses exceed the 6-hour interval allowed by our definition.

In cardiovascular sudden death, arrhythmic cardiac arrest is the main pathophysiologic mechanism (93%). Mechanical cardiac arrest (7%) caused by aortic rupture or pulmonary thromboembolism is frequent, especially in the elderly, but death is rarely instantaneous to fit the definition. Table 11-2 presents our experience of all causes of cardiovascular sudden death in the young in the Veneto region of Italy.[44]

AORTIC RUPTURE AND MECHANICAL SUDDEN CARDIAC DEATH

Spontaneous rupture of the aorta may occur in the setting of infective and degenerative disease.

Syphilis

Once a major cause of death, nowadays, this disease rarely reaches the tertiary stage to involve the aorta with mesoaortitis, so patients do not develop saccular aneurysms at risk of rupture.[45]

TABLE 11-1 • Mechanisms of Sudden Death—Study Project "Juvenile Sudden Death," Veneto Region, Italy

Mechanisms of Sudden Death	N	(%)
Cerebral	15	7.5
Respiratory	10	5.0
Cardiovascular	163	81.5
Mechanical—12		
Arrhythmic—151		
Unexplained	12	6.0
TOTAL	200	100

Data from Corrado D, Basso C, Poletti A, et al: Sudden death in the young. Is coronary thrombosis the major precipitating factor? Circulation 90:2315, 1994
N = number of cases.

TABLE 11-2 • Cardiovascular Causes of Sudden Death—Study Project "Juvenile Sudden Death," Veneto Region, Italy

Cardiovascular Causes of Sudden Death	N	%
Obstructive coronary atherosclerosis	37	23.0
Arrhythmogenic right ventricular cardiomyopathy	20	12.0
Mitral valve prolapse	17	10.5
Conduction system abnormalities	17	10.5
Congenital coronary anomalies	14	8.5
Myocarditis	12	7.0
Hypertrophic cardiomyopathy	9	5.5
Aortic rupture	9	5.5
Dilated cardiomyopathy	8	5.0
Nonatherosclerotic, acquired coronary artery disease	6	3.5
Postoperative congenital heart disease	5	3.0
Aortic stenosis	3	2.0
Pulmonary thromboembolism	3	2.0
Other	3	2.0
TOTAL	163	

Data from Corrado D, Basso C, Poletti A, et al: Sudden death in the young. Is coronary thrombosis the major precipitating factor? Circulation 9:2315, 1994
N = number of cases.

Infectious Aortic Aneurysms

These are a consequence of a localized bacterial aortitis and may develop unexpectedly in patients with septicemia, even in the absence of valve endocarditis.[46] Bacteria enter the vessel wall through the vasa vasorum, settle, and destroy the media, leading to abscess and aneurysm formation. Such aneurysms may be located in the ascending aorta within the pericardial sac, so that their rupture leads to cardiac tamponade and instantaneous death (Fig. 11-2).

Aortic Dissection

The pathology of this condition is discussed in Chapter 5. The dissection usually occurs as a "bolt from the blue." Tearing of the intima is followed by splitting of the media. The dissection may involve the entire aorta (type I), the ascending segment (type II), or the descending thoracic aorta (type III).[47] The location of dissection in the outer media, close to the adventitia, makes the intramural hematoma prone to external rupture. Hemopericardium and cardiac tamponade occur with rupture into the pericardial cavity and hemothorax, particularly of the left pleural cavity, develops when rupture involves the descending thoracic aorta. Retrograde dissection toward the aortic root may give rise to other mechanisms of sudden death. For example, the coronary ostia may be involved with abrupt obstruction, myocardial ischemia, and ventricular fibrillation, with or without evidence of a myocardial infarction. Acute aortic valve incompetence resulting from commissural dehiscence of the cusps may induce acute ventricular volume overload and pulmonary edema. A retrograde dissecting hematoma may also extend to the atrial septum through the aortoatrial space and may spread to the coronary sinus and surround the AV node, thereby creating atrionodal discontinuity with the onset of AV block and cardiac arrest.[48]

Aortic dissection in the elderly is mostly a complica-

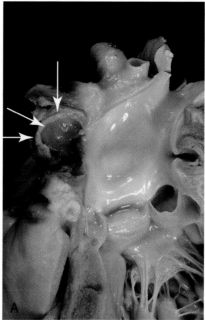

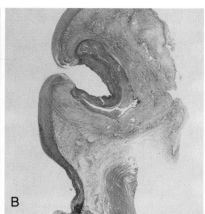

Figure 11-2 • Mycotic aneurysm of the ascending aorta and mechanical sudden cardiac death in a 3-year-old child. *A,* Saccular aneurysm of the ascending aorta (defined by arrows) 1 cm above the sinotubular junction, leading to rupture, cardiac tamponade and sudden death. *B,* Histology showing complete aortic wall destruction and pseudoaneurysm. (Heidenhain trichrome.)

tion of systemic hypertension,[49] and the intimal tear is a consequence of a hypertensive attack. Whether the tunica media exhibits significant changes in terms of medionecrosis, severe disruption of elastic fibers, loss of smooth muscle cells, and accumulation of proteoglycan pools among hypertensive subjects when compared with those of controls, is a controversial matter, because these changes are not unique to that condition.[50] When aortic dissection occurs in the young, these abnormalities are a constant microscopic feature.[51] A genetic or congenital anomaly underlies aortic dissection in the young (e.g., familial miopragia,[52] Marfan syndrome,[53] isthmal coarctation,[54, 55] or a bicuspid aortic valve.[56–58])

Although many cases have an equal severity of medionecrosis, only in Marfan syndrome has a genetic defect been discovered, mapping to chromosome 15q15-q21.3.[59, 60] The disease is familial in the majority of patients, whereas 30% of cases are sporadic. The defective gene encodes fibrillin-1, which is the major constituent of microfibrils of the extracellular matrix. The heart in Marfan patients who die suddenly because of aortic dissection (usually type I or II, with rupture within the pericardial cavity) exhibits typical cardiovascular features consisting of mitral valve prolapse, annuloaortic ectasia, with or without fusiform aneurysm of the ascending aorta, and aortic incompetence[53] (Fig. 11-3). Nonetheless, aortic dissection in Marfan syndrome may also be observed without dilatation of the aorta, its occurrence being unpredictable on clinical grounds.[53]

Familial aortic dissection in the absence of Marfan stigmata and hypertension has been reported rarely,[52] and no defective gene has yet been identified.

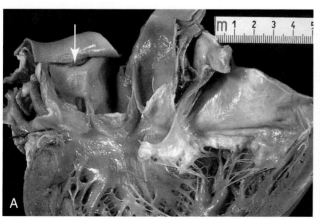

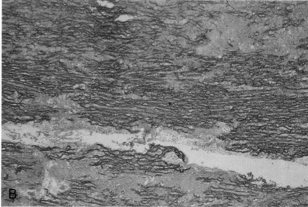

Figure 11-3 • Aortic dissection, Marfan syndrome, and mechanical sudden cardiac death in a 31-year-old man. *A,* View of the left side of the heart and the aortic valve with annuloaortic ectasia and transverse intimal tear (arrow) located 2 cm beyond the sinotubular junction. Note mitral valve prolapse. *B,* Histology of the aortic wall showing hemorrhagic dissection of the tunica media affected by elastic disruption and severe cystic medionecrosis (Weigert-van Gieson).

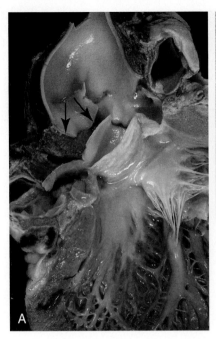

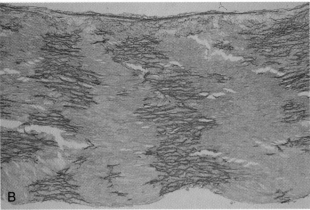

Figure 11-4 • Aortic dissection, isolated bicuspid aortic valve, and mechanical sudden cardiac death in a 24-year-old man. *A,* Spontaneous intimal laceration (arrows) and dissection of the ascending aorta in a heart with a pliable bicuspid aortic valve. *B,* Massive atrophy of elastic lamellae of the aortic tunica media (Weigert-van Gieson).

Bicuspid Aortic Valve and Aortic Dissection

The association between an isolated bicuspid valve and aortic dissection is not incidental (see Chapter 13 also). Indeed, the rate of bicuspid aortic valve among those with aortic dissection is significantly higher than in the normal population (12% vs. 1%).[51, 56, 57, 61–63] The rupture involves a severely degenerated ascending aorta, with or without dilatation, in the setting of a normally pliable bileaflet valve (Fig. 11-4). Although dissections have been reported among the offspring of individuals with a bicuspid aortic valve, familial sudden death has not been proved.[64, 65] Considering the frequency of a bicuspid aortic valve among the general population, the risk of dissection is quite low. Most probably, medionecrosis is present only in a subpopulation of patients with a bicuspid aortic valve. Echocardiographic monitoring of the aortic root in individuals with this anomaly may detect progressive aortic dilatation as a marker of underlying vessel wall degeneration and impending rupture.[58] Of course, this provides indirect evidence of aortic wall fragility. An ultrasonographic technique has been tested in vitro that is clearly able to distinguish aortic walls with regular elastic lamellae units from those with medionecrosis.[66] One may wonder whether a bicuspid aortic valve and medionecrosis are the phenotypic expressions of the same genetic disease or simply a congenital heart disease complex in which the maldevelopment involves either the aortic valve or the wall, which both derive from the neural crest.[67, 68]

This seems to be the case in isthmal coarctation (so-called adult coarctation), also associated with a bicuspid aortic valve in 50% of cases, and in which aortic dissection is an unexpected fatal outcome in its natural history[69] (Fig. 11-5). An equal severity of medionecrosis in spontaneous aortic rupture has been reported in those with Marfan syndrome, or isolated bicuspid aortic valve or isthmal coarctation, with or without a bicuspid valve.[51, 62] A relationship between the development of the aortic arch and the neural crest has been proved by experimental embryologists.[68]

Table 11-3 reports cases of spontaneous aortic rupture in the Juvenile Sudden Death project from the Veneto Region of Italy.[51] Aortic dissection was quite prevalent, displaying a congenital or genetic milieu in all.

Atherosclerosis

Aortic rupture in the setting of an atherosclerotic aneurysm is not a rare event in the elderly (see Chapter 4 also). Such aneurysms are located more frequently in the abdominal infrarenal aorta than in the thoracic aorta. They develop as a consequence of aortic medial atrophy and degeneration with wall thinning. Medial atrophy may be caused by intimal atherosclerosis, but the cause of both wall thinning and intimal atherosclerosis remains to be established.[70, 71] An abdominal aneurysm exceeding 5 cm in diameter is considered at high risk of impending rupture and is an indisputable indication for surgery, because of the high wall tension according to the Laplace law ($T = p \times r/2s$, [T = tension, p = pressure, r = radius and s = wall thickness]).[72–74]

TABLE 11-3 • **Aortic Rupture—Study Project "Juvenile Sudden Death," Veneto Region, Italy**

Type	N
Mycotic Aneurysm	2
Aortic Dissection associated with:	7
Bicuspid aortic valve and isthmic coarctation	3
Isolated bicuspid aortic valve	2
Marfan syndrome	2
TOTAL	9

Data from Basso C, Frescura C, Corrado D, et al: Congenital heart disease and sudden death in the young. Hum Pathol 26:1065, 1995
N = number of cases.

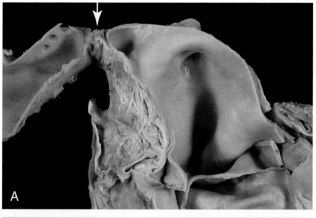
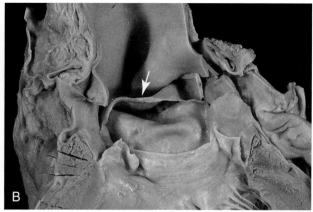
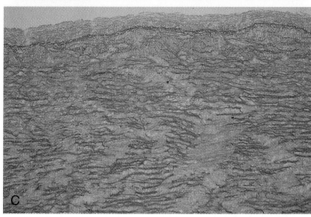

Figure 11-5 • Aortic dissection, isthmic coarctation, and bicuspid aortic valve with mechanical sudden cardiac death in a 17-year-old boy. *A,* Coarctation of the aortic isthmus (arrow). *B,* Large intimal tear (arrow) in the ascending aorta; note the bicuspid aortic valve. *C,* Histology shows disruption of the elastic lamellae in the tunica media (Weigert-van Gieson).

CORONARY ARTERY DISEASE AND ARRHYTHMIC SUDDEN CARDIAC DEATH

Atherosclerotic Coronary Artery Disease

Although instantaneous deaths complicating myocardial infarction in intensive care units are usually ascribable to cardiac rupture, and although historically most cases reported in Lancisi's "De subitaneis mortibus"[75] and Morgagni's "De Sedibus"[76] were explained by this complication, death under these circumstances is not compatible with the definition of an *unexpected event,* and nowadays is not considered a sudden one. The patient is usually hospitalized and clearly recognized to have a myocardial infarction, rupture of which is a predictable, mechanical, fatal complication.[77]

Sudden cardiac death in the setting of ischemic heart disease is almost invariably arrhythmic. Clinical studies conducted on patients rescued from cardiac arrest, including ECG recordings, enzyme test, and follow-up, demonstrate that aborted sudden death occurs in a variable framework that includes the following conditions.

Acute Myocardial Infarction

Cardiac arrest may be the earliest manifestation of an acute myocardial infarction. Nearly 40% of patients who are resuscitated after the arrest develop overt signs of a myocardial infarction, with Q wave and serum enzyme elevations.[78] Most deaths related to myocardial infarction,

either first or recurrent episode, occur within the first hour of the onset of an anginal attack and are a consequence of an ischemic, life-threatening arrhythmia. Either of these conditions usually develops before the patient is admitted to an intensive coronary care unit. The coronary artery pathology consists of single-, double-, or triple-vessel atherosclerotic disease and usually includes a thrombotic occlusion of a coronary segment, which produces a sharp interruption of regional myocardial blood flow.[79-83] Immediate coronary angiography in survivors of out-of-hospital cardiac arrests disclosed significant coronary artery disease in 70% of patients and coronary artery occlusion in nearly half.[83] Thrombus may precipitate onto a ruptured atherosclerotic plaque or an endothelial erosion[84-87] (Fig. 11-6). Rupture affects plaque with lipid-rich cores and thin fibrous caps. Erosion is usually the consequence of inflammation and may involve a fibrocellular plaque devoid of lipids.[85, 86] Acute myocardial damage accounts for automaticity or, most probably, for slow conduction, priming unidirectional blocks, reentry circuits, and the onset of ventricular tachyarrhythmias. High-frequency ventricular tachycardia as well as ventricular fibrillation are the terminal arrhythmias recorded by ECG.

If the coronary thrombosis affects the right coronary artery in a right dominant circulation or the left circumflex artery in a left dominant pattern, blood supply to the sinus and AV nodes may be jeopardized.[88-90] In those circumstances, cardiac arrest may result in asystole caused either by sinus arrest or AV block. Although conducting tissues are resistant to ischemia, temporary dysfunction of

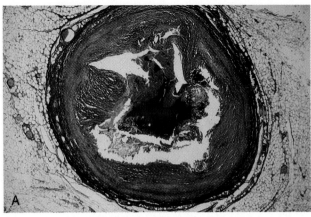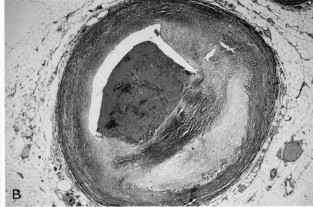

Figure 11-6 • Arrhythmic sudden cardiac death caused by occlusive thrombosis of the left anterior descending coronary artery. *A,* The acute thrombosis is related to a ruptured atherosclerotic plaque from a 35-year-old man. *B,* Acute thrombosis associated with an eccentric plaque with a thick fibrous cap. Thrombus probably caused by an endothelial erosion; from a 33-year-old man. (Both, Heidenhain trichrome.)

the origin and transmission of the electric impulse may occur and be fatal.

It is worth stressing that in this setting myocardial infarction, although clearly diagnosed in vivo by ECG abnormalities (Q wave, ST segment–T wave changes) and enzyme elevation, may not be obvious pathologically because of the short time elapsing between onset of symptoms and death, even if the triphenyl tetrazolium chloride (TTC) test or another gross histochemical technique test is employed. The histology of the myocardium in early infarction may be negative as far as classical findings are considered (e.g., coagulative necrosis, wavy fibers, granulocyte infiltrates).[91–94] A thorough microscopic examination, however, allows detection of very early damage in terms of contraction band necrosis or anisoinotropism of cross striations, which both indicate breaking of the sarcolemma barrier and flooding of the sarcoplasm with conduction disturbances provoked by Ca^{++}.[94] However, the specificity of these lesions is questionable, because they may also be explained by reperfusion damage after resuscitation.

Healed Myocardial Infarction

Life-threatening ventricular tachyarrhythmias arise in patients with myocardial scars from previous infarction and result from a slowing of conduction and the onset of reentry circuits at the border between normal myocardium and scar,[81, 95–100] as well as a zigzag propagation of the impulse within the fibrotic area (Fig. 11-7). Postmortem studies of sudden cardiac death report an incidence of healed myocardial infarction in up to two thirds of adult cases.[101] Neurovegetative influences, whether stemming from emotion or effort, may have a triggering role.[102] Late potentials detected by signal-averaged ECG may reflect this intraventricular conduction defect and the risk of reentrant ventricular arrhythmias, and they represent a prognostic clinical marker for ventricular electrical instability. Warning ventricular arrhythmias in the form of premature ventricular beats or ventricular tachycardia (nonsustained or sustained), may be recorded by 24-hour Holter monitoring and be induced by programmed ventricu-

lar stimulation. Decreased left ventricular ejection fraction, mitral incompetence, left ventricular aneurysm, and residual myocardial ischemia are all poor predictors of survival and help to define risk stratification of sudden death, which, by the way, remains the main mode of death in the long term after a myocardial infarction.

Transient Ischemia

Temporary myocardial ischemia, occurring in the setting of stable or unstable and vasospastic angina pectoris, may trigger fatal arrhythmias in the absence of overt myocardial damage, or, more probably, in the presence of patchy contraction band necrosis sufficient to account for slow conduction unidirectional block and reentry phenomena.[92, 103–106] This may be the mechanism of sudden death in the young with early obstructive coronary atherosclerosis, in whom occlusive thrombosis or a healed myocardial infarction are rarely observed. Indeed, whereas coronary sudden death in adult and elderly patients is mostly associated with multivessel disease and an occlusive or mural

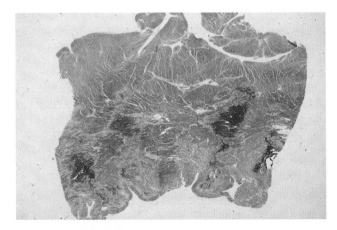

Figure 11-7 • Arrhythmic sudden cardiac death in a healed myocardial infarction. Spots of replacement-type fibrosis are scattered in the anteroseptal wall of the left ventricle accounting for a zigzag intraventricular impulse propagation. (Heidenhain trichrome.)

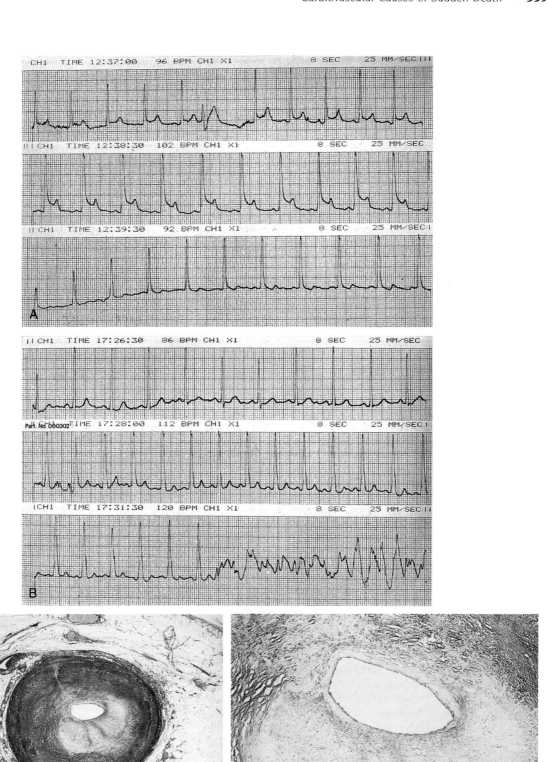

Figure 11-8 • Arrhythmic sudden cardiac death in a 54-year-old man with variant angina. *A,* Holter monitor strips recorded a few hours before sudden death reveal episodes of ST segment elevation in keeping with transient ischemia. *B,* Holter strips recorded at the time of sudden death showing the onset of fatal ventricular fibrillation. *C,* At postmortem examination, a single obstructive atherosclerotic plaque was found in the proximal left anterior descending coronary artery (Heidenhain trichrome). *D,* Details of the plaque showing its nonatheromatous, fibrocellular, myxoid nature (Heidenhain trichrome).

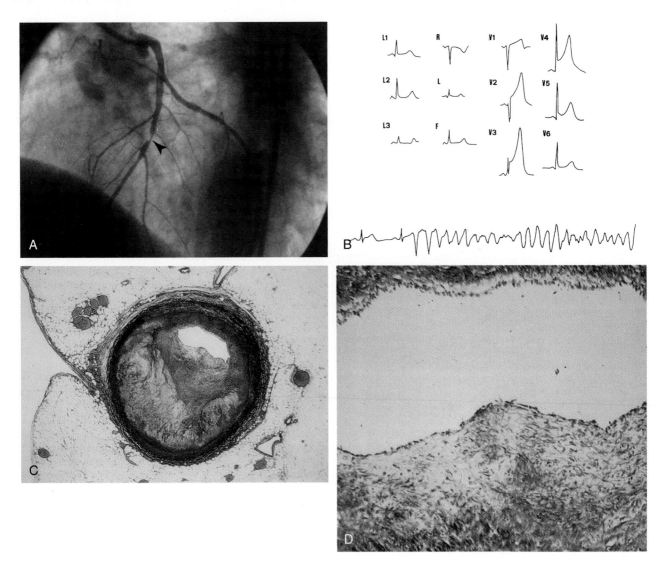

Figure 11-9 • Arrhythmic sudden cardiac death in a 45-year-old man with variant angina. *A,* Selective left coronary angiography showing a single obstructive plaque in the mid part of the left anterior descending coronary artery (arrow). *B,* Electrocardiographic tracing showing marked ST segment elevation followed by ventricular fibrillation. *C,* Histology of the plaque demonstrating severe eccentric stenosis of the left anterior descending coronary artery. *D,* Recent intimal proliferation by smooth muscle cells enmeshed within myxoid tissue. (*C* and *D,* Heidenhain trichrome.)

thrombus,[38, 80, 81, 91, 95, 107–111] coronary sudden death in young patients is rarely precipitated by coronary thrombosis.[44] Rather, the pathology usually consists of a single subobstructive plaque, located at the first part of the left anterior descending coronary artery. The plaque is mainly fibrocellular and devoid of atheroma, fissuring, or thrombosis.[44, 112, 113] Preservation of the tunica media, absence of thrombosis, and frequent occurrence of unexpected death at rest after episodes of variant angina are all features in keeping with a transient ischemic episode, most probably attributable to coronary vasospasm[44, 114] (Figs. 11-8 and 11-9). The observation of contraction band necrosis in the myocardium related to the obstructed artery also favors a transient ischemia followed by reperfusion (Fig. 11-10).

Another feature that distinguishes sudden coronary death in the young from that in the adult, is the infrequency of a previous myocardial infarction in the former,

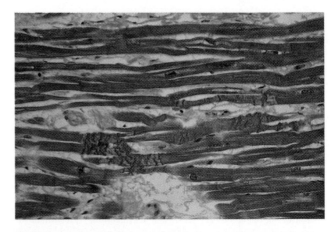

Figure 11-10 • Arrhythmic sudden cardiac death in a 30-year-old man caused by obstructive coronary atherosclerosis in the absence of thrombosis. Early signs of ischemic injury with contraction band necrosis are in keeping with transient ischemia (Heidenhain trichrome).

NORMAL

ORIGIN OF THE RIGHT CORONARY

ARTERY FROM THE LEFT SINUS

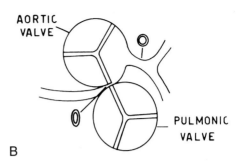

A

B

Figure 11-11 • Diagram illustrating normal origin of coronary arteries (*A*) and anomalous origin of the right coronary artery from the left sinus (*B*). In the latter condition, note the abnormal proximal course between aorta and pulmonary trunk with a slit-like lumen.

and the frequent observation of postinfarction scars in the latter. Sudden death is the sword of Damocles for those who have suffered a myocardial infarction caused either by recurrence of a coronary thrombosis or by the arrhythmogenicity of myocardial scars.[81, 101]

Congenital Coronary Artery Anomalies

The normal pattern of the coronary arterial tree is characterized by two coronary arteries, left and right, which arise from left and right anterior aortic sinuses, respectively, at the sinotubular junction. They arise perpendicular to the aortic root with widely patent ostia and have no relation to the pulmonary trunk in their proximal course (Fig. 11-11). A separate origin within the proper sinus of the conal artery from the right coronary artery or of the left circumflex branch from the left anterior descending coronary artery should be considered variants of normal. Right dominant, left dominant, and balanced patterns of circulation are also individual variations and are within the normal range. The main stems of the coronary arteries run in the subepicardium before branching into perforating, intramural arteries (see Chapter 6 also).

Coronary artery anomalies observed in patients who died suddenly relate to an anomalous origin or course or to both.

Aortic Plication

Coronary ostial malformations include severe stenosis of the lumen caused by a plication of the aortic wall that produces a valve-like ridge (Fig. 11-12). This effectively blocks an ostium during diastolic filling, thus causing transient ischemia and, if prolonged, life-threatening arrhythmias and sudden death.[51, 115] Both left and right coronary ostia may manifest such plications.

Macaroni Disease

Another severe form of coronary ostial obstruction is observed in cases of hyperelastosis of the aortic wall ("macaroni disease").[116, 117] In this condition, the coronary ostium and the vessel's proximal course demonstrate severe obstruction along their intramural course. This malformation may be observed in supravalvular aortic stenosis (William syndrome), in which the coronary ostia may also be totally or partially isolated from the aortic lumen because of fusion of the aortic cusps with the vessel wall.[117]

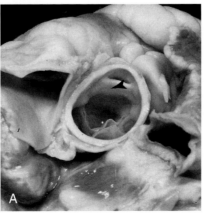

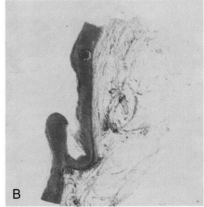

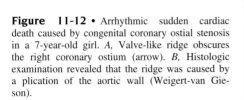

Figure 11-12 • Arrhythmic sudden cardiac death caused by congenital coronary ostial stenosis in a 7-year-old girl. *A,* Valve-like ridge obscures the right coronary ostium (arrow). *B,* Histologic examination revealed that the ridge was caused by a plication of the aortic wall (Weigert-van Gieson).

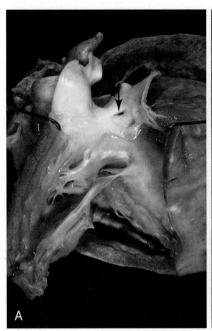
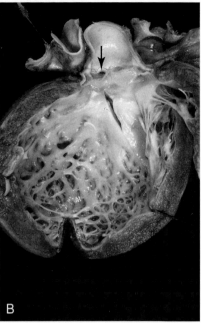

Figure 11-13 • Arrhythmic sudden cardiac death caused by the anomalous origin of the left coronary artery from the pulmonary trunk in a 4-month-old infant. *A,* View of the right ventricle and the pulmonary artery; note a coronary ostium located in the pulmonary root (arrow). *B,* View of the left ventricle and aorta; only the right coronary artery ostium is visible at the aortic root (arrow). Note the remarkable left ventricular dilatation resulting from ischemic heart disease and fibroelastic endocardial thickening.

Origin from Pulmonary Artery

Anomalous origin of a coronary artery from the pulmonary trunk, usually the left coronary stem (Fig. 11-13), is symptomatic in infancy because of coronary blood steal from the aorta to the pulmonary artery, with resultant severe myocardial ischemia and necrosis.[118, 119] Congestive heart failure rather than sudden death is the usual clinical manifestation.

Origin from Coronary Sinus/Aorta

Subjects with anomalous coronary artery origin from the aorta itself have a greater risk of arrhythmic cardiac arrest.

Origin from Wrong Aortic Sinuses

The most common, life-threatening anomaly is an origin of a coronary artery from a wrong aortic sinus, either the right coronary artery from the left sinus (Fig. 11-14; see also Fig. 11-11) or the left vessel from the right coronary sinus (Fig. 11-15).[120] In both situations, the proximal tract of the anomalous artery courses between the pulmonary artery and aorta.[121–123] Because of an oblique origin, the lumen of the anomalous vessel is slit-like.[121, 122] A flap-like closure of its orifice has been postulated,[124] and the vessel's proximal course within the aortic media further aggravates the obstruction.[51, 125] Both right and left coronary artery origins from the contralat-

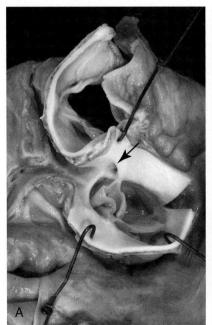
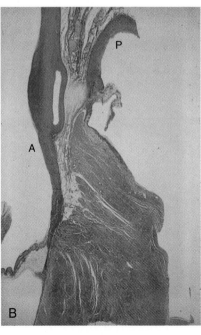

Figure 11-14 • Arrhythmic sudden cardiac death caused by the anomalous origin of the right coronary artery from the left aortic sinus in a 22-year-old soccer player. *A,* View of the aortic root held open by black hooks and showing the origin of both the left and right (arrow) coronary arteries from the left aortic sinus. *B,* Histology of the root of the aorta (**A**) and pulmonary artery (**P**) reveal the intramural aortic course of the anomalous right coronary artery with its slit-like lumen (Weigert-van Gieson).

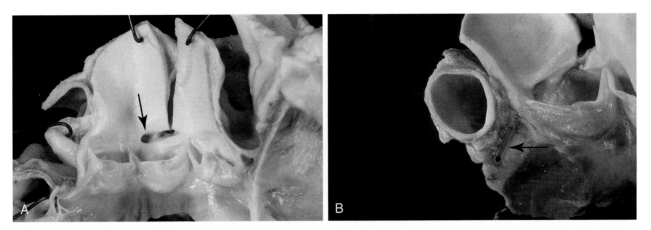

Figure 11-15 • Arrhythmic sudden cardiac death caused by the anomalous origin of the left coronary artery from the right aortic sinus. *A,* An 11-year-old girl who died suddenly. Note the origin of both left (arrow) and right coronary ostia from the right aortic sinus. *B* An 11-year-old boy who died suddenly during a soccer game. Note the course of the left main trunk (arrow) between aorta and pulmonary artery.

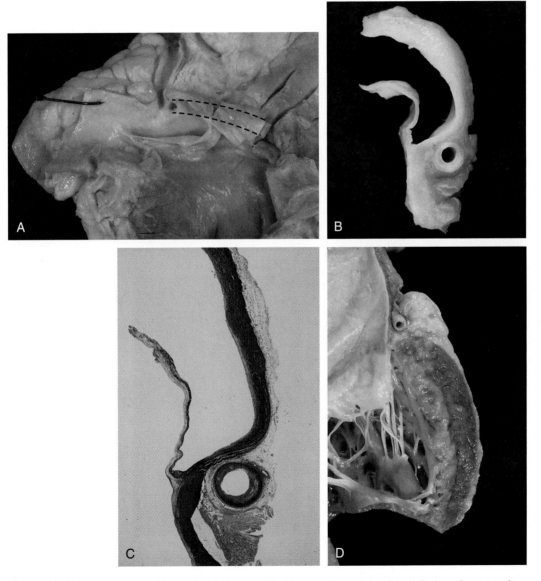

Figure 11-16 • Arrhythmic sudden cardiac death caused by the anomalous origin of the left circumflex artery from the right aortic sinus in a 53-year-old man. *A,* Dotted lines indicate the retroaortic course of the anomalous artery. *B,* Longitudinal section of the posterior aortic sinus showing the circumflex artery located behind the sinus. *C,* Histology of *B,* Note the absence of significant coronary artery disease (Heidenhain trichrome). *D,* Gross view of the lateral wall of the patient's left ventricle showing a healed subendocardial myocardial infarction.

eral sinus raise the risk of sudden death. Origin of the left artery from the right sinus is considered the more malignant condition, having been reported mostly in cases of sudden death or myocardial infarction. This is probably because of the large amount of left ventricle at risk of ischemia.[120] In a review by Barth and Roberts[122] of 38 necropsy patients with a left coronary artery arising from the right aortic sinus and coursing between the aorta and pulmonary trunk, 61% died suddenly in the first two decades of life, and all but one during, or shortly after, vigorous exercise. On the other hand, origin of the right coronary artery from the left sinus may be an incidental observation on angiography or autopsy. Ischemia is usually precipitated by strenuous, prolonged effort, and this explains why a basal ECG or even a stress test ECG may be negative.[125, 126] Syncopal episodes are the only prodromal symptoms. Repetitive ischemic episodes may cause patchy myocardial necrosis and fibrosis as well as ventricular hypertrophy, which eventually can elicit arrhythmias because of the malignant combination of acute and chronic substrates. This may explain why sudden death, associated with an anomalous origin of a coronary artery from the wrong sinus, may occur in adults even though the anomaly has been present since birth.

As for an anomalous origin of the left coronary artery from the posterior aortic sinus, the situation is exceedingly rare and may be associated with sudden death.[121, 127, 128] An anomalous origin of the left circumflex artery from the right coronary artery, or from the right coronary sinus itself with a separate ostium, has also been described in victims of unexpected arrhythmic sudden death. After the anomalous take-off, the left circumflex coronary artery has an abnormal retroaortic course and then reaches the left AV groove by crossing the mitral-aortic fibrous continuity[129] (Fig. 11-16). This anomaly was considered a benign condition[118, 127, 130] until cases were reported, both clinically and pathologically, with evidence of myocardial ischemia in the absence, of obstructive coronary atherosclerosis or any other cause but the malformation itself.[131–133]

High Take-Off

A high take-off of coronary arteries has also been observed in otherwise unexplained sudden cardiac deaths. Nevertheless, in hearts from patients dying of noncardiac causes, the location of coronary ostia in the aorta (within 2 to 3 mm of the sinotubular junction) has been accepted as normal.[134] In the first instance, a higher take-off may result in a vertical intramural aortic course before reaching the aortic root and then the AV sulcus. A funnel-like ostium with a slit-like lumen along the intramural aortic course has been reported to account for myocardial ischemia.[126]

Clinical Diagnosis

To identify these anomalous origins in the clinical setting, transthoracic two-dimensional echocardiography has been used, although it is not very effective in the nonpediatric population.[135] Transesophageal echocardiography is much more sensitive, but is a semi-invasive tool.[136, 137]

Magnetic resonance angiography has been proposed as a gold standard for the noninvasive identification of an anomalous coronary artery origin and its proximal course.[138, 139]

Myocardial Bridges

Most of the previously described conditions combine both anomalous origin and course of a coronary artery. A condition of purely anomalous course is the so-called *myocardial bridge*. An epicardial stem, usually the left anterior descending coronary artery, may run within the myocardium, demonstrating an intramural course (Fig. 11-17). In postmortem studies, thin loops of myocardium surrounding the vessel have been reported in as many as 70% of hearts of patients dying of different causes. Thus, these myocardial bridges should be considered a variant of normal.[140–142] However, clinical cases have been reported in patients with angina and myocardial infarction[143–145] in whom coronary angiography detected nothing but a myocardial constriction ("milking effect"). Surgical debridging was effective in relieving both symptoms and signs of ischemia.[146] Moreover, sudden cardiac death has been described in patients with a myocardial bridge as the only plausible substrate for death.[125, 147] Detailed histopathologic analysis has established that this anomaly is of likely pathologic significance when a coronary artery has a long (2 to 3 cm), deep (2 to 3 mm) intramural course and the myocardium encircling the intramural segment has the features of a sheath acting as a sphincter.[125, 148] Moreover, the surrounding myocardium shows architectural

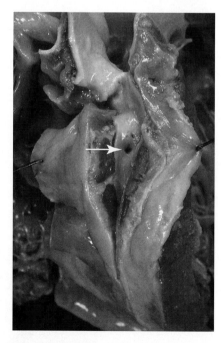

Figure 11-17 • Arrhythmic sudden cardiac death associated with intramural course of the left anterior descending coronary artery in a 35-year-old male runner. Note the deep intramyocardial course of the proximal vessel; the arrow indicates the origin of the first septal perforating branch.

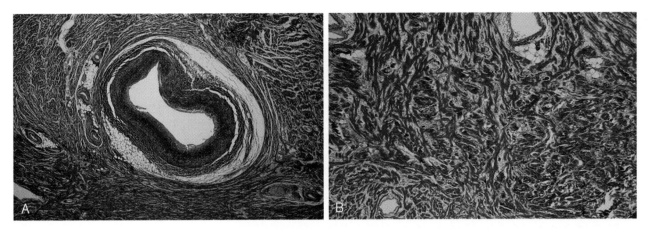

Figure 11-18 • Arrhythmic sudden cardiac death with intramural course of the left anterior descending coronary artery in a 29-year-old man who died at rest. *A,* At histologic examination, the left anterior descending coronary artery manifests a deep intramural course and is encircled by a myocardial sheath. *B,* Close-up of surrounding myocardium showing marked myocardial disarray. (Both, Heidenhain trichrome.)

disarray and fibrosis (Fig. 11-18). Intramural courses of coronary arteries have been reported in cases of hypertrophic cardiomyopathy with sudden death.[147, 149] All these features are in keeping not only with a systolic lumen obliteration, but also with persistent occlusion during diastole, when coronary blood filling occurs as a result of impaired relaxation of myocardium surrounding the anomalous segment, a mechanism recently proven in vivo.[150]

Nonatherosclerotic, Acquired Coronary Artery Disease

Myocardial ischemia may spring from acquired coronary artery diseases other than atherosclerosis, even though the latter is by far the leading cause (see Chapter 8 also).

Coronary Embolism

Coronary embolism induces abrupt coronary occlusion (Fig. 11-19), frequently of the left common coronary trunk. Sudden death, more than regional myocardial infarction, is the classic clinical presentation.[151-153] Mural thrombosis in a left-side cardiac chamber is the usual source of the embolism, occurring in the setting of symptomatic cardiac disease such as previous myocardial infarction, dilated cardiomyopathy, rheumatic mitral valve disease or atrial fibrillation. Infective endocarditis with friable septic vegetations is frequently another cause of embolism to the coronary arterial tree. Rarely, coronary embolism may be the first manifestation of underlying disease. This is the case with occult endocardial tumors, such as myxoma (Fig. 11-20) or papilloma, or of nonbacterial thrombotic endocarditis, or as a complication of occult adenocarcinomas.[152, 154, 155] Embolism of myocardial tissue is a very rare complication of cardiac surgery.[155a]

Coronary Artery Dissection

A well-known complication of invasive procedures (e.g., coronary angiography, balloon angioplasty), coronary artery dissection is caused by mechanical invasion of

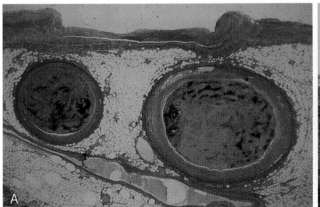
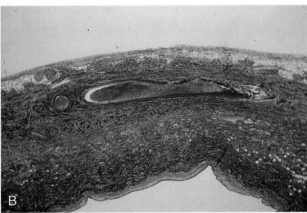

Figure 11-19 • Arrhythmic sudden cardiac death by coronary thromboembolism in a 42-year-old woman. No source of embolism was found at autopsy. *A,* Histology of the right coronary artery and acute marginal branch occluded by thromboembolism. *B,* The thromboembolism also involved the sinus node artery, leading to massive infarction of the sinus node and the crista terminalis. (Both, Heidenhain trichrome.)

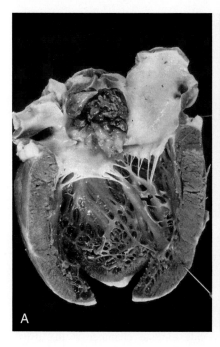
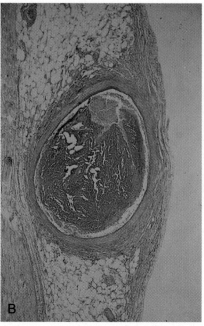

Figure 11-20 • Arrhythmic sudden cardiac death caused by embolizing left atrial myxoma in a 15-year-old boy. *A,* Villous myxoma of the left atrium attached to the atrial septum on the left side. *B,* Histology of the posterior descending coronary artery, which is occluded by myxoid neoplastic tissue (Alcian PAS).

the vessel wall. However, dissections may also occur spontaneously with sudden death the first and last symptom.[156–159] Major subepicardial coronary arteries are involved, usually the left common trunk or the anterior descending coronary artery (Fig. 11-21). The dissecting hematoma is located in the outer third of the tunica media and produces luminal occlusion by forcing the inner media against the opposing wall. Blood filling the false lumen may simulate a coronary thrombosis to the naked eye, masking the dissection. Thus, the real incidence of this entity may be underestimated at autopsy, unless careful histologic examination of the coronary artery is done. In comparison with aortic dissections, an intimal tear is rarely observed in spontaneous cases,[160] suggesting that

the source of blood may be through vasa vasorum bleeding.[161] Associated microscopic features that have been reported sporadically include cystic medial necrosis,[162, 163] eosinophilic infiltrates,[164–166] and angiomatosis of the adventitia.[156] However, and again differing from an aortic dissection, a histologic substrate favoring dissection is absent in the majority of cases. An association with pregnancy or the peripartum period was reported,[167–171] but in most cases no risk factors are identifiable.[156] The coronary arteries are free from atherosclerosis, the patient is not hypertensive, and the dissection occurs mostly in healthy women. Thus, the event is unpredictable and, in most cases, death is instantaneous because of ventricular fibrillation.

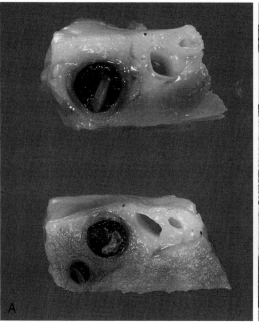
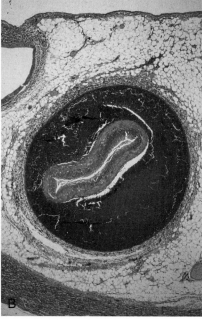

Figure 11-21 • Arrhythmic sudden cardiac death caused by coronary artery dissection in a 23-year-old man. *A,* Cross-sections of the left anterior descending coronary artery showing an intramural hematoma and a virtual true lumen. *B,* Histology discloses the coronary inner walls flattened by the hemorrhagic dissection located between the tunica media and the adventitia (Heidenhain trichrome).

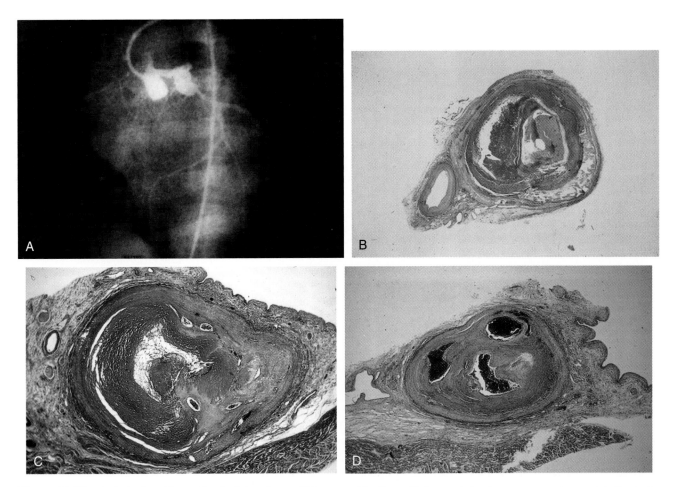

Figure 11-22 • Arrhythmic sudden cardiac death in a 6-year-old boy caused by Kawasaki disease. *A,* In vivo coronary angiogram: injection in the aortic root reveals a huge aneurysm at the bifurcation of the left main trunk. *B,* Histology reveals the aneurysm involving the proximal left circumflex artery. *C,* Right coronary artery showing aneurysmal dilation. *D,* Left anterior descending coronary artery with recanalized luminal thrombotic occlusion. (*B–D,* Heidenhain trichrome.)

Coronary Arteritis

Kawasaki Disease

Originally known as infantile polyarteritis nodosa and then as mucocutaneous lymph node syndrome, Kawasaki disease is a necrotizing arteritis that involves the subepicardial coronary tree of infants and children, especially in Eastern countries. Affected vessels have a tendency to develop aneurysms (Fig. 11-22). Death rarely occurs in the acute stage, most fatalities being reported in the subacute/healing stages.[172, 173] Myocardial ischemia, aneurysm rupture, and myocarditis are the most frequent causes of death.[174] Thrombosis within the aneurysm may occlude the lumen and precipitate myocardial infarction and sudden death many years after the initial clinical manifestations.[175]

Takayasu Arteritis

This is a chronic inflammatory disease of unknown etiology that usually affects young women.[176] Elastic arteries such as the ascending aorta, aortic arch, brachiocephalic branches (Fig. 11-23), and pulmonary arteries are typical locations for the disease. Coronary artery ostia are involved as extensions of aortic root inflammatory disease[177, 178] (Fig. 11-24). Sudden cardiac arrest has been reported as the first manifestation, so that the diagnosis of the arteritis was made at autopsy.[179] Histology of the involved vascular segment discloses disruption of the elastic tunica media by necrotizing angiitis and intimal obstructive proliferation, mononuclear inflammatory infiltrates with rare giant cells, and fibrous thickening of the adventitia.

Giant Cell Arteritis

This disease very rarely involves the coronary arteries. It usually affects older people and is the equivalent of temporal Horton arteritis or giant cell aortitis. Histology reveals granulomatous arteritis of epicardial coronary arteries and intramural branches.[180]

Other Arteritides

Coronary artery involvement has been reported in other types of arteritis, including polyarteritis nodosa[181] and thromboangiitis obliterans.[182, 183] In the former condition, selective angiitis of sinus and AV node arteries may be additional features.[184]

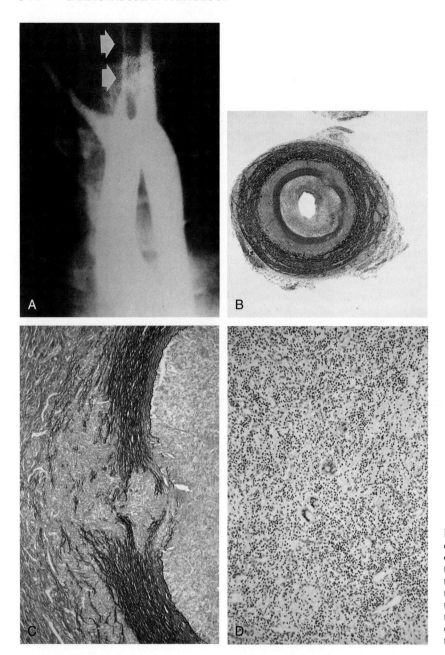

Figure 11-23 • Arrhythmic sudden cardiac death caused by Takayasu disease in a 14-year-old girl. *A,* Aortography shows severe stenosis of the left carotid artery (arrows). *B,* Histology of the left carotid artery discloses concentric obstructive intimal proliferation, focal disruption of the tunica media, and remarkable adventitial fibrotic thickening. *C,* Close-up of disrupted tunica media (*B* and *C,* Weigert-van Gieson). *D,* The inflammatory infiltrate includes giant cells. (H&E stain.)

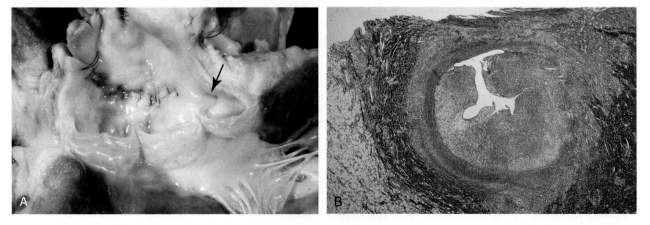

Figure 11-24 • Same case as in Figure 11-23. *A,* The aortic root showing thickened aortic wall and stenosed coronary ostia (arrow). *B,* Histology of the left main coronary artery stenosed by intimal proliferation (Weigert-van Gieson).

HEART MUSCLE DISEASE AND ARRHYTHMIC SUDDEN CARDIAC DEATH

"Electric" cardiac arrest may develop in the absence of an ischemic milieu. This is the case in some myocarditides and cardiomyopathies in which the prime myocardial abnormalities may be arrhythmogenic (see Chapters 9 and 10 also).

Cardiomyopathies

Dilated Cardiomyopathy

The natural history of dilated cardiomyopathy demonstrates that death not only occurs as a consequence of progressive congestive heart failure or as a complication of thromboembolism but also abruptly because of arrhythmic cardiac arrest.[185–187] In this circumstance, death is obviously expected and, according to definition, should not strictly be considered a true sudden death. However, in a few cases of dilated cardiomyopathy, arrhythmic sudden death may be the first manifestation of the disease, and the diagnosis is achieved only at postmortem examination by observing a heavy heart with dilated chambers and no inflammatory or coronary artery disease.

Hypertrophic Cardiomyopathy

The natural history of hypertrophic cardiomyopathy is often marked by sudden death. Heart dysfunction appears more in the form of electrical instability than impaired contractility, which, to the contrary, may be enhanced. The reported incidence of sudden death is 2 to 4% annually in adults and 4 to 6% annually in children and adolescents.[188, 189] Typically, the victim is a previously asymptomatic adolescent or young adult who was not performing strenuous activity.[190, 191] Risk factors are considered to be young age,[188–192] previous syncopal episodes,[190, 193] a malignant family history,[194] myocardial

ischemia,[195] sustained ventricular tachycardia on electrophysiologic testing,[196] and ventricular tachycardia on Holter monitoring.[197] Molecular genetic studies demonstrate that hypertrophic cardiomyopathy is a heterogeneous disease, with several missense mutations in genes encoding for proteins of the cardiac sarcomere, namely, β-myosin heavy chain, cardiac troponin T, α-tropomyosin, and myosin-binding protein C.[198] Some mutations seem to have a benign significance, with a low risk of sudden death, whereas others are associated with a poor prognosis, explaining the existence of subgroups of families with a malignant history.[199–204] (See Chapter 24 also.)

A complex interaction occurs between left ventricular hypertrophy, left ventricular outflow pressure gradient, diastolic dysfunction, and myocardial ischemia, which accounts for the great variability of clinical findings. The clinical picture varies considerably, ranging from asymptomatic patients to those with end-stage dyspnea on effort, angina, syncope, and arrhythmias, and to rare cases with congestive heart failure.

On chest radiography, the cardiac silhouette may be normal or markedly increased. When enlarged, it is normally the result of left ventricular dilation, left atrial enlargement, or both.

The basal ECG is usually abnormal, with the most common changes being ST segment and T wave abnormalities and high QRS voltage resulting from left ventricular hypertrophy. Giant T waves seem characteristic of apical forms. Ventricular arrhythmias occur in most patients with hypertrophic cardiomyopathy during 24-hour Holter monitoring, and atrial fibrillation may be present in about 10%.

The echocardiogram is vital in identifying and quantifying morphological (site and extent of hypertrophy), functional (hypercontractile left ventricle), and hemodynamic features (degree of outflow gradient). Left ventricular hypertrophy is the crucial echocardiographic feature for diagnosing hypertrophic cardiomyopathy. Considerable variability exists in its degree and patterns (from very

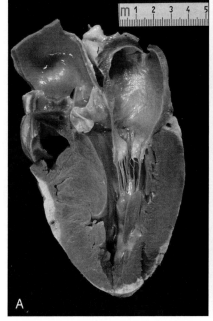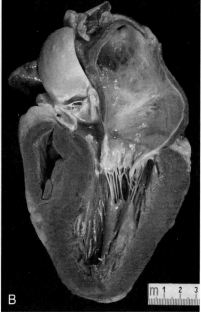

Figure 11-25 • Arrhythmic sudden cardiac death in hypertrophic cardiomyopathy. *A,* Asymmetric septal hypertrophy in a 31-year-old man. *B,* Asymmetric septal hypertrophy in a 54-year-old man; note in this case the endocardial plaque superimposed on the septal myocardial bulge and the thickening of the anterior mitral leaflet that mirrors the plaque. The two were in contact, aggravating outflow tract obstruction.

mild hypertrophy [13 to 15 mm] to massive hypertrophy [up to 50 mm]). However, the finding of a septal thickness that is at least 1.3 to 1.5 times the posterior wall thickness measured in diastole is a major criterion for diagnosis. Other frequent echocardiographic markers of hypertrophic cardiomyopathy are a narrowing of the left ventricular outflow tract accounting for obstruction and systolic pressure gradient and an abnormal systolic anterior motion of the anterior mitral valve leaflet, leading to mitral incompetence. Diastolic abnormalities in terms of

impaired ventricular relaxation may be detectable by echocardiography and Doppler investigation in about 80% of cases.

At postmortem examination, the heart shows asymmetric left ventricular hypertrophy, usually in the basal portion of the ventricular septum (Fig. 11-25A) but also in the anterior free wall and apex. The septal bulging, which may be aggravated by a septal endocardial plaque and anterior mitral valve leaflet thickening, representing friction lesions, may create subaortic obstruction, and account

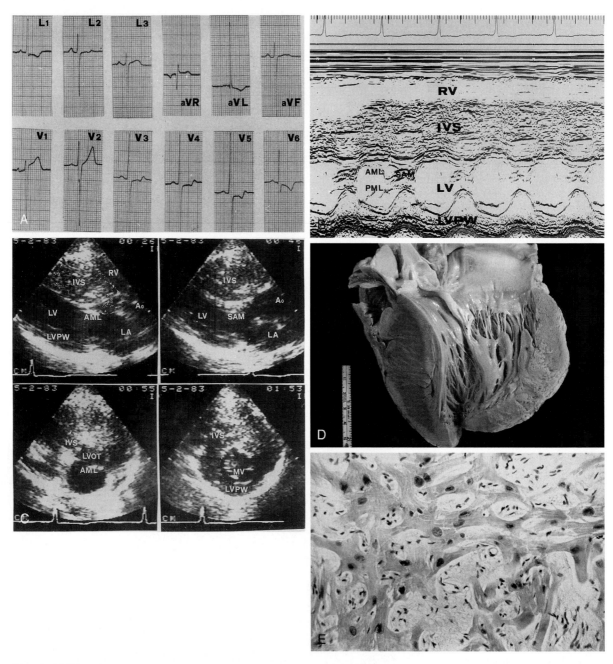

Figure 11-26 • Arrhythmic sudden cardiac death caused by hypertrophic cardiomyopathy in a 29-year-old man with diagnosis made in life. *A,* Basal electrocardiogram (ECG) showing left ventricular hypertrophy and inverted T waves in lateral precordial leads. *B,* Monodimensional echocardiogram showing asymmetric septal hypertrophy and systolic anterior motion of the mitral valve. *C,* Two-dimensional echocardiography showing asymmetric septal hypertrophy with systolic anterior motion of the anterior mitral valve leaflet (Ao = aorta, AML = anterior mitral leaflet, IVS = interventricular septum, LA = left atrium, SAM = systolic anterior motion, LVPW = left ventricular posterior wall, LVOT = left ventricular outflow tract, RV = right ventricle). *D,* Heart specimen with massive asymmetric septal hypertrophy. *E,* Histology of ventricular septum showing myocardial disarray and interstitial fibrosis (H&E stain).

for the left ventricular outflow gradient (Figs. 11-25*B* and 11-26). The dysplastic histologic features of the myocardium in the form of disarray, with myocytes spatially arranged in a chaotic manner, and interstitial fibrosis, represent an ideal substrate of inhomogeneous intraventricular conduction with potential reentry phenomena[205, 206] (Fig. 11-26*E*). However, detailed pathologic studies on subjects who died suddenly demonstrate the superimposition of ischemic damage on the dysplastic myocardium in the form of myocyte necrosis and large fibrous scars mimicking healed infarction.[51, 207] The ischemic damage occurs in the absence of significant epicardial coronary artery disease, although small-vessel disease as well as an intramural course of the left anterior descending coronary artery have been noted.[207, 208] Elevated intramyocardial diastolic pressure may restrict intramural arteries during diastolic coronary filling, thus impairing myocardial perfusion. The combination of myocardial disarray and replacement fibrosis has to be considered as the malignant arrhythmogenic substrate in hypertrophic cardiomyopathy. An association of accessory pathways with hypertrophic cardiomyopathy has been advocated as a mechanism of cardiac arrest, especially in the presence of atrial fibrillation.[209]

Restrictive Cardiomyopathy

Primary restrictive cardiomyopathy is marked by normal or nearly normal ventricles and dilated atria. Cardiac dysfunction is a result of impaired ventricular compliance hindering diastolic filling.[210, 211] The clinical course is characterized by progressive congestive heart failure; ventricular arrhythmias and sudden death are exceedingly rare. This is surprising because microscopic features may be similar to those of hypertrophic cardiomyopathy in terms of myocardial disarray and interstitial fibrosis, which, as previously noted, are potentially arrhythmogenic.[210] The absence of hypertrophy and myocardial ischemia may account for the lack of electrical instability.

Arrhythmogenic Cardiomyopathy

This condition, also known as right ventricular dysplasia,[212] and arrhythmogenic right ventricular cardiomyopathy was reported in Italy as a leading cause of sudden death in the young.[213] It is characterized by a peculiar myocardial atrophy with fibrofatty substitution, very often of the right ventricular free wall (Fig. 11-27).

At gross examination, heart weight is usually within normal limits (less than 400 g) and the right ventricle

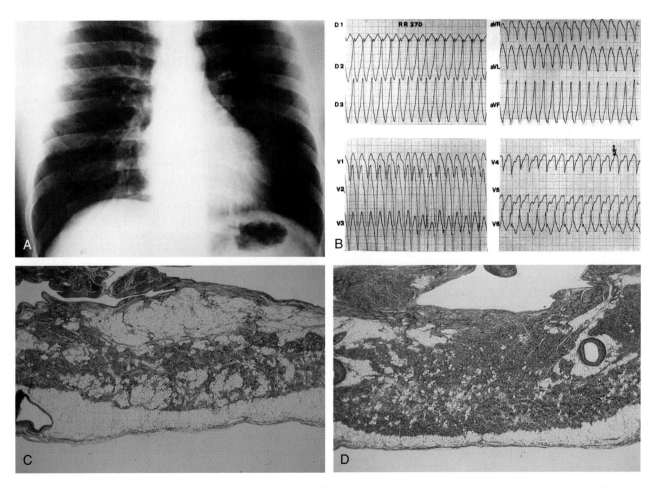

Figure 11-27 • Arrhythmic sudden cardiac death during effort in a 26-year-old male runner, with arrhythmogenic right ventricular cardiomyopathy. *A,* Chest radiograph with normal cardiothoracic ratio. *B,* Sustained ventricular tachycardia on effort with left bundle branch block morphology suggesting origin from the right ventricle. *C,* Histology of the pulmonary infundibulum with massive fibrofatty replacement. *D,* Histology of the right ventricular free wall with massive fibrofatty replacement (*C* and *D,* Heidenhain trichrome.)

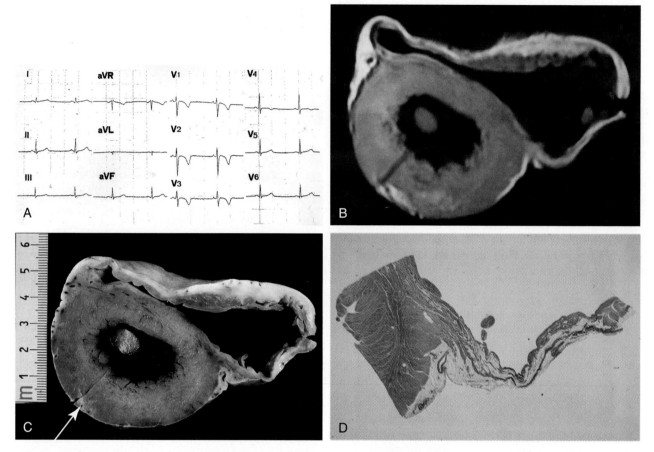

Figure 11-28 • Arrhythmic sudden cardiac death in a 17-year-old boy with arrhythmogenic right ventricular cardiomyopathy. *A,* Basal electrocardiogram showing inverted T wave in right precordial lead up to V4. *B,* Postmortem nuclear magnetic resonance image, in cross-section view, showing transmural bright signal of right ventricle and aneurysms in the anterior and posterior walls, with spotty involvement of the left ventricle and intact ventricular septum. *C,* Equivalent gross cross-section of the heart with obvious fatty replacement and infundibular and posterior aneurysms of the right ventricle. Arrow indicates spotty left ventricular involvement. *D,* Histology of the posterior right ventricular free wall corresponding to aneurysmal dilatation, with remarkable fatty replacement (Heidenhain trichrome).

appears yellow or whitish with a thinned wall. Right ventricular aneurysms are present in nearly 50% of cases, typically located in the posteroinferior wall but also located at the apex and infundibulum (triangle of dysplasia) (Fig. 11-28).[213–216] When confined to the right ventricle, the septum is often spared by the disease, probably because of the preferential involvement of the subepicardial layers of the right ventricular free wall. However, the left ventricle may be affected, especially in older patients, as a sign of disease progression.[216, 217, 217a] Histology discloses the disappearance (atrophy) of the right ventricular myocardium with a fibrofatty or fatty replacement and with a wave-front extension from the epicardium toward the endocardium. Focal myocarditis with myocyte death was observed in all cases with the fibrofatty variant (Fig. 11-29); whether inflammation is primary or secondary to cell death remains to be established.[216, 218] Apoptosis has been postulated to account for cell death, and evidence supporting this viewpoint has been demonstrated in both autopsy and biopsy material.[219, 220]

A familial relationship has been demonstrated in nearly 50% of cases[221, 222] and, even though a defective gene has not been yet identified, gene loci have been mapped to three different chromosomes (14, 1, and 2).[223–226] A ge-

netically determined atrophy may explain this cardiomyopathy, which could then be considered a myocardial dystrophy.[216, 227] The histologic similarities to some skeletal muscular dystrophies, such as those of Duchenne and Becker, favor this hypothesis. Focal, progressive cell death may lead to either fibrous or fatty replacement, with adipocytes taking the place of dying myocytes (see Fig. 11-29). Evidence of an acquired, progressive cell death excludes the hypothesis of congenital heart disease (dysplasia = maldevelopment) and points to a true cardiomyopathy. The disease is now listed among cardiomyopathies in the World Health Organization (WHO) revised classification.[211]

Intraventricular conduction delay, consequent to fibrofatty replacement, is a source of electrical instability caused by reentrant phenomena. It takes the form of ventricular arrhythmias (e.g., premature ventricular beats, nonsustained or sustained ventricular tachycardia) with left bundle branch block morphology (see Fig. 11-27B), indicating a right ventricular origin. Focal myocarditis, bouts of apoptosis, right ventricular aneurysms, and left ventricular involvement most probably worsen ventricular electrical vulnerability and lower the ventricular fibrillation threshold.[216–218]

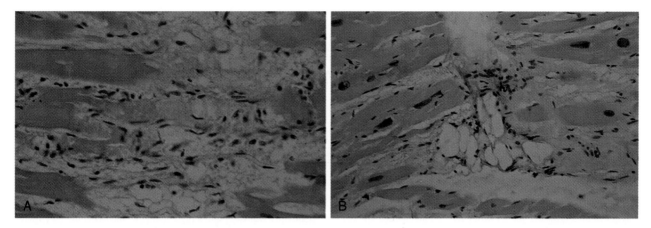

Figure 11-29 • Cell death and fibrofatty replacement in arrhythmogenic right ventricular cardiomyopathy. *A,* Histologic features consist of myocyte death, inflammatory infiltrates, and early scarring. *B,* Adipocytes replace dead myocytes; note the coexistence of lymphocytic infiltrates. (Both H&E stain.)

Arrhythmogenic right ventricular cardiomyopathy may be an occult abnormality in apparently healthy subjects. In terms of contractility, heart performance is preserved because the left ventricle is usually spared. This explains why the disease is observed in sports champions who manifest only minor symptoms such as palpitations or lipothymia, and why the diagnosis is frequently missed in preparticipation screenings.[228, 229]

In these subjects, the presence of ECG abnormalities, such as an inverted T wave in the right precordial leads (V1-V3); increased QRS duration (more than 110 msec); late potentials detected by high resolution ECG; and ventricular arrhythmias, even single premature ventricular beats with left bundle branch block morphology, should raise suspicion of the disease and lead to further investigation.[214, 222, 230–232] Imaging procedures, whether noninvasive, such as echocardiography,[233, 234] or invasive such as cineangiography,[235, 236] help to detect structural and functional abnormalities of the right ventricle, such as bulging, wall motion abnormalities, and dilatation. Nuclear magnetic resonance, furthermore, is a very effective tool for tissue characterization and may help to detect the fatty myocardial infiltration.[237–240] Endomyocardial biopsy can

be useful in achieving an in vivo diagnosis, because the dystrophic process is frequently transmural and then detectable through an endocardial approach.[241, 242]

Myocarditis

Myocarditis usually appears with clinical signs of pump failure and ventricular dilatation. Nonetheless, ventricular arrhythmias have been described in patients with myocarditis and an apparently normal heart.[243, 244] Sudden death may occur in both the active or healed phases as a consequence of life-threatening ventricular arrhythmias that develop mostly in the setting of an unstable myocardial substrate, namely inflammatory infiltrate (Fig. 11-30), interstitial edema, myocardial necrosis, and fibrosis.[79, 245, 246] Prodromes may consist of a flu-like illness a few days before death, syncopal episodes, and premature ventricular beats. (See further discussion in Chapter 9.)

The gross appearance of the heart is not distinctive and its weight may be within normal values. Histology invariably discloses a patchy inflammatory infiltrate, sometimes with no more than three foci at magnification 6× and not necessarily associated with myocardial necro-

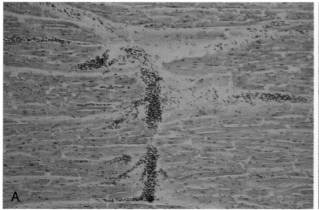
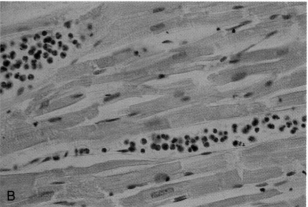

Figure 11-30 • Arrhythmic sudden cardiac death in a 25-year-old man with myocarditis. *A,* Multiple foci of inflammatory infiltrates. *B,* Higher power showing polymorphous infiltrates and no evidence of myocardial necrosis. (Both H&E stain.)

sis. The inflammatory infiltrate is usually polymorphous and, less frequently, is purely lymphocytic. Sudden death as a consequence of patchy giant cell myocarditis as well as eosinophilic myocarditis in the setting of allergic conditions, have also been reported. Rheumatic myocarditis is nowadays an exceptional finding. Evidence of viral myocardial infection is often found by employing molecular biology techniques. Noteworthy is the report of an increased sudden cardiac death rate among young Swedish elite orienteers with histopathologic evidence of myocarditis and serologic demonstration of antibodies to *Chlamydia pneumoniae*.[247]

Sudden death caused by myocarditis is not rare, particularly in the young,[15, 246, 248–251] according to the Veneto Region experience[44] (see Table 11-2). The strongest evidence that subclinical myocarditis can cause ventricular fibrillation comes from an autopsy series on United States army recruits in which 40% of those who died suddenly had histologic evidence of myocarditis.[250] Thus, myocarditis in conjunction with sudden death is usually associated with an acute patchy, polymorphous infiltrate with scarce myocardial necrosis and with a grossly normal heart. This subtle substrate, together with possible inflammatory involvement of the conduction system, is highly arrhythmogenic, accounting for unexpected arrhythmic cardiac arrest.

Idiopathic Left Ventricular Hypertrophy

This condition, which has been described in young people and athletes who died suddenly, is characterized by concentric left ventricular hypertrophy. The degree of hypertrophy is beyond that seen in the cardiac hypertrophy of the trained athlete, with left ventricular thickness exceeding 15 or 16 mm.

The affected individuals demonstrate no conditions that would predispose them to left ventricular hypertrophy (e.g., aortic valve stenosis, isthmal coarctation, systemic hypertension). Unlike findings in classic hypertrophic cardiomyopathy, the myocardial hypertrophy in these cases is concentric and symmetric; there is no evidence of subaortic plaque and mitral valve disease; and, above all, histology does not reveal myocardial disarray. Moreover, a genetic transmission has not been reported. Idiopathic concentric left ventricular hypertrophy is considered a potential cause of sudden death in athletes. In the series reported by Maron and associates,[252] of 29 cases of competitive athletes who died suddenly, 5 were affected by idiopathic left ventricular hypertrophy.

We are inclined to consider such cases as hypertrophic cardiomyopathy because this is a primary muscle disease of unknown etiology with hypertrophy. Whether this condition should be considered a genetic and sporadic form of hypertrophic cardiomyopathy, in other words, a sarcomere disease, remains to be proven.

VALVULAR HEART DISEASE AND ARRHYTHMIC SUDDEN CARDIAC DEATH

Three valve diseases are associated with sudden death: aortic stenosis, mitral valve prolapse, and Ebstein malformation of the tricuspid valve. In all, the mechanism of cardiac arrest is arrhythmic, not mechanical.

Aortic Stenosis

In aortic stenosis (see Chapter 13 also), the area of the valve orifice is so restricted that it creates a significant gradient between the left ventricle and the aorta, with resultant systolic overload and compensatory left ventricular hypertrophy.[253] The hypertrophy may be so massive that it hugely increases left ventricular wall thickness and mass with a severe reduction of cavity volume. Elevated ventricular systolic pressure as well as increased myocardial mass may account for both raised oxygen consumption and reduced coronary reserve and provide a substrate for myocardial ischemia, particularly in the subendocardium and even in the absence of coronary artery disease.[254] By Holter monitoring, complex ventricular arrhythmias have been detected with high frequency in affected patients. The risk of sudden death is usually confined to those with a left ventricular/aortic gradient above 50 mmHg[255, 256]. Sudden death occurs in as many as 20% of patients with aortic stenosis.[117] However, nowadays aortic stenosis is an uncommon cause of sudden death because of improved identification of patients at risk, sports restriction, and timely surgical intervention.

Pathologic study of these sudden death cases usually discloses subendocardial ischemia in terms of myocytosis and scarring, both well-known arrhythmogenetic substrates[245, 246, 257] (Fig. 11-31). Exercise increases oxygen demand and the blood perfusion discrepancy with the risk of onset of lethal ventricular tachyarrhythmias.

In the elderly, aortic stenosis is usually the result of senile dystrophic calcification of the aortic valve or of a calcified bicuspid valve.[258, 259] Calcification may extend to the aortic annulus, the membranous septum, and the crest of the ventricular septum, and may involve the conduction axis with risk of AV block. In these circumstances cardiac arrest may occur in asystole. Moreover, in the elderly, aortic stenosis and obstructive coronary artery disease are a frequent malignant combination that worsens the coronary flow impairment and the ischemic substrate.

In the young, aortic stenosis is mostly related to congenital valvular malformations such as unicuspid or bicuspid conditions with dysplastic stiff cusps[260–262] (see Fig. 11-31A). Supravalvular aortic stenosis, observed in the Williams syndrome, presents an hourglass obstruction of the ascending aorta and left ventricular hypertrophy. It is marked by elastosis of the aortic tunica media, intimal thickening, and dysplastic aortic valve cusps. Isolation of the coronary ostia, because of fusion of semilunar cusps with the aortic wall, is a feature that further aggravates coronary ischemia in these patients.[263, 264]

Mitral Valve Prolapse

Mitral valve prolapse (see Chapter 14 also) has been reported to occur in 1% of males and 6% of females.[265] However, associated sudden death is rare, especially in people younger than 20 years old. Unexpected death may be a mechanical complication of valve function, for example, chordal rupture with pulmonary edema. However,

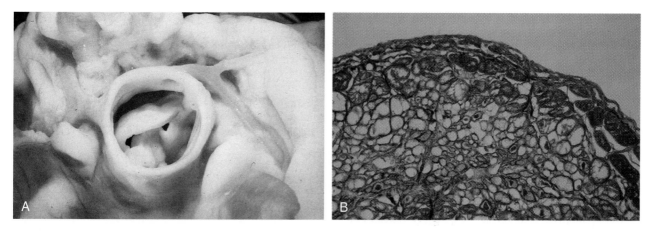

Figure 11-31 • Arrhythmic sudden cardiac death in a 9-year-old girl during gymnastic activity. *A,* View of the aortic root shows bicuspid aortic valve stenosed by thickened and dysplastic cusps. *B,* Histology of the subendocardium of the left ventricle reveals ischemic damage in the form of colliquative myocytolysis (Heidenhain trichrome).

more frequently, it is a consequence of an abrupt electrical disorder in the form of ventricular tachycardia and fibrillation. It was postulated that elongated chordae or redundant valve leaflets, by rubbing against the ventricu-

lar endocardium, could elicit ventricular electrical instability and promote cardiac arrest.[266–268] Hemodynamically significant mitral valve regurgitation,[269] autonomic nervous system dysfunction,[270, 271] conduction system abnormalities,

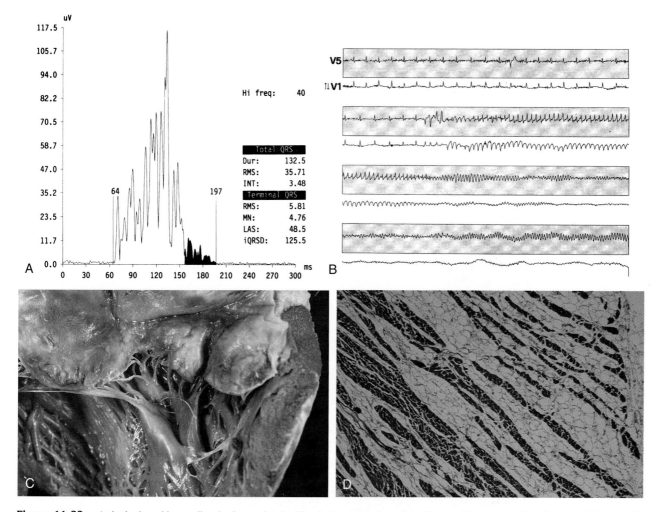

Figure 11-32 • Arrhythmic sudden cardiac death associated with mitral valve prolapse in a 42-year-old woman. *A,* Signal-averaged electrocardiogram (ECG) shows late potentials. *B,* Final ECG tracing at Holter monitoring: ventricular fibrillation is initiated by late diastolic couplets followed by ventricular tachycardia. *C,* Mitral valve shows thickening and prolapse of the three scallops of the posterior leaflet. *D,* Histology of the pulmonary infundibulum discloses marked fatty infiltration (trichrome Heidenhain).

and focal myocarditis[272–276] have also been advanced as possible etiopathogenetic mechanisms. Recently, histologic studies of the right ventricular myocardium disclosed significant fatty infiltration, especially at the infundibular level, in a subset of patients who died suddenly[276–278] (Fig. 11-32). This observation fits the frequent ECG recording of ventricular arrhythmias of right ventricular origin with a pattern of left bundle branch block. Thus, mitral valve prolapse may entail a potential electrical disorder of the ventricular myocardium related to fatty dystrophy of the right ventricle.

Ebstein Malformation

Ebstein anomaly (see Chapter 14 also), the most common dysplastic condition of the tricuspid valve, consists of an abnormal development of the septal and posterior leaflets and tensor apparatus, with downward displacement and a partial atrialization of the right ventricular cavity. Besides valve dysfunction in terms of incompetence or stenosis with incompetence, the condition is associated with a risk of supraventricular tachyarrhythmias, namely, atrial fibrillation and reciprocating supraventricular tachycardia.[279] The malformation of the septal leaflet with apical displacement promotes a maldevelopment of both the central fibrous body and the fibrous ring[280, 281] (Fig. 11-33). Atrial and ventricular musculatures are not separated on the right side of the ventricular septum, thus delineating a potential septal Kent fascicle and ventricular preexcitation. The risk of sudden death is particularly high, taking into consideration the adverse association of atrial fibrillation and preexcitation. Ebstein malformation

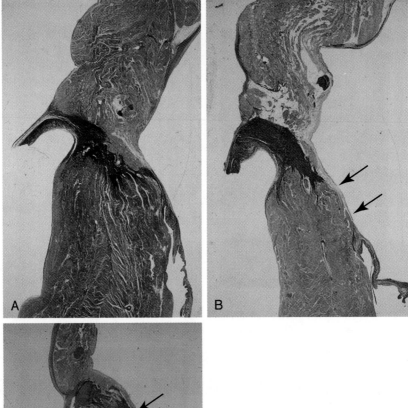

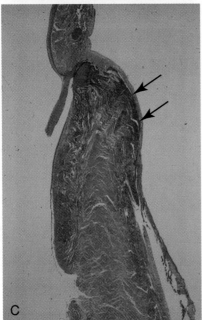

Figure 11-33 • Arrhythmic sudden cardiac death in microEbstein malformation. *A,* Normal heart; note a regular insertion of the septal leaflet of the triscupid valve and the continuity of the central fibrous body and atrioventricular (AV) ring. *B,* Mild downward displacement of the triscupid valve septal leaflet with a gap between the fibrous ring and the central fibrous body (arrows) in a 25-year-old woman who died suddenly at rest. *C,* Moderate lowering of the septal leaflet of tricuspid valve in an 11-year-old girl who died suddenly during gymnastic exercise at school. Note that an atrial myocardial fascicle bypasses the AV node and makes contact directly with the ventricular myocardium (arrows). (All, Heidenhain trichrome.)

may entail no hemodynamic dysfunction and may appear only as a microscopic defect with a mild lowering of the septal attachment of the tricuspid septal leaflet (micro-Ebstein).[282, 283]

CONDUCTION SYSTEM INNERVATION AND ARRHYTHMIC SUDDEN CARDIAC DEATH

Anatomy

The electrical function of the heart is under the control of the conduction system (see Chapter 20 also), a specialized myogenic tissue that originates and transmits the electrical impulse like a power plant. Normally, the sinus node, located in the right atrium at the root of the superior vena cava, is the pacemaker. The electrical impulse then spreads to the atria through preferential pathways to excite the myocardium and ensure atrial systole. The impulse converges on the AV node, located near the coronary sinus, where, before passing to the ventricles, it is slowed, thereby allowing ventricular blood filling to occur during atrial emptying. The electrical impulse is then transmitted to the ventricles via the His bundle, which is the only pathway connecting atria to ventricles, and spreads through the right and left bundle branches to ultimately excite the ordinary ventricular myocardium through the Purkinje network.

Myocyte-to-myocyte transmission allows excitation of all the ventricular mass in a wave-front manner, leaving unexcitable myocardium during repolarization until the following regular impulse occurs. The electrical activity, recorded by a surface ECG, consists of a P wave (excitation of the atrial musculature), the PR interval (time of conduction delay at the AV node level), a QRS complex (ventricular depolarization), and a T wave (ventricular repolarization).

Moreover, the heart is influenced by its innervation, which is both extrinsic and intrinsic.[284] The extrinsic cardiac plexus comprises the mediastinal nerve ganglia and paraganglia (bodies) located in aortopulmonary, intertruncal, and intercarotid areas. The sympathetic cardiac nerves have their center in the intermediolateral neuronal column at T1–T5 thoracic level, leave it by the anterior roots of the upper thoracic nerves, synapse in stellate and caudal cervical ganglia, and converge into, and anastomose variably with, the vagus cardiac nerves. Atrial innervation (especially sinoatrial) is mainly parasympathetic (vagal), whereas the ventricular innervation is sympathetic in nature. It should be emphasized that precise sympathovagal identifications are extremely difficult by light microscopy.

Intrinsic cardiac innervation can be schematically subdivided into a gross subepicardial ganglionated plexus, which is rich in the atrium (right atrium and sinus node area) and AV sulcus, and poor in the ventricles; a fine intramural plexus (especially along the coronary tree); and a "terminal" plexus (intramural, subendocardial, and epicardial).

The so-called cardiovascular centers in the brain, to which afferent impulses from intracardiac, mediastinal, and intercarotid, as well as peripheral, receptors are conveyed by neuronal circuits elaborating afferent reflexogenesis, are located in the brain stem, partially coincident with the respiratory reticular formation and tightly linked with the sympathetic nuclei of the intermediolateral neurons in the thoracic (T1–T5) cord as well as descending mesencephalic-hypothalamic and cortical impulses. The central integration of reflexes encompasses the neuronal circuit of the nucleus solitarius and nucleus ambiguus (vagal-glossopharyngeal) and also involves the spinal trigeminal nucleus and nuclei of the ventrolateral reticular formation.

Pathology

With the notable exception of Rossi[285] and a very few other authors, little attention has been paid to intracardiac nerves and ganglia in cases of sudden unexpected death.

Theoretically, any severe electrical disorder of the heart, particularly those inducing cardiac arrhythmic arrest, should involve the conduction system and intrinsic cardiac innervation. However, this is only partially true, because the most frequent life-threatening arrhythmias arise from abnormalities at the very periphery of the conduction system, namely, the ordinary myocardium, in the setting of ischemic, inflammatory (myocarditis), or dystrophic-dysplastic (cardiomyopathy) substrates. Nonetheless, some morbid entities primarily involve the conduction system and intrinsic cardiac innervation and may induce cardiac arrest.

Pathology of the Sinoatrial Node

Heart standstill may be a consequence of sinus arrest because of a sudden "blackout" of sinus node activity. Sudden ischemia may develop during a posteroseptal myocardial infarction following coronary thombosis of the right coronary artery, proximal to the origin of the sinus node artery, 1 to 2 cm from the right coronary ostium.[88, 89, 286] It should be noted that conducting tissues are highly resistant to ischemia; thus, sinus arrest does not necessarily imply histologic damage of the sinus node. Indeed, infarction of both the sinus node and the sinoatrial approaches is extremely rare. It is usually associated with an embolic occlusion of the distal sinus node artery (see Fig. 11-19). Ganglionitis (Fig. 11-34) and neuronal depletion of sinoatrial intrinsic cardiac ganglia caused by satellite cell proliferation (Terplan nodules) have been reported in sinoatrial block.[92, 287]

The peculiar topography of the sinus node, which is located in the sulcus terminalis just deep to the epicardium, renders it vulnerable to inflammatory infiltrates in the setting of acute pericarditis. The inflammatory cells may infiltrate both the sinus node itself and the ganglionated plexus with neuroganglionitis, accounting for the onset of even life-threatening arrhythmias.[288]

Pathology of the Specialized AV Junction

Sudden asystole may also be ascribed to ischemia of the AV node in the early phase of a posteroseptal myocardial infarction, when the coronary thrombotic occlu-

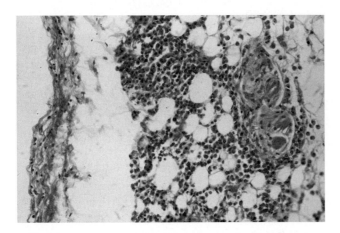

Figure 11-34 • Arrhythmic sudden cardiac death caused by cardioneuropathology. Inflammatory infiltrates of an autonomic nervous ganglion close to the sinus node (H&E stain).

counts for only a functional disorder of the AV node. If prolonged enough to generate complete AV block, it may result in cardiac arrest in the absence of a junctional or ventricular escape rhythm. In an acute anteroseptal myocardial infarction, proximal bundle branches may be involved by ischemic injury producing bundle branch block.[291–293]

The most frequent cause of AV block, requiring pacemaker implantation, is degeneration of the bifurcating bundle and proximal bundle branches in the absence of ischemia.[294, 295] The histopathologic substrate consists of elective atrophy of the conducting tissues, with fibrotic disruption and discontinuity of the His bundle and bundle branches (Figs. 11-35 and 11-36). The ECG manifestations of a discontinuity of the specialized AV axis ranges from prolongation of the PR interval (first-degree AV block); occasionally, nonconducted P waves (second-degree AV block); or complete dissociation between atrial and ventricular activity (third-degree AV block). The idioventricular rhythm, which takes over pacemaker function in cases of complete AV block, may be so slow that cardiac output is inadequate, leading to sudden death.

Primary and metastatic tumors can be associated with electrical instability and conduction block. A cystic tumor of the AV node (Tawarioma) represents an embryonal

sion of the dominant right coronary artery is located proximal to the crux cordis, where the AV node artery takes origin.[88–90, 289, 290] Again, with the exception of its occurrence in coronary embolism, infarction of the AV node and His bundle is quite rare.[291] The ischemia ac-

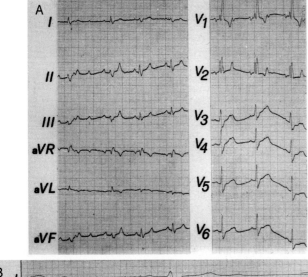

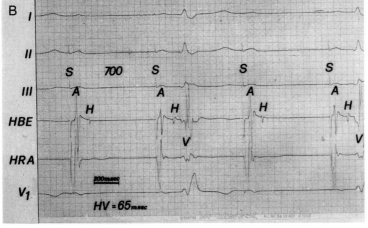

Figure 11-35 • Arrhythmic sudden cardiac death caused by atrioventricular (AV) block in a 55-year-old man. *A,* An electrocardiogram (ECG) shows complete AV block in peripheral leads and second-degree AV block in precordial leads. *B,* Endocavitary electrophysiologic study showing 2/1 infraHissian AV block during atrial pacing.

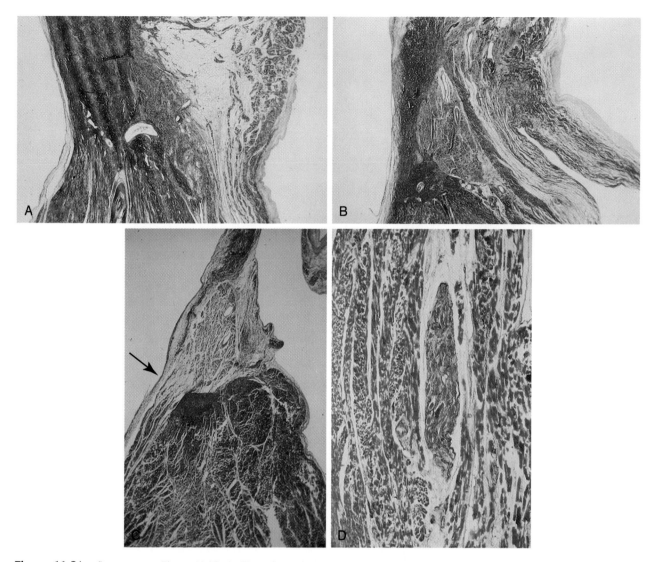

Figure 11-36 • Same case as Figure 11-35. *A,* The atrioventricular (AV) node is normal. *B,* The His bundle is also normal. *C,* There is scleroatrophy of the branching bundle at the beginning of the left bundle branch stem (arrow). *D,* The intramyocardial tract of the right bundle branch shows almost complete replacement by fibrous tissue. (All, Heidenhain trichrome.)

inclusion in the heart's center of mesodermal tissue, which grows more or less rapidly with tubulocystic features and produces congenital, juvenile, or adult complete AV block with sudden death[92] (Fig. 11-37). The Purkinje-like (oncocytic) lesion reported in infants consists of hamartoma-like myocyte aggregation, often connected to the conduction system, a feature that may underlie lethal brady- and tachyarrhythmias.[296] (See Chapter 10 also.) A cardiac fibroma that is located in the central fibrous body may compress the His bundle and induce AV block.[297, 298] Sudden death has been reported in lipomatous hypertrophy of the interatrial septum (see Chapter 19 also).

Ventricular Preexcitation

Ventricular preexcitation is the opposite of AV block and is usually a congenital disorder defined by rapid impulse transmission to the ventricles.[297]

Figure 11-38 summarizes the accessory AV connec-

tions that predispose to ventricular preexcitation and sudden death. They may be subdivided into two main types:

1. *Direct AV connections:* These are located outside the specialized AV junction, either in the lateral or septal AV rings, and consist of ordinary myocardium directly connecting working atrial and ventricular myocardium (Kent fascicle). They do not possess decremental (delay) properties.
2. *Mediated AV connections:* They involve the specialized AV junction, with decremental conduction, either connecting the septal atrial myocardium with the His bundle (AV inlet James[299] or Brechenmacher[300] fibers) or the Tawarian system with the ventricular myocardium (outlet Mahaim fibers[301]).

Direct AV Connections

In Wolff-Parkinson-White syndrome, an aberrant myocardial fascicle joins the atria to the ventricles beyond the

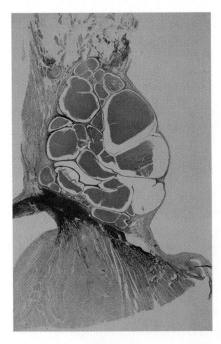

Figure 11-37 • Arrhythmic sudden cardiac death by Tawarioma (celothelioma) of the atrioventricular (AV) node. Note a tumor with multiple cysts at the AV junction with atrophy of the AV node (Heidenhain trichrome).

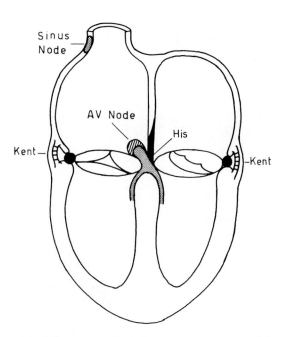

Figure 11-39 • Diagram illustrating the normal anatomy of the conduction system and Kent fascicles located in the lateral atrioventricular rings.

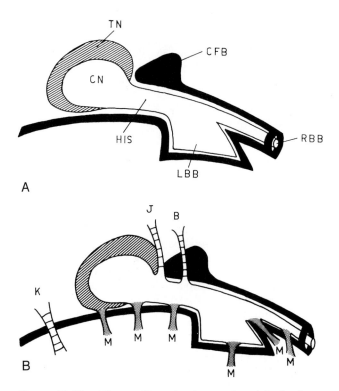

Figure 11-38 • Diagrams illustrating the normal specialized atrioventricular (AV) junction (*A*) (CFB = central fibrous body; CN = compact node; TN = transitional node; LBB = left bundle branch; RBB = right bundle branch.) and the AV junction with accessory AV connections at the septal level (*B*). Mediated AV connections involve the specialized AV junction joining the septal atrial myocardium with the His bundle (James [**J**] or Brechenmacher [**B**] fibers = inlet fibers) or the Tawarian system with the septal ventricular myocardium (Mahaim (**M**) fibers = outlet fibers). Kent fascicle (**K**) may be situated also at the septal level and represents a direct AV connection.

specialized AV junction (Fig. 11-39). Known as the Kent fascicle or bundle, it consists of a thin structure (200 to 400 μ), directly connecting the atrial with the ventricular musculature[302-304] (Fig. 11-40). Usually located in the lateral rings, especially the left, where it is related to the attachment of the mural mitral leaflet, it consists of ordinary myocardium that does not possess the decremental properties of specialized conducting tissues of the AV node. Thus, the atrial impulse excites the ventricles earlier through the accessory pathway. This is recorded on an ECG as a short PR interval with a delta wave of the QRS complex, the latter corresponding to early ventricular excitation. The aberrant fascicle may serve not only as an AV bypass tract for ventricular preexcitation, but also as a limb for an AV reentry circuit (usually retrograde), accounting for a reciprocating supraventricular tachycardia.[305] The accessory fascicle is located in the AV sulcus, only 0.5 to 1 mm from the endocardium. The size and site are such that the Kent bundle is easily subject to endocardial transcatheter ablation, the current procedure to treat the syndrome and reestablish AV electrical connection only through the His bundle. Wolff-Parkinson-White ventricular preexcitation is an uncommon congenital heart disease that affects 0.5 to 1% of live births.[306-308] The risk of sudden death in patients is low and mainly related to the occurrence of atrial fibrillation. This may convert to ventricular fibrillation because of the short refractoriness of the AV accessory pathway, which allows transmission of more than 300 impulses per minute to the ventricles.[309-313] A focal myocarditis affecting the atrial musculature may be an acute substrate triggering atrial fibrillation and sudden cardiac death in previously asymptomatic Wolff-Parkinson-White patients.

Mahaim fibers, which connect the AV junction to the

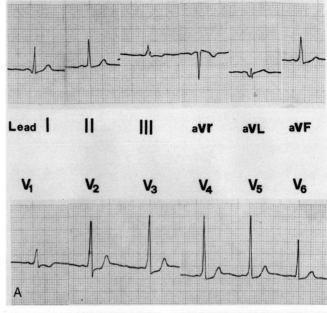

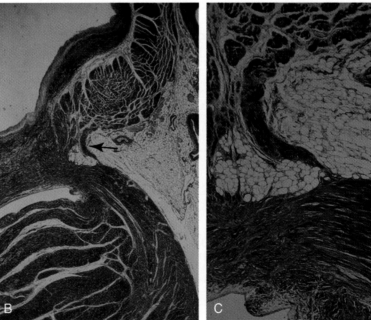

Figure 11-40 • Arrhythmic sudden cardiac death caused by ventricular preexcitation (Wolff-Parkinson-White syndrome) in a 30-year-old man who died during sleep. *A*, Basal ECG shows short PR interval with delta wave. *B*, Histology of the left atrioventricular groove discloses a Kent fascicle (arrow) connecting the left atrial and the ventricular musculature. *C*, Close-up of the Kent fascicle. (*B* and *C*, Heidenhain trichrome.)

upper ventricular septum,[301] may also participate in ventricular preexcitation.

Mediated AV Connections

Another rare condition promoting early ventricular excitation is so-called enhanced AV conduction, also known as the Lown-Ganong-Levine syndrome.[314] The impulse runs through the His bundle branches very quickly, with a short PR interval and a normal QRS complex. Two histologic backgrounds explain the absent delay at the AV node. One is a congenitally hypoplastic node, so that a lessened bulk of specialized tissue is present to delay impulse transmission from atria to ventricles[315] (Figs. 11-41 and 11-42). The second is an atrio-Hisian bundle that bypasses the AV node and transmits the activation signal directly to the His bundle, avoiding a delay at the AV node.[299, 300] In both substrates, the onset of atrial fibrillation may precipitate ventricular fibrillation with a mechanism identical to that in the Wolff-Parkinson-White syndrome.

ARRHYTHMIC SUDDEN CARDIAC DEATH IN INDIVIDUALS WITH A NORMAL HEART

There are patients who have a cardiac arrest resulting from ventricular fibrillation in whom clinical identification of either subtle structural abnormality or functional causes are lacking.[316] Whether these cases are truly idiopathic, or unexplained because of a clinical inability to identify

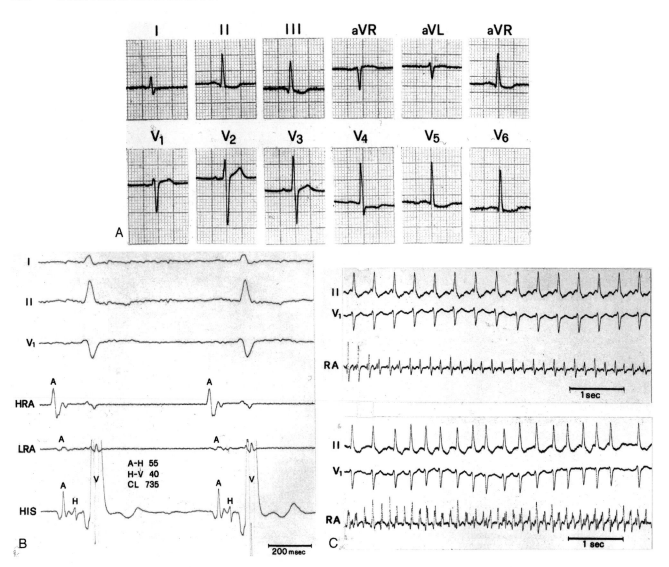

Figure 11-41 • Arrhythmic sudden cardiac death caused by enhanced atrioventicular (AV) conduction (Lown-Ganong-Levine syndrome) in a 34-year-old man who died at rest. *A,* Basal electrocardiogram (ECG) shows sinus rhythm, short PR interval (0.12 sec) with normal QRS complex. *B,* Electrophysiologic study revealed accelerated AV conduction was caused by short AH interval, namely, rapid conduction at the AV node level. *C,* Atrial flutter (upper tracings) and atrial fibrillation (lower tracings) with high-rate ventricular response.

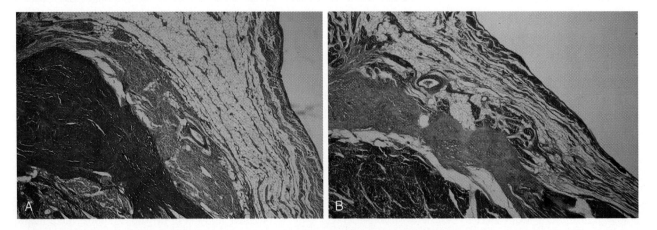

Figure 11-42 • Same case as Figure 11-41. Comparison of a control subject atrioventricular (AV) node (*A*) with that of the sudden death patient (*B*); note the extreme hypoplasia of the latter (Heidenhain trichrome).

pathologic substrates, remains to be determined. Maybe the structural abnormality resides at a molecular level. Having excluded an extracardiac cause of death, gross examination fails to show any cardiac cause, such as obstructive coronary atherosclerosis, congenital coronary anomaly, cardiomyopathy, valve disease, or aortic dissection, in nearly one third of juvenile sudden cardiac deaths.[317] In 75% of them, evidence of a concealed "arrhythmic" substrate is found at histopathologic investigation and consists of focal myocarditis, segmental arrhythmogenic right ventricular cardiomyopathy, or abnormalities of the conduction system. Overall, sudden cardiac death remains unexplained in 5 to 10% of cases, even after a thorough macroscopic and microscopic examination including the conduction system and cardiac innervation. In other words, no apparent organic substrate is detected by traditional investigations ("mors sine materia"), and death is ascribable merely to an abrupt functional disorder.[318, 319]

Recognized Genetic Abnormalities

The Long QT Syndrome

This is the best known congenital cause of arrhythmic sudden death in which structural cardiac pathology is absent.[320] It is a familial disease with high cardiac electrical instability, presenting with syncope caused by ventricular tachyarrhythmias or with cardiac arrest on exercise or emotional stress, often in patients younger than 15 years of age. The cause of death at necropsy cannot be ascertained unless there are previous ECG data. Genetic analysis has revealed multiple abnormalities in four different chromosomes (11, 7, 3, and 4), with genes related both to potassium and sodium cardiac channels.[321-323] Alterations of ion pumps and current account for the lengthened action potential and prolonged QT interval on ECG and the propensity to ventricular fibrillation. The mortality in untreated symptomatic cases exceeds 60% within 15 years.[320] Clearly ECG screening of surviving relatives is

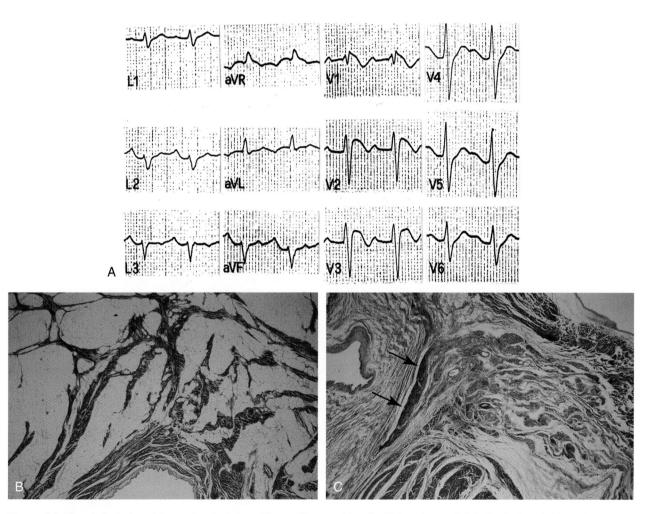

Figure 11-43 • Arrhythmic sudden cardiac death in a 35-year-old man with a familial syndrome of right bundle branch block, ST segment elevation, and sudden death. *A,* Basal ECG showing prolonged PR interval, right bundle branch block, and ST segment elevation in right precordial leads. *B,* Histology of the right ventricular free wall shows remarkable myocardial atrophy with fatty replacement and slight interstitial fibrosis. *C,* Severe fibrosis of the bifurcating bundle with sclerotic interruption of the right bundle branch (arrows). (*B* and *C,* Heidenhain trichrome.)

the best way to establish the diagnosis in asymptomatic carriers. (See Chapter 24 also.)

Right Bundle Branch Block With Right Precordial ST Segment Elevation

A clinical and ECG syndrome characterized by right bundle branch block with right precordial ST segment elevation and an apparently normal heart has been described in cases of sudden death by Brugada and Brugada, unfortunately without postmortem reports.[324] Noteworthy mutations in cardiac sodium channels gene SCN5A have been identified to contribute to the risk of developing idiopathic ventricular fibrillation.[325] Actually, Martini and colleagues[326] previously reported similar cases with apparent idiopathic ventricular fibrillation in which there was evidence of concealed right ventricular pathology. By studying a family with a case of sudden death, confirmation of an organic substrate was given by Corrado and coworkers,[327] who reported not only fibrofatty dystrophy in the right ventricular free wall but also involvement of the conduction system with sclerotic interruption of the right bundle branch (Fig. 11-43). The coexistence of both septal and parietal right conduction defects might account for the ECG pattern of right bundle branch block and persistent ST segment elevation as well as ventricular electrical instability.

Other Conditions

Unsuspected ventricular preexcitation caused by occult accessory AV connections is another theoretical cause of "mors sine materia." However, the absence of a positive ECG neither allows a clinical diagnosis nor helps indicate the presence and topographical site of anomalous connections. Incidentally, considering their small size (200 to 400 μ) histologic search without an ECG is like looking for a needle in a haystack. On the other hand, the finding of an accessory AV connection on histologic examination does not allow any surmises about electrical or clinical significance in the absence of an ECG recording.

Finally, sudden unwitnessed deaths have been reported in people with a history of epilepsy in the presence of a normal heart at postmortem examination. Possibly, in some circumstances, epileptic seizures involve the brain stem and are liable to provoke a violent cardioinhibitory-vasodepressor effect, with prolonged vagal cardiac syncope and irreversible cardiac arrest.[23, 24]

Saunas have been reported to precipitate cardiac arrest in patients with coronary artery disease; changes in their blood pressure and serum electrolyte concentrations have been postulated as potential mechanisms. Sauna bathing, even in combination with heavy alcohol intake, does not appear to provoke cardiac arrhythmias in healthy young men with normal hearts.[328] However, circulatory regulation seems to be more difficult to achieve in children during sauna, which has been proved particularly risky for children who have disorders of the sinus node.[329]

Life-threatening ventricular arrhythmias may also occur (mostly as a consequence of hypokalemia) in other clinical settings, such as anorexia nervosa, bulimia, or excessive dieting.[330] (See Chapter 16 also.)

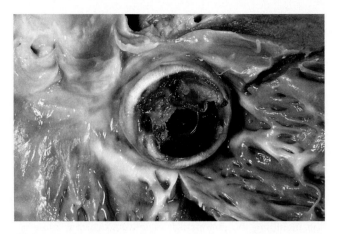

Figure 11-44 • Sudden death after mitral valve replacement with Björk-Shiley tilting-disc mechanical prosthesis. Massive thrombosis caused poppet entrapment, lumen occlusion, and acute pulmonary edema.

SUDDEN DEATH AFTER HEART SURGERY

Sudden death may occur in adult patients who have undergone cardiac surgery.

For those with coronary artery bypass surgery, the presence of myocardial scars, the progression of the native atherosclerotic disease in nonrevascularized vessels, and the onset of obstructive disease in a vascular graft, whether saphenous vein or internal mammary artery, are all potential explanations for triggering arrhythmic cardiac arrest.[331]

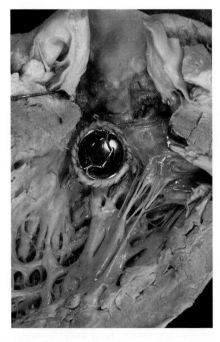

Figure 11-45 • Sudden death following aortic valve replacement with Björk-Shiley tilting-disc mechanical prosthesis. Sudden detachment of annular suture anchorage caused acute left ventricular failure.

Sudden death has been reported also in cardiac transplantation, either early, during acute rejection involving the conduction system,[332] or late, because of obstructive vasculopathy of coronary arteries as a result of chronic rejection.[333] (See Chapter 23 also.)

Sudden death may also occur in patients after heart valve replacement and may be related to prosthesis dysfunction (see also Chapter 21)[334]. In cases of mechanical valve prostheses, massive thrombosis with poppet block (Fig. 11-44), embolization of valve thrombosis, anticoagulation-related hemorrhage, abrupt detachment of annular suture anchorage (Fig. 11-45), and strut fracture (Fig. 11-46) are the main reported causes. In bioprostheses, sudden commissural tearing, either primary (Fig. 11-47) or related to calcification, is the equivalent of a strut fracture. These causes usually account for acute pump failure and pulmonary edema. However, sudden death in patients

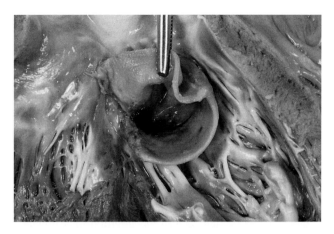

Figure 11-47 • Sudden death after mitral valve replacement with a unicusp pericardial prosthesis. An abrupt cuspal tear at one commissure led to severe mitral incompetence and pulmonary edema.

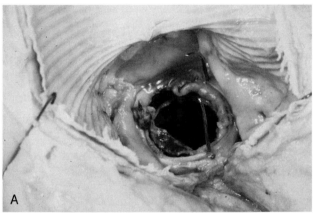

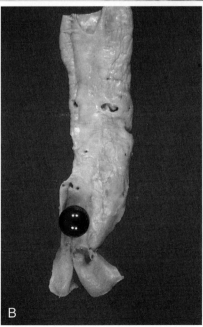

Figure 11-46 • Sudden death caused by strut fracture after aortic valve replacement with a De Bakey caged-ball mechanical prosthesis in the setting of chronic aortic dissection. *A,* View of the aortic root showing disappearance of one stent and of the poppet from the prosthesis. *B,* The ball was found at the bifurcation of the abdominal aorta.

with heart valve replacement may be unrelated to valve prostheses and otherwise explained by arrhythmias in the setting of concomitant severe cardiac hypertrophy or coronary atherosclerosis, with acute or old myocardial infarction.

Finally, aortic rupture may occur subsequent to aortic valve replacement at the site of an aortotomy if cystic medial necrosis accompanies native valve disease. This is particularly true in cases of noninflammatory aortic incompetence with degeneration of the aortic wall as in those with bicuspid aortic valve and annuloaortic ectasia.

CONGENITAL HEART DISEASE AND SUDDEN DEATH

In dealing with the various causes of sudden cardiac death, we mentioned many substrates that are congenital in nature—for example, bicuspid aortic valve, Marfan syndrome, aortic coarctation, aortic valve stenosis, coronary artery anomalies, hypertrophic cardiomyopathy and Wolff-Parkinson-White syndrome. Overall, sudden cardiac death in the young is ascribable to congenital heart defects in nearly one third of cases.[51] The abnormalities are mostly concealed, while signs and symptoms may be scarce or even absent. Sudden death is truly unexpected and often the first manifestation of disease.

A quite different problem is presented by sudden death in patients who have previously undergone operation to repair highly symptomatic cardiac malformations.[249, 335-339] They are recognized subjects at risk of cardiac arrest in whom surveillance is considered mandatory through periodic examination. Surgical repair may add to the risk of cardiac arrest by two main mechanisms:

1. *Injury to the conduction system.* While closing a ventricular or AV septal defect, a suture may damage the AV bundle, which is usually located in the posteroinferior rim with resultant onset of early or late AV block.[340-342] In the atrial repair of a complete transposition of the great arteries (especially the Mustard op-

eration), resection of the atrial septum and insertion of a baffle to switch the venous drainage may injure the sinus node, the crista terminalis, and the AV node itself, leaving room for a potential substrate for electrical instability. Arrhythmias and sudden death have been reported with an alarming rate after atrial repair of complete transposition.[51, 338, 343]

2. *Ventriculotomy.* Right ventriculotomy is a frequent approach used to repair many congenital heart diseases; for example, in tetralogy of Fallot, with infundibular resection and insertion of a transannular patch (Fig. 11-48), and in malformations characterized by right ventricle–pulmonary artery discontinuity, such as truncus arteriosus and pulmonary atresia with ventricular septal defect, which require the insertion of a conduit between the right ventricle and pulmonary trunk for

total correction.[344–347] In the past, even isolated perimembranous ventricular septal defects were closed by a ventriculotomy.[348] The subsequent scarring after this procedure may be so extensive that it becomes the substrate for ominous ventricular arrhythmias. Ventricular tachycardia is a well-known sequel some time after repair of tetralogy of Fallot and a proven risk for postoperative sudden cardiac death, which, unfortunately, also occurs without previous ventricular arrhythmias.[349, 350]

The increasing number of living patients successfully operated on for congenital heart disease raises important questions about the need to control their cardiac electrical vulnerability.[343–345, 351] Surgeons are fully aware of the need to avoid damaging the conduction system as well as

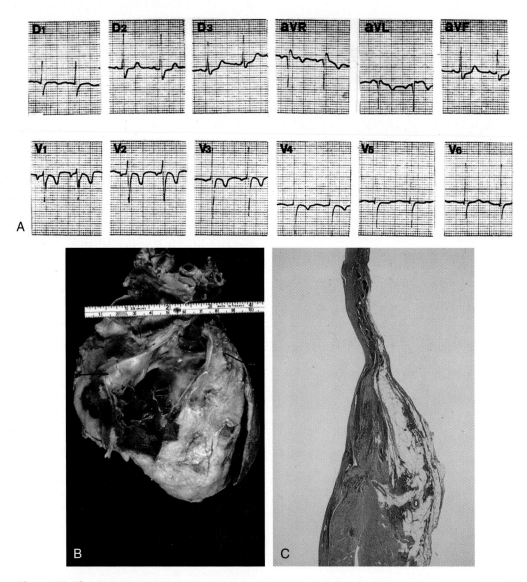

Figure 11-48 • Arrhythmic sudden cardiac death in a 12-year-old girl, 7 years after repair of tetralogy of Fallot. *A,* Basal electrocardiogram (ECG) shows inverted T waves in right precordial leads without conduction disturbances or ventricular arrhythmias. *B,* Gross view of the heart showing infundibular dilatation caused by infundibulectomy and transannular patch insertion. *C,* Histology of the infundibulum with extensive fibrofatty replacement (Weigert-van Gieson).

limiting ventriculotomy to cases in which it is strictly necessary. Both ventricular septal defects and tetralogy of Fallot are nowadays repaired through an atrial approach to avoid ventricular myocardial scarring. (See Chapter 22 also.)

SUDDEN DEATH IN YOUNG ATHLETES

Sudden death in athletes is a special issue in that it threatens the lives of apparently normal subjects capable of an extraordinary exercise performance. It is an amazing example of dissociation between myocardial contractility, which is preserved or even increased, and electrical stability, which is highly vulnerable.

Several cardiac diseases have been discovered at postmortem examination in athletes who died suddenly. In the United States, hypertrophic cardiomyopathy is by far the leading cause (as many as 36% of cases), followed by congenital coronary artery anomalies, aortic rupture, and coronary atherosclerosis.[252, 352, 353] In the Veneto Region of Italy, in comparison, arrhythmogenic right ventricular cardiomyopathy is the primary cause, followed by either congenital or acquired coronary artery disease (Table 11-4).[228, 229] This difference may be related to genetic or ethnic factors. However, in contrast to practice in the United States, competitive athletes in Italy undergo obligatory preparticipation screening. Therefore, most subjects with hypertrophic cardiomyopathy are disqualified from participation on the basis of ECG and two-dimensional echocardiographic findings.[354] This may account for a smaller number of sudden deaths from hypertrophic cardiomyopathy among Italian athletes.

The question is whether particular cardiac diseases exist in which exercise raises the risk of cardiac arrest.[229, 354, 355] A recent study compared the prevalence of sport as opposed to nonsport-related sudden deaths in various morbid entities within a large population of juvenile sudden deaths.[229, 354] Only deaths from arrhythmogenic right ventricular cardiomyopathy and congenital anomalies of coronary arteries, particularly those with origin from the wrong sinus, were found to be significantly associated with exercise. In arrhythmogenic right ventricular cardiomyopathy, electrical instability may be triggered by ventricular dilation and autonomous nervous system influences occurring during effort. In an anomalous origin of a coronary artery from a wrong sinus, exercise clearly exacerbates myocardial ischemia by the potentially obstructive effect of an intramural aortic course and a slit-like lumen. Oddly enough, sudden death resulting from coronary atherosclerosis in the young is not significantly related to effort.[44] In these subjects, cardiac arrest occurs as frequently when they are at rest. The unique shape of a single eccentric plaque located in the proximal left descending coronary artery with preserved tunica media, a most probable site of coronary vasospasm, may explain the phenomenon.

Arrhythmogenic right ventricular cardiomyopathy may be a more frequent cause of death than previously thought, because it is often misdiagnosed at postmortem examination.[213] Forensic pathologists are not familiar with this disease, because they usually concentrate on the left ventricle when looking for an explanation of an unexpected death (e.g., left ventricular hypertrophy, myocardial infarction or scars, mitral valve prolapse, aortic valve disease, coronary artery disease). Moreover, right ventricular abnormalities in arrhythmogenic right ventricular cardiomyopathy may not be striking on gross examination.[216] Nevertheless, more cases may be diagnosed if the right ventricle is transilluminated during postmortem examination in cases of sudden death. It is a common belief that fatty infiltration of the right ventricular free wall is normal. This is true in adults or elderly people but not in the young. Arrhythmogenic right ventricular cardiomyopathy has prodromal symptoms (syncope, lipothymia, palpitations) and signs (basal ECG abnormalities such as right precordial T wave inversion, premature ventricular beats, and ventricular tachycardia of left bundle branch block morphology) that help to identify apparently healthy subjects at risk and lead to their disqualification from sports in Italy. Unfortunately, this is not true of coronary artery anomalies, which, although being significantly related to effort as a risk for sudden death, rarely induce symptoms or signs during preparticipation screening to raise suspicion and allow diagnosis.[228, 229, 354]

IN VIVO DIAGNOSIS OF CONCEALED DEFECTS, TREATMENT, AND PREVENTION

Most of the previously mentioned cardiac diseases that promote sudden death do not manifest cardiomegaly or a heart murmur. Thus, chest radiography and cardiac auscultation, although vital in any medical examination, rarely allow diagnosis or raise suspicion of an underlying abnormality. On the other hand, only noninvasive investigations can be reasonably employed at screening.[354, 356–358]

The clinical history is a fundamental source of infor-

TABLE 11-4 • **Causes of Sudden Death in 49 Young Competitive Athletes**

Causes	N
Arrhythmogenic right ventricular cardiomyopathy	11
Atherosclerotic coronary artery disease	9
Congenital anomalies of coronary arteries	8
Mitral valve prolapse	5
Conduction system pathology	4
Myocarditis	3
Cerebral embolism	2
Hypertrophic cardiomyopathy	1
Dilated cardiomyopathy	1
Aortic dissection	1
Cerebral aneurysm	1
Pulmonary thromboembolism	1
Long QT syndrome	1
Unexplained	1
TOTAL	49

N = number of cases
Data from Corrado D, Basso C, Schiavon M, Thiene G: Screening for hypertrophic cardiomyopathy in young athletes. N Engl J Med 339:364, 1998

mation. Palpitations, dizziness, lipothymia, and syncope are frequent complaints of unsuspected carriers, although often their significance is underestimated. They should cause alarm and prompt other clinical investigations. This, of course, is obligatory after an episode of cardiac arrest or aborted sudden death. Oddly enough, loss of consciousness is frequently interpreted as a transient ischemic cerebral attack or a primary neurologic defect such as epilepsy, thus diverting attention from the heart to the brain or the carotid arteries.

An ECG represents the first of any noninvasive examinations aimed to detect heart diseases that induce the risk of electrical instability. Relevant ECG features include changes in ventricular depolarization (QRS complex) or repolarization (ST segment, T waves, QT interval) as well as rhythm and conduction abnormalities. For instance, both the long QT and Wolff-Parkinson-White syndrome are easily diagnosed on the basis of their distinctive ECG findings. Abnormalities of ventricular depolarization or repolarization are observed in acute or chronic ischemia. However, the ECG is neither highly specific nor sensitive for myocardial ischemia,[229] because T wave inversion is frequently observed in nonischemic conditions such as cardiomyopathies.[232, 358] Severe coronary artery disease, whether congenital or acquired, may escape detection in an ECG done at rest or during effort.[354] Twenty-four-hour Holter monitoring is very important in registering warning rhythm and conduction abnormalities.

Two-dimensional echocardiography allows a superb in vivo investigation of both cardiac shape and function. It may be considered the gold-standard for detecting most heart disease with structural abnormalities, having a sensitivity and specificity comparable to those of postmortem examination. Most patients who have cardiac diseases associated with sudden death have gross structural abnormalities, potentially visible at echo scanning.[51] The diagnosis of hypertrophic cardiomyopathy, mitral valve prolapse, bicuspid aortic valve, annuloaortic ectasia, or cardiac masses is nowadays easily achieved by echocardiography. Even the anomalous origin of a coronary artery may be diagnosed by a skillful practitioner.[135] The right ventricle, because of its anterior substernal position and thin wall, is less easily investigated; however, aneurysms and dilation, such as those present in arrhythmogenic right ventricular cardiomyopathy, may be seen and are easily interpreted through proper views.[233, 234] The sensitivity of two-dimensional echocardiography has been greatly increased by the transesophageal approach.

Tissue characterization is almost exclusively attainable by magnetic resonance, which is of particular value in detecting fatty infiltration of ventricular walls, as in arrhythmogenic right ventricular cardiomyopathy.[237–240] Cinemagnetic resonance is currently employed as an alternative to cineangiography for exploring cardiac shape and function. Unfortunately, magnetic resonance studies are expensive and cannot be contemplated as a first-level investigation. This is also true for radionuclide angiography and for scintigraphy, which are aimed to detect perfusion defects, and for positron emission tomography, which is capable of investigating metabolic disorders.

Invasive investigations are deemed necessary when interventional or surgical treatments are planned. Intracavi-

tary electrophysiology helps to diagnose rhythm and conduction abnormalities by assessing conduction times and refractoriness as well as by testing inducibility of either atrial or ventricular arrhythmias after programmed stimulation. Moreover, a transcatheter endocardial approach is currently employed to map and ablate accessory pathways; AV junction or arrhythmogenic circuits; and focuses, whether atrial or ventricular.[319] Coronary cineangiography is essential for visualizing the coronary arterial tree, with the aim of detecting stenosis, anomalous origin, or myocardial bridges.[359] Coronary angioplasty and stenting are currently performed to relieve arterial stenosis. A nonsurgical reduction of the basal interventricular septum has been performed in obstructive hypertrophic cardiomyopathy by a selective injection of alcohol into the first septal coronary artery.[360] Finally, surgical repair, either through bypass grafting or conservative procedures (coronary ostioplasty, myocardial debridging), requires thoracotomy, now feasible by minimally invasive methods.[359] Left stellate ganglia sympathetic denervation has been accomplished in cases with long QT interval syndrome, although its efficacy has been questioned.[361]

Prophylactic pharmacologic therapy is indicated in cases of either disabling or life-threatening arrhythmias. The most effective drugs include flecainide and propafenone, amiodarone and sotalol, β-blockers and calcioantagonists.[362, 363] However, the risk/benefit ratio of antiarrhythmic therapy has to be evaluated carefully because most of these drugs can produce serious side-effects or have a paradoxical proarrhythmic consequence. When the risk of ventricular fibrillation is very high, particularly in patients who survive aborted sudden death, the implantation of a ventricular defibrillator (Fig. 11-49) is mandatory to prevent cardiac arrest.[363] In cases of symptomatic bradyarrhythmias, pacemaker implantation is also a well-established, lifesaving procedure.

It is well known that effort and emotion may trigger arrhythmic cardiac arrest.[354] When a condition at risk of sudden death is diagnosed, patients should be advised to avoid strenuous exercise regardless of the type of treatment; competitive sport activity should be prohibited. Although this may entail economic and psychological drawbacks, sedentary activity is the simplest preventive measure available.

THE PATHOLOGIST'S ROLE IN FAMILIAL SUDDEN DEATH

A sudden death has a tragic impact on families. An autopsy in such cases should not only be used to write a correct death certificate, or establish whether death was the result of natural or unnatural causes and whether there are associated legal implications. The autopsy is also the source of vital information for the community, for the relatives of the deceased person, and for future generations.

An accurate diagnosis of the underlying morbid entity and the ultimate cause of death is a prerequisite for establishing whether the disease is hereditary. The final pathologic diagnosis may serve as the starting point for a

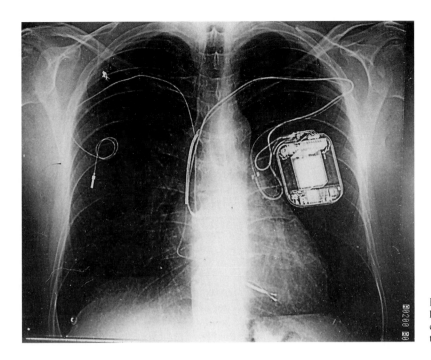

Figure 11-49 • Chest radiogram of a patient with hypertrophic cardiomyopathy and recurrent episodes of cardiac arrest. A ventricular defibrillator was implanted to prevent sudden death.

widespread investigation of the family, to detect asymptomatic carriers, to reassure noncarriers, to adopt therapeutic and preventive measures, or to assess the magnitude of risk of sudden death in an individual.

A full family history, including the ages and causes of death of members with subsequent construction of a genealogical tree, is critical.[364] ECG and echocardiographic studies are essential preliminary investigations that should be made for all first-degree family members. Unfortunately, these tests can detect only a small proportion of gene carriers, particularly in children, in whom phenotypic expression may still be absent.

Genetic screening is, theoretically, the most effective tool in the early recognition of asymptomatic genetic carriers. Its potential benefit for patients and family members is self-evident, because, in most cases, sudden death may be the first and only manifestation of a familial disease. Moreover, the risk of cardiac arrest is demonstrably higher with some specific mutations. Another advantage is the extension of scientific knowledge, which is likely in the future to benefit all individuals with the abnormal gene. Only within large families can abnormal genes be identified by linkage analysis, which becomes an extremely valuable research tool.

However, there are concerns about genetic screening. First, it is an expensive procedure at present, mostly limited to large families with several affected individuals, and it can be performed only at a few tertiary referral centers with a specific research interest in molecular genetics. There are pressures to study families because of competition in science. Some people question whether genetic knowledge is beneficial, neutral, or harmful, and whether parents have the right to make decisions for their children, especially if a disease is not apparent until middle age and if little can be offered in terms of treatment. The potential for eugenic abuse should also be consid-

ered. For example, in 1995, China passed a law prohibiting marriage of a couple who carry genetic disorders.[357]

Pathologists, who see most of the index cases, have a great responsibility. If nothing is done and another sudden death occurs, the family rightly feels aggrieved. If the pathologic diagnosis is wrong, many expensive and time-consuming investigations are conducted without benefit. This implies that all sudden deaths should undergo autopsy by expert pathologists. When a precise diagnosis is made and a potentially hereditary disease is recognized as the cause of death, it is advisable to inform the family through their general practitioner. That should start a sequence of investigations from a detailed family history to referral of parents, siblings, and offspring to a cardiologist for screening. Whether such screening should go beyond ECG and echocardiography is questionable. A full genetic study should be performed if the family asks for it. Research should ultimately be assumed by the National Health Service or insuring agencies. Hypertrophic cardiomyopathy, the long QT syndrome, Marfan syndrome, and arrhythmogenic right ventricular cardiomyopathy are, at present, cardiac familial diseases that carry risk of sudden death; all are amenable to genetic screening. All have the potential to devastate families by expected sudden death, and families have a right to the best available advice. A close collaboration of pathologist, cardiologist, and geneticist is strongly advised. (See discussion in Chapter 24 also.)

•••••

APPENDIX: STUDY METHOD

1. Collect the patient's history before dissection, with special reference to the occurrence of familial sudden death, symptoms and signs in life, and diagnostic procedures; retrieve all available ECG tracings.

2. Inquire about the circumstances of death, whether witnessed or unwitnessed, to rule out any suspicion of an unnatural death or to point to a specific mode of death (respiratory, cerebral, cardiac).

3. Take blood and urine samples or other organic fluids for toxicologic investigation, to exclude drug addiction or doping.

4. Inspect the cadaver to detect peculiar stigmata or possible injuries; record weight and height.

5. Make a thorough postmortem examination, including brain, lungs and abdominal viscera, to exclude an extracardiac cause of death such as a stroke, airway obstruction, gastrointestinal hemorrhage, pancreatitis, or adrenal apoplexy; inspect the peritoneal and pleural spaces to detect blood.

6. Open the pericardial sac and exclude cardiac tamponade; open the pulmonary artery and exclude pulmonary embolism; remove the heart from the arterial and venous pedicles and open the aortic arch in search of isthmal coarctation. In a case of aortic dissection, remove the heart together with the aorta and main branches to the ileofemoral arteries. Open the aorta to display intimal tears, a false lumen, collateral artery occlusion, reentry, and external rupture. Check the aortic root to ascertain whether a bicuspid valve exists.

7. Weigh the heart and compare the usual values for height, gender, and age. Take transverse and longitudinal axis measurements.

8. Look at the epicardial surface of the ventricles and see whether aneurysms, scars, or fatty infiltration are present, particularly in the right ventricle.

9. Inspect the Valsalva sinuses to check whether coronary ostia are rightly located and whether they show stenosis or obstructions.

10. Cut transversally with a scalpel the coronary arterial tree at 3- to 5-mm intervals, starting from the left main trunk and the left anterior descending coronary artery. Pay attention to the existence of plaque, embolism, dissection, or aneurysm. Decalcify vessels, if indicated, before instituting this procedure.

11. Open the left atrium and the left auricle to see whether thrombi are present; inspect the mitral leaflet to exclude redundancy and prolapse. In the right atrium, avoid cutting the sinus node when opening the chamber.

12. If there is any suspicion of myocardial infarction, cut the heart in the short axis two thirds of the distance toward the apex; for hypertrophic cardiomyopathy, cut in the long axis parasternal view; for arrhythmogenic right ventricular cardiomyopathy, cut in the four-chamber view.

13. Measure the maximal wall thickness of the right and left ventricles as well as of the ventricular septum.

14. Observe the ventricular myocardium and look for acute myocardial infarction, scarring, or adiposis. Transilluminate the ventricular free wall to detect translucent areas.

15. In a case of ventricular preexcitation, do not cut through the AV grooves where accessory AV fascicles may be located.

16. All heart cavities, both atrial and ventricular, should be inspected for masses (tumors, thrombi). Observe the endocardium and look for possible small endocardial papillomas.

17. Take relevant gross pictures and await their return before proceeding to remove histologic samples.

18. In cases of alleged ischemic heart disease, besides coronary artery segments, take myocardial samples, possibly all around the ventricular cavities: anteroseptal, anterolateral, inferolateral, and inferoseptal for the left ventricle; anterior, lateral, and inferior for the right ventricle. In hypertrophic cardiomyopathy, take transverse tissue sections from the septum, perpendicularly to the long axis cut made in the heart. In arrhythmogenic right ventricular cardiomyopathy, take samples from any translucent areas and all around the free wall and the septum in the four-chamber cut and from the inferior and anterior walls from the base to the apex, including the pulmonary infundibulum.

19. Conduct a microscopic examination of coronary artery segments to establish the type and severity of atherosclerotic plaques and the presence of thrombosis and inflammation. Hematoxylin-eosin, Heidenhain trichrome, and elastic van Gieson stains are the routine ones we employ. An immunohistochemical panel of antibodies for inflammatory infiltrates and smooth muscle cells should be used routinely. The same histologic and immunohistochemical stains are applicable to the normal myocardium.

20. Investigate the conduction system and innervation, at least when both gross and histologic examinations of the myocardium do not reveal any plausible explanation of death. The sinus node and AV junction should be removed, each in a single block, to ensure investigation of the continuity of the conduction system. By rule, serial histologic sections should be studied and hematoxylin-eosin and trichrome stains should be used; see Chapter 20 for details. Representative sections are *not* considered sufficient. Methods for neurofilaments (monoclonal antibodies S-100) and Bielschowsky argyrophil method for ganglia are recommended to study the intrinsic innervation.[92]

21. In a case of preexcitation syndrome, the AV septal and lateral rings should be investigated. Blocks of the lateral rings should include atrial and ventricular myocardium and be cut serially, retaining and staining every 10th section. The site of block removal is usually indicated by the ECG. For this purpose, the presence of an electrophysiologist is recommended when the specimen is inspected, to define the most plausible site of the accessory pathway.

22. Clinical and pathologic findings should be correlated and a final diagnosis advanced. In cases of potential familial disease, information must be made available for the family doctor to institute clinical and genetic screening.

Acknowledgments

The investigation has been supported by the Veneto Region, Venice and National Council for Research, Rome, Italy.

The authors are deeply indebted to Agostino Leorin

for photograph assistance and Anna Saracino for excellent technical histologic work.

REFERENCES

1. Goldstein S: The necessity of a uniform definition of sudden coronary death: Witnessed death within 1 hour of the onset of acute symptoms. Am Heart J 103:156, 1982
2. Manolio TA, Furberg CD: Epidemiology of sudden cardiac death. In: Akhtar M, Myerburg RJ, Ruskin JN: Sudden Cardiac Death. Baltimore, Williams & Wilkins, 1994
3. Gillum RF: Sudden coronary death in the United States: 1980–1985. Circulation 79:756, 1989
4. Schatzkin A, Cupples LA, Heeren T, et al: The epidemiology of sudden unexpected death: Risk factors for men and women in the Framingham Heart Study. Am Heart J 107:1300, 1984
5. Elveback LR, Connolly DC, Kulrand LT: Coronary heart disease in residents of Rochester, Minnesota: II. Mortality, incidence, and survivorship, 1950–1975. Mayo Clin Proc 56:655, 1981
6. Chiang BN, Perlman LV, Fulton M, et al: Predisposing factors in sudden cardiac death in Tecumseh, Michigan. Circulation 41:31, 1970
7. Kuller LH, Lilienfeld AM, Fisher R: An epidemiological study of sudden and unexpected deaths in adults. Medicine 46:341, 1967
8. Hagstrom RM, Federspiel CF, Ho YC: Incidence of myocardial infarction and sudden death from coronary heart disease in Nashville, Tennessee. Circulation 44:884, 1971
9. Gillum RF, Folsom A, Luepker RV, et al: Sudden death and acute myocardial infarction in a metropolitan area. 1970–1980. N Engl J Med 309:1353, 1983
10. Kannel WB, Doyle JT, McNamara PM, et al: Precursors of sudden coronary death. Circulation 51:606, 1975
11. Goldberg RJ, Gore JM, Alpert JS, Dalen JE: Incidence and case fatality rates of acute myocardial infarction (1975–1984): The Worcester Heart Attack Study. Am Heart J 115:751, 1988
12. Myocardial Infarction Community Registers: Public Health in Europe 5. Copenhagen, Regional Office for Europe, World Health Organization, 1976
13. Suhonen O, Reunanen A, Knekt P, Aromaa A: Risk factors for sudden and nonsudden coronary death. Acta Med Scand 223:19, 1988
14. Silka MJ, Kron J, Walance CG, et al: Assessment and follow-up of pediatric survivors of sudden cardiac death. Circulation 82:341, 1990
15. Driscoll DJ, Edwards WD: Sudden unexpected death in children and adolescents. J Am Coll Cardiol 5(suppl B):118B, 1985
16. Shen WK, Edwards WD, Hammil SC, et al: Sudden unexpected non-traumatic death in 54 young adults: A 30 year population-based study. Am J Cardiol 76:148, 1995
17. Kuller L: Sudden death: Definition and epidemiologic considerations. Prog Cardiovasc Dis 23:1, 1980
18. Feinleib M, Simon AB, Gillum RF, et al: Prodromal symptoms and signs of sudden death. Circulation 52(6 suppl 3): 155, 1975
19. Kuller L: Sudden and unexpected non-traumatic deaths in adults: A review of epidemiological and clinical studies. J Chronic Dis 19:1165, 1966
20. Schievink WI, Wijdicks EFM, Parisi JE, et al: Sudden death from aneurysmal subarachnoid hemorrhage. Neurology 45:871, 1995
21. Sacco RL, Wolf PA, Bharicha NE, et al: Subarachnoid and intracerebral hemorrhage: Natural history, prognosis and precursive factors in the Framingham Study. Neurology 34:847, 1984
22. Schievink WI: Intracranial aneurysms. N Engl J Med 336:28, 1997
23. Johnston SC, Horn JK, Valente J, Simon RP: The role of hypoventilation in a sheep model of epileptic sudden death. Ann Neurol 37:531, 1995
24. Nashef L, Walker F, Allen P, et al: Apnoea and bradycardia during epileptic seizures: Relation to sudden death in epilepsy. J Neurol Neurosurg Psychiatry 60:297, 1996
25. Molfino NA, Nannini LJ, Martelli AN, Slutsky AS: Respiratory arrest in near-fatal asthma. N Engl J Med 324:285, 1991
26. Kikuchi Y, Okabe S, Tamura G, et al: Chemosensitivity and perception of dyspnea in patients with a history of near-fatal asthma. N Engl J Med 324:285, 1991
27. Saetta M, Thiene G, Crescioli S, Fabbri LM: Fatal asthma in a young patient with severe bronchial hyperresponsiveness but stable peak flow records. Eur Respir J 2:1008, 1989
28. Isselbacher EM, Cigarroa JE, Eagle KA: Cardiac tamponade complicating proximal aortic dissection. Is pericardiocentesis harmful? Circulation 90:2375, 1994
29. Adelson L, Hirsch CS: Sudden and unexpected death from natural causes in adults. In: Spitz WV, Fisher RS (eds): Medicolegal Investigations of Death. 2nd ed. Springfield, IL, Charles C Thomas, 1980, p 88
30. Bohm N: Adrenal cutaneous and myocardial lesions in fulminating endotoxinemia. Pathol Res Pract 174:92, 1982
31. Schwartz HJ, Yunginger JW, Schwrtz LB: Is unrecognized anaphylaxis a cause of sudden unexpected death? Clin Exp Allergy 25:866, 1995
32. Breckenridge RT, Ratnoff OD: Pulmonary embolism and unexpected death in supposedly normal individuals. N Engl J Med 270: 298, 1964
33. Nelson DA, Ray CD: Extracardiac thrombotic embolic and hemorrhagic causes of sudden death. Cardiovasc Pathol 3:129, 1994
34. Fozzard HA: Electromechanical dissociation and its possible role in sudden cardiac death. J Am Coll Cardiol 5:318, 1985
35. Goldstein S, Friedman L, Hutchinson R: Timing mechanism and clinical setting of witnessed deaths in post-myocardial infarction patients. J Am Coll Cardiol 3:1111, 1984
36. Goldstein S, Landis R, Leighton R, et al: Characteristics of resuscitated out-of-hospital cardiac arrest victim with coronary heart disease. Circulation 64:977, 1981
37. Kempf FC, Josephson ME: Cardiac arrest recorded on ambulatory electrocardiograms. Am J Cardiol 53:1577, 1984
38. Liberthson RR, Nagel EL, Hirshman JC, et al: Pathophysiologic observations in pre-hospital ventricular fibrillation and sudden cardiac death. Circulation 49:790, 1974
39. Myerburg R, Conde C, Sung R, et al: Clinical, electrophysiologic and hemodynamic profile of patients resuscitated from prehospital cardiac arrest. Am J Med 68:568, 1980
40. Nikolic G, Bishop RL, Singh JB: Sudden death recorded during Holter monitoring. Circulation 66:218, 1982
41. Raizes G, Wagner GS, Hackel DB: Instantaneous non-arrhythmic cardiac death in acute myocardial infarction. Am J Cardiol 39:1, 1973
42. Greene HL. Sudden arrhythmic cardiac death—mechanisms, resuscitation and classification: The Seattle perspective. Am J Cardiol 65:4B, 1990
43. Pole JE, Bardy GH: Sudden cardiac death. In: Zipes DP, Jalife J. (eds): Cardiac Electrophysiology: From Cell to Bedside. 2nd ed. Philadelphia, WB Saunders, 1995, p 812
44. Corrado D, Basso C, Poletti A, et al: Sudden death in the young. Is coronary thrombosis the major precipitating factor? Circulation 90:2315, 1994
45. Heggtveit HA: Syphilitic aortitis: A clinicopathologic autopsy study of 100 cases, 1950 to 1960. Circulation 29:346, 1964
46. Virmani R, McAllister HA: Pathology of the aorta and major arteries. In: Lande A, Berkmen YN, McAllister HA (eds): Aortitis. Clinical pathologic and radiographic aspects. New York, Raven Press, 1986
47. De Bakey ME, Hehly WSM, Cooley DD, et al: Surgical management of dissecting aneurysm of the aorta. J Thorac Cardiovasc Surg 49:130, 1965
48. Thiene G, Rossi L, Becker A: The atrioventricular conduction system in dissecting aneurysm of the aorta. Am Heart J 98:447, 1979
49. Larson EW, Edwards WD: Risk factors of aortic dissection: A necropsy study of 161 cases. Am J Cardiol 53:849, 1984
50. Schlatmann TJM, Becker AE: Histologic changes in the normal aging aorta: Implications for dissecting aortic aneurysm. Am J Cardiol 39:13, 1977
51. Basso C, Frescura C, Corrado D, et al: Congenital heart disease and sudden death in the young. Hum Pathol 26:1065, 1995
52. Disertori M, Bertagnolli C, Thiene G, et al: Aneurisma dissecante dell'aorta a carattere familiare. G Ital Cardiol 21:849, 1991
53. Roberts WC, Honig HS: The spectrum of cardiovascular disease in the Marfan syndrome: A clinicopathologic study of 18 necropsy patients and comparison to 151 previously reported necropsy patients. Am Heart J 104:115, 1982
54. Edwards JE: Aneurysms of the thoracic aorta complicating coarctation. Circulation 48:195, 1973
55. Cohen M, Fuster V, Steele PM, et al: Coarctation of the aorta.

Long-term follow-up and prediction of outcome after surgical correction. Circulation 80:840, 1989

56. Edwards WD, Leaf DS, Edwards JE: Dissecting aortic aneurysm associated with congenital bicuspid aortic valve. Circulation 57: 1022, 1978

57. Roberts CS, Roberts WC: Dissection of the aorta associated with congenital malformation of aortic valve. J Am Coll Cardiol 17: 712, 1991

58. Pachulski RT, Weinberg AL, Chan KW: Aortic aneurysm in patients with functionally normal or minimally stenotic bicuspid aortic valve. Am J Cardiol 67:781, 1991

59. Kaimaulainen K, Pulkkinen K, Savolainem A, et al: Location on chromosome 15 of the gene defect causing Marfan syndrome. N Engl J Med 323:935, 1990

60. Dietz HC, Outting GR, Pyeritz RE, et al: Marfan syndrome caused by a recurrent de novo missense mutation in the fibrilline gene. Nature 352:337, 1991

61. Giusti S, Cocco P, Thiene G: Valvola aortica bicuspide: Una cardiopatia congenita "minore" a rischio di catastrofiche complicanze. G Ital Cardiol 21:189, 1991

62. Stefani G, Cocco P, Sans-Coma V, et al: Morte improvvisa giovanile da rottura spontanea dell'aorta. G Ital Cardiol 23:55, 1993

63. McKusick VA, Logue RB, Bahnson HT: Association of aortic valvular disease and cystic medial necrosis of the ascending aorta. Report of four instances. Circulation 16:188, 1957

64. Emanuel R, Withers R, O'Brien K, et al: Congenitally bicuspid aortic valves. Clinicogenetic study of 41 families. Br Heart J 40: 1402, 1978

65. Godden DJ, Sandhu PS, Kerr F: Stenosed bicuspid aortic valves in twins. Eur Heart J 8:316, 1987

66. Recchia D, Sharkey AM, Bosner MS, et al: Sensitive detection of abnormal aortic architecture in Marfan syndrome with high-frequency ultrasonic tissue characterization. Circulation 91:1036, 1995

67. Lindsay J. Coarctation of the aorta, bicuspid aortic valve and abnormal ascending aortic wall. Am J Cardiol 61:182, 1988

68. Kappetein AP, Gittenberger-de Groot AC, Zwinderman AH, et al: The neural crest as a possible pathogenetic factor in coarctation of the aorta and bicuspid aortic valve. J Thorac Cardiovasc Surg 102: 830, 1991

69. Abbott ME: Coarctation of the aorta of the adult type: A statistical study and historical retrospect of 200 recorded cases with autopsy of stenosis or obliteration of the descending aorta in subjects over the age two years. Am Heart J 3:574, 1928

70. Eagle KA, De Sanctis RW: Diseases of the aorta. In: Braunwald E (ed): Heart Disease. 4th ed. Philadelphia, WB Saunders, 1992, p 1528

71. Zarins CK, Glagov S, Vesselinovitch D, Wissler RW: Aneurysm formation in experimental atherosclerosis: Relationship to plaque evolution. J Vasc Sug 12:246, 1990

72. Nevitt MP, Ballard DJ, Hallett JW: Prognosis of abdominal aortic aneurysms. A population-based study. N Engl J Med 321:1009, 1989.

73. Ernst CB: Abdominal aortic aneurysm. N Engl J Med 328:1167, 1993

74. Johansson G, Nydahl S, Olofsson P, Swedenborg J: Survival of patients with abdominal aortic aneurysms: Comparison between operative and non-operative managements. Eur J Vasc Surg 4:497, 1990

75. Lancisi GM: De subitaneis mortibus. Venezia, 1708

76. Morgagni GB: De sedibus et causis morborum per anatomen indagatis. Venezia, 1761

77. Lavie CJ, Gersh BJ: Mechanical and electrical complications of acute myocardial infarction. Mayo Clin Proc 65:709, 1990

78. Cobb L, Baum R, Alvarez H, Schaffer WA: Resuscitation from out-of-hospital ventricular fibrillation: 4 years follow-up. Circulation 52: (6 suppl) III−223, 1975

79. Davies MJ: Pathological view of sudden cardiac death. Br Heart J 45:88, 1981

80. Davies MJ, Thomas A: Thrombosis and acute coronary artery lesions in sudden cardiac ischemic death. N Engl J Med 310:1137, 1984

81. Davies MJ, Bland JM, Hangartner JRW, et al: Factors influencing the presence or absence of acute coronary artery thrombi in sudden ischaemic death. Eur Heart J 10:203, 1989

82. DeWood MA, Spores J, Notske R: Prevalence of total coronary occlusion during the early hours of transmural myocardial infarction. N Engl J Med 303:897, 1980

83. Spaulding CM, Jaly LM, Rosenberg A, et al: Immediate coronary angiography in survivors of out-of-hospital cardiac arrest. N Engl J Med 336:1629, 1997

84. Davies MJ: Stability and instability: Two faces of coronary atherosclerosis. The Paul Dudley With Lecture 1995. Circulation 94: 2013, 1996

85. Burke AP, Farb A, Malcom GT, et al: Coronary risk factors and plaque morphology in men with coronary disease who died suddenly. N Engl J Med 336:1276, 1997

86. Van der Wal AC, Becker AE, van der Loos CM, Das PK: Site of intimal rupture or erosion of thrombosed coronary atherosclerotic plaques is characterized by an inflammatory process irrespective of the dominant plaque morphology. Circulation 89:36, 1994

87. Moreno PR, Bernardi VH, López-Cuéllar J, et al: Macrophages, smooth muscle cells, and tissue factor in unstable angina. Implications for cell-mediated thrombogenicity in acute coronary syndromes. Circulation 94:3090, 1996

88. Hackel DB, Estes EH: Pathologic features of atrioventricular and intraventricular conduction disturbances in acute myocardial infarction. Circulation 43:977, 1971

89. James TW: The coronary circulation and conduction system in acute myocardial infarction. Prog Cardiovasc Dis 10:410, 1968

90. Lev M, Kihane SG, Pick A: The pathogenesis of atrioventricular block in coronary artery disease. Circulation 42:409, 1970

91. Baroldi G, Falzi G, Mariani F: Sudden coronary death. A postmortem study in 208 selected cases compared to 97 "control" subjects. Am Heart J 98:20, 1979

92. Rossi L, Thiene G: Arrhythmologic pathology of sudden cardiac death. Milan, Casa Editrice Ambrosiana, 1983

93. Bouchardy B, Majno G: Histopathology of early myocardial infarcts. Am J Pathol 74:301, 1974

94. Rossi L, Matturri L: Anisoinotropismo miocardiocitico: Quadro istologico elementare della dis-energia ischemica precoce. G Ital Cardiol 17:479, 1987

95. Friedman M, Manwaring JH, Roseman RH, et al: Instantaneous and sudden deaths. Clinical and pathologic differentiation in coronary artery disease. JAMA 225:1319, 1973

96. Lie JT, Titus JL. Pathology of the myocardium and conduction system in sudden coronary death. Circulation 52-III:41, 1975

97. Newman WP, Tracy RE, Strong JP, et al: Pathology of sudden cardiac death. N Y Acad Sci 382:39, 1982

98. Rosenthal ME, Oseran DS, Gang E, Peter T: Sudden cardiac death following acute myocardial infarction. Am Heart J 109:865, 1985

99. Perper JA, Kuller LH, Cooper M: Arteriosclerosis of coronary arteries in sudden unexpected death. Circulation 51 (suppl 3):199, 1975

100. Reichenbach DD, Moss NS, Meyer E: Pathology of the heart in sudden cardiac death. Am J Cardiol 39:865, 1977

101. Lovergrove T, Thompson P: The role of acute myocardial infarction in sudden cardiac death: A statistician's nightmare. Am Heart J 96:711, 1978

102. Schwartz PJ, Billman GE, Stone HL: Autonomic mechanism in ventricular fibrillation induced by myocardial infarction. An experimental preparation for sudden cardiac death. Circulation 69:790, 1984

103. Maseri A, Chierchia S: Coronary artery spasm: Demonstration, definition, diagnosis and consequences. Prog Cardiovasc Dis 25: 169, 1982

104. Myerburg RJ, Kessler KM, Mallon SM, et al: Life-threatening ventricular arrhythmia in patients with silent myocardial ischemia due to coronary artery spasm. N Engl J Med 326:1451, 1992

105. Flugelman MY, Virmani R, Correa R, et al: Smooth muscle cell abundance and fibroblast growth factors in coronary lesions of patients with nonfatal unstable angina: A clue to the mechanism of tranformation from the stable to the unstable clinical state. Circulation 88:2493, 1993

106. Rossi L: Pathologic changes in the cardiac conduction and nervous system in sudden coronary death. Ann N Y Acad Sci 382:50, 1982

107. Spain DM, Brodness VA, Mohr C: Coronary atherosclerosis as a cause of unexpected and unexplained death: Autopsy study from 1949–1959. JAMA 174:384, 1960

108. Kuller L: Sudden death in arteriosclerotic heart disease. Am J Cardiol 24:617, 1969

109. Falk E: Plaque rupture with severe pre-existing stenosis precipitating coronary thrombosis: Characteristics of coronary atherosclerotic plaques underlying fatal occlusive thrombi. Br Heart J 50:127, 1983

110. Warnes CA, Roberts WC: Sudden coronary death: Comparison of patients with to those without coronary thrombus at necropsy. Am J Cardiol 54:1206, 1984

111. Falk E: Unstable angina with fatal outcome: Dynamic coronary thrombosis leading to infarction and/or sudden death: Autopsy evidence of recurrent mural thrombosis with peripheral embolization culminating in total vascular occlusion. Circulation 71:699, 1985

112. Klein LW, Agarwal JB, Herlich MB, et al: Prognosis of symptomatic coronary artery disease in young adults aged 40 years or less. Am J Cardiol 60:1269, 1987

113. Johnson WD, Strong JP, Oalmann MC, et al: Sudden death from coronary artery disease in young men. Arch Pathol Lab Med 105:227, 1981

114. Corrado D, Thiene G, Buja GF, et al: The relationship between growth of atherosclerotic plaques, variant angina and sudden death. Int J Cardiol 26:361, 1990

115. Virmani R, Chun PKC, Goldstein RE, et al: Acute takeoffs of the coronary arteries along the aortic wall and congenital coronary ostial valve-like ridges: Association with sudden death. J Am Coll Cardiol 3:766, 1984.

116. Beuren AJ, Hort W, Kalbfleisch H, et al: Dysplasia of the systemic and pulmonary arterial system with tortuosity and lengthening of the arteries. Circulation 38:109, 1969

117. Thiene G, Ho SY: Aortic root pathology and sudden death in youth: Review of anatomical varieties. Appl Pathol 4:237, 1986

118. Virmani R, Rogan K, Cheitlin MD: Congenital coronary artery anomalies: Pathologic aspects. In: Virmani R, Forman MB (eds). Nonatheroselerotic ischemic heart disease. New York, Raven Press, 1989, p 153

119. Moodie DS, Fyfe D, Gill CC, et al: Anomalous origin of the left coronary artery from the pulmonary artery (Bland-White-Garland syndrome) in adult patients: Long-term follow-up after surgery. Am Heart J 106:381, 1983

120. Cheitlin MD: Sudden death as a complication of anomalous left coronary origin from the anterior sinus of Valsalva. A not-so-minor congenital anomaly. Circulation 50:780, 1974

121. Taylor AJ, Rogan K, Virmani R: Sudden cardiac death associated with isolated congenital coronary artery anomalies. J Am Coll Cardiol 20:640, 1992

122. Barth CW III, Roberts WC: Left main coronary artery originating from the right sinus of Valsalva and coursing between the aorta and pulmonary trunk. J Am Coll Cardiol 7:366, 1986

123. Liberthson RR, Dinsmore RE, Fallon JT: Aberrant coronary artery origin from the aorta: Report of 18 patients, review of the literature and delineation of natural history and management. Circulation 59:748, 1979

124. Steinberger J, Lucas RV, Edwards JE, Titus JL: Causes of sudden unexpected cardiac death in the first two decades of life. Am J Cardiol 77:992, 1996

125. Corrado D, Frescura C, Cocco P, Thiene G: Non-atherosclerotic coronary artery disease and sudden death in the young. Br Heart J 68:601, 1992

126. Frescura C, Basso C, Thiene G, et al: Anomalous origin of coronary arteries and risk of sudden death: A study based on an autopsy population of congenital heart disease. Hum Pathol 29:689, 1998

127. Roberts WC: Major anomalies of coronary arterial origin seen in adulthood. Am Heart J 111:941, 1986

128. Lipsett J, Byard RW, Carpenter BF, et al: Anomalous coronary arteries arising from the aorta associated with sudden death in infancy and early childhood. Arch Pathol Lab Med 115:770, 1991

129. Page HL, Engel HJ, Campbell WB, Thomas CS: Anomalous origin of the left circumflex coronary artery: Recognition, angiographic demonstration and clinical significance. Circulation 50:768, 1974

130. Chaitman BR, Lespérance J, Saltiel J, Bourasse MG: Clinical, angiographic and hemodynamic findings in patients with anomalous origin of the coronary arteries. Circulation 53:122, 1976

131. Murphy D, Roy D, Sohal M, Chandler B: Anomalous origin of the left main coronary artery from anterior sinus of Valsalva with myocardial infarction. J Thorac Cardiovasc Surg 75:282, 1978

132. Corrado D, Pennelli T, Piovesana P, Thiene G: Anomalous origin of the left circumflex coronary artery from the right aortic sinus of Valsalva and sudden death. Cardiovasc Pathol 3:269, 1994

133. Piovesana P, Corrado D, Contessotto F, et al: Echocardiographic identification of anomalous origin of the left circumflex coronary artery from the right aortic sinus of Valsalva. Am Heart J 119:205, 1990

134. Muriago M, Sheppard MN, Ho SY, Anderson RH: The location of the coronary arterial orifices in the normal heart. Clin Anat 10:1, 1997

135. Pelliccia A, Spataro A, Maron BJ: Prospective echocardiographic screening for coronary artery anomalies in 1,360 elite competitive athletes. Am J Cardiol 72:978, 1993

136. Giannoccaro PJ, Sochowski RA, Morton BC, Chan KL: Complementary role of transesophageal echocardiography to coronary angiography in the assessment of coronary artery anomalies. Br Heart J 70:70, 1993

137. Fernandez F, Alan M, Smith S, Khaja F: The role of transesophageal echocardiography in identifying anomalous coronary artereis. Circulation 88:2532, 1993

138. McConnell MV, Ganz P, Selwyn AP, et al: Identification of anomalous coronary arteries and their anatomic course by magnetic resonance coronary angiography. Circulation 92:3158, 1995

139. Post JC, Van Rossum AC, Bronzwear JFC, et al. Magnetic resonance angiography of anomalous coronary arteries: A new gold standard for delineating the proximal course? Circulation 92:3163, 1995

140. Geiringer E: The mural coronary. Am Heart J 41:359, 1951

141. Angelini P, Trivellato M, Donis J, Leachman RD: Myocardial bridges: A review. Prog Cardiovasc 26:75, 1983

142. Polacek P: Relation of myocardial bridges and loops on the coronary arteries to coronary occlusions. Am Heart J 61:44, 1961

143. Feldman AM, Baughman KL: Myocardial infarction associated with a myocardial bridge. Am Heart J 111:784, 1986

144. Vasan RS, Bahl VK, Rajani M: Myocardial infarction associated with a myocardial bridge. Int J Cardiol 25:140, 1989

145. Ciampricotti R, El Gamal M: Vasospastic coronary occlusion associated with a myocardial bridge. Cathet Cardiovasc Diagn 14:118, 1988

146. Faruqui AM, Maloy WC, Felner JM, et al: Symptomatic myocardial bridging of coronary artery. Am J Cardiol 41:1305, 1978

147. Morales AR, Romanelli R, Boucek RJ: The mural left anterior descending coronary artery, strenuous exercise and sudden death. Circulation 62:230, 1980

148. Ferreira AG, Trotter SE, Konig B, et al: Myocardial bridges: Morphological and functional aspects. Br Heart J 66:364, 1991

149. Gori F, Basso C, Thiene G: Myocardial infarction in a patient with hypertrophic cardiomyopathy. N Engl J Med 342:593, 2000

150. Ge J, Erbel R, Rupprecht HJ, et al: Comparison of intravascular ultrasound and angiography in the assessment of myocardial bridging. Circulation 89:1725, 1994

151. Prizel KR, Hutchins GM, Bulkley BH: Coronary artery embolism and myocardial infarction. A clinicopathologic study of 55 patients. Ann Intern Med 88:155, 1978

152. Roberts WC: Coronary embolism: A review of causes, consequences and diagnostic considerations. Cardiovasc Med 3:699, 1978

153. Basso C, Thiene G, Dalla Volta S: Embolia coronarica: Una causa spesso dimenticata di infarto miocardico e morte improvvisa. G Ital Cardiol 22:751, 1992

154. Valente M: Structural profile of cardiac myxoma. Appl Pathol 1:251, 1983

155. Valente M, Basso C, Thiene G, et al: Fibroelastic papilloma: A not so benign cardiac tumor. Cardiovasc Pathol 1:161, 1992

155a. Chan S, Silver MD: Fatal myocardial embolus after myectomy. Can J Cardiol 15:1239, 2000

156. Basso C, Morgagni GL, Thiene G: Spontaneous coronary artery dissection: A neglected cause of acute myocardial ischemia and sudden death. Heart 75:451, 1996

157. Thayer JO, Healy RW, Maggs PR: Spontaneous coronary artery dissection. Ann Thorac Surg 44:97, 1987

158. De Maio S J, Kinsella SH, Silverman ME: Clinical course and long-term prognosis of spontaneous coronary artery dissection. Am J Cardiol 64:471, 1989

159. Jorgensen MB, Aharonian V, Mansukhani P, Mahrer P: Spontaneous coronary dissection: A cluster of cases with this rare finding. Am Heart J 127:1382, 1994

160. Claudon DG, Claudon DB, Edwards JE: Primary dissecting aneurysm of coronary artery. Circulation 45:259, 1972

161. Nalbandian RM, Chason JL: Intramural (intramedial) dissecting hematomas in normal or otherwise unremarkable coronary arteries. Am J Clin Pathol 43:348, 1965

162. Boschetti AE, Levine A: Cystic medionecrosis with dissecting aneurysm of coronary arteries. Arch Intern Med 102:562, 1958

163. Kaufman G, Englebrecht WJ: Hemorrhagic intramedial dissection of coronary artery with cystic medial necrosis. Am J Cardiol 24:409, 1969

164. Barrett DL: Isolated dissecting aneurysm of the coronary artery: Report of a case apparently due to hypersensitivity angiitis. Ohio State Med J 65:830, 1969

165. Robinowitz M, Virmani R, McAllister H: Spontaneous coronary artery dissection and eosinophilic inflammation: A cause and effect relationship? Am J Med 72:923, 1982

166. Dowling GP, Buja LM: Spontaneous coronary artery dissection occurs with and without periadventitial inflammation. Arch Pathol Lab Med 111:470, 1987

167. Ascuncion CM, Hyun J: Dissecting intramural hematoma of the coronary artery in pregnancy and the puerperium. Obstet Gynecol 40:202, 1972

168. Shaver PJ, Carring TF, Baker WP: Postpartum coronary artery dissection. Br Heart J 40:83, 1978

169. Jewitt JF: Two dissecting coronary artery aneurysms postpartum. N Engl J Med 298:1255, 1979

170. Palomino SJ: Dissecting intramural hematoma of the left coronary artery in the puerperium. Am J Clin Pathol 51:119, 1969

171. Bac DJ, Lotgering FK, Verkaaik APK, Deckers JW: Spontaneous coronary artery dissection during pregnancy and postpartum. Eur Heart J 16:136, 1995

172. Melish ME: Kawasaki syndrome (the mucocutaneous lymph node syndrome). Ann Rev Med 33:569, 1982

173. Byard RW, Jimenez CL, Carpenter BF, et al: Four unusual cases of sudden and unexpected cardiovascular death in infancy and childhood. Med Sci Law 31:157, 1991

174. Fujiwara H, Fujiwara T, Ohshio G, Hamashima Y: Pathology of Kawasaki disease in the healed stage: Relationships between typical and atypical cases of Kawasaki disease. Acta Pathol Jpn 36:857, 1986

175. Wreford FS, Conradi SE, Cohle SD, et al: Sudden death caused by coronary artery aneurysms: A late complication of Kawasaki disease. J Forensic Sci 36:51, 1991

176. Lupi-Herrera E, Sanchez-Torres G, Marcushamer J, et al: Takayasu's arteritis: Clinical study of 107 cases. Am Heart J 93:94, 1977

177. Amano J, Suzuki A: Coronary artery involvement in Takayasu's arteritis. Collective review and guidelines for surgical treatment. J Thorac Cardiovasc Surg 102:554, 1991

178. Cipriano PR, Silverman JF, Perlroth MG, et al: Coronary arterial narrowing in Takayasu's aortitis. Am J Cardiol 39:744, 1977

179. Basso C, Baracca E, Zonzin P, Thiene G: Sudden cardiac arrest in a teenager as first manifestation of Takayasu's disease. Int J Cardiol 43:87, 1994

180. Lie JT, Failoni DD, Davis DC: Temporal arteritis with giant cell aortitis, coronary arteritis and myocardial infarction. Arch Pathol Lab Med 110:857, 1986

181. Holsinger DR, Osmundson PJ, Edwards JE: The heart in periarteritis nodosa. Circulation 25:610, 1962

182. Ohno H, Matsuda Y, Takashiba K, et al: Acute myocardial infarction in Buerger's disease. Am J Cardiol 57:690, 1986

183. Donatelli F, Triggiani M, Nascimbene S, et al: Thromboangiitis obliterans of coronary and internal thoracic arteries in a young woman. J Thorac Cardiovasc Surg 113:800, 1997

184. Thiene G, Valente M, Rossi L: Involvement of the cardiac conduction system in panarteritis nodosa. Am Heart J 95:716, 1978

185. Hofmann T, Meinertz T, Kasper W, et al: Mode of death in idiopathic dilated cardiomyopathy: A multivariate analysis of prognostic determinants. Am Heart J 116:1455, 1988

186. Roberts WC, Siegel RJ, McManus: Idiopathic dilated cardiomyopathy: Analysis of 152 necropsy patients. Am J Cardiol 60:1340, 1987

187. Fuster V, Gersh BJ, Giuliani ER, et al: The natural history of idiopathic dilated cardiomyopathy. Am J Cardiol 47:525, 1981

188. McKenna WJ, Goodwin JF: The natural history of hypertrophic cardiomyopathy. In: Harvey P (ed): Current Problems in Cardiology. Vol 6. Chicago, Year Book Medical Publishers, 1981, p 5

189. McKenna WJ, Camm AJ: Sudden death in hypertrophic cardiomyopathy: Assessment of patients at high risk. Circulation 80:1489, 1989

190. Maron BJ, Roberts WJ, Epstein SE: Sudden death in hypertrophic cardiomyopathy: A profile of 78 patients. Circulation 67:1388, 1982

191. McKenna WJ, Deanfield J, Faruqui A, et al: Prognosis in hypertrophic cardiomyopathy: Role of age and clinical, electrocardiographic and hemodynamic features. Am J Cardiol 47:532, 1981

192. Maron BJ, Fananapazir L: Sudden death in hypertrophic cardiomyopathy. Circulation 85:I:57, 1992

193. McKenna WJ, Deanfield JE: Hypertrophic cardiomyopathy. An important cause of sudden death. Arch Dis Child 59:971, 1984

194. Maron BJ, Lipson LC, Roberts WC, et al: Malignant hypertrophic cardiomyopathy: Identification of a subgroup of families with unusually frequent premature death. Am J Cardiol 41:1133, 1978

195. Dilsizian V, Bonow RO, Epstein SE, Fananapazir L: Myocardial ischemia detected by thallium scintigraphy is frequently related to cardiac arrest and syncope in young patients with hypertrophic cardiomyopathy. J Am Coll Cardiol 22:796, 1993

196. Fananapazir L, Chang AC, Epstein SE, McAreavy D: Prognostic determinants in hypertrophic cardiomyopathy: Prospective evaluation of a therapeutic strategy based on clinical, holter, hemodynamic and electrophysiological findings. Circulation 86:730, 1992

197. Maron BJ, Savage DD, Wolfson JK, Epstein SE: Prognostic significance of 24 hour ambulatory electrocardiographic monitoring in patients with hypertrophic cardiomyopathy: A prospective study. Am J Cardiol 48:252, 1981

198. Spirito P, Seidman CE, McKenna WJ, Maron BJ: The management of hypertrophic cardiomyopathy. N Engl J Med 336:775, 1997

199. Marian AJ, Mares A Jr, Kelly DP, et al: Sudden cardiac death in hypertrophic cardiomyopathy: Variability in phenotypic expression of beta-myosin heavy chain mutations. Eur Heart J 16:368, 1995

200. Marian AJ, Roberts WC: Recent advances in the molecular genetics of hypertrophic cardiomyopathy. Circulation 92:1336, 1995

201. Marian AJ: Sudden cardiac death in patients with hypertrophic cardiomyopathy: From bench to bedside with an emphasis on genetic markers. Clin Cardiol 18:189, 1995

202. Watkins H, Rosenzweig A, Hwang D, et al: Characteristics and prognostic implications of myosin missense mutations in familial hypertrophic cardiomyopathy. N Engl J Med 326:1108, 1992

203. Epstein ND, Cohn GM, Cyran F, Fananapazir L: Differences in clinical expression of hypertrophic cardiomyopathy associated with two distinct mutations in the beta myosin heavy chain gene: A 908 Leu-Val mutation and a 403 Arg-Gln mutation. Circulation 86:345, 1992

204. Fananapazir L, Epstein ND: Genotype-phenotype correlations in hypertrophic cardiomyopathy: Insights provided by comparisons of kindreds with distinct and identical beta-myosin heavy chain gene mutations. Circulation 89:22, 1994

205. Maron BJ, Roberts WC: Quantitative analysis of cardiac muscle cell disorganization in the ventricular septum of patients with hypertrophic cardiomyopathy. Circulation 59:689, 1979

206. Maron BJ, Anan TJ, Roberts WC: Quantitative analysis of the distribution of cardiac muscle cell disorganization in the left ventricular wall of patients with hypertrophic cardiomyopathy. Circulation 63:882, 1981

207. Maron BJ, Epstein SE, Roberts WC: Hypertrophic cardiomyopathy and transmural myocardial infarction without significant atherosclerosis of the extramural coronary arteries. Am J Cardiol 43:1086, 1979

208. Maron BJ, Wolfson JK, Epstein SE, Roberts WC: Intramural ("small vessel") coronary artery disease in hypertrophic cardiomyopathy. J Am Coll Cardiol 8:545, 1986

209. Krikler DM, Davies MJ, Rowland E, et al: Sudden death in hyper-

trophic cardiomyopathy: Associated accessory atrioventricular pathways. Br Heart J 43:245, 1980

210. Angelini A, Calzolari V, Thiene G, et al: Morphologic spectrum of primary restrictive cardiomyopathy. Am J Cardiol 80:1046, 1997

211. Richardson P, McKenna WJ, Bristow M, et al: Report of the 1995 WHO/ISFC Task Force on the definition and classification of cardiomyopathies. Circulation 93:841, 1996

212. Nava A, Rossi L, Thiene G. (eds): Arrhythmogenic right ventricular cardiomyopathy/dysplasia. Amsterdam, Elsevier, 1997

213. Thiene G, Nava A, Corrado D, et al: Right ventricular cardiomyopathy and sudden death in young people. N Engl J Med 318:129, 1988

214. Marcus FI, Fontaine G, Guiraudon G, et al: Right ventricular dysplasia. A report of 24 adult cases. Circulation 65:384, 1982

215. Lobo FV, Heggtveit HA, Butany J, Silver MD, Edwards JE: Right ventricular dysplasia: Morphological findings in 13 cases. Can J Cardiol 8:261, 1992

216. Basso C, Thiene G, Corrado D, et al: Arrhythmogenic right ventricular cardiomyopathy: Dysplasia, dystrophy, or myocarditis? Circulation 94:983, 1996

217. Corrado D, Basso C, Thiene G, et al: The spectrum of clinico-pathologic manifestations of arrhythmogenic right ventricular cardiomyopathy/dysplasia. A Multicenter Study. J Am Coll Cardiol 30:1512, 1997

217a. Lobo F, Silver MD, Butany J, Heggtviet HA: Left ventricular involvement in right ventricular dysplasia/cardiomyopathy. Can J Cardiol 15:139, 1999

218. Thiene G, Corrado D, Nava A, et al: Right ventricular cardiomyopathy: Is there evidence of an inflammatory aetiology? Eur Heart J 12(suppl D):22, 1991

219. Mallat Z, Tedgui A, Fontaliran F, et al: Evidence of apoptosis in arrhythmogenic right ventricular dysplasia. N Engl J Med 335:1190, 1996

220. Valente M, Calabrese F, Thiene G, et al: In vivo evidence of apoptosis in arrhythmogenic right ventricular cardiomyopathy. Am J Pathol 152:479, 1998

221. Nava A, Scognamiglio R, Thiene G, et al: A polymorphic form of familial arrhythmogenic right ventricular dysplasia. Am J Cardiol 59:1405, 1987

222. Nava A, Thiene G, Canciani B, et al: Familial occurrence of right ventricular dysplasia. A study involving nine families. J Am Coll Cardiol 12:122, 1988

223. Rampazzo A, Nava A, Danieli GA, et al: The gene for arrhythmogenic right ventricular cardiomyopathy maps to chromosome 14q23–q24. Hum Mol Genet 3:959, 1994

224. Rampazzo A, Nava A, Erne P, et al: A new locus for arrhythmogenic right ventricular cardiomyopathy (ARVD2) maps to chromosome 1q42–q43. Hum Mol Genet 4:2151, 1995

225. Rampazzo A, Nava A, Miorin M, et al: ARVD4 a new locus for arrhythmogenic right ventricular cardiomyopathy, maps to chromosome 2 long arm. Genomics 45:259, 1997

226. Severini GM, Krajinovic M, Pinamonti B, et al: A new locus for arrhythmogenic right ventricular dysplasia on the long arm of chromosome 14. Genomics 31:193, 1996

227. Thiene G, Basso C, Danieli GA, et al: Arrhythmogenic right ventricular cardiomyopathy: A still underrecognized clinical entity. Trends Cardiovasc Med 7:84, 1997

228. Corrado D, Thiene G, Nava A, et al: Sudden death in young competitive athletes: Clinico-pathologic correlations in 22 cases. Am J Med 89:588, 1990

229. Corrado D, Basso C, Thiene G: Pathological findings in victims of sport-related sudden cardiac death. Sports Exerc Injury 2:78, 1996

230. Frank R, Fontaine G, Vedel J, et al: Electrocardiologie de quatre cas de dysplasie ventriculaire droite arythmogène. Arch Mal Coeur Vaiss 71:963, 1978

231. Marcus FI, Fontaine G: Arrhythmogenic right ventricular dysplasia/cardiomyopathy: A review. Pacing Clin Electrophysiol 18:1298, 1995

232. McKenna WJ, Thiene G, Nava A, et al: Diagnosis of arrhythmogenic right ventricular dysplasia/cardiomyopathy. Br Heart J 71:215, 1994

233. Blomström-Lundqvist C, Beckman-Surküla M; Wallentin I, et al: Ventricular dimensions and wall motion assessed by echocardiog-

raphy in patients with arrhythmogenic right ventricular dysplasia. Eur Heart J 9:1291, 1988

234. Scognamiglio R, Fasoli G, Nava A, et al: Contribution of cross-sectional echocardiography to the diagnosis of right ventricular dysplasia at the asymptomatic stage. Eur Heart J 10:538, 1989

235. Daubert C, Descaves C, Foulgoc JL, et al: Critical analysis of cineangiographic criteria for diagnosis of arrhythmogenic right ventricular dysplasia. Am Heart J 115:448, 1988

236. Daliento L, Rizzoli G, Thiene G, et al: Diagnostic accuracy of right ventriculography in arrhythmogenic right ventricular cardiomyopathy. Am J Cardiol 66:741, 1990

237. Menghetti L, Basso C, Nava A, et al: Spin-echo nuclear magnetic resonance for tissue characterization in arrhythmogenic right ventricular cardiomyopathy. Heart 76:467, 1996

238. Auffermann W, Wichter T, Breithhardt G, et al: Arrhythmogenic right ventricular disease: MR imaging vs angiography. Am J Radiol 161:549, 1993

239. Ricci C, Longo P, Pagnan L, et al: Magnetic resonance imaging in right ventricular dysplasia. Am J Cardiol 70:1589, 1992

240. Blake LM, Sheinmann MM, Higgins CB: Magnetic resonance features of arrhythmogenic right ventricular dysplasia. Am J Radiol 162:809, 1994

241. Angelini A, Thiene G, Boffa GM, et al: Endomyocardial biopsy in right ventricular cardiomyopathy. Int J Cardiol 40:273, 1993

242. Angelini A, Basso C, Nava A, Thiene G: Endomyocardial biopsy in arrhythmogenic right ventricular cardiomyopathy. Am Heart J 132:203, 1996

243. Frustaci A, Bellocci F, Olsen EGJ: Results of biventricular endomyocardial biopsy in survivors of cardiac arrest with apparently normal hearts. Am J Cardiol 74:890, 1994

244. Zeppilli P, Santini C, Palmieri V, et al: Role of myocarditis in athletes with minor arrhythmias and/or echocardiographic abnormalities. Chest 106:373, 1994

245. Virmani R, Roberts WC: Sudden cardiac death. Hum Pathol 18:485, 1987

246. Topaz O, Edwards JE: Pathologic features of sudden death in children, adolescents, and young adults. Chest 87:476, 1985

247. Wesslén L, Pahlson C, Lindquist O, et al. An increase in sudden unexpected cardiac deaths among young Swedish orienteers during 1979–1992. Eur Heart J 17:902, 1996

248. Neuspiel DR, Kuller LH: Sudden and unexpected natural death in childhood and adolescence. JAMA 254:1321, 1985

249. Molander M: Sudden natural death in later childhood and adolescence. Arch Dis Child 57:572, 1982

250. Phillips MP, Robinowtz M, Higgins JR, et al: Sudden cardiac death in Air Force recruits. JAMA 256:2696, 1986

251. Shirani J, Freant LJ, Roberts WC: Gross and semiquantitative histologic findings in mononuclear cell myocarditis causing sudden death, and implications for endomyocardial biopsy. Am J Cardiol 72:952, 1993

252. Maron BJ, Roberts WC, McAllister MA, et al: Sudden death in young athletes. Circulation 62:218, 1980

253. Wood P: Aortic stenosis. Am J Cardiol 1:553, 1958

254. Marcus ML, Doty DB, Hiratzka LF, et al: Decreased coronary reserve: A mechanism for angina pectoris in patients with aortic stenosis and normal coronary arteries. N Engl J Med 307:1362, 1982

255. Doyle EF, Aurumugham P, Lara E, et al: Sudden death in young patients with congenital aortic stenosis. Pediatrics 53:481, 1974

256. Klein CR: Ventricular arrhythmias in aortic valve disease: Analysis of 102 patients. Am J Cardiol 53:1079, 1984

257. Schwarts LS, Goldfischer J, Sprague GJ, Schartz SP: Syncope and sudden death in aortic stenosis. Am J Cardiol 23:647, 1969

258. Turri M, Thiene G, Bortolotti U, et al: Surgical pathology of aortic valve disease. A study based on 602 specimens. Eur J Cardiothorac Surg 4:556, 1990

259. Angelini A, Basso C, Grassi G, et al: Surgical pathology of valve disease in the elderly. Aging Clin Exp Res 6:225, 1994

260. Cheitlin MD, Fenoglio JJ, McAllister HA, et al: Congenital aortic stenosis secondary to dysplasia of congenital bicuspid aortic valve without commissural fusion. Am J Cardiol 42:102, 1978

261. Ellis FH, Kirklin JW: Congenital valvular aortic stenosis: Anatomic findings and surgical techniques. J Thorac Cardiovasc Surg 43:199, 1962

262. Pomerance A: Pathogenesis of aortic stenosis and its relation to age. Br Heart J 34:569, 1972

263. Williams JCP, Barratt Boyes BG, Lowe JB: Supravalvular aortic stenosis. Circulation 24:1311, 1961

264. Morrow AG, Waldhausen JA, Peters RL, et al: Supravalvular aortic stenosis. Clinical, hemodynamic and pathologic observations. Circulation 20:1003, 1959

265. Jeresaty RM: Mitral valve prolapse: Definition and implications in athletes. J Am Coll Cardiol 7:231, 1986

266. Cobbs BW, King SB: Ventricular buckling: A factor in the normal ventriculogram and peculiar hemodynamics associated with mitral valve prolapse. Am Heart J 93:741, 1977

267. Criley JM, Zeilinga DW, Morgan MT: Mitral dysfunction: A possible cause of arrhythmias in the prolapsing mitral leaflet syndrome. Trans Am Clin Climatol Assoc 85:44, 1973

268. Salazar AE, Edwards JE: Friction lesions of ventricular endocardium: Relation to chordae tendineae of mitral valve. Arch Pathol 90:364, 1970

269. Kligfield P, Levy D, Devereux RB, Savage DD: Arrhythmias and sudden death in mitral valve prolapse. Am Heart J 113:1316, 1987

270. Boudoulas H, Kolibash AJ, Baker P, et al: Mitral valve prolapse and the mitral valve prolapse syndrome: A diagnostic classification and pathogenesis of symptoms. Am Heart J 118:796, 1989

271. Puddu PE, Pasternac A, Tubau JF, et al: QT interval prolongation and increased plasma catecholamine levels in patients with mitral valve prolapse. Am Heart J 105:422, 1983

272. Crawford MH, O'Rourke RA: Mitral valve prolapse: A cardiomyopathic state? Prog Cardiovasc Dis 27:133, 1984

273. Scamparadonis G, Yang SS, Maranhas V: Left ventricular abnormalities in prolapsed mitral leaflet syndrome: A review of 87 cases. Circulation 48:287, 1973

274. Gulotta SJ, Guico L, Padmanabhman V, Miller S: The syndrome of systolic click, murmur and mitral valve prolapse-cardiomyopathy. Circulation 49:717, 1974

275. Bharati S, Granston AS, Liebson PR, et al: The conduction system in mitral valve prolapse syndrome with sudden death. Am Heart J 101:667, 1981

276. Bharati S, Rosen KM, Miller LB, et al: Sudden death in three teenagers (abstract). Circulation 64(suppl IV):72, 1981

277. Corrado D, Basso C, Nava A, et al: Sudden death in young people with apparently isolated mitral valve prolapse. G Ital Cardiol 27:1097, 1997

278. Martini B, Basso C, Thiene G: Sudden death in mitral valve prolapse with Holter monitoring-documented ventricular fibrillation: evidence of coexisting arrhythmogenic right ventricular cardiomyopathy. Int J Cardiol 49:274, 1995

279. Watson H: Natural history of Ebstein's anomaly of tricuspid valve in childhhod and adolescence: An international cooperative study of 505 cases. Br Heart J 36:417, 1974

280. Lev M, Gibson S, Miller R: Ebstein's disease with Wolff-Parkinson-White syndrome. Report of a case with histopathologic study of possible conduction patways. Am Heart J 49:724, 1955

281. Smith WM, Gallagher JJ, Kerr CR, et al; The electrophysiologic basis and management of symptomatic recurrent tachycardia in patients with Ebstein's anomaly of the tricuspid valve. Am J Cardiol 49:1223, 1955

282. Thiene G, Pennelli N, Rossi L: Cardiac conduction system abnormalities as a possible cause of sudden death in young athletes. Hum Pathol 14:704, 1983

283. Rossi L, Thiene G: Mild Ebstein's anomaly associated with supraventricular tachycardia and sudden death: Clinicomorphologic features in 3 patients. Am J Cardiol 53:332, 1984

284. Rossi L: Neuroanatomopathology of the cardiovascular system. In: Kulbertus H, Franck G (eds): Neurocardiology. Mount Kisko, NY, Futura, 1988, p 25

285. Rossi L: Histopathology of Cardiac Arrhythmias. 2nd ed. Milan, Casa Editrice Ambrosiana, 1978

286. Kyrickidis M, Barbetseas J, Antonopoulos A, et al: Early atrial arrhythmias in acute myocardial infarction: Role of the sinus node artery. Chest 101:944, 1992

287. Rossi L, Thiene G, Caregaro L, et al: Dysrhythmias and sudden death in acromegalic heart disease. A clinicopathologic study. Chest 72:495, 1977

288. James TN: Pericarditis and the sinus node. Arch Intern Med 110:301, 1962

289. Kostuk WJ, Beanlands DS: Complete heart block associated with acute myocardial infarction. Am J Cardiol 26:380, 1970

290. Mavric Z, Zaputovic L, Matana A, et al: Prognostic significance of complete atrioventricular block in patients with acute inferior myocardial infarction with and without right ventricular involvement. Am Heart J 119:823, 1990

291. Becker AE, Lie KI, Anderson RH: Bundle-branch block in the setting of acute anteroseptal myocardial infarction. Clinico-pathologic correlation. Br Heart J 40:773, 1978

292. Hindman MC, Wagner GS, Jaro M, et al: The clinical significance of bundle branch block complicating acute myocardial infarction. 1. Clinical characteristics, hospital mortality and 1 year follow-up. Circulation 58:679, 1978

293. Rossi L: Occurrence and significance of coagulative myocytolysis in the specialized conduction system: Clinicopathologic observations. Am J Cardiol 45:757, 1980

294. Lenegre T: Aetiology and pathology of bilateral bundle branch fibrosis in relation to complete heart block. Prog Cardiovasc Dis 6:409, 1964

295. Lev M, Bharati S: Lesions of the conduction system and their functional significance. Pathol Annu 9:157, 1974

296. Rossi L, Piffer R, Turolla E, et al: Multifocal Purkinje tumor of the heart. Occurrence with other anatomic abnormalities in the atrioventricular junction of an infant with junctional tachycardia, Lown-Ganong-Levine Syndrome and sudden death. Chest 87:340, 1985

297. James TN, Carlson DJL, Marshall TK: De subitaneis mortibus. I. Fibroma compressing His bundle. Circulation 48:428, 1973

298. James TN: Chance and sudden death. J Am Coll Cardiol 1:164,1983

299. James TW. Morphology of the human atrioventricular node, with remarks pertinent to its electrophysiology. Am Heart J 62:756, 1961

300. Brechenmacher C. Atrio-His bundle tracts. Br Heart J 37:853, 1975

301. Mahaim U, Benatt A: Nouvelles recherches sur les connexions superieures de la branche gauche du faisceau de His-Tawara avec le cloison interventriculaire. Cardiologia 1:161, 1938

302. Kent AFS: Research on the structure and function of the mammalian heart. J Physiol 14:233, 1893

303. Anderson RH, Becker AF, Brechenmacher C, et al: Ventricular preexcitation. A proposed nomenclature for its substrates. Eur J Cardiol 3:27, 1975

304. Wood BC, Wolferth CC, Geckeler GD: Histologic demonstrations of accessory muscular connections between auricle and ventricle in a case of short PR interval and prolonged QRS complex. Am Heart J 25:454, 1943

305. Wolff L, Parkinson J, White PD: Bundle branch block with short PR interval in healthy young people prone to paroxysmal tachycardia. Am Heart J 5:685, 1930

306. Hiss RG, Lamb LE: Electrocardiographic findings in 122,043 individuals. Circulation 25:947, 1962

307. Guize L, Soria R, Chaouat JC, et al: Prevalence and course of Wolff-Parkinson-White syndrome in a population of 138,048 subjects. Ann Med Interne (Paris) 136:474, 1985

308. Munger TM, Packer DL, Hammil SC, et al: A population study of the natural history of Wolff-Parkinson-White syndrome in Olmsted County Minnesota, 1953–1989. Circulation 87:866, 1993

309. Klein GJ, Prystowsky EN, Yee R, et al: Asymptomatic Wolff-Parkinson-White: Should we intervene? Circulation 80:1902, 1989

310. Leitch JW, Klein GJ, Yee R, et al: The prognostic value of electrophysiologic testing in asymptomatic patients with Wolff-Parkinson-White pattern. Circulation 82:1718, 1989

311. Klein GJ, Bashore TM, Sellers TD, et al: Ventricular fibrillation in the Wolff-Parkinson-White syndrome. N Engl J Med 301:1080, 1979

312. Wellens HJJ, Durrer D: Wolff-Parkinson-White syndrome and atrial fibrillation. Am J Cardiol 34:777, 1974

313. Wellens HJJ, Bar FW, Farre J, et al: Sudden death in the Wolff-Parkinson-White syndrome. In: Kulbertus H, Wellens HJJ (eds): Sudden Death. Boston, Martinus Nijhoff, 1980, p 392

314. Lown B, Ganong WF, Levine SA: The syndrome of short PR

interval QRS complex and paroxysmal rapid heart action. Circulation 5:693, 1952

315. Ometto R, Thiene G, Corrado D, et al: Enhanced AV nodal conduction (Lown-Ganong-Levine syndrome) by congenitally hypoplastic AV node. Eur Heart J 13:1579, 1992

316. Consensus statement of the Joint Steering Committees of the UCARE and of the Idiopathic Ventricular Fibrillation Registry of the United States. Survivors of out-of-hospital cardiac arrest with apparently normal heart. Need for definition and standardized clinical evaluation. Circulation 95:265, 1997

317. Corrado D, Basso C, Angelini A, Thiene G: Sudden arrhythmic death in young people with apparently normal heart. Eur Heart J 17:589, 1996

318. Trappe HJ, Brugada P, Talajic M, et al: Prognosis of patients with ventricular tachycardia and fibrillation: Role of underlying etiology. J Am Coll Cardiol 12:166, 1988

319. Poole JE, Mathisen TL, Kudenchuk PJ, et al: Long-term outcome in patients who survive out of hospital ventricular fibrillation and undergo electrophysiologic studies: Evaluation by electrophysiologic subgroups. J Am Coll Cardiol 16:657, 1990

320. Schwartz PJ, Locati EH, Napolitano C, Priori SG: The long QT syndrome. In: Zipes DP, Jalife J (eds): Cardiac Electrophysiology: From Cell to Bedside. 2nd ed. Philadelphia, WB Saunders, 1995, p 788

321. Keating M, Atkinson D, Dunn C, et al: Linkage of a cardiac arrhythmia, the long QT syndrome and the Harvey ras-1 gene. Science 252:704, 1991

322. Jiang C, Atkinson D, Towbin JA, et al: Two long QT syndrome loci map to chromosomes 3 and 7 with evidence for further heterogeneity. Nature Genet 8:141, 1994

323. Schott JJ, Charpantier F, Pettier S, et al: Mapping of a gene for long QT syndrome to chromosome 4q25-27. Am J Hum Genet 57: 1114, 1995

324. Brugada P, Brugada J: Right bundle branch block, persistent ST segment elevation and sudden cardiac death: A distinct clinical and electrocardiographic syndrome. J Am Coll Cardiol 20:1391, 1992

325. Chen Q, Kirsch GE, Zhang D, et al: Genetic basis and molecular mechanism for idiopathic ventricular fibrillation. Nature 392:293, 1998

326. Martini B, Nava A, Thiene G, et al: Ventricular fibrillation without apparent heart disease: Description of six cases. Am Heart J 118: 1203, 1989

327. Corrado D, Nava A, Buja G, et al: Familial cardiomyopathy underlies syndrome of right bundle branch block, ST segment elevation and sudden death. J Am Coll Cardiol 27:443, 1996

328. Roine R, Luurila OJ, Suokas A, et al: Alcohol and sauna bathing: Effects on cardiac rhythm, blood pressure, and serum electrolyte and cortisol concentrations. J Intern Med 231:333, 1992

329. Jokinen E, Valimaki I: Children in sauna: Electrocardiographic abnormalities. Acta Paediatr Scand 80:370, 1991

330. Rajs J, Rajs E, Lundman T: Unexpected death in patients suffering from eating disorders. Acta Psychiatr Scand 74:587, 1986

331. Kambara H, Kinoshita M, Nakagawa M, et al: Sudden death among 1000 patients with myocardial infarction: Incidence and contributory factors. J Cardiol 25:55, 1995.

332. Calzolari V, Angelini A, Basso C, et al: Histologic findings in the conduction system after cardiac transplantation and correlation with electrocardiographic findings. Am J Cardiol 84:765, 1999

333. Gallo P, Agozzino L, Arbustini E, et al: Immediate causes of death in short term surviving heart transplant recipients. Cardiovasc Pathol 3:273, 1994

334. Burke AP, Farb A, Sessums L, et al: Causes of sudden cardiac death in patients with replacement valves: An autopsy study. J Heart Valve Dis 3:10, 1994

335. Dunningan A, Pritzker MR, Benditt DG, et al: Life threatening ventricular tachycardia in late survivors of surgically corrected tetralogy of Fallot. Am J Cardiol 46:635, 1980

336. Deanfield JE, Ho SY, Anderson RH, et al: Late sudden death after repair of tetralogy of Fallot: A clinicopathologic study. Circulation 67:626, 1983

337. Murphy JG, Gersh BJ, Mair DD, et al: Long-term outcome in patients undergoing surgical repair of tetralogy of Fallot. N Engl J Med 329:593, 1993

338. Gillette PC, Kugler, JD, Garson A, et al: Mechanism of cardiac

339. Stelling JA, Danford DA, Kugler JD, et al: Late potentials and inducible ventricular tachycardia in surgically repaired congenital heart disease. Circulation 82:1690, 1990

340. Thiene G, Wenink AG, Frescura C, et al: Surgical anatomy and pathology of the conduction tissue in atrioventricular defects. J Thorac Cardiovasc Surg 82:928, 1981

341. Titus JL, Daugherty GW, Edwards JE: Anatomy of the atrioventricular conduction system in ventricular septal defect. Circulation 28:72, 1963

342. Okoroma EO, Guller B, Maloney JD, Weidman WH: Etiology of right bundle branch block pattern after surgical repair of ventricular septal defects. Am Heart J 90:14, 1975

343. Anderson RH, Ho SY: The morphologic substrates for pediatric arrhythmias. Cardiol Young 1:159, 1991

344. Garson A, Randall DG, McVery P, et al: Prevention of sudden death after repair of tetralogy of Fallot: Treatment of ventricular arrhythmias. J Am Coll Cardiol 6:221, 1985

345. Janosek J, Paul T, Bartakova H: Role of late potentials in identifying patients at risk for ventricular tachycardia after surgical correction of congenital heart disease. Am J Cardiol 75:146, 1995

346. Vetter VL, Horowitz LN: Electrophysiologic residua and sequelae of surgery for congenital heart defects. Am J Cardiol 50:588, 1982

347. Rosing DR, Borer JS, Went KM, et al: Long term hemodynamic and electrocardiographic assessment following operative repair of tetralogy of Fallot. Circulation 58:1, 1978

348. Kirklin JW, Barratt-Boyes BG (eds): Cardiac Surgery. New York, Wiley & Sons, 1986

349. Horowitz LN, Vetter VL, Harken AH, Josephson ME: Electrophysiologic characteristics of sustained ventricular tachycardia after repair of tetralogy of Fallot. Am J Cardiol 46:436, 1980

350. Garson A, Porter CBJ, Gillette PC, McNamara DG: Induction of ventricular tachycardia during electrophysiologic study after repair of tetralogy of Fallot. J Am Coll Cardiol 1:1493, 1983

351. Daliento L, Caneve F, Turrini P, et al: Clinical significance of high-frequency, low-amplitude electrocardiographic signals and QT dispersion in patients operated on for tetralogy of Fallot. Am J Cardiol 76:408, 1997

352. Maron BJ, Epstein SE, Roberts WC: Causes of sudden death in competitive athletes. J Am Coll Cardiol 7:204, 1986

353. Maron BJ, Shirani J, Poliac LC, et al: Sudden death in young competitive athletes. Clinical, demographic, and pathological profiles. JAMA 276:199, 1996.

354. Corrado D, Basso C, Schiavon M, Thiene G: Screening for hypertrophic cardiomyopathy in young athletes. N Engl J Med 339:364, 1998

355. Burke AP, Farb A, Virmani R, et al: Sports-related and non-sports-related sudden cardiac death in young adults. Am Heart J 121:568, 1991

356. Pelliccia A, Maron BJ: Preparticipation cardiovascular evaluation of the competitive athlete: Perspectives from the 30-year Italian experience. Am J Cardiol 75:827, 1995

357. Maron BJ, Mitchell JH: 26th Bethesda Conference recommendations for detecting eligibility for competition in athletes with cardiovascular abnormalities. J Am Coll Cardiol 24:845, 1994

358. Maron BJ, Pelliccia A, Spirito P: Cardiac disease in young trained athletes. Insights into methods for distinguishing athlete's heart from structural heart disease, with particular emphasis on hypertrophic cardiomyopathy. Circulation 82:1995, 1990

359. O'Rourke RA: Coronary artery surgery for the prevention and treatment of sudden cardiac death. In: Akhtar M, Myerburg RJ, Ruskin JN (eds): Sudden Cardiac Death. Philadelphia, Williams & Wilkins, 1994

360. Sigwart U: Non-surgical myocardial reduction for hypertrophic obstructive cardiomyopathy. Lancet 346:211, 1995

361. Moss AJ, McDonald J: Unilateral cervicothoracic sympathetic ganglionectomy for the treatment of long QT interval syndrome. N Engl J Med 285:903, 1970

362. Prystowski EN, Knilans TK: Serial electrophysiological-electropharmacological testing in survivors of cardiac arrest. In: Akhtar M, Myerburg RJ, Ruskin JN (eds): Sudden Cardiac Death. Philadelphia, Williams & Wilkins, 1994

363. Lehmann MH, Steinman RT, Meissner MD: Comparison of therapeutic modalities for preventing sudden cardiac death in patients with sustained ventricular tachyarrhythmias. In: Akhtar M, Myerburg RJ, Ruskin JN (eds): Sudden Cardiac Death. Philadelphia, Williams & Wilkins, 1994

364. Burn J, Camm J, Davies MJ, et al: The phenotype/genotype relation and the current status of genetic screening in hypertrophic cardiomyopathy, Marfan syndrome and the long QT syndrome. Heart 78:110, 1997

Chapter 12

The Pericardium and Its Diseases

. . . . .
J. Butany • A. Woo

The pericardium forms a fibrous sac in which the heart is suspended (Fig. 12-1). Hippocrates first described the normal pericardium as "a smooth mantle surrounding the heart and containing a small amount of fluid resembling urine."[1] It does not appear to be essential for life, since its congenital absence or surgical removal does not usually produce significant adverse effects. Yet, laboratory studies provide convincing evidence that the pericardium influences the heart's function. It serves as a barrier against infection or neoplasm spreading from adjacent organs, holds the heart in a fixed geometric position, prevents acute dilation of cardiac chambers, and plays a role in the distribution of hydrostatic forces on the heart and the diastolic coupling of the cardiac chambers.[2] The stabilizing influence of the pericardium and the effects of changes in its structure on cardiac function are related to its anatomic structure, relations, and attachments and the fact that it is composed of relatively inextensible tissues.

This chapter presents the anatomy and histology of the pericardium (see Chapters 1 and 2 also), and discusses pericardial fluid, the response of the pericardium to injury, and specific pathologic conditions.

ANATOMY

The pericardium is a two-layered sac composed of a thick, fibrous outer layer and a thin, inner serous layer.

The serous layer consists of a single layer of mesothelial cells. It encases the outer surface of the heart to form the visceral pericardium and is separated from the myocardium in some areas (e.g., atrioventricular and interventricular sulci) by a layer of fibrofatty tissue of variable thickness. With increasing body weight, fat deposition becomes prominent in these areas and may extend over the adjacent surface of the heart. The mesothelial cell layer reflects upon itself, lines the outer fibrous layer, and forms the parietal pericardium. This is so because the heart invaginates the pericardial sac during fetal development. The pericardial sac normally contains 15 to 50 ml of clear, straw-colored serous fluid.

The reflection of the pericardium onto the great vessels forms two sinuses (Fig. 12-2; see Fig. 1-1): (1) the *oblique* sinus, a blind space bounded by the left atrium, the four pulmonary veins, and the inferior vena cava, and (2) the *transverse* sinus, which lies between the aorta and pulmonary artery anteriorly and the atria posteriorly.[3] The parietal pericardium may extend 3 to 4 cm along the great vessels and covers the main pulmonary artery, veins, and vena cava. Its fibrous component becomes continuous with the adventitia of the vessels. Its thickness can range from 0.1 cm to a maximum of 0.35 cm, with the variation mainly resulting from a varying thickness of fibrous tissue. The sac is thickest over thinner parts of the heart (e.g., atria, right ventricle). In mammals, the pericardium has pores, less than 50 μm in diameter, which connect it to the pleural cavity.[4]

The parietal pericardium is anchored anteriorly to the manubrium and xyphoid processes of the sternum by the superior and inferior pericardiosternal ligaments, respectively. It is attached posteriorly to the vertebral column and caudally to the tendinous portion of the diaphragm, its most extensive attachment. The pericardial blood supply anteriorly is from small branches arising from the internal thoracic arteries and posteriorly from the aorta; the venous return is probably to the veins accompanying the internal thoracic artery. Its nerve supply is largely on the diaphragmatic surface and is derived primarily from phrenic, left recurrent laryngeal, and vagus nerves and the esophageal plexus. Sympathetic innervation is from the stellate and first dorsal ganglion as well as the aortic, cardiac, and diaphragmatic plexuses (Fig. 12-3).

HISTOLOGY

Chapter 2 contains some discussion of pericardial histology.

Mesothelial Cells

The single layer of mesothelial cells interdigitate and overlap, permitting changes in surface configuration (see Fig. 12-3A). Their cytoplasm contain mitochondria, lysosomes, Golgi bodies, actin filaments that actively alter cell shape, and a cytoskeleton that provides structural support. Mesothelial cells sit on a basal lamina and change their shape and size with the different phases of the cardiac cycle. They tend to be relatively perpendicular during systole and become oblique during diastole. Ultrastructurally, mesothelial cells possess microvilli up to 3 μm long and 0.1 μm wide (Fig. 12-4). The microvilli often completely cover a cell's surface, although some cells may have a relatively smooth cell membrane with only their central portions showing a concentration of microvilli. The microvilli diminish friction, increase surface area, and facilitate an exchange of fluid and ions. A few mesothelial cells have single large cilia, which are thicker and longer than microvilli.

Collagen

Collagen is the major component of parietal pericardium. It is stiff and relatively inexpansile and gives the

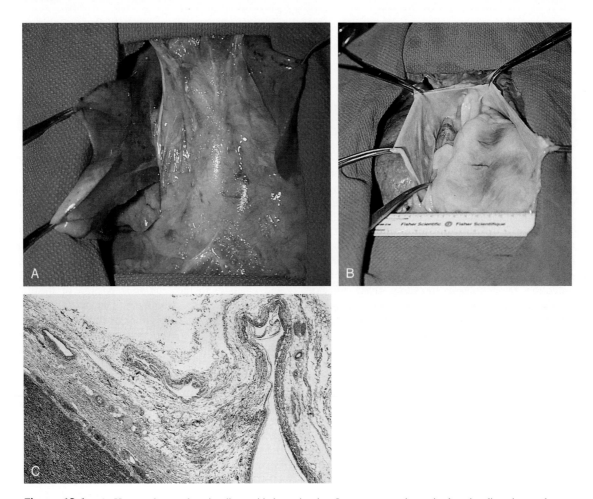

Figure 12-1 • *A,* Unopened normal pericardium with heart in situ. In most cases the parietal pericardium is translucent, except where covered by a layer of adipose tissue. The pericardium can be seen extending over the superior vena cava, pulmonary artery, and ascending aorta. The close proximity of the lungs and the pleural cavities, as well as the rib cage, is easily appreciated. *B,* Gross relationships of the pericardium (the surrounding ribs have been covered with green towels). The parietal pericardium is lifted off with hemostats. It is composed of a thick fibrosa, lined on its inner surface by a mesothelial cell layer. The latter reflects onto the visceral pericardium, which covers the surface of the heart and great vessels. The visceral pericardium is transparent under normal circumstances but becomes thickened and fibrotic after episodes of pericarditis (see Fig. 12-15). *C,* Histologic section of the aorta on the left, showing medial muscle, adventitia, and the pericardial reflection to the right (Elastic trichrome).

pericardium little elasticity. Although collagen fibers run through the pericardium in various directions as wavy bands,[4] three main layers form a wide, meshed net. The superficial and middle collagen layers have thick fibers, and the deep layer is composed of thinner ones. These layers are oriented at approximately 120 degrees to one another. The deeper ones form a basket-weave pattern with collagen fiber bundles running in apparently random directions. Elastic fibers are interspersed among the collagen bundles and modify the viscoelastic properties of the pericardium. The elastic fibers are small and often oriented at right angles to collagen bundles (see Fig. 12-4*A*).

Increased tension in the pericardial sac (e.g., from an increasing fluid volume within it) leads to a gradual straightening of the wavy collagen bundles and associated stretching of elastic fibers. Once straightened, collagen stiffens and offers marked resistance to further stretching or elongation. Studies indicate that the stress-strain curve of fibrous pericardium is similar to its pressure-volume curve. This curve is initially flat, when strain is increased

without increased stress, but it becomes extremely steep as total intrapericardial volume increases. The mechanism by which the pericardium expands in response to chronic cardiac dilation and volume overload is controversial. However, it is generally believed this adaptation is achieved by pericardial hypertrophy and an increased compliance of the pericardial chamber[5] or by the tensile viscoelastic properties of human pericardial tissue.[2, 6]

The wavy collagen bundles of youth tend to straighten with increasing age. This probably reduces pericardial compliance. Another feature seen with age is an increased strength of the loose connective tissue of the epicardium deep to the mesothelial cell layer. Further changes that occur with age are discussed in Chapter 3.

Pericardial Fluid and Pressures

Mesothelial cells do not offer much resistance to the to-and-fro passage of fluid, electrolytes, or proteins between pericardial and interstitial spaces. Fluid from capil-

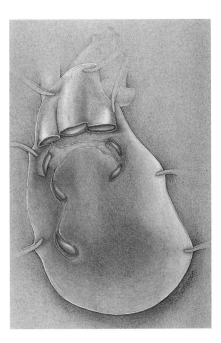

Figure 12-2 • Schematic representation of the inner aspect of the parietal pericardium, after heart is removed. The aorta and pulmonary artery are seen at the top, the pulmonary veins just below them, and the inferior vena cava further down. See text for description of oblique and transverse sinuses and Fig. 1-1 also.

laries adjacent to the pericardial space easily diffuses into these compartments.[7] Similarly, pericardial fluid may diffuse back through the interstitium into capillaries. Protein-rich fluid accumulates in the interstitial spaces and is continually drained by lymphatics.[8] Drainage of the pericardial space occurs both by the thoracic duct via the parietal pericardium and through the right lymphatic duct via the right pleural space. The protein content of normal pericardial fluid is lower than that of plasma. However, albumin is present in a relatively higher ratio than other proteins, probably because of its low molecular weight and ease of transport. Pericardial fluid has a lower osmo-

lality than plasma. All of these features suggest that it is an ultrafiltrate. Pericardial fluid is present in the pericardial space of fetuses as early as the second half of gestation.[9] Some muscle fiber–related enzymes are often present in it, and their levels may be increased in pathologic states.

Intrapericardial pressure is believed to be 0 to 2 mm Hg during diastole (right ventricular pressure is 1 to 2 mm Hg) and less than zero during systole. In animals with an intact pericardium, pericardial pressures varied from -3 to -5 mm Hg during quiet respiration and reached -9 mm Hg during deep inspiration,[10] a finding confirmed by Morgan and coworkers[11] and Kenner and Wood.[12] In addition, there are differences in hydrostatic pressure within the pericardial sac related to effects of adjoining structures. Intrapericardial pressure is maximal during middle to late diastole and falls sharply during systolic ejection.

CONGENITAL ABNORMALITIES

Congenital pericardial abnormalities may manifest as partial or complete defects of the pericardium or as cysts, diverticula, or benign teratomas. These abnormalities are rare in the adult population.

Congenital Absence and Defects of the Pericardium

Although these congenital abnormalities were recognized centuries ago, the first large series of pleuropericardial defects was reported by Saint-Pierre in 1970.[13] They have a male/female ratio of approximately 3:1, and approximately one third of cases are associated with congenital anomalies of the left side of the heart and/or lungs. These include patent ductus arteriosus, atrial septal defect, mitral stenosis, bronchogenic cysts, and pulmonary sequestration. The origin of pericardial defects is not certain. They may result from premature atrophy of the left

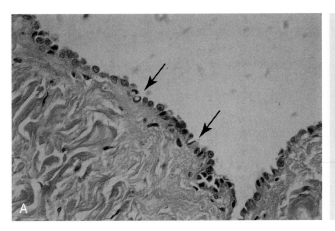

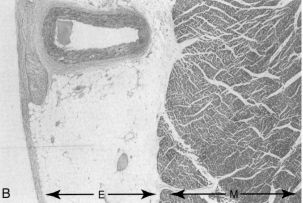

Figure 12-3 • Normal visceral pericardium. *A,* Normal epicardium with single layer of mesothelial cells (arrows). *B,* Epicardium mesothelial cells not obvious here, with peripheral nerves, adipose tissue, and blood vessels of varying sizes. E, epicardium; M, myocardium. (Both, H&E stain.)

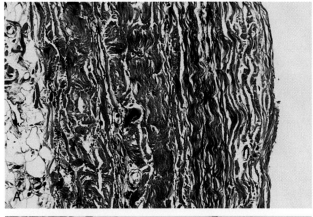

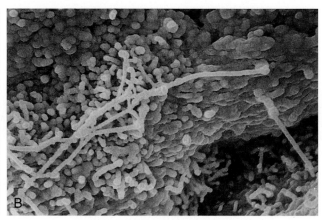

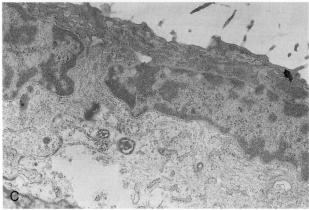

Figure 12-4 • *A,* Histologic section of the visceral pericardium showing an intact layer of mesothelial cells on the surface (to right) with underlying collagen and interspersed elastic fibers. Underlying this is adipose tissue in which blood vessels (arteries and veins) are evident (Elastic-trichrome). *B,* Scanning electron micrograph of the surface of the mesothelial layer showing projecting microvilli. (Courtesy of D.H. Spodick, MD, Worcester, Massachusetts.) *C,* Transmission electron micrograph of the parietal pericardium showing mesothelial cells. A few longitudinally cut microvilli are seen on their surface.

duct of Cuvier. This results in a loss of blood supply to the pleuropericardial membrane, which eventually becomes the pericardium.

Complete Absence of Pericardium

Patients with no associated congenital lesions are usually asymptomatic. However, the most common symptom is vague chest pain, which is probably caused by torsion of the great vessels due to excess mobility of the heart and absence of the stabilizing forces of the pericardium (Fig. 12-5A–C). Occasionally, a portion of the heart herniates through the defect and incurs ischemic damage.[14] A similar situation can develop after lung surgery.[15]

Patients often have a widened splitting of the second heart sound, leftward displacement of the apical impulse, and a systolic murmur at the upper left sternal border, probably related to turbulent blood flow caused by an unusually mobile heart. Chest roentgenography reveals marked displacement of the cardiac silhouette, a prominent main pulmonary artery, and interposition of the lung between the left hemidiaphragm and inferior border of the heart. Echocardiographic findings simulate abnormalities seen in right ventricular volume overload, including right ventricular dilation and paradoxic motion of the interventricular septum. Abnormal systolic motion is induced by anteroposterior displacement of the left ventricle.[16, 17] Computerized tomography and magnetic resonance imaging can demonstrate the absence of the pericardium and the abnormal presence of a wedge of lung between the aorta and pulmonary artery.[18] No specific therapy is required.

Partial Defects of Pericardium

Partial left-sided pericardial defects may be complicated by partial cardiac herniation and compression of the epicardial coronary arteries[19–21] (see Fig. 12-5C). Partial right-sided defects are rare and can be associated with inspiratory chest discomfort secondary to herniation of the right atrium or ventricle through the defect or herniation of lung into the pericardial cavity. Surgical treatment is done both to prevent cardiac strangulation and relieve symptoms.

Congenital Pericardial Cysts

These rare developmental abnormalities form between 4 and 7% of all congenital thoracic cysts.[22] They are most commonly situated at the right costophrenic angle and are more common in men (reported male/female ratio, approximately 3:2). Although pericardial cysts occur at all ages, the majority are detected in the fourth decade. Their cause is uncertain. The most accepted theories are the lacuna theory and the weakness theory. Under the *lacuna theory,*[23] the pericardium is derived from lacunae that join to form the pericardial cavity. Failure of union of some lacunae could be manifested subsequently as a cyst or diverticulum. Under the *weakness theory,*[24] areas of potential pericardial weakness exist where vessels and nerves enter or leave the pericardium. These would be preferential sites of pericardial diverticulum or cyst formation.

Patients with pericardial cysts are usually asymptomatic. However, chest pain may occur secondary to tor-

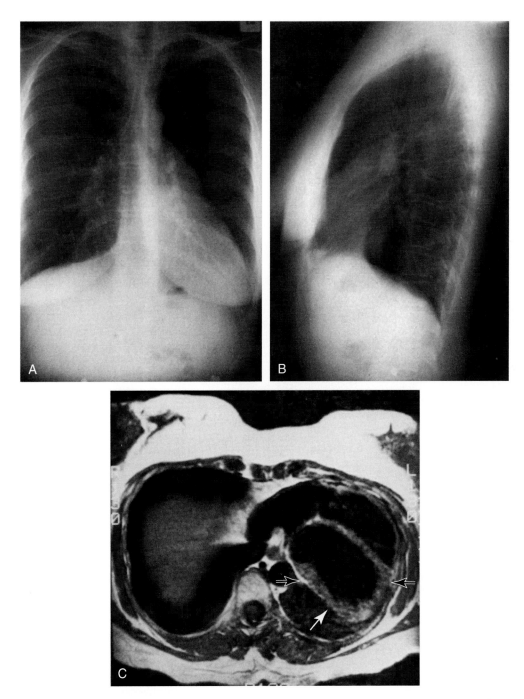

Figure 12-5 • Posteroanterior (A) and lateral (B) chest radiographs showing the elongated, pear-shaped heart resulting from a congenital absence of the parietal pericardium. (Courtesy of L. Zelowitsky, MD, Toronto, Ontario.) *C*, Magnetic resonance imaging scan showing congenital absence of the left hemipericardium with herniation of the ventricles (left and right) through the defect. The cardiac chambers are displaced to the left with torsion around the great vessels. The anterior pericardium is present (black arrows), and the posterior is absent (arrow). The patient underwent surgical repair of the defect. (Courtesy of P. Liu, MD, Toronto, Ontario.)

sion. Cysts can be differentiated from solid tumors by two-dimensional echocardiography or computed tomographic scanning. Pericardial cysts vary in size and range in weight from 100 to 300 g (Fig. 12-6). A cyst containing 1 L of fluid and measuring 25.0 × 37.0 cm has been reported.[23] Cyst fluid is usually a clear transudate. The cyst wall has fibrous connective tissue and an inner lining of a single layer of flattened cells, similar to serosal or endothelial cells.

Teratomas

Intrapericardial teratomas are rare and almost invariably benign, receiving their blood supply from either the root of the aorta or the pulmonary artery. They are usually found in children and have a strong female predominance. A teratoma is the most likely diagnosis in a child who has a recurrent nonbloody pericardial effusion. These tumors grow up to 15.0 cm in diameter and can cause

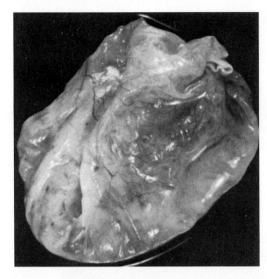

Figure 12-6 • A congenital pericardial cyst, removed incidentally during insertion of aortocoronary bypass grafts. The cyst measured 6.5 cm in diameter and contained 40 to 50 ml of clear serous fluid.

compression of cardiac chambers. Cases can be detected in utero by fetal echocardiography.[24, 25] Histologic features and management are similar to those of teratomas at other sites (see Chapter 19). Surgical excision is usually curative.

PERICARDIAL EFFUSION

Pericardial effusions may be acute or chronic, serous, serosanguineous, or sanguinous. Pericardial fluid is rarely composed of lymph or chyle. Serous effusions are usually related to a decreased return of pericardial fluid or to decreased serum osmolality, as in hypoproteinemia. They are seen in a variety of conditions (Tables 12-1 and 12-2). Serosanguineous effusions are often associated with inflammatory pericardial lesions. Inflammatory effusions are often purulent. Sanguinous effusions are usually related to trauma, including surgical trauma, myocardial rupture, neoplasm, or pericarditis associated with uremia or infection.

Several factors determine the intrapericardial pressure that develops secondary to a pericardial effusion. They include (1) the volume of the effusion, (2) the rate of fluid accumulation, and (3) the physical characteristics of the pericardial cavity. The rapid accumulation of an effusion in excess of 150 ml in a normal pericardial sac

TABLE 12-1 • Causes of Acute Pericardial Effusion

Cause	Type of Fluid
Congestive heart failure	Clear/pale straw-colored
Postmyocardial infarction	Serous/blood-tinged or hemorrhagic
Viral infection	Serous/serosanguineous/sanguinous
Bacterial infection	Purulent/serosanguineous
Myocardial (free wall) rupture	Sanguinous
Trauma	Sanguinous/serosanguineous
Drugs (e.g., minoxidil)	Serous

TABLE 12-2 • Chronic Pericardial Effusion

Cause	Type of Effusion
Cardiac causes	
Congestive heart failure	Serous
Postmyocardial infarction syndrome	Serous/serosanguineous
Cardiomyopathy, obstructive	Serous
Cor pulmonale	Serous/serosanguineous
Left ventricular hypertrophy	Serous
Rheumatic heart disease	Serosanguineous
Myocarditis	Serous/serosanguineous
Post-heart transplantation	Serous/serosanguineous
Trauma	Sanguinous
Collagen vascular diseases	Serous
Chronic infections	
Mycobacterium tuberculosis	Serosanguineous
Fungi	Serous/serosanguineous
Parasites	Serous/serosanguineous
Acquired immunodeficiency syndrome	
Infection	Serous/serosanguineous
Kaposi sarcoma	Sanguinous
Chronic renal disease	Serosanguineous/fibrinous
Neoplasms	
Cardiac	
Atrial myxoma	Serous
Malignant (e.g., mesothelioma, atrial angiosarcoma)	Serosanguineous/sanguinous
Metastatic	
Solid tumors (e.g., lung, breast)	Serosanguineous/sanguinous
Leukemia/lymphomas	Serous/serosanguineous
Radiotherapy	Serous
Other causes	
Pregnancy (usually self-limiting)	Serous
Drug-related (e.g., procainamide)	Serous
Lymphopericardium (e.g., pericardial lymphangioma, lymphangiectasia)	Serous (lymph)
Chylopericardium (primary or secondary)	Chyle
Myxedema	Serous
Clotting disorders	Sanguinous
Idiopathic pericarditis	Serous/serosanguineous
Cause unknown	Usually serous

results in a marked increase in intrapericardial pressure. However, gradual accumulation causes pericardial stretching, and the cavity can accommodate more than 2 L without elevating the intrapericardial pressure significantly. The most common causes of large pericardial effusions are postmyocardial infarction, malignant neoplasm, collagen vascular diseases, and, occasionally, chemotherapeutic agents.[26, 27]

Clinical Features

A pericardial effusion in the absence of raised intrapericardial pressure may be completely asymptomatic. The symptoms and signs caused by large pericardial effusions are listed in Table 12-3. Echocardiography is the most rapid and accurate technique used to evaluate pericardial effusions; M-mode echocardiography may detect as little as 20 ml of fluid in the pericardial cavity.[28] Two-dimensional echocardiography is indicated clinically to define its presence, amount, and distribution.[29] It may also help determine the cause of the effusion and identify other

TABLE 12-3 • **Pericardial Effusion: Clinical Symptoms**
Mild chest discomfort
Mechanical compression of adjacent structures
Diminished intensity of heart sounds
Enlarged cardiac silhouette on chest radiography
Reduced QRS voltage

Echocardiographic changes
    M-mode—detects as little as 20 ml of fluid
    Two-dimensional—helps detect presence, amount, and distribution

TABLE 12-4 • **Pericardium: Reaction to Injury**
Acute inflammatory infiltrate
Fibrinous exudate with acute inflammatory cells
(Combination of above)
Increased transudation of fluid (serous)
(Combination of the above)

pericardial abnormalities, such as fibrous strands, tumor masses, and blood clots (Fig. 12-7).[30] In addition, echocardiography has an important role in the recognition of cardiac tamponade[31] and in providing visual guidance during pericardiocentesis.

Chronic Pericardial Effusion

Chronic pericardial effusions persisting for longer than 6 months may develop from any cause of pericarditis. They are most common in patients with serous effusions secondary to congestive heart failure, previous idiopathic or viral pericarditis, uremic pericarditis, or malignant effusions. Such chronic effusions produce significant fibrous thickening of the pericardium and a mild-to-moderate chronic inflammatory cell infiltrate. In the developing world, chronic pericardial effusions are often infectious and particularly caused by tuberculosis (see Table 12-2). In such cases, the pericardium may show mild or no thickening with a mild lymphocytic infiltrate in the epicardium or the patient may develop chronic constrictive pericarditis.

REACTION OF THE PERICARDIUM TO INJURY

With acute injury, the pericardium shows an acute inflammatory infiltrate, an increased transudation of fluid, an exudation of fibrin and acute inflammatory cells, or a combination of these reactions (Table 12-4). The type of fluid (whether an exudate or a transudate) and the type of inflammatory cells found in the exudate depend on the cause of the pericardial disease. The presence of serum or blood, per se, in the pericardial sac does not incite a significant tissue response in the normal pericardium. However, if it is also injured, the pericardium responds by producing fibrous adhesions (Fig. 12-8A), which often result in loculated accumulations of fluid.[32]

In infectious pericarditis, the reaction depends on the causative organism (see Fig. 12-8B,C). Bacteria induce an acute polymorphonuclear cell response that may produce a fibrinous exudate, the classic "bread and butter" pericarditis, leading subsequently to fibrous thickening with or without pericardial constriction. Acid-fast bacilli incite a chronic granulomatous response that leads to severe fibrous pericardial thickening. Calcification often develops and may be extensive. Viruses generally produce a transient pericardial reaction that resolves. However, they

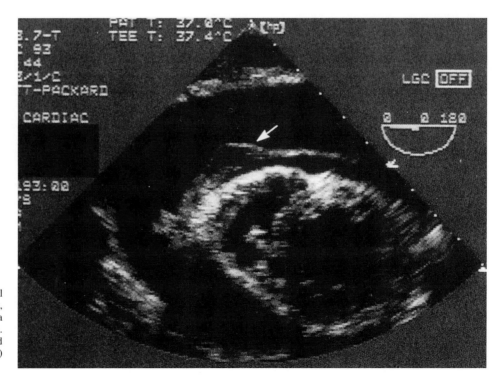

Figure 12-7 • Transesophageal echocardiogram, short access view, of a 50-year-old woman with a large malignant pericardial effusion. The effusion is circumferential, and visible fibrin strands (white arrow) extend from the epicardial surface.

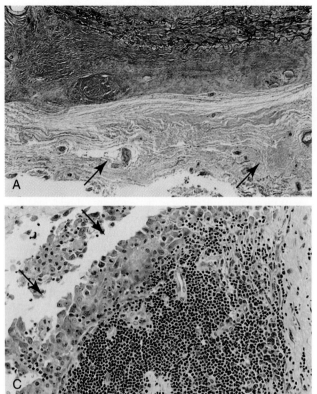

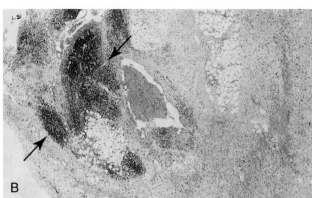

Figure 12-8 • *A,* Thickened pericardium with fibrous adhesions (arrows). *B* and *C,* Sections from a surgically excised pericardium showing marked chronic inflammation (arrows). *B,* The surface shows prominent mesothelial cells (arrows) and clusters of these cells, the result of the inflammatory process (*A,* Elastic trichrome; *B* and *C,* Hematoxylin and eosin).

may invoke a significant fibrous reaction leading to constrictive pericarditis. Calcification may develop in this fibrotic pericardium.

There may be a proliferation of mesothelial cells after acute or chronic injury (see Fig. 12-8*A, B*). Occasionally, the proliferating cells develop a papilliform arrangement associated with mitotic figures. At times this histologic appearance is difficult to differentiate from that of malignant neoplasms, especially a metastatic adenocarcinoma invading the pericardium or even a mesothelioma.[33] Immunoperoxidase stains that help differentiate these cell types include keratin, vimentin, carcinoembyronic antigen (CEA), and LEU-M1. Keratin and vimentin are positive in mesothelial cells, whereas CEA and LEU-M1 are positive in adenocarcinomas.[33] Ultrastructural examination of mesothelial cells may identify numerous long, complex microvilli, which are not found on adenocarcinoma cells.

CARDIAC TAMPONADE

Tamponade, a French word of German origin, means compression of the heart. Cardiac compression may result from accumulation of fluid, blood, or air in the pericardial cavity. Rarely, it is caused by large volumes of blood in the mediastinum. There may be regional tamponade, caused by a loculated collection of fluid overlying a chamber (Fig. 12-9). This often occurs in the oblique sinus and can compress the left atrium.

The accumulation of fluid in the pericardial sac and an associated rise in intrapericardial pressure increases, and equalizes, the intraventricular diastolic pressures of both ventricles and causes a significant decrease in the trans-

mural distending pressures and their filling during diastole.[34] There is an ultimate fall in ventricular stroke volume and cardiac output. In acute cardiac tamponade, the pericardium is unlikely to show significant pathologic change, except for fluid in the pericardial cavity and fibrin on lining surfaces.

Clinical features that suggest acute cardiac tamponade are listed in Table 12-5. Beck's triad[35] is typically ob-

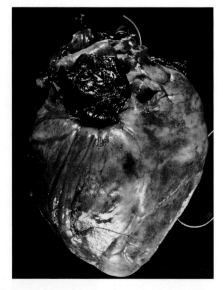

Figure 12-9 • "Regional" tamponade. A large hematoma overlies the left atrium and the oblique sinus in this postoperative case, leading to atrial tamponade and sudden death. The patient had undergone open heart surgery.

TABLE 12-5 • **Acute Cardiac Tamponade: Clinical Features**

Pulsus paradoxus

Beck's triad
  Hypotension
  Raised jugular venous pressure
  Diminished heart sounds

Tachycardia

Low-output state

Features of cerebral hypoperfusion

served in acute tamponade from sudden intrapericardial hemorrhage. With a tamponade that develops slowly, such as in malignant pericardial effusions, patients generally have dyspnea and chest discomfort. Physical findings in a series of 56 patients[36, 37] were as follows: elevated systemic venous pressure (100%), pulsus paradoxus (98%), respiratory rate more than 20 breaths/minute (80%), heart rate more than 100 beats/minute (77%), and systolic blood pressure more than 100 mm Hg (64%). Pericardiocentesis can be lifesaving in acute tamponade. More definitive therapies include making a pericardial window and surgical pericardiotomy. The former has the advantage of allowing a pericardial biopsy, which may define the underlying disease and allow treatment.

TYPES OF EFFUSION

Hemopericardium and Serosanguineous Effusions

A hemopericardium is an acute sanguineous effusion that has a hematocrit virtually identical to that of blood. It is always significant because it generally signifies frank bleeding into the pericardial space. It is seen acutely in myocardial rupture secondary to trauma or myocardial infarction, intrapericardial rupture of an aortic aneurysm (usually a dissecting one), coronary artery rupture, and coagulation disorders (Fig. 12-10).

Malignant neoplasms and tuberculosis are common causes of chronic sanguinous or serosanguineous effusions. They also develop under other circumstances, including idiopathic pericarditis, systemic lupus erythematosus (SLE) and other collagen vascular disorders, rheumatic fever, uremia (see later), and Dressler syndrome. Kaposi sarcoma involving the pericardium with an associated sanguinous pericardial effusion has been reported.[37] Sanguinous fluid generally remains fluid owing to the anticoagulant properties of the pericardial serous lining and the constant movement of the heart, which effectively defibrinates the blood. Long-term sequelae include the potential to produce significant fibrous adhesions and loculation of fluid.

Chylopericardium

Accumulation of chylous fluid in the pericardium is usually idiopathic, but occasionally it occurs secondary to surgery,[38] traumatic injury to the thoracic duct, or lymphatic occlusion by parasites or metastatic tumor. Diagno-

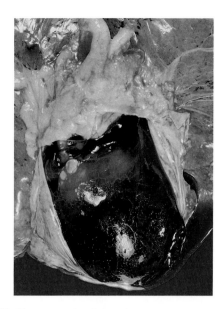

Figure 12-10 • The pericardial sac has been opened to reveal a large (>300 g) hematoma that developed secondary to a ruptured myocardial infarction. It caused cardiac tamponade.

sis is confirmed by the aspiration of milky-white pericardial fluid that clears on the addition of ether. A chylopericardium is usually large and chronic and often has an associated element of chronic tamponade (Fig. 12-11). It rarely causes a constrictive pericarditis. Treatment consists of draining the fluid and/or repairing the thoracic duct.

Cholesterol Pericarditis

Cholesterol pericarditis, often termed "golden pericarditis" because of its gross appearance, is characterized by a high concentration of cholesterol and other lipids in the pericardial fluid and the presence of cholesterol crystals in pericardial tissue. A cholesterol-rich effusion is usually turbid, brown, yellow, amber, or opalescent. Typical crystalline structures are found in it. Cholesterol crystals give

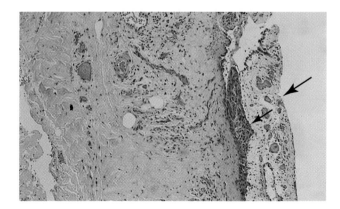

Figure 12-11 • Surgically excised pericardium in which the pericardial sac contained chylous fluid, the effusion having developed postoperatively. Significant inflammatory infiltrate is seen in the parietal pericardium, as is thickening of the fibrous layer. Mesothelial cells are proliferating (small arrow) and the free surface shows a fibrinous exudate (large arrow) (H&E stain).

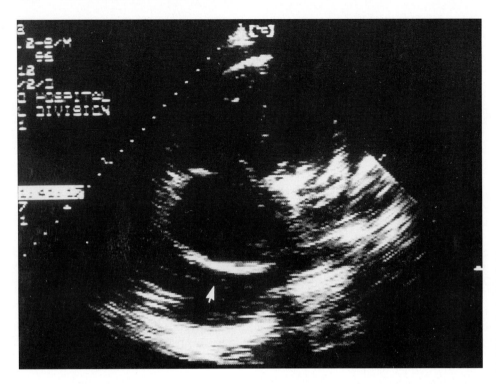

Figure 12-12 • Postpericardiotomy syndrome. Transthoracic echocardiogram in the apical four-chamber view, 3 weeks after a prosthetic mitral valve replacement in a 65-year-old woman with rheumatic heart disease and multiple previous surgical procedures; there is a small pericardial effusion and a thickened visceral pericardial layer (white arrow).

the pericardium a gold-painted appearance and incite a marked cellular reaction that in turn increases the pericardial effusion and leads to pericardial thickening and fibrosis. The pericardium may show fibrin, yellowish nodules or plaques, or atheromatous masses of cholesterol on its inner surface. The epicardium often shows inflammation, and constrictive epicarditis may occur. Histologic examination reveals severe fibrosis, inflammation, and numerous cholesterol or other lipid crystals. In addition, foam cells and macrophages containing iron pigment are often present.

Cholesterol-rich effusions tend to be large and chronic; they have many causes. All myxedematous effusions contain cholesterol, without associated crystal formation (see later discussion).

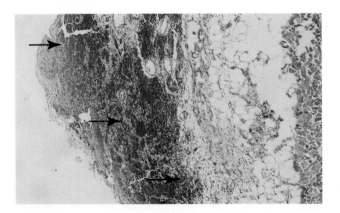

Figure 12-13 • This visceral pericardium shows a significant acute hemorrhage (arrows). The postoperative pericardium often shows patchy areas of mild hemorrhage, associated with a mild acute inflammatory exudate. Regional fibrous pericardial adhesions may be seen in late postoperative periods (Elastic trichrome).

Pericardial Effusions After Cardiac Surgery

Cardiac surgery is associated with a significant incidence of pericardial effusions. Two-dimensional echocardiography is more sensitive in detecting them than are most other investigations (Fig. 12-12). They are most often seen after significant postoperative bleeding (Fig. 12-13). Although the majority of these effusions are benign, up to 6% in one series were associated with cardiac tamponade in the early postoperative period. Early postcardiotomy tamponade, occurring in the first few postoperative days, has been reported and is likely to be related to anticoagulant therapy, excess mediastinal drainage, bleeding disorders, or the postpericardiotomy syndrome.[39] Insertion of a pericardial drain does not necessarily inhibit fluid accumulation. Late postoperative tamponade is even less common[40] and is usually related to the postpericardiotomy syndrome.[41]

Pneumopericardium

The accumulation of air in the pericardium is an uncommon event. It usually occurs after penetrating or nonpenetrating chest trauma. Mechanisms include (1) a direct tracheobronchial-pericardial communication, (2) pneumothorax with a pleuropericardial tear, or (3) penetration of the long pulmonary vein's perivascular sheath from ruptured alveoli with extension of the air to the pericardium. Pneumopericardium occasionally induces cardiac tamponade in the absence of trauma.[42, 43] It may also occur after fistula formation between pericardium and an adjacent organ (Fig. 12-14). Patients receiving mechanical ventilation are at risk due to alveolar rupture by high-pressure oxygen dissecting into the pericardium at weak points in

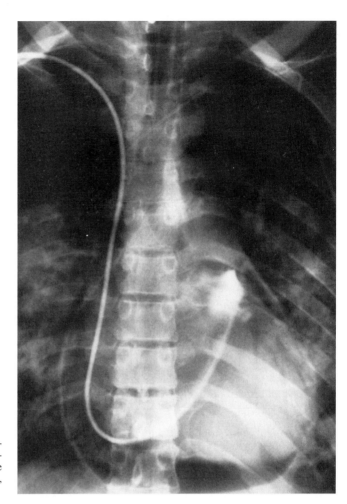

Figure 12-14 • Chest radiograph showing a large pneumopericardium. A Swan-Ganz catheter is in place. This iatrogenic pneumopericardium apparently developed during an endobronchial biopsy. The outcome was favorable. (Courtesy of L. Zelitowsky, MD, Toronto, Ontario.)

the pericardial reflection of great vessels. Abdominal laparoscopic procedures may also be followed by air in the pericardium, probably as a result of communication through embryonic pericardioperitoneal channels. Rarely it may arise from a gas-forming infection, typically by *Peptostreptococcus, Bacteroides, Escherichia coli,* or *Klebsiella* species.[44]

Chest radiography demonstrates the pneumopericardium (see Fig. 12-14). Occasionally it is associated with fluid accumulation, giving rise to a pneumohydropericar-

dium. Echocardiographic examination may reveal hyperechoic floating particles, which have been called "intrapericardial spontaneous contrast echoes."[45, 46] In this life-threatening condition, the pericardium may show no significant abnormality histologically.

PERICARDITIS

Clinical Features

Acute pericarditis classically manifests with precordial chest pain aggravated by deep respiration, a pericardial friction rub, and serial electrocardiographic abnormalities.[47] Other clinical features depend on the presence and amount of pericardial fluid and the severity of the inflammatory process (Table 12-6). All types of pericarditis are more common in men than in women.[47]

Pathogenesis

Acute pericarditis has many causes (Table 12-7). Infectious microorganisms gain access by hematogenous dissemination, spread from contiguous structures (e.g., lungs, pleura, mediastinum), or by penetrating trauma including the trauma of surgery, or extension from a perivalvular

---

TABLE 12-6 • **Classification of Pericarditis**

Infectious

Idiopathic

Associated with acute myocardial infarction

Iatrogenic and traumatic, related to
    Cardiovascular surgery
    Complications of cardiac catheterization
    Irradiation
    Chemical agents
    Penetrating/nonpenetrating injury

Associated with systemic diseases

Associated with malignant neoplasms

Associated with endocrine diseases

TABLE 12-7 • **Classification of Infectious Pericarditis**

Bacterial pericarditis
    Gram-positive
    Gram-negative
    Mycobacterial

Fungal pericarditis
    Histoplasmosis
    Candidiasis

Acute nonspecific pericarditis

Viral pericarditis

Protozoal pericarditis (e.g., ameba, toxoplasmosis, echinococcus, trypanosomiasis, filariasis)

Pericarditis and the acquired immunodeficiency syndrome

Lyme disease

TABLE 12-8 • **Acute Pericarditis: Morphologic Features and Sequelae**

Acute inflammatory infiltrate

Fibrinous exudate with acute inflammatory cells

Increased pericardial vascularity

Sequelae
    No residual lesions
    Fibrous adhesions
    Pericardial fibrosis and thickening (white patches)

abscess in infective endocarditis. Viral pericarditis is associated with antibody reactions to the sarcolemmal membranes of myocardial fibers. Much of the damage is thought to be caused by the cytotoxic and fibrinolytic effects of mononuclear cells. Drug-induced pericarditis probably occurs via allergic or delayed hypersensitivity mechanisms. In radiation-induced pericarditis, direct tissue injury is probably the inciting mechanism. Pericarditis is the most common cardiac manifestation of collagen vascular diseases.

Acute pericarditis in the setting of a viral infection, after myocardial infarction, or after cardiac surgery is usually self-limited. Significant complications include (1) recurrent episodes of pericarditis[48]; (2) development of a large pericardial effusion under pressure, resulting in cardiac tamponade; (3) constrictive pericarditis; and (4) a combination of effusive and constrictive pericardial disease. Tamponade occurs in approximately 15% of patients with acute pericarditis.[47] Recurrent pericarditis affected more than 20% in some series.[48, 49] It has been observed that about 9% of patients with acute idiopathic pericarditis and pericardial effusion develop evidence, either by clinical examination or through noninvasive investigations, of mild transient pericardial constriction, occurring

within the first month.[50] This typically resolves spontaneously within 3 months and suggests that transient constrictive physiology may occur during a resolving episode of acute pericarditis.

Pathology and Management

The pathologic changes of acute pericarditis are listed in Table 12-8. Many cases of pericarditis resolve without residual damage. In other instances, the fibrin deposits (see Fig. 12-8A) organize and form adhesions between pericardium and epicardium and between pericardium and adjacent sternum and pleura. Pericardial fibrosis is generally seen as white patches on the epicardial surface (Fig. 12-15).

The principles of management of acute pericarditis include determining the underlying cause and controlling symptoms. The pain of acute pericarditis usually responds to nonsteroidal anti-inflammatory agents (e.g., aspirin, indomethacin). Short-term corticosteroid therapy is reserved for patients with refractory severe pain.

TYPES OF PERICARDITIS

Bacterial Pericarditis

Bacterial pericarditis occurs more commonly in children than in adults. Its incidence is far less common

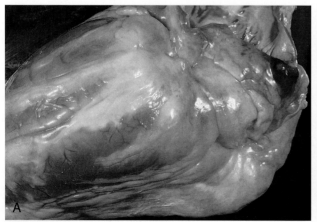 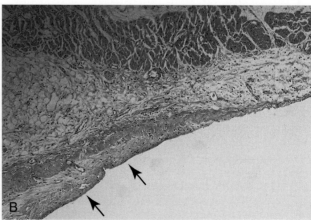

Figure 12-15 • *A,* Epicardial surface of a heart with a large white patch of visceral pericardial thickening. *B,* Histologic section showing localized area of pericardial thickening and fibrosis with minimal lymphocytic infiltrate (H&E stain).

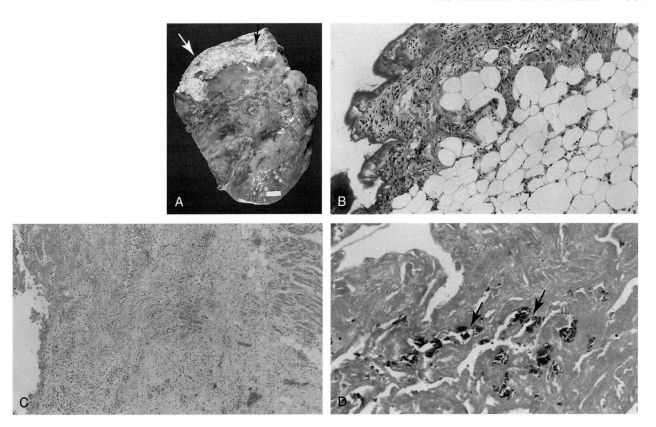

Figure 12-16 • Acute pericarditis. *A* through *D,* From a case of postoperative acute infective endocarditis. *A,* The right atrial epicardium has a thick layer of creamy yellow material deposited on its surface (arrows). Adhesions between the visceral and the parietal pericardium have been lysed and the parietal pericardium has been excised. *B,* Fibrinous exudate with an admixture of polymorphonuclear leukocytes. The epicardium shows thickening, edema, proliferation of capillaries and small blood vessels, and a significant acute inflammatory infiltrate. Small colonies of microorganisms may also be seen. *C,* Surface of the visceral pericardium showing fibrinous exudate and blue colonies of cocci which on culture proved to be *Staphylococcus aureus. D,* Fibrinous pericardial exudate with colonies of gram-positive cocci (arrows) (*A, B, C,* H&E stain; *D,* Gram stain).

today than in the preantibiotic era.[3, 51] It is typically a fulminant acute illness. Grossly, both layers of pericardium appear thickened (Fig. 12-16) and are covered by a fibrinopurulent exudate. An infiltrate of polymorphonuclear leukocytes is seen, with the cells abundant in the epicardium. The pericardial space may be filled by an exudate which is serous, serosanguineous, or turbid and yellow-green. It contains abundant polymorphonuclear leukocytes. In the absence of prior antimicrobial therapy, microorganisms can be demonstrated by a Gram stain of the pericardial fluid. Untreated purulent pericarditis is associated with a high mortality rate. Medically treated cases have been associated with a mortality rate as high as 77%.[52] Bacterial pericarditis may be associated with underlying myocardial infections, especially the ring abscesses of infective endocarditis of native or prosthetic valves (see Chapter 14). The sequelae of bacterial pericarditis include cardiac tamponade, loculated collections of exudate that require surgical drainage, fibrous adhesions, areas of calcification, and constrictive pericarditis.

Gram-Positive Infections

Staphylococci, streptococci, and pneumococci are the gram-positive organisms most commonly associated with acute pericarditis. Staphylococcal pericarditis is a life-threatening condition that may be complicated by cardiac tamponade (see Fig. 12-16). Recently it has been associated with human immunodeficiency virus (HIV) infection.[53] Risk factors for *Staphylococcus aureus* infection in HIV-positive patients include a high rate of skin and nasal colonization,[54] frequent dermatologic disease,[55] and the use of intravenous catheters. Pneumococcal pericarditis previously accounted for half of the cases but comprises fewer than 10% today. It is usually the result of direct extension from adjoining lung or pleural infection. Only a few cases of primary pneumococcal pericarditis are reported.[56]

Gram-Negative Infections

Common gram-negative bacilli causing pericarditis include the *Neisseria* species, *Haemophilus influenzae, E. coli, Pseudomonas aeruginosa,* and *Klebsiella pneumoniae. H. influenzae* was the second most common cause of purulent pericarditis in children.[57] Meningococcal pericarditis was responsible for 2 to 4% of adult cases.[58, 59] Meningococcal pericarditis was found in 6 of 32 patients who had meningococcal meningitis.[60] Primary involvement of the pericardium, a rare phenomenon, is usually seen during epidemics. Meningococcal pericarditis is fairly common in children, accounting for approximately

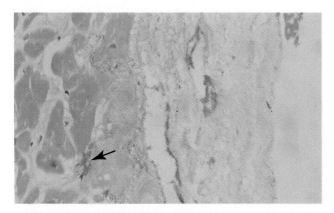

Figure 12-17 • This visceral pericardium and underlying tissues show colonies of bluish bacilli. The surrounding tissue shows no inflammatory infiltrate, edema, or pericardial exudate. These microorganisms proliferated after death. (H&E stain.)

one third of all cases.[61] Postmortem growth of bacteria can occur on the pericardium. In this instance, the associated microscopic features of an acute infection are not seen (Fig. 12-17).

Other Bacterial Infections

Cases of pericarditis have been reported secondary to infection from *Legionella pneumophila*,[62] *Campylobacter*,[63] *Listeria monocytogenes*,[64] *Neisseria mucosa*,[65] *Nocardia asteroides*,[66] and *Chlamydia*.[67] Anaerobic bacteria, such as *Bacteroides fragilis* and the clostridia organisms, are occasionally associated with acute pericarditis.[68]

Lyme Disease

Lyme disease is caused by *Borrelia burgdorferi*, a spirochete transferred by the bite of the *Ixodes dammini* tick. It occurs in several clinical stages (Table 12-9). Cardiac involvement is a feature of the second stage and is characterized by arrhythmias (atrioventricular nodal block), myopericarditis, and pancarditis. Pericardial involvement is the major clinical cardiac manifestation. Cardiac involvement, characterized by myopericarditis, mild interstitial fibrosis, a lymphocytic infiltrate, and conduction abnormalities, may be the only indication of an underlying *B. burgdorferi* infection.[69] (See discussion in Chapter 9.)

Tuberculous Pericarditis

Mycobacterium tuberculosis is a frequent cause of infectious pericarditis worldwide.[70] Its incidence has declined dramatically in the industrialized world in the past four decades but is rising again because of multidrug-resistant organisms. Tuberculous pericarditis develops by spread from mediastinal, peribronchial, or paratracheal lymph nodes or by early hematogenous dissemination. Less commonly, it is a result of contiguous spread from a pulmonary lesion or from the adjacent sternum or spine.[71] Fewer than 10% of patients with systemic tuberculosis develop tuberculous pericarditis. Granulomatous epicarditis without demonstrable bacterial infection may also occur.[72]

Tuberculous pericarditis is generally characterized by three stages: acute, subacute, and chronic (Table 12-10).

TABLE 12-9 • Lyme Disease: Morphologic and Clinical Features of *Borrelia burgdorferi* Infestation

	Morphologic Features	Clinical Features
Stage 1:	Lymphoplasmocytic infiltrate at site of bite	Fever
	Redness	
	? Pale center	
	Induration	
	Lymphadenopathy	
Stage 2:	Early disseminated stage	Joint and muscle
	Secondary skin lesions	pains
	Lymphadenopathy	
	Antibodies to spirochaetal flagellar proteins	
	Myopericarditis or cardiac arrhythmias	
	Pancarditis	
	Cranial nerve involvement	Meningitis
	Synovial	
Stage 3:	Late disseminated stage	
	Chronic arthritis	Joint pains
	Arteritis with "onion skin–like" lesions	
	Encephalitis	Restriction of
	Destruction of articular cartilage	movement

Acute involvement can be further subdivided into fibrinous and effusive stages. The morphologic features are similar to those of mycobacterial infection at any other site (Fig. 12-18).

The clinical presentation of tuberculous pericarditis is variable, with patients usually presenting either in the early effusive stage or after developing constrictive pathology. Clinical features in the effusive stage can be nonspecific and include fever, night sweats, dyspnea, abdominal discomfort, and jugular venous distension.[73, 74] The acute chest pain characteristically seen in viral pericarditis is uncommon in tuberculous pericarditis. If tuberculous pericarditis manifests with chronic constrictive pericarditis, its clinical features are predominantly those defined in Table 12-10 and muscle wasting.

A definitive diagnosis is established by isolating the organism from pericardial fluid or pericardial biopsy. The probability of obtaining a diagnosis is greatest if both fluid and biopsy specimens are examined in the early effusive stage.[75] Other diagnostic techniques include measuring adenosine deaminase activity (more than 40 U/L) in pleural or pericardial fluid,[76] polymerase chain reaction (PCR),[77] and pericardioscopy.[78, 79] Constrictive pericarditis develops ultimately in almost all patients with

TABLE 12-10 • Stages of Tuberculous Pericarditis

Stage	Morphologic Features
Acute	Fibrinous pericarditis: serosanguineous effusion, lymphocytic infiltrate, ?immune mediated
	Effusion: Lymphocytes in pericardial fluid (mycobacteria rarely seen/recovered)
Subacute	Granulomatous inflammation with or without caseous necrosis (mycobacteria usually seen on special stains)
Chronic	Pericardial fibrosis and thickening, marked
	Pericardial calcification—patchy or diffuse
	Obliteration of pericardial cavity
	Constrictive pericarditis (mycobacteria usually not demonstrable)

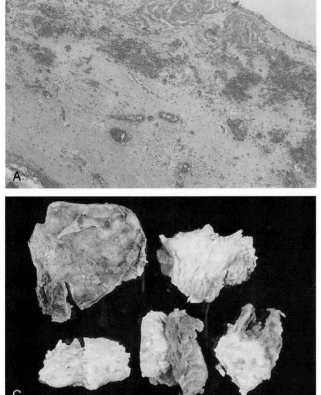

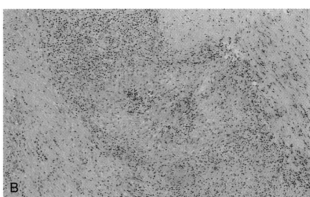

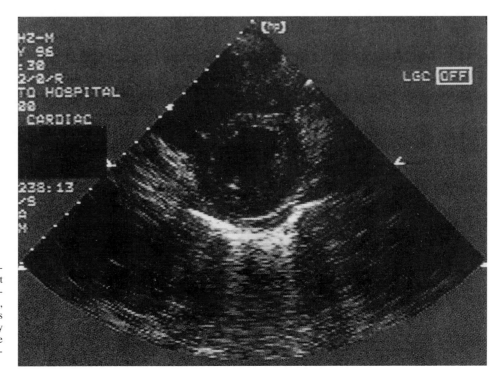

Figure 12-18 • Granulomatous pericarditis. *A* and *B,* histologic sections of the pericardium showing marked thickening, areas of fibrosis, and an infiltrate of mononuclear cells (lymphocytes, macrophages, and occasional plasma cells). Several necrotizing granulomatous lesions are seen in *B.* (Both, H&E stain.) *C,* Pieces of heavily calcified, markedly thickened parietal pericardium excised from a patient who had constrictive pericarditis and a past history of tuberculosis. In most such cases, it is virtually impossible to demonstrate any classic lesions of tuberculous infection, or causative microorganisms.

untreated tuberculous pericarditis.[80] In a series of 294 consecutive patients with acute pericarditis, 13 had a tuberculous infection (Fig. 12-19). Seven of these patients developed constrictive pericarditis requiring pericardiec-

tomy.[81] A trial of 143 patients with tuberculous pericarditis and constrictive physiology demonstrated that combined treatment with antituberculous chemotherapy and steroids decreased mortality and the requirement for peri-

Figure 12-19 • Constrictive pericardium in a 67-year-old patient with a remote history of tuberculosis. Transthoracic echocardiogram, parasternal long axis view. There is a significant increase in reflectivity from the marked calcification of the parietal as well as the visceral pericardia.

cardectomy and resulted in more rapid clinical improvement.[82]

Other Mycobacterial Infections

Pericardial involvement by mycobacteria other than *M. tuberculosis* has been reported. Endocarditis and pericarditis associated with infection by *Mycobacterium chelonei* was initially described in 1979.[83] Pericarditis associated with disseminated *Mycobacterium avium intracellulare* infection has been reported in patients with HIV infection.[84]

Viral Pericarditis

Most cases of viral pericarditis are caused by enteroviral infections, for example, with coxsackievirus A and B, echovirus, or polioviruses. They are usually associated with myocarditis. Other viruses implicated in acute pericarditis include those associated with influenza, measles, mumps, chickenpox, hepatitis B, and herpes simplex. A specific viral cause is difficult to demonstrate because positive viral cultures are rarely obtained. However, a significant (four-fold) rise in viral titers during convalescence may help establish the diagnosis. In experimental studies, Tsui and Burch showed that coxsackievirus B4 infection is initiated by viral invasion of the lung and mesothelial cells with their resultant degeneration and an accompanying inflammatory response.[85] A pericardial effusion subsequently appears. It may be serous, suppurative, or hemorrhagic. In general, viral pericarditis resolves with complete recovery in a few weeks. Occasionally, recurrence occurs and fibrous organization of inflammatory exudate leads to fibrous adhesions and constrictive pericarditis. Pericarditis related to coxsackievirus (A and B) is associated with a significant incidence of postinfectious dilated cardiomyopathy.

Fungal Pericarditis

Primary fungal pericarditis is rare. It is usually associated with spread from adjoining structures, especially the lungs and pleural cavities, and with advanced malignancy or immunodeficiency states. Fungal infections that commonly cause pericarditis are histoplasmosis, blastomycosis, cryptococcosis, coccidioidomycosis, and *Candida* species.

Pericardial actinomycosis, cryptococcosis, and coccidioidomycosis are rare. They are usually associated with a serosanguineous effusion and often heal by fibrosis and adhesions. The specific organisms can be demonstrated histologically.

Histoplasmosis

Pericarditis caused by *Histoplasma capsulatum* is rare and most commonly occurs in endemic areas.[86] It usually provokes a fibrinous exudate, may be associated with a serosanguineous effusion, and histologically shows a mixed inflammatory cell infiltrate of polymorphonuclear leukocytes and lymphocytes. Granulomas may be associated with cell necrosis. Organization with fibrosis and patchy calcification occurs and may lead to constrictive

pericarditis. The diagnosis is confirmed by histologic demonstration of microorganisms from pericardial fluid or in pericardial biopsy. Histoplasma skin tests and histoplasma complement fixation tests are available. Treatment is indicated in cases of disseminated histoplasmosis.

Candidiasis

Candida species typically cause pericarditis in susceptible individuals such as immunodeficient or immunosuppressed patients, particularly those with depressed T-cell function (Fig. 12-20). *Candida* pericarditis also occurs in patients with *Candida* endocarditis, especially after prosthetic valve surgery. Purulent cases of *Candida* pericarditis generally have a poor prognosis.[87] Some authors suggest that treatment should include a combination of amphotericin B and surgical pericardiectomy.[88]

Parasitic Pericarditis

Parasitic infections of the pericardium are rare. The most commonly associated organisms are *Entamoeba histolytica*, *Toxoplasma gondii*, *Trypanosoma cruzi*, and echinococcus.

Amebic Pericarditis

An adjacent unruptured amebic hepatic abscess may produce a serous pericardial effusion caused by pericardial irritation. This resolves with successful treatment of the abscess and uncommonly progresses to constrictive pericarditis.[89] However, when a hepatic abscess ruptures into the pericardial cavity, an amebic pericarditis results with the pericardium showing a characteristic brownish-purulent exudate ("anchovy sauce pus"). This can cause cardiac tamponade. Histologic examination shows an acute inflammatory infiltrate and trophozoites of *E. histolytica* in pericardial tissue. The pericardium may also be secondarily infected with bacteria. There was a 1.3% incidence of amebic pericarditis in a review of 2000 cases of

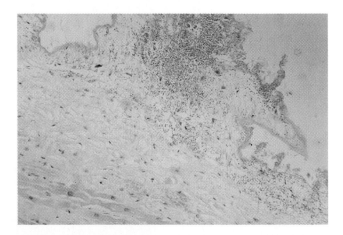

Figure 12-20 • Fungal pericarditis. Pericardium showing infection with pale blue fungal *Candida* species (upper middle region). The patient was a 54-year-old man with acute lymphoblastic leukemia and a systemic fungal infection (H&E stain).

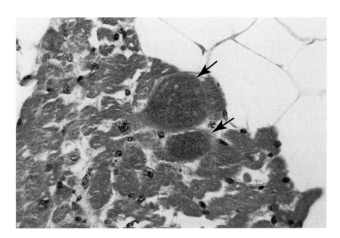

Figure 12-21 • Toxoplasmosis with associated pericarditis. This myocardium shows two muscle fibers (arrow) which are distended and contain the typical *Toxoplasma gondii* parasite. The patient had acquired immunodeficiency syndrome (H&E stain).

hepatic amebiasis, with a mortality rate of 29.6%.[90] Patients treated with a combination of chemotherapy, pericardiocentesis, and surgical aspiration of fluid had a better prognosis.

Toxoplasmosis

Pericarditis associated with *T. gondii* infection may be congenital or acquired. An increasing number of cases have been reported because of the increased incidence of acquired immunodeficiency syndrome (AIDS). A history of exposure to raw meats or cats is suggestive.[91] The parasite is associated with meningoencephalitis, myocarditis, lymphadenitis, and liver and skin lesions. The pericardium shows an infiltrate of plasma cells and lymphocytes, fibrosis, and occasional epithelioid granulomas. Pericardial effusion, constrictive pericarditis, and cardiac tamponade are possible complications. The trophozoite is rarely seen in the pericardial fluid, and the diagnosis is generally made by serology or by finding the microorganism in the myocardium (Fig. 12-21).

Echinococcosis

Cardiovascular involvement in hydatid disease is rare. It is most frequent in sheep-rearing areas of Uruguay, Australia, New Zealand, and Mediterranean countries. Hydatid disease predominantly affects the liver and lungs; cardiovascular involvement is seen in 0.5 to 2% of cases. It most commonly occurs in men in the second to fifth decade. Infestation starts in the myocardium. Fifty percent of hydatid cysts are located in the free wall of the left ventricle, with clinical widening of the interventricular septum.[92] The cyst may rupture into a cardiac cavity or pericardium.

Pericardial involvement develops in approximately 40% of patients with cardiac echinococcal disease and is characterized by a clear and serous effusion that may contain hydatid sand, germinal epithelium, and daughter cysts. The pericardium shows an intense inflammatory response with a significant infiltrate of eosinophils and lymphocytes. Secondary pericardial infection by bacteria may develop. Late complications include fibrinous pericarditis, tamponade, and constrictive pericarditis.

Chagas Disease

Chagas disease is endemic in parts of South America. Generally, the heart shows the classic signs of Chagas cardiomyopathy and the patient has clinical manifestations of congestive heart failure, ventricular arrhythmias, or sudden death. The myocardium demonstrates multifocal areas of scarring and persistent chronic inflammatory infiltrates. The epicardium shows patchy areas of fibrosis and thickening due to previous inflammation. Pericardial findings are nonspecific, with mild thickening of both pericardial layers and a mild lymphocytic infiltrate in the epicardium.[93]

Filariasis

Infection with *Wuchereria bancrofti* produces inflammation of the lymphatics and subsequent lymph stasis leading to "elephantiasis" of the limbs, the scrotum, and, occasionally, the breasts. Pericarditis is an uncommon complication. Morphologically, it is associated with a mild lymphocytic infiltrate and pericardial thickening and fibrosis. Pericardial effusions and constrictive pericarditis may also occur. Microfilaria can be found in the pericardial fluid. Specific symptoms related to the inflammation are rare.

AIDS AND PERICARDIAL DISEASE

Approximately 50% of patients with AIDS have a mild, nonspecific pericarditis at postmortem examination.[94, 95] The causes have included endocarditis,[96] Kaposi sarcoma (Fig. 12-22), mycobacteria,[97] cytomegalovirus,[98] bacterial pericarditis, and lymphoma.[99] The prevalence of pericardial effusions in AIDS has ranged from 5 to 30%.

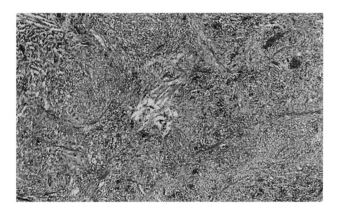

Figure 12-22 • Kaposi sarcoma involving the visceral pericardium as well as underlying myocardium. The patient had acquired immunodeficiency syndrome, and the photomicrograph shows the classic spindle-shaped cells. Mitoses are infrequent. Kaposi sarcoma was found at numerous other sites (Elastic trichrome stain).

In a prospective echocardiographic study of 231 subjects, 80% of effusions were small and caused no symptoms.[100] The survival of AIDS patients with effusions was 36% at 36 months and was significantly shorter for those without effusions (93% at 6 months).[100–102] This shortened survival was independent of CD4 count and serum albumin level.

ACUTE NONSPECIFIC PERICARDITIS

This is also known as benign, idiopathic, relapsing, or primary pericarditis of unknown origin. Viral, tuberculous, autoimmune, and toxic causes have been invoked.[47, 103] Patients most commonly present in the fourth decade, with a male/female ratio of 10:1.[103] Clinical features include a preceding upper respiratory tract infection and symptoms and signs related to congestive heart failure. Pleural-pericardial effusions are seen fairly often. A leukocytosis and an elevated erythrocyte sedimentation rate are generally present. There is frequently an associated perimyocarditis.

The clinical course is generally benign. Symptoms usually subside in a few days and resolve completely in a few weeks. This course can be modified by the administration of corticosteroids. Approximately one third of patients experience a recurrence. Constrictive pericarditis is a rare late development.[104]

Acute nonspecific pericarditis typically causes a fibrinous exudate. The pericardial surface has an initial shaggy appearance, followed later by fibrous adhesions. Histologic examination reveals pericardial congestion and a mixed inflammatory infiltrate. Associated involvement of the sinoatrial nodal region can cause arrhythmias. Pericardial effusions, either serous or serosanguineous, may occur. Cardiac tamponade can result if fluid accumulates rapidly and in large quantities.

PERICARDITIS ASSOCIATED WITH ACUTE MYOCARDIAL INFARCTION

The incidence of early postmyocardial infarction pericarditis varies from 28 to 40% of fatal infarcts studied at autopsy.[105] Its incidence has decreased by 50% in the thrombolytic era.[106] Postmyocardial infarction syndrome, or Dressler syndrome, manifests with chest pain, a pericardial friction rub, pleurisy, fever, and leukocytosis.[107] It may be caused by a combination of viral activation and antimyocardial antibodies[108] (see later discussion).

Transmural myocardial infarction is usually associated with a variable degree of fibrinous pericarditis (Fig. 12-23). The pericarditis may involve only the area overlying the infarct or a larger pericardial surface, and it can be associated with a serous or serosanguineous effusion.[109] As the pericarditis organizes, the two pericardial layers gradually adhere, especially in the region of a transmural infarct. There may be subsequent calcification of this region.

The pericardium shows variable deposits of fibrin between its two layers. This is followed by a proliferation of capillaries and fibroblasts. An infiltrate of macrophages

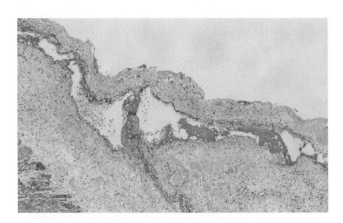

Figure 12-23 • This patient had an acute myocardial infarction and died approximately 36 hours later. The epicardium shows edema and a brightly eosinophilic fibrinous exudate. (H&E stain).

is often present, generally in association with fat necrosis. A variable lymphocytic infiltrate is also observed, although the explanation for this finding is not certain. The inflammatory process generally resolves, producing fibrous adhesions between the pericardial layers. The parietal pericardium is often thickened. Echocardiographic studies demonstrate a mild pericardial effusion in up to 17% of patients.[109]

Focal pericardial adhesions occasionally localize the extravasation of blood that follows a postinfarction free wall rupture. A pseudoaneurysm may develop. Histologically, its wall is partly or completely formed by thickened pericardial fibrous tissue and its lumen is filled by laminated thrombus. These lesions rarely rupture to cause tamponade[110] (see Chapter 8).

IATROGENIC AND TRAUMATIC PERICARDITIS

Pericardial injury of any kind leads to a reactive pericarditis.[111–113] The underlying mechanism is a loss of mesothelial cells from the pericardial surfaces,[32, 114] which leads to an effusion of fibrin. As the damaged pericardium heals, fibrin is gradually organized and replaced by adhesions.[111] The parietal pericardium is rarely thickened in traumatic pericarditis. The release of blood and blood products into the pericardial space and their contact with damaged pericardial cells culminates in fibrous adhesions and more significant pericardial thickening.[114] The intentional or unintentional deposition of foreign material also results in pericardial inflammation and fibrosis (Fig. 12-24).

Nonpenetrating and penetrating chest trauma can induce similar fibrinous pericardial reactions.[107] Other early complications of chest trauma are pericardial laceration or rupture, hemopericardium, and acute tamponade[108] (see Chapter 18). The mortality rate of pericardial rupture exceeds 60%, because it is usually associated with other major cardiovascular injuries. Late complications are rare but include postpericardiotomy syndrome, constrictive pericarditis, and cardiac herniation.

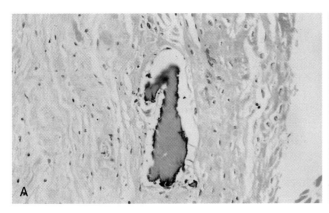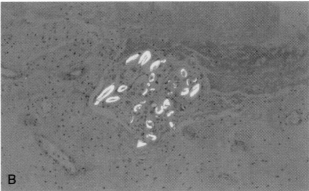

Figure 12-24 • Artefacts. *A,* This patient had open heart surgery 6 months before death. The pericardium is thickened by fibrous tissue and in the center is a fragment of dead bone. This was probably deposited during the previous surgical procedure. *B,* This patient also underwent open heart surgery. The pericardium contains a cluster of cotton fibers, with associated mild fibrotic reaction (both, H&E stain; with *B,* under polarized light).

Cardiovascular Surgery

A mild pericarditis and a low-grade fever are common during the first few days after open heart surgery.[115] The extent of pericardial inflammation depends on the manipulation of the heart and the amount of blood spilled into the pericardial cavity. Some hemorrhage is seen in virtually every case. Initially, a thin layer of fibrin with a mild infiltrate of polymorphonuclear leukocytes is seen in the epicardium (Fig. 12-25). Epicardial fat necrosis may be seen. There is gradual organization of this reaction, and the heart subsequently shows a variable degree of fibrous pericardial adhesions.

When open heart surgery was first introduced, the pericardial sac was left open at the end of the operative procedure. Adhesions frequently developed between epicardium and the sternum.[115] This fixation of the heart could lead to graft occlusion[116] and the risk of heart or aortic rupture at a subsequent sternal split (see also Chapter 18).

Postoperative constrictive pericarditis can occur.[117, 118] The time for development ranges from a few weeks to 34

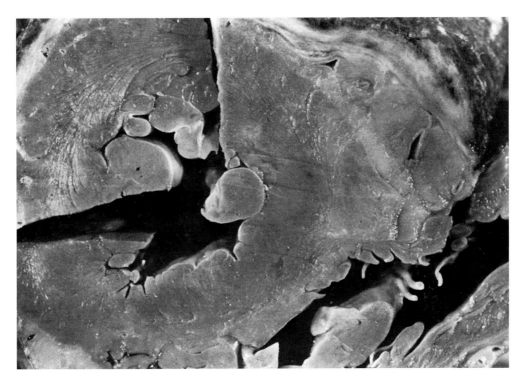

Figure 12-25 • Postoperative pericardial thickening and adhesions caused by fibrosis involving both the parietal and visceral layers. The patient had open heart surgery 2 years previously. Here in this view of the sectioned heart, fibrosis is seen over the right and left ventricles.

months, with a median of 23 months in one series.[118] Most patients experience significant symptomatic improvement after pericardiectomy. A few develop severe generalized or loculated pericardial effusions after surgery.

Postpericardiotomy Syndrome

The postpericardiotomy syndrome is a group of symptoms characterized by chest discomfort, fever, clinical evidence of pericarditis, pleuritis, and an increased erythrocyte sedimentation rate. It was first recognized after surgery for rheumatic mitral stenosis in the 1950s[119, 120] and was initially called the postcommissurotomy syndrome. Other causes of a postoperative pyrexia, such as infective endocarditis, osteomyelitis, pulmonary embolism, pneumonia, and infectious pericarditis, must be excluded before this diagnosis is made. Its reported incidence varies widely among institutions and ranges from 1.6% to more than 30%.[121]

Symptoms are usually seen in the first 10 days to 2 months after open heart surgery. They last from a few days to a few weeks, and about 30% of patients have recurrences. A few develop cardiac tamponade and may require pericardiocentesis or surgical drainage.[122]

Morphologic findings are nonspecific. Early stages show fibrin and polymorphonuclear leukocytes and later mononuclear cells. Fibrous pericardial adhesions develop gradually. Constrictive pericarditis and cardiac tamponade are rare complications.[121]

The pathogenic mechanism underlying this syndrome is not known, but immune-mediated damage is suspected.[123] A similar syndrome is seen after myocardial infarction (see earlier discussion) or after penetrating or blunt chest trauma.[122] Engle and colleagues noted a correlation with the presence of antiheart antibodies and a rise in viral titers with the subsequent development of clinical symptoms of this syndrome.[123] The viruses found were coxsackieviruses B4, B3, B2, and B5, adenoviruses, and cytomegalovirus.

RADIATION

Radiation for thoracic neoplasms may injure the pericardium, myocardium, and endocardium, as well as surrounding vascular structures. Mediastinal irradiation of rabbits given in doses equivalent to 4000 rad to humans produces an initial polymorphonuclear pericardial reaction that is followed, 1 or 2 days later, by a mononuclear cell infiltrate. Endothelial cells in lymphatics and capillaries are damaged, leading to pericardial effusion. Cardiac tamponade can occur. Later, the pericardium is thickened by fibrous tissue and the two layers adhere. Fibroblasts may have bizarre nuclei and small vessels sclerose. Epicardial coronary arteries can be damaged, promoting a rapid progression of atherosclerosis and subsequent myocardial infarction. Fat necrosis is often seen in the pericardium associated with radiation-associated changes.

PERICARDITIS ASSOCIATED WITH SYSTEMIC DISEASES

Rheumatic Fever

Acute rheumatic fever is rare in North America today but still relatively common in developing countries. It is associated with a fibrinous pericarditis and a mild mononuclear cell infiltrate. This reaction usually resolves, and patients with rheumatic valvular disease seldom show significant pericardial disease at autopsy or initial surgery. Small focal areas of pericardial calcification or lymphocytic infiltration may be seen but are extremely rare (see Chapter 13).

Rheumatoid Arthritis

Cardiac involvement is estimated to occur in 1 to 3% of patients. In an autopsy series, pericarditis was found in 41% of 148 such cases. Men and women are equally affected. Other rheumatic disorders, including juvenile rheumatoid arthritis, Still disease, Felty syndrome, ankylosing spondylitis, psoriatic arthritis, and the arthritis associated with inflammatory bowel disease, may all be associated with similar cardiac involvement (see Chapter 16).

Systemic Lupus Erythematosus

Cardiovascular manifestations are common in SLE, and the pericardium is the most commonly involved tissue. Pericardial effusions were observed in 27% of patients in one prospective study.[124] Acute, subacute, or chronic inflammation of the serosal membranes was found.[125] This includes involvement of the pericardium. In the acute phase, the mesothelium is covered by a fibrinous exudate that gradually becomes thicker, opaque, and shaggy. This gradually leads to partial or complete obliteration of the pericardial cavity. Parts of the pericardial sac that appear grossly normal usually show edema, focal areas of vasculitis, an inflammatory infiltrate, and fibrinoid necrosis on histologic examination. Hematoxylin bodies may be seen in areas of fibrinoid necrosis. Pericarditis may be associated with an effusion that is usually thick and hemorrhagic, contains polymorphonuclear leukocytes, and often has a high level of protein and gammaglobulins. Cardiac tamponade may occur. Constrictive pericarditis is a rare complication. At autopsy, patchy areas of pericardial fibrosis and thickening and calcification are seen (see Chapter 16).

Scleroderma

Pericarditis is found in 50 to 70% of cases at autopsy.[125, 126] The significant abnormality is an activation of fibroblasts, which synthesize more collagen than their normal counterparts. The collagen produced is normal. The pericarditis is most often chronic. The pericardial fluid has a high specific gravity, is protein-rich, has normal glucose levels, and contains few polymorphonuclear

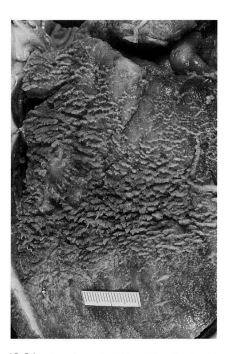

Figure 12-26 • Uremic pericarditis. This 57-year-old man had chronic renal failure. Both surfaces of the pericardium were covered by a fibrinous exudate, of shaggy "bread and butter" appearance. The layers peeled apart easily.

cells. Immune complexes have not been demonstrated. Many patients present with arrhythmias, and involvement of the sinoatrial node has been found[126] (see Chapter 16).

Vasculitides

Pericardial involvement is relatively uncommon. There may be an associated pericardial effusion. In Kawasaki syndrome, rupture of a coronary aneurysm may lead to hemopericardium.

Uremic Pericarditis

Before the use of dialysis, Richter and O'Hare were quoted as describing the ominous prognosis of a pericardial rub in association with uremic pericarditis as follows[127]: "The diagnostic rub is one of the very few single signs in medicine which enables the physician to prognosticate the death of his patient within a few days or weeks." Treatment is by management of renal function (failure) and of uremia. A fibrinous (bread and butter) pericarditis has long been recognized clinically and at autopsy in patients dying of acute or chronic renal disease with uremia (Fig. 12-26). Uremic pericarditis is still seen with chronic renal failure and chronic dialysis therapy. Its cause is not certain, but it is believed to be initiated by a chemical reaction to retained metabolic products or to be the result of a hemorrhage diathesis, the introduction of a living agent during hemodialysis, or an immune response to a component of the hemodialysis fluid or equipment.[127] The pericarditis may be hemorrhagic and lead to constrictive pericarditis.

Pericarditis with Endocrine and Metabolic Disorders

Pericardial effusions in myxedema may be large and can cause cardiac tamponade.[128] The fluid has a high specific gravity, is rich in protein and cholesterol, and is distinctly yellow. A mild degree of chronic pericarditis is usually seen, and cholesterol deposits may be evident. A pericardial effusion associated with voice changes, a low pulse rate, and diminished tendon reflexes should suggest this diagnosis. Endomyocardial biopsy may show vacuolated muscle fibers.[120]

Diabetes mellitus[130] and gout[131] may involve the pericardium, leading to a mild pericarditis. Gout pericarditis is probably related to hyperuricemia, and the pericardial fluid is rich in uric acid. Gout crystals are occasionally seen in the myocardium or heart valves.

Pericarditis Associated with Metastatic Malignant Neoplasms

Pericardial metastases are most common in leukemia, lymphomas, metastatic melanoma, and neoplasms of adjacent organs (Fig. 12-27). The majority of malignant neoplasms involving the heart have pericardial involvement. Malignant neoplasms are almost always associated with a serosanguineous pericardial effusion (see Chapter 19).

CONSTRICTIVE PERICARDITIS

Constrictive pericarditis is the result of a thickened, fibrotic, often calcified and adherent pericardium that restricts diastolic filling of the heart (Fig. 12-28).[131-134] There are many causes (Table 12-11); tuberculosis was previously the most common. Since its incidence has declined, the underlying cause for constriction is usually idiopathic pericarditis. Mycobacteria were demonstrable in only 6% of a series of 231 patients who underwent pericardectomy for chronic constrictive pericarditis.[133] At surgery and autopsy, the pericardial space is obliterated and both pericardial layers are thickened, with diffuse (occasionally localized) fibrous adhesions and variable degrees of calcification. Clinical features suggestive of constrictive pericarditis include dyspnea and abdominal distention. Investigative findings are listed in Table 12–11.

TABLE 12-11 • **Constrictive Pericarditis**

Clinical Features	Investigation
Rapid x and y descents on jugular venous pressure	Echocardiography
Jugular venous distention	Pericardial thickening
Kussmaul sign	Abnormal septal motion
Pericardial knock (on auscultation)	Atrial enlargement, mild
	Ventricles normal
	Inferior vena cava enlarged
	Doppler
	Characteristic patterns across atrioventricular valves, pulmonary veins and venae cavae

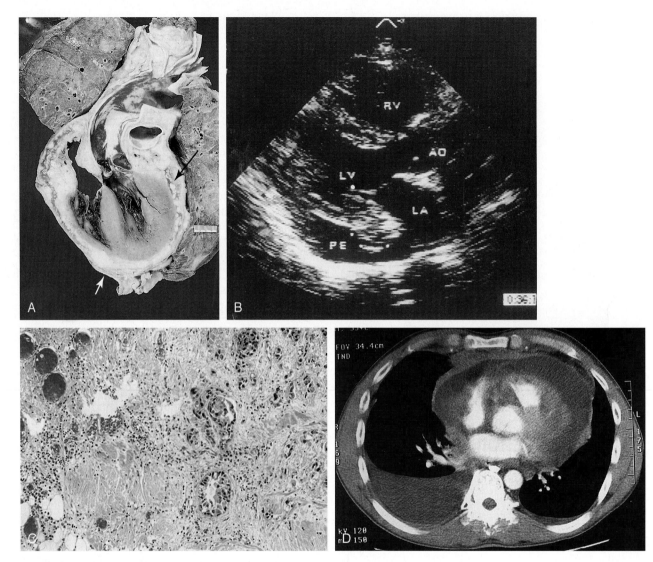

Figure 12-27 • *A,* The pericardium is diffusely thickened owing to spread of metastatic adenocarcinoma from the lungs. A minimal amount of serosanginous fluid was seen in the pericardial sac. *B,* Pericarditis associated with malignant neoplasm. Transthoracic echocardiogram in the parasternal long-axis view in a 75-year-old woman with adenocarcinoma of unknown source. A small pericardial effusion and small nodules on the epicardial surface suggest neoplastic involvement. *C,* Histologic appearance of the pericardium showing marked pericardial thickening with fibrosis, metastatic adenocarcinoma, and some chronic inflammation (H&E stain). *D,* This 64-year-old man had stage IV non-Hodgkin lymphoma. A computed tomographic scan of the chest demonstrates a large pericardial effusion, a pericardial mass, and extensive mediastinal lymphadenopathy.

PERICARDIAL TUMORS

Metastatic tumors of the heart occur 20 to 40 times more commonly than primary tumors. Primary pericardial tumors are rare. Of benign tumors, pericardial or mesothelial cysts are the most common. Other benign tumors include angiomas, lymphangiomas, fibromas, teratomas, and lipomas (see Chapter 19 for details.) They have similar clinical manifestations. Surgical excision is generally curative.

Other benign tumor and tumor-like conditions are incidental mesothelial cardiac excrescences (called MICE) and mesothelial papillomas of the pericardium. MICE are small collections of mesothelial cells mixed with fat cells and macrophages, with no intervening stroma; they are of no clinical significance and are probably artefacts. The mesothelial papilloma manifests as a cuboidal/epithelioid cell papillary tumor arising from the pericardial (or peritoneal or pleural) surface. The tumor is also called an adenomatoid tumor. It is not certain whether this is a true benign tumor or a reactive proliferation of mesothelial cells. It is usually an incidental finding at autopsy.[135, 136]

Malignant pericardial tumors are generally sarcomas.[137]

Malignant Mesothelioma

These malignant neoplasms arise from pericardial mesothelial cells. By definition the patient must have no similar tumor elsewhere. Pericardial mesotheliomas are the third most common primary malignant tumor of the heart and pericardium, but they are, nevertheless, rare[138-140]; only about 200 cases have been reported worldwide.[141, 142]

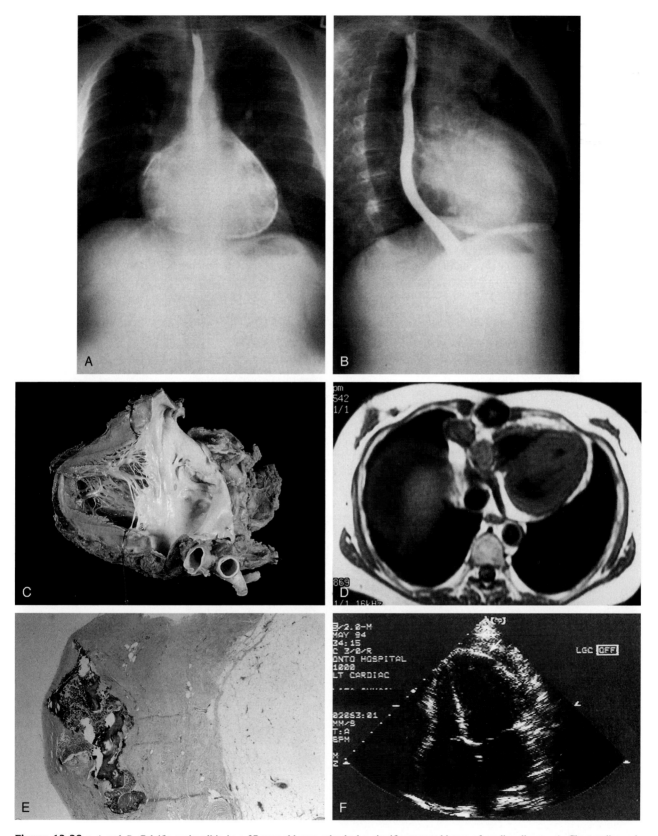

Figure 12-28 • *A* and *B*, Calcific pericarditis in a 37-year-old man who had a significant past history of cardiac disease. *A,* Chest radiograph (posteroanterior view) shows the enlarged heart and an almost circumferential rim of calcification. *B,* A barium swallow (lateral view) shows contrast material in the esophagus and indentation (notching) of the esophagus. (*A* and *B,* Courtesy of L. Zelowitsky, MD, Toronto, Ontario). *C,* Constrictive pericarditis. This heart, here photographed with the free wall of the left ventricle downward, shows diffuse thickening of the parietal and visceral pericardium and diffuse adhesions between the two layers. No pericardial fluid was present. The atria were dilated and the ventricles relatively small. *D,* Computed tomographic scan of the chest of a 75-year-old woman with constrictive pericarditis of unknown origin. The pericardium is thickened. No pericardial fluid is seen. A small right pleural effusion and right lower lobe atelectasis are evident. *E,* Excised pericardial fragment showing marked fibrosis and thickening of parietal pericardium with a central nodular area of calcification (H&E stain). *F,* This transthoracic echocardiogram in the apical four-chamber view from a 60-year-old man with constrictive pericarditis demonstrates the characteristic features of biatrial enlargement, normal ventricular size, and thickened adherent pericardial layers (white arrow). During the actual recording, abnormalities of septal wall motion were seen, suggesting abnormal diastolic filling.

They represent about 0.7% of all malignant mesotheliomas, with the majority of those tumors arising from the peritoneal and pleural surfaces. Their link with asbestosis is established: there is an increased incidence among individuals who have been exposed to that material. The mean age of affected patients is 46 years (range, 2 to 78 years). Presenting features include pericarditis and features of constriction. The tumors usually appear as firm gray-white nodules of varying size on the pericardial surface and often fill the pericardial cavity. Nevertheless, hemorrhagic, cystic, and necrotic areas are frequently present. Aspirated pericardial fluid is generally sanguinous. The tumor may encircle great vessels. Myocardial infiltration is rare, although extension to the tricuspid valve has been reported.[143] Microscopically, the tumor resembles pleural mesotheliomas and has the same epithelial, biphasic, and sarcomatoid patterns.[144]

A malignant mesothelioma must be differentiated from metastatic adenocarcinoma. This is achieved by histochemical, ultrastructural, and immunohistologic studies. The periodic acid–Schiff (PAS) stain with diastase pretreatment is the simplest to apply. Intracytoplasmic PAS-positive vacuoles are rarely (if ever) found in mesotheliomas but are found in more than two thirds of adenocarcinomas. Alcian blue is another useful stain. Ultrastructurally, intracytoplasmic lumens and cytoplasmic vacuoles are usually absent, whereas more than 50% of adenocarcinomas of the lung show these features. On the other hand, most mesothelioma cells have abundant microvilli; characteristically, they are long as compared to those seen on adenocarcinoma cells. CEA is positive in a majority of adenocarcinomas but in only a very small number of mesotheliomas.[145] Leu-M1, a glycoprotein associated with the cell membrane, is present in most if not all

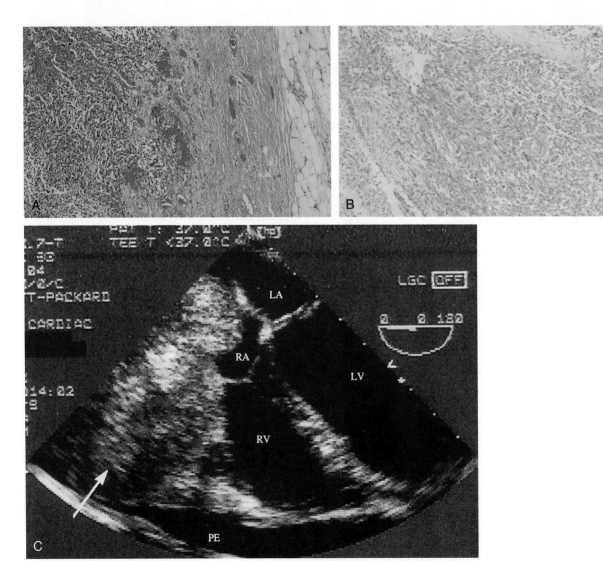

Figure 12-29 • Angiosarcoma. This 37-year-old, obese white man was in good health until 2 months before death. He developed tachycardia (120/minute), shoulder tendinitis, swelling of the ankles, and bleeding per rectum. Diagnosis of cardiac tamponade was considered, but the patient died within 1 day after admission. *A,* At necropsy, the pericardium was thickened and the pericardial space was filled by a gray-black tumor as well as fresh and old blood (H&E stain). *B,* A spindle-celled vascular tumor with occasional mitoses and vascular spaces. Positive staining for factor VIII, confirming that all cells stained like endothelial cells (Factor VIII stain). *C,* Transesophageal echocardiogram from a 40-year-old woman who presented with cardiac tamponade. Four-chamber view demonstrates a soft tissue cardiac mass in the right atrium and extending into the pericardial space (white arrow). There is an associated pericardial effusion (PE). The patient underwent surgical excision of the mass and was found to have an angiosarcoma.

adenocarcinomas of the lung but is demonstrable in only a very small percentage of mesotheliomas. Other markers that help differentiation are BER-EPS and MOC-31.[146]

Pericardial Angiosarcoma

Angiosarcomas, like mesotheliomas, involve the pericardium diffusely. However, this tumor produces a thickened, dark, gray-black pericardium (Fig. 12-29). Histologically, it is composed of endothelium-lined channels. Immunologic stains for factor VIII–related antigen and cytokeratin help differentiate it from mesothelioma[140] (see Chapter 19).

CONCLUDING REMARKS

The diagnosis of pericardial disease can be difficult and frustrating. Surgically excised and formalin-fixed pieces of calcified, thickened, and leathery pericardium often show nonspecific changes of old fibrosis, chronic inflammation, and thickening. Seldom is an acute inflammatory process evident. Despite special stains, one can usually, at best, only allude to the underlying cause of the findings. Mueller and associates prospectively performed diagnostic tests on the tissue and pericardial fluid at the time of surgery.[147] Of 92 patients, a specific etiologic diagnosis was reached in 20, of whom 12 had neoplasms, 5 infections (4 tuberculous and 1 bacterial), 2 chyloperi-cardia, and 1 amyloidosis.[147] Eleven of these were clinically unsuspected diagnoses. It is essential to perform such planned and detailed studies on excised pericardium to ensure a full and complete diagnosis.

REFERENCES

1. Spoddick DH: Medical history of the pericardium: The hairy hearts of hoary heroes. Am J Cardiol 26:447, 1970
2. Holt JP, Rhode EA, Kines H: Pericardial and ventricular pressure. Circ Res 8:1171, 1960
3. Holt JP: The normal pericardium. Am J Cardiol 26:455, 1970
4. Lee JM, Boughner DR: The mechanics of canine pericardium in different test environments: Evidence for time dependent accommodation, absence of plasticity and new roles for collagen and fibrosis. Circ Res 49:533, 1981
5. Freeman GL, LeWinter MM: Pericardial adaptations during chronic cardiac dilation in dogs. Circ Res 54:292, 1984
6. Lee JM, Boughner DR: Mechanical properties of human pericardium: Differences in viscoelastic response when compared with canine pericardium. Circ Res 55:474, 1985
7. Fukuo Y, Nakatani T, Shinohara H, Matsuda T: Pericardium of rodents: Pores connect the pericardial and pleural cavities. Anat Res 220:132, 1988
8. Hollenberg N, Dougherty J: Lymph flow and 131 I-albumin absorption from pericardial effusions in man. Am J Cardiol 24:514, 1969
9. Shenker L, Reed KL, Anderson CF, Kern W: Fetal pericardial effusion. Am J Obstet Gynecol 160:1505, 1989
10. Adamkiewica A, Jacobson H: Ueber den Druck im Herzbeutel. Centralbl Med Wissensch 11:483, 1973 (1873)
11. Morgan BC, Gunteroth WG, Dillard SH: Relationship of pericardial to pleural pressure during quiet respiration and cardiac tamponade. Circ Res 16:493, 1965
12. Kenner HM, Wood EH: Intrapericardial, intrapleural and intracardiac pressures during acute heart failure in dogs studied without thoracotomy. Circ Res 19:1071, 1966

13. Saint-Pierre A, Froemont R: Absenses totales et partielles du pericardes. Arch Mal Coeur Vaiss 63:638, 1970
14. Nasser WK: Congenital absence of the left pericardium. Am J Cardiol 26:466, 1970
15. Dippel WF, Ehrenhaft JL: Herniation of the heart after pneumonectomy. J Thorac Cardiovasc Surg 65:207, 1973
16. Candan I, Erol C, Sonel A: Cross-sectional echocardiographic appearance in presumed congenital absence of the left pericardium. Br Heart J 55:405, 1986
17. Oki T, Tabata T, Yamada H, et al: Cross sectional echocardiographic demonstration of the mechanisms of abnormal interventricular septal motion in congenital total absence of the left pericardium. Heart 77:247, 1997
18. Gutieerrez FR, Shaackelford GD, McKnight RC, et al: Diagnosis of congenital absence of left pericardium by MR imaging. J Comput Assist Tomogr 9:551, 1985
19. Saito R, Hotta F: Congenital pericardial defect associated with cardiac incarceration: Case report. Am Heart J 100:866, 1980
20. Jones JW, McManus BM: Fatal cardiac strangulation by congenital partial pericardial defect. Am Heart J 107:183, 1984
21. Wolff F, Fritz A, Dumeny P, Eisenmann B: Diastolic coronary prolapse in partial left pericardial agenesis. Arch Mal Coeur Vaiss 80:206, 1987
22. Rubush JL, Gardner IR, Boyd WD, et al: Mediastinal tumours: A review of 186 cases. J Thorac Cardiovasc Surg 65:126, 1973
23. Lambert AV: Etiology of thin-walled thoracic cysts. J Thorac Surg 10:1, 1940
24. Haas L: Diverticulum pericardii. Acta Radiol 220:228, 1939
25. DeGreeter B, Kretz JG, Nisand I, et al: Intrapericardial teratoma in a newborn infant: Use of fetal echocardiography. Ann Thorac Surg 35:664, 1983
26. Illan Y, Oren R, Ben-Chetrit E: Etiology, treatment, and prognosis of large pericardial effusions. Chest 100:958, 1991
27. Angelucci E, Mariotti E, Lucarelli G, et al: Sudden cardiac tamponade after chemotherapy for marrow transplantation in thalassemia. Lancet 339:287, 1992
28. Horowitz MS, Schultz CS, Stinson EB: Sensitivity and specificity of echocardiographic diagnosis of pericardial effusion. Circulation 50:239, 1974
29. Cheitlin MD (Chair): ACC/AHA guidelines for the clinical application of echocardiography: Executive summary. J Am Coll Cardiol 29:4:862, 1997
30. Hinds SW, Reisner SA, Amico AF, Meltzer RS: Diagnosis of pericardial abnormalities by 2D-echo: A pathology-echocardiography correlation in 85 patients. Am Heart J 123:143, 1992
31. Levine MJ, Lorell BH, Diber DJ, Come PC: Implications of echocardiographically assisted diagnosis of pericardial tamponade in contemporary medical patients: Detection before hemodynamic embarrassment. J Am Coll Cardiol 17:59, 1991
32. Cliff WJ, Grobety J, Ryan GB: Post-operative pericardial adhesions: The role of mild serosal injury and spilled blood. J Thorac Cardiovasc Surg 65:744, 1973
33. Ordones NG: The immunohistochemical diagnosis of mesothelioma: Differentiation of mesothelioma and lung adenocarcinoma. Am J Surg Pathol 13:276, 1989
34. Reddy PS, Curtiss EI, O'Toole JD, Shaver JA: Cardiac tamponade: Hemodynamic observations in man. Circulation 58:265, 1978
35. Beck CS: Two cardiac compression triads. JAMA 104:714, 1935
36. Guberman BA, Fowler NO, Engel PJ, et al: Cardiac tamponade in medical patients. Circulation 64:633, 1981
37. Stotka JL, Good CB, Downar WR, Kapoor WN: Pericardial effusion and tamponade due to Kaposi's sarcoma in acquired immunodeficiency syndrome. Chest 95:1359, 1989
38. Deloney A, Daicoff GR, Hess PJ, Victoria B: Chylopericardial with cardiac tamponade after cardiovascular surgery in two patients. Chest 69:381, 1976
39. Maronas JM, Otero-Coto, Cafferena JM: Late cardiac tamponade after open heart surgery. J Cardiovasc Surg 28:89, 1987
40. Merrill W, Donakov JS, Brawley RK, Taylor D: Late cardiac tamponade: A potentially lethal complication of open heart surgery. J Thorac Cardiovasc Surg 72:929, 1976
41. Ofori-Krakye SK, Tyberg TI, Geha AS, et al: Late cardiac tamponade after open heart surgery: Incidence, role of anticoagulants in the pathogenesis and its relationship to the post-pericardiotomy syndrome. Circulation 63:1323, 1981
42. Costa IV, Soto B, Diethelm L, Zarco T: Air pericardial tamponade. Am J Cardiol 60:1421, 1987

43. Johnston SL, Oliver RM: Cardiac tamponade due to pneumopericardium. J Thorac Cardiovasc Surg 43:482, 1988

44. Tsai WC, Lin LJ, Chen JH, Wu MH: Afebrile spontaneous pneumopyopericardium. Int J Cardiol 54:69, 1996

45. Hsu TL, Chen CC, Lee GW, et al: Intrapericardial spontaneous contrast echoes in pneumopyopericardium due to gas-forming organism. Am J Cardiol 58:1143, 1986

46. Matana A, Marvric Z, Vukas D, Beg-Zec Z: Spontaneous contrast echoes in pericardial effusion: Sign of gas-producing infection. Am Heart J 124:521, 1992

47. Permanyer-Miralda G, Sagrista-Sauleda J, Soler-Soler J: Primary acute pericardial disease: A prospective series of 231 consecutive patients. Am J Cardiol 56:623, 1985

48. Fowler NO, Harbin AD: Recurrent pericarditis: Follow-up of 31 patients. J Am Coll Cardiol 7:300, 1986

49. Adler Y, Zandman-Goddard G, Ravid M, et al: Usefulness of colchicine in preventing recurrences of pericarditis. Am J Cardiol 73:916, 1994

50. Sagrista-Sauleda J, Permanyer-Miralda G, Candell-Riera J, et al: Transient cardiac constriction: An unrecognized pattern of evolution in effusive acute idiopathic pericarditis. Am J Cardiol 59:961, 1987

51. Klacsmann PG, Bulkley BM, Hutchins GM: The changed spectrum of purulent pericarditis: An 86-year autopsy experience in 200 patients. Am J Med 63:666, 1977

52. Rubin RH, Moellering RC Jr: Clinical, microbiologic and therapeutic aspects of purulent pericarditis. Am J Med 59:68, 1975

53. Decker CF, Tuazon CU: *Staphylococcus aureus* pericarditis in HIV-infected patients. Chest 105:615, 1994

54. Raviglione MP, Mariuz P, Pablos-Mendez A, et al: High *Staphylococcus aureus* nasal carriage rate in patients with acquired immunodeficiency syndrome or AIDS-related complex. Am J Infect Control 18:64, 1990

55. Fisher BK, Warner LC: Cutaneous manifestations of the acquired immunodeficiency syndrome. Int J Dermatol 26:615, 1987

56. Schlossberg D, Zocarias F, Shulman JA: Primary pneumococcal pericarditis. JAMA 2334:853, 1975

57. Cheatam JE Jr, Grantham RN, Peyton MD, et al: *Hemophilus influenzae* purulent pericarditis in children. J Thorac Cardiovasc Surg 79:933, 1980

58. Beahl LR, Ustach TJ, Forker AD: Meningococcemia without meningitis presenting as cardiac tamponade. Am J Med 74:212, 1971

59. Pierce HI, Cooper EB: Meningococcal pericarditis: Clinical features and therapy in 5 patients. Arch Intern Med 129:918, 1972

60. Morse JR, Oretsky MI, Hudson JA: Pericarditis is a complication of meningococcal meningitis. Ann Intern Med 74:212, 1971

61. Okaroma EO, Perry LW, Scott LP III: Acute bacterial pericarditis in children: Report of 25 cases. Am Heart J 90:709, 1975

62. Feinstein V, Musher DM, Young EJ: Purulent pericarditis in a patient with Legionnaire's disease. Arch Intern Med 142:1234, 1982

63. Lieber CH, Rensimer ER, Ericson CD: *Campylobacter* pericarditis and myocardial abscess. Am Heart J 92:18, 1981

64. Tice AD, Nelson JS, Visconti EB: *Listeria monocytogenes* pericarditis and myocardial abscess. R I Med J 62:135, 1979

65. Feldman WE: Bacterial etiology and mortality of purulent pericarditis in pediatric patients. Am J Dis Child 133:641, 1979

66. Hornick P, Harris P, Smith P: Nocardia asteroides purulent pericarditis. Eur J Cardiothorac Surg 9:468, 1995

67. Sutton GC, Morrissey RA, Tobin JR, Anderson TO: Pericardial and myocardial disease associated with serological evidence of infection by the agents of psittacosis: Lymphogranuloma venerum group (Chlamydiaceae). Circulation 36:830, 1987

68. Guerin JM: Pericarditis purulentes a anaerobies: Revue de la literature a propos d'un cas. Sem Hop (Paris) 57:707, 1981

69. Nagi KS, Joshi R, Thakur RK: Cardiac manifestations of Lyme disease: A review. Can J Cardiol 12:503, 1996

70. Susman S: Tuberculous pericardial effusion. Br Heart J 5:19, 1943

71. Peel AAF: Tuberculous pericarditis. Br Heart J 19:195, 1948

72. Morgas A, Vidal M: Granulomatous eosinophilic epicarditis in the newborn: Report of 3 cases. Arch Pathol 88:459, 1969

73. Schepers GWH: Tuberculous pericarditis. Am J Cardiol 9:248, 1962

74. Strang JIG: Tuberculous pericarditis in Transkei. Clin Cardiol 5:667, 1984

75. Barr JF: The use of pericardial biopsy in establishing etiologic diagnosis in acute pericarditis. Arch Intern Med 96:693, 1955

76. Koh KK, Kim EJ, Cho CH, et al: Adenosine deaminase and carcinoembryonic antigen and pericardial effusion diagnosis, especially in suspected tuberculous pericarditis. Circulation 89:2728, 1994

77. Seino Y, Ikeda U, Kawaguchi K, et al: Tuberculous pericarditis presumably diagnosed by polymerase chain reaction analysis. Am Heart J 126:249, 1993

78. Selig MB: Percutaneous transcatheter pericardial interventions: Aspiration, biopsy, and pericardioplasty. Am Heart J 125:269, 1993

79. Nugue O, Millaire A, Porte H, et al: Pericardioscopy in the etiologic diagnosis of pericardial effusion in 141 consecutive patients. Circulation 94:1635, 1996

80. Hageman JH, D'Esopo ND, Glenn WW: Tuberculosis of the pericardium: A long-term analysis of forty-four cases. N Engl J Med 270:327, 1964

81. Sagrista-Sauleda J, Permanyer-Miralda G, Soler-Soler J: Tuberculous pericarditis: Ten-year experience with a prospective protocol for diagnosis and treatment. J Am Coll Cardiol 11:724, 1988

82. Strang JI, Kakaza HH, Gibson DG, et al: Controlled trial of prednisone as adjuvant in the treatment of tuberculous constrictive pericarditis in Transkei. Lancet 2:1418, 1987

83. Valinski E: Non-tuberculous mycobacteria and associated diseases. Am Rev Respir Dis 119:107, 1979

84. Butany J, Silver MD: Cardiovascular findings in AIDS: A report of 45 cases. Lab Invest 61:13A, 1989

85. Tsui C, Burch GE: Coxsackie virus B4 pericarditis in mice. Br J Exp Pathol 52:47, 1971

86. Piccardi JL, Kauffman CA, Schwartz J, et al: Pericarditis caused by *Histoplasma capsulatum*. Am J Cardiol 37:82, 1976

87. Kaufman LD, Seifert FC, Elliott DJ, et al: *Candida* pericarditis and tamponade in a patient with SLE. Arch Intern Med 148:715, 1988

88. Kraus WE, Valentin PN: Purulent pericarditis caused by candida: Report of three (3) cases and identification of high risk populations as an aid to early diagnosis. Rev Infect Dis 10:34, 1988

89. Bard CS, Varma AR, Lakhotin M: A case of subacute effusive constrictive pericarditis with a probable amoebic etiology. Br Heart J 58:296, 1987

90. Adams EB, MacLeod IN: Invasive amoebiasis II: Amoebic liver abscess and its complications. Medicine 56:325, 1977

91. Theoglides A, Kennedy BV: Toxoplasmic myocarditis and pericarditis. Am J Med 45:169, 1969

92. Dighiero J, Canabal EJ, Aguirre CV, et al: Echinococcal disease of the heart. Circulation 17:127, 1958

93. Rocha A, deMeneses AC, daSilva AM, et al: Pathology of patients of Chagas disease and AIDS. Am J Trop Med Hyg 50:261, 1994

94. Anderson DW, Virmani R: Emerging patterns of heart disease in human immunodeficiency virus infection. Hum Pathol 21:253, 1990

95. Malu K, Lango-M'benza B, Lushauma Z, Odlo W: Pericarditis and acquired immunodeficiency syndrome. Arch Mal Coeur Vaiss 81:2, 1988

96. Eisenberg MJ, Gordon AS, Schiller NB: HIV-associated pericardial effusions. Chest 102:956, 1992

97. Sunderam G, McDonald RJ, Maniatis T, et al: Tuberculosis as a manifestation of AIDS. JAMA 256:362, 1986

98. Nathan PE, Arsura EL, Zappi M: Pericarditis with tamponade due to cytomegalovirus in the acquired immunodeficiency syndrome. Chest 99:765, 1991

99. Kelsey RC, Saker A, Morgan M: Cardiac lymphoma in a patient with AIDS. Ann Intern Med 115:370, 1991

100. Heidenreich PA, Eisenberg MJ, Kee LL, et al: Pericardial effusion in AIDS: Incidence and survival. Circulation 92:3229, 19915

101. Nash G, Said JW, Nash WV, DeGirolami U: The pathology of AIDS. Mod Pathol 8:199, 1995

102. Ferguson DW, Volpp BD: Cardiovascular complications of AIDS. 3:388, 1994

103. Scherl ND: Acute non-specific pericarditis: A survey of the literature and study of thirty additional cases. J Mt Sinai Hospital 23:83, 1956

104. Rabinex SF, Spectos L, Ripstein CB, Schlecker AA: Chronic constrictive pericarditis as a sequel to acute benign pericarditis. N Engl J Med 251:425, 1954

105. Oliva PB, Hammill SC, Talano JV: The effect of definition on incidence of post myocardial infarction pericarditis: Is it time to redefine post infarction pericarditis? Circulation 90:1537, 1994

106. Van der Wert F: Lessons from the European Cooperative Recombinant Tissue-type Plasminogen Activator versus Placebo trial. J Am Coll Cardiol 12:14A, 1988

107. Dressler W: The post-myocardial infarction syndrome. JAMA 160:1379, 1970

108. Kossowsky WA, Lyon AF, Spain DM: Reappraisal of the post myocardial infarction Dressler's syndrome. Am Heart J 102:954, 1981

109. Charlap S, Greenberg S, Greengart A, et al: Pericardial effusion in acute myocardial infarction. Clin Cardiol 12:252, 1989

110. Ersek RA, Chesler E, Korns ME, Edwards JE: Spontaneous rupture of a false left ventricular aneurysm following myocardial infarction. Am Heart J 77:677, 1969

111. Fulda G, Braithwaite CE, Turney SZ, et al: Blunt traumatic rupture of the heart and pericardium: A ten year experience. J Trauma 31:167, 1991

112. Gallego GM, Lopez-Cambra MJ, Fernandez-Acenero MJ, et al: Traumatic rupture of the pericardium: Case report and literature review. J Cardiovasc Surg 37:187, 1996

113. Goodkind MJ, Bloomer WE, Goodyear AVN: Recurrent pericardial effusion after non-penetrating trauma. N Engl J Med 26:874, 1950

114. Cliff WJ, Grobetz J, Ryan GB: Post-operative pericardial adhesions: The role of mild serosal injury and spilled blood. J Thorac Cardiovasc Surg 65:744, 1973

115. Burch GE, Colcolough HL: Post-cardiotomy and post-infarction syndromes: A theory. Am Heart J 80:290, 1970

116. Urschl HC, Razzuk MA, Gardner N: Coronary artery bypass occlusion secondary to post-cardiotomy syndrome. Am J Thorac Surg 22:538, 1972

117. Kutcher MA, King SB III, Alimurung BN, et al: Constrictive pericarditis as a complication of cardiac surgery: Recognition of an entity. Am J Cardiol 50:742, 1982

118. Killian DN, Furiasse JG, Scanlon PJ, et al: Constrictive pericarditis after cardiac surgery. Am Heart J 118:563, 1989

119. Soloff LA, Zatulchli J, Janton OH, et al: Reactivation of rheumatic fever following mitral commissurotomy. Circulation 8:481, 1953

120. Kaminsky NE, Rodan DA, Osborne DR, et al: Post-pericardiotomy syndrome. AJR Am J Roentgenol 138:503, 1982

121. Toom TE Jr, Selzmer TJ, Sahn SA: Cardiac tamponade complicating the postpericardiotomy syndrome. Chest 83:500, 1983

122. Segal F, Padatznik B: Postpericardiotomy syndrome following penetrating stab wound of the chest: In comparison with the post-commissurotomy syndrome. Am Heart J 59:175, 1960

123. Engle MA, Ehler KH, O'Loughlin JE Jr, et al: The post pericardiotomy syndrome: Iatrogenic illness and immunological and virologic components. Cardiovasc Clin 11:2, 1981

124. Cervera R, Font J, Pare C, et al: Cardiac disease in SLE. Ann Rheum Dis 51:156, 1992

125. D'Angelo WA, Fries JS, Masi AT, Shulman LE: Pathological observations in systemic sclerosis (scleroderma): A study of 58 autopsy cases and 58 matched controls. Am J Med 46:428, 1969

126. James TN: De subitaneis mortibus. VIII. Coronary arteries and conduction system in scleroderma heart disease. Circulation 50:844, 1974

127. Compty CM, Cohen SL, Shapiro FL: Pericarditis in chronic uremia and its sequelae. Ann Intern Med 75:173, 1973

128. Smolar EN, Rubin JE, Avramides A, et al: Cardiac tamponade and primary myxedema: A review of the literature. Am J Med Sci 272:345, 1976

129. Fujimoto K, Tagata M, Nagao M, et al: [A case of myxedema heart with serial endomyocardial biopsy]. Kokyo To Junkan (Respiration and Circulation) 40:1019, 1992

130. Campbell IW, Duncan LJP, Clarke BF: Pericarditis in diabetes ketoacidosis. Br Heart J 39:110, 1977

131. Polay JW, Barlow Ke, Kating PEJ, Stevens J: Acute gouty pericarditis. Lancet 1:21, 1963

132. Arthur A, Oskrig R, Basta LL: Calcific rheumatoid constrictive pericarditis with cardiac failure treated by pericardiectomy. Chest 64:769, 1973

133. McLaughlin BC, Schaff HV, Piehler JM, et al: Early and late results of pericardiectomy for constrictive pericarditis. J Thorac Cardiovasc Surg 89:340, 1985

134. Oh JK, HaHe LK, Seward JB, et al: Diagnostic role of Doppler echocardiography in constrictive pericarditis. J Am Coll Cardiol 23:154, 1994

135. Luthringer DJ, Virmani R, Weiss SW, Rosai J: A distinctive cardiovascular lesion resembling histiocytoid (epithelioid) hemangioma: Evidence suggesting mesothelial participation. Am J Surg Pathol 14:993, 1990

136. Hanson RM, Caya JG, Clowry LJ Jr, Anderson T: Benign mesothelial proliferation with effusion: Clinicopathologic entity that may mimic malignancy. Am J Med 77:887, 1984

137. Pamella JS, Paige ML, Victor TA, et al: Angiosarcoma of the heart: Diagnosis by echocardiography. Chest 76:21, 1979

138. Suzuki Y: Pathology of human malignant mesothelioma. Semin Oncol 8:268, 1981

139. Suzuki Y, Chury J, Kannerslein M: Ultrastructure of human diffuse mesothelioma. Am J Pathol 85:241, 1976

140. Burke A, Virmani R: Atlas of Tumor Pathology. Tumors of the Heart and Great Vessels. Fasicle 16 (Series 3). Washington, DC, Armed Forces Institute of Pathology, 1996

141. Hillerdal G: Malignant mesotheliomas 1982: Review of 4710 published cases. Br J Dis Chest 77:321, 1983

142. Turk J, Kenda M, Kranjec I: Primary malignant pericardial mesothelioma. Klin Wochenschr 69:674, 1991

143. Walters LL, Taxy JB: Malignant mesotheliomas of the pleura with extensive cardiac invasion and tricuspid orifice occlusion. Cancer 52:1736, 1983

144. Sytman AL, McAlpine RN: Primary pericardial mesothelioma: Report of 2 cases in review of the literature. Am Heart J 81:760, 1971

145. Hoffler H, Schmidt P, Tscheliessnigg KH: Malignes Angioblastisches Mesotheliom tes Perikards. Zentralbl Allg Pathol 1979; 123:344

146. Wick MR, Mills SE, Swanson PE: Expression of myelomonocytic antigens in mesotheliomas and adenocarcinomas involving the serosal surfaces. Am J Clin Pathol 94:18, 1990

147. Mueller XM, Tevaerai HT, Humi M, et al. Etiologic diagnosis of pericardial disease: The value of routine tests during surgical procedures. J Am Coll Surg 184:645, 1997

Chapter 13

Valvular Heart Disease: General Principles and Stenosis

.....

Frederick J. Schoen • William D. Edwards

The clinical outcome of patients with valvular heart disease has improved substantially over the last several decades. This favorable trend has resulted principally from the combination of increasingly effective noninvasive assessment of valve dysfunction and monitoring of ventricular function, development of guidelines for choosing the proper timing of surgical intervention, less invasive surgical approaches, improvements in prosthetic valves, and advances in valve reconstruction techniques.[1-3] Owing to the success of surgical treatment, there are fewer patients seen at autopsy whose valvular heart disease has followed its natural course, whereas increasing numbers of patients have had a heart valve prosthesis inserted or have undergone repair procedures. Thus, at present, in centers where cardiovascular surgery is performed, whole specimens or fragments of diseased heart valves are frequently available for pathologic examination in the surgical pathology laboratory, and valvular heart disease is rarely encountered in the autopsy suite. In contrast, in underdeveloped countries, recognition and treatment of valvular heart disease has had a lesser impact on the huge reservoir of individuals with rheumatic valvular disease. They are more likely to die of complications from their valvular disease than their counterparts in the industrialized world.

In this chapter, we present concepts that are applicable to the many varieties of valvular heart disease, followed by a detailed discussion of specific pathologic processes that produce obstruction to blood flow at the valvular, subvalvular, and supravalvular levels of the four cardiac valves. Pathologic anatomy, clinicopathologic correlations, treatment, specimen evaluation and, to the extent known, pathogenesis are summarized, and the most common conditions are emphasized. Consistent with the general theme of this book, which favors conditions found in the adult, we discuss in detail only congenital valvular lesions that permit survival to adulthood; comprehensive information on pediatric valvular pathology can be found elsewhere.[4] Dysfunction with stenosis or regurgitation of substitute heart valves is discussed in detail in Chapter 21.

FUNCTIONAL VALVE ANATOMY

Normal cardiac valves permit unidirectional flow of blood without obstruction or regurgitation, trauma to molecular or formed blood elements, thromboembolism, or excessive mechanical stress in the cusps and leaflets. Valve function requires interactions among several anatomic components. For the atrioventricular (mitral and tricuspid) valves, these elements include the annulus, leaf-

lets, commissures, chordae tendineae (tendinous cords), papillary muscles, and atrial and ventricular myocardium. For the semilunar (aortic and pulmonary) valves, the key structures are the annulus, cusps, commissures, and their supporting structures in the great arteries and subjacent ventricular myocardium (see Table 14-1).

Mitral Valve

As depicted in Figure 13-1, the mitral valve has an anterior (also called septal, or aortic) leaflet and a posterior (also called mural, or ventricular) leaflet.[5-7] The anterior leaflet is deeper (in the radial dimension) and has a roughly semicircular shape, with the base inserting along approximately one third of the annulus. The posterior leaflet, although shallower, is attached to about two thirds of the annulus and typically has a scalloped appearance. The mitral leaflets have a combined area approximately twice that of the orifice; they meet during systole, with coaptation comprising the distal 50% of the posterior leaflet and the distal 30% of the anterior leaflet. The anterolateral and posteromedial papillary muscles are positioned directly distal to their respective commissures so that the approximately 120 tendinous cords extend from and anchor both leaflets to each of the two muscles.

The mitral annulus is shaped like the letter D. The flat anteromedial portion comprises the anterior leaflet attachment to noncontractile subaortic fibrous tissue. In contrast, the semicircular posterolateral portion of the annulus comprises the posterior leaflet attachment to the contractile left ventricular free wall. Thus, during systole, left ventricular contraction constricts this muscular portion of the annulus, thereby reducing the area of the orifice. The edges of the mitral leaflets are held at or below (i.e., distal to) the plane of the orifice by the tendinous cords, pulled from below by the contraction and foreshortening of the papillary muscles.[8] Contraction of the papillary muscles during systole tends to draw the two leaflets together and thereby promotes valve closure and maintains competence. In contrast to the mitral valve, the tricuspid valve has three leaflets (anterior, posterior, and septal), with a larger and less distinct orifice and larger but thinner leaflets.[9]

Aortic Valve

Extending from the apex of the heart to the aortic valve, the left ventricular outflow tract is shaped like a gently inverted letter S. Its borders are defined by the ventricular septum, the anterior portion of the free wall,

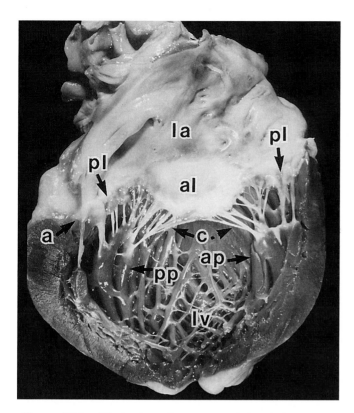

Figure 13-1 • Mitral valve and components of the mitral apparatus, shown in opened left ventricle of normal heart. al = anterior leaflet; pl = posterior leaflet; a = annulus; c = chordae tendineae (tendinous cords); ap = anterior papillary muscle; pp = posterior papillary muscle; la = left atrium; lv = left ventricle. (From Schoen FJ: Interventional and Surgical Cardiovascular Pathology: Clinical Correlations and Basic Principles. Philadelphia, WB Saunders, 1989.)

and the anterior mitral leaflet and its subjacent chordae and papillary muscles. Motion of the anterior mitral leaflet during the cardiac cycle alters the caliber of the sub-aortic outflow tract. Thus, in ventricular diastole, when the mitral valve opens, the tract is narrowed as the ante-

rior leaflet moves toward the ventricular septum. Conversely, during ventricular systole, the outflow tract becomes larger as the anterior leaflet moves away from the septum to close the mitral valve orifice. The lower border of the aortic sleeve, attached to the ventricular septum and the base of the anterior mitral leaflet, is, anatomically, the narrowest portion of the aortic valve complex.

The aortic valve annulus forms part of the fibrous cardiac skeleton and is surrounded by, and in direct contact with, the annulus of each of the other three cardiac valves and with the membranous septum. The gross anatomy of the aortic valve is illustrated in Figure 13-2. The aortic valve cusps attach to the aortic wall in a crescentic or semilunar fashion, ascending to the commissures and descending to the trough or base of each cusp.[10] The line of attachment of the cusps forms a fibrous nonplanar structure shaped like a triradiate crown. It also abuts the ventricular septum below and the atrial septum above. Accordingly, calcific or infective processes of the valve cusps may extend onto any of these adjacent structures and can produce functional impairment. Also potentially involved are the atrioventricular (His) bundle and the left bundle branch of the specialized conduction system (see Fig. 14-14). Furthermore, during surgical excision of the aortic valve, these structures may be injured. The three commissures occupy the three points of the annular crown and represent the sites of separation of one cusp from its adjacent cusps. Commissures are spaced circumferentially approximately 120 degrees apart, although there is substantial individual variability. The sinuses of Valsalva are dilated pockets of the aortic root behind the valve cusps that bulge with each systolic ejection of blood. The aortic valve cusps and their respective sinuses are named for their relationship to the coronary artery ostia that arise from them. Thus, a normal valve is said to have left, right, and noncoronary (or posterior) cusps and corresponding aortic sinuses. The coronary arterial orifices typically arise from the right and left aortic sinuses immediately distal to the cuspal free edges.

Aortic valve cusps must open toward the aortic wall

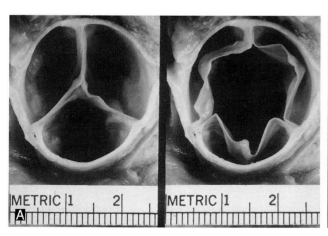
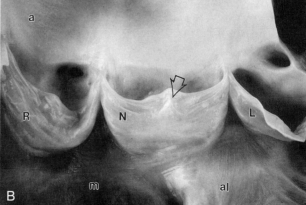

Figure 13-2 • Aortic valve. *A*, View from distal aspect in closed (left) and open (right) phases. The closed cusps are closely apposed during ventricular diastole and virtually completely open against the aortic wall during systole. *B*, Aortic valve after dissection with incision of the left ventricular outflow tract, revealing left (L), right (R), and noncoronary (N) cusps. a = aortic wall; m = left ventricular outflow tract myocardium; al = anterior mitral leaflet, ventricular side. The nodule of Arantius of the noncoronary cusp is designated by an open arrow.

during ventricular systole and close rapidly and completely under minimal reverse pressure, maintaining full competency throughout diastole (see Fig. 13-2). Each has a similar half-moon (semilunar) shape, but the three are usually of somewhat unequal size. Although the pressure differential across the closed valve induces a large load on the cusps, prolapse of the cusps into the left ventricular outflow tract does not normally occur because of the substantial area of coaptation and the fibrous network that effectively transfers the cuspal stresses to the annulus (see later). Located along the ventricular aspect of each cusp, between its free edge and its closing edge, are two crescentic regions, termed lunulas. During valve closure, the two lunular areas of one cusp contact the corresponding regions of both adjacent cusps and thereby effect a competent seal. In the middle of the free edge of each cusp, on its ventricular surface, is a fibrous mound, the nodule of Arantius. Coaptation of the three nodules ensures complete central closure of the valve orifice during ventricular diastole. The collective coaptation area of the aortic valve is substantial and can be as much as 50% of the total surface area of the loaded cusp. The structure of the pulmonary valve and its surrounding tissues is similar to that of the aortic valve, except that the former has a more delicate structure and absence of coronary arterial origins. The pulmonary valve is cradled somewhat by a collar of myocardium in the right ventricular outflow tract.

Valve Histology and Biology

The aortic valve serves as the paradigm for valvular microstructural adaptation to the essential requirements of function. The complex, repetitive, and substantial changes in shape and dimension of natural aortic valve cusps during the cardiac cycle are accomplished by a highly specialized inhomogeneous structure composed of three histologically well-defined tissue layers, whose major distinguishing features are related to their extracellular matrix (Table 13-1 and Figs. 13-3 and 13-4).[11–13] From proximal to distal, the layers are: (1) the ventricular layer (*ventricularis*) facing the inflow surface, composed predominantly of collagen with radially aligned elastic fibers

TABLE 13-1 • The Layers of the Aortic Valve

Layer	Predominant Extracellular Matrix Component	Function
Ventricular	Elastin	Extend in diastole, contract in systole
Spongy	Glycosaminoglycans	Absorb shear forces and cushion shock between ventricular and fibrous layers during cyclic valve motion
Fibrous	Collagen	Provide strength and stiffness to maintain coaptation during diastole

Modified from Schoen FJ: Aortic valve structure-function correlations: Role of elastic fibers no longer a stretch of the imagination. J Heart Valve Dis 6:1, 1997.

lined by endothelial cells; (2) the subjacent spongy layer (*spongiosa*), composed of loosely arranged collagen and abundant proteoglycans; and (3) the fibrous layer (fibrosa) facing the outflow surface, composed predominantly of circumferentially aligned, densely packed collagen fibers, largely arranged parallel to the cuspal free edge. There is a poorly demarcated fourth layer immediately below the aortic surface (aortalis), which contains scant collagen and elastin and which is lined by endothelial cells.

Some histologic aspects of atrioventricular and semilunar valves are dissimilar, reflecting different embryogenesis and closure mechanisms. However, the similarities are more important for consideration of valvular function and disease progression.[14] The mitral and tricuspid valves have analogous components: atrial (*atrialis*), spongy, fibrous, and ventricular layers (from inflow to outflow, respectively). Their tendinous cords have a densely collagenous core, with a thin endocardial lining but no consistent spongy layer.

For all four valves, the fibrous layer provides strength to maintain structural integrity. The spongy layer, in contrast, has negligible structural strength but appears to allow gliding (shear) between the fibrous and elastic layers to permit (1) moldability and interdigitation of apposing

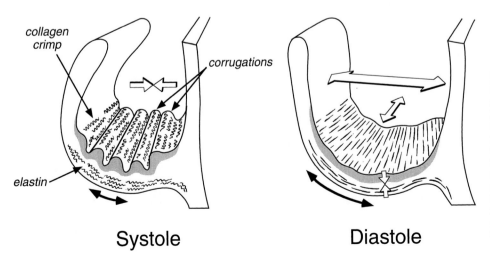

collagen crimp

corrugations

elastin

Systole

Diastole

Figure 13-3 • Schematic representation of dynamic aortic valve cuspal architecture and configuration of collagen and elastin in systole and diastole. (Modified from Schoen FJ: Pathology of bioprostheses and other tissue heart valve replacements. In: Silver MD [ed]: Cardiovascular Pathology, 2nd ed. New York, Churchill Livingstone, 1991, p. 1547. From Schoen FJ: Aortic valve structure-function correlations: Role of elastic fibers no longer a stretch of the imagination. J Heart Valve Dis 6:1, 1997.)

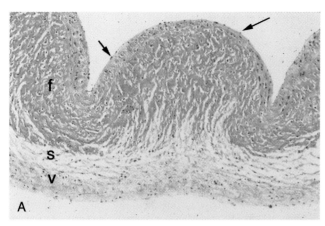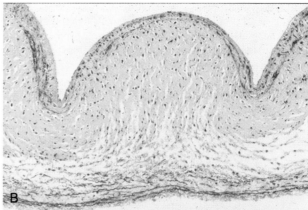

Figure 13-4 • Aortic valve histology, shown as low-magnification photomicrographs of cross-section cuspal configuration in the nondistended state, emphasizing three major layers: ventricularis (v), spongiosa (s), and fibrosa (f). A, Overall architecture, with superficial endothelial cells (arrows) and diffusely distributed deep interstitial cells. B, Section stained for elastin, emphasizing the dense, laminated elastic tissue, particularly in the ventricularis. In both A and B, the outflow surface is at the top. A, H&E stain; B, Verhoeff–van Gieson stain (elastin is black). (B, From Schoen FJ: Aortic valve structure-function correlations: Role of elastic fibers no longer a stretch of the imagination. J Heart Valve Dis 6:1, 1997.)

leaflets in forming a competent seal, (2) the dynamic changes in shape of the cusps during the cardiac cycle, and (3) to dissipate energy by acting as a shock absorber during closure. The rich elastin of the ventricular layer of the aortic valve facilitates contraction of the cusps, producing minimal surface area when the valve is open but stretching to form a large coaptation area when back pressure is applied during closure.[15, 16]

The cardiac valves have cells of two types: interstitial and endothelial. The interstitial cell population has morphologic and functional features characteristic of fibroblasts, smooth muscle cells, and myofibroblasts.[17–23] They are believed to continuously synthesize, remodel, and replenish the connective tissue matrix in valvular homeostasis and may play an important role in disease.[24] Interstitial cells respond to vasoactive agents by contraction, growth, and collagen synthesis.[25, 26] Moreover, valves have been shown to contain nerves, a recent finding that suggests a physiologic role for contraction of interstitial cells.[27, 28] This finding is particularly relevant in view of data suggesting that the onset of aortic valve opening precedes the development of the required transvalvular pressure gradients. Moreover, in calcific degeneration, mineral is initially deposited in interstitial cells, in both normal and bioprosthetic valves.[29–31] Endothelial cells coat all surfaces of the valve cusps. Evidence suggests that valvular endothelial cells may express different genes and respond differently to injury than endothelial cells at other sites, but the nature and extent of those differences remain to be determined.[32, 33] For example, experimental and human heart transplants with massive myocardial rejection show little inflammation in the valves, and fresh porcine valves are not rejected in primates.[33–35]

The origins of valvular cells in development and their replenishment during normal valvular function are areas of great interest. Considerable data show that some valvular endothelial cells undergo an epithelial-to-mesenchymal transformation during developmental valvulogenesis, yield-

ing an important source of interstitial cells.[36] Other data suggest that this process of "transdifferentiation" continues postnatally.[37]

Complex microstructural rearrangements and several specializations of collagen accommodate the cyclic response to transvalvular pressure.[38–40] Despite a substantial pressure differential across the closed aortic valve, which induces a large load on the cusps, their fibrous network effectively transfers the resultant stresses to the annulus and aortic wall. This ensures that excessive stress is not concentrated at the commissures, provided that normal coaptation is maintained.

During opening, as each cusp moves toward the aortic wall, the ventricular layer must stretch while the fibrous layer undergoes compression. Stresses caused by this differential movement are largely dissipated in the spongiosa. Moreover, with the capacity of extending in a radial direction, both collagen corrugations, which produce a grossly visible surface rippling and microscopic crimp (folding) of collagen fibers, enable cusps to be extremely soft and pliable when unloaded. However, cusps have low compliance when loaded (when the corrugations and crimp are extended), allowing cuspal shape and dimension to vary during different phases of the cardiac cycle. The fibrous layer is also reinforced by the presence of cords within the layer, composed of focal thickenings of collagen fibers arranged in bundles, oriented (circumferentially) toward the commissures and points near the cuspal base. These cords assist in transferring the stresses of the closed portion of the cycle to the aortic wall. Through the stiffening induced by extended collagen crimp, flattened corrugations, and taut collagen cords, exaggerated sag of the cusp centers is prevented when the valve is shut, thereby preserving maximum coaptation.

The prevailing view maintains that normal human semilunar and atrioventricular valve cusps and leaflets are nearly avascular but may contain a few capillaries in the proximal third of their cusps and leaflets.[41] Presumably, the mobile structures are sufficiently thin to be perfused from the heart's blood. However, a recent examination of porcine heart valves using a novel perfusion protocol suggests that the functional valvular vasculature may be more extensive than previously thought.[42]

Age-Related Changes in the Cardiac Valves

The general morphologic changes that occur during the aging of heart valves have been widely described (see Chapter 3).[43-48]

Age-related changes of the mitral valve may be functionally important. The mitral leaflets thicken progressively with each decade, particularly along their closure margins.[49] Collagen deposition and degeneration, lipid accumulation, and dystrophic calcification, particularly in the annulus, can be observed histologically. Extensive mitral annular calcification can cause functional impairment, usually mitral insufficiency, but, occasionally, stenosis (see later). Moreover, shortening of the overall base-to-apex length of the left ventricle may cause the mitral tendinous cords to appear relatively longer than necessary and allow mild hooding of the posterior leaflet, simulating mitral valve prolapse.

Age-related degenerative changes may also appreciably alter aortic valve anatomy and function and should be taken into account during evaluation of aortic valve disease. The weight and area of the individual aortic valve cusps increase with age, accompanied by stretching, fibrosis, and accumulation of lipid.[50] With increasing age, there is a progressive increase in the diameter of the aortic root and valvular annulus, with the diameter of the aortic annulus approaching that of the mitral annulus in elderly individuals.[51, 52] Indeed, idiopathic dilation of the aortic annulus is now reported to be the most common cause of symptomatic aortic regurgitation.[53] Moreover, with increasing age, and especially in patients older than 65 years, the annular tissue tends to thicken and to acquire calcific deposits. Degenerative calcification of an otherwise normal-appearing aortic valve with three cusps may result in progressive aortic stenosis (see later). Although fenestrations (holes) within the lunulas near the free edges as an age-related degenerative abnormality are common, they generally have no functional significance, because the lunular tissue lies above the closing edge of each cusp. In contrast, fenestrations below the lunula not only cause incompetence but may also suggest previous or active infection. With increasing age, fibrous, whisker-like projections known as Lambl's excrescences may form along the closing edge, the free edge, and the nodule of Arantius. Amyloid deposits are also found in aging and calcified aortic valves.[54-56]

Although the various age-related changes that affect the cardiac valves and alter the geometry of the heart may be responsible in part for the low-grade systolic ejection murmurs commonly noted in elderly individuals, it is not known whether normal age-related changes in the cardiac valves increase the risk of infective endocarditis. Two competing factors play a role. Alterations that produce turbulence favor the development of valve injury, thrombotic vegetations, and infection. However, beyond a point of maximal susceptibility, the more heavily calcified, stenotic, and, consequently, flow-limiting a valve becomes, the less likely it is to become infected.

PRINCIPLES OF VALVULAR HEART DISEASE

Pathologic Anatomy

The major functional abnormalities of the cardiac valves are *stenosis* (i.e., obstruction caused by failure of a valve to open completely, thereby inhibiting forward flow), and *regurgitation* (i.e., reversed flow caused by failure of a valve to close completely, also called valvular insufficiency or incompetence). Valve dysfunction can be due to disorders affecting the valve cusps/leaflets, their supporting structures, or both. Stenosis generally results from fibrous and calcific distortion of valvular cusp/leaflet anatomy and, hence, usually develops relatively slowly, as a chronic process. In contrast, insufficiency not only results from either intrinsic disease of the valve cusps/leaflets or damage to associated structures (e.g., the aorta, the left ventricular myocardium, or the chordae), but it also may develop acutely or slowly. Stenosis and insufficiency may coexist in the same valve (*combined dysfunction*), but usually one predominates. If stenosis or insufficiency alone is present, the valvular disease is called *pure*. Involvement of a single valve is known as *isolated* valvular disease, and that of more than one valve is termed *multivalvular* disease.

Valvular abnormalities may be caused by congenital disorders or by a variety of acquired diseases. The most important causes of acquired heart valve dysfunction are summarized in Table 13-2. In contrast to the many potential causes of valvular insufficiency, only a relatively few conditions commonly produce acquired valvular stenosis.

The clinical picture of valve stenosis can result from obstruction at the valvular, subvalvular, or supravalvular levels (Table 13-3). Nevertheless, stenosis occurs most frequently at the level of the valve. The two most common causes of valvular stenosis are fibrous or calcific stiffening of the cusps or leaflets and commissural fusion, either alone or in combination. Rarely, the orifice is stenosed by a mass (vegetation, thrombus, or neoplasm) or by external compression. Like their valvular counterparts, subvalvular and supravalvular obstructions may be congenital or acquired.

Overall, stenotic valves are encountered more often in the surgical pathology laboratory than purely regurgitant ones, as emphasized by the experience from one institution that is summarized in Table 13-4.[57] However, the data presented in Table 13-4 were obtained over several decades before 1980, and contemporary surgical pathology practice in North America may now be modified. Aortic stenosis continues to be the most common lesion. Indeed, as a condition most prominent in older individuals, aortic stenosis is becoming more prevalent as the population ages.[58, 59] Moreover, because repair of aortic valve stenosis remains an unsuccessful surgical option,

TABLE 13-2 • **Most Common Causes of Acquired Heart Valve Disease**

Mitral Valve	Aortic Valve
Mitral Stenosis	**Aortic Stenosis**
Postinflammatory scarring (rheumatic heart disease)	Degenerative calcific aortic stenosis
	Calcification of congenitally deformed valve
	Postinflammatory scarring (rheumatic heart disease)
Mitral Regurgitation	**Aortic Regurgitation**
Abnormalities of leaflets and commissures	Intrinsic valvular disease
Mitral valve prolapse	Bicuspid aortic valve
Infective endocarditis	Infective endocarditis
Postinflammatory scarring (rheumatic heart disease)	Postinflammatory scarring (rheumatic heart disease)
Abnormalities of tensor apparatus	Aortic disease
Rupture of tendinous cords	Degenerative aortic dilation
Rupture of papillary muscle	Giant cell aortitis
Papillary muscle dysfunction (fibrosis)	Ankylosing spondylitis
Abnormalities of annulus	Rheumatoid arthritis
Mitral annular calcification	Marfan syndrome
Abnormalities of left ventricular cavity and/or annulus	Syphilitic aortitis
LV enlargement (myocarditis, congestive cardiomyopathy)	
Calcification of mitral ring	

LV = left ventricular.

Modified from Schoen FJ: Surgical pathology of removed natural and prosthetic valves. Hum Pathol 18:558, 1987.

and although repair for aortic valve regurgitation can be done in some cases,[60] pathologists will frequently continue to encounter specimens of excised aortic valves in the surgical pathology laboratory. However, because of the decline in rheumatic heart disease in the past several decades, the importance of rheumatic mitral stenosis has diminished greatly.[61] Pure mitral regurgitation (most frequently due to myxomatous degeneration) and pure aortic insufficiency (most frequently due to aortic dilation) are next in frequency (over mitral stenosis, tricuspid stenosis, and pulmonary stenosis). However, as a consequence of the increasing prominence of reparative mitral valve surgery,[62, 63] only a portion of many such valves may be

TABLE 13-4 • **Functional Distribution of Operatively Excised Cardiac Valves From Patients Aged 15 Years or Older**

Lesion	Number (%)	
	Patients	Valves
Aortic stenosis (AS)	491 (35)	491 (28)
Mitral stenosis (MS)	404 (28)	404 (23)
AS + MS	254 (18)	508 (29)
Mitral regurgitation (MR)	121 (8)	121 (7)
Aortic regurgitation (AR)	82 (6)	82 (5)
MS + AR	28 (2)	56 (3)
MS + tricuspid regurgitation (TR)	14 (1)	28 (2)
AR + MR	13 (0.9)	26 (2)
MS + AS + tricuspid stenosis (TS)	4 (0.2)	10 (0.6)
TR	1 (0.1)	1 (0.1)
Other mixed lesions	2 (0.1)	6 (0.4)
Total	1414 (100)	1733 (100)

Modified from Waller BF, Bloch T, Barker BG, et al: Evaluation of operatively excised cardiac valves: Etiologic determination of valvular heart disease. Cardiol Clin 2:687, 1984.

available for study by pathologists.[64] Because careful gross inspection is often the most informative step in the pathologic/etiologic diagnosis of cardiac valves (as emphasized later in this chapter), diagnostic difficulties may arise in cases where only fragments of a dysfunctional valve are available for study.[65]

Replacement of one valve occurs more commonly than multiple valve replacement. When multivalvular lesions are present, the lesions can be either *concordant* (i.e., all stenotic or all purely regurgitant, usually of the same etiology) or *discordant* (i.e., combinations such as a stenotic bicuspid aortic valve coexisting with a regurgitant myxomatous mitral valve, or rheumatic mitral stenosis coexisting with tricuspid regurgitation due to pulmonary hypertension).

Clinicopathologic Correlations

The signs, symptoms, and functional consequences of valvular disease depend on which cardiac valve or valves are involved and to what degree. They may vary from slight and physiologically unimportant to severe. The clinical syndromes of mitral and aortic stenosis imply a

TABLE 13-3 • **Location, Frequency, and Mechanisms of Obstruction to Blood Flow Through the Heart**

Mechanisms of Obstruction	Frequency	Example
Valvular		
Congenital deformity	Uncommon	Congenital AS
Leaflet or cusp thickening, fibrosis, calcification	Common	Degenerative calcific AS, rheumatic AS
Commissural fusion	Common	Rheumatic MS
Filling of valve lumen	Uncommon	Vegetations, tumor, prosthetic heart valve thrombus
External compression of lumen	Uncommon	Tumor
Subvalvular and Supravalvular		
Filling orifice	Uncommon	Tumor, aortic atherosclerotic plaque
Originating from wall components	Uncommon	Membranous subaortic stenosis, muscular subaortic stenosis, atrial myxoma, aortic wall abnormalities (e.g., Williams syndrome)
External compression	Rare	Tumor, constrictive pericarditis

AS = aortic stenosis; MS = mitral stenosis.

substantial impairment of valve orifice area.[3] The normal aortic orifice area is approximately 2.6 to 4.0 cm² in adults. Consideration of hemodynamic and natural history data lead to an approximate sorting of the degree of aortic stenosis into mild (area > 1.5 cm²), moderate (1.0–1.5 cm²), and severe (< 1.0 cm²). In severe stenosis, the transvalvular gradient is usually greater than 50 mm Hg when the cardiac output is normal. The normal mitral orifice area is 3.0 to 5.0 cm²; symptoms occur on stress or exertion with a valve area less than 2 to 2.5 cm² and at rest with a valve area approximately 1.5 cm². Severe mitral stenosis generally indicates a valve area less than 1.0 cm². Valve orifice sizes increase with greater age and body size, and atrioventricular valve annuli enlarge in cardiac failure, but stiffening of cusps may inhibit their motion; therefore, the normal valve areas should be viewed as general approximations. Males generally have larger valve areas than females.

In many cases, valvular lesions require surgical intervention, or they may ultimately become lethal. Furthermore, the degree of tolerable dysfunction, and thus the course and prognosis for an individual patient, vary secondary to both the degree and the rate of development of the hemodynamic abnormality. For example, sudden destruction of an aortic valve by infective endocarditis can cause rapidly fatal cardiac failure, whereas clinically significant mitral stenosis usually takes several decades to become symptomatic. Depending upon extent, duration, and etiology, valvular dysfunction may produce secondary changes in the heart, blood vessels, and other organs, both proximal and distal to the valvular lesion. These include cardiac hypertrophy and dilation (see later), visceral congestion, inadequate downstream perfusion with potential ischemic injury and fibrosis, and embolism. A more detailed list is presented as Table 13-5.

The clinical significance of valvular disease results from its anatomic and physiologic consequences, especially ventricular dysfunction, atrial fibrillation, pulmonary venous hypertension, pulmonary edema, or sudden death. Aortic valvular dysfunction places a hemodynamic burden on the left ventricular myocardium, which is initially tolerated as the cardiovascular system compensates for the overload. However, sustained pressure or volume overload eventually leads to myocardial dysfunction, congestive heart failure, and, in some cases, sudden death.[1, 2, 66] Indeed, some valve lesions yield a prolonged latent period in which morbidity and mortality are very low. The most important consequence of mitral stenosis is left atrial hypertension, which in turn elevates pressures in the pulmonary vascular system and is largely responsible for dyspnea, the principal cause of the patient's disability.

The poor long-term survival of untreated severe aortic stenosis provides the rationale for operative intervention to provide relief of the hemodynamic abnormality. Unoperated symptomatic aortic stenosis has a 3- to 5-year survival of greater than 50% owing to the failure of myocardial compensatory mechanisms that causes symptoms and indicates the need for surgery.[67–69] Nevertheless, potential problems associated with the surgery itself and postoperative complications require that surgery not be undertaken prematurely (see Chapter 21). In most cases, surgery or other nonmedical treatments for stenotic

TABLE 13-5 • Secondary Anatomic Changes in Valvular Heart Disease

Heart
Left ventricular hypertrophy ± dilation*
Myocardial ischemia
Left atrial hypertrophy ± dilation†
Poststenotic dilation of aorta
Right ventricular hypertrophy ± dilation

Lungs
Congestion and edema with hemosiderin-laden macrophages
Brown induration‡
Fibrosis
Venous and arterial hypertensive vascular changes

Systemic—Venous
Chronic passive liver congestion
Centrilobular necrosis
Central vein sclerosis ("cardiac" cirrhosis)
Splenic congestion ± enlargement
Peripheral edema
Pleural effusions
Ascites

Systemic—Arterial
Depressed organ perfusion
Emboli ± infarction

---

* Except in mitral stenosis.
† Most pronounced in mitral stenosis, often associated with atrial fibrillation.
‡ Particularly in long-standing mitral valve disease.

valvular disease can be delayed until symptoms appear, attesting to the remarkable capacity of the ventricular myocardium to accommodate and compensate for pressure and volume overload.[70, 71] Symptoms generally herald the onset of myocardial dysfunction. However, sometimes in aortic stenosis, but more frequently in regurgitant valvular heart disease, prognostically important left ventricular dysfunction can develop in the absence of symptoms. Thus, valve surgery may be appropriate for some asymptomatic patients.

Myocardial Changes: Hypertrophy and Dysfunction

To compensate for the increased pressure or volume workload that accompanies valvular dysfunction, the myocardium undergoes *hypertrophy,* consisting of augmentation of muscle cell size but not number; *hyperplasia* of nonmuscular interstitial cellular components; and increased synthesis of extracellular connective tissue. Cardiac myocytes are terminally differentiated cells that are incapable of substantial, if any, division. Therefore, functionally important hyperplasia of myocytes does not occur in the adult heart. Because the pathobiology of myocardial dysfunction is a key element of the clinicopathologic picture of valvular and other cardiac disease, a brief discussion of the cellular and molecular progression of cardiac hypertrophy and myocardial failure follows.

Cardiac myocytes are normally approximately 15 μm in diameter; their size can increase to 25 μm or larger in hypertrophy that results from valvular disease, yielding a heart weight approximately two to three times greater

TABLE 13-6 • **Myocardial Hypertrophy in Valvular Heart Disease***

	Normal	*Pressure Overload*	*Volume Overload*	*All*
Mean heart weight (g)	230–415†	642	584	615
Mean myocyte diameter (μm)	15	25.9	20.4	23.4

* Early postoperative deaths of six patients with AS or AS/AI and 5 patients with AI or MR. (AS = aortic stenosis; AI = aortic insufficiency and MR = mitral regurgitation). Data from Schoen FJ, Lawrie GM, Titus JL: Left ventricular cellular hypertrophy in pressure- and volume-overload valvular heart disease. Hum Pathol 15: 860, 1984.

† Dependent on sex and body size. Data from Kitzman DW, Scholz DG, Hagen PT, et al: Age related changes in normal human hearts during the first 10 decades of life. Part II (Maturity): A quantitative anatomic study of 765 specimens from subjects 20 to 99 years old. Mayo Clin Proc 63:137, 1988.

than normal (Table 13-6).[72] Unfortunately, the myocardial vasculature does not proliferate commensurate with the increased cardiac mass. Thus, the hypertrophied myocardium, with its high wall stress (a major determinant of myocardial oxygen need) and inadequate vasculature, is often underperfused relative to its needs. This yields some degree of ischemia, particularly in the subendocardium. Moreover, myocardial fibrous tissue is often increased.

The general changes in myocardial structure and function in response to certain stimuli are often referred to as "remodeling," with features largely dependent on the nature of the underlying stimulus (Fig. 13-5).[73] In conditions of left ventricular pressure overload (e.g., accompanying aortic stenosis or systemic hypertension), *concentric or pressure hypertrophy* develops, with an increased ventricular thickness and increased mass and ratio of wall thickness to cavity radius and without appreciable dilation. With pressure-overload hypertrophy, the left ventricular wall is thickened concentrically and the enlarged papillary muscles and muscular trabeculations compromise the left ventricular chamber, which may seem small (Fig. 13-6). The hypertrophied septum often bulges into, and encroaches on, the right ventricular cavity. In contrast, volume-overloaded ventricles (e.g., aortic or mitral regurgitation) develop hypertrophy with chamber dilation in which both ventricular radius and wall mass are increased (*eccentric or volume hypertrophy*).[74] In volume hypertrophy, dilation may mask the degree of hypertrophy, and wall thickness may or may not be increased; indeed, it may be normal or even decreased. The gross patterns reflect the predominant augmentation of cell width (parallel addition of sarcomeres) induced by pressure hypertrophy and augmentation of both cell width and length (parallel and series addition of sarcomeres) stimulated by volume overload.[75] Histologically, in either pattern, left ventricular myocytes are hypertrophied.

Hypertrophy induced by valvular disease is initially adaptive and helpful, improving contractility and enhancing sensitivity to catecholamines. However, prolonged hyperfunction may give rise to impaired performance. Although myocardial remodeling is a normal feature during maturation and a useful adaptation to increased demands in the adult (e.g., athletic training), the myocardial remodeling that occurs in response to pathologic stimuli (e.g., abnormal wall stresses) is maladaptive over the long term and often induces further myocardial dysfunction (Fig. 13-7).[73, 75, 76] Ventricular hypertrophy, coexistent myocardial fibrosis, or both increase diastolic stiffness and further impair ventricular filling. Late stages are also often

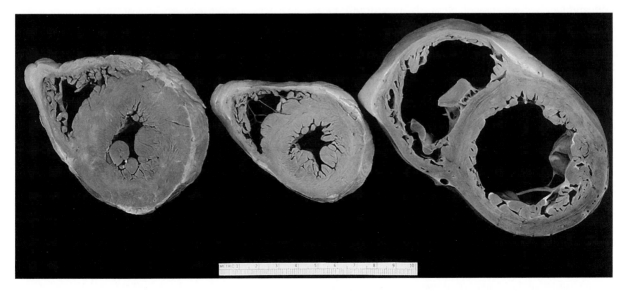

Figure 13-5 • Altered cardiac configuration in left ventricular hypertrophy, without and with dilation, viewed in transverse heart sections. Compared with a normal heart (center), the pressure hypertrophied heart (left) has increased mass and a thick left ventricular wall, but the hypertrophied and dilated heart (right) has increased mass but a diminished wall thickness. (From Edwards D: Cardiac anatomy and examination of cardiac specimens. In: Gutgessel HP, Emmanouilides GC, Riemenschneider PA, Allen HD [eds]: Moss and Adams' Heart Disease in Infants, Children and Adolescents: Including the Fetus and Young Adults, 5th ed. Baltimore, Williams and Wilkins, 1995, p 86.)

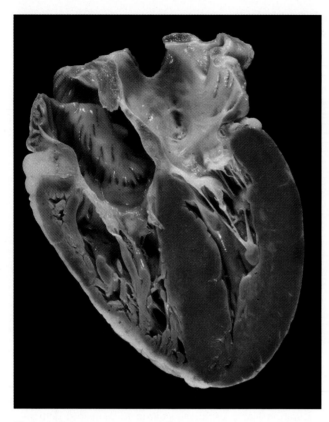

Figure 13-6 • Pressure hypertrophy owing to left ventricular outflow tract obstruction. Both the septum and free wall of the left ventricle are markedly thickened and the left ventricular chamber is very small. Left ventricle is at right of photo. (From Schoen FJ: The heart. In: Cotran RS, Kumar V, Collins T [eds]: Robbins Pathologic Basis of Disease, 6th ed. Philadelphia, WB Saunders, 1999, p 543.)

of providing adequate myocardial perfusion to a massively hypertrophied heart. Moreover, chronic ultrastructural alterations in hypertrophied myocardium from valvular disease are more pronounced in patients with mitral or aortic regurgitation than in patients with mitral or aortic stenosis.[81] This suggests a partial explanation for the generally poorer short- and long-term prognosis in patients who undergo surgery for regurgitant lesions. Changes in the quality and nature of the extracellular matrix may be particularly important in determining the myocardial response to pathologic stimuli.[82, 83]

At the molecular level, ventricular remodeling (hypertrophy and failure) involves a reinduction of fetal genes that are not normally expressed in adult myocardium and a reciprocal decrease in some adult muscle-specific genes.[76-79] The patterns of gene expression may differ in the remodeling induced by different stimuli (pressure vs. volume overload, compensated hypertrophy vs. decompensated heart failure). Prominent changes relate to both abnormal calcium regulation and the composition of pro-

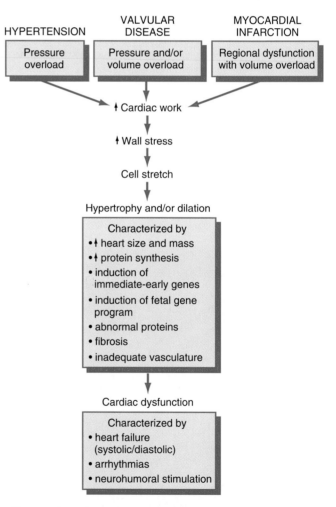

Figure 13-7 • Schematic representation of the sequence of events in cardiac hypertrophy and its progression to heart failure, emphasizing cellular and extracellular changes. (From Schoen FJ: The heart. In: Cotran RS, Kumar V, Collins T [eds]: Robbins Pathologic Basis of Disease, 6th ed. Philadelphia, WB Saunders, 1999, p 543.)

associated with depressed myocardial contractility. Thus, in response to valvular disease, the left ventricle may progress through a compensated phase of hypertrophy to a decompensated state of failure. However, the precise trigger to the transition from compensated hypertrophy to failure, as well as the molecular/biochemical/structural markers, are uncertain.

At the tissue level, the process of myocardial remodeling comprises molecular and cellular changes that include not only hypertrophy of individual myocytes, as mentioned above, but also alterations in gene expression and death of some cardiac myocytes by apoptosis and changes in both the quantity and quality of the extracellular matrix.[73, 76-79] From a morphologic, molecular, and functional perspective, myocardial changes accompanying valvular disease are largely identical to those that occur in idiopathic dilated cardiomyopathy. Myocardial hypertrophy and interstitial fibrosis in valvular heart disease are illustrated in Figure 13-8. Because perfusion of the subendocardium is reduced in the pressure or volume-overloaded left ventricle, myocyte vacuolization (as evidence of chronic sublethal ischemia) or myocardial necrosis or fibrosis may be seen in this zone.[80] Patients with aortic stenosis may be at particular risk for myocardial injury during valve replacement surgery owing to the difficulty

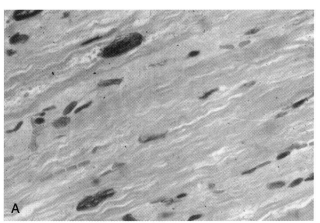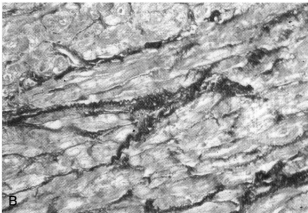

Figure 13-8 • Myocardial hypertrophy (*A*) and interstitial fibrosis (*B*) in valvular heart disease. *A*, H&E stain; *B*, Masson trichrome stain (collagen blue).

teins that regulate formation of the contractile apparatus. Although the most common identifiable stimulus for myocardial hypertrophy is hemodynamic overload (acting on individual cardiac myocytes through circumferential wall stress), extrinsic factors such as the sympathetic nervous system, the renin-angiotensin system, endothelin, peptide growth factors, oxidative stress, inflammatory cytokines, and nitric oxide provide additional, and potentially important, causes and modifiers of the mechanisms of myocardial hypertrophy and failure.

There is evidence that pathologic remodeling also involves the death of myocytes by apoptosis, or programmed cell death.[84, 85] Apoptosis has been demonstrated in human dilated cardiomyopathy adjacent to a recent myocardial infarction, as well as after other insults in animal models and in vitro systems.[86, 87] However, its pathophysiologic significance in myocardial failure is unknown. It has been hypothesized that progressive myocardial failure reflects a continuing loss of viable muscle cells, and that apoptosis of cardiac myocytes may be the result of an aborted growth response to pathophysiologic stimuli reactivating a dormant fetal growth program in cells no longer capable of progressing through the cell cycle.

Moreover, there has been interest in the observation that myocyte hypertrophy is associated with the elevation of, or enhanced sensitivity to, intracellular calcium. Calcineurin is a calcium-dependent phosphatase that activates the NF-AT transcription factors to enhance the hypertrophic response. Because the immunosuppressant cyclosporin A is an inhibitor of calcineurin activity, there is considerable interest in determining whether pharmacologic inhibition of the calcineurin pathway may be useful in the prevention or treatment of cardiac hypertrophy; as yet, the results are conflicting.[88–90]

We now turn our attention to the pathologic anatomy, the clinical features and pathogenesis of specific valve abnormalities related to stenosis. Some of the lesions that are described here superficially were discussed in detail in the previous edition of this book.[91, 92]

PRINCIPLES OF RHEUMATIC HEART DISEASE

Acute Rheumatic Fever

Acute rheumatic fever is an immunologically mediated, multisystem, inflammatory disease that occurs approximately 10 days to 6 weeks after an episode of group A (β-hemolytic) streptococcal pharyngitis.[93] Acute rheumatic carditis is its most important manifestation. Often potentiated by repeated attacks of acute rheumatic fever, chronic rheumatic heart disease can develop over time and is characterized principally by deforming fibrotic or fibrocalcific valvular lesions and progressive valvular dysfunction, most frequently mitral stenosis. Severe, sometimes fatal, cardiac dysfunction can result. This generally occurs decades after attacks of rheumatic fever in patients in developed countries, but it often occurs after a shorter interval among those in developing countries.

The incidence and mortality rate of patients with acute rheumatic fever have declined remarkably in many parts of the world since the middle of the 20th century, owing to improved socioeconomic conditions, rapid diagnosis and treatment of streptococcal pharyngitis, and an unexplained decrease in the virulence of group A streptococci. Nevertheless, acute rheumatic fever and chronic rheumatic heart disease continue to be major public health problems in the developing world. In North America, the disease still occasionally occurs in overcrowded areas of major cities and in areas populated by those low on the socioeconomic ladder, and isolated outbreaks in the United States have been recorded in recent years.[94, 95] Whether new cases in the industrialized world are caused by a particularly virulent new strain of streptococcus or whether there is another explanation is uncertain.[96]

As an autoimmune disease, acute rheumatic fever induces exudative and proliferative inflammatory reactions in connective tissue, particularly in the heart, joints, brain, and skin. The condition is characterized by a variable

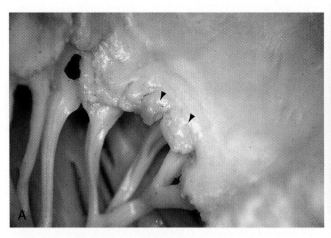
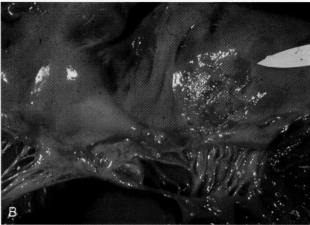

Figure 13-9 • Gross pathologic features of acute rheumatic carditis. *A,* Valvulitis manifested as small vegetations (verrucae) are visible along the line of closure of the mitral valve leaflet (arrowheads) superimposed on chronic rheumatic mitral valve thickening. Previous episodes of rheumatic valve have caused fibrous thickening and fusion of the tendinous cords. *B,* McCallum plaque (highlighted by large arrow) in the left atrium adjacent to the posterior leaflet of the mitral valve. This valve shows underlying features of chronic rheumatic valvulitis. (*A,* From Schoen FJ: The heart. In: Cotran RS, Kumar V, Collins T [eds]: Robbins Pathologic Basis of Disease, 6th ed. Philadelphia, WB Saunders, 1999, p 543.)

constellation of clinical findings among five major manifestations in these systems: carditis, migratory polyarthritis of the large joints, subcutaneous nodules, cutaneous erythema marginatum, and Sydenham chorea; and three minor (and nonspecific) manifestations of fever, arthralgia, and elevated acute-phase reactants. The diagnosis of acute rheumatic fever is established by the Jones criteria (revised); namely, evidence of a preceding group A streptococcal infection accompanied by either two of the major manifestations listed above or by one major and two minor manifestations.[97] Although pharyngeal cultures for streptococci are usually negative by the time acute rheumatic fever begins, antibodies to one or more streptococcal enzymes, such as streptolysin O and DNAse B, continue to be present and can be detected in the sera of most patients. Rheumatic polyarthritis is more common in adults than in children and is typically associated with involvement of one large joint after another for a period of days, followed by spontaneous remittance, leaving no residual disability. Clinical features related to acute carditis include pericardial friction rubs, weak heart sounds, tachycardia, and arrhythmias. Rheumatic myocarditis may cause cardiac dilation that evolves to functional mitral insufficiency or heart failure. Overall, the primary attack generally has a good prognosis, with only 1% mortality.

Acute rheumatic fever occurs with greatest frequency, and usually for the first time, in children between 5 and 15 years of age. However, approximately 20% of first attacks occur in middle to later life, and a person who has had one bout of acute rheumatic fever is prone to others. Indeed, after an initial attack, vulnerability to reactivation of the disease with subsequent pharyngeal infections may be increased, and the same manifestations are likely to appear with each recurrence. Valvular damage is often cumulative. Recurrent attacks diminish with age, but a recurrence may elicit an unusual manifestation in an older patient. Although there is no gender difference in the attack rate of the acute disease, mitral stenosis affects women twice as frequently as men, and aortic stenosis affects men twice as frequently as women.

Inflammatory lesions may be found in any of the three layers of the heart—pericardium, myocardium, or endocardium—representing a *pancarditis.* The cardiac lesions are sterile. In the pericardium, they are accompanied by a fibrinous or serofibrinous exudate, described as a "bread-and-butter" pericarditis, which generally resolves without sequelae.

Characteristic gross and microscopic features of acute rheumatic carditis are illustrated in Figures 13-9 and 13-10, respectively. In the acute phase, valvular endocardial lesions are found most commonly on the mitral valve and next in frequency on the aortic valve. Initially, they are small, translucent, beadlike vegetations (*verrucae*) 1 to 2 mm in diameter, which subsequently become gray-

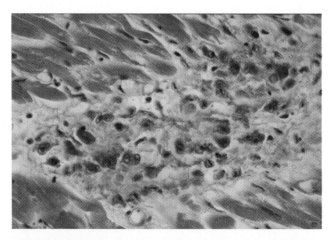

Figure 13-10 • Aschoff body, the characteristic microscopic lesion in acute rheumatic carditis (H&E stain). (From Schoen FJ: The heart. In: Cotran RS, Kumar V, Collins T [eds]: Robbins Pathologic Basis of Disease, 6th ed. Philadelphia, WB Saunders, 1999, p 543.)

brown. They adhere firmly to the leaflet along the line of closure on the atrial aspect of the atrioventricular valves and on the ventricular aspect of the semilunar valves. In rare instances, they may extend onto the tendinous cords of the atrioventricular valves or be associated with chordal rupture. The vegetations rarely embolize.

MacCallum described a characteristic left atrial endocardial lesion in acute rheumatic fever containing Aschoff nodules. The rough, patchlike thickening, 2 to 3 cm in diameter, near the annulus of the posterior mitral leaflet (MacCallum patch) may become a site of secondary infective endocarditis.[98] It should not be confused with endocardial lesions elsewhere that represent jet lesions from regurgitant valves.

Histologically, verrucae consist of platelets and fibrin and usually overlie an inflammatory reaction with fibrinoid necrosis (degenerating collagen), mononuclear cells, fibroblasts, and occasional giant cells in the adjacent valve. It is presumed that the verrucae develop as a result of damage to the connective tissue as part of an immune reaction, followed by ulceration of the surface endothelium, with or without extrusion of damaged collagen and subsequent thrombus formation. The relative frequency of valvular lesions correlates to their closing pressures (mitral > aortic > tricuspid > pulmonary).

Aschoff bodies (or nodules) are the most characteristic microscopic lesions within the heart in acute rheumatic fever.[99] The myocardial involvement of rheumatic fever—myocarditis—takes the form of scattered, often perivascular, Aschoff bodies within the interstitial connective tissue. The earliest lesions are found in the heart several weeks after the onset of a clinical attack and are characterized by focal swelling, edema, and eventual fibrinoid necrosis of the connective tissue. Subsequent accumulation of inflammatory cells produces the granulomatous stage of the Aschoff nodule, constituting central foci of fibrinoid degeneration surrounded by lymphocytes (primarily T cells), occasional plasma cells, and plump macrophages called Anitschkow cells. These distinctive cells have abundant amphophilic cytoplasm and central round-to-ovoid nuclei in which the chromatin is disposed in a central, slender, wavy ribbon (hence the designation "caterpillar" cells when they are cut longitudinally, and "owl-eye" nuclei when they are cut in cross section). Some of the larger altered histiocytes become multinucleated to form Aschoff giant cells. Aschoff nodules are found 1 month or more after an acute attack and are likely to remain in the tissue for 3 to 6 months or even longer. They often persist long after clinical symptoms of an acute attack have subsided. Acute pericarditis is common in acute or recurrent attacks of acute rheumatic fever, and Aschoff nodules may be found in epicardial or pericardial tissue. Similar lesions may also occur in the joints, skin, and connective tissue, brain, and vessels of the lung.

Pathogenesis of Rheumatic Fever

An antibody and/or T cell−mediated immune response occurs during the interval between a sore throat caused by group A streptococci (usually 2 to 3 weeks) and the initial or recurrent attack of acute rheumatic fever. Evidence based on clinical, epidemiologic, and immunologic studies strongly indicates that acute rheumatic fever is a consequence of an abnormal humoral and cellular response to streptococcal antigens that cross-react with tissues antigens of the host, initiating an autoimmune response in about 3% of patients with untreated group A streptococcal pharyngitis (Fig. 13-11). Nevertheless, despite decades of investigation, the exact pathogenesis remains uncertain.

Streptococci are absent from tissue lesions, although components of the cell wall and extracellular products have already induced immune reactions in a susceptible host. Antibodies directed against cell wall proteins of certain strains of streptococci cross-react with tissue glycoproteins in the heart, joints, skin, and other affected tissues.

The general concept is that mimicry of specific epitopes of the streptococcal M protein may induce cross-reactive autoimmune responses to epitopes in myocardium and valve, joint, and neuronal tissues of susceptible individuals.[100] The streptococcal M protein, a major component of the streptococcal cell surface, is highly immunogenic; it is also the major virulence factor because it confers antiphagocytic properties.[101] More than 80 recognized serotypes of group A streptococci are distinguished on the basis of antigenic differences in M proteins. Several lines of evidence suggest that the immunologic response is directed primarily against M protein. Specific M types have been associated with outbreaks of rheumatic fever and accordingly have been labeled rheumatogenic. M protein also shares structural homology and antibody cross-reactivity with proteins such as myosin, tropomyosin, and vimentin in cardiac myocytes, and endothelial cell basement membrane and elastin from extracellular matrix; antibodies against streptococcal proteins can lead to cytotoxic reactions against cardiac myocyte and heart valve endothelium.[102−104] Moreover, the group-specific carbohydrate moiety in the streptococcal cell wall has a high concentration of N-acetylglucosamine found in valvular tissue, and valvular glycoproteins cross-react with serum to group A carbohydrate.[105, 106] Moreover, lymphocytes, particularly CD4+ T cells, which simultaneously recognize streptococcal M and heart proteins, are also present at lesion sites, suggesting a direct role for cell-mediated immunity in the pathogenesis of acute rheumatic fever.[107]

Because only a minority of infected patients develop rheumatic fever, it is suspected that genetic susceptibility regulates the hypersensitivity reaction. The association of specific HLA antigens with several other autoimmune disorders has provoked a search for analogous associations in acute rheumatic fever. Although several investigators have found an increased frequency of HLA-DR4 in white patients in Utah and elsewhere, the results worldwide are highly variable.

Chronic Rheumatic Valvular Disease

Chronic rheumatic heart disease evolves through organization of the acute inflammation of acute rheumatic fever, with subsequent thickening and retraction of leaf-

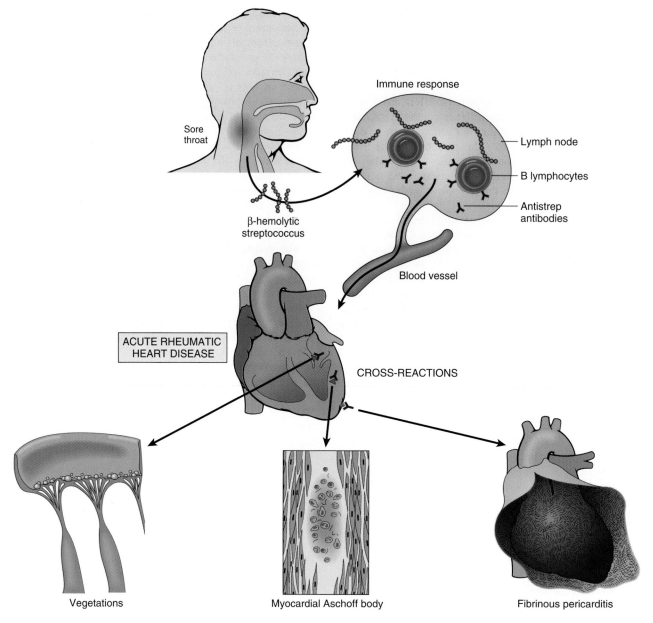

Figure 13-11 • Pathogenetic sequence and key morphologic features of acute rheumatic heart disease. (From Schoen FJ: The heart. In: Cotran RS, Kumar V, Collins T [eds]: Robbins Pathologic Basis of Disease, 6th ed. Philadelphia, WB Saunders, 1999, p 543.)

lets and cusps and shortening of chordae, fusion of chordae and commissures, and secondary damage caused by altered hemodynamics. Additional damage may accrue through minute thrombi on the valve surfaces, with their subsequent organization and scarring of the valve. The end result is a deforming valvular fibrosis. In some patients, calcification may be extensive, especially at the commissures. In chronic disease, the mitral valve is virtually always deformed. Thus, the diagnosis of rheumatic heart disease is tenuous in the presence of an anatomically normal mitral valve. In some patients, however, involvement of the aortic or another valve may be more important clinically than mitral valve involvement.

The mitral valve alone is involved in 65 to 70% of cases, and the mitral and aortic valves in about 25%. Similar but generally less severe fibrous thickenings and

stenoses can occur in the tricuspid valve and, rarely, in the pulmonary valve.[108] With tight mitral stenosis, the left atrium progressively dilates and may harbor thrombi either in its appendage or attached to its wall. The longstanding congestive changes in the lungs may induce pulmonary vascular and parenchymal changes (see Chapter 7) and, in time, lead to right ventricular hypertrophy. With isolated pure mitral stenosis, the left ventricle is usually normal.

Chronic rheumatic carditis usually does not cause clinical manifestations for years or even decades after the initial episode of rheumatic fever. In countries with a high standard of living, a period as long as 40 to 50 years may elapse between the acute attacks and evolution of severe valve dysfunction. However, in other countries, the latent period is shorter, probably as a result of the

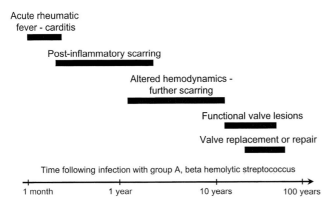

Acute rheumatic
fever - carditis

Post-inflammatory scarring

Altered hemodynamics -
further scarring

Functional valve lesions

Valve replacement or repair

Time following infection with group A, beta hemolytic streptococcus

1 month   1 year   10 years   100 years

Figure 13-12 • Temporal progression of the various clinical and pathologic features of rheumatic heart disease. As emphasized by the logarithmic time axis, the responsible and initiating sequence of events occurs in a very short time span (weeks to months) while the onset of clinically important chronic rheumatic heart disease typically takes at least several decades to become manifest.

greater risk of repeated attacks, and critical mitral stenosis may occur before the age of 20 years. In the very large clinical study of Clawson, the death rate for acute rheumatic fever peaked in the first and second decades of life, whereas death caused by chronic rheumatic valvular deformities was maximal in the fifth decade. The typically protracted natural history of rheumatic heart disease is illustrated in Figure 13-12.

LEFT VENTRICULAR INFLOW TRACT OBSTRUCTION (AT OR RELATED TO THE MITRAL VALVE)

Rheumatic Mitral Stenosis

Mitral stenosis is overwhelmingly caused by chronic rheumatic heart disease. Other causes are unusual (Table 13-7).

The cardinal anatomic changes of rheumatic mitral valve stenosis are leaflet thickening; commissural fusion; and shortening, thickening, and fusion of the tendinous cords (Fig. 13-13). At an early stage, these changes cause obliteration of the clefts defining the scallops of the posterior mitral leaflet. As a result, the leaflet is shortened and puckered and appears to have only one scallop instead of the usual three. After this or concomitant with it, the leaflets thicken and the adjacent surfaces of both mitral valve leaflets fuse in the commissural area. When marked, this ultimately produces an oval or slitlike, stenosed orifice, termed "fishmouth" or "buttonhole." When the accompanying changes cause shortening, thickening, and fusion of both leaflets and cords, a funnel-shaped stenosis may result, with stiff, rigid leaflets seemingly attached to the apices of the papillary muscles. Such cases are said to represent subvalvular mitral stenosis (Fig. 13-14). Dystrophic calcification often appears in the stenosed leaflet and chordal tissue, prominent as nodules within the thickened valve substance or as large yellow masses that ulcerate the leaflet

surface, particularly on the inflow aspect, and especially in commissural areas. These ulcerated lesions tend to accumulate thrombotic material, which can embolize, and may, in rare instances, be a source of emboli of calcific material, a site for infection or a source of hemolysis. Lambl's excrescences or papillary tumors may develop on such deformed valves in adults. The functional end result of all of the processes discussed may be either pure stenosis, stenosis and insufficiency, or pure insufficiency. Insufficiency predominates when leaflet retraction is the major feature of the process.

Histologically, there is diffuse fibrosis, which eradicates the originally layered leaflet architecture, and, often, prominent neovascularization with thick-walled, irregular blood vessels, microfocal lymphocytic aggregates, and superficial thrombus (Fig. 13-15). However, there is considerable variability noted in the morphology of valves from patients with chronic rheumatic heart disease, and not all the features described are seen in all such specimens. Stenotic mitral valves examined many years after the last attack of acute rheumatic fever usually do not show verrucae. Aschoff bodies generally are replaced by fibrous scar and, accordingly, are rarely seen in surgical specimens of valves or myocardium obtained at autopsy.[109]

Clinicopathologic Correlations

Mild stenosis occurs when the mitral orifice is reduced to less than 2.0 to 2.5 cm² (normal mitral orifice area equals 3.0–5.0 cm²). Valve areas of 1.0 to 1.5 cm² constitute moderate mitral stenosis. When the opening is reduced to 1.0 cm², severe (critical) mitral stenosis is generally present, and the left atrial pressure is sufficiently elevated to induce atrial hypertrophy and dilation. The endocardium of the left atrial wall thickens, and egg shell–like plaques of calcium may develop in it over time; presumably these plaques derive from mural thrombi and their organization. Calcification can be visible on plain-film radiographs and is usually seen in patients with severe, long-standing mitral stenosis. The natural history of mitral stenosis is highly variable and dependent on specific complications (Fig. 13-16). Patients

TABLE 13-7 • **Causes of Mitral Stenosis (With or Without Regurgitation)**

Postinflammatory scarring—rheumatic heart disease (about 95% of cases)
Massive mitral annular calcification
Ergotamine-induced or methysergide-induced disease
Congenital (parachute valve, supravalvular stenosis)
Infective endocarditis with obstructive vegetations
Systemic lupus erythematosus
Antiphospholipid antibody syndrome
Rheumatoid arthritis
Gout
Amyloidosis
Whipple disease
Carcinoid heart disease
Mucopolysaccharidosis
Fabry disease
Pseudoxanthoma elasticum

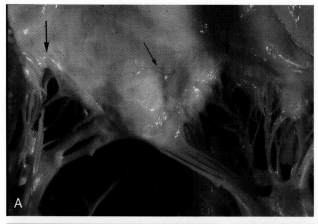

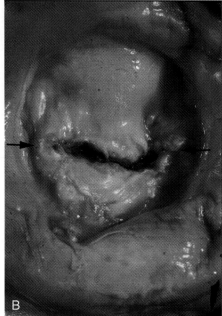

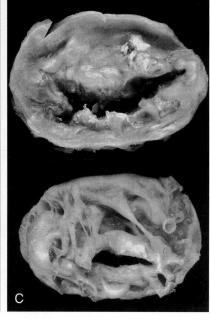

Figure 13-13 • Chronic rheumatic heart disease, manifest as mitral stenosis. *A,* Opened mitral valve of one lesion. *B* Left atrial view of another heart. *C,* Valve surgically removed for severe mitral stenosis from yet another patient (inflow aspect at top, outflow at bottom). Each specimen demonstrates diffuse fibrous thickening and distortion of the valve leaflets, commissural fusion (arrows in *A* and *B*) and thickening and shortening of the tendinous cords. *A,* Emphasizes neovascularization of the anterior mitral leaflet (small arrow). In *C,* leaflet calcification is evident. (*A* and *B* From Schoen FJ: The heart. In: Cotran RS, Kumar V, Collins T [eds]: Robbins Pathologic Basis of Disease, 6th ed. Philadelphia, WB Saunders, 1999, p 543.)

with chronic rheumatic heart disease may suffer from, and become worse in association with, arrhythmias (particularly atrial fibrillation in the setting of mitral stenosis with enlarged atria), thromboembolic complications, and infective endocarditis (Fig. 13-17). Some patients develop a giant left atrium that can extend into the hilum of each lung.

However, because secondary effects occur early, particularly elevated pulmonary venous and capillary pressures, rheumatic mitral stenosis usually leads to symptoms, including exertional dyspnea, soon after the valve area becomes critically diminished. Patients with mitral stenosis usually have not only dyspnea on exertion but also orthopnea and paroxysmal nocturnal dyspnea, which are pulmonary congestive symptoms typical of left-sided heart failure. The first episodes of dyspnea are usually precipitated by exercise or other enhanced physical activity, pregnancy, emotional stress, infection, or atrial fibrillation, all of which promote increased cardiac output and thereby increase the rate of blood flow across the mitral orifice, resulting in further elevation of the left atrial pres-

sure. Less frequently, hemoptysis or hoarseness (due to pulmonary hypertension) or symptoms of right ventricular failure are present. In some cases, a patient remains asymptomatic until atrial fibrillation intervenes.

On physical examination, mitral stenosis is characterized by an opening snap followed by a classic diastolic rumble. The opening snap results from rapid flexion of the anterior leaflet. Thus, as this leaflet becomes calcified, the opening snap becomes softer and eventually disappears. Chronic pulmonary venous hypertension may also be associated with a loud sound (P_2), right ventricular lift, distended neck veins, congestive hepatomegaly, ascites, and generalized edema (anasarca), the signs and symptoms of pulmonary arterial and systemic venous hypertension. The degree of pulmonary hypertension is directly related to the prognosis and the risk associated with surgery.

Echocardiography is used to assess the severity of mitral stenosis and to plan the approach to intervention. Because patients with mitral stenosis are at risk for infective endocarditis, they should receive antibiotic prophy-

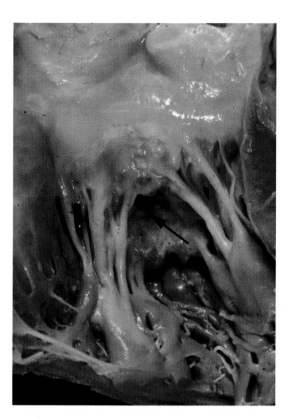

Figure 13-14 • Severe subvalvular obstruction in mitral stenosis caused by dense fusion with thickening and shortening of the tendinous cords. The left ventricular inflow orifice is indicated by an arrow. The anterior mitral leaflet is visible near the top of the photograph. A portion of the aortic valve can be seen at the upper edge.

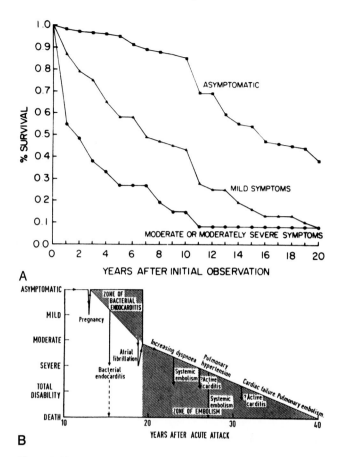

Figure 13-16 • Natural history of mitral stenosis without surgical treatment. *A,* Variability of the prognosis of patients with mitral stenosis and dependence on the level of symptoms. *B,* Schematic representation of an individual patient's course with mitral stenosis, emphasizing that there is commonly a period of several years without symptoms and often no history of rheumatic fever; symptoms then begin gradually, the principal one being dyspnea. The course tends to be gradually downhill, punctuated by crises induced by pregnancy, infective endocarditis, atrial fibrillation, systemic embolism, or pulmonary hypertension. (*A,* Modified from Rowe JC et al: The course of mitral stenosis without surgery: 10 and 20 year perspectives. Ann Intern Med 52:741, 1960. Reproduced from Kirklin JW, Barratt-Boyes BG: Cardiac Surgery. New York, John Wiley, 1986, p 327. *B,* From Goodwin JF: The indications for surgery in acquired heart disease. Proc Roy Soc Med 60:1009, 1967.)

laxis for dental care and other situations in which bacteremia is anticipated. Anticoagulation therapy is required for patients with atrial fibrillation and mitral stenosis, owing to their high risk of embolism.[110] Patients with valve areas less than 1.4 cm^2 constitute the population from which surgical candidates are selected.

Nonrheumatic Acquired Mitral Stenosis

Many individuals whose hearts have morphologic features of rheumatic heart disease do not have a history of acute rheumatic fever. However, cases of nonrheumatic mitral stenosis in which the etiology is well documented are uncommon; most result from leaflet stiffening.

Three causes of nonrheumatic mitral stenosis are illustrated in Figure 13-18. The overuse of ergot alkaloids (ergotamine and methysergide) for migraine headaches may cause the development of plaquelike lesions on the mitral valve (Fig. 13-18A).[111, 112] An association has been drawn between the chronic use of certain appetite suppressants (phentermine, fenfluramine, and dexfenfluramine) and lesions that are in many respects similar to those that form with ergot use and in patients with carcinoid valvular disease that causes mitral regurgitation or,

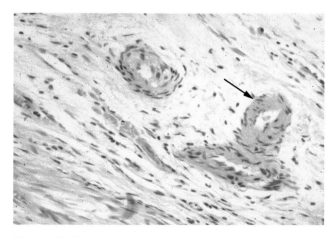

Figure 13-15 • Neovascularization in chronic rheumatic heart disease, manifested by small, thick walled arterial vessels (arrow). (H&E stain)

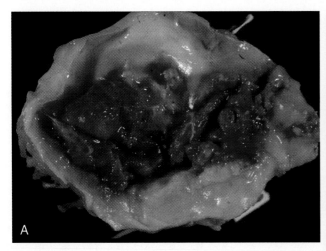

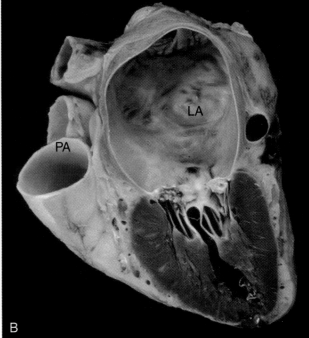

Figure 13-17 • Complications of mitral stenosis. *A*, Infective endocarditis with large vegetations superimposed on valve with rheumatic postinflammatory scarring. *B*, Large left atrium (LA) and pulmonary artery (PA) in mitral stenosis.

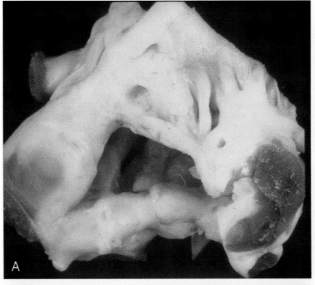

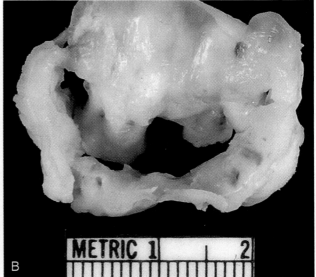

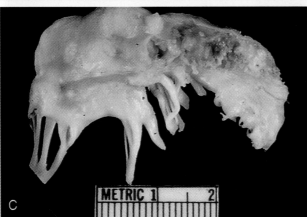

Figure 13-18 • Nonrheumatic causes of mitral stenosis observed in surgically excised valves. *A*, Stenosis associated with use of ergot medications. *B*, Mixed mitral stenosis/insufficiency, owing to use of fenfluramine/phentermine. *C*, Stenosis and severe mitral regurgitation after irradiation for breast cancer.

occasionally, stenosis (Fig. 13-18*B*).[113] (See also Chapter 17.) Therapeutic mediastinal irradiation may result in fibrocalcific valve disease, including mitral stenosis with or without regurgitation (Fig. 13-18*C*).[114] Infrequently, mitral stenosis is a complication of systemic lupus erythematosus or the antiphospholipid syndrome (or both), rheumatoid arthritis, or the mucopolysaccharidoses (such as Hunter-Hurley or Maroteaux-Lamy), tophaceous gout, or other metabolic abnormalities.[115–118] Mitral stenosis may also develop in a patient with carcinoid syndrome who has an interatrial communication or a pulmonary carcinoid tumor.[119] Also, mitral stenosis has been reported in patients with familial pseudoxanthoma elasticum, in which histologic sections of the valve show irregular, coarse-fibered, abnormally fragmented elastic fibers similar to those seen in skin lesions.[120] Another reported cause of mitral stenosis is Whipple disease, in which characteristic PAS-positive macrophages and gram-positive, rod-shaped bacteria (named *Tropheryma whippelii* and identical to those found in the mucosa of the small intestine of such patients) are seen in the valvular lesions.[121] (See also Chapter 16.)

Although calcification of the mitral annulus usually results in mitral regurgitation by splinting the physiologic contraction of the mitral annulus during systole, mitral annular calcification can cause stenosis by inhibiting the mobility of the valve leaflets or being marked by subvalvular or intravalvular extension of calcific deposits.[122] Large vegetations of infective endocarditis, particularly from fungal infections, rarely induce mitral stenosis. A left atrial myxoma or other tissue mass may also project into the valve orifice and produce the symptoms of mitral stenosis. It is unresolved whether nonrheumatic infectious diseases (e.g., with viruses, brucellosis, Q fever) can produce valvular lesions morphologically indistinguishable from those caused by rheumatic valvular disease, as has been suggested by some authors.[123]

Congenital Mitral Stenosis

Congenital fusion of mitral commissures or accessory mitral valve tissue, often with dysplastic leaflet and chordal thickening, are uncommon causes of mitral stenosis that may appear in infancy, childhood, or adolescence.[124] Two other congenital causes of mitral stenosis include a so-called supravalvular ridge (which is actually either annular or subannular) and a parachute mitral valve with only one well-formed papillary muscle (see later). These two may be part of the Shone syndrome, which also includes subaortic stenosis and coarctation of the aorta.[125–127]

Supravalvular and Subvalvular Mitral Stenosis

Triatrial heart (cor triatriatum) is a rare congenital anomaly in which a membranous ridge or diaphragm containing variable numbers of myocardial fibers and fibroelastic tissue divides the left atrium into two chambers. It is usually apparent in childhood, either as an isolated abnormality or associated with other congenital heart defects.[128, 129] The age of onset and severity of symptoms are determined by the extent of obstruction within the left atrium. In adults, the perimeter of the membrane may become calcified. Usually, the mitral valve is normal, although regurgitation may develop. The degree of obstruction caused by the membrane varies with the number and size of perforations. In children, the membrane may or may not contain small perforations. In adults, perforations are usually large, and occasional patients are asymptomatic until the third decade. Symptoms are similar to those of mitral stenosis. Surgical correction of cor triatriatum is undertaken if the patient develops symptoms or if pulmonary hypertension becomes prominent.[130]

Because blood must flow through the chordae tendineae and past the papillary muscles in its passage into the left ventricle, congenital or acquired lesions of these structures may cause a subvalvular obstruction to blood flow. With parachute mitral valve, only one papillary muscle is present in the left ventricle, or two are very close together, and tendinous cords pass to both mitral valve leaflets. As a result, interchordal spaces are effectively narrowed, producing a subvalvular obstruction. In neonates or children, this abnormality is more often associated with other congenital cardiac anomalies, whereas in adults it may occur as an isolated phenomenon. Acquired subvalvular stenosis occurs most frequently as a complication of rheumatic valvular disease in which chordal fusion is a prominent feature.

Treatment of Mitral Stenosis

The mechanical treatment of rheumatic mitral stenosis includes one interventional procedure, balloon valvuloplasty, and three different surgical approaches: (1) closed mitral valvotomy; (2) open valvotomy, carried out under direct vision during cardiopulmonary bypass; and (3) mitral valve replacement.[131, 132] Valvuloplasty and the first two surgical approaches are discussed in this section, and valve replacement is discussed in Chapter 21.

Balloon Valvuloplasty

Balloon valvuloplasty is an alternative to surgical treatment of mitral stenosis.[133, 134] In this technique, a catheter is introduced into the systemic venous circulation and advanced across the interatrial septum via a trans-septal puncture. One large or two small balloons are passed across the mitral orifice and inflated. The hemodynamic results have been quite favorable in several series, with reduction of the transmitral pressure gradient from an average of approximately 18 to 6 mm Hg, a small (average 20%) increase in cardiac output, and, on the average, a doubling of the calculated mitral valve area from 1.0 to 2.0 cm². Balloon valvotomy for mitral stenosis provides excellent mechanical relief that usually results in prolonged benefit, unlike valvotomy in aortic stenosis (see later). The presence of heavy valvular calcification, severe subvalvular distortion, or more than mild mitral regurgitation mitigates against the use of balloon valvotomy. In such cases, open commissurotomy, valve reconstruction, or mitral valve replacement improves survival and reduces symptoms. The reported procedural mortality for balloon valvuloplasty is approximately 0.5%.

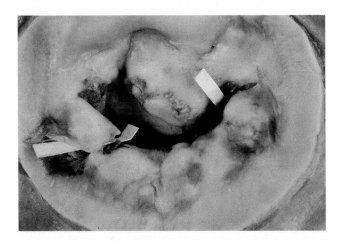

Figure 13-19 • Findings following balloon valvuloplasty for mitral stenosis. Commissural fractures and splits are indicated by tapes.

The mechanisms responsible for improving function after balloon valvuloplasty for mitral stenosis include commissural separation and fracture (Fig. 13-19). Results are especially impressive in younger patients without valvular thickening or calcification and have been less successful in those who have valves with fluoroscopically detectable commissural calcium. Approximately 10% of patients are left with a small atrial septal defect (due to perforation during the trans-septal approach), but in most, this subsequently closes or decreases in size.

Complications include cerebral embolic events (despite an absence of detectable thrombus on two-dimensional echocardiography before valvular dilation) and cardiac perforation, each occurring at approximately 1% frequency, and the development of mitral regurgitation severe enough to require operation in another 2% (approximately 15% develop lesser but still undesirable degrees of regurgitation).

In follow-up studies over 3 years, hemodynamic benefit was maintained in the majority of patients, and they did not require surgical treatment. Approximately 10% developed restenosis resulting from thrombosis, fibrosis,

and eventual calcification along the sites of balloon-induced valvular fracture, particularly at the commissures.[135] The best candidates are patients with symptomatic, hemodynamically severe stenosis but without leaflet rigidity, valvular calcification or thrombus, subvalvular disease, or left atrial thrombus.[136]

Surgical Valvotomy

The mortality rate after mitral valvotomy, whether open or closed, ranges from 1 to 3%, depending on the condition of the patient and the skill and experience of the surgical team. Five-year survival rates are 90 to 96%, and event-free survival rates are 72 to 94%. In general, by allowing relatively greater control to produce clean commissural incisions (Fig. 13-20), open valvotomy provides better hemodynamic relief of mitral valve obstruction and less risk of dislodging thrombi from the atrium or calcium from the mitral valve than the closed procedure. Left atrial enlargement, the need for mitral or tricuspid annuloplasty, and the presence of left atrial thrombus are all risk factors for a less than optimal outcome. Surgical valvulotomy does not produce a structurally normal mitral valve, but it does result in a better functioning one, essentially resembling its appearance perhaps a decade earlier. A stenosed mitral valve may restenose after open or closed surgical commissurotomy. Organization of fibrin microthrombus is believed to play an important role in restenosis.[137] The incidence of restenosis is 18 to 35% at follow-up of at least 5 years.[138, 139]

LEFT VENTRICULAR OUTFLOW TRACT OBSTRUCTION (AT OR RELATED TO THE AORTIC VALVE)

Obstruction to blood flow in the vicinity of the aortic valve can occur at subvalvular, valvular, or supravalvular levels (Fig. 13-21).[140] Lesions causing the clinical picture of aortic stenosis may be congenital or acquired and may induce clinical manifestations at any age. In adults, aortic

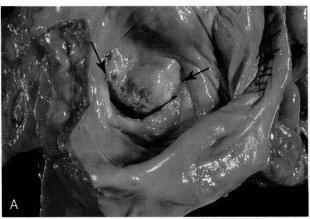

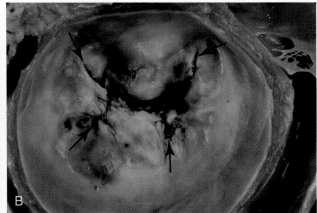

Figure 13-20 • Open surgical mitral commissurotomy. *A,* Pure mitral stenosis. Incised commissures are indicated by arrows. *B,* Mitral commissurotomy with repair, for mixed stenosis/regurgitation. Incised commissures are indicated by arrows. (*A,* From Schoen FJ, Sutton MS: Contemporary issues in the pathology of valvular heart disease. Hum Pathol 18:568, 1987.)

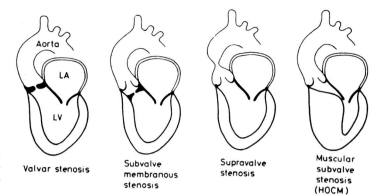

Figure 13-21 • Diagrammatic representation of various levels of left ventricular outflow tract obstruction. HOCM, hypertrophic obstructive cardiomyopathy. (From Davies MJ: Pathology of Cardiac Valves. London, Butterworth Scientific, 1980.)

valvular stenosis occurs far more frequently than subvalvular and supravalvular stenoses. Aortic stenosis occurs most often in middle-aged or elderly adults and has potentially serious consequences.

Acquired valvular stenosis may be caused by (1) cusp stiffening and immobility, either through cuspal fibrosis or deposition of material in the cusp parenchyma (usually nodular calcium phosphate mineral) or both, (2) commissural fusion, or (3) a combination of these changes. The common feature is obstruction to left ventricular outflow, resulting in a pressure gradient across the valve during systole. Largely based on gross examination, stenotic aortic valves can be classified etiologically as degenerative, postinflammatory, congenitally bicuspid, or other.

An ongoing Mayo Clinic study of the temporal changes in relative frequency of the etiologic categories of valvular disease emphasizes several important trends pertinent to aortic valve stenosis. Although several investigators in North America showed that calcification of a congenitally bicuspid aortic valve was the predominant cause of acquired aortic stenosis in the mid-20th century,[140–143] degeneration of a previously anatomically normal aortic valve with three cusps is the most common cause in older patients and overall, became the most common cause in the 1980s (Fig. 13-22 and Table 13-8).[53–58, 141] The

increasing incidence of degenerative aortic valve disease is not surprising in view of aging trends in the United States that show a shift toward an elderly population and increasing longevity. Indeed, the ages of patients having surgery for aortic stenosis is increasing; among 236 stenotic aortic valves surgically excised at the Mayo Clinic in 1990, the mean patient age was 76 years compared with a mean age of 54 years in 1965. In this study, stenotic valves accounted for 65% of the total group with aortic valve disease; 25% were purely regurgitant and 10% were both stenotic and insufficient.[143, 144]

In contemporary surgical pathology studies, congenitally bicuspid aortic valves comprise the second most common lesion causing aortic valve stenosis.[53, 58, 143] Bicuspid valves are most often stenotic (68%) but can become regurgitant (19%) or be both stenotic and regurgitant (13%). Postinflammatory (rheumatic) disease continues to decline as a cause of aortic valve dysfunction—58% of cases in 1965, but only 11% in 1990.

Degenerative Aortic Stenosis

Degenerative (or senile) calcific aortic stenosis results principally from an age-related deposition of calcium phosphate mineral in the three cusps of a valve that was

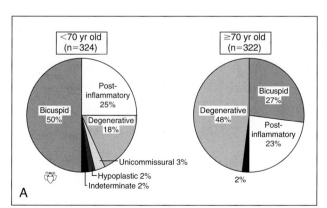

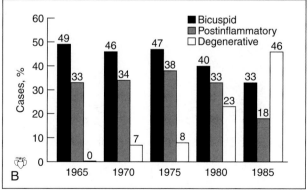

Figure 13-22 • Causes of aortic stenosis, by age group and year of surgery. *A,* By age group amongst patients younger than 70 years of age, calcification of congenitally bicuspid valves accounted for half of the surgical cases. In contrast, in those 70 years of age or older, degenerative calcification of a previously normal valve causes almost half of the cases. *B,* Temporal changes in later years of aortic stenosis in a surgical population (488 cases) from 1965 to 1985. The relative frequency of bicuspid and postinflammatory cases decreased, and that of degenerative cases increased. (From Passik CS, Ackermann DM, Pluth JR, Edwards WD: Temporal changes in the causes of aortic stenosis: A surgical pathologic study of 646 cases. Mayo Clin Proc 62:119, 1987.)

TABLE 13-8 • **Etiologic Distribution of Aortic Stenosis***

Etiology	No. of Cases (% of group)	Gender		Mean Age, Yr (range)
		M	F	
Aortic Stenosis				
Degenerative	79 (51)	49	30	74 (49–92)
Bicuspid	55 (36)	32	23	65 (20–84)
Postinflammatory	14 (9)	7	7	70 (49–80)
Other and indeterminate	6 (4)	3	3	50 (34–79)
Total	154 (100)	91	63	70 (20–92)
Mixed Aortic Stenosis and Insufficiency				
Degenerative	11 (46)	7	4	74 (64–84)
Bicuspid	4 (17)	4	0	70 (54–82)
Postinflammatory	4 (17)	3	1	58 (42–64)
Other and indeterminate	5 (20)	3	2	66 (39–79)
Total	24 (100)	17	7	69 (39–84)

* From the Mayo Clinic, 1990.

Data from Dare AJ, Veinot JP, Edwards WD: New observations on the etiology of aortic valve disease: A surgical pathologic study of 236 cases from 1990. Hum Pathol 24:1330, 1993.

originally anatomically normal. Calcification is progressive with age, and calcific stenosis affects men and women equally, occurring most commonly in patients older than 65 years. The morphologic hallmark is heaped-up, archlike calcified masses along the aortic aspects of the cusps, which become anchored to the annulus, thereby preventing opening of the cusps (Fig. 13-23).[145] The calcific deposits distort cuspal architecture, primarily at their bases, whereas their free edges are usually uninvolved. Notably, and in contrast to rheumatic aortic stenosis, commissural fusion is usually absent or only minimal in degenerative aortic stenosis, and the valve orifice is triradiate. This process does not involve the mitral valve independently. Thus, the mitral valve is generally normal in patients with degenerative aortic stenosis, other than their having some mitral annular calcification or direct extension of aortic valve calcific deposits onto the anterior mitral leaflet. As previously mentioned, this contrasts with rheumatic aortic stenosis, in which characteristic primary structural abnormalities of the mitral valve are generally present.

In most cases of degenerative calcific aortic stenosis, the calcific process begins in, and is largely centered on, the fibrosa layer of the valve cusps, at the points of maximal cusp flexion (the margins of attachment), but the microscopic layered architecture is largely preserved (Fig. 13-24). The early fibrocalcific changes (called aortic valve sclerosis) are common in elderly patients (29% in those >age 65 years) but are not usually associated with a significant gradient across the valve.[146] Larger calcific deposits impair the opening of the aortic valve cusps and may become transmural within the valve wall. They frequently ulcerate at their distal aspect and occasionally fragment spontaneously, producing both emboli and a roughened surface. Moreover, calcium emboli may also be dislodged from calcified stenosed aortic valves during cardiac catheterization, balloon valvuloplasty, or corrective surgery. Bland thrombi related to such ulcers may raise suspicion of infective endocarditis on gross examination of a valve specimen. Calcification may also extend from the valve cusps into the ventricular septum and damage or destroy the His bundle or left bundle branch,

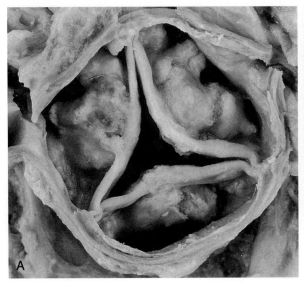

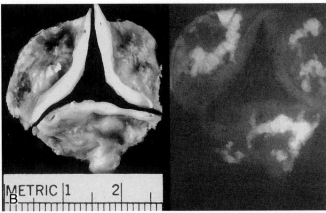

Figure 13-23 • Severe degenerative calcification of a previously anatomically normal valve, the predominant cause of aortic stenosis in the elderly and overall. *A*, Autopsy specimen. *B*, Excised surgical pathology specimen shown with its radiograph at right.

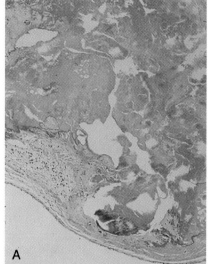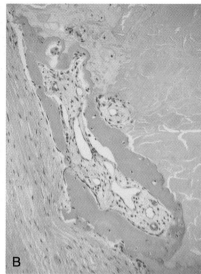

Figure 13-24 • Microscopic appearance of calcific deposits in degenerative aortic stenosis. *A,* Typical case. Deposits begin in the fibrosa layer and grow predominantly distally (top); the underlying layered architecture of the cusps is largely intact. *B,* Osseous degeneration of calcific deposits with formation of bone and poorly organized marrow elements. (*A* and *B,* H&E stain.)

inducing complete heart block in some. Hemolysis can be a feature. Metaplastic cartilage or bone, sometimes with bone marrow (cartilaginous, osseous, and myeloid metaplasia, respectively), not uncommonly develop within the calcium deposits. It has been suggested that metaplastic changes may be potentiated by balloon valvuloplasty.[147–150] "Kissing" of cusps may induce traumatic perforation of an uncalcified area by an adjacent calcific nodule, causing valve incompetence.

Stenosis of Bicuspid Aortic Valves

A bicuspid aortic valve is a common congenital cardiac anomaly that occurs in 1 to 2% of the population and affects men 3 to 4 times as frequently as women (Fig. 13-25).[151, 152] Bicuspid valves usually exhibit normal function at birth and during early life. By age 60 years, however, few of these valves are functioning normally. Overall, about 85% develop stenosis with or without insufficiency, and 15% become purely regurgitant. Causes of stenosis include calcification and fibrosis, whereas the causes of regurgitation encompass annular dilation, cusp prolapse, rupture of an atypical (fenestrated) raphe, infective endocarditis, and acute aortic dissection (see Chapter 14). Calcification associated with this congenital anomaly generally becomes clinically important 10 to 15 years earlier than degenerative aortic stenosis on a valve with three cusps. Thus, calcification of a congenitally bicuspid aortic valve is the most frequent cause of isolated aortic stenosis in patients who are 50 to 70 years old.

The cusps of a congenitally bicuspid aortic valve may be of equal size and have commissures opposite each other (180-degree circumferential amplitude between commissures); more often, however, one cusp is larger than the other. In the latter instance, the larger conjoined cusp represents absent or aborted development at one commissure or fusion of two cusps during fetal life. The two fused cusps tend to be smaller than normal in aggregate and the nonconjoined cusp larger than normal. Unlike normal aortic valve cusps, the larger conjoined cusp of a congenitally bicuspid aortic valve is often 3.5 to

4.0 cm wide along the free margin. Because surgeons generally remove bicuspid valves in only one or two pieces, the large size of the conjoined cusp, when seen in the surgical pathology laboratory, may be a clue to this anomaly. Valves with cusps of equal or unequal size are prone to similar complications.

Usually, the location of the aborted third commissure, or *raphe,* is obvious along the aortic aspect of the conjoined cusp, but it is not always present. The morphology of a raphe presents a spectrum of abnormal development. It can be shallow or tall, solid or fenestrated.[153] In addition, it may extend a varying distance from the aortic sinus toward the cusp, vary in its height related to the free edge of the cusp, and show partial separation of its free margin into cusp margins. In general, the combina-

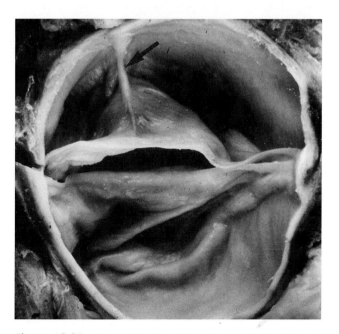

Figure 13-25 • Congenitally bicuspid aortic valve (without stenosis or regurgitation). A raphe is present (arrow). Tissue at the base of both nonconjoint cusp and adjacent sinus wall is folded.

tion of grossly unequal cusp size and a shallow raphe serves to distinguish congenital from acquired fusions.[154] Sometimes, in acquired cuspal fusion, separate valve fibrosa from each of the two commissures can be traced near to the point of valve attachment to the annulus; distinct sets of cusp structures are generally not apparent in congenitally fused cusps. However, although some investigators have suggested that histologic sections of commissural areas help in some cases to distinguish between congenital and acquired commissural fusion in valves distorted by calcification or infection, most cardiac pathologists do not find that microscopic sections serve to distinguish bicuspid from tricuspid valves.[155]

Theoretically, the commissures of a congenitally bicuspid aortic valve may be located anywhere around the circumference of the aortic root. In about 75% of cases, however, the right and left cusps are conjoined, and both coronary arteries arise from the two aortic sinuses above this cusp.[154] If the noncoronary cusp is fused to either the right or left cusp, one coronary artery arises from the aorta above the conjoined cusp, and the other originates above the nonconjoined cusp.

Calcification characteristically occurs first along the raphe, forming an immobile strut that hinders motion of the conjoined cusp, as well as motion along the aortic aspect of the nonconjoined cusp.[152] Calcification of the raphe, calcification in the cuspal sinuses, cusp fibrosis, and secondary acquired fusion of one or both true commissures may all contribute to stenosis (Fig. 13-26). Ultimately, progressive stenosis results in an obstructed orifice that is shaped like a boomerang, a tear drop, or an ellipse.

Although a bicuspid aortic valve is usually an isolated lesion, it may occasionally be associated with other congenital cardiovascular anomalies, particularly coarctation of the aorta. About 50% of the patients with aortic coarctation also have a bicuspid aortic valve, but the converse is not true. The presence of a bicuspid aortic valve also increases the risk of infective endocarditis. Moreover, aortic dilation and dissection are more likely in patients with congenitally bicuspid valves than in those with degenerative or rheumatic aortic stenosis, suggesting an inherently weaker aorta in patients with malformed aortic valves.[156, 157] The cause of the aortic wall abnormalities,

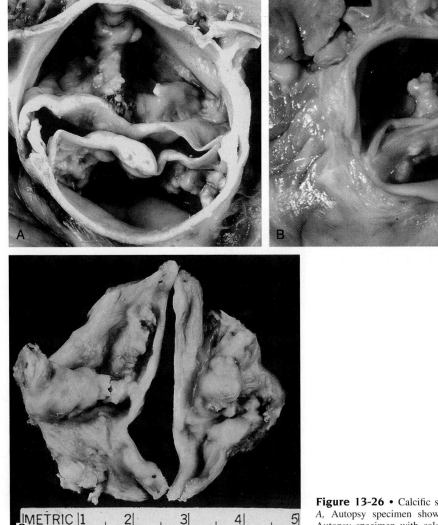

Figure 13-26 • Calcific stenosis of congenitally bicuspid aortic valves. *A,* Autopsy specimen showing calcified bicuspid valve with raphe. *B,* Autopsy specimen with calcified symmetrical bicuspid valve cusps without a raphe. *C,* Surgical pathology specimen.

which manifest morphologically as augmented degenerative changes similar to those of cystic medial degeneration, is uncertain.[158]

Pathogenesis of Aortic Valve Calcification

Age-related calcification of the aortic valve has generally been attributed to a progressive degeneration involving dystrophic calcification, which results from injury, induced by a lifetime of continuous mechanical stress. Like other pathologic calcification processes, the deposition of calcium mineral in the aortic valve is dependent on the structure and biochemistry of the substrate tissue and the composition of the chemical environment to which the tissue is exposed, although the specific events and regulatory factors remain subjects of active investigation and controversy.

Calcification occurs in a pattern that reflects regions of increased mechanical stress. The smallest and earliest deposits are found at the cusp attachments and along the line of cusp coaptation, the sites of greatest bending and unbending during valve opening and closing.[159] Whether the valve is bicuspid or tricuspid, variation in cusp size and hemodynamic forces experienced by the cusps may be important factors increasing wear and tear on their tissue. Deformed aortic valves, such as congenitally bicuspid valves, have abnormal sharing of stress between the cusps and the aortic wall, leading to enhanced attachment and coaptation stresses, and they have accelerated calcification compared with valves having normal structure. Conditions with a chronically elevated stroke volume or altered calcium metabolism (Paget's disease or renal failure) are believed to potentiate aortic stenosis.[160, 161]

The mechanisms involved in calcific aortic valve degeneration are generally considered distinct from those causing atherosclerosis per se, and risk factors for atherosclerosis (including systemic hypertension) and aortic stenosis are only weakly associated.[162] Nevertheless, some features of the pathogenesis of atherosclerosis and calcific valvular disease are shared, and some authors have hypothesized a close relationship between the two disease processes.[163] Studies suggest that the formation of calcific deposits is associated with lipid accumulation in aging aortic valves, particularly in the valvular fibrosa, where aging of fibroblasts is accelerated and their numbers are diminished. Both lipid deposition and early calcification are localized to the fragments of degenerating fibroblasts.[29] Interestingly, mice fed an atherogenic diet accumulate macrophages and lipoproteins at sites that correspond to the distribution of hemodynamic forces.[164] Moreover, there is evidence that a gradual impairment of ionic calcium regulation occurs in aging cells.[165] Such dysregulation of ion fluxes may allow extracellular calcium to react with membrane phospholipids of deteriorating cells to nucleate early formation of calcium phosphate crystals.[166] The process of valve calcification is considered somewhat analogous to calcification occurring in tissue heart valve substitutes and other biomaterials, and, indeed, has many similarities to cell-oriented physiologic mineralization of the skeleton.[30, 31, 167, 168] Similar mechanisms of pathologic calcification have also been described in noncardiovascular tissues.[169]

However, the view that aortic valve calcification is merely a passive consequence of cellular aging has been challenged recently. A growing body of evidence suggests that native aortic valve and other cardiovascular calcification may be regulated via noncollagenous extracellular matrix proteins, analogous to physiologic musculoskeletal calcification.[170, 171] For example, osteopontin is one of a group of noncollagenous matrix proteins of bone that has been implicated in cell adhesion, spreading, and cycling. Osteopontin binds readily to hydroxyapatite and may play a role in cardiovascular calcification.[172, 173] Several studies have shown correlations among calcification, macrophage accumulation, and the expression of osteopontin in both aortic valvular stenosis and arterial atherosclerosis.[174-177] Nevertheless, it is unclear whether osteopontin promotes or inhibits calcification in this context. The lipids that are naturally present in this matrix and that accumulate with aging also foster calcification.[178] Additional details on the current concepts of the pathogenesis of cardiovascular calcification are summarized in the context of tissue valve substitutes in Chapter 21.

Postinflammatory (Rheumatic) Aortic Stenosis

Like rheumatic mitral valve disease, rheumatic aortic valvular deformities are characterized by diffuse cuspal thickening that extends to their free edges and by commissural fusion (Fig. 13-27). Calcification may occur secondarily. These features contrast with the principal morphologic features in degenerative aortic stenosis, which is marked by basal calcific nodules and no involvement of the free edge or commissures. Although sclerosis and shortening (i.e., retraction) of the cusps predominate in rheumatic aortic incompetence, fusion of adjacent sides of the cusps in the commissural areas, with or without cusp sclerosis, is of greater importance in potentiating stenosis. The acquired commissural fusion in rheumatic aortic valve disease, which may affect one, two, or all three commissures can generally be distinguished from the commissural fusion of congenital valve abnormalities. In advanced cases, rheumatic postinflammatory scarring may affect each commissural area equally, producing a small circular or triangular valve orifice that is both stenotic and regurgitant. As previously mentioned, aortic rheumatic valvular disease is not usually isolated; rather, rheumatic aortic stenosis is virtually always associated with mitral valve deformities, even though mitral dysfunction may be less important clinically. Rheumatic valvular disease may affect not only an initially anatomically normal aortic valve but also a congenitally bicuspid or other deformed aortic valve.

Histologically, the cusps of a valve having chronic rheumatic aortic stenosis show diffuse, transmural fibrosis and, frequently, neovascularization with thick-walled small vessels, variable collections of chronic inflammatory cells, and transmural calcification similar to that of rheumatic mitral stenosis.

Aortic cusps damaged by rheumatic disease without calcification may remain quite pliable for extended periods. However, rheumatic aortic stenosis may progress

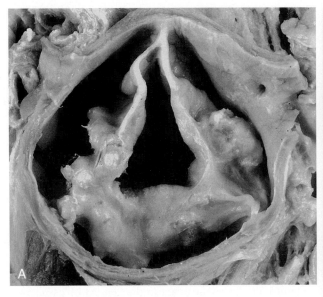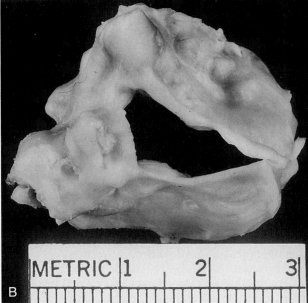

Figure 13-27 • Rheumatic aortic stenosis demonstrating diffuse cuspal fibrosis and commissural fusion with secondary calcification. *A,* Autopsy specimen. *B,* Surgical pathology specimen.

rapidly, typically in Third World countries, when cusps are heavily sclerosed and only mildly calcified. In the industrialized world, rheumatic aortic stenosis has decreased in frequency in surgical cases during the last several decades following the decline of rheumatic fever that began about 1950.

Other Causes of Acquired Aortic Stenosis

Young adults with type II hyperlipidemia can develop marked lipid deposits in their aortic valve cusps, and secondary dystrophic calcification may cause aortic stenosis. The family history, associated clinical findings, and marked deposits of atheromatous material in the cusps permit diagnosis.

Large vegetations of infective endocarditis may cause acute aortic stenosis and, rarely, healed calcified vegetations can induce chronic aortic stenosis. Rheumatoid nodules in the aortic annulus may encroach upon the valve lumen and cause aortic stenosis in patients with rheumatoid arthritis. In patients with systemic lupus erythematosus, aortic fibrosis may be caused by massive Libman-Sacks thrombosis on the valves by postinflammatory (rheumatic-like) cusp fibrosis and commissural fusion.[115] Patients with a glycogen storage disease or ochronosis may develop secondary calcification and stenosis of the aortic valve.[179] Aortic valvular disease can also occur in gout. (See Chapter 16 also.)

Clinicopathologic Correlations

The overall pathophysiology of the consequences of aortic stenosis is summarized in Figure 13-28.

Obstructions to left ventricular outflow worsen gradually and stimulate progressive concentric left ventricular hypertrophy. Often, the hypertrophied ventricle can sustain and adapt to a substantial pressure gradient across an obstruction for many years without any reduction in cardiac function. However, the onset of symptoms marks the loss of compensation and from this point on, the patient's prognosis is especially poor unless the obstruction is relieved.

Symptoms and Signs

The classic symptoms of aortic stenosis are exertional angina, syncope, and dyspnea. Angina develops in part because of reduced coronary flow reserve and in part because of increased myocardial oxygen demand caused by high workload. Heart failure can be caused by diastolic dysfunction, systolic dysfunction, or both. Diastolic dysfunction results from increased left ventricular wall thickness and increased collagen content, whereas systolic dysfunction results from excess afterload, decreased contractility, or a combination of these factors. The most common sign of aortic stenosis is a systolic ejection murmur radiating to the neck. The carotid upstroke classically becomes diminished in amplitude and delayed in time.

Epidemiology and Natural History

Studies of autopsy material and clinical studies of elderly institutionalized and unselected people suggest a prevalence of at least moderate aortic stenosis in about 5% and critical stenosis in approximately 3% of individuals between 75 and 86 years of age.[46, 180, 181] Approximately half of persons in this age range have some degree of calcification demonstrable by echocardiography.

There is considerable variability in the rate of hemodynamic progression among adults with valvular aortic ste-

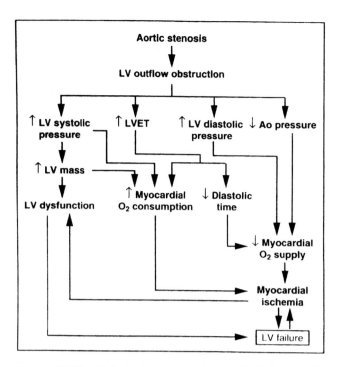

Figure 13-28 • Pathophysiology of aortic stenosis. Left ventricular (LV) outflow obstruction results in an increased LV systolic pressure, increased LV ejection time (LVET), increased LV diastolic pressure, and decreased aortic pressure. Increased LV systolic pressure with LV volume overload increases LV mass, which may lead to myocardial dysfunction and failure. Increased LV systolic pressure, increased LV mass, and increased ejection time increase myocardial oxygen consumption—a major determinant of perfusion demand. Concurrent with increased LVET is a decrease in diastolic time available for myocardial perfusion. The combination of increased LV diastolic pressure and decreased aortic diastolic pressure serves to decrease coronary perfusion pressure, which, coupled with increased LV mass produces myocardial ischemia that is further deleterious to LV function. (From Boudoulas H, Gravanis MB: Valvular heart disease. In: Gravanis MB [ed]: Cardiovascular Disorders: Pathogenesis and Pathophysiology. St. Louis, CV Mosby, 1993.)

nosis. The rate of progression is generally considered slow, with the exception of a subgroup of elderly patients, most frequently female, whose course may accelerate from mild to severe over a 2- to 3-year period.[182] Among 142 patients with mild stenosis (aortic valve orifice area >1.5 cm²), clinical progression within 10 years of initial diagnosis occurred in only 12%.[183] Twenty-five years after diagnosis, the severity of aortic stenosis was clinically unchanged in 38%, whereas 25% had developed moderate stenosis and 38% had required valve replacement. Progression of moderate stenosis (aortic orifice area between 0.8 and 1.5 cm²) was variable but could be more rapid than that of mild disease. The average interval between manifestations of moderate stenosis and surgery was 13 years. However, in another study, 74% of those with an average valve area of 1.3 cm² had undergone valve replacement or died within 5 years.[184] Studies of patients with mild to moderate stenosis suggest that the average decrease in valve area is approximately 0.1 cm² per year.[185] One study estimated a progression of the aortic valve pressure gradient of approximately 18 mm Hg per decade in patients with bicuspid valves.[186]

In contrast to mitral stenosis, in which symptoms occur almost immediately after valve obstruction ensues, patients with aortic stenosis may be asymptomatic for many years despite the presence of severe obstruction. The mean systolic pressure gradient across a stenotic aortic valve can exceed 150 mm Hg, and the maximum instantaneous systolic pressure can reach approximately 300 mm Hg. The pressure overload hypertrophy that occurs in aortic stenosis may lead to relatively little increase in overall heart size on radiographic examination, and such a heart may maintain normal left ventricular end-diastolic and end-systolic volumes for a long time. Indeed, patients with severe aortic stenosis are frequently asymptomatic until relatively late in the course of the disease. Generally, asymptomatic patients have a good prognosis.[186-189] Nevertheless, it has recently been demonstrated that aortic stenosis is associated with a 50% increased risk of death from cardiovascular disease and myocardial infarction, even in the absence of hemodynamically significant obstruction.[190] In symptomatic patients with severe aortic stenosis, sudden death, like syncope, may occur.[191-193]

The timing of aortic valve replacement in adults with aortic stenosis is based strictly on the development of symptoms, which heralds exhaustion of compensatory myocardial hyperfunction. Thus, once symptoms develop, the cumulative mortality in patients with unoperated aortic stenosis is high: with angina or syncope, the average survival is 2 to 4 years, whereas with congestive heart failure it is 1.5 years (Fig. 13-29).[191-193] Rapaport's series showed that only 38% of patients who received medical treatment for symptomatic aortic stenosis survived for 5 years, and only 20% were alive 10 years after diagnosis.[191] In a group of elderly patients with severe aortic stenosis and heart failure who declined surgery, 50% had died by 18 months of follow-up, and the ejection fraction correlated inversely with survival.[194] Thus, the natural history of symptomatic aortic stenosis is considerably more severe than that of symptomatic aortic regurgitation, mitral stenosis, or mitral regurgitation. Nevertheless, patients

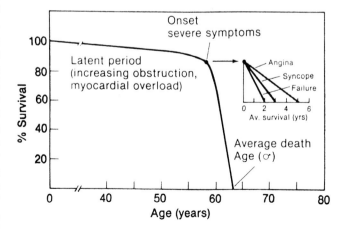

Figure 13-29 • Natural history of aortic stenosis without operative treatment in a typical patient, emphasizing the rapid downhill course that often occurs after onset of symptoms. (From Ross J, Braunwald E: Aortic stenosis. Circulation 38 [suppl V]:61, 1968.)

with aortic stenosis are usually dramatically improved by aortic valve replacement, which is performed with low mortality, even in the elderly.[112, 195, 196]

Left Ventricular Hypertrophy

Aortic stenosis is usually associated with the development of concentric left ventricular hypertrophy. Occasionally, disproportionate septal hypertrophy occurs and may mimic hypertrophic cardiomyopathy. Microscopically (as previously discussed in this chapter), myocytes show increased cell size, and interstitial collagen is increased, particularly subendocardially. Scarring may be more prominent in the setting of coexistent coronary atherosclerosis. In the elderly, senile amyloid can also affect the left ventricle and contribute to wall thickening. Acute subendocardial ischemia may develop readily during hypotensive or hypoxemic episodes; it may also occur during anesthesia induction or surgical procedures or during an acute exacerbation of chronic obstructive pulmonary disease.

Pulmonary Vascular Disease (Secondary to Left-Sided Valvular Disease)

The hypertrophied and poorly compliant (stiff) left ventricle is associated with an elevated end-diastolic pressure. Accordingly, pressures become elevated in the left atrium, pulmonary vascular bed, and right ventricle. This pressure elevation constitutes chronic pulmonary venous hypertension. Its microscopic counterparts include dilation and medial hypertrophy of pulmonary veins and congestion of the pulmonary microcirculation; focal alveolar edema, hemorrhages, or clusters of siderophages; edema of interlobular septa (the source of Kerley B lines radiographically); dilation of pleural and septal lymphatics; and, ultimately, medial hypertrophy and secondary eccentric intimal fibrosis of muscular pulmonary arteries. This constellation of findings is generally less extensive in patients with aortic stenosis than in those with mitral stenosis.

Other features associated with chronic pulmonary venous hypertension include hypertrophy and dilation of the left atrium, right ventricle, and right atrium. Mediastinal pulmonary veins and arteries may be dilated, as may the pulmonary and tricuspid valve annuli.

Poststenotic Dilation of the Ascending Aorta

Poststenotic dilation of the ascending aorta caused by a high-pressure jet of blood is a common finding in patients with valvular aortic stenosis, particularly of the rheumatic type. A plaque of thickened intima can develop in the vessel wall at the site of jet impaction. Moreover, a localized jet may, in rare instances, produce an aneurysm. Histologically, the aorta may show focal cystic medial degeneration, with elastic tissue disruption and an increased accumulation of glycosaminoglycans. These changes are like those found in older persons or in individuals with systemic hypertension. Poststenotic dilation may weaken the ascending aorta and render it prone to intimal tears and medial dissections.

Endocarditis and Emboli

Infective endocarditis may develop on calcified, stenotic aortic valves, but the risk is low. Rather, the risk is greatest in younger patients with mild, subclinical valvular dysfunction (such as early valvular calcification or noncalcified bicuspid valve) and in those with established aortic incompetence. Cerebral emboli may originate from infected or thrombotic vegetations or from calcific nodules on stenotic aortic valves.

Coronary Insufficiency

Myocardial ischemia may be multifactorial in patients with valvular heart disease. Left ventricular chamber enlargement, increased wall thickening and wall stress, and right ventricular hypertrophy may contribute. Thus, angina is a poor marker of coronary artery disease in patients with aortic stenosis. Atherosclerotic coronary artery disease is prevalent in a population of individuals with aortic valve disease, and more than half of patients having valve replacement for aortic stenosis have simultaneous coronary bypass surgery (personal communication, Gregory Cooper MD, Brigham and Women's Hospital, Boston, MA).[197] Coronary artery disease is less prevalent in patients with aortic regurgitation and mitral stenosis than in those with aortic stenosis. However, because mitral regurgitation is a common manifestation of coronary artery and ischemic heart disease, the relationship between mitral regurgitation and coronary artery disease is more complex.

Coronary blood flow is impaired by the elevated left ventricular end-diastolic pressure and the shortened diastolic phase of hearts with aortic stenosis (due to prolonged ejection time). In aortic insufficiency, coronary blood flow is particularly impaired by the rapid loss of pressure in the aortic root during diastole. In addition, the hypertrophied left ventricular muscle mass and elevated systolic pressure increase the myocardial oxygen requirement. Thus, the myocardium is prone to ischemia, making the patient with aortic stenosis liable to myocardial injury and subsequent fibrosis; ventricular arrhythmias; and, potentially, sudden death. Patients with aortic stenosis who have atherosclerotic coronary arterial obstructions are particularly at increased risk.

Aortic Stenosis and Colonic Angiodysplasia

An arteriovenous malformation (also known as angiodysplasia), most commonly in the right colon, is a potential cause of recurrent gastrointestinal bleeding in elderly patients who have valvular aortic stenosis, an association known as the Heyde syndrome.[198] The frequency of aortic stenosis in patients with angiodysplasia is variably reported as 10 to 60%. Although the mechanism of the association is unknown, surgical alleviation of a patient's aortic stenosis generally cures the gastrointestinal hemorrhage.

Congenital Aortic Stenosis

Congenitally malformed aortic valves may be acommissural (dome-shaped), unicommissural, bicuspid, tricuspid, or quadricuspid and may present with calcific or

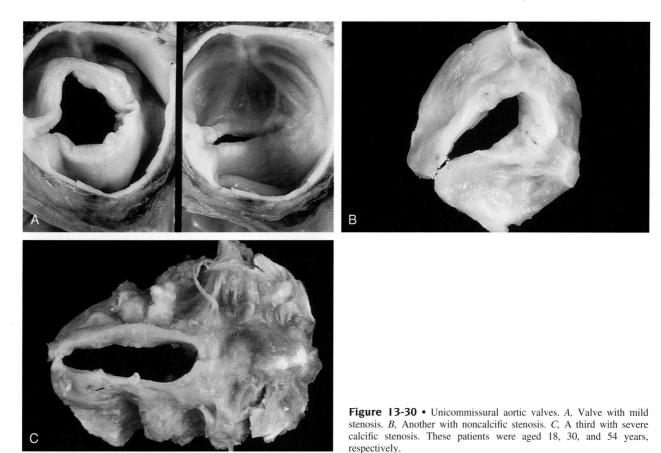

Figure 13-30 • Unicommissural aortic valves. *A,* Valve with mild stenosis. *B,* Another with noncalcific stenosis. *C,* A third with severe calcific stenosis. These patients were aged 18, 30, and 54 years, respectively.

noncalcific aortic stenosis in adults (Fig. 13-30).[199] Congenital aortic stenosis generally is the result of diffuse or nodular dysplasia and annular hypoplasia, regardless of the number of cusps. Severely stenotic valves are also commonly associated with hypoplastic left ventricle, secondary endocardial fibroelastosis, hypoplastic ascending aorta, coarctation of the aorta, patent ductal artery, and mitral valve dysfunction.

Critical aortic stenosis in infancy is usually associated with a hypoplastic and dysplastic unicommissural valve or, less commonly, a bicuspid valve. In contrast, mild to moderate congenital stenosis most frequently is the result of a bicuspid valve with only mildly dysplastic and hypoplastic features. To put this in perspective, however, recall that the vast majority of bicuspid aortic valves are neither stenotic nor regurgitant at birth and only become dysfunctional later in life as a result of calcification, infection, annular dilation, or cusp prolapse.

Subvalvular Aortic Stenosis

Theoretically, an excess or redundancy of any of the structures forming the boundaries of the outflow tract of the left ventricle or their congenital malposition may cause subvalvular obstruction. In the young, fixed subaortic stenosis is commonly associated with other congenital cardiac anomalies, and without surgery, adult survival is exceptional. A pathologist may encounter subvalvular stenosis in teenagers and young adults who died suddenly or as surgically excised fragments of tissue in known causes of outflow tract obstruction. Isolated aortic subvalvular obstruction may be fibrous or muscular.

Discrete Subaortic Stenosis

Also called discrete membranous subaortic stenosis, this anomaly is characterized by a tough, gray-white fibroelastic endocardial ridge that obstructs the outflow tract of the left ventricle approximately 1 to 2 cm proximal to the aortic valve, often extending onto the anterior mitral leaflet (Fig. 13-31). The tissue varies in width (2 to 4 mm) and forms a C-shaped or O-shaped obstructive ridge. The outflow tract of the left ventricle does not appear narrowed, except at the site of the fibrous ridge. The ridge varies from thin and membranous to thick and fibromuscular, and contains smooth muscle cells but not cardiac myocytes. The septum shows malalignment in 40% and prominent hypertrophy in 25% of the cases. Aortic coarctation or a ventricular septal defect may coexist.[200] Discrete subaortic stenosis accounts for 8 to 10% of all cases of congenital left ventricular outflow obstruction and affects males twice as frequently as females.

Usually, the aortic annulus is of normal size, and the aortic valve has three cusps. If the cusps are injured by a high-pressure jet of blood passing through the membranous subvalvular obstruction, they may become thickened and distorted, leading to aortic incompetence. Damaged

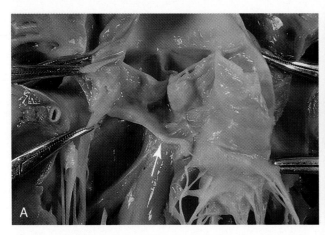
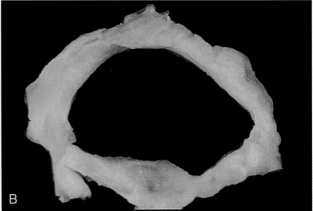

Figure 13-31 • Discrete membranous subaortic stenosis. *A*, Autopsy specimen: arrow denotes subvalvular membrane. *B*, Surgical specimen.

aortic cusps are also prone to infective endocarditis. In general, subvalvular obstructions do not cause poststenotic dilation of the aorta, but there may be dilation in the area between membrane and aortic valve cusps. Small intramyocardial vessels and the septal muscle may show changes similar to those noted in hypertrophic cardiomyopathy (see Chapter 10).

Surgical resection, with or without replacement of the aortic or mitral valve, is the usual mode of therapy. However, restenosis may occur after surgery.

Tunnel Subaortic Stenosis

Tunnel subaortic stenosis is a fibrous endocardial lesion, like discrete subaortic stenosis. The entire left ventricular outflow tract is narrowed by a thick and irregular sleeve of fibrotic endocardium that can involve the aortic valve and may also produce mitral regurgitation. Restenosis can occur postoperatively.

Muscular Subaortic Stenosis

Muscular subaortic stenosis (MSS) involves the ventricular septal myocardium rather than the endocardium. Hypertrophic cardiomyopathy is the most common form. It has a particular microscopic morphology and is described in detail in Chapter 10. A form of MSS with similar gross if not microscopic characteristics may occur in infants of diabetic mothers.

Congenital forms of MSS are often associated with malalignment ventricular septal defects so that the outlet (infundibular) septum is shifted leftward. As a result, the left ventricular outflow tract is narrowed. Because of diminished blood flow, the aortic valve and aortic arch may be hypoplastic, and coarctation of the aorta or interruption of the aortic arch is a relatively common association. MSS is also a feature of Shone syndrome (see earlier description of congenital mitral stenosis). It is generally due to exaggerated bulging of the subaortic septum, although in some hearts it may resemble hypertrophic cardiomyopathy.

In some adults with valvular aortic stenosis or chronic hypertension, the left ventricle generally shows concentric pressure hypertrophy in which there is disproportionate septal hypertrophy. Age-related angulation of the septum (so-called sigmoid septum) can accentuate the asymmetric process.[201] The importance of this age-related phenomenon is twofold. First, such hearts may be misdiagnosed as having hypertrophic cardiomyopathy. Second, after surgical relief of valvular aortic stenosis in some patients, dynamic outflow tract obstruction may develop if a septal myectomy is not also performed. In addition, amyloid and metabolic products in storage diseases may be deposited preferentially in the inferoseptal region of the left ventricle, in some cases causing asymmetry,[202, 203] and possibly producing appreciable outflow tract obstruction.

Supravalvular Aortic Stenosis

Supravalvular aortic stenosis, the least common form of left ventricular outflow tract obstruction, represents a form of arterial dysplasia. Stenosis may result from discrete narrowing at the aortic sinotubular junction or diffuse narrowing of the entire ascending aorta and aortic arch. Involved areas show marked wall thickening and luminal narrowing. The aortic sinuses are usually not dilated in supravalvular aortic stenosis, nor is poststenotic dilation common. Indeed, the aorta beyond a localized obstruction may be relatively hypoplastic.

The coronary arteries in this condition are subject to systolic hypertension and are perfused primarily during systole. Of large diameter and tortuous configuration, they show intimal thickening and are prone to premature atherosclerosis. Indeed, the severity of clinical disease in adults often correlates better with abnormalities of the coronary arteries than with the severity of the supravalvular obstruction, although both may be significant.

Usually, the aortic valve has three cusps that may become thickened and incompetent. Also, the free margin of an aortic valve cusp can adhere to the ascending aorta and may obstruct a coronary ostium. Microscopically, thickened arterial walls are affected by fibromuscular dysplasia, with merging of the medial and intimal layers and with whirled and haphazard, rather than parallel, arrangement of the smooth muscle cells and elastic fibers.[204]

Supravalvular aortic stenosis may be inherited as an autosomal dominant trait with variable penetrance, or it

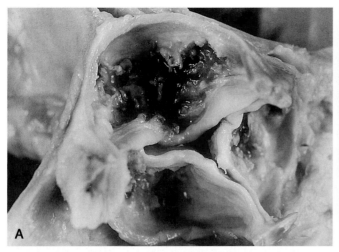
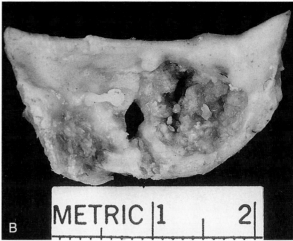
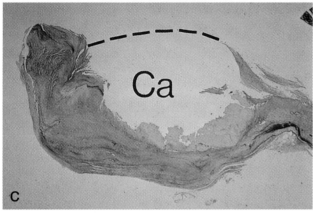

Figure 13-32 • Operative decalcification of the aortic valve. A, Aortic valve after mechanical decalcification. B, Perforated aortic cusp following decalcification procedure. C, Histologic cross section of aortic valve cusp after decalcification with lithotripter. (Weigert elastic stain). Ca = calcium.

may occur sporadically. It is more common in males than in females. Supravalvular aortic stenosis may be part of the hypercalcemic Williams-Beurens syndrome, in which the affected person may have a characteristic elfin facies, mental retardation, dysplastic supravalvular pulmonary stenosis, inguinal hernia, strabismus, and abnormalities of dental development.[205] Rarely, mitral valve prolapse and mitral insufficiency are complications. The genetic form of supravalvular aortic stenosis is the result of mutation or deletion of the elastin gene.[206] Supravalvular aortic stenosis may also be part of the congenital rubella syndrome.

Acquired supravalvular aortic stenosis is an extremely rare condition. Patients with homozygous type II hyperlipoproteinemia can develop severe calcific atherosclerosis in the ascending aorta that may cause supravalvular stenosis. Secondary nodular calcification of healed aortitis may also lead to obstruction.

As with other forms of left ventricular outflow tract obstruction, the usual symptoms at presentation are angina pectoris and congestive heart failure. Symptoms usually indicate a poor prognosis, and sudden death can occur.

Treatment

Patients with symptomatic aortic stenosis most commonly require valve replacement (see Chapter 21) but

balloon aortic valvuloplasty, in which dilation catheters are advanced along a guidewire positioned at the left ventricular apex, is an increasingly attractive alternative to aortic valvotomy in children, adolescents, and young adults with congenital noncalcific aortic stenosis.[207] However, the value of balloon valvotomy is limited in adults with calcific aortic stenosis.

Operative decalcification procedures have also been used without much success.[208, 209] They leave an ulcerated cuspal surface with exposed collagen and calcium that are highly thrombogenic. Also, because of the depth of degenerative calcific deposits within the cusps, such procedures frequently leave regions of markedly thinned cusp, which can tear or perforate (Fig. 13-32).

Balloon Aortic Valvotomy

Balloon aortic valvotomy for adult-acquired aortic stenosis is used only for palliation of the disease.[210] Balloon dilation of calcified stenotic aortic valves primarily causes fracture of calcified nodules, providing the main mechanism for amelioration (Fig. 13-33).[211] Additional mechanisms involving separation of fused commissures and stretching of the aortic valve ring may be involved, but they are probably of only limited extended benefit and often result in restenosis.[212–214]

Despite a considerable variation in response, most patients have an initial relief of obstruction after balloon

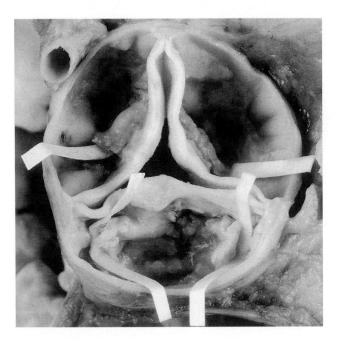

Figure 13-33 • Aortic valve balloon valvuloplasty for degenerative calcific aortic stenosis, demonstrating fractures of calcific deposits, highlighted by tapes.

aortic valvuloplasty. In a report of a multicenter registry involving 674 elderly (average age, 78 years) and seriously ill patients treated at 24 centers, the procedural mortality was 3%, the 30-day mortality was 14%, and the 1-year mortality was 45%.[215] Valve area initially increased from 0.50 to 0.80 cm², and the mean gradient declined from approximately 55 to 29 mm Hg. Another 6% developed serious complications such as myocardial perforation, myocardial infarction, stroke, aortic rupture, vascular injury, and severe aortic regurgitation.[216, 217] The

major disadvantage of balloon valvuloplasty in adults with critical calcific aortic stenosis is restenosis due to scarring. Symptoms lessen in severity in the majority of those treated but recur in approximately 30% by 6 months. In most series, patients have been elderly, have had heart failure, and have been considered poor operative risks. Although the procedure is not lifesaving, it may be useful in alleviating symptoms in patients who, because of other medical problems, are clearly not candidates for aortic valve replacement.

RIGHT VENTRICULAR INFLOW TRACT OBSTRUCTION (AT OR RELATED TO THE TRICUSPID VALVE)

In the adult, acquired tricuspid stenosis is much less frequent than mitral or aortic stenosis but more common than pulmonary stenosis. Rheumatic disease is the main cause of pure tricuspid stenosis.[218] Combined tricuspid stenosis and regurgitation are most commonly secondary to rheumatic postinflammatory scarring or carcinoid heart disease.

Rheumatic Tricuspid Stenosis

Rarely an isolated lesion, rheumatic tricuspid stenosis usually accompanies mitral, and often aortic, stenosis. Although found anatomically at autopsy in 15% of patients with rheumatic heart disease, tricuspid stenosis is clinically important in only about 5%.[219] Organic tricuspid disease is more common in India and elsewhere in the world than in North America or Europe, in the former instance, possibly affecting more than one third of patients with rheumatic heart disease coming to autopsy.[220]

In patients with advanced rheumatic tricuspid stenosis, the valve is nearly always incompetent as well, with leaf-

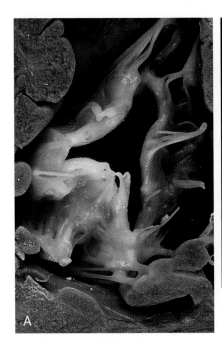

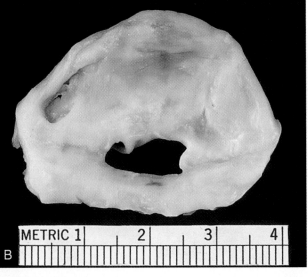

Figure 13-34 • Rheumatic tricuspid stenosis/insufficiency. *A,* Autopsy specimen (from ventricular aspect). *B,* Surgical pathology specimen from inflow aspect.

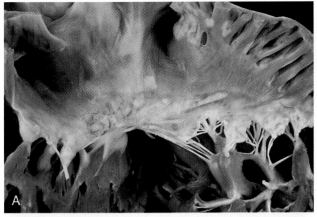
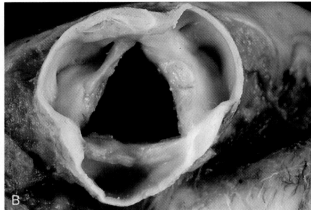
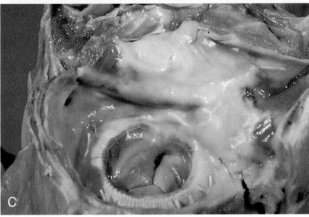

Figure 13-35 • Carcinoid heart disease. *A,* Plaques on the right atrium and tricuspid valve causing tricuspid stenosis and insufficiency. *B,* Plaque on the pulmonary valve causing pulmonary stenosis and insufficiency. *C,* Plaque involving the right atrium and a tricuspid porcine bioprosthetic valve. (*C,* From Schoen FJ, Hausner RJ, Howell JF, et al: Porcine heterograft valve replacement in carcinoid heart disease. J Thorac Cardiovasc Surg 81:100, 1981.)

let thickening, commissural fusion, and chordal thickening (Fig. 13-34). Commissural fusion is usually most marked at the anteroseptal commissure. The shortened, thickened, and retracted leaflets, fused at their commissures, produce a diaphragm-like impediment to flow, funneling toward the right ventricle with a fixed round, oval, or triangular orifice. In contrast to the heavy calcification often associated with mitral stenosis, secondary calcification of the stenosed tricuspid valve is rare (see also Fig. 14-5).

Carcinoid and Other Acquired Causes of Tricuspid Stenosis

Clinically important endocardial and valvular lesions of carcinoid heart disease are usually limited to the right side of the heart. Carcinoid heart disease occurs frequently in patients who have carcinoid tumors of the gastrointestinal tract with hepatic metastases or such tumors at other sites (such as an ovary) that drain directly into the systemic venous circulation.[221-223] Tricuspid regurgitation and pulmonary stenosis are the predominant valvular abnormalities, although there is usually some accompanying tricuspid stenosis and pulmonary regurgitation. The combination of pulmonary stenosis and tricuspid regurgitation is particularly deleterious to right-sided cardiac function because the former exacerbates the latter. Carcinoid heart disease, if unoperated, is frequently fatal.

Carcinoid-induced valve lesions consist of endocardial fibrous thickenings that are rich in smooth muscle cells

and devoid of elastic fibers. They generally occur on the ventricular aspect of the tricuspid valve and the arterial (outflow) aspect of the pulmonary valve (Figs. 13-35 and 13-36).[224] The underlying valvular architecture is otherwise normal. Fibrous tissue thickens the valve cusps and reduces their mobility, whereas deposits in the pulmonary sinuses tend to contract the valvular ring, contributing to stenosis. The extracellular matrix of young carcinoid plaques is rich in proteoglycans, whereas that of older lesions is more densely collagenous. Calcification is not a feature.

Although the development of carcinoid heart disease appears unrelated to the duration of symptoms of the carcinoid syndrome, groups of patients with valvular lesions have higher levels of plasma serotonin (5-hydroxytryptamine) and urinary 5-HIAA (5-hydroxy-indole acetic acid, the principal metabolite of serotonin) than those without symptoms.[225-227] Other circulating vasoactive substances are also elevated in patients with carcinoid heart disease, including neuropeptide K, substance P, and atrial natriuretic peptide. Nevertheless, the specific pathogenesis of the intracardiac fibrous lesions is uncertain. Interestingly, the morphology is similar to that of the fibrous lesions that develop in some patients who take methylsergide or ergot derivatives or fenfluramine and phentermine, drugs that elevate plasma serotonin and its metabolites (see earlier in this chapter).

The leaflets of the tricuspid valve may also become thickened and stenotic as a result of metabolic or enzymatic abnormalities, for example in Fabry or Whipple

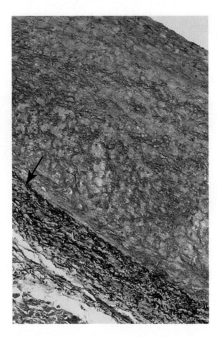

Figure 13-36 • Histology of plaque in carcinoid heart disease (Movat stain) demonstrating intact elastic lamina of normal cardiac structures (arrow) and extracellular matrix-rich plaque containing spindle cells superimposed on the normal structures.

disease. Occasionally, right-sided endocarditis can yield large infected vegetations which may fill the lumen and cause transient valvular stenosis. This is especially likely in patients with intravenous drug addiction (see Chapter 14).

Secondary tumor invasion of the pericardium, usually from a primary tumor in lung or breast, can also cause obstruction by external compression of the tricuspid valve or right atrium or ventricle. Rarely, obstruction to right ventricular inflow is caused by endomyocardial fibrosis.

Congenital Tricuspid Atresia

In tricuspid atresia, no communication exists between the right atrium and ventricle, and all right atrial blood must be shunted through a patent foramen ovale (most frequently) or an atrial septal defect to reach the left heart. In 85%, the right atrioventricular connection is absent, and in 15% a fibrous plug, representing the imperforate valve, is present. Associated anomalies include transposition of the great arteries, subpulmonary stenosis, a muscular ventricular septal defect (present in 90% and usually restrictive), and a mildly malformed mitral valve.

Congenital tricuspid stenosis is an extremely rare, isolated anomaly. More commonly, it occurs with pulmonary atresia and an intact ventricular septum and is associated with a hypoplastic tricuspid annulus, Ebstein features, and hypoplastic right ventricle.

Clinicopathologic Correlations

Tricuspid stenosis causes a rise in right atrial pressure, inducing dilation and hypertrophy. The elevated intralu-

minal pressure causes dilation of the veins draining into the right atrium and congestion of the liver and spleen. Severe and prolonged valve disease can produce in centrilobular fibrosis (so-called cardiac sclerosis) and hepatic dysfunction, ultimately with a cirrhosis-like picture in some.

The low cardiac output and elevated systemic venous pressure associated with tricuspid stenosis cause progressive fatigue, peripheral edema, anorexia, and, often, abdominal discomfort due to hepatomegaly and splenomegaly, abdominal swelling, or ascites. Reflecting the right-sided disease, these symptoms and signs are out of proportion with the degree of dyspnea. Indeed, orthopnea and paroxysmal nocturnal dyspnea are both minimal and unusual, and pulmonary edema and hemoptysis are typically rare, even if mitral stenosis coexists.

Patients with tricuspid stenosis are wasted, with peripheral cyanosis, often prominent neck vein distention, and visible V waves. There is a right ventricular lift and a holosystolic murmur heard best at the left lower sternal border. Electrocardiograms show full right atrial P waves and no right ventricular hypertrophy. Radiographs reveal marked cardiomegaly with a dilated right atrium and without an enlarged pulmonary artery segment. Imaging by two-dimensional echocardiography shows diastolic doming of the valve leaflets, with thickening and restriction of motion and reduced separation of leaflet tips.

As indicated above, most patients with tricuspid stenosis have coexistent, clinically significant, left-sided valve disease. When multivalvular disease is present, the diagnostic features of tricuspid valve disease may be overshadowed by those of mitral stenosis. Surgical valve replacement is generally done when the mean diastolic pressure gradient exceeds 5 mm Hg and the valve orifice is less than 2.0 cm². Balloon dilation and commissurotomy have been attempted but are usually not efficacious because of preexisting and concomitant valvular regurgitation.

Supravalvular Obstruction

The clinical impression of a supravalvular obstruction of the tricuspid valve could be caused by the uncommon congenital abnormality known as cor triatriatum dexter, in which the right atrial chamber appears to be divided into two parts, probably due to anomalous development or prominence of the eustachian valve of the inferior vena cava.[228] The surgical correction of certain congenital anomalies can produce a small right atrial chamber that may behave similarly to a supravalvular stenosis. Several acquired lesions, including an aneurysm of the fossa ovalis,[229] a right atrial myxoma, other primary or secondary tumors that invade the right atrium or venae cavae (e.g., primary angiosarcoma, leiomyosarcoma, or renal carcinoma extending through the inferior vena cava), and a large mural thrombus or aneurysm of the sinus of Valsalva, may all bulge into the right atrium and, potentially, the tricuspid valve, to cause supravalvular (or valvular) stenosis. Obstructing thrombus or pseudocyst may be associated with the use of right atrial catheters.[230–232]

RIGHT VENTRICULAR OUTFLOW TRACT OBSTRUCTION (AT OR RELATED TO THE PULMONARY VALVE)

Acquired Pulmonary Stenosis

Carcinoid plaques may cause pulmonary stenosis, usually also with regurgitation (see earlier).

Although acute rheumatic fever often involves the pulmonary valve microscopically, rheumatic post-inflammatory scarring causing pulmonary stenosis is uncommon and invariably associated with rheumatic disease affecting other cardiac valves.[233] Usually, there is slight commissural fusion with noncalcific cusp thickening, and the overall deformity is not severe. The vegetations of infective endocarditis can rarely cause stenosis. Cardiac tumors or aneurysms of the sinus of Valsalva can stenose the subvalvular or valvular area, as may external pressure induced by calcification from tuberculous pericarditis.[234]

Clinicopathologic Correlations

Pulmonary stenosis of either congenital or acquired etiology causes hypertrophy and variable dilation of the right ventricle (Fig. 13-37). Marked infundibular hypertrophy can add to right ventricular outflow tract obstruction. Secondary endocardial fibroelastosis can develop in the right ventricle, particularly in the outflow tract, and patchy fibrosis of the right ventricle is a common finding at autopsy. Moreover, the jet of blood forced through the stenosed valve can produce an intimal jet lesion or cause poststenotic dilation of the pulmonary artery. Myocardial hypertrophy decreases the compliance of the right ventricle and impedes right atrial emptying. If right atrial pressure is increased markedly, it may cause a right-to-left shunt through a patent foramen ovale.

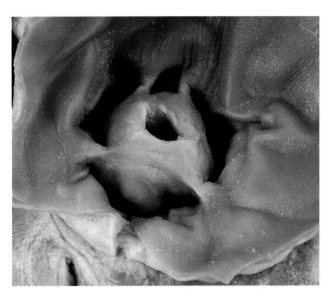

Figure 13-38 • Severe congenital pulmonary stenosis with acommissural, dome-shaped valve.

Nevertheless, most patients with mild pulmonary stenosis are asymptomatic. Severe stenosis eventually induces functional tricuspid valve regurgitation with its associated symptoms, right heart failure and occasionally sudden death. On physical examination, a systolic murmur and thrill may be obvious in the pulmonary area. Echocardiography helps define both the pathology and the physiologic importance of pulmonary stenosis. Percutaneous balloon valvuloplasty is often a safe and effective treatment; alternatively, valvulectomy may be required. Often, the valve is excised but *not* replaced by a prosthetic valve.

Congenital Pulmonary Stenosis

The majority of cases of isolated right ventricular outflow tract obstruction occur at the valvular level and are congenital.[235]

Accounting for approximately 8% of all cases of congenital heart disease, isolated pulmonary stenosis (Fig. 13-38) is one of the common congenital cardiac anomalies in which adult survival is expected. Pulmonary valvular stenosis associated with tetralogy of Fallot is most frequently associated with a bicuspid valve with variable annular hypoplasia. In isolated pulmonary stenosis, the valve is commonly either dome-shaped and acommissural or thickened and tricuspid (Fig. 13-39). Isolated stenosis of the pulmonary valve is also the most common cardiac anomaly encountered in the LEOPARD syndrome[236] and Noonan syndrome.[237] Stenotic pulmonary valves may undergo calcification after several decades or after an episode of infective endocarditis.[238] Otherwise, congenitally bicuspid or quadricuspid pulmonary valves rarely become stenotic as a result of calcification and fibrosis. Balloon valvuloplasty has been used to manage congenital pulmonic stenosis, particularly in children.[239]

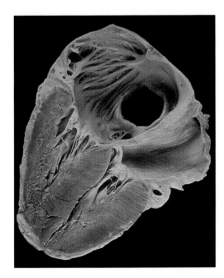

Figure 13-37 • Severe congenital pulmonary stenosis in a 73-year-old man with marked right ventricular hypertrophy and right atrial dilation (seen in four-chamber projection), right ventricle at left.

Congenital Subvalvular Pulmonary Stenosis

Most congenital anomalies cause clinical problems in infancy or childhood and are now usually corrected surgically early in life, but minor forms could permit long-term survival. Isolated infundibular stenosis is a rare congenital anomaly. Like subaortic obstruction, right ventricular outflow tract obstruction may result from a fibrous band at the junction of the main cavity of the right ventricle and the infundibulum or by muscle impinging on the lumen and narrowing it over a long or short segment. In contrast, infundibular stenosis caused by the myocardium impinging on the lumen most commonly occurs as part of tetralogy of Fallot. Right ventricular outflow tract obstruction can also be caused by aneurysms of the membranous septum.

Congenital Supravalvular Pulmonary Stenosis

Congenital supravalvular stenosis can occur in the pulmonary trunk, in its main branches, or in the intrapulmonary arteries. Pulmonary arterial stenosis may be isolated or, more often, associated with other congenital cardiac anomalies. The stenosis may be single or multiple, localized or segmental, or may be due to a generalized (diffuse) hypoplasia of the vessels. It may coexist with supravalvular aortic stenosis. Demonstration at autopsy may be facilitated by postmortem angiography.

APPROACH TO THE PATHOLOGIC ANALYSIS OF VALVES WITH STENOSIS

The primary goals of the surgical pathologist in studying excised natural heart valves are to document the severity and etiologic nature of the disease and to reveal unanticipated pathology, such as infective endocarditis.

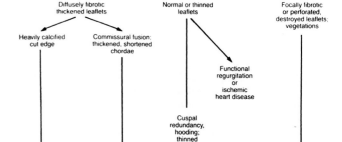

Figure 13-39 • Protocols for valve diagnoses for (*A*) mitral and (*B*) aortic valve disease. (From Schoen FJ: Evaluation of surgically removed natural and prosthetic heart valves. In: Virmani R, Atkinson JB, Fenoglio JJ [eds]: Cardiovascular Pathology. Philadelphia, WB Saunders, 1991, p 399.)

TABLE 13-9 • **Gross Morphologic Comparison Between Stenotic and Regurgitant Valves**

Pathologic Feature	Stenotic Valve	Purely Regurgitant Valve
For All Valves		
Valve weight	Increased	Normal, or slightly increased or decreased
Fibrous thickening	Diffuse	Diffuse, focal, or none
Calcific deposits	None to heavy	Minimal (if any)
Tissue loss (perforation, indentation)	None	May be present
Vegetations	Minimal	May be present
Commissural fusion	May be present	Minimal (if any)
Annular circumference	Normal	Normal or increased
For Aortic Valves		
Number of cusps	1–3	2–4
For Mitral (or Tricuspid) Valves		
Abnormal papillary muscles	No	May be present
Tendinous cords		
Fusion	Usually present	Absent
Elongation	Absent	May be present
Shortening	Usually present	May be present
Rupture	Absent	May be present

TABLE 13-10 • Aortic Valve Stenosis: Gross Diagnostic Features by Etiologic Category

Degenerative ("Senile")

Arch-shaped calcification along aortic aspect (usually sparing free edge)
Variable amounts of diffuse fibrosis
No or minimal commissural fusion

Postinflammatory (Most Commonly Postrheumatic)

Commissural fusion (1 to 3 commissures may be involved)
Variable amounts of fibrosis, often diffuse ("dripped candle wax" appearance common)
Variable amounts of nodular calcification (may involve free edge)

Congenitally Bicuspid

Two cusps usually of unequal size
Raphe frequently calcified (with stenosis)
Mild to moderate annular dilation

Post-therapeutic ("Iatrogenic")

Most frequently has features of either degenerative or postinflammatory valve
Can be difficult, without history, to distinguish from postinflammatory valve

Modified from Tazelaar H: Surgical pathology of the heart: Endomyocardial biopsy, valvular heart disease, and cardiac tumors. In: Schoen FJ, Gimbrone MA Jr (eds): Cardiovascular Pathology: Clinicopathologic Correlations and Pathogenetic Mechanisms. Philadelphia, Williams & Wilkins, 1995, p 81.

Determination of etiology in an individual patient helps to predict natural history, surgical risks, postoperative prognosis, and potential complications, as well as revealing the presence of unsuspected or unproved systemic disease. In addition, careful examination of diseased valves may serve to correlate pathologic anatomy with preoperative diagnoses, hemodynamic findings, and complications; assist in the validation of new diagnostic imaging techniques; assess whether indications for conservative surgery might be applied to similar future patients (i.e., whether valve reconstruction rather than replacement could have been done); and elucidate the pathobiology of valve diseases.

Valves are often removed intact by a surgeon, but the requirements of the surgical procedure may lead to a fragmented specimen, especially with heavily calcified valves. Most aortic valves are removed in two or three pieces, and some mitral valves are only partially excised, without papillary muscles. Microbiologic cultures of valves with suspected infective endocarditis are best taken in the operating room by the surgical team.

Precise diagnosis and understanding of valvular diseases result primarily from careful gross inspection of the specimen.[65, 240, 241] Close-range photographs (and, occasionally, specimen radiographs) provide the most effective record of pathologic findings and permit correlations between pathologic anatomy and clinical, hemodynamic, and operative findings. For an atrioventricular valve, both atrial and ventricular aspects should be shown; for an aortic valve, the outflow aspect is usually more informative. Functional and etiologic classification of operatively excised valves may, in some cases, require data from preoperative echocardiography or cardiac catheterization, or information from the surgeon or an operative report about the structural and functional status of a valve that has been examined but not removed.

Inspection and description of the specimen should provide the anatomic site, degree, and location of calcification and other cuspal and leaflet abnormalities; presence of vegetations; and nature of the functional abnormality (i.e., appearance of the valve as incompetent or stenotic) (Table 13-9). Separate considerations of annulus, leaflets, tendinous cords, or papillary muscles of an atrioventricular valve are useful. For aortic valves, documentation of the number and relative size of the valve cusps is important. The specific questions to be answered by gross inspection are the following: Are the cusps/leaflets fibrotic, calcified, perforated, immobile, shortened, stretched, redundant (ballooned), or normal? Is the abnormality focal or diffuse, situated at the leaflet margins, on one surface or both? If vegetations are present, are they single or multiple, large or small, firm or friable? Do calcific de-

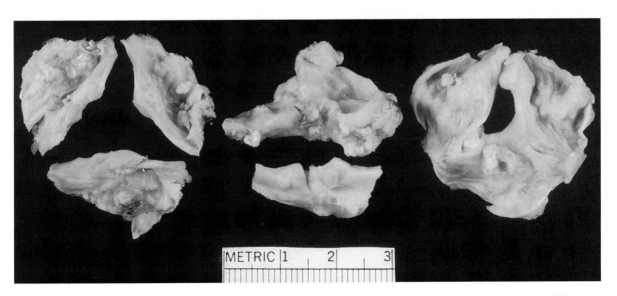

Figure 13-40 • Aortic valve stenosis resulting from three major etiologies: aortic stenosis affecting a tricuspid valve (left); aortic stenosis of a congenitally bicuspid valve (middle); rheumatic changes after inflammatory scarring (right).

posits predominate at the free edges or at the margin of resection? Is vascularity noted grossly? Are the commissures fused, either completely or partially? Are the tendinous cords intact, ruptured, shortened, elongated, fused, or normal? Are the papillary muscles or their fragments normal, infarcted, scarred, hypertrophied, or elongated?

Table 13-10 summarizes the major etiologic categories and salient diagnostic features. Careful gross examination of a valve that has been obtained at autopsy or that has been surgically excised allows the diagnosis of etiology in approximately 90% of cases. The protocols illustrated in Figure 13-39 may be helpful. In the majority, histology is unnecessary, adding only time and cost to the examination; gross examination alone is usually sufficient for diagnosis. Figure 13-40, for example, offers a comparison of the gross features of aortic stenosis caused by degenerative calcification (three cusps) at left, congenital bicuspid calcific valve at center, and rheumatic heart disease at right. However, histologic examination is required when infective endocarditis or an active inflammatory process is suspected clinically or by gross examination. It is useful to confirm features of the diagnosis and to identify other conditions, such as amyloid, found histologically in some calcified, stenosed aortic valve cusps. Microscopic analysis may be useful in some cases to document primary myxomatous degeneration or tissue accumulations of metabolic diseases, and to distinguish congenital from acquired valvular lesions.

Because infective endocarditis may occur on either anatomically normal or previously diseased valves,[242] the underlying anatomic state of the valve (i.e., before infection) should be ascertained in addition to confirming or ruling out endocarditis. If gross inspection alone is insufficient for determining whether an aortic valve is bicuspid or tricuspid, a microscopic section may be taken at the site of the presumed commissural fusion (see earlier discussion of bicuspid aortic valve).

Representative sections of valve leaflets or cusps should include tissue from the annulus to the free edge. In determining whether to section a valve, the pathologist should consider whether microscopic study justifies destruction of the specimen, precluding correlation of valvular pathology with preoperative clinical, hemodynamic, and radiographic findings.

REFERENCES

1. Rahimtoolah SH: Perspective on valvular heart disease: An update. J Am Coll Cardiol 14:1, 1989
2. Carabello BA, Crawford FA: Valvular heart disease. N Engl J Med 337:32, 1997
3. Bonow RO, Carabello BA, de Leon AC Jr, et al: ACC/AHA guidelines for the management of patients with valvular heart disease: Executive summary. A report of the American College of Cardiology/American Heart Association Task Force on Practice Guidelines (Committee on Management of Patients With Valvular Heart Disease). Circulation 98:1949, 1998
4. Edwards WD: Congenital heart disease. In: Damjanov I, Linder J (eds): Anderson's Pathology, 10th ed. St. Louis, Mosby, 1996, p 1339
5. Ranganathan N, Lam JHC, Wigle ED, Silver MD: Morphology of human mitral valve. II. The valve leaflets. Circulation 41:459, 1970
6. Roberts WC: Morphologic features of the normal and abnormal mitral valve. Am J Cardiol 51:1005, 1983
7. Edwards WD: Applied anatomy of the heart. In: ER Giuliani (ed): Mayo Clinic Practice of Cardiology, 3rd ed. St Louis, Mosby, 1996, p 422
8. Lam JHC, Ranganathan N, Wigle ED, Silver MD: Morphology of the human mitral valve. I. Chordae tendineae: A new classification. Circulation 41:449, 1970
9. Seccombe JF, Cahill DR, Edwards WD: Quantitative morphology of the normal human tricuspid valve: Autopsy study of 24 valves. Clin Anat 6:203, 1993
10. Sutton JP, Ho SY, Anderson RH: The forgotten interleaflet triangles: A review of the surgical anatomy of the aortic valve. Ann Thorac Surg 59:419, 1995
11. Ferrans VJ, Spray TL, Billingham ME, Roberts WC: Structural changes in glutaraldehyde-treated porcine heterografts used as substitute cardiac valves. Am J Cardiol 41:1159, 1978
12. Schoen FJ: Aortic valve structure-function correlations: Role of elastic fibers: No longer a stretch of the imagination. J Heart Valve Dis 6:1, 1997
13. Peskin CS, McQueen DM: Mechanical equilibrium determines the fractal fiber architecture of aortic heart valve leaflets. Am J Physiol 266:H319, 1994
14. Gross L, Kugel MA: Topographic anatomy and histology of the valves in the human heart. Am J Pathol 7:445, 1931
15. Vesely I: The role of elastin in aortic valve mechanics. J Biomech 31:115, 1998
16. Adamczyk MM, Lee TC, Vesely I: Biaxial strain properties of elastase-digested porcine aortic valves. J Heart Valve Dis 9:445, 2000
17. Lester W, Rosenthal A, Granton B, Gotlieb AI: Porcine mitral valve interstitial cells in culture. Lab Invest 59:710, 1988
18. Messier RH, Bass BL, Aly AM, et al: Dual structural and functional phenotypes of the porcine aortic valve interstitial population: Characteristics of the leaflet myofibroblast. J Surg Res 57:1, 1994
19. Mulholland DL, Gotlieb AI: Cell biology of valvular interstitial cells. Can J Cardiol 12:231, 1996
20. Mulholland DL, Gotlieb AI: Cardiac valve interstitial cells: Regulator of valve structure and function. Cardiovasc Pathol 6:167, 1997
21. Taylor PM, Allen SP, Yacoub MH: Phenotypic and functional characterization of interstitial cells from human heart valves, pericardium and skin. J Heart Valve Dis 9:150, 2000
22. Powell DW, Mifflin RC, Valentich JD, et al: Myofibroblasts. I. Paracrine cells important in health and disease. Am J Physiol 277:C1, 1999
23. Roy A, Brand NJ, Yacoub MH: Molecular characterization of interstitial cells isolated from human heart valves. J Heart Valve Dis 9:459, 2000
24. Tamura K, Jones M, Yamada I, Ferrans VJ: Wound healing in the mitral valve. J Heart Valve Dis 9:53, 2000
25. Fitzgerald LW, Burn TC, Brown BS, et al: Possible role of valvular serotonin 5-HT$_{2B}$ receptors in the cardiopathy associated with fenfluramine. Mol Pharmacol 57:75, 2000
26. Hafizi S, Taylor PM, Chester AH, et al: Mitogenic and secretory responses of human valve interstitial cells to vasoactive agents. J Heart Valve Dis 9:454, 2000
27. Yacoub MH, Kilner PJ, Birks EJ, Misfeld M: The aortic outflow and root: A tale of dynamism and crosstalk. Ann Thorac Surg 68:S37, 1999
28. Marron K, Yacoub MH, Polak JM, et al: Innervation of human atrioventricular and arterial valves. Circulation 94:368, 1996
29. Kim KM, Huang S-H: Ultrastructural study of calcification of human aortic valve. Lab Invest 25:357, 1971
30. Schoen FJ, Levy RJ, Nelson AC, et al: Onset and progression of experimental bioprosthetic heart valve calcification. Lab Invest 52:523, 1985
31. Mohler ER, Chawla MK, Chang AW, et al: Identification and characterization of calcifying valve cells from human and canine aortic valves. J Heart Valve Dis 8:254, 1999
32. Johnson CM, Fass DN: Porcine cardiac valvular endothelial cells in culture. Lab Invest 49:589, 1983
33. Mitchell RN, Jonas RA, Schoen FJ: Pathology of explanted cryopreserved allograft heart valves: Comparison with aortic valves from orthotopic heart transplants. J Thorac Cardiovasc Surg 115:118, 1998
34. Chen RH, Mitchell RN, Kadner A, Adams DH: Differential galac-

tose a(1,3) galactose expression by porcine cardiac vascular endothelium. Xenotransplantation 6:169, 1999

35. Chen RH, Kadner A, Mitchell RN, Adams DH: Fresh porcine cardiac valves are not rejected in primates. J Thorac Cardiovasc Surg 119:1216, 2000

36. Eisenberg LM, Markwald RR: Molecular regulation of atrioventricular valvuloseptal morphogenesis. Circ Res 17:1, 1995

37. Arciniegas E, Sutton AB, Allen TD, Schor AM: Transforming growth factor beta 1 promotes the differentiation of endothelial cells into smooth muscle-like cells in vitro. J Cell Sci 103:521, 1992

38. Hilbert SL, Barrick MK, Ferrans VJ. Porcine aortic valve bioprostheses: A morphologic comparison of the effects of fixation pressure. J Biomed Mater Res 24:773, 1990

39. Flomenbaum MA, Schoen FJ: Effects of fixation back pressure and antimineralization treatment on the morphology of porcine aortic bioprosthetic valves. J Thorac Cardiovasc Surg 105:154, 1993

40. Sacks MS, Smith DB, Hiester EK: The aortic valve microstructure: Effects of transvalvular pressure. J Biomed Mater Res 41:131, 1998

41. Ferrans VJ, Butany J: Ultrastructural pathology of the heart. In: Trump BJ, Jones RT (eds): Diagnostic Electron Microscopy, Vol 4. New York, John Wiley & Sons, 1983, p 421

42. Weind KL, Ellis CG, Boughner DR: The aortic valve blood supply. J Heart Valve Dis 9:1, 2000

43. Angrist A: Aging heart valves and a unified pathological hypothesis for sclerosis. J Gerontol 19:135, 1964

44. McMillan JB, Lev M: The aging heart, II. The valves. J Gerontol 19:1, 1964

45. Sell S, Scully RE: Aging changes in the aortic and mitral valves. Histologic and histochemical studies, with observations on the pathogenesis of calcific aortic stenosis and calcification of the mitral annulus. Am J Pathol 46:345, 1965

46. Pomerance A: Ageing changes in human heart valves. Br Heart J 29:222, 1967

47. Waller BF, Bloch T, Barker BG, et al: The old-age heart: Aging changes of the normal elderly heart and cardiovascular disease in 12 necropsy patients aged 90 to 101 years. Cardiol Clin 2:753, 1984

48. Kitzman DW, Edwards WD: Age-related changes in the anatomy of the normal human heart. J Gerontol 45:M33, 1990

49. Sahasakul Y, Edwards WD, Naessens JM, Tajik AJ: Age-related changes in aortic and mitral valve thickness: Implications for two-dimensional echocardiography based on an autopsy study of 200 normal human hearts. Am J Cardiol 62:424, 1988

50. Silver MA, Roberts WC: Detailed anatomy of the normally functioning aortic valve in hearts of normal and increased weight. Am J Cardiol 55:454, 1985

51. Westaby S, Karp RB, Blackstone EH, Bishop SP: Adult human valve dimensions and their surgical significance. Am J Cardiol 53:552, 1984

52. Kitzman DW, Scholz DG, Hagen PT, et al: Age related changes in normal human hearts during the first 10 decades of life. Part II (Maturity): A quantitative anatomic study of 765 specimens from subjects 20 to 99 years old. Mayo Clin Proc 63:137, 1988

53. Dare AJ, Veinot JP, Edwards WD, et al: New observations on the etiology of aortic valve disease: A surgical pathologic study of 236 cases from 1990. Hum Pathol 24:1330, 1993

54. Falk E, Ladefoged C, Christensen HE: Amyloid deposits in calcified aortic valves. Acta Pathol Microbiol Scand 89:23, 1981

55. Cooper JH: Localized dystrophic amyloidosis of heart valves. Hum Pathol 14:649, 1983

56. Goffin YA, Gruys E, Sorenson GD, Wellens F: Amyloid deposits in bioprosthetic cardiac valves after long-term implantation in man. A new localization of amyloidosis. Am J Pathol 114:431, 1984

57. Waller BF, Bloch T, Barker BG, et al: Evaluation of operatively excised cardiac valves: Etiologic determination of valvular heart disease. Cardiol Clin 4:687, 1984

58. Passik CS, Ackermann DM, Pluth JR, Edwards WD: Temporal changes in the causes of aortic stenosis: A surgical pathologic study of 646 cases. Mayo Clin Proc 62:119, 1987

59. Foot DK, Lewis RP, Pearson TA, Beller GA: Demographics and cardiology, 1950–2050. J Am Coll Cardiol 35:1067, 2000

60. David TE: Aortic valve repair for management of aortic insufficiency. Adv Card Surg 11:129, 1999

61. Olson LJ, Subramanian R, Ackermann DM, et al: Surgical pathol-

ogy of the mitral valve: A study of 712 cases spanning 21 years. Mayo Clin Proc 62:22, 1987

62. Lawrie GM: Mitral valve repair vs. replacement. Current recommendations and long-term results. Cardiol Clin 16:437, 1998

63. Espada R, Westaby S: New developments in mitral valve repair. Curr Opin Cardiol 13:80, 1998

64. Dare AJ, Harrity PJ, Tazelaar HD, et al: Evaluation of surgically excised mitral valves: Revised recommendations based on changing operative procedures in the 1990s. Hum Pathol 24:1286, 1993

65. Roberts WC, Morrow AG: Cardiac valves and the surgical pathologist. Arch Pathol 82:309, 1966

66. Katz AM: The cardiomyopathy of overload: An unnatural growth response in the hypertrophied heart. Ann Intern Med 121:363, 1994

67. Ross J, Braunwald E: Aortic stenosis. Circulation 38(suppl 5):V-61, 1968

68. Frank S, Johnson A, Ross J: Natural history of valvular aortic stenosis. Br Heart J 35:41, 1973

69. Chizner MA, Pearle DL, deLeon AC: The natural history of aortic stenosis in adults. Am Heart J 99:419, 1980

70. Schoen FJ, St John Sutton M: Contemporary issues in the pathology of valvular heart disease. Hum Pathol 18:568, 1987

71. Braunwald E: Valvular heart disease. In: Braunwald E, Zipes DP, Libby P (eds): Heart Disease: A Textbook of Cardiovascular Medicine, 6th ed. Philadelphia, WB Saunders, 2000, p 1643

72. Schoen FJ, Lawrie GM, Titus JL: Left ventricular cellular hypertrophy in pressure-and volume-overload valvular heart disease. Hum Pathol 15:860, 1984

73. Cohn JN, Ferrari R, Sharpe N: Cardiac remodeling—concepts and clinical implications: A consensus paper from an International Forum on Cardiac Remodeling. J Am Coll Cardiol 35:569, 2000

74. Grossman W, Jones D, McLaurin LP: Wall stress and patterns of hypertrophy in the human left ventricle. J Clin Invest 56:56, 1975

75. Grossman W: Cardiac hypertrophy: Useful adaptation or pathologic process. Am J Med 69:576, 1980

76. Colucci WS: Molecular and cellular mechanisms of myocardial failure. Am J Cardiol 80:15, 1997

77. Schwartz K, Mercadier J-J: Molecular and cellular biology of heart failure. Curr Opin Cardiol 11;227, 1996

78. Bristow MR: Why does the myocardium fail? Insights from basic science. Lancet 352:8, 1998

79. Hunter JJ, Chien KR: Signaling pathways for cardiac hypertrophy and failure. New Engl J Med 341:1276, 1999

80. Geer JC, Crayo CA, Little WC, et al: Subendocardial ischemic myocardial lesions associated with severe coronary atherosclerosis. Am J Pathol 98:663, 1980

81. Maron BJ, Ferrans VJ, Roberts WC: Myocardial ultrastructure in patients with chronic aortic valve disease. Am J Cardiol 35:725, 1975

82. Swan HJC: Left ventricular dysfunction in ischemic heart disease: Fundamental importance of the fibrous matrix. Cardiovasc Drugs Ther 8:305, 1994

83. Weber KT. Extracellular matrix remodeling in heart failure: A role for de novo angiotensin II generation. Circulation 96:4065, 1997

84. Anversa P, Leri A, Beltrami A, et al: Myocyte death and growth in the failing heart. Lab Invest 78:767, 1998

85. Haunstetter A, Izumo S: Apoptosis: Basic mechanisms and implications for cardiovascular disease. Circ Res 82:1111, 1998

86. Narula J, Haider N, Virmani R, et al: Apoptosis in myocytes in end-stage heart failure. N Engl J Med 335:1182, 1996

87. Olivetti G, Abb R, Quani F, et al: Apoptosis in the failing human heart. N Engl J Med 336:1131, 1997

88. Sussman MA, Lim W, Gude N, et al: Prevention of cardiac hypertrophy in mice by calcineurin inhibition. Science 281:1690, 1998

89. Molkentin JD, Lu JR, Antos CL, et al: A calcineurin-dependent transcriptional pathway for cardiac hypertrophy. Cell 93:215, 1998

90. Fatkin D, McConnell BK, Mudd JO, et al: An abnormal Ca^{2+} response in mutant sarcomere protein-mediated familial hypertrophic cardiomyopathy. J Clin Invest 106:1351, 2000

91. Silver MD: Blood flow obstruction related to tricuspid, pulmonary, and mitral valves. In: Silver Md (ed): Cardiovascular Pathology, 2nd ed. New York, Churchill Livingstone, 1991, p 933

92. Silver MD: Blood flow obstruction related to the aortic valve. In: Silver MD (ed): Cardiovascular Pathology, 2nd ed. New York, Churchill Livingstone, 1991, p 985

93. Barlow JB: Aspects of active rheumatic carditis. Aust N Z J Med 22:592, 1992

94. Veasy LG, Wiedmeier SE, Orsmond GS, et al: Resurgence of

acute rheumatic fever in the inter-mountain area of the United States. N Engl J Med 316:421, 1987

95. Hosier DM, Craenen JM, Teske DW, Wheeler JJ: Resurgence of acute rheumatic fever. Am J Dis Child 141:730, 1987

96. Bronze MS, Dale JB: The reemergence of serious group A streptococcal infections and acute rheumatic fever. Am J Med Sci 311:41, 1996

97. Guidelines for the diagnosis of rheumatic fever. Jones Criteria, 1992 update. Special Writing Group of Committee on Rheumatic Fever, Endocarditis, and Kawasaki Disease of the Council on Cardiovascular Disease in the Young of the American Heart Association. J Am Med Assoc 268:2069, 1992

98. MacCallum WG: Rheumatic lesions of the left auricle of the heart. The Johns Hopkins Hosp Bull 35:329, 1924

99. Gross L, Ehrlich JC: Studies on the myocardial Aschoff body. Am J Pathol 10:467, 1934

100. Davies JM: Molecular mimicry: Can epitope mimicry induce autoimmune disease? Immunol Cell Biol 75:113, 1997

101. Veasy LG, Hill HR: Immunologic and clinical correlations in rheumatic fever and rheumatic heart disease. Pediatr Infect Dis J 16:400, 1997

102. Kaplan MH, Meyeserian M: Immunologic cross reaction between group A streptococcal cells and human heart tissue. Lancet 1:706, 1962

103. Zabriskie JB, Freimer EH: An immunologic relationship between the group A Streptococcus and mammalian muscle. J Exp Med 124:661, 1966.

104. Cunningham MW, Antone SM, Gulizia JM, et al: Cytotoxic and viral neutralizing antibodies cross react with streptococcal M protein, enteroviruses, and human cardiac myosin. Proc Natl Acad Sci U S A 89:1320, 1992

105. Gulizia JM, Cunningham MW, McManus BM: Immunoreactivity of anti-streptococcal monoclonal antibodies to human heart valves. Evidence of multiple cross-reactive epitopes. Am J Pathol 138:285, 1991

106. Appleton RS, Victorica BE, Tamer D, Ayoub E: Specificity of persistence of antibody to the streptococcal group A carbohydrate in rheumatic valvular disease. J Lab Clin Med 105:114, 1985

107. Guilherme L, Cunha-Neto E, Coelho V, et al: Human heart-infiltrating T-cell clones from rheumatic heart disease patients recognize both streptococcal and cardiac proteins. Circulation 92:415, 1995

108. Clawson BJ: Rheumatic heart disease. An analysis of 796 cases. Am Heart J 20:454, 1940

109. Virmani R, Roberts WC: Aschoff bodies in operatively excised atrial appendages and in papillary muscles. Frequency and clinical significance. Circulation 55:559, 1977

110. Wolf PA, Abbott RD, Kannel WB: Atrial fibrillation as an independent risk factor for stroke: The Framingham Study. Stroke 22:983, 1991

111. Hauck AJ, Edwards WD, Danielson GK, et al: Mitral and aortic valve disease associated with ergotamine therapy for migraine. Arch Pathol Lab Med 114:62, 1990

112. Redfield MM, Nicholson WJ, Edwards WD, Tajik AJ: Valve disease associated with ergot alkaloid use: Echocardiographic and pathologic correlations. Ann Intern Med 117:50, 1992

113. Connolly HM, Crary JL, McGoon MD, et al: Valvular heart disease associated with fenfluramine-phentermine. N Engl J Med 337:581, 1997

114. Veinot JP, Edwards WD: Pathology of radiation-induced heart disease: A surgical and autopsy study of 27 cases. Hum Pathol 27:766, 1996

115. Alameddine AK, Schoen FJ, Yanagi H, et al: Aortic or mitral valve replacement in systemic lupus erythematosus. Am J Cardiol 70:955, 1992

116. Hojnik M, George J, Ziporen L, Shoenfeld Y: Heart valve involvement (Libman-Sacks endocarditis) in the antiphospholipid syndrome. Circulation 93:1579, 1996

117. Tan CTT, Schaff HV, Miller FA, et al: Valvular heart disease in four patients with Maroteaux-Lamy syndrome. Circulation 85:188, 1992

118. Scalapino JN, Edwards WD, Steckelberg JM, et al: Mitral stenosis associated with valvular tophi. Mayo Clin Proc 59:509, 1984

119. Horstkottke D, Hiehus R, Strauer BE: Pathomorphologic aspects,

aetiology and natural history of acquired mitral valve disease. Eur Heart J 12(suppl B): 55, 1991

120. Fukuda K, Uno K, Fujii T, et al: Mitral stenosis in pseudoxanthoma elasticum. Chest 101:1706, 1992

121. McAllister HA Jr, Fenoglio JJ Jr: Cardiac involvement in Whipple's disease. Circulation 52:152, 1975

122. Korn D, DeSanctis RW, Sell S: Massive calcification of the mitral annulus. N Engl J Med 267:900, 1962

123. Burch GE, Giles TD: The role of viruses in the production of heart disease. Am J Cardiol 29:231, 1972

124. Ruckman RN, Van Praagh R: Anatomic types of congenital mitral stenosis: Report of 49 autopsy cases with consideration of diagnosis and surgical implications. Am J Cardiol 42:592, 1978

125. Shone JD, Sellers RD, Anderson RC, et al: The developmental complex of "parachute mitral valve," supravalvular ring of left atrium, subaortic stenosis, and coarctation of aorta. Am J Cardiol 11:714, 1963

126. Tandon R, Moller JH, Edwards JE: Anomalies associated with the parachute mitral valve: A pathologic analysis of 52 cases. Can J Cardiol 2:278, 1986

127. Bolling SF, Iannettoni MD, Rosenthal A, Bove EL: Shone's anomaly: Operative results and late outcome. Ann Thorac Surg 49:887, 1990

128. Marin-Garcia J, Tandon R, Lucas RV, Edwards JE: Cor triatriatum: Study of 20 cases. Am J Cardiol 35:59, 1975

129. van Son JAM, Danielson GK, Schaff HV, et al: Cor triatriatum: Diagnosis, operative approach and late results. Mayo Clin Proc 68:854, 1993

130. Rodefeld MD, Brown JW, Heimansohn DA, et al: Cor triatriatum: Clinical presentation and surgical results in 12 patients. Ann Thorac Surg 50:562, 1990

131. John S, Bashi VV, Jairaj PS, et al: Closed mitral valvotomy: Early results and long-term follow-up of 3724 consecutive patients. Circulation 68:891, 1983

132. Cohn LH, Allred EN, Cohn LA, et al: Long-term results of open mitral valve reconstruction for mitral stenosis. Am J Cardiol 55:731, 1985

133. Glazier JJ, Turi ZG: Percutaneous balloon mitral valvuloplasty. Prog Cardiovasc Dis 40:5, 1997

134. Bruce CJ, Nishimura RA: Newer advances in the diagnosis and treatment of mitral stenosis. Curr Probl Cardiol 23:125, 1998

135. Cohen DJ, Kuntz RE, Gordon SPF, et al: Predictors of long-term outcome after percutaneous balloon mitral valvuloplasty. N Engl J Med 327:1329, 1992

136. Palacios IF, Tuzeu ME, Weyman AE, et al: Clinical follow-up of patients undergoing percutaneous mitral balloon valvotomy. Circulation 91;671, 1995

137. Dekker A, Black H, von Lichtenberg F: Mitral valve restenosis. A pathologic study. J Thorac Cardiovasc Surg 55:434, 1968

138. Logan A, Lowther CP, Turner RWD: Reoperation for mitral stenosis, Lancet 1:443, 1962

139. Keith TA, Fowler NO, Helmsworth JA, Gralnick H: The course of surgically modified mitral stenosis: Study of ninety-four patients with emphasis on the problem of restenosis. Am J Med 34:308; 1963

140. Edwards JE: Pathology of left ventricular outflow tract obstruction. Circulation 31:586, 1965

141. Roberts WC: The structure of the aortic valve in clinically isolated aortic stenosis: An autopsy study of 162 patients over 15 years of age. Circulation 42:91, 1970

142. Pomerance A: Pathogenesis of aortic stenosis and its relation to age. Br Heart J 34:569, 1972

143. Subramanian R, Olson LJ, Edwards WD: Surgical pathology of pure aortic stenosis: A study of 374 cases. Mayo Clin Proc 59:683, 1984

144. Subramanian R, Olson LJ, Edwards WD: Surgical pathology of combined aortic stenosis and insufficiency: A study of 213 cases. Mayo Clin Proc 60:247, 1985

145. Roberts WC, Perloff JK, Costantino T: Severe valvular aortic stenosis in patients over 65 years of age. Am J Cardiol 27:497, 1971

146. Otto CM, Lind BK, Kitzman DW, et al: Association of aortic-valve sclerosis with cardiovascular mortality and morbidity in the elderly. N Engl J Med 341:142, 1999

147. Groom DA, Starke WR: Cartilaginous metaplasia in calcific aortic valve disease. Am J Clin Pathol 93:809, 1990

148. Arumugam SB, Sankar NM, Chyerian KM: Osseous metaplasia with functioning marrow in a calcified aortic valve. J Card Surg 10:610, 1995

149. Fernandez Gonzalez AL, Montero JA, Martinez Monzonis A, et al: Osseous metaplasia and hematopoietic bone marrow in a calcified aortic valve. Tex Heart Inst J 24:232, 1997

150. Feldman TC, Glagov S, Carroll JD: Restenosis following successful balloon valvuloplasty: Bone formation in aortic valve leaflet. Cathet Cardiovasc Diagn 29:1, 1993

151. Walley VM, Antecol DH, Kyrollos AG, Chan KL: Congenitally bicuspid aortic valves: Study of a variant with fenestrated raphe. Can J Cardiol 10:535, 1994

152. Waller BF, Carter JB, Williams HJ Jr, et al: Bicuspid aortic valve: Comparison of congenital and acquired types. Circulation 48:1140, 1973

153. Isner JM, Chokshi SK, DeFranco A, et al: Contrasting histoarchitecture of calcified leaflets from stenotic bicuspid versus stenotic tricuspid aortic valves. J Am Coll Cardiol 15:1104, 1990

154. Sabet HY, Edwards WD, Tazelaar HD, Daly RC: Congenitally bicuspid aortic valves: A surgical pathology study of 542 cases (1991–1996) and a literature review of 2715 additional cases. Mayo Clin Proc 74:14, 1999

155. Roberts WC: The congenitally bicuspid aortic valve: A study of 85 autopsy cases. Am J Cardiol 26:72, 1970

156. Larson EW, Edwards WD: Risk factors for aortic dissection: A necropsy study of 161 cases. Am J Cardiol 53:849, 1984.

157. Roberts CS, Roberts WC: Dissection of the aorta associated with congenital malformation of the aortic valve. J Am Coll Cardiol 17:712, 1991

158. de Sa M, Moshkovitz Y, Butany J, David TE: Histologic abnormalities of the ascending aorta and pulmonary trunk in patients with bicuspid aortic valve disease: Clinical relevance to the Ross procedure. J Thorac Cardiovasc Surg 118:588, 1999

159. Thubrikar MJ, Aouad J, Nolan SP: Patterns of calcific deposits in operatively excised stenotic or purely regurgitant aortic valves and their relation to mechanical stress. Am J Cardiol 58:304, 1986

160. Strickberger SA, Schulman SP, Hutchins GM: Association of Paget's disease of bone with calcific aortic valve disease. Am J Med 82:953, 1987

161. Maher ER, Pazianas M, Curtis JR: Calcific aortic stenosis: A complication of chronic uraemia. Nephron 47:119, 1987

162. Hoagland PM, Cook F, Flatley M, et al: Case-control analysis of risk factors for presence of aortic stenosis in adults (age 50 years or older). Am J Cardiol 55:744, 1985

163. Wierzbicki A, Shetty C: Aortic stenosis: An atherosclerotic disease? J Heart Valve Dis 8:416, 1999

164. Mehrabian M, Demer LL, Lusis AJ: Differential accumulation of intimal monocytemacrophages relative to lipoproteins and lipofuscin corresponds to hemodynamic forces in cardiac valves in mice. Arterioscler Thromb 11:947, 1991

165. Peterson C, Goldman JE: Alterations in calcium content and biochemical processes in cultured skin fibroblasts from aged and Alzheimer donors. Proc Natl Acad Sci U S A 83:2758, 1986

166. Schoen FJ, Tsao JW, Levy RJ: Calcification of bovine pericardium used in cardiac valve bioprostheses: Implications for the mechanisms of bioprosthetic tissue mineralization. Am J Pathol 123:134, 1986

167. Anderson HC: Mechanisms of pathologic calcification. Rheum Dis Clin North Am 14:303, 1988

168. Schoen FJ, Harasaki H, Kim KM, et al: Biomaterial-associated calcification: Pathology, mechanisms, and strategies for prevention. J Biomed Mater Res 22(A1 suppl):11, 1988

169. Kim KM: Apoptosis and calcification. Scanning Microsc 9:1137, 1995

170. Giachelli CM, Steitz S, Jono S: Potential roles of bone matrix proteins in vascular calcification. Clinical Calcium 9:208, 1999

171. Demer L, Yin T: Osteopontin: Between a rock and a hard plaque. Circ Res 84:250, 1999

172. Giachelli CM, Schwartz SM, Liaw L: Molecular and cellular biology of osteopontin. Potential role in cardiovascular disease. Trends Cardiovasc Med 5:88, 1995

173. Donley GE, Fitzpatrick LA: Noncollagenous matrix proteins controlling mineralization: Possible role in pathologic calcification of vascular tissue. Trends Cardiovasc Med 8:199, 1998

174. Otto CM, Kuusito J, Reichenbach DD, et al: Characterization of the early lesion of "degenerative" valvular aortic stenosis. Histological and immunohistochemical studies. Circulation 90:844, 1994

175. Fitzpatrick LA, Severson A, Edwards WD, Ingram RT: Diffuse calcification in human coronary arteries. Association of osteopontin and atherosclerosis. J Clin Invest 94:1597, 1994

176. O'Brien KD, Kuusito J, Reichenbach DD, et al: Osteopontin is expressed in human aortic valvular lesions. Circulation 92:2163, 1995

177. Srivatsa SS, Harrity PJ, Maercklein PB, et al: Increased cellular expression of matrix proteins that regulate mineralization is associated with calcification of native human and porcine xenograft bioprosthetic heart valves. J Clin Invest 99:996, 1997

178. Demer LL: Lipid hypothesis of cardiovascular calcification. Circulation 95:297, 1997

179. Zimmerman B, Lally EV, Sharma SC, et al: Severe aortic stenosis in systemic lupus erythematosus and mucopolysaccharidosis Type II (Hunter's syndrome). Clin Cardiol 11:723, 1988

180. Lindroos M, Kupari M, Heikkila J, Tilvis R: Prevalence of aortic valve abnormalities in the elderly: An echocardiographic study of a random population sample. J Am Coll Cardiol 21:1220, 1993

181. Aronow WS, Kronzon I: Prevalence and severity of valvular aortic stenosis determined by Doppler echocardiography and its association with echocardiographic and electrocardiographic left ventricular hypertrophy and physical signs of aortic stenosis in elderly patients. Am J Cardiol 67:776, 1991

182. Cagner S, Selzer A: Patterns of progression of aortic stenosis. A longitudinal hemodynamic study. Circulation 65:709, 1982

183. Horstkotte D, Loogen F: The natural history of aortic valve stenosis. Eur Heart J 9:57, 1988

184. Otto CM, Burwash IG, Legget ME, et al: Prospective study of asymptomatic valvular aortic stenosis. Clinical, echocardiographic, and exercise predictors of outcome. Circulation 95:2262, 1997

185. Jonasson R, Jonsson B, Nolander R, et al: Rate of progression or severity of valvular aortic stenosis. Acta Med Scand 213:51, 1983

186. Beppu S, Suzuki S, Matsuda H, et al: Rapidity of progression of aortic stenosis in patients with congenital bicuspid aortic valves. Am J Cardiol 71:322, 1993

187. Kelly TA, Rothbart RM, Cooper CM, et al: Comparison of outcome of symptomatic to asymptomatic patients older than 20 years of age with valvular aortic stenosis. Am J Cardiol 61:123, 1988

188. Pellikka PA, Nishimura RA, Bailey KR, Tajik AJ: The natural history of adults with asymptomatic, hemodynamically significant aortic stenosis. J Am Coll Cardiol 15:1012, 1990

189. Kennedy KD, Nishimura RA, Holmes DRJ, Bailey KR: Natural history of moderate aortic stenosis. J Am Coll Cardiol 17:313, 1991

190. Otto CM, Lind BK, Kitzman DW, et al: Association of aortic-valve stenosis with cardiovascular mortality and morbidity in the elderly. N Engl J Med 341:142, 1999

191. Rapaport E: Natural history of aortic and mitral valve disease. Am J Cardiol 35:221, 1975

192. Ross J Jr, Braunwald E: The influence of corrective operations on the natural history of aortic stenosis. Circulation 37:61, 1968

193. Frank S, Johnson A, Ross J Jr: Natural history of valvular aortic stenosis. Br Heart J 35:41, 1973

194. Aronow WS, Ahn C, Kronson I, Nanna M: Prognosis of congestive heart failure in patients aged ≥62 years with unoperated severe valvular aortic stenosis. Am J Cardiol 72:846, 1993

195. Roberts DL, DeWeese JA, Mahoney EB, Yu PN: Long-term survival following aortic valve replacement. Am Heart J 91:311, 1976

196. Cohn LH: The long-term results of aortic valve replacement. Chest 85:387, 1984

197. Gall S, Lowe JE, Wolfe WG, Oldham HN, et al: Eficacy of the internal mammary artery in combined aortic valve replacement–coronary artery bypass grafting. Ann Thorac Surg 69:524, 2000

198. Heyde E: GI bleeding with aortic stenosis. N Engl J Med 259:196, 1958

199. Edwards WD: Surgical pathology of the aortic valve. In: Waller BF (ed): Pathology of the Heart and Great Vessels. New York, Churchill Livingstone, 1988, p 43

200. Maizza AF, Ho SY, Anderson RH: Obstruction of the left ventricular outflow tract: Anatomical obstructions and surgical implications. J Heart Valve Dis 2:66, 1993

201. Dalldorf FG, Willis PW 4th: Angled aorta ("sigmoid septum") as a cause of hypertrophic subaortic stenosis. Hum Pathol 16:457, 1985

202. Edwards WD: Cardiomyopathies. In: Virmani R, Atkinson JB, Fenoglio JJ (eds): Cardiovascular Pathology. Philadelphia, WB Saunders, 1991, p 257

203. Colucci WS, Lorell BH, Schoen FJ, et al: Hypertrophic obstructive cardiomyopathy due to Fabry's disease. N Engl J Med 307:926, 1982

204. von Son JAM, Edwards WD, Danielson GK: Pathology of coronary arteries, myocardium, and great arteries in supravalvular aortic stenosis: Report of five cases with implications for surgical treatment. J Thorac Cardiovasc Surg 108:21, 1994

205. Jones KL: Williams syndrome: An historical perspective of its evolution, natural history, and etiology. Am J Med Genet Suppl 6: 89, 1990

206. Morris CA: Genetic aspects of supravalvular aortic stenosis. Curr Opin Cardiol 13:213, 1998

207. Brickner ME, Hillis LD, Lange RA: Medical progress: Congenital heart disease in adults: First of two parts. N Engl J Med 342:256, 2000

208. Dahm M, Dohmen G, Groh E, et al: Decalcification of the aortic valve does not prevent early recalcification. J Heart Valve Dis 9: 21, 2000

209. Freeman WK, Schaff HV, Orszulak TA, Tajik AJ: Ultrasonic aortic valve decalcification: Serial Doppler echocardiographic follow-up. J Am Coll Cardiol 16:623, 1990

210. Wang A, Harrison JK, Bashore TM: Balloon aortic valvuloplasty. Prog Cardiovasc Dis 40:27, 1997

211. Kennedy KD, Hauck AJ, Edwards WD, et al: Mechanism of reduction of aortic valvular stenosis by percutaneous transluminal balloon valvuloplasty: Report of five cases and review of literature. Mayo Clin Proc 63:769, 1988

212. Safian RD, Mandell VS, Thurer RE, et al: Postmortem and intraoperative balloon valvuloplasty of cardiac aortic stenosis in elderly patients: Mechanisms of successful dilation. J Am Coll Cardiol 9: 655, 1987.

213. Beatt KJ: Balloon dilation of the aortic valve in adults: A physician's view. Br Heart J 73:207, 1990

214. Robicsek F, Harbold NB, Scotten LN, Walker DK: Balloon dilatation of the stenosed aortic valve: How does it work? Why does it fail? Am J Cardiol 65:761, 1990

215. Otto CM, Mickel MC, Kennedy JW, et al: Three-year outcome after balloon aortic valvuloplasty: Insights into prognosis of valvular aortic stenosis. Circulation 89:642, 1994

216. Isner JA and the Mansfield Scientific Aortic Valvuloplasty Registry Investigators: Acute catastrophic complications of balloon aortic valvuloplasty. J Am Coll Cardiol 17:1436, 1991

217. Holmes DR Jr, Nishimura RA, Reeder GS: In-hospital mortality after balloon aortic valvuloplasty: Frequency and associated factors. J Am Coll Cardiol 17:189, 1991

218. Hauck AJ, Freeman DP, Ackermann DM, et al: Surgical pathology of the tricuspid valve: A study of 363 cases spanning 25 years. Mayo Clin Proc 63:851, 1988

219. Kitchin A, Turner R: Diagnosis and treatment of tricuspid stenosis. Br Heart J 26:354, 1964

220. Ewy GA: Tricuspid valve disease. In: Chatterjee K, Cheitlin MD, Karliner J, et al (eds): Cardiology: An Illustrated Text Reference, Vol 2. Philadelphia, JB Lippincott 1991, p 991

221. Roberts WC, Sjoerdsma A: The cardiac disease associated with the carcinoid syndrome (carcinoid heart disease). Am J Med 36:5, 1964

222. Pellikka PA, Tajik AJ, Khandheria KK, et al: Carcinoid heart disease. Clinical and echocardiographic spectrum in 74 patients. Circulation 87:1188, 1993

223. Roberts WC: A unique heart disease associated with a unique cancer: Carcinoid heart disease. Am J Cardiol 80:251, 1997

224. Ross EM, Roberts WC: The carcinoid syndrome: Comparison of 21 necropsy subjects with carcinoid heart disease to 15 necropsy subjects without carcinoid heart disease. Am J Med 79:339, 1986

225. Himelman RB, Schiller NB: Clinical and echocardiographic spectrum in 74 patients. Circulation 87:1188, 1993

226. Lundin L, Norheim I, Landelius J, et al: Carcinoid heart disease: Relationship of circulating vasoactive substances to ultrasound-detectable cardiac abnormalities. Circulation 77:264, 1988

227. Ribiolio PA, Rigolin VH, Wilson JS, et al: Carcinoid heart disease. Correlation of high serotonin levels with valvular abnormalities detected by cardiac catheterization and echocardiography. Circulation 92:790, 1995

228. Hudson REB: Cardiovascular Pathology, Vols. 1 and 3. Baltimore, Williams & Wilkins, 1965 and 1970

229. Silver MD, Dorsey JS: Aneurysm of septum primum in adults. Arch Pathol Lab Med 102:62, 1978

230. Chakravarthy A, Edwards WD, Fleming CR: Fatal tricuspid valve obstruction due to a large infected thrombus attached to a Hickman catheter. JAMA 257:801, 1987

231. Foster-Smith K, Edwards WD, O'Murchu B, et al: Severe tricuspid stenosis: An unusual and unique case. Am Heart J 130:621, 1995

232. Loh E, Rabbani LE, Lee RT, et al: Giant right atrial LeVeen shunt pseudocyst. Am J Cardiol 63:1289, 1989

233. Edwards WD, Peterson K, Edwards JE: Acute valvulitis associated with chronic rheumatic valvulitis and active myocarditis. Circulation 57:181, 1978

234. Seymour J, Emanuel R, Patterson N: Acquired pulmonary stenosis. Br Heart J 30:776, 1968

235. Altrichter PM, Olson LJ, Edwards WD, et al: Surgical pathology of the pulmonary valve: A study of 116 cases spanning 15 years. Mayo Clin Proc 64:1352, 1989

236. Seuanez H, Maine-Garzon F, Kolski R: Cardio-cutaneous syndrome (the "LEOPARD" Syndrome). Review of the literature and a new family. Clin Genet 9:266, 1976

237. Noonan JA, Ehmke DA: Associated noncardiac malformations in children with congenital heart disease. J Pediatr 63:468, 1963

238. Roberts WC, Mason DT, Morrow AG, Braunwald E: Calcific pulmonic stenosis. Circulation 37:973, 1968

239. Chen C-R, Cheng TO, Huang T, et al: Percutaneous balloon valvuloplasty for pulmonic stenosis in adolescents and adults. N Engl J Med 335:21, 1996

240. Davies MJ: Pathology of Cardiac Valves. London, Butterworths, 1980

241. Pomerance A: Pathogenesis of aortic stenosis and its relation to age. Br Heart J 34:569, 1972

242. Buchbinder NA, Roberts WC: Left-sided valvular active infective endocarditis. A study of forty-five necropsy patients. Am J Med 53:20, 1972

Chapter 14

Valvular Heart Disease—Conditions Causing Regurgitation

Malcolm D. Silver • Meredith M. Silver

The anatomy of native heart valves is presented in Chapters 1 and 13, their histology in Chapters 2 and 13, and their biology in Chapter 13. Despite two other viewpoints that are contrary to each other and differ from that which follows,[1, 2] we continue the convention of previous chapters in describing semilunar valves as having cusps and atrioventricular valves as having leaflets.

Closure of native heart valves involves the sequential and integrated function of those anatomic structures listed in Table 14-1 (see also Chapter 13). Thus, closure of an atrioventricular valve occurs when blood flow brings the leaflets together, contraction of the annulus narrows the valve lumen, and a synchronous and effective contraction of both papillary muscles and adjacent ventricular wall produces tension on chordae tendineae to keep leaflets and their commissures closed during systole. Semilunar valve cusps are brought together by a reverse flow of blood in the proximal ascending aorta or pulmonary artery that fills the sinuses of Valsalva; blood pressure then maintains cusp apposition. Also, contraction of the annulus and subjacent ventricular myocardium helps to reduce the valve lumen.

When closed, a native valve's cusps or leaflets do not meet at the tips of their free margins. Rather, their distal parts come together, with the main zone of contact marked by ridges on their flow surfaces—the lines of closure. Each cusp has two semilunar ridges or linea alba that are placed just short of their free margin on the flow surface; these ridges meet the central nodule of Arantius (see Figs. 3-3 and 13-2), and each atrioventricular leaflet or part of a leaflet (e.g., the scallops of the posterior mitral leaflet) shows a line of closure that follows the curvature of the free margin a short distance from it (see Figs. 1-11 and 1-16). Chapter 13 provides more details about the areas of cusp leaflet contact during systole and the mechanisms of both their opening and closure. Age changes that affect both valves and lines of closure are discussed in Chapters 3 and 13.

Heart valve prostheses belong to two families. Mechanical valves have occluders constructed of plastic with metal components that govern their movements. Their closure depends on changes in blood flow and pressure that bring the occluder over the valve orifice and hold it there during systole. The occluder may be ball-shaped, with its movement restrained within a cage-like structure (Fig. 21-3A); more often, it is diskoid, and its tilting movement is controlled by projections from the luminal surface (see Figs. 21-3B and 3C). Some mechanical valves have bileaflet occluders (see Figs. 21-3D and 3F). The fixed and moving parts of many types of mechanical

prostheses are coated by a layer of black, pyrolytic carbon, which is tough and inhibits thrombosis (see Figs. 21-2B, 2C, 2D, and 2E). The moving parts of bioprosthetic valves, in contrast, are constructed of tissue, usually semilunar valves obtained from animal hearts (see Fig. 21-4). Like native valves, bioprosthetic valve cusps are brought together and maintained in apposition by changes in blood flow and pressure differentials. In most prostheses, the annulus is fixed and has no role in aiding valve closure. See Chapter 21 for more details.

The valvular dysfunction discussed in this chapter is defined as a "backward flowing of blood in the heart or between the chambers of the heart when a valve is incompetent." In discussing regurgitation of specific heart valves, the definition adds "owing to imperfect functioning (insufficiency or incompetence) of that valve."[3] This definition applies to both native and prosthetic heart valve regurgitation. Throughout the text, the terms *insufficiency* and *incompetence* are used as synonyms for regurgitation. Valvular regurgitation may be *isolated,* if it affects only one valve, or *multivalvular,* if it affects several.

MECHANISMS OF VALVULAR REGURGITATION

A native valve may leak because a congenital anomaly or acquired pathology affects its function, producing *pathologic regurgitation*; it can also reflux blood without its structures exhibiting any such lesions, which is called *functional regurgitation.* The latter affects atrioventricular valves much more often than semilunar ones, and the tricuspid more often than the mitral valve. Functional regurgitation should resolve once the factors inducing it—for example, chamber dilation caused by heart failure—are relieved. Nevertheless, surgeons often perform annuloplasty, using either sutures or a cloth-covered ring, to hasten the recovery of functionally insufficient atrioventricular valves.

On occasion, a native valve becomes incompetent because a lesion obstructs its lumen proximal or distal to the valve orifice. Such intraluminal lesions are rare compared with the much more common congenital or acquired changes that affect the valve components themselves. When lesions interfere with the function of the anatomic structures involved in valve closure, they may affect one component alone or several in concert. The final mechanisms that interfere with leaflet or cusp coaptation and promote valvular regurgitation in both native and bioprosthetic valves are listed in Table 14-2.

TABLE 14-1 • **Anatomic Structures Involved in Native Heart Valve Closure**

Atrioventricular Valves	Semilunar Valves
Distal atrial wall	Subjacent ventricular myocardium
Valve annulus	Valve annulus
Valve leaflets (including commissures)	Cusps (including commissures)
	Sinus walls
Chordae tendineae	Proximal great vessels
Papillary muscles and adjacent ventricular wall	

Components are listed from proximal to distal.

TABLE 14-3 • **Mechanisms Inducing Regurgitation of Mechanical Prosthetic Valves**

Occluder cannot close (most frequent cause) for the following reasons:
    External components impinge on lumen or cage (rare); this may involve long sutures, tags of severed chordae tendineae, or other heart components
    Tissue (e.g., bland or infected thrombus or pannus) encroaches on lumen (most frequent cause)
    Thrombus may actually encase the occluder, entrapping it in a semi-open position
Prosthesis inserted upside down (extremely rare)
Structural abnormality (either metal or plastic fatigue with subsequent fracture) allows occluder to escape from its cage (rare)

Table 14-3 presents reasons why mechanical prostheses become incompetent.

The causes of acquired regurgitation that affect individual native valves are listed in Tables 14-4 through 14-7 (see also Table 13-2). In the subsequent discussion, we deal first with conditions that induce regurgitation of any heart valve by one or several mechanisms and then those that are likely to affect a particular valve.

PATHOLOGY AND CLINICOPATHOLOGIC CORRELATIONS

The pathologic anatomy found in valvular heart disease, whether stenotic or regurgitant, is discussed in Chapter 13. The secondary anatomic changes that may be observed are listed in Table 13-5. Congenital or acquired lesions of native valves can induce pure valvular stenosis, pure valvular incompetence, or a combined dysfunction. Usually, when there is combined dysfunction, either stenosis or insufficiency predominates. Table 13-9 provides gross morphologic comparisons between a regurgitant and a stenosed heart valve.

The pathologic mechanisms listed earlier may induce acute, chronic, or acute on chronic valvular regurgitation, with a patient's symptoms and signs reflecting the rate at which regurgitation develops, the severity of the leak, the progression of the pathology causing it, and other cardiac factors. For example, mild regurgitation may cause no symptoms, whereas acute mitral or aortic regurgitation is life-threatening because the chamber into which the blood leaks usually has normal compliance, resulting in sudden and severe pulmonary congestion and edema. In general, left-sided valvular regurgitation is more serious than right-sided regurgitation because of the pressure difference.

If a patient survives the acute onset of mitral incom-

petence and severe regurgitation continues, the left atrium hypertrophies, and pulmonary arteries may develop hypertensive changes (see Chapter 7). If regurgitation develops less rapidly, the left atrium enlarges to enormous size and may compress surrounding anatomic structures; at this point, the vascular changes of pulmonary hypertension are uncommon. In these circumstances, the atrial wall adjusts by dilation and hypertrophy, with eventual replacement of hypertrophied myocardium by fibrous tissue that may contain areas of calcification. Atrial fibrillation may ensure, but it has less clinical significance than if it develops in mitral stenosis.

In explaining the progression of mitral insufficiency and why some patients who have tolerated the condition for years suddenly develop severe symptoms, Edwards and Burchall emphasized that "mitral insufficiency begets mitral insufficiency."[4] By this, they meant that with such valvular dysfunction, the inferior wall of the enlarged left atrium is displaced posteriorly and inferiorly, inducing an effective rotation of the posterior mitral annulus so that the posterior leaflet is pulled backward and inferiorly. Because this leaflet is attached through chordae to the apex of the papillary muscle, it becomes immobilized and can no longer coapt effectively with the anterior leaflet, thus aggravating regurgitation. In addition, the tensed

TABLE 14-2 • **Final Mechanisms Inducing Regurgitation of Native Valves and Bioprostheses**

Luminal Obstruction
Prevention of cusp or leaflet coaptation by:
Prolapse
Real or apparent shortening
Stiffening
Ulceration of free margin
Perforation or shredding

TABLE 14-4 • **Causes of Acquired Tricuspid Valve Regurgitation**

Heart failure
Trauma and iatrogenic causes
Conditions affecting structures involved in valve closure
  Annulus
    Marfan syndrome (also affects leaflets and chordae)
    Rheumatoid heart disease
  Leaflets/chordae
    Rheumatic carditis and valvular disease
    Infective endocarditis and its complications
    Myxomatous degeneration (also affects annulus)
    Carcinoid heart disease and endocardial disease induced by drugs
    Trauma, including surgical excision to treat infective endocarditis
    Radiation therapy
    Endomyocardial fibroelastosis
    Systemic lupus erythematosus
  Myocardium/papillary muscles
    Cardiomyopathy
    Ischemia or infarction
Extravalvular pathology
  Primary or secondary tumor mass impinging on valve
  Pulmonary hypertension

TABLE 14-5 • **Causes of Acquired Pulmonary Valve Regurgitation**

Heart failure
Trauma and iatrogenic causes
Conditions affecting structures involved in valve closure
    Annulus
        Rheumatoid heart disease
        Annular dilation associated with pulmonary hypertension
    Valve cusps
        Infective endocarditis and its complications
        Myxomatous degeneration (also affects annulus)
        Cardinoid syndrome
    Sinuses and main pulmonary trunk
        Aneurysm or dissection, whether or not associated with Marfan syndrome
Extravalvular pathology
    Primary or secondary tumor mass impinging on valve
    Pulmonary hypertension

TABLE 14-6 • **Causes of Acquired Mitral Valve Regurgitation**

Heart failure
Trauma and iatrogenic causes
Conditions affecting structures involved in valve closure
    Left atrial wall
        Dilation of left atrium
    Annulus
        Calcification
        Acute rheumatic fever
        Rheumatoid heart disease (also affects leaflets)
        Subvalvular aneurysm
    Leaflets/chordae
        Rheumatic carditis and valvular disease
        Infective endocarditis and its complications
        Mitral valve prolapse
        Ehlers-Danlos syndrome
        Carcinoid heart disease and endocardial disease induced by drugs
        Radiation therapy
        Endomyocardial fibroelastosis and hypereosinophilic syndromes
        Systemic lupus erythematosus
        Pseudoxanthoma elasticum
    Myocardium/papillary muscles
        Ischemia
        Infarction and its complications
            Acute infarction
            Chordal avulsion
            Papillary muscle rupture
            Ventricular aneurysm
            Fibrosis and papillary muscle atrophy
            Dyssynchronous electrical activity reaching papillary muscles
Extravalvular pathology
    Primary or secondary tumor mass impinging on valve
    Subaortic stenosis

chordae in this situation (and in others, such as a prolapsed mitral valve) may rub against the adjacent left ventricular endocardium and either produce a friction lesion (see Fig. 3-2) or become incorporated into the endocardium. The regurgitant blood can cause a jet lesion (see Chapter 3) on the left atrial wall, usually its inferior one.

Aortic regurgitation can be asymptomatic for years, but it gradually produces left ventricular hypertrophy. Where regurgitant blood under high pressure impinges on an endocardial surface, it may induce a localized jet lesion. These are found on the septal wall of the left ventricular outflow tract (see Fig. 1-17) or on the ventricular surface of the anterior mitral leaflet. Sometimes, by examining the direction of the pocket formed by the jet lesion, a pathologist can localize the site of valve leakage. In practice, because most patients with aortic incompetence now receive surgical treatment for their valvular disease, such jet lesions are an uncommon finding at autopsy.

Both tricuspid and pulmonary valve regurgitation may be asymptomatic for years in the absence of pulmonary hypertension, with gradual hypertrophy of the right ventricle.

If regurgitation has been long-standing, affected native valves show a fibrous thickening and rolling of their free edges, a change especially noticeable in aortic valve cusps (Figs. 14-1A and B).

As might be expected, valvular regurgitation is marked clinically by heart murmurs and may induce symptoms and signs of congestive cardiac failure. Regurgitation is well demonstrated by echocardiography and can be measured by other invasive or noninvasive cardiologic techniques.[5]

OVERVIEW OF DISEASE FREQUENCY

Pathologists at several centers have studied the pathology of heart valves excised surgically from adults to determine the causes of valvular disease and assess their frequency.[6-12] The results are interesting but biased, in that they reflect the situation at a particular institution in a particular city and country during a particular period,

even though some studies have included groups of valves collected over a protracted period. Furthermore, they are a product of differing definitions of cause, dissimilar methods of pathologic diagnosis, and changing modes of clinical practice. Therefore, one study cannot be compared with another, nor can the results be applied to the

TABLE 14-7 • **Causes of Acquired Aortic Valve Regurgitation**

Heart failure
Trauma and iatrogenic causes
Lesions affecting structures involved in valve closure
    Annulus/sinuses and ascending aorta
        Aortitis and aortopathies
        Conditions causing annuloaortic ectasia
            Hypertension
            Aneurysm of the sinus of Valsalva
            Rheumatoid heart disease (also affects cusps)
            Dissecting aneurysm
            Marfan syndrome
            Ankylosing spondylitis
            Ehlers-Danlos syndrome
            Pseudoxanthoma elasticum
    Cusps
        Rheumatic valvular disease
        Infective endocarditis and its complications
        Myxomatous degeneration (also affects annulus)
        Whipple disease
Extravalvular pathology
    Primary or secondary tumor mass impinging on valve
    Cusp damage/prolapse associated with congenital anomalies, such as discrete subaortic stenosis or ventricular septal defect

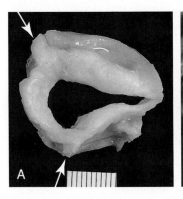
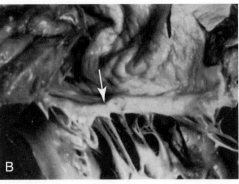

Figure 14-1 • *A*, Congenitally unicuspid aortic valve with raphes marked by arrows. This valve was mildly stenosed and severely regurgitant. Note the cusp's thickened free margin rolled toward the ventricular aspect. *B*, Mitral valve affected by rheumatic heart disease producing valvular regurgitation. Arrow defines posteromedial commissural area. Note the shortened, thickened posterior leaflet, showing a rolled edge and cleft fusion (right of arrow). In this instance, chordal changes are not marked. (Note that the scale in *A*, and in subsequent figures, is metric.)

general population. The trends that emerge from these investigations seem to be intuitive, and what one might expect in the face of an aging population, an expansion of indications for valvular surgery and changes in the prevalence of rheumatic valvular disease. Because of these reservations, no statistics on valvular disease frequency from those investigations are cited in this chapter. Rather, general statements about the frequency of valvular disease are provided.

RHEUMATIC VALVULAR DISEASE

The pathogenesis and pathology of acute rheumatic fever are discussed in Chapter 13, with an emphasis on its cardiac complication: rheumatic valvular disease causing stenosis. Here we confine the discussion to rheumatic valvular disease that induces regurgitation. It should be noted that functional regurgitation, especially of the mitral valve, is common during acute attacks of rheumatic fever and that functional tricuspid regurgitation often occurs as a result of mitral, or combined mitral and aortic, rheumatic valvular disease.

Pathologic regurgitation may be the sole result of rheumatic valvular disease. It can affect any valve, although the mitral, aortic, and tricuspid valves (in that

order) are involved more often than the pulmonary valve. However, pulmonary valve incompetence is not uncommon when rheumatic disease occurs in the tropics or at high altitudes. Isolated or multivalvular incompetence can be a direct result of leaflet or cusp shortening caused by scarring when acute rheumatic lesions heal. This change is best appreciated on the posterior mitral valve leaflet, where it is usually associated with obliteration of clefts due to fusion of leaflet scallops on their adjacent sides (see Fig. 14-1*B*) or in aortic valve cusps. Cusps or leaflets are shortened and thickened and, as indicated earlier, if the incompetence is of long standing, the cusps have thickened free margins rolled in the direction of regurgitant blood flow (see Fig. 14-1*B*). However, rheumatic valvular regurgitation is more often associated with rheumatic valve stenosis caused by fusion of adjacent sides of cusps or leaflets at one or more commissures, often producing a diaphragm-like valve with a fixed orifice that is both stenosed and incompetent. If this process takes years to evolve, the markedly fibrosed and thickened aortic cusps or mitral leaflets and their fused commissural areas usually develop secondary calcification and, rarely, bony metaplasia. Ulcerated calcium nodules may induce peripheral calcium emboli or tiny thrombi and some hemolysis. When they are very large, the nodules may directly ulcerate adjacent cusps or leaflets. In these circumstances, the resultant perforation has a jagged edge that may be rimmed by a ridge of thrombus. Usually, in autopsy cases, the cause of the perforation is obvious. However, that differentiation may not be so simple in surgical pathology specimens. It is best to regard the rimming thrombus as infected until proved otherwise.

In countries where socioeconomic circumstances are poor, repeated attacks of rheumatic fever may induce severe valvular disease in a relatively short period. Then, leaflets or cusps are sclerosed, and commissures are fused by fibrous tissue; neither is calcified. In the mitral valve, a fixed valve orifice is often the result of fusion in only one commissure. Alternatively, chordal shortening can be so marked that it tethers thickened leaflets to the apices of the left ventricular papillary muscles, prohibiting leaflet coaptation during systole (Fig. 14-2). The aortic valve may also develop an acquired bicuspidization, but, more often, all commissures are fused, resulting in a narrowed and incompetent triangular valve orifice. Nevertheless, even if all three aortic valve commissures are fused, one or more may show more severe change (Fig. 14-3*A* and *B*).

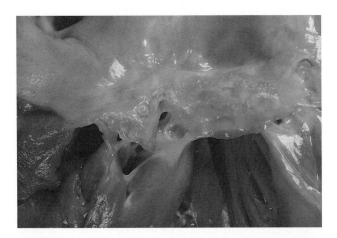

Figure 14-2 • Mitral valve affected by rheumatic valvular disease. Note shortening of leaflets and chordae, with the latter tethering the former to the apices of the papillary muscle, causing leaflet fixation. Clinically, the patient had mild mitral stenosis and severe regurgitation.

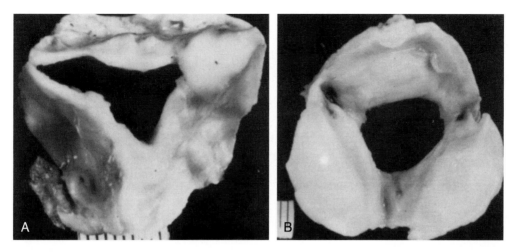

Figure 14-3 • Aortic (*A*) and ventricular (*B*) aspects of two different surgically excised aortic valves affected by rheumatic valvular disease. *A,* Two commissures are fused, with that to the right showing a nodule of calcification. *B,* Fusion at all three commissures has produced a fixed, triangular orifice. Clinically, both patients had both valvular stenosis and regurgitation.

Tricuspid valves that are both stenosed and incompetent have fibrosed and thickened leaflets, usually with no secondary calcification and little obvious shortening or fusion of the related chordae tendineae (Fig. 14-4).

NONBACTERIAL THROMBOTIC ENDOCARDITIS

Nonbacterial thrombotic endocarditis (NBTE) rarely causes valvular dysfunction. The condition is discussed here, before infective endocarditis, because the two may be confused on gross examination. Whether they are related, with lesions of NBTE subsequently becoming infected, is debatable.[13]

In NBTE, thrombotic vegetations that do not contain microorganisms develop on heart valves that usually have no underlying pathology.[13, 14] Present in 1 to 2 of patients at autopsy, the vegetations are usually larger (3 to 4 mm diameter) than those of 1 to 2 mm that are found in patients with acute rheumatic fever (see Chapter 13). They are most frequently attached to the flow surfaces along

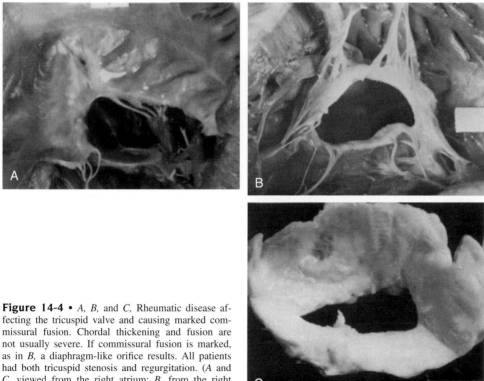

Figure 14-4 • *A, B,* and *C,* Rheumatic disease affecting the tricuspid valve and causing marked commissural fusion. Chordal thickening and fusion are not usually severe. If commissural fusion is marked, as in *B,* a diaphragm-like orifice results. All patients had both tricuspid stenosis and regurgitation. (*A* and *C,* viewed from the right atrium; *B,* from the right ventricle. *C* is a surgically excised valve.)

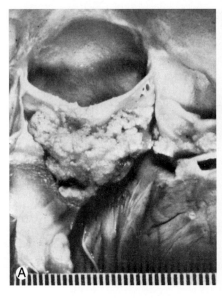
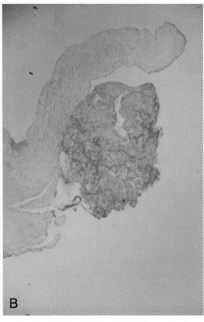

Figure 14-5 • Gross (*A*) and histologic (*B*) appearance of nonbacterial thrombotic endocarditis on an aortic valve cusp from a 68-year-old woman with metastatic adenocarcinoma of the pancreas (*B*, H&E stain). She had cerebral symptoms thought to be caused by emboli 7 days before she died. (Courtesy of M. M. Silver, MD.)

the lines of closure and often to the nodule of Arantius of an aortic cusp. They are smooth-surfaced and firmly attached (Fig. 14-5*A*), or they may become bulky, nodular, and friable, producing emboli. They can spread over the surface of adjacent cusps or leaflets, producing "kissing" lesions. The mitral valve is most often affected singly, followed in frequency by the aortic and tricuspid valves, but multiple valve involvement is not infrequent. When NBTE is associated with indwelling catheters, right-sided lesions are more common (see Chapter 18). NBTE may occur at any age, but it most often affects patients in their fourth through eighth decades. It afflicts the sexes equally.

Histologically, early vegetations consist of platelets admixed with fibrin and red blood cells (Fig. 14-5*B*). The adjacent valve is usually normal but can contain a little fibrin and, rarely, a few polymorphonuclear leukocytes. Subsequently, vegetations lyse or, in healing, organize and become endothelialized; vegetations may also calcify. The healing of NBTE lesions may produce Lambl's excrescence (see Chapters 3 and 19). If, as a result of abnormal blood flow or other factors, the deposition or healing process becomes repetitive, this, over time, thickens heart valves, stenoses a previously damaged valve, or restenoses one that had undergone commissurotomy or surgical repair.[15] The organization of mitral valve NBTE lesions in patients who have systemic lupus erythematosus (SLE) and are treated with steroids may tether leaflets or chordae to the adjacent mural endocardium, thereby inducing mitral incompetence (see Chapter 16). A similar mechanism causes chordae to adhere to endocardial friction lesions (see Fig. 3-2).

Approximately 50% of NBTE cases occur in patients who are in a hypercoagulable state or who have disseminated intravascular coagulation, suggesting a causal relationship. The lesions are not infrequent in those with terminal malignant disease, especially mucin-producing adenocarcinoma of the lung, pancreas, or colon, or lymphomas. In a group of cancer patients with NBTE and peripheral embolism, the plasma D-dimer level was significantly increased.[16] Rarely, valvular NBTE lesions in patients with malignant disease contain tumor cells. NBTE also occurs in those with acquired immunodeficiency syndrome (AIDS) and other clinical conditions.[17]

Many examples of NBTE found incidentally at autopsy likely developed during the terminal part of the patient's life. However, such vegetations may arise before death and give origin to bland thromboemboli that produce symptoms or kill.[13, 18] Cerebral complications of NBTE are discussed in Chapter 15. The systemic effects of emboli from NTBE can be the presenting manifestations of a malignancy. Whether NBTE vegetations are a likely site of infection is uncertain, but that seems possible in light of animal experiments (see later discussion).

The verrucae of acute rheumatic fever (see Chapter 13) and of Libman-Sacks endocarditis in SLE (see Fig. 16-17 and Chapter 16) are examples of NBTE, although they rarely give rise to emboli. Except in these circumstances, a pathologist finding NBTE lesions at autopsy should assume that they are infected until proved otherwise by both culture and histologic examination.

Although its exact pathogenesis is uncertain, NBTE may have several causes. For example, it can develop as a result of direct trauma associated with the insertion of intracardiac catheters (see Chapter 18), implying endothelial cell damage with superimposed thrombus formation on cusps or leaflets. Also, as discussed earlier, the condition is found in those who are in hypercoagulable states or who have certain malignancies in which the antiphospholipid syndrome (APLS) develops.[14, 16] Although there is dissenting opinion, APLS, whether primary or secondary, has been linked to valvular heart disease in SLE (see also Chapter 16).[19, 20] Indeed, some authors have found an association between APLS and other forms of valvular heart disease.[21] They believe that NBTE lesions are organized to cause valve thickening. Damaged valves in SLE contain deposits of immunoglobulins, including anticardiolipin antibody and complement components.[22] Furthermore, the demonstration that a subset of antiphospholipid antibodies reacts with the complex of phospholipid and the serum protein B2 glycoprotein 1, which inhibits factor XII and platelet activation as well as prothrombinase activity, provides a potent way by which antiphospholipid antibodies could promote a prothrombotic diathesis.[23] A link between valvular "injury" and related thrombosis in APLS comes from the investigations of Afek and colleagues.[24] They recorded a prominent deposition of immunoglobulins in the valves of patients with APLS and observed endothelial activation marked by expression of $\alpha_3 \beta_1$ integrin. Pierangeli and colleagues also observed that antiphospholipid antibodies from patients with APLS activate endothelial cells both in vitro and in vivo.[25]

INFECTIVE ENDOCARDITIS

This infection is caused by microorganisms that become incorporated into, and proliferate in, thrombotic vegetations attached to the endocardium. It usually involves a heart valve—one that often, though not invariably, has a congenital anomaly or acquired pathology. There the microorganisms induce an inflammatory reaction in both the vegetation and the adjacent valve.

Infective endocarditis can occur at any age but is rare in infancy. In general, males are more often affected than females. Usually the disease involves left-sided heart valves, with mitral valve endocarditis being more common than aortic valve disease. If a patient's valves were previously damaged by rheumatic disease, the mitral, aortic, tricuspid, and pulmonary valves are affected (in order of decreasing frequency). In these circumstances, single valve infections are more frequent that those affecting two or more valves. Nevertheless, an infection involving both mitral and aortic valves is not uncommon. Right-sided heart valve infections are overwhelmingly associated with intravenous drug abuse. Ramadan and colleagues reported a case of isolated pulmonary valve endocarditis affecting the normal heart of an individual who was not a drug addict. The authors reviewed the literature associated with this rare condition.[25a]

In countries where rheumatic heart disease is now uncommon and where congenital cardiac anomalies are treated surgically, the disease is less frequently observed than in the past. In these circumstances, perhaps one third of infections develop on valves that most pathologists would regard as normal, with aortic valves becoming infected more often than mitral valves. Patients whose normal native valves become infected may have other predisposing factors, such as intravenous drug abuse, chronic alcoholism, or chronic dialysis. Davies questioned

whether such valves were actually normal before becoming infected.[26] In these countries, the disease is mainly one of older adults with degenerative valvular disease. Furthermore, nosocomial infections are often a problem. Tricuspid endocarditis may occur in neonates subjected to intravenous right heart catheterization. In them, it often involves a structurally normal heart. Neonatal, infantile, and childhood endocarditis also occurs in individuals with congenital cardiac anomalies or in those who have had corrective or palliative cardiac surgery. Young adults who are intravenous drug addicts develop infections of both right- and left-sided heart valves, although some developing only right-sided infections. In the latter case, the tricuspid valve is infected more often than the pulmonary valve. In countries where rheumatic heart disease is still prevalent, infective endocarditis remains a disease of older children and young adults.

Much less often, an infection occurs on mural endocardium, where a high-pressure blood jet impacts (mural endocarditis). This occurs, for example, in the right ventricle in association with a ventricular septal defect, or on endocardium that bears the brunt of a jet passing through a regurgitant mitral or aortic valve. We have seen septic myocarditis impinge on an endocardial surface and produce similar lesions (Fig. 14-6). Rarely, infection affects the lining of a blood vessel, for example, distal to a coarctation of the aorta or associated with a patent ductus arteriosus (infective intimitis). A thrombus located in a vascular aneurysm (see discussion in Chapter 4) or in a myocardial aneurysm may also become infected.

Infections also occur on heart valve prostheses, in conduits, or on patches used to bypass or obliterate congenital or acquired cardiac defects, or they may be related to catheters that have been inserted into the cardiovascular system for diagnosis, monitoring purposes, or treatment. Table 14-8 lists conditions that may be associated with infections of heart valves or vessel linings. Durack presents this information in a different manner, listing con-

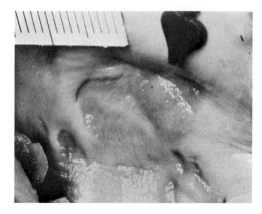

Figure 14-6 • Yellow-brown plaque of mural endocarditis (at tip of arrow), thickening the endocardium and situated on the septal wall of the left atrium in a 29-year-old woman with leukemia and disseminated candidiasis. Mural endocarditis developed by spread of infection from an intramyocardial abscess, with formation of overlying infected thrombotic vegetations.

TABLE 14-8 • **Cardiovascular Conditions Associated With Infective Endocarditis or Intimitis**

Frequently Associated	Infrequently Associated
Congenital	
Tetralogy of Fallot	Large ventricular septal defect
Ventricular septal defect	Isolated atrial septal defect
Patent ductus arteriosus	
Coarctation of aorta	
Subvalvular membranous aortic stenosis	
Anomalies of heart valves (e.g., congenitally bicuspid aortic valve, pulmonary stenosis)	
Primum-type atrial septal defect	
Arteriovenous fistula	
Hypertrophic cardiomyopathy	
Acquired	
Conditions causing valve incompetence	Mitral valve prolapse without regurgitation
Conditions causing valve stenosis	Conditions causing pure valve stenosis
Mitral valve prolapse with regurgitation	
Calcification of mitral valve annulus	
Conditions causing combined valve stenosis and incompetence	
Previous endocarditis	
Miscellaneous	
Prosthetic heart valves	Mural thrombi in aneurysm or associated with myocardial infarcts
Arteriovenous fistula	Pacemaker wires
Cardiac surgery with residual hemodynamic abnormality	Bypass vein grafts

ditions associated with infective endocarditis as having high, intermediate, or low risk.[27]

Clinical Features

The infection produces clinical effects that are essentially the result of microorganisms proliferating in the blood stream and both local and systemic complications.[28] However, a particular patient may not manifest all clinical features, nor does the mode of presentation necessarily follow any particular sequence. Traditionally, clinicians classified the disease as acute or subacute, depending on the course: rapid and fulminant, or indolent with inconspicuous symptoms. Infection with certain microorganisms— for example, coagulase-positive staphylococci, β-hemolytic streptococci, *Neisseria meningitidis,* or *Haemophilus influenzae*—is often associated with acute symptoms. In contrast, α-hemolytic streptococci or coagulase-negative staphylococci usually cause subacute infections. This differentiation may have merit in defining a clinical course, but it is not fundamental; a continuum exists between the two extremes of presentation.

Diagnosis is suspected clinically if patients have suggestive clinical symptoms, especially if they are from a group at increased risk (see Table 14-8). Furthermore, because the disease may have an indolent course, manifesting vague symptoms, clinicians must maintain a high index of suspicion. Diagnosis is confirmed if (1) microorganisms are recovered from blood cultures or are demonstrated by polymerase chain reaction (PCR) techniques; (2) serologic changes occur; or (3) microorganisms are demonstrated in vegetations, abscess tissue, or in emboli that have been examined histologically. In the future, the identification of genes specifically induced in the host during endocarditis may aid in diagnosis.[29] When microorganisms are not recovered after repeated blood sampling and prolonged culture, the disease may be inferred by (1) echocardiographic findings (transesophageal studies are best) revealing vegetations 3 to 5 mm in diameter; or (2) sinuses or fistulas induced by annular abscesses, as demonstrated by Doppler flow techniques. These considerations have led to a redefinition of major and minor diagnostic criteria.[30] Healed endocarditis may be inferred if the effects of local cardiac complications produce changes in intracardiac pressures, oxygen tensions, or echocardiographic, angiographic, or pathologic findings.

Pathogenesis

In considering the pathogenesis of this disease, explanations must be found for (1) the genesis of infected thrombotic vegetations found attached to heart valves and other sites, (2) the propensity of certain microorganisms to cause endocarditis frequently, (3) the location of vegetations on heart valves, and (4) the frequent association of endocarditis with certain congenital or acquired heart diseases. The subsequent discussion of pathogenesis is general in nature, but the reader is referred to other sources that provide greater detail.[31-40]

Current concepts regarding the pathogenesis of infective endocarditis are based on observations from human autopsies and experimental studies. Normal endocardial and endothelial cells form a relatively impermeable barrier to blood and resist invasion by microorganisms. Nevertheless, in vitro, certain microorganisms both adhere to, and are engulfed by, endothelial cells that subsequently die.[41, 42]

In vivo, endothelial loss can predispose to localized thrombus formation, or the defect may heal rapidly (see Chapter 4). Experimentally, in rabbits, sterile thrombotic vegetations (i.e., NBTE) induced on heart valves or the aortic wall become infected if a bacteremia is induced by staphylococci.[43, 44] However, human NBTE vegetations do not necessarily become infected in the presence of a bacteremia. Then, microorganisms adhere to and are engulfed by leukocytes and blood platelets, with the platelet aggregation-associated protein having an important role.[40, 45] Thus, adherence mechanisms could involve (1) a direct attachment of microorganisms to endothelial cells, (2) the infection of NBTE vegetations, (3) the precipitation on endothelial surfaces of aggregates of microorganisms, (4) endothelial invasion by infected leukocytes, or (5) infection via blood vessels in the valves. Normal heart valves contain minute blood vessels, with their number increasing and extending further toward the free margins of a pathologically thickened valve. However, it is unlikely that many cases of infective endocarditis are caused by infected material being carried into and lodging within them. Rather, the first four mechanisms listed, acting either alone or in combination, are thought to be the main mechanisms of adhesion and invasion, which in all probability are multifactorial phenomena. This would explain why infections develop on both normal and diseased heart valves.

Theoretically, any microorganism or blood-borne parasite can induce infective endocarditis. Practically, Gram-positive cocci do so with much greater frequency than other organisms. For infective endocarditis to develop, an organism must gain entry to the blood stream, circumvent host defense mechanisms, adhere to the endocardium or intima, and find there a satisfactory milieu in which to proliferate, again circumventing body defense mechanisms.

Usually, microorganisms enter the blood stream through lymphatics or by crossing a vessel wall. In fact, spontaneously occurring and transient bacteremias are a recurrent event in all human beings, but the body has efficient defense mechanisms to overcome them. Blood stream entry is enhanced during infection (e.g., an infected mural thrombus acting as the source), whereas the injection of contaminated material explains the frequency of infective endocarditis among intravenous drug addicts. Any patient with a preexisting infection, such as decubitus ulcer, burn, or peritonitis, is at risk. So, too, are those who have procedures done in which microorganisms are normally found—for example, tooth extraction, sigmoidoscopy, and urinary tract procedures. Rarely, infective endocarditis follows an invasive diagnostic or treatment modality such as cardiac catheterization, hemodialysis, or hyperalimentation. Also, alcoholism, an altered immune state, or treatment with corticosteroids or chemotherapy makes patients prone to the disease. Nevertheless, in some cases, no obvious underlying promoting factor or source of infection is apparent.

To survive in the blood stream and induce an infection, a microorganism must be able to deal with both humoral (e.g., complement) and cellular host defense mechanisms and circumvent its clearance from the blood stream as a single structure or after incorporation into an immunoglobulin complex or as a platelet-microorganism mass. Here the glycocalyx of an invading organism is important. A concept gaining favor is that blood stream

pathogens with an innate or acquired resistance to platelet microbiocidal proteins—small cationic peptides released at sites of endovascular damage to kill common blood stream pathogens—gain an advantage in survival, allowing both induction and progression of endovascular infections.[32]

The exact mechanism of microorganism adherence to endothelial or intimal cells or extracellular matrix is still unknown. Adherence may be direct or involve a step-by-step process with interactions among microorganism, blood components, and endothelial cells. Chapter 4 discusses the complexity of interactions between endothelial cells and blood components. The cell membrane (e.g., adhesion molecules) of an infecting organism, its cellular products (e.g., dextran), and its ability to interact with platelets and blood products (e.g., fibronectin) either directly or indirectly by interaction with host cells are all important. The presence or absence of some of these components also determines the virulence, and thus the frequency, with which a particular microorganism induces infective endocarditis. Once encased within a thrombus on an endocardial or intimal surface, a proliferating microorganism may promote further thrombus formation, with the vegetation affording protection from body defense mechanisms by its mass. This also hinders the entry of antibiotics used in treatment.

Vegetations of infective endocarditis are most commonly found attached to native valves—on the atrial aspect of atrioventricular valves (Fig. 14-7) or on the ventricular aspect of semilunar ones. In either instance, they are related to the lines of closure on these flow surfaces. Rarely, they are located away from a line of closure, but, if so, a pathologic reason is usually obvious. For example, those on the ventricular surface of the anterior mitral leaflet and located near its base or midpoint develop when an infection spreads from the aortic valve in a regurgitant flow or to a jet lesion. Alternatively, a perforation at the base of this leaflet, which is best seen on its flow surface with surrounding infected vegetations (see Fig. 14-14A), is usually caused by an aortic annular abscess extending to or rupturing at that site. Vegetations found near the base of the posterior mitral leaflet on its flow surface occur in cases of infection associated with a calcified mitral valve annulus (Fig. 14-8).

The explanation for the usual sites of infection seems related to hemodynamic factors. Lepeschkin, in a study of autopsy cases, correlated the impact pressure on heart valves with the frequency with which individual valves showed infective endocarditis.[46] This revealed that the mitral valve was most frequently infected, followed by the aortic, tricuspid, and pulmonary valves. The argument was proposed that mechanical stress is an important factor influencing the location of infection, because the average blood pressure on the mitral valve is 116 mm Hg and on the pulmonary valve 5 mm Hg. These studies were done in 1952, when many of the infected valves were probably damaged by rheumatic valvular disease. Thus, turbulent blood flow associated with a heart valve affected by a congenital or acquired condition could also increase the likelihood of endocardial damage and thus infection, an association that is well recognized in clinical practice. Robard observed that when infected fluid is forced at

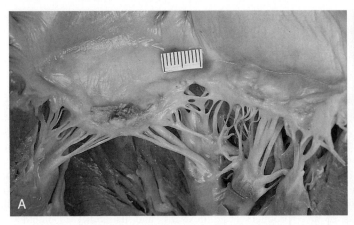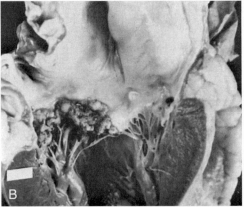

Figure 14-7 • Vegetations of infective endocarditis on mitral valves. *A,* Small lesions extending from the line of closure on the anterior leaflet; valve shows rheumatic valvular disease. Note the "kissing" lesion on the posterior leaflet (at right). *B,* Large vegetations (at left) located on adjacent sides of anterior and posterior leaflets, again presenting kissing lesions. This 63-year-old man had bilateral aortoiliac vascular grafts inserted and developed wound sepsis. (*B,* From Mambo N, Silver MD, Brunsdon DFV: Bacterial endocarditis of the mitral valve associated with annular calcification. Reprinted from Can Med Assoc J, by permission of the publishers, CMAJ, 1978; 119(4), pp 323–326. © 1978 Canadian Medical Association.)

high pressure through a constriction, microorganisms settle maximally in a collar-like arrangement in the low-pressure "sink" immediately beyond the constriction, which would explain why microorganisms settle preferentially where infected vegetations are usually found.[47] Robard thought that his observations also explained the sites of infected lesions found elsewhere in the vascular system, particularly on the downstream wall of the aorta in coarctation and on the pulmonary artery wall immediately distal to the ostium of a patent ductus arteriosus.

Microbiology

Theoretically, any microorganism may cause disease on native or prosthetic valves. Nevertheless, certain microorganisms induce infection frequently. We make no attempt to provide a comprehensive list of infecting agents, because new ones are constantly being reported. Rather, we describe the common causes of infection encountered in particular circumstances, reflecting our own experience.

Among vulnerable infants, such as those who are preterm or neonates with various indwelling lines and tubes, coagulase-negative staphylococci and *S. aureus* are the principal causes of infective endocarditis, with coliforms and *Candida* causing fewer cases. Among children, in whom the disease is uncommon, except for those with congenital cardiac abnormalities, streptococcal infections predominate, with *S. aureus* infections the next most common. Children and young adults with rheumatic valvular disease are still prone to α-hemolytic streptococcal infections, but the frequency of staphylococcal infections is rising. Intravenous drug abusers develop both right- and left-sided infective endocarditis. Their infections are most commonly caused by *S. aureus,* with enterococci, streptococci, and coliform bacteria, usually of the HACEK group (*Haemophilus parainfluenzae, Haemophilus aphrophilus, Actinobacillus actinomycetemcomitans, Cardiobacterium hominis, Eikenella* species, and *Kingella*

species) as less frequent pathogens. *Candida* endocarditis and polymicrobial infections also occur. These patients often have infections caused by unusual agents. Among adults with degenerative heart disease, streptococci and *S. aureus* cause equal numbers of cases, with enterococcal infections and those induced by coagulase-negative staphylococci less common. Nosocomial infective endocarditis is mainly the result of *S. aureus* or coagulase-negative staphylococci; enterococci, streptococci, and *Candida* cause fewer of cases.

Gram-negative organisms, particularly *Salmonella* species, may infect mural thrombi found in aortic or cardiac aneurysms.

Pathology

The vegetations of infective endocarditis on native valves vary in size, with fungal infections often causing large ones (Fig. 14-7).[48-50] Transesophageal echocardiography demonstrates lesions 3 to 5 mm in diameter and has a sensitivity of approximately 60% but lacks specificity; vegetations are not usually visualized during the first 2 weeks of an infection and often retain the same size during therapy and for many months thereafter.[51, 52] It seems that vegetations larger than 1 cm in diameter have the greatest risk of embolization, especially if they are located on the mitral valve. Small vegetations or those remaining after embolization of their superficial parts are often overlooked by pathologists because they produce a local irregularity or thickening along the line of closure Vegetations may be gray-pink, soft, and friable or gray, yellow-brown, and quite firm. They can have a smooth surface, but more often it is irregular or bosselated and granular. The underlying valve may show a preexisting congenital anomaly or acquired pathology or have a normal appearance.

Histologically, recent vegetations consist of platelet and fibrin thrombi containing polymorphonuclear leukocytes (PMNs) and lesser numbers of other white blood

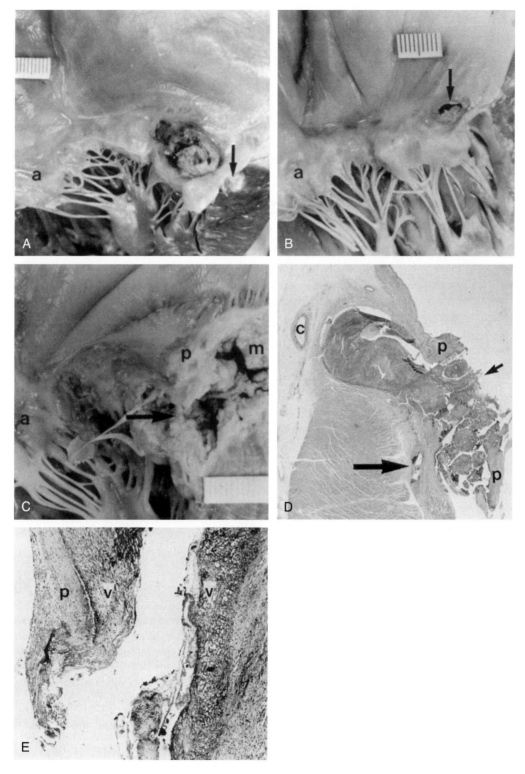

Figure 14-8 • Infective endocarditis associated with calcification of the mitral valve annulus. *A,* Infected vegetations at base of posterior mitral leaflet (characteristic location) related to calcium deposit in the annulus (arrow). *B,* Vegetations at base of leaflet with perforation, a common associated finding. *C,* Large infected annular calcium mass (m) extends into adjacent base of left ventricle. Note that the posterior leaflet was stretched over the calcium mass and tethered to it, causing valve incompetence. Overlying infected endocardial vegetation is not present in this section, but breakdown of the underlying tissue is caused by pus, with ulceration of the abscess into ventricular cavity (arrow). Such events give rise to systemic emboli of calcium and other debris. In these cases, infection is usually due to staphylococci. *D,* Annular abscess extending into epicardial fat adjacent to circumflex coronary artery (c) from infection associated with annular calcification. The posterior mitral leaflet is perforated (small arrow). This section shows only a little of the calcification in the annular region (large arrow). *E,* Infected vegetation (v) on both ventricular aspects of the posterior mitral leaflet and adjacent mural endocardium of the left ventricle (*D* and *E,* H&E stain). a, anterior leaflet; p, posterior leaflet. (From Mambo N, Silver MD, Brunsdon DFV: Bacterial endocarditis of the mitral valve associated with annular calcification. Can Med Assoc J 119:323, 1978.)

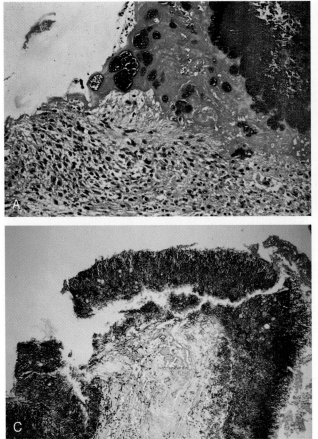

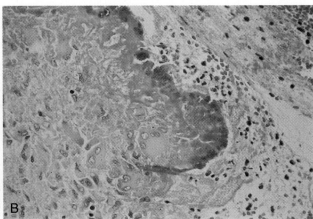

Figure 14-9 • Histology of vegetations in infective endocarditis. *A,* Indolent infection caused by *Streptococcus viridans,* showing clumps of coccal organisms in the thrombus to the upper right. Note the chronic inflammatory reaction in the adjacent mitral valve. *B,* Giant cell reaction in vegetation associated with an enterococcal infection (*A* and *B,* H&E stain). *C, Candida albicans* infective endocarditis (Gomori methenamine silver stain).

cells. Later the thrombus may hyalinize; in this case, PMNs are more numerous at the vegetation's edges and in surrounding valve tissue. Chronic inflammatory cells or giant cells also occur (Fig. 14-9). Giant cells are a feature of vegetations in patients with endocarditis caused by *Coxiella burnetti* and certain fungi. Bacterial colonies or fungal hyphae may be found at the edge and within the vegetation but are not always demonstrable by special stains, particularly if a patient has received antibiotic therapy. In an indolent infection, vegetations often show a varying degree of organization or calcification. Changes found in adjacent cusp or leaflet tissue are determined by preexisting lesions and are affected by the duration of infection, the virulence of the infecting microorganism, and the resulting complications. In an acute infection, local tissue may become necrotic, there is an acute inflammatory reaction with edema and a PMN infiltrate. Alternatively, in a long-standing infection, evidence of both inflammation (acute, subacute, chronic, or rarely, granulomatous) and repair may be observed.

A pathologist finding thrombotic vegetations attached to a heart valve in surgical pathology or at autopsy is never certain whether the vegetations are infected. They should be regarded as infected until proved otherwise by microbiologic and histologic examination. Such vegetations must always be sampled for microbiologic culture. Swabbing them may yield a causative organism, but definitive results are more likely if a portion of the vegetation is forwarded for culture. Part of the vegetation must

be removed and smeared on a glass slide for special stains or sent as a block for histologic examination. We prefer the latter action and employ both Gram and Gomori methenamine silver (GMS) stains. The combination is useful because a GMS stain not only defines fungal spores and hyphae but also may reveal coccal organisms that do not react to Gram stain as a result of alterations in their surface coating or because they are dead. The Macchiavello stain may be indicated if infections by organisms such as rickettsiae is suspected. The presence of many giant cells in an inflammatory exudate should raise suspicion that the causative microorganism is an unusual one. Electron microscopy may reveal microorganisms, particularly if the infection is caused by those with a deficient cell wall that is not revealed by Gram stain. With time, a thrombotic vegetation of infective endocarditis may calcify, as may dead microorganisms. Care must be taken to distinguish between the irregularly sized granules of calcium and smaller, regularly sized, calcified cocci. If a vegetation recovered surgically is not immediately placed in formaldehyde solution, its surface may become contaminated. In that instance, microorganisms are found only on its surface and are not associated with an acute inflammatory reaction in the vegetation. Even in the absence of demonstrable microorganisms, a presumptive diagnosis of healed endocarditis is possible if gross or microscopic examination reveals complications of the disease (Fig. 14-10). Furthermore, pathologists must maintain a high index of suspicion in dealing with pe-

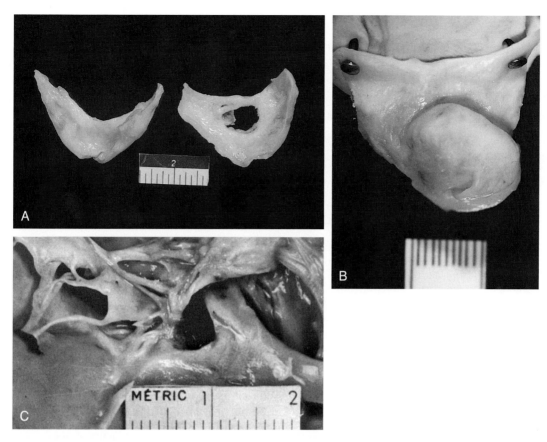

Figure 14-10 • *A* and *B*, Surgically excised aortic valve cusps showing lesions that allow a presumptive diagnosis of healed infective endocarditis. *A*, Congenitally bicuspid valve with one cusp showing a perforation. Note its smooth, rounded edges. *B*, Aneurysm on one cusp (pinned to a board) from an aortic valve that had three. No active inflammation or microorganisms related to the lesions could be demonstrated histologically; there was only evidence of a healed process. No other pathology could explain these findings. Both patients had vague histories until they developed heart failure. *C*, Healed fistula orifice opening into the right ventricle at autopsy in a patient with a Starr-Edwards aortic prosthesis and a past history of infective endocarditis. The lesion was presumably caused by an annular abscess. (*C*, Courtesy of H. S. Asseltine, MD.)

ripheral thromboemboli recovered surgically, especially if the patient has a prosthetic heart valve or if the clinical history suggests the diagnosis of infective endocarditis.

Complications

Table 14-9 lists the complications of infective endocarditis, which may be grouped into those that are local and those that are systemic.

Local Interference of Valve Function

The physical bulk of infected vegetations can temporarily or permanently affect native, or especially prosthetic, valve function and induce valvular stenosis or regurgitation with transient or persistent heart murmurs. They can also occlude a valve orifice acutely.[53]

Local Destruction

With tissue necrosis caused by infection, the edge of a cusp or leaflet may ulcerate (Fig. 14-11*A*), becoming ragged or irregular, or its body may be perforated (see Fig.

14-10*A*; Fig. 14–11*B*; see Fig. 14-20). Either lesion may induce or aggravate valvular regurgitation.

If an infection weakens valvular tissue fabric, an aneurysm may result. This usually occurs as a late complica-

---

TABLE 14-9 • **Complications of Infective Endocarditis**

Local

Interference with valve function by vegetations
Destruction of cusp/leaflet tissue with:
    Ulceration or perforation
    Aneurysm
Local spread of infection with:
    Annular abscess
    Sinus and fistula formation
    Ruptured chordae tendineae or papillary muscle

Systemic

Related to microorganisms proliferating in the blood stream
    Bacteremia and septicemia
    Changes in blood proteins
    Immune-mediated conditions (e.g., vasculitis or glomerulonephritis)
Systemic embolization of bland or infected thrombi
    Organ ischemia, infarction, or atrophy
    Infective vasculitis with or without aneurysm formation

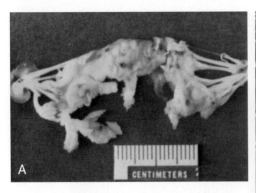

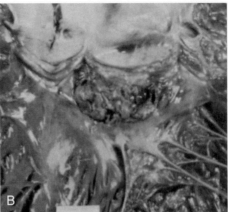

Figure 14-11 • *A,* Surgically excised anterior mitral leaflet showing ulceration of its free margin and destruction caused by a group A streptococcal endocarditis that developed on a normal valve. *B,* Acute *Staphylococcus aureus* infection of a normal aortic valve, causing cusp perforation. The specimen is from a 23-year-old man who had jabbed a skin pimple with a pin 5 days before presenting with acute, lethal aortic regurgitation.

tion (Fig. 14-12; see also Fig. 14-10*B* and Fig. 14-16). Aneurysms are not common, but those affecting mitral valves occur most frequently. Aortic and tricuspid valve aneurysms are much less common. No matter where they are located, these smooth-surfaced lesions usually cause valvular regurgitation. Lesions on aortic cusps are often 2 to 3 mm in diameter but may be larger and bulge toward the left ventricle. Mitral valve aneurysms can affect either leaflet, but more often they affect the anterior one and are located near its midpoint or base.[54, 55] They may be associated with aortic valve endocarditis. Aneurysms on all valves bulge toward the flow surface. On the anterior mitral leaflet, they often assume a "windsock" appearance, having an ostium 2 to 3 mm in diameter on the leaflet's ventricular surface, and extending conically up to several centimeters from that site on the leaflet's flow surface. Histologically, the aneurysm wall is connective tissue that may contain valve remnants, as revealed by special stains. It is unusual for the wall to show signs of acute infection or to have thrombus in its lumen. Also, the apex of an aneurysm can perforate, worsening regur-

gitation (Fig. 14–12*A*). Nowadays, these lesions are more often seen in surgical pathology than at autopsy.

Local Spread

Vegetations may extend to involve contiguous structures, producing kissing lesions on adjacent cusps or leaflets or chordae tendineae in direct contact with a vegetation (see Fig. 14-7). If an infected aortic valve was regurgitant before infection or has become so as a result of cusp or leaflet perforation or ulceration, the regurgitant blood jet carrying microorganisms may impinge on the septal wall of the left ventricle or the ventricular aspect of the anterior mitral leaflet. These sites, or any jet lesions preexisting there, may then become infected, producing satellite lesions. The latter also develop de novo or are associated with jet lesions on the left atrial wall when a mitral valve is infected.

An infection can also extend into annular tissue, producing an annular or ring abscess.[56, 57] Those associated with native heart valves are uncommon. Aortic annular

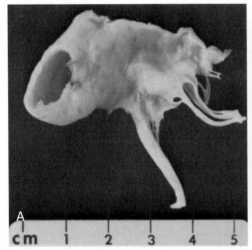

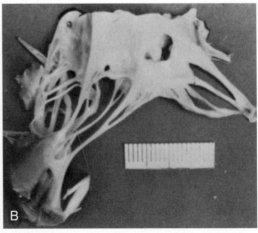

Figure 14-12 • Surgically excised mitral valves with aneurysms following infective endocarditis. *A,* "Windsock" aneurysm of the anterior leaflet excised surgically 1 month after an attack of infective endocarditis. The perforation at its apex was increased in size during excision. *B,* Ostium of a similar lesion viewed from the ventricular aspect of the anterior leaflet. (*A,* Courtesy of A. Gotleib, MD. *B,* Courtesy of N. Ranganathan, MD.)

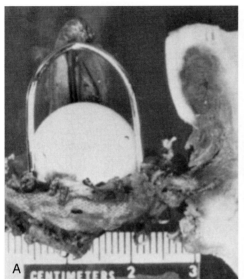

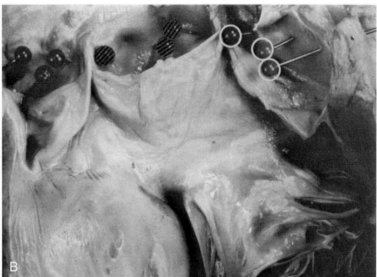

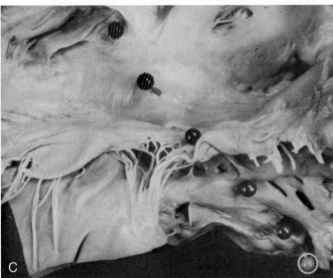

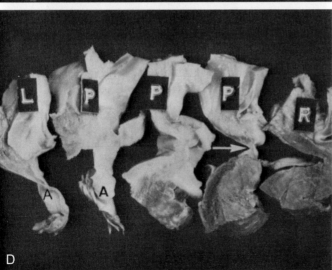

Figure 14-13 • Routes of spread of annular abscesses after infective endocarditis of the aortic valve (extending aneurysms of the sinuses of Valsalva may follow comparable lateral or distal pathways). *A, Staphylococcus aureus* annular abscess extending distally from an aortic Starr-Edwards valve into the aortic wall. This rarely occurs but can induce pericarditis, aortic rupture with hemopericardium, or aortic–left ventricular fistulas and paravalvular regurgitation. *B* and *C,* Lateral relationships of sinuses of Valsalva and the pathway of sinus tracts or fistulas produced by annular abscesses. *B* shows the outflow tract of the left ventricle. Note the close relationship between the anterior mitral leaflet and both posterior and left aortic valve cusps, which facilitates spread of infection from an incompetent aortic valve to the leaflet or adjacent ventricular septal wall. Note, too, that the membranous interventricular septum is related to the right and posterior cusps. Pins have been placed laterally through the annular region in each third of the sinus, related to the commissures and midportions, respectively, to help define the direction of ring abscess spread. *C,* Lateral spread from the left sinus of Valsalva (pins with white circles) may reach the pericardium, inducing pericarditis or cardiac tamponade after rupture or sinuses or fistulas passing to the outflow tract of the right ventricle, the infundibulum, or the pulmonary trunk (not shown). Abscesses from the posterior sinus (crosshatched pins) pass toward the right or left atria (latter not illustrated), while spread from the right sinus (black pins) extends into the right atrium or ventricle. The latter may produce an acquired ventricular septal defect, which, depending on the site of abscess tract rupture, may pass into the right atrium, right ventricle, or both chambers. *D,* Relationships of the aortic annulus and sinuses of Valsalva and structures affected by annular abscesses extending toward the heart's apex. Thus, an infection may extend into the left ventricular myocardium or the anterior mitral leaflet (A), where fistulas are found at the base or midregion of the leaflet, and rupture into the left atrium or onto the leaflet's flow or nonflow surfaces or destroy the membranous interventricular septum (white arrow) and adjacent conducting system, causing compete heart block. L, left sinus; R, right sinus; P, posterior sinus. (*B, C,* and *D,* From Silver FMD: Infectious endocarditis as seen by the pathologist in 1974. In: Russek HI [ed]: Cardiovascular Problems: Perspectives and Progress. Baltimore, University Park Press, 1976.)

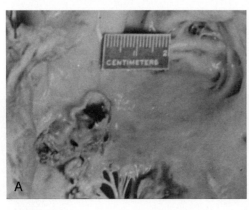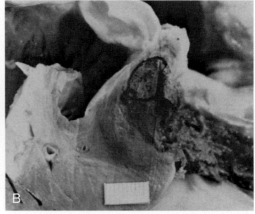

Figure 14-14 • *A,* Fistula opening at the base of the anterior mitral leaflet and into the right atrium following spread of an annular abscess caused by *Staphylococcus pyogenes* from the right sinus of Valsalva region. *B,* Annular abscess extending toward the outflow tract of the right ventricle from an enterococcal annular abscess associated with an aortic bioprosthetic valve (removed for photography). The endocardium overlying the abscess bulges and is reddened.

abscesses predominate in frequency, with the infection spreading from the cusps. The anatomic relationships of this valve must be understood to appreciate the path of extension when abscesses burrow proximally, laterally, or distally away from the annulus. In doing so, they can induce sinus tracts or fistulas that pass into the proximal aorta (Fig. 14-13*A*), into any heart chamber (Figs. 14-13 and 14-14), or into the pericardium, or that induce complete heart block. Dean and colleagues reported a case of myocardial infarction after left coronary artery compression by an aortic root abscess.[58] An extending sinus may produce a reddish nodular endocardial elevation. Also, some annular abscesses produce several sinuses or fistulas. Many annular aneurysms, even large ones, are now excised surgically, often requiring a surgical tour de force in reconstruction.[59, 60]

Annular abscesses associated with mitral valve infection are much less common. They may extend proximally in the left atrial wall or interatrial septum, distally into the left ventricle, or laterally (Fig. 14-15; see also Fig. 14-8*D*). In the last instance, they may (1) induce myocardial ischemia or infarction by compressing a coronary artery or by promoting an arteritis in the circumflex coronary vessel with associated thrombosis; (2) erode into the vessel; (3) elicit a pericarditis; or (4) on rupture, produce a hemopericardium. A healed lesion may induce a mitral subannular aneurysm.[61]

Annular abscesses complicating right heart valve endocarditis are rare.[62] Again, an understanding of the anatomic relationships of the annulus of these valves is important in tracing the pathway of any resultant sinuses or fistulas.

The sinuses or fistulous tracts produced by burrowing annular abscesses, irrespective of their origin, contain or are lined by thrombus. Microorganisms may be demonstrated but are usually not if the patient has been treated with antibiotics before excision or if the lesion has healed. Figure 14-10*C* shows such a healed fistula opening into the right ventricle.

If an infection extends onto adjacent chordae tendineae or papillary muscles, either structure can rupture (Fig. 14-

16), but these are rare events. Chordal rupture caused by infective endocarditis usually affects anterior mitral leaflet chordae. Papillary muscle rupture also occurs from direct extension of the infection or if the myocardium is infarcted after coronary artery embolism.

Systemic Complications Caused by Proliferation

Microorganisms in the blood stream cause a bacteremia or, if they multiply there, a septicemia—important

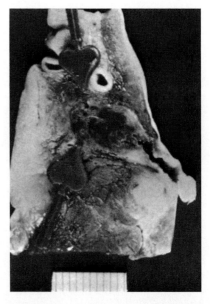

Figure 14-15 • Annular abscess of the mitral valve (defined by markers developed in association with annular calcification (white myocardial nodule to the right). The abscess had burrowed laterally toward the endocardium where it induced pericarditis. Cardiac tamponade would have resulted if this abscess had ruptured. Note the close anatomic relationship with the circumflex coronary artery. In this situation, it may be compressed or develop an arteritis with subsequent thrombosis. Either event could induce myocardial ischemia or infarction. Such an abscess can also erode the artery.

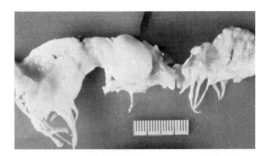

Figure 14-16 • Surgically excised mitral valve showing aneurysm (marker) on the posterior leaflet after infective endocarditis. The infection spread to the adjacent chordae and caused their rupture. Both lesions contributed to the patient's mitral regurgitation. (From Silver MD: Infectious endocarditis as seen by the pathologist in 1974. In: Russek HI [ed]: Cardiovascular Problems: Perspectives and Progress. Baltimore, University Park Press, 1976.)

determinants in establishing a clinical diagnosis by blood culture. A septicemia causes a patient's systemic symptoms[28] and sometimes may stimulate disseminated intravascular coagulation. Bacterial proliferation in the blood stream also induces specific and nonspecific antibody formation; immune-mediated disease can follow, producing, for example, small vessel vasculitis or focal (Fig. 14-17) or diffuse glomerulonephritis. Despite extensive glomerular damage in the acute phase, substantial recovery of renal function occurs.

Systemic Embolization and Sequelae

The vegetations of infective endocarditis are a source of emboli, particularly during the active phase of the disease, when they are friable.[30] Usually they are composed of bland thrombus or thrombus admixed with mi-

croorganisms; rarely, fragments of damaged heart valve tissue embolize.

Emboli from right-sided endocarditis pass into the pulmonary circulation and cause complications in the lungs. Repeated pulmonary infections or infarcts may be signs of tricuspid valve infection. Those from left-sided endocarditis pass into the systemic circulation, with the brain (see Chapter 15), heart (Fig. 14-18), spleen, and kidney being common target organs. However, if an intracardiac shunt exists or develops as a complication of the infection, paradoxical embolism is possible, or emboli from left-sided infections may pass into the lung.

The clinical effects of an embolus are related to (1) its size, (2) whether it contains microorganisms or is bland, (3) the size of the vessel occluded, (4) whether the organ has a good collateral arterial supply, and (5) whether vascular spasm is an associated factor. Many emboli in infective endocarditis are small and produce subclinical effects. Indeed, the extent of embolization found at autopsy is usually more marked than is suggested by clinical manifestations. Some emboli cause minor symptoms that are transient; others can have more severe and permanent effects; still others, especially those to the brain or heart, can kill. Recurrent embolic episodes may be the first manifestation of infective endocarditis. In such cir-

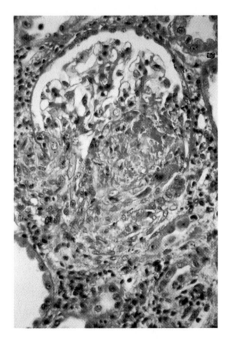

Figure 14-17 • Segmental glomerulonephritis developed in association with an indolent *Streptococcal viridans* infection on a mitral valve affected by rheumatic disease.

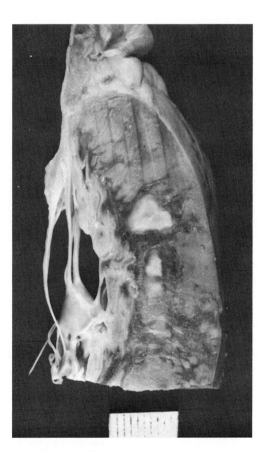

Figure 14-18 • Case illustrated in Figure 14-11*B* showing myocardial necrosis and abscesses developed as a result of emboli from *Staphylococcal aureus* endocarditis of the aortic valve. (From Silver MD: Infectious endocarditis as seen by the pathologist in 1974. In: Russek HI [ed]: Cardiovascular Problems: Perspectives and Progress. Baltimore, University Park Press, 1976.)

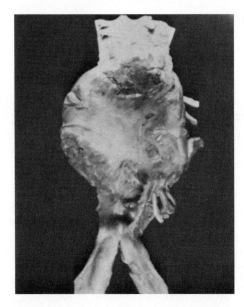

Figure 14-19 • Infectious (mycotic) aneurysm on the proximal part of the superior mesenteric artery. Its rupture 3 months after mitral valve endocarditis had been successfully treated medically but caused this 63-year-old woman's death.

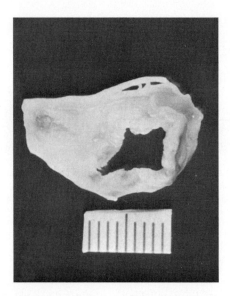

Figure 14-20 • One of three surgically excised aortic valve cups from a patient with *Staphylococcal aureus* endocarditis who developed acute valvular regurgitation. Note the infected vegetations rimming this acute perforation and its irregular outline. Compare with morphology of healed perforation shown in Figure 14-10*A*.

cumstances, surgically recovered emboli must be examined with great care, using special stains to demonstrate microorganisms. We cannot overemphasize this point, especially if a patient has a heart valve prosthesis. A surgical pathologist may be the first to diagnose the disease.

Pathologically, an embolus can cause ischemia or tissue infarction (see Fig. 14-18) or, if it occurs in a younger person, lead to organ atrophy. Infected emboli may induce a localized infection where they impact, producing a vasculitis that leads to vessel thrombosis and occlusion or an infectious (mycotic) aneurysm (Fig. 14-19, see also Fig. 5-30); if the inflammation spreads locally, an abscess may form (see Fig. 14-18). Infectious aneurysms are discussed in Chapter 5. They occur on cerebral, mesenteric, splenic, coronary, and pulmonary vessels in particular and may be multiple. Most develop at vessel bifurcations peripherally and may or may not induce symptoms. They may cause death through rupture long after the valvular infection has been cured. Infective endocarditis is the most frequent cause of infectious aneurysms.

Healed Lesions

The successful medical treatment of infective endocarditis means that pathologists now see healed lesions more frequently both in surgical pathology and at autopsy.[63] They result from the healing of the complications discussed earlier. Their presence allows a presumptive diagnosis of past disease. Here, we can draw a comparison between a healed cusp or leaflet perforation (see Fig. 14-10*A*), which generally has a smoothly rounded and thickened margin devoid of vegetations, and an acute perforation (Fig. 14-20; see also Figs. 14-11*B* and 14-14*A*), where infected, brownish vegetations usually rim its irregular and nonthickened margin.

Endocarditis Affecting Prosthetic Heart Valves

Some aspects of the disease occurring in patients with prosthetic heart valves have already been discussed. Overall, infectious endocarditis is not a common complication of prosthetic valves, each year occurring in approximately 1% of those bearing them, but it is a dreaded one. Some infections manifest soon after a valve is inserted and are the result of contamination of the valve from the heart-lung machine or from infection spreading from an adjacent site. Their frequency is diminishing. Alternatively, infective endocarditis may develop on a heart valve prosthesis at a later stage, generally 2 months or more after insertion, and is the result of microorganisms entering the blood stream in the manner described earlier for infection of native valves. This late form of endocarditis is not diminishing in frequency.

Aortic and mitral valve prostheses are affected with about equal frequency, but infections on the aortic valve produce clinical symptoms more often and are likely to be more destructive. Infections on mechanical valves usually begin in association with thrombi attached to the sewing ring or extending across the valve lumen; infections on tissue valves usually begin on their cusps.[57] The latter phenomenon could reduce the risk of spread into annular tissue. Nevertheless, annular abscesses occur more frequently with both types of prostheses than with infections of native valves.

Staphylococci are a frequent cause of perioperative infections, whereas staphylococci, streptococci, and fungal infections produce most of the late ones.

Bulky vegetations may interfere with the closure of mechanical prostheses, and tissue valves are subject to ulceration of their free margins or perforations. Other local complications may develop. Where an annular abscess develops, mild or severe perivalvular leaks can re-

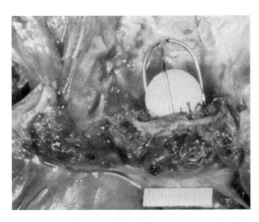

Figure 14-21 • Annular abscess associated with a *Candida* species infection on an aortic Starr-Edwards prosthesis and causing its dehiscence.

sult, because retaining sutures separate from the infected tissue, allowing partial or complete valve dehiscence (Fig. 14-21; see also Fig. 14-13A).

Again, pathologists in autopsy or surgical pathology practice must maintain a high index of suspicion when dealing with any thrombus recovered from a heart valve prosthesis, considering it infected until proved otherwise.

Prosthetic valve endocarditis is also discussed in Chapter 21 and further illustrated in Figures 21-12 and 21-13.

Endocarditis in Hypertrophic Cardiomyopathy

In a clinical study, Spirito and colleagues[64] found that in a group of 810 patients with hypertrophic cardiomyopathy, endocarditis was virtually confined to patients who had left ventricular outflow tract obstruction under basal conditions. The risk of this complication was highest among those who had both outflow tract obstruction and marked left atrial dilation. Among the 10 cases studied, mitral valve infections occurred in seven, and combined mitral and aortic valve infections in three. Microorganisms were recovered from six individuals, with staphylococci and streptococci organisms causing the infection in equal numbers.

TRICUSPID REGURGITATION

Functional Regurgitation

Tricuspid regurgitation is more often functional than pathologic and is associated with right ventricular failure. The latter is most often related to pulmonary hypertension, whether caused by left ventricular failure (common) or by pulmonary vascular or interstitial disease (uncommon). Stenosis of the outflow tract of the right ventricle rarely causes functional tricuspid insufficiency in adults; the exceptions are those with congenital stenosis of the pulmonary valve or those born with tetralogy of Fallot who have had anomalies corrected and develop this complication later in life.

Pathologic Regurgitation

Congenital Anomalies

Among congenital conditions associated with this valvular dysfunction in which survival to adulthood occurs, the Ebstein anomaly shows a displacement of fused or malformed tricuspid valvular tissue—usually the posterior and septal leaflets—into the right ventricular cavity so that the basal attachments of the leaflets are to the right ventricular wall distal to the true annulus of the valve (Fig. 14-22). However, from their studies, Schreiber and colleagues concluded that the anomaly is more than a simple "downward displacement" of the leaflets.[65] The authors suggested that, "in essence, the valvular orifice is formed within the ventricular cavity at the junction of the atrialized inlet and functional ventricular components." This anomaly is commonly associated with a patent valvular foramen ovale or fossa ovalis–type atrial septal defect, but it may occur as part of a complex congenital cardiac anomaly. The abnormal valve may be incompetent or stenosed but is often neither. The Ebstein anomaly is also discussed in Chapter 11, where the associated risk of supraventricular arrhythmias and sudden death is emphasized and the histology, found in overt cases and in those with no gross abnormality but microscopic findings, is illustrated (see Fig. 11-33).

Tricuspid valve regurgitation also occurs when a ventricular septal defect heals spontaneously, to produce an aneurysm of the ventricular septum. Closure of the defect is achieved by proliferation of connective tissue extending across it from its perimeter, by tricuspid leaflet tissue occluding the lesion, or by a combination of these processes (Fig. 14-23).

Acquired Lesions

Many of the acquired conditions inducing tricuspid regurgitation were discussed earlier in this chapter (see Table 14-4) or in preceding chapters—myocardial ischemia and infarction in Chapter 8; endomyocardial fibroelastosis and cardiomyopathy in Chapter 10; rheumatic disease and carcinoid heart disease in Chapter 13; rheumatoid heart disease, SLE, and pseudoxanthoma elas-

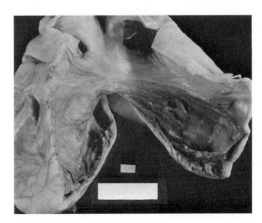

Figure 14-22 • The Ebstein anomaly of the tricuspid valve in a 27-year-old woman with a valvular patent foramen ovale. Note attachment of leaflets to the right ventricular wall (Courtesy of M. Lipa, MD.)

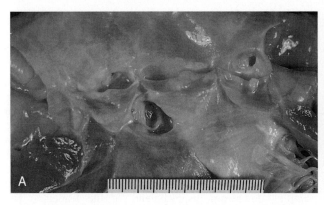
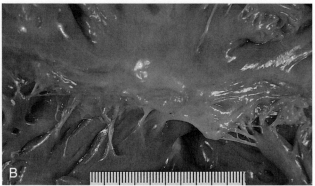

Figure 14-23 • Spontaneous closure of a ventricular septal defect. *A,* Ostium viewed from left ventricular aspect. *B,* Anterior tricuspid valve leaflet occludes right ventricular ostium and bulges aneurysmally into the ventricular chamber, causing tricuspid regurgitation.

ticum in Chapter 16; endocardial disease induced by drugs in Chapter 17; trauma, radiation therapy, and iatrogenic causes in Chapter 18; and cardiac tumors in Chapter 19. Myxomatous degeneration may be a cause of tricuspid valve regurgitation. The whole tricuspid valve may be excised to treat infective endocarditis. It is surprising, considering how often tricuspid valve leaflets and chordae tendineae become intimately adherent to pacemaker leads passing through the valve, that these attachments rarely induce tricuspid regurgitation.

PULMONARY REGURGITATION

Pulmonary regurgitation is uncommon, and its clinical effects, if isolated, may not be marked. Table 14-5 lists possible causes affecting native valves. In fact, pulmonary valve incompetence is most often functional and a result of valve annulus dilation associated with pulmonary hypertension, whatever the cause. Dilation of the pulmonary trunk induced by Marfan syndrome or aneurysm also produces this valvular dysfunction. Among pathologic causes, infective endocarditis and iatrogenic damage produced during repair of isolated pulmonary valve stenosis or tetralogy of Fallot are seen, the latter becoming more frequent as treated children become adults.

MITRAL REGURGITATION

Many conditions that cause mitral insufficiency, whether functional or pathologic, have been discussed earlier (see Table 14-6) or in other chapters—Chapter 3 (mitral annular calcification), Chapter 10 (cardiomyopathies, including the association with hypertrophic cardiomyopathy), Chapter 16 (systemic diseases), Chapter 17 (effects of drugs), and Chapter 19 (tumors and tumor-like conditions).

Congenital Anomalies

Individuals with congenital clefts or fenestrations in their mitral valves may reach adulthood. In corrected transposition of the great vessel, the tricuspid valve is the left-sided atrioventricular valve. In this circumstance, valve design or deficiency does not permit it to function normally during a patient's lifetime, and mitral insufficiency can result.

Acquired Lesions Affecting the Annular Region

Mitral, subvalvular, annular aneurysms extending from the left ventricle were once thought to be most common among blacks in sub-Saharan Africa, but they are now reported in all races and in adults and children.[66-69] The lesion rarely causes mitral incompetence thought to be caused by a defect in the posterior mitral valve annulus tissue. Similar lesions, although usually smaller, can be induced by tearing the mitral valve annulus during mitral valve replacement (Fig. 14-24), other trauma,[70] or after healing of a mitral valve annular abscess associated with infective endocarditis. Similar congenital or acquired lesions occur in the subaortic region, producing aortic incompetence.[71] At either valvular location, aneurysms may be multiple. Deshpande and colleagues reviewed 19 subvalvular aneurysms in 16 cases. Subaortic ones, in their series, were associated with infective endocarditis, and 5 cases of subvalvular mitral aneurysm were associated with aneurysm of a sinus of valsalva.[71a]

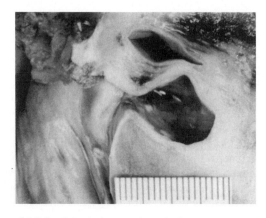

Figure 14-24 • Subvalvular, annular, mitral aneurysm resulting from annular injury induced during mitral valve replacement 4 years before patient's death.

Mitral annular calcification and its complications, including valve regurgitation, are discussed in Chapters 3 and 13.

Acquired Lesions Affecting Leaflets, Chordae, and Papillary Muscles

Mitral Valve Prolapse

The mitral valve prolapse syndrome (MVPS), which has many synonyms, is one of the more prevalent cardiac valvular abnormalities. MVPS has many pathologic causes, ranging from myxomatous degeneration of valve tissue and other mitral valve abnormalities to dysfunctional papillary muscles.

Braunwald indicates that during contraction, mitral valve leaflets normally billow slightly into the left atrium.[5] Clinicians who study valve movement by echocardiography speak of leaflets "billowing" when that movement is exaggerated or of the valve being "floppy" when billowing is extreme. Furthermore, mitral valve prolapse occurs when leaflet edges do not coapt, causing mitral regurgitation; leaflets become "flail" if chordal or papillary muscle rupture allows prolapse. Braunwald acknowledges that these conditions blend with one another clinically and are often difficult to distinguish.

Pathologists do not have the benefit of leaflet movement at autopsy or in a specimen excised surgically but they can distinguish some of these clinical findings. Nevertheless, clinicopathologic correlations are not ideal.[72] Thus, a pathologist may find the free margin of a mitral leaflet between chordal insertions bulging toward the left atrium (Fig. 14-25). We do not know whether this corresponds exactly to the clinical definition of leaflet billowing, but the change is not usually associated with symptoms, and the affected parts of the valve may or may not show myxomatous degeneration. Edwards considered this finding within the range of normal morphology; he called it "interchordal hooding" and noted that it affected both rough and clear zones of a leaflet; was less than 4 mm high and involved only one third or less of a leaflet's free margin.[73] In contrast, he diagnosed a floppy mitral valve

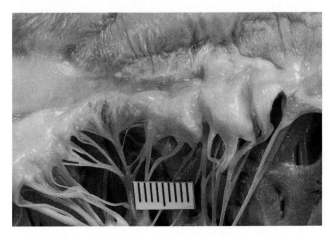

Figure 14-25 • Free margin of the middle scallop of the posterior mitral valve leaflet bulging between chordal insertions. This patient had no heart murmur or other clinical symptoms of mitral valve disease caused by this "interchordal hooding."

when such hooding was greater than 4 mm in height, it involved a leaflet's rough and clear zones, and at least half the anterior leaflet or two thirds of the posterior leaflet showed this morphology. Practically, the leaflets of a floppy mitral valve usually show the histologic changes of myxomatous degeneration, often with similar changes in valve annulus and chordae. Full-blown mitral valve prolapse and flail leaflets are not difficult to recognize pathologically. When MVPS is of long standing, leaflets are voluminous and bulge markedly toward the left atrium (see Fig. 14-27), with their free margins markedly hooded. Examination of autopsy cases leaves no doubt that the leaflets' free margins would not coapt. When prolapse is acute in origin and due to ruptured chordae or ruptured papillary muscles, the flail leaflet usually has the ruptured structure attached to it if the leaflet itself shows no other gross pathology. Conversely, if chordae rupture in MVPS, producing acute or chronic mitral insufficiency, they are usually associated with voluminous prolapsed leaflets.

Myxomatous Degeneration

Myxomatous degeneration affects up to 5% of the population and is more common in young females than males. It is the most frequent cause of mitral valve prolapse and, in most cases, is clinically benign. Its most obvious histologic finding is an excessive accumulation of glycosaminoglycan material distributed within the cusp or leaflet structure and separating other tissue components. The deposits may represent a genetic condition or be secondary to a preexisting lesion.

Pathogenesis

Certain pointers provide insight into pathogenesis. For example, myxomatous degeneration is often related to Marfan syndrome or the forme fruste of that condition, in which mutations in the gene that encodes fibrillin-1 on chromosome 15 are recorded (see Chapters 5 and 16). Myxomatous degeneration, particularly of the mitral valve, is reported in Ehlers-Danlos syndrome and in other conditions in which collagen formation is affected (see Chapter 16). What is uncertain is whether the functional mechanism of the genetic abnormalities is direct, affecting and weakening valve structures themselves, or indirect, altering muscular contraction, some other cardiac function, or the integrity of the cusp or leaflet structure, thus putting stress on the valves and inducing myxomatous change secondarily. In inherited myxomatous degeneration, the deposits are usually generalized throughout the valve structure. They may be marked and can involve the annulus of affected valves and the chordae tendineae of atrioventricular ones. Theoretically, such genetic abnormalities could be associated with myxomatous changes that affect all heart valves. In some cases this is so, but, practically, left-sided valves are most often affected—in particular, the mitral valve. We note at this point that many cases of myxomatous degeneration of the mitral valve are familial with a dominant inheritance. A genetic abnormality, mapped to Xq28, has been reported in one cohort but not yet in others.[74]

Secondary myxomatous degeneration is often focal in nature but can be generalized. It is considered a manifestation of cusp or leaflet adaptation or repair—the accu-

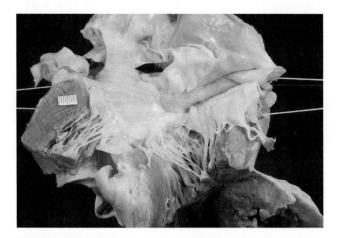

Figure 14-26 • Prolapsed posterior mitral valve as part of the Eisenmenger reaction. Marker defines a valvular patent foramen ovale.

mulation of proteoglycans being a manifestation of adaptation or repair in many parts of the cardiovascular system. This mechanism may explain myxomatous degeneration found in tricuspid or pulmonary valves associated with pulmonary hypertension, the prolapsed mitral valve

in the Eisenmenger reaction (Fig. 14-26), or those cases of mitral valve prolapse associated with an anomalous insertion of mitral valve chordae tendineae or reported as "postinflammatory" and related to acute rheumatic fever.[75-77] All these conditions place excess stress or strain on parts of a leaflet. In secondary myxomatous degeneration, only one valve is usually affected, with the mitral valve commonly involved.

Pathology

The gross and microscopic morphology of the myxomatous valve varies from case to case and from valve to valve.[72, 78]

With focal deposits, cusps or leaflets often show evidence of preexisting disease or associated anomalies. That may also apply when generalized myxomatous changes exist, but usually not. When deposits are generalized, semilunar valve cusps may be thinner than normal and semitranslucent. This makes them prone to aneurysm, spontaneous rupture, or shredding.

More often, both semilunar valves and the leaflets of atrioventricular valves are thickened (Fig. 14-27), presenting on cut section a moist, grayish, gelatinous morphology (see Fig. 14-29A). Examination may also reveal some

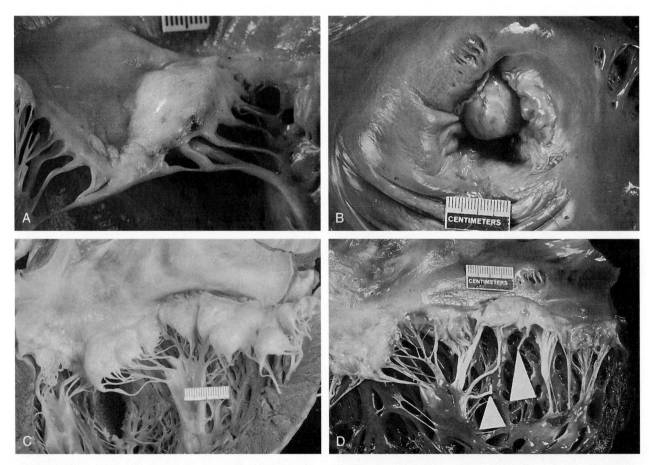

Figure 14-27 • Varying gross morphology in mitral valve prolapse syndrome (MVPS) caused by myxomatous degeneration. *A,* Prolapse of posteromedial half of the anterior leaflet. *B,* Left atrial view of partially prolapsed posterior leaflet. Note linear recent thrombus at its base. *C,* Severe prolapse affecting both leaflets. *D,* Hooded, prolapsed, flail middle scallop of posterior leaflet associated with a ruptured chorda. Its free edges are defined by markers. Note thickened chordae in *A* and *D,* without evidence of the commissural fusion which occurs in rheumatic valvular disease.

TABLE 14-10 • **Complications of Mitral Valve Myxomatous Degeneration**	
Clinical	**Pathologic**
Acute, chronic, or acute on chronic mitral regurgitation	Affecting leaflets
	Aneurysm
Stroke (controversial)	Prolapse
Sudden death	Annular calcification
	Infective endocarditis
	Endocardial thrombus
	Affecting chordae
	Thickening
	Elongation
	Rupture
	Affecting annulus
	Ectasia

of the complications listed in Table 14-10. When prolapse results, part or all of a cusp or leaflet bulges anatomically toward the associated ventricle or atrium (Figs. 14-27 and 14–28). In the latter instance, a prolapsed mitral valve may have a distinctly hooded appearance. Both prolapse and hooding are better appreciated at autopsy but may be noted in some surgical pathology specimens. Overlying endocardium on the flow surfaces is usually thickened, and tiny thrombi may be attached to leaflets or chordae. Linear thrombus may be present at the base of a prolapsed mitral leaflet in the angle between it and the adjacent left atrial wall, presumably arising in an area of relative blood stasis between the two (see Fig. 14-27B and C). If the thrombus is subsequently organized, connective tissue obliterates that angle. Chordae tendineae of atrioventricular valves are often elongated (see Fig. 14-28) and may be reduced in diameter and rupture (see Fig. 14-27D). However, chordae can also be thickened (see Fig. 14-27A and D) and not rupture. If thickened, they do not often fuse together, nor is there evidence of commissural fusion. These findings help to differentiate changes related to a myxomatous valve from those caused by rheumatic valvular disease.

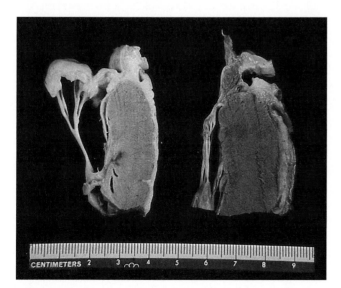

Figure 14-28 • Histologic block of prolapsed mitral valve caused by myxomatous degeneration (to left) compared with normal valve. Note elongated chordae and accentuation of prolapse between leaflet's free margin and line of closure but also affecting the leaflet elsewhere.

As emphasized in Chapter 1, the ends of chordae tendineae attached to surgically excised floppy mitral valves must be examined closely with a magnifying glass to determine whether any were ruptured. We also examine ruptured chordae found at autopsy in this manner. If chordae were recently ruptured, their ends may be expanded by a tiny thrombus. Subsequently, that thrombus may organize. Other ruptured chordae are whisker-like, or they may recurve and become reattached to the undersurface of the leaflet. We embed both ends of any definite or suspected ruptured chordae and cut the histologic block at several depths through it, using hematoxylin-eosin, an elastic-trichrome stain, and the Movat pentachrome stain at each level. This can reveal much pathology, with the findings often indicating the age of the rupture and its cause.

In diagnosing myxomatous degeneration histologically, pathologists must remember that the spongiosa of cusps and leaflets normally contains loosely arranged tissue rich in proteoglycans and that it expands in width toward the free margins of the cusps or leaflets (see Chapter 2). This normal morphology must not be mistaken for myxomatous change.

Small secondary accumulations of proteoglycans are common in the connective tissue of valve cusps or leaflets from the aged or in association with other diseases (e.g., rheumatic valvular disease). Such deposits should be noted in reports and referred to as minor and focal. If they are generalized but minor in degree, they are not likely to be associated with any of the complications listed in Table 14-10.

In cases in which myxomatous change is often associated with these complications, the key histologic findings are an excess of proteoglycans within cusp or leaflet tissue extending into the fibrosa, widening it, and particularly extending toward the base of the cusps or leaflets (Fig. 14-29). The proteoglycan deposit is associated with degeneration and loss of collagen and elastic tissue. Lester described biochemical findings in floppy valves, and Tamura and colleagues indicated the ultrastructural abnormalities of elastic fibers and other connective tissue components.[79, 80] Akhtar and associates discussed the immunolocalization of extracellular matrix components in normal and myxomatous heart valves.[81] Ancillary changes often include a fibroelastic endocardial thickening on the flow surface of a prolapsed leaflet (see Fig. 14-29B) or encasing the thickened chordae, as well as myxomatous deposits in both annulus and chordae tendineae. Tiny thrombi may be present on prolapsed leaflets or their chordae (see Fig. 14-29D). When the condition is full blown, histologic changes are very obvious, and diagnosis is not a problem. In daily use, we find the Movat pentachrome stain best in defining proteoglycans and aiding diagnosis.

Some mitral valve components that are excised surgically to treat a patient with a prolapsed valve do not show much myxomatous change or may be normal. In this case, the surgical pathologist is probably dealing with a cause of mitral regurgitation other than myxomatous degeneration and must make clinicopathologic correlations before issuing a report.

The question of whether myxomatous degeneration can heal, with the myxomatous deposits disappearing but

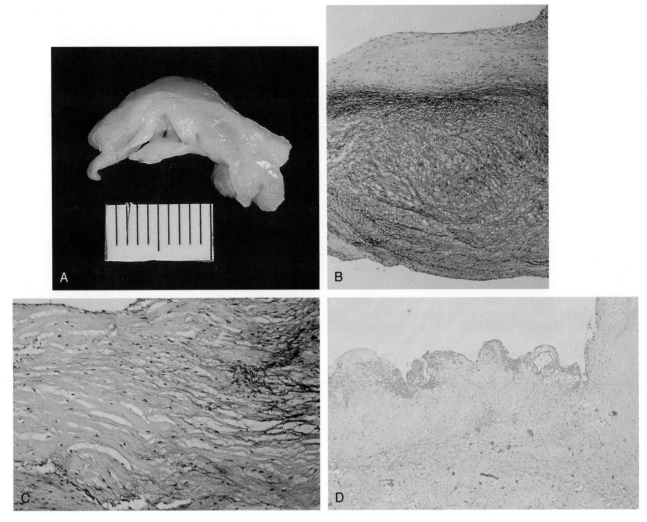

Figure 14-29 • Gross and histologic morphology of MVPS caused by myxomatous degeneration. *A,* Thickened, moist, grayish, gelatinous appearance of sectioned posterior leaflet. *B,* Endocardial thickening on flow surface. *C,* Greenish proteoglycan material extending between yellowish collagen fibers of the fibrosa. *D,* Tiny thrombi on leaflet's endocardial surface. (*B,* Elastic trichrome stain; *C,* Movat pentachrome stain; *D,* H&E stain.)

leaving thickened cusps or leaflets and chordal changes, is an intriguing one. We believe that it occurs.

Complications

Patients with mitral valve prolapse caused by myxomatous degeneration are prone to the complications listed in Table 14-10.[73] An association with sudden death is described in Chapter 11, and the occurrence of stroke in younger patients is covered in Chapter 15. The latter is controversial, because some studies do not demonstrate an association.[82, 83] As discussed earlier, individuals with this condition also have an increased risk of infective endocarditis. Annular calcification extending into the base of the prolapsed leaflet can develop in long-standing cases.

Rupture of the chordae tendineae is another complication of myxomatous degeneration either inducing mitral regurgitation or aggravating preexisting insufficiency. Akhtar and colleagues presented the ultrastructural abnormalities in proteoglycans, collagen fibrils, and elastic fibers found in the chordae of myxomatous mitral valves.[84]

Ruptured Chordae Tendineae

Chordal rupture can have many causes, including trauma, infective endocarditis, or fraying caused by calcium nodules in the mitral annulus, but these are all uncommon. In our experience, the greatest number are associated with myxomatous changes in their substance as part of a myxomatous valve. We stress that careful examination of chordal ends is essential both in establishing the possibility of rupture and in determining its cause. Pathologists must remember that the free ends of chordae may recurve and reattach to the ventricular surface of leaflets. Because we have retrieved and cut chordae for histologic section, we have concluded that there is no such thing as idiopathic chordal rupture and suspect that most cases formerly classified as such were not studied with enough attention to gross and histologic examination.

We note that ruptured chordae may be replaced surgically with cloth cords. They become encased in fibroelastic tissue, but with time, they may fray and rupture.

Ruptured Papillary Muscle

This condition is discussed in Chapter 8 (myocardial ishemia and infarction) and Chapter 18 (trauma and iatrogenic conditions). The clinical effects of a ruptured papillary muscle depend on the site of its rupture and the number of chordae released.

With avulsion of chordae tendineae after a myocardial infarction (often erroneously called ruptured chordae tendineae), careful gross examination usually reveals a tiny fleck of infarcted myocardium or fibrous tissue from the tip of the papillary muscle attached to the one or two chordae released. If the lesion is fresh, thrombus or fibrin may be attached to those tiny remnants; later, they become encased in a nubbin of connective tissue. Histologically, leaflets and chordae are normal. The resultant mitral valve prolapse and valvular regurgitation are not great. A patient may survive initial rupture and, with time, develop a leaflet that is thickened and hooded but one that like the associated thickened chordae, does not show myxomatous changes.

When the body of a papillary muscle is ruptured, chordae attached to the freed end and passing to contiguous sides of anterior and posterior mitral valve leaflets are released, with resultant severe valvular regurgitation. This is often life-threatening and kills unless the valve is soon replaced by a prosthesis. At gross examination, the freed chordae are often twisted about their long axis and have a large chunk of infarcted papillary muscle attached to them. Gross and histologic examination reveals no abnormality of leaflets or chordae.

Papillary Muscle Dysfunction

Myocardial ischemia and infarction and their sequelae are common causes of both functional and pathologic mitral regurgitation, with the condition coming on acutely (within a few days) or as a late complication (see Chapter 8). In this setting, papillary muscle dysfunction may be a result of ischemia; acute infarction; infarct scarring involving a papillary muscle and adjacent ventricular wall; papillary muscle atrophy; a dyssynchronous electrical impulse from the conducting system activating the papillary muscles; mechanical separation of the papillary muscles, as may result with an aneurysm, and worsening congestive cardiac failure.

It is of interest that Gorman and colleagues suggested that after an acute posterior left ventricular infarction induced in sheep, papillary muscle discoordination with minimal annular dilation distorted leaflet coaption sufficiently to produce severe mitral regurgitation, formerly attributed to annular dilation in the animal.[85]

AORTIC REGURGITATION

Congenital Anomalies

Acommissural, Unicommissural, and Bicuspid Aortic Valves

The frustrum shape and configuration of a congenitally acommissural or unicuspid valve favor development of stenosis (see Chapter 13). However, once a valve's orifice becomes fixed, as may be present at birth or develop after sclerosis or calcification, combined stenosis and regurgitation result (Fig. 14-30).

The commissures of a congenitally bicuspid valve may be located, anteriorly and posteriorly (one third of cases), producing medial and lateral cusps; alternatively, one is placed medially and the other laterally, with associated anterior and posterior cusps (two thirds of cases). In the former instance, one coronary artery usually arises from each sinus; in the latter, both arteries are likely to arise from the anterior sinus. Although it often becomes stenosed once it is thickened by connective tissue or calcification, the congenitally bicuspid valve is also prone to incompetence once its orifice is fixed. However, a con-

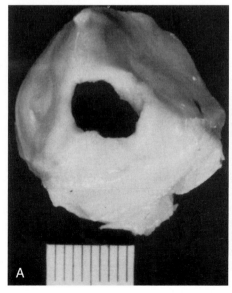
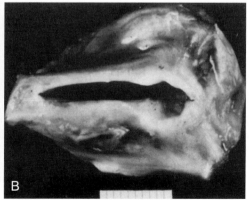

Figure 14-30 • Congenitally acommissural (*A*) and unicuspid (*B*) aortic valves that were stenosed and became incompetent once they developed fixed orifices. Note in *A* the acommissural valve's dome-shaped and rounded orifice and the raphes or ridges marking aborted commissure formation, and in *B*, the single commissure and orifice that suggest the shape of an exclamation point. Two raphes, representing aborted commissures, are seen to the right of this photograph.

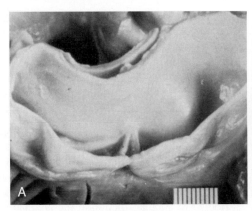
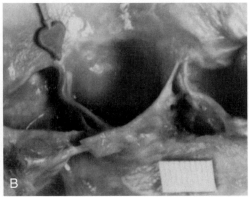

Figure 14-31 • Reduced height of a conjoined cusp of a congenitally bicuspid aortic valve with low attachment of raphe fostering aortic regurgitation. Note rolled, everted edge of cusp at site of reflow.

genitally bicuspid valve may also produce isolated aortic incompetence. As Schoen and Edwards pointed out (see Chapter 13), the morphology of a raphe presents a spectrum of abnormal development, being shallow, tall, or fenestrated. In addition, it may extend a varying distance from the aortic sinus toward the cusp, vary in its height in relation to the cusp's free edge, and show partial separation of its free margin into cusp margins. Also, the height of a conjoined cusp is often least in its midregion adjacent to a raphe, if one is present. Certain features within this spectrum of variation promote the risk of isolated aortic regurgitation. Thus, when raphe attachment and cusp height are low toward the center of a conjoined cusp, conditions exist for cusp prolapse and chronic aortic regurgitation to evolve (Fig. 14-31). This is a frequent cause of regurgitation.[86] Again, when a raphe is fenestrated, the cusp is tethered to the aortic wall by a strand of tissue. If it should rupture spontaneously, acute cusp prolapse results, with the sudden onset of valvular incompetence.[87] This is a rare cause of regurgitation. In either of the last two instances, the incompetent cusp is usually supple and not calcified.

Ventricular Septal Defect

When a supracristal (less often an infracristal) ventricular septal defect is closely related to the aortic root, the right aortic cusp (less often the left one) may prolapse into the defect, with the valve becoming incompetent. Presumably, the aortic root in the vicinity is not adequately attached to the cardiac skeleton (Fig. 14-32).

Acquired Lesions

Some of the causes of aortic regurgitation affecting native valves were discussed earlier (see Table 14-7). Others are covered in Chapter 5 (aortitis and annuloaortic ectasia), Chapter 13 (left-sided carcinoid disease and aortic incompetence associated with discrete membranous subaortic stenosis), Chapter 16 (systemic diseases), Chapter 17 (drugs affecting the cardiovascular system), Chapter 18 (trauma and iatrogenic lesions), and Chapter 19 (tumor and tumor-like conditions).

Laceration of the Aorta

Lacerations of the aorta develop after trauma (see Chapter 18), occur with or without an associated dissecting aneurysm, or, rarely, complicate an aortitis (see Chapter 5). In these instances, the laceration may involve a commissural region of the aortic valve. Tissue retraction after the laceration produces acute aortic regurgitation and, if the patient survives the acute event, chronic valvular insufficiency.

Whipple Disease

This condition is discussed in Chapter 13. It is a cause of aortic insufficiency and has induced valvular insufficiency by affecting the leaflets of a bioprosthetic mitral valve.

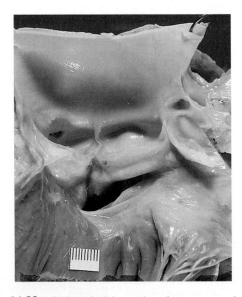

Figure 14-32 • Prolapsed right aortic valve cusp associated with supracristal ventricular septal defect.

Fenestrations of Aortic Valve Cusps

Most of these lesions, which increase in frequency with age (see Chapter 3), do not cause functional abnormality because they are located above the line of closure. Rarely, one extends beyond that line, with resultant valvular incompetence.

Thickening of Nodules of Arantius

Shapira and colleagues[88] described 11 cases of aortic insufficiency resulting from fibrosis and thickening of the nodules of Arantius in otherwise normal aortic valves. The condition was treated by sculpting the involved cusps.

REFERENCES

1. Nomina Anatomica. 5th ed. Baltimore, Williams & Wilkins, 1980, pp A48-A49
2. Angelini A, Ho SY, Anderson RH, et al: The morphology of the normal aortic valve as compared with the aortic valve having two leaflets. J Thorac Cardiovasc Surg 98:362, 1989
3. Dorland's Illustrated Medical Dictionary. 29th ed. Philadelphia, WB Saunders, 2000
4. Edwards JE, Burchall HB: Pathologic anatomy of mitral insufficiency. Mayo Clin Proc 33:497, 1958
5. Braunwald E: Valvular heart disease. In: Braunwald E (ed): Heart Disease: A Textbook of Cardiovascular Medicine. 4th ed. Philadelphia, WB Saunders, 1992, p 1007
6. Subramanian R, Olson LJ, Edwards WD: Surgical pathology of combined aortic stenosis and insufficiency: A study of 213 cases. Mayo Clin Proc 4:247, 1985
7. Olson LJ, Subramanian R, Ackermann DM, et al: Surgical pathology of the mitral valve: A study of 712 cases spanning 21 years. Mayo Clin Proc 62:22, 1987
8. Angelini A, Basso C, Grassi G, et al: Surgical pathology of valve disease in the elderly. Aging 6:225, 1994
9. Dare AJ, Veinot JP, Edwards WD, et al: New observations on the etiology of aortic valve disease: A surgical pathological study of 236 cases from 1990. Hum Pathol 24:1330, 1993
10. Becker AE: Acquired heart valve pathology: An update for the millennium. Herz 23:415, 1998
11. Turri M, Thiene G, Bortolotti U, et al: Surgical pathology of aortic valve disease: A study based on 602 specimens. Eur J Cardiothorac Surg 4:556, 1990
12. Agnozzino L, Falco A, de Vito F, et al: Surgical pathology of the mitral valve: Gross and histological study of 1288 surgically excised valves. Int J Cardiol 37:79, 1992
13. Steiner I: Nonbacterial thrombotic versus infective endocarditis: A necropsy study of 320 cases. Cardiovasc Pathol 4:207, 1995
14. Lopez JA, Ross RE, Fishbein MC, Seigel RJ: Nonbacterial thrombotic endocarditis: A review. Am Heart J 113:773, 1987
15. Magarey FR: Pathogenesis of mitral stenosis. BMJ 1:856, 1951
16. Edoute Y, Haim N, Rinkevich D, et al: Cardiac valvular vegetations in cancer patients: A prospective echocardiographic study of 200 patients. Am J Med 102:252, 1997
17. Schafer AI, Kroll MH: Nonatheromatous arterial thrombosis. Annu Rev Med 44:155, 1993
18. Kuramoto K, Matsushita S, Yamanouchi H: Nonbacterial thrombotic endocarditis as a cause of cerebral and myocardial infarction. Jpn Circ J 46:1000, 1984
19. Gabrielli F, Alcini E, Di Prima MA, et al: Cardiac valve involvement in systemic lupus erythematosus and primary antiphospholipid syndrome: Lack of correlation with antiphospholipid antibodies. Int J Cardiol 51:117, 1995
20. Hojnik M, George J, Ziporen L, Schoenfeld Y: Heart valve involvement (Libman-Sacks endocarditis) in the antiphospholipid syndrome. Circulation 93:1579, 1996
21. Ford SE, Ford PM: The cardiovascular pathology of phospholipid antibodies: An illustrative case and review of the literature. Cardiovasc Pathol 4:111, 1995
22. Ziporen L, Goldberg I, Arad M, et al: Libman-Sacks endocarditis in the antiphospholipid syndrome: Immunopathologic findings in deformed heart valves. Lupus 5:196, 1996
23. McNeil HP, Simpson RJ, Chesterman CN, Krilis SA: Antiphospholipid antibodies are directed against a complex antigen that includes a lipid-binding inhibitor of coagulation: Beta 2-glycoprotein I (apolioprotein H). Proc Natl Acad Sci U S A 87:4120, 1990
24. Afek A, Shoenfeld Y, Manor R, et al: Increased endothelial cell expression of alpha3beta1 integrin in cardiac valvulopathy in the primary (Hughes) and secondary antiphospholipid syndrome. Lupus 8:502, 1999
25. Pierangeli SS, Colden-Stanfield M, Xiaowei L, et al: Antiphospholipid antibodies from antiphospholipid syndrome patients activate endothelial cells in vitro and in vivo. Circulation 99:1997, 1999
25a. Ramadan FB, Beanlands DS, Burwash IG: Isolated pulmonic valve endocarditis in healthy hearts: A case report and review of the literature. Can J Cardiol 10:1282, 2000
26. Davies MJ: Pathology of Cardiac Valves. London, Butterworths, 1980
27. Durack DT: Prevention of infective endocarditis. N Engl J Med 332:32, 1995
28. Korzniowski OM, Kaye D: Infective endocarditis. In: Braunwald E (ed): Heart Disease: A Textbook of Cardiovascular Medicine. 4th ed. Philadelphia, WB Saunders, 1992
29. Kili AO, Herzberg MC, Meyer MW, et al: Streptococcal reporter gene-fusion vector for identification of in vivo expressed genes. Plasmid 42:67, 1999
30. Bayer AS, Bolger AF, Taubert, KA, et al: Diagnosis and management of infective endocarditis and its complications. Circulation 98:2936, 1998
31. Auclair F: Update on pathogenesis of infective endocarditis. Cardiovasc Pathol 4:265, 1995
32. Bayer AS, Cheng D, Yeaman MR, et al: In vitro resistance to thrombin-induced platelet microbicidal proteins among clinical bacteremic isolates of *Staphylococcus aureus* correlates with an endovascular infectious source. Antimicrob Agents Chemother 432:3169, 1998
33. Vriesma AJ, Beekhuizen H, Hamdi M, et al: Altered gene expression in *Staphylococcus aureus* upon interaction with human endothelial cells. Infect Immun 68:1756, 2000
34. Vriesma AJ, Dankert J, Zaat SA: A shift from oral blood pH is a stimulus for adaptive gene expression of *Staphylococcus gordonii* CH1 and induced protection against oxidative stress and enhanced bacterial growth by expressions of msrA. Infect Immun 68:1061, 2000
35. Xiong YQ, Vasil ML, Johnson Z, et al: The oxygen- and iron-dependent sigma factor pvdS of *Pseudomonas aeruginosa* is an important virulence factor in experimental infective endocarditis. J Infect Dis 181:1020, 2000
36. Ochiai K, Kikuchi K, Fukushima K, Kurita-Ochiai T: Co-aggregation as a virulent factor of *Streptococcus sanguis* isolated from infective endocarditis. J Oral Sci 41:117, 1999
37. Okada Y, Kitada K, Tagagaki M, et al: Endocardiac infectivity and binding to extracellular matrix proteins of oral *Abiotrophia* species. FEMS Immunol Med Microbiol 27:257, 2000
38. Peacock SJ, Foster TJ, Cameron BJ, Berendt AR: Bacterial fibronectin-binding proteins and endothelial cell surface fibronectin mediate adherence of *Staphylococcus aureus* to resting human endothelial cells. Microbiology 145:3477, 1999
39. Ellmerich S, Djouder N, Scholler M, Klein JP: Production of cytokines by monocytes, epithelial and endothelial cells activated by *Streptococcus bovis*. Cytokine 12:26, 2000
40. Herzberg MC: Platelet-streptococcal interactions in endocarditis. Crit Rev Oral Biol Med 7:222, 1996
41. Rotrosen D, Edwards JE Jr, Gibson TR, et al: Adherence of *Candida* to cultured vascular endothelial cells: Mechanism of attachment and endothelial cell penetration. J Infect Dis 152:1264, 1985
42. Hamil RJ, Vann JM, Proctor RA: Phagocytosis of *Staphylococcus aureus* by cultured bovine aortic endothelial cells: Model for post adherence events in endovascular infections. Infect Immun 54:833, 1986

43. Ferguson DJP, McColm AA, Savage TJ: A morphologic study of experimental rabbit staphylococcal endocarditis and aortitis. I. Formation and effect of infected and uninfected vegetations on the aorta. Br J Exp Pathol 67:667, 1986

44. Ferguson DJP, McColm AA, Savage TJ: A morphologic study of experimental rabbit staphylococcal endocarditis and aortitis. II. Interrelationship of bacteria, vegetation and cardiovasculature in established infections. Br J Exp Pathol 67: 679, 1986

45. Manning JE, Geyelin AJ, Ansmits LM, et al: A comparative study of the aggregation of human, rat and rabbit platelets by members of the *Streptococcus sanguis* group. J Med Mircrobiol 41:10, 1994

46. Lepeschkin E: On the relation between the site of valvular involvement in endocarditis and the blood pressure resting on the valve. Am J Med Sci 2243:318, 1952

47. Robard S: Blood velocity and endocarditis. Circulation 27:18, 1963

48. Roberts WC, Buchbinder NA: Right sided valvular infective endocarditis: A clinicopathologic study of twelve necropsy patients Am J Med 53:7, 1972

49. Buchbinder NA, Roberts WC: Left-sided valvular active endocarditis: A study of forty-five necropsy patients. Am J Med 53:20, 1972

50. Fernicola DJ, Roberts WC: Clinicopathological features of active infective endocarditis isolated to the native mitral valve. Am J Cardiol 71:1186, 1993

51. Dillon JC, Feigenbaum H, Konecke LL, et al: Echocardiographic findings in bacterial endocarditis. Am Heart J 86:698, 1973

52. Editorial: Vegetations, valves and echocardiography. Lancet 2:1118, 1988

53. Prasquier R, Gilbert C, Wichitz S, et al: Acute mitral valve obstruction during infective endocarditis BMJ 1:9, 1978

54. Li YH, Lin JM, Lei MH, et al: Mitral valve aneurysm and infective endocarditis: Report of four cases. J Formos Med Assoc 8:499, 1995

55. Vilacosta I, San Roman JA, Sarria C, et al: Clinical, anatomic and echocardiographic characteristics of aneurysms of the mitral valve. Am J Cardiol 84:110 1999

56. Arnett EN, Roberts WC: Valve ring abscess in active infective endocarditis: Frequency, location and clues to clinical diagnosis from the study of 95 necropsy patients. Circulation 54:1450, 1979

57. Fernicola DJ, Roberts WC: Frequency of ring abscesses and cuspal infection in active endocarditis involving bioprosthetic valves Am J Cardiol 72:314, 1993

58. Dean JW, Kuo J, Wood AJ: Myocardial infarction due to coronary artery compression by aortic root abscess. Int J Cardiol 41:165, 1993

59. Glazier JJ, Verwilghen J, Donaldson RM, Ross DN: Treatment of complicated prosthetic aortic valve endocarditis with annular abscess formation by homograft aortic root replacement. J Am Coll Cardiol 17:1177, 1991

60. David TE, Kuo J, Armstrong S: Aortic and mitral valve replacement with reconstruction of the intervalvular fibrous body. J Thorac Cardiovasc Surg 114:766, 1997

61. Fiorelli R, Tomasco B, Tesler UF: Pseudoaneurysm of the left ventricle: A rare sequel of mitral valve endocarditis. Tex Heart Inst J 26:309, 1999

62. van der Westhuizen NG, Rose AG: Right sided valvular infective endocarditis: A clinicopathological study of 29 patients. S Afr Med J 71:25, 1987

63. Roberts WC, Buchbinder NA: Healed left sided endocarditis: A clinicopathological study of 59 patients. Am J Cardiol 40:876, 1976

64. Spirito P, Rapezzi C, Bellone P, et al: Infective endocarditis in hypertrophic cardiomyopathy: Prevalence, incidence, and indications for antibiotic prophylaxis. Circulation 99:3132, 1999

65. Schreiber C, Cook A, Ho SY, Anderson RH: Morphologic spectrum of Ebstein's malformation: Revisitation relative to surgical repair. Thorac Cardiovasc Surg 117:148, 1999

66. Poltera AA, Jones AW: Subvalvular left ventricular aneurysm: A report of 5 Ugandan cases. Br Heart J 35:1085, 1973

67. Sharma S, Daxini BV, Loya YS: Profile of submitral left ventricular aneurysms in Indian patients. Indian Heart J 42:153, 1990

68. Grossi EA, Colvin SB, Galloway AC, et al: Repair of posterior left ventricular aneurysm in a six-year-old boy. Ann Thorac Surg 51: 484, 1991

69. Esposito F, Renzulli A, Festa M, et al: Submitral left ventricular aneurysm: Report of 2 surgical cases. Tex Heart Inst J 23:51, 1996

70. Matthews RV, French WJ, Criley JM: Chest trauma and subvalvular left ventricular aneurysm. Chest 95:474, 1989

71. Olowoyeye JO, Thadani U, Charrette EJ, et al: Subaortic annular left ventricular aneurysm: An unusual cause of aortic regurgitation. Cathet Cardiovasc Diagn 6:285, 1980

71a. Deshpande J, Valdeeswar P, Sivaraman A: Subvalvular left ventricular aneurysms. Cardiovasc Pathol 9:276, 2000

72. Barlow JB: Mitral valve billowing and prolapse—an overview. Aust N Z J Med 22:541, 1992

73. Edwards JE: Floppy mitral valve syndrome. In: Waller BF (ed): Contemporary Issues in Cardiovascular Pathology. Philadelphia, FA Davis, 1988, p 249

74. Trochu JN, Kyndt F, Schott JJ, et al: Clinical characteristics of a familial inherited myxomatous valvular dystrophy mapped to Xq28. J Am Coll Cardiol 35:1890, 2000

75. van der Bel-Kahn J, Duren DR, Becker AE: Isolated mitral valve prolapse: Chordal architecture as an anatomic basis in older patients. J Am Coll Cardiol 5: 1335, 1985

76. Wu MH, Lue HC, Wang JK, Wu JM: Implications of mitral valve prolapse in children with rheumatic mitral regurgitation. J Am Coll Cardiol 23:1199, 1994

77. Zhou LY, Lu K: Inflammatory valve prolapse produced by acute rheumatic carditis: Echocardiographic analysis of 66 cases of acute rheumatic carditis. Int J Cardiol 58:175, 1997

78. Angelini A, Becker AE, Anderson RH, Davies MJ: Mitral valve morphology: Normal and mitral valve prolapse. In: Boudoulas H, Wooley CF (eds): Mitral Valve Prolapse and the Mitral Valve Prolapse Syndrome. Mt Kisco, NY, Futura, 1988

79. Lester WM: Myxomatous mitral valve disease and related entities: The role of matrix in valvular heart disease. Cardiovasc Pathol 4: 256, 1995

80. Tamura K, Fukuda Y, Ishizaki M, et al: Abnormalities in elastic fibers and other connective tissue components of floppy mitral valve. Am Heart J 129:1149, 1995

81. Akhtar S, Meek KM, James V: Immunolocalization of elastin, collagen type I and type III, fibronectin, and victonectin in extracellular matrix components of normal and myxomatous mitral heart valves. Cardiovasc Pathol 8:203, 1999

82. Egeblad H, Soelberg Sorensen P: Prevalence of mitral valve prolapse in younger patients with cerebral ischemic attacks: A blinded controlled study. Acta Med Scand 216:385, 1984

83. Gilon D, Buonanno FS, Joffe MM, et al: Lack of evidence of an association between mitral-valve prolapse and stroke in young patients. N Engl J Med 341:8, 1999

84. Akhtar S, Meek KM, James V: Ultrastructure abnormalities in proteoglycans, collagen fibrils, and elastic fibers in normal and myxomatous mitral valve chordae tendineae. Cardiovasc Pathol 8:191, 1999

85. Gorman JH 3rd, Jackson BM, Gorman RC, et al: Papillary muscle discoordination rather than increased annular area facilitates mitral regurgitation after acute posterior myocardial infarction. Circulation 96 (suppl 11):124, 1997

86. Sadee AS, Becker AE, Verheul HA, et al: Aortic valve regurgitation and the congenitally bicuspid valve: A clinico-pathological correlation. Br Heart J 67:439, 1992

87. Walley VM, Antecol DH, Kyrollos AG, Chan KL: Congenitally bicuspid aortic valves: Study of a variant with fenestrated raphe. Can J Cardiol 10:535, 1994

88. Shapira N, Fernandez J, McNicholas KW, et al: Hypertrophy of nodules of Arantius and aortic insufficiency: Pathophysiology and repair. Ann Thorac Surg 51:969, 1991

Chapter 15

Interactions Between Heart and Brain

· · · · ·

Harry V. Vinters • Reza Jahan

This chapter deals with the clinicopathologic effects that lesions of the heart and great vessels have on the central nervous system (CNS), including brain and spinal cord, and the effects of encephalic lesions on the heart. The former are more extensively documented than the latter, both in this chapter and in the literature. Several terms merit definition and explanation. *Stroke* denotes a clinical syndrome characterized by a sudden, nonconvulsive focal neurologic deficit; that is, a stroke is *not* necessarily caused by vascular disease, and the term defines a clinicopathologic spectrum rather than a unique pathologic entity.[1] Clinicians often use stroke as a synonym for cerebrovascular accident (CVA), an even less optimal but nonetheless widely used name for a group of clinical conditions. Strokes or CVAs are usually caused by cerebral infarction or hemorrhage or a combination of the two events. Illustrative cases presented throughout this chapter emphasize CNS lesions rather than causal cardiovascular ones, which are discussed extensively throughout this book. Because pathologists are now often called upon to compare anatomic specimens with neuroimaging studies, selected examples of computed tomography (CT) and magnetic resonance imaging (MRI) scans and angiograms of lesions are presented for comparison with pathologic specimens. Readers interested in an in-depth approach to clinicopathologic features of stroke and cerebrovascular disease in general are referred to other sources.[2-6] In any stroke patient who comes to autopsy, the detective work involved in finding the cause of a cerebral infarct must include thorough and detailed examination of the carotid and vertebral arteries throughout their length, as well as of the heart and the great vessels.

CEREBRAL AND GENERALIZED ATHEROSCLEROSIS

Of particular interest to the neuropathologist is an understanding of the degree of atherosclerosis that may impact on the brain in relation to systemic atherosclerotic disease. Based on a meticulous autopsy study of the extent and severity of carotid and vertebrobasilar atherosclerosis in almost 180 patients, Fisher and colleagues concluded that extracranial atherosclerosis of the carotid artery was usually less severe than that of the aorta but more severe than that of the vertebral and intracranial cerebral arteries.[7] The cervical great vessels often showed severe, sometimes occlusive atherosclerosis, which was commonly asymptomatic during life. Symptomatic occlusive atherosclerosis usually affected the carotid arteries extracranially and the vertebrobasilar system intracranially. Hypertension was found to aggravate cerebral ather-

osclerosis, especially that involving the basilar artery. Atherosclerosis increased significantly in patients older than 50 years of age, although more slowly in the carotid arteries than in the aorta, to the extent that lesion progression can be judged from necropsy material. Epidemiologic investigations such as the Framingham Study suggest that hypercholesterolemia is less predictive of cerebral than of coronary atherosclerosis.[8] Atherosclerosis of the ascending aorta appears to be an independent risk factor for cerebrovascular events, possibly as a potential source of microemboli in the brain or as a marker for generalized atherosclerosis.[9]

Coronary and cerebrovascular atherosclerosis often coexist; thus, coronary artery disease is frequently a cause of death in patients with cerebrovascular disease. Atherosclerosis of intracranial arteries tends to lag behind coronary artery disease by 5 to 10 years, although coronary atherosclerosis may occur simultaneously with *extra*cranial carotid atherosclerosis.[10] Among patients undergoing cerebrovascular surgical procedures such as carotid endarterectomy, operative mortality is relatively high in those with symptomatic coronary artery disease. The most common cause of death among patients with cerebral infarcts or transient ischemic attacks (TIAs) is myocardial infarction, not neurologic disease.[11] Stroke occurs in fewer than 5% of patients after coronary artery bypass graft placement. Furthermore, asymptomatic unilateral internal carotid artery stenosis of less than 90% does not increase stroke risk during coronary artery bypass surgery.[12]

CARDIOEMBOLIC STROKE

The two major subtypes of stroke are cerebral ischemic infarct and encephalic or intracranial hemorrhage. Cardioembolic infarcts or strokes constitute one further subset of ischemic infarcts as defined by etiology; the other subset is infarcts caused by in situ arterial thrombosis. The distinction between cerebral hemorrhages and infarcts may be further blurred in a hemorrhagic infarct (Fig. 15-1), which often results from an embolic cerebral arterial occlusion[13-17] and may, especially if large, mimic primary intracerebral hemorrhage (Fig. 15-2). Data from stroke banks and registries suggest that embolic infarcts are less common than thrombotic infarcts,[18, 19] although how much less common is difficult to ascertain, in large part because of the biases inherent in various studies and existing at the various stroke centers. Data from large registries and multicenter studies suggest that cardioembolic strokes make up 5 to 25% of all ischemic strokes.[20, 21] A patient at risk for thrombotic occlusion of a cerebral or cervical artery is also at risk for a cardiac

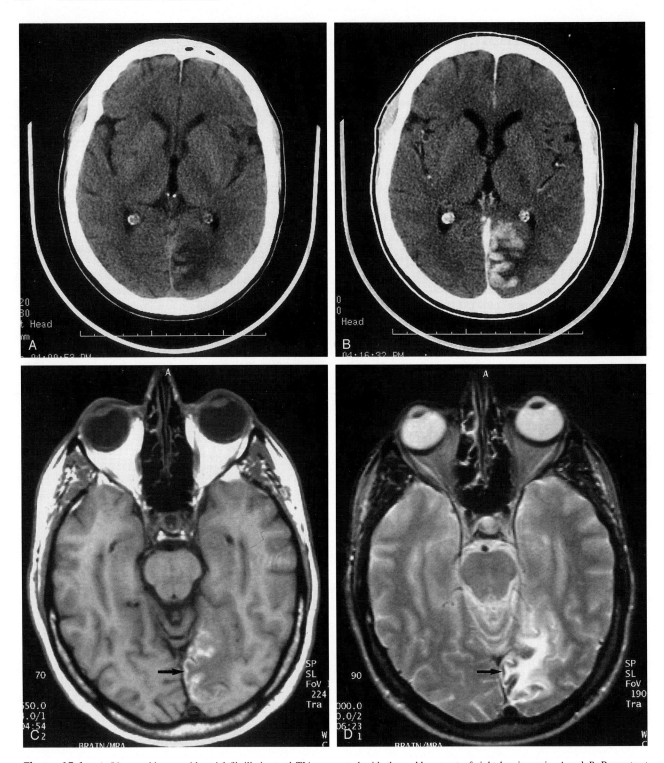

Figure 15-1 • A 56-year-old man with atrial fibrillation and TIAs presented with the sudden onset of right hemianopsia. *A* and *B,* Precontrast and postcontrast CT scans show area of hypodensity in the left occipital and posterior left temporal lobes consistent with an infarct in the distribution of the left posterior cerebral artery. On postcontrast images, gyriform enhancement of the infarcted region is present. *C* and *D,* T1- and T2-weighted MRIs of the brain show the infarcted region as hypointensity on T1 and hyperintensity on T2. T1 hyperintensity and T2 hypointensity (arrows) are present along the medial aspect of the left occipital lobe, consistent with gyriform petechial hemorrhage.

lesion; that is, a hypokinetic ventricular wall segment with cardiac mural thrombus consequent to a myocardial infarct that may predispose to an embolic event (see later section). In general and in clinical studies, risk factors for atherosclerosis, (e.g., cigarette smoking, hypertension, diabetes mellitus, hypercholesterolemia) are relatively more common in stroke patients *without* potential cardiac sources of embolism.[20] The best available CT and MRI scans and angiographic as well as cardiac imaging modalities such as two-dimensional echocardiography may not allow a clinician to distinguish a thrombotic from a cardioembolic infarct. The occurrence of stroke in a young

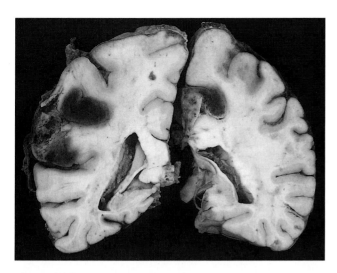

Figure 15-2 • An elderly female with multiple primary malignancies who developed NBTE and cerebral infarcts. This brain slice shows a predominantly hemorrhagic infarct in the left middle cerebral artery territory. A right medial parietal hemorrhagic infarct is approximately at the watershed between the anterior and posterior cerebral artery territories. The left cerebral hemorrhagic infarcts resemble primary cerebral hemorrhages.

person, however, tends to increase the relative likelihood of an embolic cause.[22]

Purely clinical criteria used to distinguish thrombotic from embolic stroke are, at best, inaccurate and flawed; neurologic features which suggest an embolic rather than thrombotic brain infarct include a sudden or abrupt onset of maximal neurologic deficit, headache, and loss of consciousness at onset; and clinical and imaging evidence of at least two distinct sites of embolization, either in the CNS or in the brain and at an extra-CNS site. Rapid recovery from a major hemispheric deficit—the phenomenon of spectacular shrinking deficit—strongly correlates with cardiogenic cerebral embolism, presumably because of embolus migration after it produces severe focal neurologic disability.[23] As mentioned, a hemorrhagic character to the infarct is predictive of an embolic cause[14–17] (Fig. 15-3). Nevertheless, these correlates of embolic stroke, although helpful, are not fully reliable, and the possibility of cardiogenic embolism should be considered in virtually *any* patient being investigated for cerebral ischemia.[24] Outstanding summaries of clinical pathophysiologic considerations in cardiogenic stroke are found in key texts and reviews.[25, 26]

Cardiogenic emboli usually migrate to the middle cerebral artery bifurcation in the sylvian fissure (Fig. 15-4) or to more distal middle cerebral artery branches; less often—approximately 10 to 20% of the time—they migrate to the vertebrobasilar system. These emboli often lodge at the basilar artery tip, producing occipital ischemia that results in visual complaints. In deciding whether an occluded artery has undergone in situ thrombosis or embolic occlusion, a pathologist must consider the degree of complicated atherosclerosis in the vessel; thrombus superimposed on a large, focally calcified, ulcerated plaque is more likely to be a thrombosis than is a platelet/fibrin plug in a relatively normal artery. The differential diagnosis becomes more difficult when the occlusive material is

atheromatous debris. If that occurs in an otherwise healthy artery an artery-to-artery embolus becomes an important diagnostic consideration.[27]

DeBono and Warlow[28] emphasized the etiologic diversity of cerebral or retinal ischemia in a consecutive series of patients investigated for TIAs. Cardiac workup revealed that almost a third of these patients had structural abnormalities of the heart and valves, a similar percentage had arrhythmias on 24-hour cardiac monitoring, and 15% had evidence of ischemic cardiac disease, although a surprisingly high proportion of control patients had similar abnormalities. In patients with a TIA, cardiac investigation assumes greater importance if cerebral angiography is normal.[29] Table 15-1 summarizes the major causes of cardioembolic brain infarcts; most of these are considered individually and in the same order in which they are presented in the table.

Abnormalities of Cardiac Rhythm

The arrhythmia most commonly associated with an increased incidence of embolic stroke is atrial fibrillation, in either the presence or the absence of primary valvular disease. Patients who have chronic atrial fibrillation have a five-fold greater risk of stroke than those who do not, and individuals with atrial fibrillation and rheumatic heart disease have an almost 20-fold greater risk.[30–32] This arrythmia accounts for approximately 6 to 24% of all ischemic brain infarcts and for more than one third of such events in the elderly.[21] Associated cerebral infarcts are often prominently hemorrhagic (Fig. 15-5).

"Silent," or subclinical, cerebral infarcts detected by neuroimaging studies are common in affected patients.[33] Paroxysmal atrial fibrillation is itself associated with an increased stroke risk and, of course, is often a precursor of chronic fibrillation.[34] Predictors of an increased likelihood of thromboembolism in patients with nonrheumatic atrial fibrillation include recent congestive heart failure, a history of hypertension, and previous thromboembolism.[35]

At the autopsy of a patient with a cerebral infarct thought to have been caused by atrial fibrillation, the left

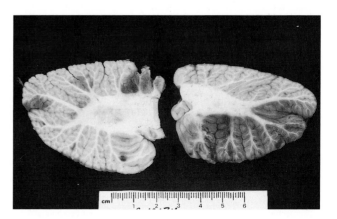

Figure 15-3 • Hemorrhagic infarcts in parasagittal sections of the cerebellar hemispheres. The patient had severe cardiomyopathy with biventricular mural thrombi and extensive endomyocardial fibrosis. Note large hemorrhagic infarcts secondary to emboli in both cerebellar hemispheres, more extensive on the right. Infarct in the right hemisphere is approximately in the posterior inferior cerebellar artery territory.

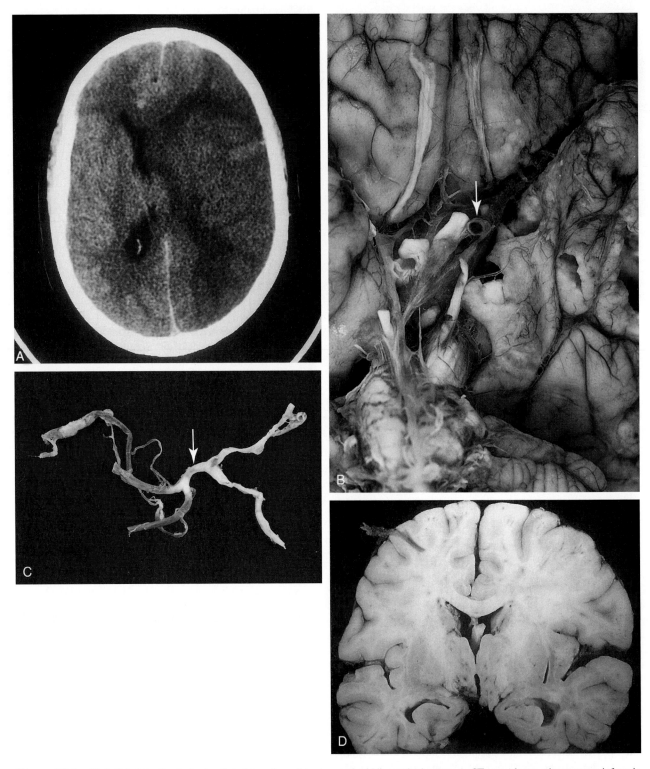

Figure 15-4 • Emboli (originating in the heart) to internal carotid artery and middle cerebral artery. *A,* CT scan shows a large recent infarct in the left middle cerebral artery territory with marked left-to-right shift of midline structures. The patient, a young woman, had a single ventricle with right-to-left shunt, suggesting that the mechanism of infarction was a paradoxical embolus. *B,* Autopsy specimen from the same patient. Note the occluded left internal carotid artery (arrow) at its cut end and left hemispheric edema. *C,* Middle cerebral artery dissected from the sylvian fissure in the brain of a patient with endocarditis. Note the pale, Y-shaped embolus (arrow) lodged at the bifurcation of the right middle cerebral artery. *D,* Resultant right cerebral hemispheric infarct, with edema and right-to-left shift of midline structures.

TABLE 15-1 • **Causes of Cardioembolic Brain Infarcts**

Clinical Condition	Potential Emboli or Other Pathogenesis
Cardiac Rhythm Abnormalities	
Atrial fibrillation (*non*valvular)	Left atrium (e.g., thrombus in appendage)
Sick sinus syndrome (multiple clinical causes)	Global brain hypoperfusion and anoxic-ischemic encephalopathy
Other and "benign" cardiac dysrhythmias	Thrombogenic valve surface in some cases
Valvular Abnormalities	
Endocarditis	
Infective (including prosthetic)	Valve surface, attachment and endocardium
Nonbacterial thrombotic	Valve surface
Rheumatic heart disease (e.g., with mitral stenosis and regurgitation)	Dilated atrium; atrial endocardial "jet" lesions
Prosthetic valve (biological or mechanical)	Site of attachment on valve surface or components
Mitral valve prolapse and myxomatous degeneration	Atrial site of valve attachment, valve surface
Mitral annular calcification	Thrombi on valve surface
Calcific aortic stenosis	Thrombi or calcified fragments
Inflammatory valvulitis (e.g., Libman-Sacks endocarditis)	
Myocardial Wall Lesions	
Ischemic heart disease	
Acute or recent	Anoxic-ischemic encephalopathy
Chronic or old	Endocardial surface, left ventricle Apical (LV), ventricular aneurysm
Ischemic Heart Disease	
Associated with investigation or treatment of ischemic heart disease	
Cardiac catheterization	
Open heart/CABG surgery	
Coronary angioplasty	
Cardiopulmonary resuscitation	
Cardiomyopathy	
Nonischemic, including hypertrophic, amyloid, hypereosinophilic, alcoholic, and neuromuscular-disorder–associated	Atrium/ventricle (usually in muscle trabeculae)
Paradoxical emboli, e.g., atrial septal defects, PFO, VSD, pulmonary arteriovenous fistula	Thrombi in (deep) venous circulation
Cardiac tumors, including atrial myxoma, papillary fibroelastoma, sarcoma	Thrombi or tumor emboli (metastases with aggressive tumors [e.g., sarcoma])
Congenital heart disease	Miscellaneous causes
Atrial septal aneurysm	Thrombi

PFO, patent foramen ovale; VSD, ventricular septal defect; CABG, coronary artery bypass graft; LV, left ventricle.

side of the heart must be examined especially carefully. Failure to demonstrate a left-sided atrial thrombus does not rule out the possibility that it was the cause of the infarct, because thrombi, especially when recently formed, may be friable and prone to embolize in their entirety to the cerebral or other distal circulation. Atrial fibrillation is associated in many patients with intrinsic cardiac disease, such as rheumatic, cardiomyopathic, and ischemic disease, and this must be carefully documented; therefore, the cardiac examination becomes as important as the neuropathologic component for the examiner who is investigating the cause of a stroke.[36]

Atrial fibrillation associated with both valvular and nonvalvular conditions is the most important disturbance of cardiac rhythm to result in stroke, but other arrhythmias have been implicated too. Sick sinus syndrome, found in patients with hypertensive, ischemic, and rheumatic heart disease, and degenerative or neuromuscular conditions such as myotonic or limb-girdle dystrophy and Friedreich ataxia (which poses a combined challenge to the neuropathologist), may produce bradycardia or alternating episodes of tachycardia and bradycardia. Diffuse cerebral hypoperfusion and ischemia rather than focal infarcts usually result, although associated dysrhythmias such as transient atrial fibrillation may cause cerebral emboli. As a cause of cardioembolic stroke, sick sinus syndrome is less than one tenth as common as atrial fibrillation.[20] Other arrhythmias that are considered benign in most circumstances may, especially when associated with a valvular abnormality, also cause cerebral infarction.[36]

Valvular Abnormalities

Endocarditis

Endocarditis may result from an infectious organism or may occur in the absence of infection. The two types of endocarditis have significant interrelationships (see Chapter 14), but are considered separately as nosologic entities.

Infective Endocarditis

Infective endocarditis (IE) may affect a native or a prosthetic heart valve, most commonly the mitral, the aortic, or both. Neurologic abnormalities are often an initial feature or they occur within 2 or 3 days after diagnosis, especially when IE is caused by a particularly virulent organism; cerebral emboli diminish in frequency within the first 2 or 3 days after diagnosis. The native valves most likely to develop IE are those that show either congenital or acquired (e.g., rheumatic) abnormalities, whereas normal valves may be colonized by microorganisms as a consequence of nosocomial infection, intravenous drug abuse, hyperalimentation, or immunosuppression.[36] As many as 15 to 25% of patients with IE experience embolic stroke. Risk for it increases with infection by *Staphylococcus aureus* and infections involving a mechanical prosthetic heart valve.[21] Most brain infarcts associated with IE are small, but those associated with *S. aureus* infection may be massive.[37] Effective control of the infection markedly diminishes the likelihood of distal emboli. Neurologic complications in this disease generally portend a worse prognosis—roughly a three-fold increase in mortality—than exists when such complications do not develop.[38]

Neurologic complications of IE include not only embolic/ischemic infarcts, the most common effect on the

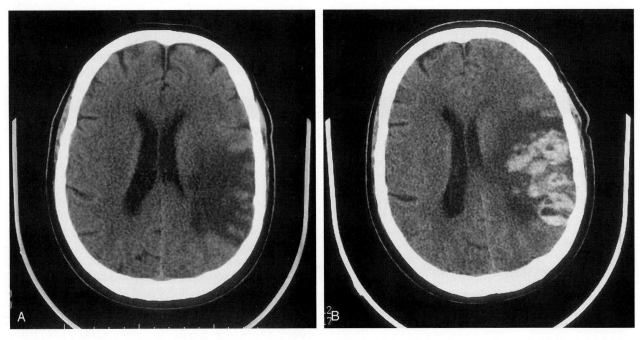

Figure 15-5 • A 67-year-old man admitted with acute-onset right-sided hemiplegia and aphasia. *A*, CT scan shows a large area of hypodensity involving the left frontal and parietal lobes in the distribution of the middle cerebral artery. Workup revealed new-onset atrial fibrillation and flutter. Echocardiogram showed no thrombus in the left atrium or ventricle, but contrast stagnation in the left atrium. Patient was started on heparin, and was found to be lethargic and poorly responsive the next day. *B*, A CT scan revealed hemorrhagic transformation of the infarct.

CNS, but also meningitis, (which occurs in 1 to 15% of patients), encephalopathy (5 to 7%), cerebral abscesses, including microabscesses (2 to 3%), mycotic aneurysm (2%), and hemorrhages (3 to 13%).[39, 40] Hemorrhages are also especially likely to occur in individuals with infection caused by *S. aureus* who develop a septic/pyogenic arteritis. Cerebral hemorrhages related to IE may be difficult to distinguish from ordinary hemorrhagic infarcts (Fig. 15-6). Arteritis in this disease is almost certainly the result of septic microemboli; they must be diligently

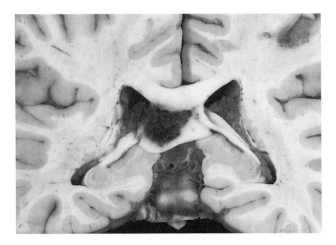

Figure 15-6 • A 17-year-old female who developed infective endocarditis in the course of pregnancy; subsequently a St. Jude valve was placed. Her stormy clinical course was complicated by multiple cerebral emboli that produced hemorrhagic infarcts, some of which (such as this lesion in the corpus callosum) resembled primary parenchymal hemorrhages.

searched for by a surgical pathologist in an evacuated cerebral hematoma, especially when they are found in an at-risk patient such as one with a suppressed immune system or one who is an abuser of intravenous drugs. Staining of clot material for microorganisms is essential and may be especially helpful in confirming the diagnosis.[41]

Infectious, or mycotic, aneurysms (the former term is more accurate) are a much less common cause of cerebral intraparenchymal or subarachnoid hemorrhage than is pyogenic arteritis, although the former probably originate from the latter.[42] Infectious aneurysms develop as a complication in approximately 2% of patients with IE and represent as many as 4 to 6% of all intracranial aneurysms; mortality is much higher in cases of infectious aneurysms caused by fungi than in those resulting from bacterial infection. Such lesions (Fig. 15-7) differ from berry or saccular aneurysms in that they usually occur in the peripheral cerebral circulation or the CNS parenchyma itself; berry aneurysms are generally situated on major branch points of the circle of Willis.

Most patients with infectious aneurysms manifest a sudden onset of subarachnoid or intraparenchymal hemorrhage, and almost half have a neurologic prodrome lasting as long as several months before hemorrhage occurs.[43] If infective endocarditis is effectively treated with antibiotics, the risk of late cerebral hemorrhage from an unsuspected infectious aneurysm is low. Infectious aneurysms develop either from focal weakening of the arterial wall caused by extension of microorganisms and inflammatory cells into it consequent to vascular occlusion by septic emboli, or from colonization of the vasa vasorum of affected arterial walls, with resultant ectasia and aneurysm formation.[40, 44, 45]

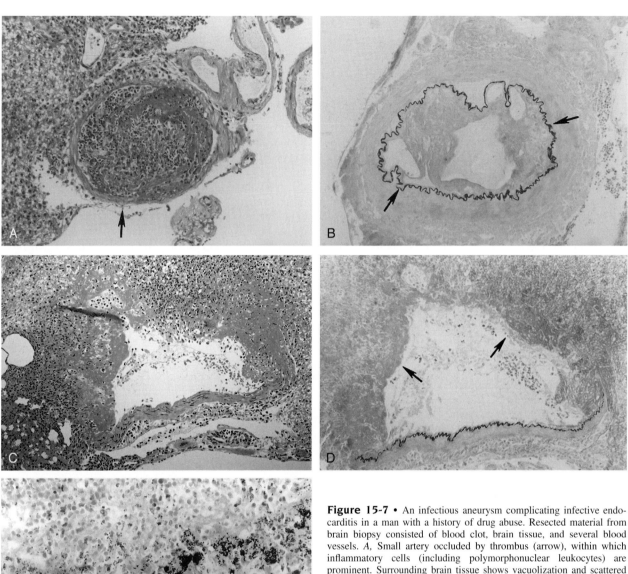

Figure 15-7 • An infectious aneurysm complicating infective endocarditis in a man with a history of drug abuse. Resected material from brain biopsy consisted of blood clot, brain tissue, and several blood vessels. *A,* Small artery occluded by thrombus (arrow), within which inflammatory cells (including polymorphonuclear leukocytes) are prominent. Surrounding brain tissue shows vacuolization and scattered inflammatory cells (H&E stain). *B,* Another small artery that has undergone thrombosis and recanalization. Elastica (arrows) is clearly visible (Elastic van Gieson stain). *C* and *D,* Parallel sections showing the intact lower portion of an artery. Superior segment (arrows in D) manifests extensive fibrinoid necrosis and surrounding acute and chronic inflammatory cells. This is an infectious aneurysm and is the presumed origin of parenchymal hemorrhage. (*C,* H&E stain; *D,* Elastic van Gieson stain). *E,* Clusters of gram-positive cocci among the inflammatory cells within the brain parenchyma and aneurysm wall (Gram stain).

Infrequently, other neurologic sequelae of infective endocarditis are observed, including meningitis; encephalopathy and seizures, probably resulting from a combination of microinfarcts and microabscesses; discitis or vertebral osteomyelitis; myelitis; and acute mononeuropathy.[39]

Nonbacterial Thrombotic Endocarditis

Nonbacterial thrombotic endocarditis (NBTE), a clinicopathologic entity of uncertain etiology and pathogenesis (see Chapter 14), may complicate a wasting disease such as widespread malignancy or autoimmune deficiency syndrome (AIDS)[46] and is found to be associated with nonneoplastic diseases affecting especially the heart, gastroin-

testinal system, or the lungs.[47] In one study of the neurologic complications of NBTE,[47] aortic and mitral valves were most commonly affected, and brain embolism was documented in one third of patients. Of 99 individuals with NBTE, 22 had coagulation abnormalities and 10 showed evidence of disseminated intravascular coagulation. Patients who come to autopsy after acute stroke in the presence of malignancies with high risk for developing NBTE, such as cancers of the lung, the pancreas or other parts of the gastrointestinal tract, or the prostate, and negligible arterial disease, must be considered to have this cause of stroke until and unless proved otherwise. It has been suggested that NBTE is an important cause in

25 to 30% of all ischemic strokes encountered in cancer patients.[21]

Rheumatic Heart Disease

Rheumatic heart disease may afflict as much as 1% of the adult population in the United States despite the declining prevalence of the disease as a result of aggressive early treatment of group A streptococcal infection. It leads to scarring and deformation (sometimes with calcification) of the mitral valve (see Chapters 13 and 14); aortic valve involvement is less common and produces neurologic impairment infrequently.[36] Cerebral emboli in patients with rheumatic heart disease usually come from the left atrium, often in association with atrial fibrillation, but thrombus or calcified material may embolize directly from the mitral valve. The incidence of embolism from rheumatic mitral stenosis is estimated to be 3 to 4% per year.

Prosthetic Cardiac Valves

Prosthetic cardiac valves, which may be mechanical or constructed from biologic materials (see Chapter 21), are a cause of significant neurologic morbidity and mortality. Mechanical valves are associated with a higher risk of thromboembolism than are bioprostheses.[36] Small fresh or organizing thrombi are often found on the surfaces or attachment sites of mechanical valves at necropsy.[48] Large thrombi of the type that occlude a major intracerebral artery are more commonly found on disk valves (Fig. 15-8). Other thrombi attached to prosthetic heart valves are illustrated in Figs. 21-10 and 21-11. Late prosthetic valve IE develops with roughly equal frequency on mechanical and bioprosthetic valves, but neurologic complications, which are associated with a higher mortality rate, are more common with mechanical valves, especially those in the mitral position; *S. aureus* is the most commonly implicated pathogen.[49]

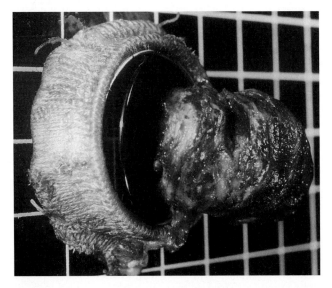

Figure 15-8 • Heart valve-prosthesis (Björk-Shiley) showing extensive large adjacent thrombus. (Courtesy of Nir Kossovsky, MD, University of California Los Angeles Medical Center, Los Angeles, California.)

Mitral Valve Prolapse

Mitral valve prolapse is estimated to affect at least 3 to 4% of males, more than 5% of females (see Chapter 14), and possibly a much larger percentage of the population. It has been associated with stroke, especially in young people, in numerous clinical investigations (for a review, see the work of Lauzier and Barnett[50]). Autopsy documentation of cerebral embolic infarcts associated with mitral valve prolapse is, however, surprisingly scarce. The valvular abnormality is identified as the putative cause of cerebral ischemia in widely varying percentages of young adult patients—the range is between 4 and 30%—probably because of the use of varying criteria in assessing echocardiographic studies and because of ascertainment bias in some of the patient populations investigated.[21] Only patients with true myxomatous degeneration of valve leaflets, chordae, and annulus appear to be at risk for cerebral or other emboli. The risk of stroke among all (i.e., unselected) individuals with mitral valve prolapse is estimated to be no greater than 1 in 11,000 per year and the risk among patients younger than 40 years of age to be 1 in 6,000 per year.[50] Stroke occurring with mitral valve prolapse is usually cardioembolic; the occurrence of a new cerebral infarct should also raise the possibility of IE superimposed upon the valvular abnormality. This likelihood is remote but must be considered. Various types of arrhythmia also occur with mitral valve prolapse and may contribute to cerebral ischemia.[50]

Neurologic complications include syncope, migraine headaches, seizures, and transient global amnesia, the last two postulated to occur because of cerebral thromboemboli arising from vegetations that form on the prolapsed valve. A suggested association between mitral valve prolapse and berry aneurysm[50] is of interest in view of possible connective tissue disorders underlying both conditions. Although mitral valve prolapse is more common in women than in men, complications are more likely to arise in the latter.[21] Embolic occlusion of arteries is frequently discovered by angiography in a subgroup of patients with documented cerebral ischemia; small and medium-sized arteries in the carotid territory are affected much more commonly than are those in the vertebrobasilar area. In familial forms of mitral valve prolapse, children can develop hemiplegia, presumably on the basis of cardioembolic events from thrombi on affected valves.[50]

Despite a clinical association of mitral valve prolapse and ischemic cardioembolic stroke, autopsy documentation of the phenomenon is extraordinarily rare; only a handful of suggestive cases have been reported. Rarely are they straightforward in documenting an ischemic infarct secondary to a thromboembolic arterial occlusion that has arisen from a mitral valve showing myxomatous degeneration. Other complicating factors, such as atrial fibrillation or NBTE affecting prolapsing mitral valve leaflets, are frequently present and cloud interpretation of the reported cases.[50]

Mitral Annular Calcification and Calcific Aortic Stenosis

Calcification of the mitral valve annulus is a common clinical and necropsy finding in elderly patients. It affects as many as 25 to 30% of those older than 90 years of

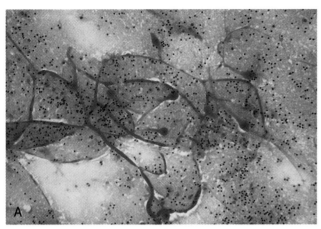
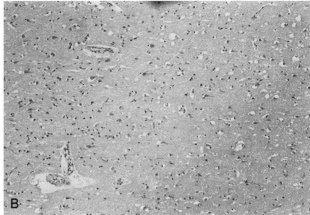

Figure 15-9 • Acute anoxic-ischemic change in cerebellum. *A,* Smear/squash preparation demonstrates numerous flask-shaped Purkinje cells with marked cytoplasmic eosinophilia. Background shows microvessels and small cells that are granule cells. *B,* A histologic section showing acute and subacute anoxic-ischemic change in the cerebral cortex. Note neuronal eosinophilia and subtle microvacuolization of the neuropil, especially in center left of the micrograph (Both H&E stain).

age, and has become the focus of increasing attention with the widespread use of echocardiography (see Chapter 3). In assigning it a causal role in a given elderly patient's stroke, keep in mind that mitral annular calcification is also a marker for generalized complicated atherosclerosis, that is, with plaque calcification.[51] Furthermore, mitral annular calcification is itself associated with other conditions that predispose to cardioembolic cerebral infarcts, such as IE and arrhythmias. Rarely, calcified cerebral embolic material, thought to originate from mitral annular calcification, is found at autopsy; given that severely calcified atherosclerotic plaque material may embolize in a similar fashion, blaming a CNS infarct on this mitral valvular lesion may be inappropriate or, at best, inaccurate.

Calcific aortic sclerosis and stenosis are noted in 0.5 to 2.5% of echocardiograms performed on patients who have experienced TIAs, or strokes. Resultant spontaneous cerebral emboli are rare and are usually tiny, producing in some patients monocular blindness secondary to occlusion of the retinal artery.[21, 52] One patient with this valvular lesion experienced multiple cerebral emboli, apparently originating from the diseased valve, immediately after cardiac catheterization.[53]

Abnormalities of the Myocardial Wall

Myocardial Ischemia

Myocardial ischemia, as well as the modern approaches to investigating and treating it, can have important sequelae that affect the CNS, whether ischemia occurs acutely or chronically. One of the most feared consequences of an acute myocardial infarct with severe arrhythmia and cardiac arrest is the occurrence of a variably severe anoxic-ischemic encephalopathy, the extent and impact of which are often difficult to gauge, assuming the patient survives the cardiac event for days or weeks. Acutely or subacutely, anoxic-ischemic encephalopathy manifests histologically as widespread neuronal eosinophilia, sometimes with associated pallor of the sur-

rounding neuropil (Fig. 15-9). Selected neuronal populations, such as hippocampal pyramidal cells and cerebellar Purkinje cells, are especially vulnerable (for a discussion of selective neuronal vulnerability, see the work of Ellison and colleagues[5]). If it is severe, anoxic-ischemic encephalopathy causes, in the long term, widespread loss of neurons, especially in the cortex and cerebellum, with resultant scarring and astrocytic gliosis.[54] The neuron loss may occur in a laminar pattern in the neocortex, with the deeper cortical layers being especially severely affected; this is described as cortical laminar necrosis (Fig. 15-10). Severe anoxic-ischemic encephalopathy often determines the quality of life of an individual who has made an otherwise successful recovery from a devastating myocardial infarct, especially if one or more episodes of cardiac arrest or severe arrhythmia have occurred.

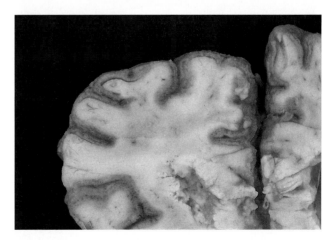

Figure 15-10 • Cortical laminar necrosis. The patient was a 41-year-old man who experienced numerous cardiac arrests and hypotensive episodes 2 and 3 days after surgery for a perforated cecum and abdominal abscess. Thereafter, he remained deeply comatose until death several days later. The neocortex shows thinning, mottling, and brown discoloration with apparent separation from the underlying white matter. Microscopic sections demonstrated pancortical necrosis, an extreme degree of laminar necrosis, and involvement of virtually all cortical layers throughout the cerebral hemispheres.

Approximately 1.5 to 3.0% of patients who have experienced an acute myocardial infarction also experience stroke, and that complication significantly worsens morbidity and mortality rates.[21, 36, 55, 56] Conversely, evidence of an old, clinically silent myocardial infarction may be discovered during the routine workup of a patient with a new stroke or even at necropsy. An estimated 80 to 90% of these strokes occur within the first month after the infarction; approximately 2 to 8% of patients experiencing acute myocardial infarction have a stroke within 2 to 4 weeks. Acute anterior wall infarcts are complicated by stroke in 4 to 12% of patients, whereas only about 1% of inferior wall infarcts are complicated by stroke.[21] Rarely, stroke occurs coincident with a myocardial infarct. In some studies, the risk for stroke appeared to increase in proportion to infarct size as judged by creatine kinase levels.[56] Most strokes that complicate myocardial infarcts are embolic in origin, although arrhythmias (especially atrial) contribute to their occurrence, and strokes onsetting coincidentally with myocardial infarcts are more likely to be related to hypoperfusion or atheroemboli dislodged from atherosclerotic carotid or vertebrobasilar arteries. Cerebral infarcts are easily visualized with use of neuroimaging modalities (Fig. 15-11).

As indicated, cerebral emboli that complicate myocardial infarcts usually occur within 1 to 2 weeks after the infarct, presumably because a ventricular thrombus forms over a hypokinetic myocardial wall segment during this period; the subsequent decrease in stroke risk may be related to organization of the thrombus as well as to the fact that a comparatively small area of thrombus is exposed to blood flow.[36] Clinically, echocardiography is used to identify the patients with left ventricular thrombus who are at increased risk for embolic cerebral infarct.

The long-term risk that a cerebral infarct will follow

an acute myocardial infarct, especially if it results from a left ventricular thrombus, is relatively low, although such thrombi may develop months after the infarct, and their occurrence has, in the past, possibly been underestimated. When a patient with a myocardial infarct develops a late complication of stroke, cerebrovascular disease should be suspected as its likely cause.

Complications Associated with Investigation/Treatment of Ischemic Heart Disease and Other Conditions

A unique set of complications is encountered in investigation into or treatment of ischemic heart disease and its major sequelae, usually acute myocardial infarction.

Atheromatous emboli are encountered in 0.5 to 1.0% of autopsies carried out on patients older than the age of 60 years.[27] Most commonly, they have been discovered in kidney and spleen, although one study[56] highlighted the relatively common occurrence of such emboli in the brain. Emboli may be discovered incidentally in many organs, but these atheroemboli, especially when they have occurred as showers into the CNS, are much more likely to produce diffuse symptoms, such as encephalopathy or confusional states in elderly patients. The common occurrence of atheroemboli even in patients who have *not* had vascular surgery or catheterization attests to the brittleness of complicated atheromatous plaques and their potential to produce distal ischemia, especially during or after surgery or instrumentation[57] (Fig. 15-12). Cardiac catheterization is rarely associated with embolization of cholesterol-containing material distally, including to the CNS.[58]

In studies conducted in the 1970s, children who had undergone cardiac surgery or catheterization were found to show intraluminal foreign particles in distal organs, including the brain, often with a giant cell reaction to the foreign body.[59] Because the material that embolizes may originate from components of drapes, caps, gowns, and masks, prevention of such iatrogenic emboli is desirable and possible.[59, 60]

Some cerebral infarcts that occur after cardiac catheterization, a rare phenomenon documented at one center in roughly 1/1000 individuals who underwent the procedure, are without doubt multifactorial in etiology. Cerebral emboli and hypotension are two major contributors to this complication.[61, 62]

Percutaneous transluminal coronary angioplasty is also associated with a low (0.1 to 0.2%) incidence of focal neurologic deficit; most cases probably result from emboli.[63]

Closed-chest cardiac massage may give rise to various types of cerebral microemboli, including those originating in bone marrow when bones are fractured during resuscitation attempts.[60, 64, 65] When such emboli are found at necropsy, they should be regarded as paradoxical and a right-to-left cardiac shunt should be sought as one factor contributing to their occurrence. For a detailed review of the various foreign materials capable of embolizing distally during cardiovascular instrumentation or open heart surgery (Fig. 15-13) see Walley and colleagues.[66]

Neurologic complications are commonly encountered in patients who have undergone open heart (see also later discussion) or aortic surgery requiring cardiopulmonary

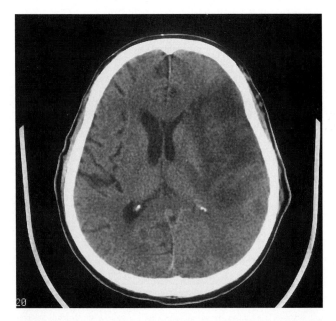

Figure 15-11 • A CT scan of a 62-year-old man admitted with acute anterolateral myocardial infarct and cardiogenic shock. During hospitalization, he developed right-sided hemiplegia. The scan shows an area of hypodensity in the territory of supply of the left middle cerebral artery, consistent with an infarct.

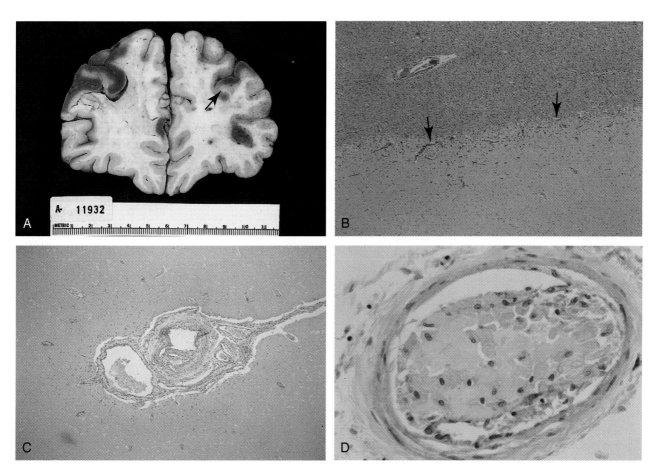

Figure 15-12 • A 58-year-old woman with hypertensive and arteriosclerotic cardiovascular disease underwent complicated coronary artery bypass that was performed over an 18-hour period. Postoperatively, she was in a coma until death several days later. At autopsy, recent and healed myocardial infarcts were identified, as were organizing mural thrombi in the left ventricle. Severe, complicated atherosclerosis was present throughout the body. *A,* Coronal section through the frontal lobes, with multiple focally hemorrhagic infarcts in both cerebral hemispheres, seen as dusky gray discoloration of the cortex. At least one infarct (arrow) is in the watershed territory between the right anterior and middle cerebral artery regions of supply. *B,* Interface between a region of cerebral infarct (lower portion of the frame) and more normal brain tissue (upper portion). Note the vascular endothelial hyperplasia (arrows) at the interface, consistent with the infarct's having occurred several days previously. *C,* Atheroembolic material was present in many meningeal arteries. Note the intraluminal lipid crystal clefts; foreign body giant cells are seen adjacent to some clefts, and some vessels had undergone recanalization. *D,* Leptomeningeal artery adjacent to the cerebellum, in which foamy macrophages, presumably originating in a proximal atherosclerotic plaque, are seen. Such atheroemboli are common in individuals who experience watershed cerebral infarcts (*B, C,* and *D,* H&E stain).

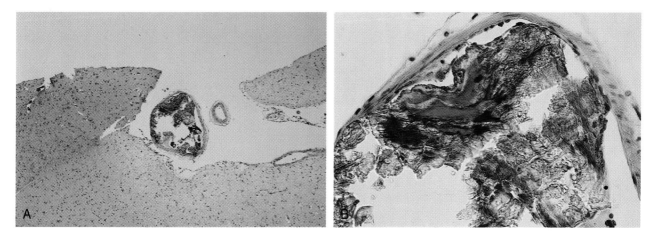

Figure 15-13 • Meningeal vessel overlying relatively intact cortex in a patient who had had cardiothoracic surgery prior to death. *A,* low magnification. *B,* high magnification. The embolic material has a solid, partly calcified appearance and is somewhat refractile (both H&E stain). (Courtesy of Virginia M. Walley, MD, Ottawa Civic Hospital and Ottawa Heart Institute, Ottawa, Canada.)

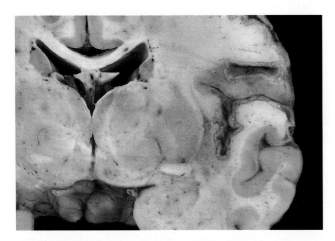

Figure 15-14 • A 15-year-old had an aortic valve replacement because of infective endocarditis. Hemiparesis was observed soon after the patient recovered from anesthesia; death occurred 6 months later. Coronal section of the brain shows extensive cortical infarct involving the right insular, inferior frontal, and superior temporal cortex. Infarct almost certainly occurred intraoperatively or soon after the procedure.

bypass. Indeed, prevention of such complications—which can dramatically worsen the quality of life in a patient with an otherwise excellent surgical outcome—is a major goal of modern cardiovascular surgical practice.[62, 67]

Clinically, neurologic dysfunction after cardiac surgery can be of varying severity such that a patient may (1) fail to regain consciousness after the procedure, (2) awaken with a focal neurologic deficit, almost always secondary to cerebral infarction, (3) recover from surgery intact neurologically but subsequently develop a neurologic deficit, or (4) awaken without focal deficit but be encephalopathic for varying intervals, sometimes indefinitely.[68] When these patients come to autopsy, defining the neuropathologic substrate of lesions[69] sometimes has direct implications for preventive measures of value in other surgical patients.

Various studies report widely differing frequencies

of neurologic complications of open heart surgery and complication rates that, as would be expected, change as techniques of cardiothoracic surgery become more refined.[70, 71] Transient neurologic complications affect 7 to 61% of patients, and permanent deficits are observed in 1.6 to 23.0%; incidence figures are higher when based on prospective than on retrospective analysis. Of patients who undergo aortocoronary artery bypass (they number approximately 150,000 per annum in the United States alone), approximately 3% experience stroke and as many as 20% become "diffusely encephalopathic."[62] Morphologic studies of the CNS of individuals who have had open heart surgery show changes that are determined by the interval between surgery and the onset of neurologic symptoms and autopsy. Ischemic and hemorrhagic CNS lesions are common and may be large or small (Fig. 15-14); late changes include abnormalities as subtle as multifocal regions of neuron or axon loss and gliosis, for example, at the depths of sulci. A pathologist may be able to explain these regions of encephalomalacia by the presence of microemboli, such as atheromatous, platelet-fibrin, calcific (from calcified valves), refractile particulate/iatrogenic, or fat, the latter demonstrable only on frozen sections at or near their centers.[69, 72]

Other contributory mechanisms that are suspected but are more difficult to verify by morphoanatomic studies are periods of hypotension, cerebral hypoperfusion, and air or gas emboli resulting from cardiopulmonary bypass.[73] One provocative autopsy study that used an alkaline phosphatase technique to highlight capillaries and arterioles in thick sections of brain[74] showed that cardiopulmonary bypass was strongly associated with the occurrence of focal small capillary and arteriolar dilations (SCADs) (Fig. 15-15), some containing birefringent material.[74] These were implicated as sites of gas bubbles or fat emboli that commonly dissolve during tissue processing. Many patients who experience neurologic deficit during or after cardiopulmonary bypass survive and develop subtle cognitive decline may have had these previously undetected microemboli, which lead to cerebral microvascular

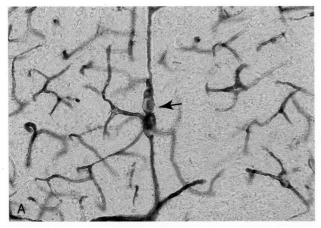
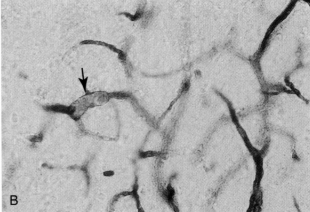

Figure 15-15 • *A* and *B,* Focal small capillary and arteriolar dilations (SCADs; indicated by arrows) in the brain of a patient who died 4 days after cardiac surgery supported by cardiopulmonary bypass. Micrographs photographed from 100-m alkaline phosphatase-stained sections without counterstain. For additional details, see the work of Moody and colleagues.[74] (Courtesy of Dixon M. Moody, MD, Bowman Gray School of Medicine, Winston-Salem, North Carolina.)

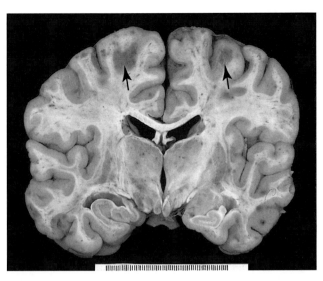

Figure 15-16 • Multiple embolic cerebral infarcts in a patient with Löffler restrictive cardiomyopathy. At autopsy, biventricular mural thrombi were seen and there was extensive myocardial fibrosis in both ventricles. A coronal section through the cerebral hemispheres shows multiple recent infarcts seen as patchy regions of gray discoloration in multiple vessel territories of both cerebral hemispheres (arrows).

abnormalities. Rare postbypass syndromes can occur. One of the authors (HVV) studied the brain of a patient who developed a clinical syndrome similar to Alzheimer disease after complicated vascular surgery. The individual had severe bilateral neuron loss in the hippocampal pyramidal cell layers but no evidence of Alzheimer changes as the primary neuropathologic abnormality.

Cardiomyopathy

Cardiomyopathy is complicated by brain embolism in as many as 10 to 15% of patients.[36] Individuals with idiopathic cardiomyopathy develop emboli at a rate of 4% per year.[21] The causal mechanism is usually assumed to be emboli from a left ventricular thrombus (Fig. 15-16) and embolic risk generally parallels the severity of the cardiomyopathy. However, atrial fibrillation (see earlier section) occurs commonly in patients with dilated cardiomyopathy. Among one large group of patients with idiopathic hypertrophic subaortic stenosis, the risk of brain infarct appeared low: none presented with stroke or cerebrovascular disease, but 3% of affected individuals experienced stroke and 4% experienced TIAs.[75] If a patient with cardiomyopathy and an embolic stroke comes to necropsy, the absence of a left ventricular thrombus may simply reflect the fact that all of it embolized to the brain.

Paradoxical Embolism

Paradoxical embolism has emerged as a putative mechanism causing stroke, especially in young people with a right-to-left shunt most commonly caused by a patent foramen ovale or an atrial septal defect (Fig. 15-17).[21, 36] Based on echocardiography, a patent foramen ovale is estimated to occur in 15% of normal people but it has a frequency of approximately 50% among young adults with otherwise unexplained strokes.[21] At autopsy, a probe-patent foramen ovale is present in about one third of individuals. The source of emboli is thought to be deep venous thrombosis in the legs or pelvis or a thrombus in the right heart. Stroke in affected patients is especially common after Valsalva-provoking activities that increase right atrial pressure. Because deep venous thrombi and even resultant pulmonary emboli may be occult, the absence of symptoms of deep venous thrombosis in a young patient with stroke of unclear cause and either a patent foramen ovale or atrial septal defect by no means excludes the diagnosis of paradoxical embolism as its cause. Should such a patient come to autopsy, the pres-

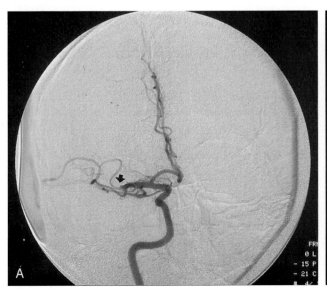
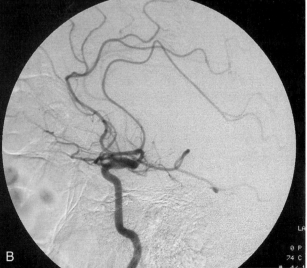

Figure 15-17 • Cerebral angiograms in a 39-year-old man with acute onset of left hemiplegia. *A,* Anteroposterior and *B,* lateral views of a right internal carotid artery injection show complete occlusion of the M2 segment (arrow in *A*) of the left middle cerebral artery. Subsequent investigations, including echocardiography, revealed an atrial septal defect.

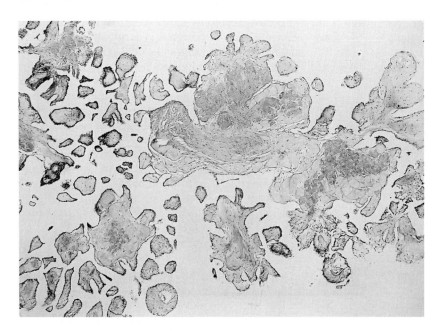

Figure 15-18 • A section of a papillary fibroelastoma from a patient who experienced embolic stroke. The tumor shows variably thickened avascular cores with overlying single layers of endothelial cells (PAS). (From Kasarskis EJ, O'Connor W, Earle G: Embolic stroke from cardiac papillary fibroelastomas. Stroke 19:1171, 1988.)

ence or absence of deep venous thrombi should be documented. Some have questioned whether paradoxical embolism is the proximate cause of stroke in patients with a patent foramen ovale.[76]

Cardiac Neoplasms

Whether primary or metastatic, cardiac neoplasms are of relatively infrequent occurrence (see Chapter 19) and must be considered a rare cause of stroke or neurologic disability. Of tumors associated with neurologic dysfunction, atrial myxoma is the most common. In one retrospective analysis, 5 of 11 patients with pathologically documented atrial myxoma had neurologic abnormalities consisting of nonhemorrhagic cerebral infarcts.[77] Neurologic problems had been the initial feature, antedating cardiac signs or symptoms, in 4 individuals. After surgical excision of a myxoma, 9 of 11 patients showed no recurrence of neurologic abnormalities. Larger series report a 25 to 30% incidence of neurologic complications with this tumor.[78] Atrial myxoma is also associated with fusiform aneurysm formation on peripheral branches of the cerebral vasculature, secondary to invasion of vessel walls, presumably by embolic myxomatous tissue.[79] Aneurysms of this type may resolve after resection of the primary tumor, although delayed aneurysm enlargement with cerebral hemorrhage has been reported.[79] Rarely, myxomas may metastasize to the CNS. Atrial myxomas also present with multiple strokes and even mimic peripheral vasculitis.[80, 81] Embolic stroke with atrial myxoma may result from tumor-fragment emboli or platelet-fibrin emboli.[36]

A neoplasm much less commonly associated with stroke secondary to cardiogenic cerebral emboli is the papillary fibroelastoma[82] (Fig. 15-18). Whereas atrial myxomas are more common in females, males predominate among the handful of cases of papillary fibroelastoma that have been described. More aggressive tumors such as sarcomas are more likely to produce cerebral metastases (Fig. 15-19) than cardioembolic infarcts, although it is assumed that the metastases most likely result from tumor emboli.

NEUROLOGIC COMPLICATIONS OF CONGENITAL HEART DISEASE

Neurologic and neuropathologic complications of congenital heart disease can be subdivided into (1) those that occur as a "natural" consequence of a given cardiac anomaly, and (2) those that result from therapeutic cardiovascular, including operative, procedures (see earlier discussion).[83] Aggressive and early treatment of most serious congenital heart disease has decreased the incidence of cerebral abscesses, infarcts, and mental retardation due to *naturally occurring,* untreated disease, but it is ironic that increasingly used novel approaches to treatment have become associated with a new and evolving set of clinical problems that affect the brain and spinal cord.

Congenital heart disease predisposes to cerebral emboli by one or more of the following mechanisms: right-to-left shunts, an increased predisposition to endocarditis, and arrhythmias, especially atrial fibrillation. Factors contributing to cerebral ischemia include hypoxemia and increased blood viscosity with peripheral sludging, as well as various clotting abnormalities.[83] Among 29 patients who experienced stroke complicating cyanotic congenital heart disease in one study,[84] the most common lesion was cerebral venous thrombosis, including thrombosis of the dural sinuses. Only 10% of stroke patients had arterial occlusions. Young cyanotic children with hypochromic microcytic anemia seemed to be at particular risk for stroke. Terplan, in a detailed necropsy analysis of approximately 500 children with congenital heart disease of various forms—shunting lesions in 172 patients, hypoplastic right heart syndrome in 125, hypoplastic left heart syndrome in 89, transposition of the great vessels in 86,

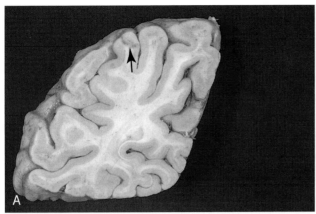

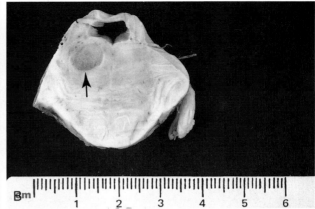

Figure 15-19 • Sections of brain from a 40-year-old male who developed a sarcoma of the left atrial endocardium. *A,* Metastases were present (arrows) in the cerebral hemispheres and *B,* the pontine tegmentum.

aortic coarctation in 26—found 17% had experienced thromboembolic infarcts. They were four to five times more common in surgical than in nonsurgical patients; 18 were noted in direct association with catheterization, whereas 21 were identified after catheterization and surgical procedures.[85] Focal or diffuse anoxic-ischemic necrosis of the cortex was four times more common in surgical than in nonsurgical patients.

A small postmortem study of cerebral complications of congenital heart disease and heart surgery carried out in eastern Europe in 1986 showed that damage to white matter was more likely in those under the age of 3 months, whereas older infants and children more commonly sustained injury to gray matter.[86] Necrosis, when detected, did not appear to be a complication of microembolization. In our autopsy experience at a large referral center for congenital heart disease, unusual cerebral hemorrhagic and necrotic lesions are frequently encountered in infants who come to autopsy (Figs. 15-20, 15-21). As discussed, patients with relatively minor congenital car-

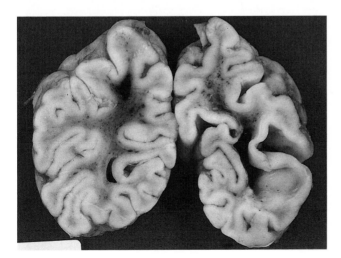

Figure 15-20 • Coronal section of brain from a 7-week-old child with transposition of the great vessels and a patent ductus arteriosus. Note extensive hemorrhage in the deep white matter. Microscopic sections showed platelet-fibrin thrombi in many of the brain's microvessels.

diac anomalies such as atrial or ventricular septal defects can present with a cerebral infarction caused by paradoxical thromboembolism. Thus, a previously undocumented congenital heart abnormality should be suspected in any young or middle-aged patient who presents with stroke (Fig. 15-22 and see Fig. 15-17).

Surgical treatment of congenital cardiac anomalies produces a spectrum of complications similar to those seen with other types of open heart surgery.[83] The Fontan procedure, for example, is associated with a 2.6% incidence of subsequent stroke.[87] Sensitive neuroimaging methods indicate that abnormal MRI scans may be seen in almost 75% of children after open heart surgery.[88] Lesions identified include diffuse findings of hypoxic-ischemic encephalopathy and focal infarcts. In that study, diffuse MRI abnormalities and various neurologic sequelae were commonly observed after prolonged hypothermic circulatory arrest.[88] As this investigation further emphasizes, modern brain imaging methods are likely to detect major brain malformations such as neuronal migration disorders that occur coincident with, though not necessarily because of, congenital cardiac lesions, an association that is increasingly well documented.[83]

Embolic stroke has been associated with aneurysm of the atrial septum.[89] This is an uncommon entity of occult origin (see Chapter 1 also); clinical examination and ECG results do not necessarily confirm the diagnosis although the lesion may be detected by two-dimensional echocardiography. Even though an atrial septal aneurysm may coexist with a stroke syndrome, a cause-and-effect relationship between the two is not well established in every case. In one review of 36 patients with echocardiographic findings typical of atrial septal aneurysm,[90] more than 25% had significant cerebrovascular events. In 5 of 10 patients with strokes, a definite embolic origin related to a septal aneurysm could be established. TIAs, probably of embolic origin, occurred in two individuals, and one experienced a peripheral embolus. The cause of the embolic events was postulated to be a thrombus associated with the septal aneurysm. Some investigators stress that atrial septal aneurysm should be considered in patients who have simultaneous emboli in both pulmonary and sys-

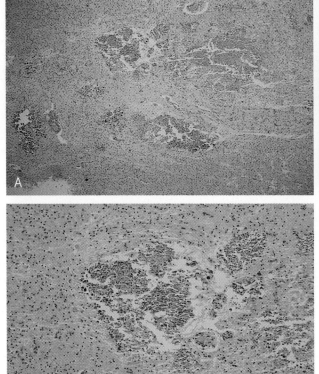

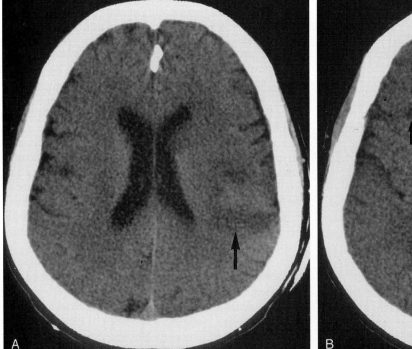

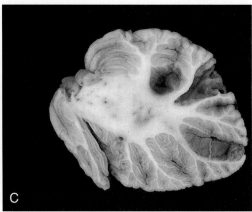

Figure 15-21 • *A* and *B,* Neuropathologic findings in a 2-month-old patient with Ebstein anomaly, including pulmonary atresia and an atrioseptal defect. A complicated clinical course followed a Blalock-Taussig procedure. Renal insufficiency, sepsis, and a seizure disorder developed, culminating in death 2 months after surgery. Numerous sections throughout the brain showed foci of necrosis and white matter calcification, as illustrated in these micrographs. *B,* Linear calcifications suggest deposition onto necrotic axons, whereas adjacent brain shows some intact neurons and astrocytic gliosis (*A* and *B,* H&E stain). *C,* Section of cerebellum from a 54-year-old patient with Ebstein anomaly. The patient had undergone numerous surgical procedures. The inferior surface of the cerebellum shows an old wedge-shaped cystic infarct and immediately adjacent to that, recent hemorrhagic infarcts.

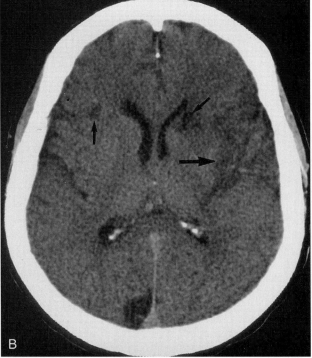

Figure 15-22 • A 30-year-old woman with severe cyanotic congenital heart disease and elevated hematocrit values presented with the sudden onset of aphasia and right-sided weakness. *A* and *B,* CT scans show hypodensity involving the left frontal lobe and insular region (large arrows in both panels) consistent with infarcts. Smaller old infarcts are seen in the left caudate head and right frontal lobe (small arrows in *B*). Angiograms showed lack of filling of many left middle cerebral artery sylvian branches.

temic circulations[91]; the only other clinicopathologic entities that apparently can produce such a syndrome are atrial septal aneurysm, biatrial myxoma, and paradoxical embolism.

Cerebral abscess remains an important potential complication of congenital heart disease, sometimes a consequence of infective endocarditis and almost always associated with a right-to-left shunt of the type seen in tetralogy of Fallot or transposition of the great vessels.[83] Approximately half of all brain abscesses result from infections in the paranasal sinuses, middle ear, or dental roots, with direct spread of infection to the nearby CNS.[5] Congenital heart disease accounts for 10 to 20% of cerebral abscesses, and such abscesses emerge as complications in as many as 2% of children with cyanotic congenital heart disease[83]; a peak incidence of abscesses occurs at age 4 to 7 years. Usually, the abscesses are solitary but in one series, 38% of patients with multiple brain abscesses had congenital heart disease as an underlying cause.[92] They result from a combination of factors: the pulmonary circulation is bypassed by septic microemboli, blood viscosity is elevated due to polycythemia, and there is cerebral hypoxia.[5] Single or multiple brain abscesses, whether secondary to congenital heart disease or resulting from any other cause such as bronchiectasis or infective endocarditis in adults, carry a mortality rate of 20 to 25%.[92] Whereas among all cerebral abscesses the most common causal pathogen is *Streptococcus milleri,* the most common bacteria isolated in patients with congenital heart disease as well as this complication are streptococcal or staphylococcal species, *Haemophilus* species, and *Neisseria gonorrhoeae.*[93]

NEUROPATHOLOGIC COMPLICATIONS OF CARDIAC TRANSPLANTATION

Orthotopic heart transplants are being used with increasing frequency to treat conditions such as coronary artery disease, cardiomyopathy, viral myocarditis, and congenital heart disease (see Chapter 23 also). As one large series indicates, the mortality rate for this procedure has been less than 10%[94] since the advent of the use of cyclosporine as an antirejection medication. Survival rates are in the range of 82% for 1 year, 60 to 70% for 5 years, and 41% for 10 years. Causes of death in the Stanford study most commonly included rejection (14% of deaths), infection (34%), graft coronary disease (18%), nonspecific graft failure (3%), malignancy (10%), and stroke and pulmonary hypertension (3% each).[94] In an autopsy study of 81 patients,[95] the most common causes of death were chronic rejection (30%), infection (usually pulmonary, 23%), and acute rejection (19%), and embolism was given as a contributory cause of death in 14% of patients. Studies focusing on neurologic and neuropathologic complications of heart transplantation are usually smaller and emphasize that neurologic disease is rarely the proximate cause of death. They suggest, however, that a high percentage (70 to 80%) of cases have significant neuropathologic findings, most commonly cerebral infarcts or regions consistent with diffuse or multifocal an-

oxic-ischemic encephalopathy. These are especially common in patients who receive a heart transplant for ischemic coronary artery disease[96] (Fig. 15-23; Table 15-2). Given the high frequency of cerebral infarcts in various conditions for which heart transplantation may be the ultimate therapy, a prosector should keep in mind that such infarcts, when discovered at necropsy, may well have antedated transplant surgery.[97, 98]

Intracranial hemorrhages in various compartments and opportunistic infections occur less frequently, the latter presenting as meningoencephalitis or brain abscess; commonly identified causal organisms include those listed in Table 15-2.[96-99] An unusual necrotizing white matter lesion that favors the pons (Fig. 15-24) is described in patients with various forms of immunosuppression, including that associated with heart transplantation.[97, 100] Infants and children undergoing such transplants have a surprisingly low incidence of severe acquired neurologic deficits despite pronounced metabolic and systemic abnormalities in the pre-, peri-, and post-transplantation periods.[101] Even the majority of infants treated before 6 months of age show normal growth, development, and neurologic outcome although postoperative seizures, which are sometimes transient, occur in as many as 20 to 25% of survivors.[102] Systemic lymphomas occur in a small percentage of adults after heart transplantation,[99] but primary CNS lymphoma or CNS involvement by disseminated lymphomatosis or related lymphoproliferative disorders are not well-documented in this patient population.

Increasingly, the more technically demanding procedure of combined heart and lung transplantation is being performed. Patients who die subsequent to this procedure overwhelmingly show cardiac or pulmonary lesions or both, for example, obliterative bronchiolitis.[103] Documented CNS infections include the spectrum of microorganisms seen in patients with heart transplantation.[104] Studies from large centers reemphasize the low frequency of CNS opportunistic infections (approximately 3%) in the cyclosporine era.[104] One heart-lung transplant recipient developed an acute disseminated encephalomyelitis of unknown cause.[105] Increasingly, idiopathic chronic CNS inflammatory foci are observed in organ transplant recipients.[106] Manifest as microglial nodules or chronic meningeal inflammatory infiltrates, they may be caused by as yet unrecognized viral opportunistic pathogens or unusual autoimmune phenomena. The identification of their origin and significance poses a major challenge to the neuropathologist.

EFFECTS OF NERVOUS SYSTEM LESIONS ON THE HEART

We now turn to the "flip side" of the heart-brain interface and examine the effects of CNS lesions on myocardial function and structure. Many effects of CNS abnormalities on the heart are better understood in physiologic and biochemical terms than in pathologic ones. The emerging field of cardiovascular neurobiology focuses on central and peripheral nervous system influences on the heart and blood vessels. It concerns itself with CNS and

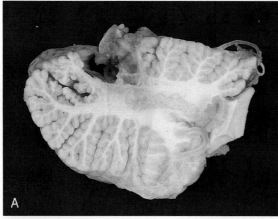

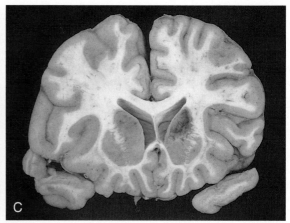

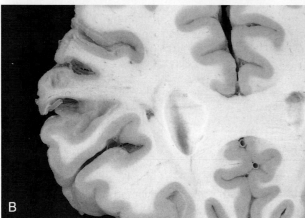

Figure 15-23 • Encephalic infarcts after orthotopic heart transplant. The patient was a 45-year-old male with familial cardiomyopathy who had undergone a transplant 14 months antemortem and had had recent acute allograft rejection. He died suddenly at home. Sections of the brain showed large, old cystic infarcts *A,* in the upper cerebellum and *B,* in the frontal lobe. *C,* In 59-year-old female, a heart transplantation 5 years prior to death had been complicated by several episodes of rejection. Two weeks prior to death, immunosuppressive therapy was changed, and she began to experience progressive dyspnea and weakness. At autopsy, multiple infarcts were found throughout the myocardium. In addition to the cystic infarct identified in the right caudate nucleus, there was focal cortical laminar necrosis.

peripheral, especially autonomic, nervous system control of heart rate and blood pressure via the balance of sympathetic and parasympathetic innervation, fundamental brainstem mechanisms of cardiovascular regulation, and autonomic interactions with neuroendocrine regulatory mechanisms, the details of which are beyond the scope of this chapter.[107-109] Important anatomic components of feedback loops between the heart and the CNS include the vagus (parasympathetic) and sympathetic nerves, which carry afferent fibers from the heart through dorsal root ganglia at the T1–T5 spinal cord levels into the cord itself.[109] Cardiac efferents include parasympathetic fibers originating in the nuclei ambiguus and sympathetic fibers originating in the upper four to five thoracic segments of the spinal cord. Entering the heart, sympathetic fibers are uniformly and widely distributed, whereas parasympathetic fibers are concentrated in the sinoatrial and atrioventricular nodes.[109] Cardiac function may be altered by surgical interruption of the cardiac nerves or by incomplete denervation, as occurs in primarily autonomic neuropathies. Although most autonomic influences on the heart and lungs are thought to originate in the brainstem or spinal cord, these structures may have significant input from limbic cortex via the hypothalamus; other basal or deep central gray matter structures, such as the basal ganglia, amygdala, and subthalamus, may be involved.[110] Furthermore, it has been suggested[107] that stimulation of the right insular cortex in humans augments sympathetic cardiovascular tone, whereas stimulation of the left insula

increases parasympathetic drive. A logical consequence of this would be that right middle cerebral artery territory infarcts disinhibit insular function which, in turn, would

TABLE 15-2 • **Neurologic and Neuropathologic Complications of Cardiac and Heart-lung Transplantation**

Vascular

Anoxic-ischemic lesions, infarcts, laminar necrosis (secondary to hypotension, loss of microvascular autoregulation)

Emboli (e.g., air, particulate, fat)

Hemorrhages (e.g., with coagulopathy, disseminated intravascular coagulation)

Infection (abscess, meningoencephalitis)

Fungal Organisms
Candida, Aspergillus, Mucormycosis, Nocardia, Cryptococcus

Parasitic Organisms
Toxoplasma gondii

Bacterial Organisms
Listeria monocytogenes, Staphylococcus aureus

Viral Organisms
Cytomegalovirus
Other herpesviruses

Lymphoma (usually outside CNS)

Metabolic Encephalopathy

Multifocal Necrotizing Leukoencephalopathy

Chronic Encephalomyelitis (with microglial nodules, demyelination)

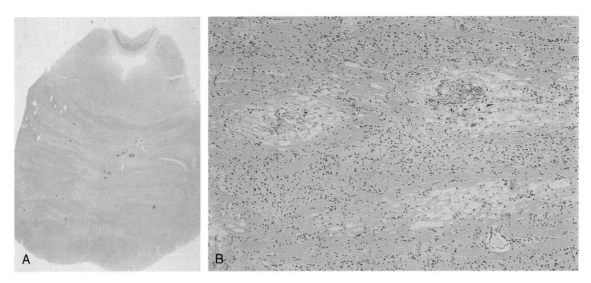

Figure 15-24 • Multifocal necrotizing leukoencephalopathy. This curious lesion, most common in the pons, is noted in individuals who manifest immunosuppression either because of naturally occurring disease such as acquired immunodeficiency syndrome (AIDS) or as a result of therapy (for heart, liver, or bone marrow transplantation; for details, see Anders and colleagues[100]). *A,* Lesions (here of the pons) can sometimes be appreciated on whole mount sections as punctate regions of microcalcification scattered throughout the basis pontis. *B,* At higher magnification, the lesions show multifocal vacuolization with neuroaxonal spheroids and, often, calcification, usually within white matter tracts, as in this section from the basis pontis (*A* and *B,* H&E stain).

produce increased sympathetic tone to mediate the cardiac manifestations of acute stroke.

It is now well established that cardiac dysfunction occurring secondary to hemorrhagic or ischemic stroke, especially subarachnoid hemorrhage, is a major contributor to stroke-related morbidity and mortality.[111] Animals with experimental subarachnoid hemorrhage develop cardiac arrhythmias; ventricular arrhythmias occur, however, only in those with intact cervical sympathetic fibers or spinal cord. Much experimental evidence (reviewed by Norris and Hachinski[111]) suggests that stimulation of various regions of the brain, including the frontal neocortex, as well as sham neurosurgical procedures in experimental animals, artificial increases in intracranial pressure, and

intracerebral infusions of blood that mimic primary intracerebral hemorrhage, all cause abnormalities that are revealed by electrocardiogram and cause microfoci of myocardial necrosis (usually contraction band necrosis). In at least some experimental paradigms, these effects appear to be mediated by increases in plasma catecholamines.

Accumulated clinical observations over the past 40 years also suggest indirectly that catastrophic stroke (e.g., subarachnoid hemorrhage, massive cerebral infarct, or intraparenchymal hemorrhage) is associated with cardiac arrhythmias and myocardial necrosis (Fig. 15-25). The frequency of these abnormalities is highest in patients with subarachnoid hemorrhage, occurring in 20% to almost 100% of afflicted individuals by various estimates,[112] but

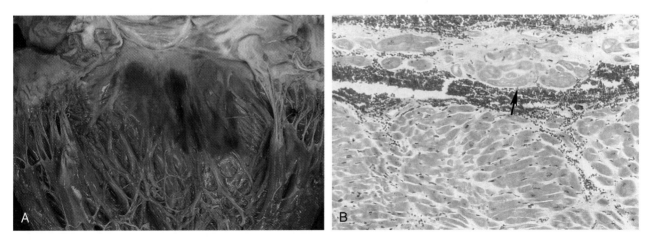

Figure 15-25 • Endocardial surface of left ventricle in a patient who died of multiple cerebral hemorrhagic metastatic tumor deposits, with raised intracranial pressure and secondary brainstem hemorrhages. *A,* Extensive subendocardial hemorrhage. *B,* Microscopic section of the endocardial surface (ventricular cavity at top) shows acute subendocardial hemorrhage. Some fibers adjacent to the hemorrhage show early necrotic change (arrow) (H&E stain).

arrhythmias occur in over 75% of those with intracerebral hemorrhage and in almost 25% of individuals with large cerebral infarcts.[111, 113] Even atrial fibrillation, a condition previously considered an important cause of ischemic stroke, has been attributed to acute stroke in some individuals.[114]

Neurogenic pulmonary edema is a well-described complication of subarachnoid hemorrhage and other catastrophic CNS lesions, including acute massive stroke (see Chapter 7 also). It may also occur, rarely, with a prolonged epileptic seizure.[111] Neurogenic pulmonary edema is usually associated with a sudden and dramatic rise in intracranial pressure, possibly resulting from hypothalamic dysfunction, with consequent autonomic discharge producing systemic and pulmonary vasoconstriction; the final pathophysiologic mechanisms are extraordinarily complex and are probably related to massive increases in pulmonary capillary pressure and changes in capillary permeability.[110, 111] Although neurogenic pulmonary edema is generally believed to be noncardiogenic, a reversible form of myocardial injury has been observed in patients with subarachnoid hemorrhage who experience such edema.[115] Finally, lung function in stroke patients may be compromised by pulmonary emboli originating from deep venous thrombosis in a paralyzed limb.[116, 117]

The unraveling of the pathophysiology of the manifestations of CNS lesions in cardiac and pulmonary circulations will begin with meticulous clinicopathologic observation that suggests experimental approaches to these extremely complex problems.

Acknowledgments

Ongoing work in one author's (HVV's) laboratory is supported by PHS Grant **P01 AG 12435**. Technical assistance in specimen preparation was provided by Alex Brooks, Yan Cheng, and Vicki Freeman. Carol Appleton assisted with the preparation of figures.

REFERENCES

1. Adams RD, Victor M, Ropper AH: Principles of Neurology. 6th ed. New York, McGraw-Hill, 1997
2. Stehbens WE: Pathology of the Cerebral Blood Vessels. St. Louis, CV Mosby, 1972
3. Barnett HJM, Mohr JP, Stein BM, Yatsu FM (eds): Stroke Pathophysiology, Diagnosis, and Management. 3rd ed. New York, Churchill Livingstone, 1998
4. Toole JF (ed): Cerebrovascular Disorders. 3rd ed. New York, Raven, 1984
5. Ellison DW, Love S, Chimelli L, et al (eds): Neuropathology. A Reference Text of CNS Pathology. London, Mosby-Wolfe, 1998
6. Batjer HH (ed): Cerebrovascular Disease. Philadelphia, Lippincott-Raven, 1997
7. Fisher CM, Gore I, Okabe N, White PD: Atherosclerosis of the carotid and vertebral arteries—extracranial and intracranial. J Neuropathol Exp Neurol 24:455, 1965
8. Wolf PA, Kannel WB, Cupples LA, D'Agostino RB: Risk factor interaction in cardiovascular and cerebrovascular disease. In: Furlan AJ (ed): The Heart and Stroke. London-Berlin, Springer-Verlag, 1987, p 331
9. Dávila-Román VG, Barzilai B, Wareing TH et al: Atherosclerosis of the ascending aorta. Prevalence and role as an independent predictor of cerebrovascular events in cardiac patients. Stroke 25: 2010, 1994
10. Moossy J: Cerebral atherosclerosis: Morphology and some relationships with coronary atherosclerosis. In Zülch KJ, Kaufmann W, Hossmann K-A, Hossmann V (eds): Brain and Heart Infarct. Berlin-Heidelberg Springer-Verlag, 1977, p 253
11. Graor RA, Hetzer NR: Management of coexistent carotid artery and coronary artery disease. Curr Concepts Cerebrovasc Dis Stroke 23:19, 1988
12. Furlan AJ, Craciun AR: Risk of stroke during coronary artery bypass graft surgery in patients with internal carotid artery disease documented by angiography. Stroke 16:797, 1985
13. Fisher CM, Adams RD: Observations on brain embolism with special reference to hemorrhagic infarction. In: Furlan AJ (ed): The Heart and Stroke. London-Berlin, Springer-Verlag, 1987
14. Hart RG, Easton JD: Hemorrhagic infarcts. Stroke 17:586, 1986
15. Lodder J, Krijne-Kubat B, van der Lugt PJM: Timing of autopsy-confirmed hemorrhagic infarction with reference to cardioembolic stroke. Stroke 19:1482, 1988
16. Lodder J, Krijne-Kubat B, Broekman J: Cerebral hemorrhagic infarction at autopsy: Cardiac embolic cause and the relationship to the cause of death. Stroke 17:626, 1986
17. Fisher CM: The history of cerebral embolism and hemorrhagic infarction. In: Furlan AJ (ed): The Heart and Stroke. London-Berlin, Springer-Verlag, 1987, p 3
18. Foulkes MA, Wolf PA, Price TR, et al: The stroke data bank: Design, methods, and baseline characteristics. Stroke 19:547, 1988
19. Mohr JP, Caplan LR, Melski JW, et al: The Harvard cooperative stroke registry: A prospective registry. Neurology 28:754, 1978
20. Bogousslavsky J, Cachin C, Regli F, et al: Cardiac sources of embolism and cerebral infarction—clinical consequences and vascular concomitants: The Lausanne Stroke Registry. Stroke 41:855, 1991
21. Cerebral Embolism Task Force: Cardiogenic brain embolism. The second report of the cerebral embolism task force. Arch Neurol 46:727, 1989
22. Furlan AJ: Stroke: The heart of the matter. Stroke 17:583, 1986
23. Minematsu K, Yamaguchi T, Omae T: "Spectacular shrinking deficit": Rapid recovery from a major hemispheric syndrome by migration of an embolus. Neurology 42:157, 1992
24. Oder W, Siostrzonek P, Lang W, et al: Distribution of ischemic cerebrovascular events in cardiac embolism. Klin Wochenschr 69: 757, 1991
25. Furlan AJ (ed): The Heart and Stroke. Exploring Mutual Cerebrovascular and Cardiovascular Issues. London-Berlin, Springer-Verlag, 1987
26. Barnett HJM: Heart in ischemic stroke—a changing emphasis. Neurol Clin 1:291, 1983
27. Kealy WF: Atheroembolism. J Clin Pathol 31:984, 1978
28. deBono DP, Warlow CP: Potential sources of emboli in patients with presumed transient cerebral or retinal ischaemia. Lancet 1: 343, 1981
29. Shuaib A, Hachinski VC, Oczkowski WJ: Transient ischemic attacks and normal cerebral angiograms: A follow-up study. Stroke 19:1223, 1988
30. Halperin JL, Hart RG: Atrial fibrillation and stroke: New ideas, persisting dilemmas. Stroke 19:937, 1988
31. Moss AJ: Atrial fibrillation and cerebral embolism. Arch Neurol 41:707, 1984
32. Sherman DG, Goldman L, Whiting RB, et al: Thromboembolism in patients with atrial fibrillation. Arch Neurol 41:708, 1984
33. Kempster PA, Gerraty RP, Gates PC: Asymptomatic cerebral infarction in patients with chronic atrial fibrillation. Stroke 19:955, 1988
34. Petersen P, Godtfredsen J: Embolic complications in paroxysmal atrial fibrillation. Stroke 17:622, 1986
35. The Stroke Prevention in Atrial Fibrillation Investigators: Predictors of thromboembolism in atrial fibrillation. I. Clinical features of patients at risk. Ann Intern Med 116:1, 1992
36. Salgado ED, Furlan AJ, Conomy JP: Cardioembolic sources of stroke. In: Furlan AJ (ed): The Heart and Stroke. London-Berlin, Springer-Verlag, 1987, p 47
37. Hart RG, Foster JW, Luther MF, Kanter MC: Stroke in infective endocarditis. Stroke 21:695, 1990
38. Le Cam B, Guivarch G, Boles JM, et al: Neurologic complications in a group of 86 bacterial endocarditis. Eur Heart J 5(suppl C):97, 1984

39. Royden Jones H Jr, Siekert RG: Neurological manifestations of infective endocarditis. Brain 112:1295, 1989
40. Tunkel AR, Kaye D: Neurologic complications of infective endocarditis. Neurol Clin 11:419, 1993
41. Hart RG, Kagan-Hallet K, Joerns SE: Mechanisms of intracranial hemorrhage in infective endocarditis. Stroke 18:1048, 1987
42. Masuda J, Yutani C, Waki R, et al: Histopathological analysis of the mechanisms of intracranial hemorrhage complicating infective endocarditis. Stroke 23:843, 1992
43. Salgado AV, Furlan AJ, Keys TF: Mycotic aneurysm, subarachnoid hemorrhage, and indications for cerebral angiography in infective endocarditis. Stroke 18:1057, 1987
44. Roach MR, Drake CG: Ruptured cerebral aneurysms caused by micro-organisms. N Engl J Med 273:240, 1965
45. Molinari GF, Smith L, Goldstein MN, Satran R: Pathogenesis of cerebral mycotic aneurysms. Neurology 23:325, 1973
46. Vinters HV, Anders KH: Neuropathology of AIDS. Boca Raton, FL, CKC, 1990
47. Biller J, Challa VR, Toole JF, Howard VJ: Nonbacterial thrombotic endocarditis. A neurologic perspective of clinicopathologic correlations of 99 patients. Arch Neurol 39:95, 1982
48. Silver MD, Butany J: Complications of mechanical heart valve prostheses. Cardiovasc Clin 18:273, 1988
49. Keyser DL, Biller J, Coffman TT, Adams HP Jr: Neurologic complications of late prosthetic valve endocarditis. Stroke 21:472, 1990
50. Lauzier S, Barnett HJM: Cerebral ischemia with mitral valve prolapse and mitral annulus calcification. In: Furlan AJ (ed): The Heart and Stroke. London-Berlin, Springer-Verlag, 1987, p. 63
51. Furlan AJ, Craciun AR, Salcedo EE, Mellino M: Risk of stroke in patients with mitral annulus calcification. Stroke 15:801, 1984
52. Brockmeier LB, Adolph RJ, Gustin BW, et al: Calcium emboli to the retinal artery in calcific aortic stenosis. Am Heart J 101:32, 1981
53. Kapila A, Hart R: Calcific cerebral emboli and aortic stenosis: Detection of computed tomography. Stroke 17:619, 1986
54. Adams JH, Brierley JB, Connor RCR, Treip CS: The effects of systemic hypotension upon the human brain. Clinical and neuropathological observations in 11 cases. Brain 89:235, 1966
55. Komrad MS, Coffey CE, Coffey KS, et al: Myocardial infarction and stroke. Neurology 34:1403, 1984
56. Thompson PL, Robinson JS: Stroke after acute myocardial infarction: Relation to infarct size. Br Med J 2:457, 1978
57. Soloway HB, Aronson SM: Atheromatous emboli to central nervous system. Report of 16 cases. Arch Neurol 11:657, 1964
58. Colt HG, Begg RJ, Saporito JJ, et al: Cholesterol emboli after cardiac catheterization. Eight cases and a review of the literature. Medicine 67:389, 1988
59. Dimmick JE, Bove KE, McAdams AJ, Benzing G III: Fiber embolization—a hazard of cardiac surgery and catheterization. N Engl J Med 292:685, 1975
60. Ghatak NR: Pathology of cerebral embolization caused by nonthrombotic agents. Hum Pathol 6:599, 1975
61. Oliva A, Scherokman B: Two cases of occipital infarction following cardiac catheterization. Stroke 19:773, 1988
62. Furlan AJ, Jones SC: Central nervous system complications related to open heart surgery. In: Furlan AJ (ed): The Heart and Stroke. London-Berlin, Springer-Verlag, 1987, p 287
63. Galbreath C, Salgado ED, Furlan AJ, Hollman J: Central nervous system complications of percutaneous transluminal coronary angioplasty. Stroke 17:616, 1986
64. Roessmann U, Zarchin LE: Cerebral bone marrow embolus after closed chest cardiac massage. Arch Neurol 36:58, 1979
65. Vagn-Hansen PL: Complications following external cardiac massage, with special emphasis on cerebral embolism. APMIS Sec. A 79:505, 1971
66. Walley VM, Stinson WA, Upton C, et al: Foreign materials found in the cardiovascular system after instrumentation or surgery (including a guide to their light microscopic identification). Cardiovasc Pathol 2:157, 1993
67. Kouchoukos NT: Adjuncts to reduce the incidence of embolic brain injury during operations on the aortic arch. Ann Thorac Surg 57:243, 1994
68. Fessatidis I, Prapas S, Hevas A, et al: Prevention of perioperative neurological dysfunction. A six-year perspective of cardiac surgery. J Cardiovasc Surg 32:570, 1991
69. Aguilar MJ, Gerbode F, Hill JD: Neuropathologic complications of cardiac surgery. J Thorac Cardiovasc Surg 61:676, 1971
70. Gilman S: Neurological complications of open heart surgery. Ann Neurol 28:475, 1990
71. Gilman S: Cerebral disorders after open-heart operations. N Engl J Med 272:489, 1965
72. Hill JD, Aguilar MJ, Baranco A, et al: Neuropathological manifestations of cardiac surgery. Ann Thorac Surg 7:409, 1969
73. Menkin M, Schwartzman RJ: Cerebral air embolism. Report of five cases and review of the literature. Arch Neurol 34:168, 1977
74. Moody DM, Bell MA, Challa VR, et al: Brain microemboli during cardiac surgery or aortography. Ann Neurol 28:477, 1990
75. Furlan AJ, Craciun AR, Raju NR, Hart N: Cerebrovascular complications associated with idiopathic hypertrophic subaortic stenosis. Stroke 15:282, 1984
76. Ranoux D, Cohen A, Cabanes L, et al: Patent foramen ovale: Is stroke due to paradoxical embolism? Stroke 24:31, 1993
77. Knepper LE, Biller J, Adams HP Jr, Bruno A: Neurologic manifestations of atrial myxoma. A 12-year experience and review. Stroke 19:1435, 1988
78. Sandok BA, von Estorff I, Giuliani ER: CNS embolism due to atrial myxoma. Clinical features and diagnosis. Arch Neurol 37:485, 1980
79. Roeltgen DP, Weimer GR, Patterson LF: Delayed neurologic complications of left atrial myxoma. Neurology 31:8, 1981
80. Thompson J, Kapoor W, Wechsler LR: Multiple strokes due to atrial myxoma with a negative echocardiogram. Stroke 19:1570, 1988
81. Huston KA, Combs JJ Jr, Lie JT, Giuliani ER: Left atrial myxoma simulating peripheral vasculitis. Mayo Clin Proc 53:752, 1978
82. Kasarskis EJ, O'Connor W, Earle G: Embolic stroke from cardiac papillary fibroelastomas. Stroke 19:1171, 1988
83. Park SC, Neches WH: The neurologic complications of congenital heart disease. Neurol Clin 11:441, 1993
84. Cottrill CM, Kaplan S: Cerebral vascular accidents in cyanotic congenital heart disease. Am J Dis Child 125:484, 1973
85. Terplan KL: Patterns of brain damage in infants and children with congenital heart disease. Association with catheterization and surgical procedures. Am J Dis Child 125:175, 1973
86. Bozóky B, Bara D, Kertész E: Autopsy study of cerebral complications of congenital heart disease and cardiac surgery. J Neurol 231:153, 1984
87. de Plessis AJ, Chang AC, Wessel DL, et al: Cerebrovascular accidents following the Fontan operation. Ped Neurol 12:230, 1995
88. Miller G, Mamourian AC, Tesman JR, et al: Long-term MRI changes in brain after pediatric open heart surgery. J Child Neurol 9:390, 1994
89. Di Pasquale G, Andreoli A, Grazi P, et al: Cardioembolic stroke from atrial septal aneurysm. Stroke 19:640, 1988
90. Belkin RN, Hurwitz BJ, Kisslo J: Atrial septal aneurysm: Association with cerebrovascular and peripheral embolic events. Stroke 18:856, 1987
91. Cheng TO, Kisslo J: Atrial septal aneurysm as a cause of cerebral embolism in young patients (letter). Stroke 19:408, 1988
92. Basit AS, Ravi B, Banerji AK, Tandon PN: Multiple pyogenic brain abscesses: An analysis of 21 patients. J Neurol Neurosurg Psychiatr 52:591, 1989
93. Kaplan K: Brain abscess. Med Clin North Am 69:345, 1985
94. Sarris GE, Moore KA, Schroeder JS, et al: Cardiac transplantation: The Stanford experience in the cyclosporine era. J Thorac Cardiovasc Surg 108:240, 1994
95. Rose AG, Viviers L, Odell JA: Autopsy-determined causes of death following cardiac transplantation. A study of 81 patients and literature review. Arch Pathol Lab Med 116:1137, 1992
96. Prayson RA, Estes ML: The neuropathology of cardiac allograft transplantation. An autopsy study of 18 patients. Arch Pathol Lab Med 119:59, 1995
97. Ang LC, Gillett JNR, Kaufmann JCE: Neuropathology of cardiac transplant: A review of 18 cases. J Neuropathol Exp Neurol 46:402, 1987
98. Adair JC, Call GK, O'Connell JB, Baringer JR: Cerebrovascular syndromes following cardiac transplantation. Neurology 42:819, 1992

99. Montero CG, Martinez AJ: Neuropathology of heart transplantation: 23 cases. Neurology 36:1149, 1986
100. Anders KH, Becker PS, Holden JK, et al: Multifocal necrotizing leukoencephalopathy with pontine predilection in immunosuppressed patients: A clinicopathologic review of 16 cases. Hum Pathol 24:897, 1993
101. Lynch BJ, Glauser TA, Canter C, Spray T: Neurologic complications of pediatric heart transplantation. Arch Pediatr Adolesc Med 148:973, 1994
102. Baum M, Chinnock R, Ashwal S, et al: Growth and neurodevelopmental outcome of infants undergoing heart transplantation. J Heart Lung Transplant 12:S211, 1993
103. Tazelaar HD, Yousem SA: The pathology of combined heart-lung transplantation: An autopsy study. Hum Pathol 19:1403, 1988
104. Hall WA, Martinez AJ, Dummer JS, et al: Central nervous system infections in heart and heart-lung transplant recipients. Arch Neurol 46:173, 1989
105. Horowitz MB, Comey C, Hirsch W, et al: Acute disseminated encephalomyelitis (ADEM) or ADEM-like inflammatory changes in a heart-lung transplant recipient: A case report. Neuroradiology 37:434, 1995
106. Ferreiro JA, Robert MA, Townsend J, Vinters HV: Neuropathologic findings after liver transplantation. Acta Neuropathol 84:1, 1992
107. Oppenheimer S: The anatomy and physiology of cortical mechanisms of cardiac control. Stroke 24[suppl I]:I3, 1993
108. Barnes KL, Ferrario CM: Role of the central nervous system in cardiovascular regulation. In: Furlan AJ (ed): The Heart and Stroke. Berlin-London, Springer-Verlag, 1987, p 155
109. Talman WT, Kelkar P: Neural control of the heart. Central and peripheral. Neurol Clin 11:239, 1993
110. Samuels MA: Neurally induced cardiac damage. Definition of the problem. Neurol Clin 11:273, 1993
111. Norris JW, Hachinski VC: Cardiac dysfunction following stroke. In: Furlan AJ (ed): The Heart and Stroke. London-Berlin, Springer-Verlag, 1987, p 171
112. Weaver JP, Fisher M: Subarachnoid hemorrhage: An update of pathogenesis, diagnosis and management. J Neurol Sci 125:119, 1994
113. Hachinski VC: The clinical problem of brain and heart. Stroke 24[suppl I]:I1, 1993
114. Vingerhoets F, Bogousslavsky J, Regli F, Van Melle G: Atrial fibrillation after acute stroke. Stroke 24:26, 1993
115. Mayer SA, Fink ME, Homma S, et al: Cardiac injury associated with neurogenic pulmonary edema following subarachnoid hemorrhage. Neurology 44:815, 1994
116. Wijdicks EFM, Scott JP: Pulmonary embolism associated with acute stroke. Mayo Clin Proc 72:297, 1997
117. Stein PD: Pulmonary embolism after acute stroke. Mayo Clin Proc 72:381, 1997

Chapter 16

Cardiovascular Effects of Systemic Diseases and Conditions

· · · · ·

Wanda M. Lester • Avrum I. Gotlieb

Many systemic disorders and conditions involve the cardiovascular system. Sometimes their effects on the heart and blood vessels are a major feature of the illness, whereas in other circumstances, involvement of the cardiovascular system is interesting but not very important. Both kinds of conditions are included here.

Metabolic, familial, endocrine, and rheumatologic disorders are considered in this chapter, in alphabetic order, with these exceptions: *anorexia nervosa* and *cachexia* are presented in the section on Malnutrition; *antiphospholipid antibody syndrome* under Systemic Lupus Erythematosus; *beriberi* under Thiamine Deficiency: *hypercalcemia* and *hypocalcemia* under Parathyroid Disorders; and *pheochromocytoma* under Adrenal Disorders.

Not discussed in this chapter are the *cardiovascular consequences of infections,* and *sarcoidosis,* found in Chapter 9. Chapter 10 covers *cardiomyopathies. Hyperlipidemia* is considered in Chapter 4; *syphilis* in Chapter 5, *carcinoid syndrome* in Chapter 13; and *nonbacterial thrombotic endocarditis* in Chapter 14.

ADRENAL DISORDERS

Addison disease causes orthostatic hypotension, hyponatremia, and hypoglycemia.[1] It is potentially lethal. The electrocardiogram may demonstrate low voltage with flat or inverted T waves and a prolonged QTc interval.[2] At autopsy, heart weight is usually decreased.[3]

Aldosterone excess resulting from either an adrenal cortical adenoma or bilateral nodular hyperplasia causes hypertension and hypokalemia.[4] Echocardiographic left ventricular hypertrophy is found[5] and may exceed that seen in patients with essential hypertension and comparable degrees of blood pressure elevation.[6] Cardiac arrest may be the presenting symptom of hyperaldosteronism.[7]

The congenital disorders of steroid synthesis that cause hypertension result from deficiencies of 11-hydroxylase, 11-hydroxysteroid oxidoreductase, or 17-hydroxylase.[8]

More than 70% of patients with *Cushing syndrome* are hypertensive.[9] Echocardiography reveals left ventricular hypertrophy in 75%, sometimes with asymmetric septal hypertrophy.[10] A few patients present with congestive heart failure.[11] Apart from hypertension, other risk factors for atherosclerosis, such as diabetes mellitus and hyperlipidemia, are common in patients, and they have excessive mortality from ischemic heart disease.[12] Cushing syndrome and/or acromegaly can be a component of the familial cardiac myxoma syndrome (see Chapter 19).[13, 14]

Pheochromocytoma

Patients with pheochromocytoma are usually hypertensive, although the hypertension is paroxysmal in about 50% of them.[15] They also risk orthostatic hypotension.[16] Death from acute hypertension or shock may be precipitated by surgery. Heart weight was increased in 92% of the 26 cases studied by Van Vliet and associates.[17] Such myocardial hypertrophy can occur secondary to hypertension or as a direct effect of catecholamines on the myocardium. The hypertrophy pattern may mimic hypertrophic cardiomyopathy clinically[18] but not histologically, with the echocardiographic features at least partly regressing after tumor removal. Characteristically, intramyocardial hemorrhages are present; histologically they reveal foci of contraction-band necrosis with mononuclear inflammation (Fig. 16-1). These lesions can occur anywhere in the heart, but they tend to be more frequent in the inner portion of the left ventricular wall.[17] Patients with a pheochromocytoma may develop congestive heart failure. Occasionally a patient has been placed on a heart transplantation list before discovery of the tumor[19]; its removal usually results in normalization of cardiac function.

Patients with normal coronary arteries and pheochromocytoma may experience myocardial infarcts, presumably caused by coronary spasm.[20] Other vascular complications of pheochromocytoma include a sometimes reversible renal artery stenosis,[21] mesenteric artery vasoconstriction causing intestinal ischemia,[22] hypertension-induced carotid artery dissection,[23] intracerebral aneurysm rupture,[24] or leukocytoclastic vasculitis.[25] Occasionally the tumor grows into the inferior vena cava and thence into the right atrium.[26]

There appears to be an association between cyanotic congenital heart disease and pheochromocytoma, neuroblastoma, and ganglioneuroma,[27] suggesting a role for chronic hypoxia in tumor development.

In addition to catecholamines, pheochromocytomas produce a newly discovered peptide called adrenomedullin which has potent vasodilating, natriuretic, and diuretic effects.[28] The functions of adrenomedullin are currently under investigation.

Cardiac paragangliomas are reviewed in Chapter 19.

ALKAPTONURIA

Alkaptonuria is an autosomal recessive disorder caused by a deficiency of the enzyme homogentisate 1,2-dioxygenase, whose gene is located on chromosome 3q2.[29]

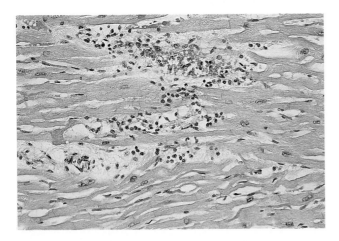

Figure 16-1 • Cardiac lesions in a patient with pheochromocytoma. There is myocardial contraction-band necrosis and a sparse mononuclear inflammatory infiltrate (H&E stain).

This deficiency results in increased homogentisic acid, a metabolite of tyrosine and phenylalanine. When secreted in the urine, it is oxidized to a melanin-like material that blackens the urine.[30] Polymerized homogentisic acid accumulates in connective tissue, where it appears blue-black grossly but histologically has a brown or ochre color. The term *ochronosis* is not specific for alkaptonuria but refers to any deposition of an ochre-colored material in connective tissue.[31]

In the cardiovascular system, polymerized homogentisic acid deposits are found in (1) the heart valves, especially valve annuli (Fig. 16-2*A*, *B*), within which they may predispose to calcific degeneration; (2) healed myocardial infarcts; (3) all three layers of arterial walls; and (4) atheromata.

The material is deposited within endothelial cells, macrophages, fibroblasts, and smooth muscle cells as well as extracellularly. The pigment is Masson-Fontana positive (argentaffin) and Prussian blue negative. Electron dense granules are seen ultrastructurally.[32]

α_1-ANTITRYPSIN DEFICIENCY

α_1-Antitrypsin deficiency is associated with a medial type of arterial fibromuscular dysplasia,[33] intracranial aneurysms, cervical internal carotid artery dissection,[34] and abdominal aortic aneurysm.[35] These vascular disorders are probably not very common in subjects with α_1-antitrypsin deficiency, but their precise frequency is not known. α_1-Antitrypsin may protect vascular tissue from enzymatic degradation.[35]

AMYLOIDOSIS–see also Chapter 3

Amyloid, a fibrillary protein with a β-pleated sheet structure, has an apple-green birefringence by Congo red stain and ultrastructurally consists of 7- to 10-nm diameter, rigid, nonbranching fibrils that can bind digoxin and calcium channel blockers.[36, 37] Because glycosaminoglycans are present in amyloid, the sulphated Alcian blue stain is useful for screening histologic material.[38] With the Gomori trichrome stain, amyloid tends to be gray-blue in contrast to the bright blue of collagen. Material suspicious for amyloid on either of these stains should be confirmed by Congo red staining. The congophilia of certain types of amyloid deposits (AA and β_2-microglobulin) is lost when the tissue is preincubated with potassium permanganate. Electron microscopy of heart biopsy material may reveal fibrils that resemble amyloid except that they have larger diameter. These tend to be associated with fibrosis. Congo red staining of the paraffin-embedded material is negative, however.[39]

A *microfibrillar cardiomyopathy* has been described in which there are deposits of eosinophilic material in subendocardial, interstitial, and perivascular sites. This material does not stain with Congo red. Ultrastructurally, it consists of bundles of microfibrils up to 17 nm wide.[40]

Amyloid may derive from several different proteins.[41] About 80% of North American patients with systemic amyloidosis have the primary (amyloid light chain, or

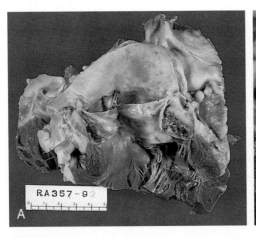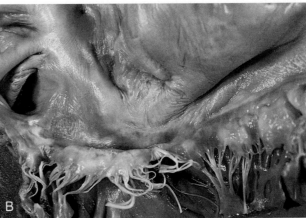

Figure 16-2 • Alkaptonuria. Gross photograph demonstrating: *A,* black discoloration of the aortic valve cusps, most prominent along the valve annulus, and *B,* black pigmentation along the mitral valve annulus, both caused by deposits of polymerized homogentisic acid.

AL) type, in which the fibrils originate from monoclonal κ or λ light chains. The λ light chains are twice as common as κ chains in patients with AL amyloidosis because λ light chains form fibrils more easily.[37] About 98% of patients with AL amyloidosis have an M protein in their serum or urine or have monoclonal plasma cells in the bone marrow. Most of the remaining patients have the secondary (amyloid A, or AA) type of amyloidosis, in which deposits derive from serum amyloid A protein. The underlying cause of AA amyloidosis is usually rheumatoid arthritis, chronic inflammatory bowel disease, tuberculosis, or leprosy. Cardiac involvement is not common in AA amyloidosis.[37] Other types that can affect the heart include senile, familial, isolated valvular, and β_2-microglobulin–related amyloidosis. Characterization of amyloid deposits as to their type is possible by use of immunohistochemistry.[41] This is important because of the possibility of treating AL amyloidosis.[42]

Clinical features of cardiac amyloidosis include heart failure, usually with restrictive physiology (see Chapter 10), and arrhythmias, especially heart block and atrial fibrillation. However angina pectoris, sudden death,[43] pericardial effusion, and even cardiac tamponade[44] have been reported. Electrocardiography tends to show a low voltage, especially in relation to cardiac mass.[45] Echocardiographic features include increased left ventricular wall thickness, sometimes mimicking gross features of hypertrophic cardiomyopathy; increased atrial septal thickness; and increased myocardial echogenicity, which may have a "sparkling" quality (Fig. 16-3A).[46] Doppler echocardiography shows impaired left ventricular diastolic filling.[47] The myocardium may take up increased amounts of technetium-99m (^{99m}Tc) pyrophosphate on scanning.[48] However, most of these techniques are of low sensitivity.[49] Scanning with iodine-123 (^{123}I)–labeled serum amyloid P component detects amyloid deposits but is reportedly less effective than echocardiography for studying cardiac involvement.[50]

Cardiac amyloid may recur in a transplanted heart.[51] There are preliminary reports of improved cardiac function when patients with AL amyloidosis were treated with melphalan[52] or bone marrow transplantation.[53]

Diagnosis may be made by heart biopsy. No practical distinction can be made among AL, senile, and familial amyloid by analysis of the extent or pattern of amyloid involvement in biopsy material.[54] It may accumulate in the endocardium or blood vessel walls, form nodules within the myocardium, or wrap around individual cardiac

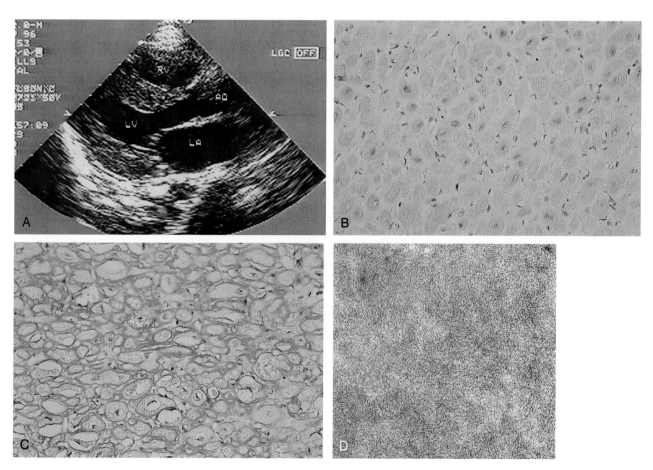

Figure 16-3 • Amyloidosis. *A,* Echocardiogram, parasternal long-axis view. The "sparkling" quality of the myocardium is strongly suggestive of amyloidosis. *B,* Amyloid deposits encircling cardiac myocytes (H&E stain). *C,* Such deposits stain green with sulfated alcian blue stain. *D,* Electron micrograph of amyloid illustrating straight, nonbranching, randomly oriented fibrils with a diameter of about 10 nm and lacking periodicity.

myocytes in an interstitial pericellular pattern (Fig. 16-3*B, C*).[54] Ultrastructural features are illustrated in Figure 16-3*D*.

At autopsy, heart weight is usually increased and the organ is firm and rubbery. Atrial dilation is common, whereas ventricles are of normal size. If the latter are dilated there is usually another explanation. The left ventricular septum is occasionally more than 1.3 times as thick as the free wall. Waxy brown amyloid deposits may be seen on the atrial endocardium or heart valves, especially the tricuspid and mitral valves[55] (see Fig. 3-1). In some cases, valvular deposits resemble candle grease droppings. Epicardial coronary artery amyloid does occur, but much less commonly than involvement of intramural coronary arteries. Often it is not clinically important.[41] Amyloid deposition within intramyocardial coronary arteries may be associated with focal myocardial infarcts that cause heart failure,[56] angina pectoris, or sudden death.[43] Amyloid is also found within the walls of myocardial lymphatics.[57] Although amyloid can be demonstrated within the cardiac conduction system, most rhythm disturbances in life are probably not caused by amyloid infiltration of the conduction tissue[58] per se. Amyloid involvement of peripheral arteries causing ischemia is occasionally reported.[41]

Familial Amyloidosis

The hereditary amyloidoses are autosomal dominant. Mutations occur in the genes for β-amyloid precursor protein, cystatin C, gelsolin, apolipoprotein A-I, lysozyme, fibrinogen α chain, or transthyretin.[59] The most common is familial amyloid polyneuropathy, which is caused by various mutations in the transthyretin gene. In this disorder, the amyloid is preferentially deposited in peripheral nerves and heart, with liver and kidney usually spared. Familial amyloidosis has been found among Portuguese, Swedish, Japanese, Jewish, Appalachian, and American black populations.[60] A late onset of symptoms is common; 44% of patients were diagnosed when 65 years old or older in one study.[61] Certain transthyretin mutations, for example Ala-60, are more often associated with cardiomyopathy than other mutations. Patients with an identical mutation may vary in their clinical features, however, and some have a mutant transthyretin but no amyloid deposits. Cardiac involvement causes heart failure and arrhythmias, especially bradyarrhythmias. Angina pectoris and sudden death also occur in some families.[62] Echocardiography may reveal ventricular hypertrophy, sometimes with disproportionate septal thickening. The myocardium may appear highly refractile[63] and show abnormal ^{99m}Tc pyrophosphate uptake.[48] Immunoelectrophoresis and immunofixation of serum, screening of a 24-hour urine specimen for monoclonal light chains, and bone marrow examination help exclude primary AL amyloidosis in these patients. Transthyretin can be demonstrated by immunohistochemical staining of deposits in biopsy material, and molecular biologic studies of blood detect transthyretin mutations.[61]

Histologic examination of hearts from a series of Swedish patients with familial amyloid polyneuropathy showed nodular amyloid deposits and amyloid encircling individual myocytes, with especially abundant deposits in the subendocardium and subepicardium and more amyloid in atria than in ventricles. Replacement and displacement of cells in the sinoatrial (SA) node by deposits were observed. Amyloid deposition also occurred in the SA node artery, although this did not narrow the vessel's lumen,[64] and in the atrioventricular (AV) conduction system.

Because transthyretin is produced in the liver, liver transplantation can eliminate abnormal transthyretin from the plasma. Some evidence of clinical improvement has been reported in patients so treated.[65]

Isolated Valvular Amyloidosis

Amyloid has been found in 15.5%[66] to 67%[67] of aortic and mitral valves removed surgically for valvular disease. It affected 14 to 45% of mitral valves and 17 to 88% of aortic valves. Deposits usually are not appreciated grossly and are detected by histologic examination. The amyloid is located in fibrotic and often calcified zones of the valve. Its congophilia is not altered by potassium permanganate treatment.[66] There is a significant association between valvular calcification and amyloid deposition,[67] with the latter thought to be a degenerative change.

Amyloid in Bioprosthetic Valves

Amyloid deposits have been found in one third of excised porcine bioprosthetic valves and also in the sewing ring of an autologous fascia lata valve.[68] The involved porcine valves had all been implanted for at least 33 months before excision for dysfunction. Amyloid deposits were small and found in the annulus, in parabasal parts of the cusps and in the spongiosa, and also occasionally in the muscle shelf of the right cusp. Sometimes deposits were found near calcification or macrophages. They were moderately to highly potassium permanganate sensitive in 60% of the affected porcine valves. In the remainder, the amyloid was resistant to potassium permanganate. It most likely derives from insudation of serum proteins.

Hemodialysis-Associated Amyloidosis

Patients receiving long-term hemodialysis therapy develop amyloidosis derived from β_2-microglobulin. Although this primarily involves joints and causes carpal tunnel syndrome, some patients develop deposits within blood vessel walls in other organs, including the heart. There may be a giant cell reaction to it. The congophilia of this form of amyloid is abolished by permanganate treatment. Cardiac involvement is asymptomatic, but vascular involvement in the gastrointestinal tract is sometimes associated with bowel perforation.[69]

ANDROGENS

Dehydroepiandrosterone and its sulfated metabolite dehydroepiandrosterone sulfate (DHEAS) are produced by the adrenal cortex. Levels are higher in men than in women and decrease with increasing age in adults. Some, but not all, studies revealed an inverse relationship between DHEAS concentration and cardiovascular mortality[70]; low levels of DHEAS have been associated with premature myocardial infarction in men.[71] In a follow-up study of 942 postmenopausal women, however, DHEAS concentration did not predict cardiovascular death.[72] An association between low levels of DHEAS and cardiac allograft vasculopathy has been reported.[73]

Serum testosterone drops during the fourth decade of life and rises again in the sixth decade in both men and women.[72] Anabolic steroids lower high-density lipoproteins (HDL) and tend to increase low-density lipoproteins (LDL). However, a small study of testosterone therapy in hypogonadal and elderly men revealed a decrease in total cholesterol and LDL cholesterol without a change in HDL cholesterol.[74] Testosterone may have a proaggregatory effect on platelets. However, testosterone can be aromatized to estradiol.[72] Studies of the relationship between estrogen level or estrogen/testosterone ratio and coronary atherosclerotic heart disease in men have generated controversy.[75–77]

Polycystic Ovaries

Women with the polycystic ovary syndrome have chronic anovulation, oligomenorrhea, hirsutism, and increased androgen levels; obesity and insulin resistance are also common. They have increased total cholesterol, LDL cholesterol, and triglycerides and lower HDL cholesterol when body mass index, age, and hormone use are controlled for. Carotid artery ultrasonography revealed significantly greater intima-media thickness in women with polycystic ovary syndrome than in control subjects,[78] suggesting increased atherosclerosis. Conversely, a study of women undergoing coronary angiography revealed an increased incidence of polycystic ovaries in those with more extensive coronary artery disease.[79]

Anabolic Steroids

Anabolic steroids, used by athletes to increase muscle mass, have deleterious effects on the cardiovascular system. They lower HDL cholesterol and may raise LDL cholesterol. They can elevate platelet counts, promote platelet aggregation,[80] and predispose to hypertension.[81] A 22-year-old weight lifter who used anabolic steroids and died of a myocardial infarction has been reported.[82] Echocardiographic studies of the effect of anabolic steroids on left ventricular morphology and function generated conflicting conclusions.[83, 84] (See Chapters 8 and 17 also.)

ANEMIA

Chronic anemia causes increased cardiac output and decreased blood viscosity.[85] At autopsy, cardiomegaly and chamber dilation are described. (See also the sections on sickle cell disease and thalassemia.)

ANKYLOSING SPONDYLITIS AND REITER SYNDROME

Ankylosing spondylitis and reactive arthritis or Reiter syndrome are spondyloarthropathies strongly associated with the human leukocyte antigen (HLA) type B27.[86] Secondary amyloidosis and cardiovascular disease are important causes of death in affected patients.[87] (See Chapter 5 also.) Typical cardiovascular disorders found in ankylosing spondylitis are aortic regurgitation and AV block; they are present in 10.1% and 8.5%, respectively, of patients who have had the disease for 30 years.[88] Both are more common in patients with peripheral joint involvement. Diastolic dysfunction of the left ventricle has also been reported. Pericarditis is uncommon.[88] AV block[89] and aortic regurgitation[90] also occur in patients with Reiter syndrome. Echocardiographic examination of patients with both conditions reveals aortic root dilation and aortic valve cusp thickening, with a subaortic fibrous ridge or bump (see Fig. 5-28) located between the anterior mitral valve leaflet and aortic valve cusps. In one series, a subaortic bump or cusp thickening was found in 11 of 36 patients in the absence of aortic regurgitation.[91]

At autopsy, patients with either ankylosing spondylitis or Reiter syndrome who had aortic regurgitation during life showed cardiomegaly, dilation of the aortic root, thickening of the sinus and proximal tubular aorta due to adventitial scar and intimal thickening, and a ridge of scar proximal to the aortic valve cusps, especially at the base of the anterior mitral valve leaflet. This latter can cause mitral regurgitation.[92] The scarring may also extend into the membranous septum, causing AV block. Aortic valve cusps are shortened, thickened, and fibrotic and tilt toward the left ventricle (Fig. 16-4). Commissural fusion is not found.

Histologically, the proximal ascending aorta shows

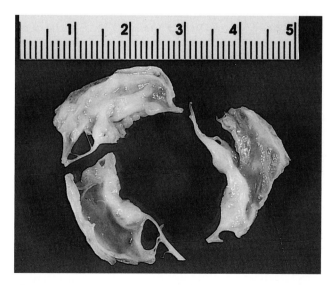

Figure 16-4 • Ankylosing spondylitis. These surgically excised aortic valve cusps demonstrate rolled edges due to valvular regurgitation caused by root dilatation. One cusp is diffusely thickened. Fenestrations are present near the free margins of the cusps. (Scale indicates centimeters.)

lymphocytes and plasma cells about the vasa vasorum, sometimes with luminal narrowing of these small vessels and medial scarring (see Fig. 5-27). The histologic features are similar to those of syphilitic aortitis. However, the process does not extend proximal to the aortic valve cusps in syphilis, and the diffuse thickening of cusps seen in ankylosing spondylitis does not occur in syphilis.[92] A mild increase in interstitial fibrous tissue was demonstrated by a morphometric study of the myocardium of patients with ankylosing spondylitis who had had no ischemic or valvular heart disease during life.[93]

BECKWITH-WIEDEMANN SYNDROME

The Beckwith-Wiedemann syndrome most commonly includes macroglossia, gigantism, and omphalocele. It predisposes to childhood tumors. Most cases are sporadic, but 15% are autosomal dominant. The disorder maps to chromosome 11p15.[94] The following cardiac anomalies have been reported: secundum atrial septal defect, ventricular septal defect, tetralogy of Fallot, patent ductus arteriosus, and hypoplastic left heart. Some patients have cardiomegaly of unknown cause.[95]

CARNITINE DISORDERS (FATTY ACID OXIDATION DEFECTS)

Carnitine deficiency is often secondary to defective fatty acid oxidation.[96] The myocardium depends on mitochondrial β oxidation of fatty acids to generate energy. To allow β oxidation, free fatty acids must be converted to acyl-coenzyme A (acyl-CoA) thioesters by acyl-CoA synthetases. Although short- and medium-chain fats directly enter the mitochondrial matrix, long-chain fats are converted to acyl-CoA forms in the cytoplasm and must be actively transported into mitochondria. The transport of long-chain acyl-CoA requires carnitine, which enters the cytoplasm via a transport protein. There is one specific carnitine transporter in the liver and another for other organs. Carnitine palmityl transferase I (CPT I), located on the inner part of the outer mitochondrial matrix, conjugates the long-chain acyl-CoA to carnitine. A translocase then moves long-chain acyl-carnitine to the inner mitochondrial membrane where CPT II removes the carnitine, so that it can shuttle back to the cytoplasm, and also releases long-chain acyl-CoA. The long-chain acyl-CoA undergoes a series of reactions that generate acetyl-CoA. These reactions involve a family of very long, long, medium, and short-chain acyl-CoA dehydrogenases.[97] (See further discussion in Chapter 10.)

Plasma Membrane Carnitine Transporter Deficiency

This prevents reabsorption of carnitine in the kidney, causing a systemic deficiency, and is an autosomal recessive condition.[96] Clinical manifestations include hydrops fetalis, hypoglycemia, childhood onset of dilated or hy-

pertrophic cardiomyopathy, muscle weakness, and lipid storage. Early treatment with carnitine is effective.[97] Systemic carnitine deficiency manifesting as familial endocardial fibroelastosis[98] was reported in 1981. More recently it was suggested that this is caused by a deficiency of the plasma membrane carnitine transporter.[99] Some patients have bizarre T waves on electrocardiography, resembling those found in posterior ischemia or hyperkalemia. Pathologic examination of the heart reveals biventricular hypertrophy, endocardial fibroelastosis, and prominent lipid deposits within cardiac myocytes. Mitochondrial atypia marked by variation in size and vacuoles is noted.

Antibiotics conjugated to pivalic acid to prolong the duration of their action may cause carnitine deficiency and a transient reduction of left ventricular mass.[100]

Carnitine/Acylcarnitine Translocase Deficiency

Deficiency of the mitochondrial membrane carnitine shuttle is rare. One reported newborn had ventricular arrhythmias, and another had paroxysmal heart block. Hypoglycemic hypoketotic episodes have been described. Carnitine levels are low in these patients.[97]

Carnitine Palmityl Transferase I and II Deficiency

Patients with CPT I deficiency may present with hypoketotic hypoglycemia and liver abnormalities.

CPT II deficiency is associated with exercise-induced myoglobinuria in adults, but there are infantile forms associated with cardiomyopathy, sudden death, and hypoketotic hypoglycemia.[101] Autopsy in a 5-day-old infant revealed neutral lipid accumulation in heart, liver, kidney, and skeletal muscle with normal mitochondrial ultrastructure.[102] There is a secondary carnitine deficiency in these patients.

Acyl-Coenzyme A Dehydrogenase Deficiencies

Deficiency of long-chain acyl-CoA dehydrogenase is associated with hypoglycemic episodes, recurrent myoglobinuria, cardiomyopathy, clinical features resembling Reye syndrome, and sudden death. Echocardiography showed features of dilated cardiomyopathy in one infant who was the subject of a case report[103]; in other reports, there was concentric hypertrophy.[101] Lipid accumulation can be found in cardiac muscle.[104, 105]

Medium-chain acyl-CoA dehydrogenase deficiency is a cause of sudden death in childhood. Episodes of hypoketotic hypoglycemia, mild hyperammonemia, and sometimes coma occur and may be misdiagnosed as Reye syndrome. There is hepatic steatosis. Patients develop secondary carnitine deficiency.[96] Cardiomyopathy is uncommon in those with medium- or short-chain acyl-CoA dehydrogenase deficiency[106]; however, lipid accumulation within cardiac myocytes was found at autopsy in a child with medium-chain acyl-CoA dehydrogenase deficiency.[104]

Multiple acyl-CoA dehydrogenase deficiency (glutaric aciduria type II), can be associated with cardiomyopathy.[107]

Possible mechanisms for cardiac damage in the disorders of fatty acid oxidation include inadequate energy provision or myocyte damage and generation of arrhythmias due to the toxic effects of accumulated intermediary metabolites.[106]

CENTRONUCLEAR/MYOTUBULAR MYOPATHY

There are two distinct hereditary types of this disorder, as well as sporadic forms. The X-linked recessive type has onset in the prenatal or perinatal period and an 82% mortality rate within the first year of life. The autosomal dominant form is less severe and manifests before 20 years of age with variable clinical features. Histologic examination of skeletal muscle reveals centrally placed nuclei, resembling fetal myotubes.[108] Central nuclei in skeletal muscle fibers are not a specific finding, however; they can be found in inflammatory myopathies and in some muscular dystrophies as well as in centronuclear myopathy.[109] Adolescent patients with centronuclear myopathy and the clinical[109] and pathologic[110] features of dilated cardiomyopathy have been reported.

CRI DU CHAT SYNDROME

Cri du chat syndrome is caused by deletions in chromosome 5p. It occurs in about 1 per 50,000 live births. Characteristic features are abnormal facies, mental retardation, and a cat-like cry. Congenital cardiac abnormalities are found in more than 25% of patients, ventricular and atrial septal defects and patent ductus arteriosus being most common.[111]

CUTIS LAXA

Cutis laxa refers to a number of congenital and acquired conditions characterized by loose skin. Hereditary cutis laxa may be autosomal dominant, X-linked, or one of three different autosomal recessive types.[112] The X-linked form is identical to type IX Ehlers-Danlos syndrome, q. v.

Pulmonary emphysema, pulmonary artery stenosis and dilation, and tortuosity and rupture of the aorta and other systemic arteries are reported.[113, 114] Histologic and ultrastructural examination of skin and affected vessels reveals loss, thinning, and fragmentation of elastic fibers and aggregates of dense granular material.[115] Loss of elastic tissue in the aorta and pulmonary arteries may be accompanied by increased amounts of glycosaminoglycan.[116]

CYSTINOSIS

Cystinosis is an autosomal recessive condition in which cystine accumulates because of defective lysosomal cystine transport. Myocardial cystine deposition is uncommon but has been reported.[117]

DIABETES MELLITUS

Diabetes mellitus is complicated by *large and small vessel arterial disease* with one or both leading to progressive renal glomerulosclerosis and Kimmelstiel-Wilson nodules,[118] retinopathy,[119] neuropathy,[120] and peripheral ischemia.[121] The large vessel complications are characterized by advanced atherosclerosis and increased medial calcification.[122, 123] A much less well-accepted notion is that a specific nonatherosclerotic disease of large vessels is associated with diabetes.[124] Extramural coronary arteries in type II diabetics are reported to have a thinner media and to contain more periodic acid–Schiff (PAS)–positive material and less acid mucopolysaccharide than normal. The content of connective tissue was increased compared with that of age-matched controls. Small vessel complications of diabetes are the result of hyaline arteriosclerosis and a microangiopathy[125] that involves small arterioles, capillaries, and venules. An infrequent small artery and arteriolar intraluminal proliferative change reported by some is considered by most others to be an artifact. In addition, a diabetic cardiomyopathy has been described to explain cardiac congestive failure, although its nature is still controversial.[126]

Small Vessel Diseases

Hyaline Arteriosclerosis

Mild hyalinization of arterioles, especially in the kidney, may occur in nonhypertensive, nondiabetic individuals generally after the age of 50 years.[127] Hyalinization of arterioles is the characteristic feature of arteriolosclerosis associated with benign hypertension. The hyaline material is deposited initially in the subintimal region. With progressive accumulation, medial smooth muscle cells are trapped within the hyaline and undergo atrophy. There is an associated fraying and reduplication of the internal elastic lamina, thickening of the vessel wall, and narrowing of the lumen, which may become totally occluded. Hyaline is a homogenous, strongly eosinophilic, PAS-positive material (Fig. 16-5). Ultrastructurally, it is a finely granular osmiophilic material with no characteristic periodicity. In renal arteriolosclerosis, the endothelial basement membrane is thickened and split and contains fine, granular, osmiophilic material.[128] These observations suggest that hyaline may be derived from serum constituents and imply that there is increased permeability or actual endothelial cell injury in the initial stages of hyaline deposition. Immunoglobulin M and the third compo-

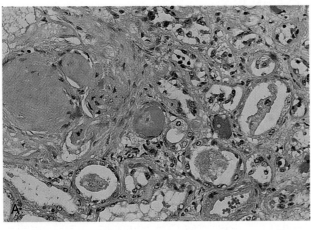
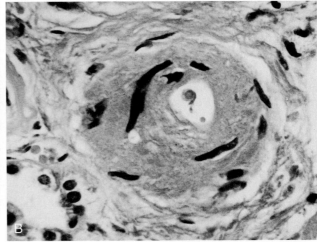

Figure 16-5 • *A,* Hyaline, a homogeneous, strongly eosinophilic material is present in the media of the vessel walls of a kidney. *B,* Capillary from skeletal muscle biopsy in diabetes showing a severely thickened basement membrane with a well-defined outer boundary. (Both H&E stain.) (Courtesy of J. Bilbao, MD, Toronto, Ontario.)

nent of complement (C3) have been demonstrated by immunofluorescence in the walls of affected arterioles.[129] The C3b binds via an ester linkage to the hydroxyl groups on the disaccharide units of hyaluronic acid, a major constituent of arteriolar hyaline.[130] Diabetic patients without hypertension also show hyaline arteriosclerosis in the kidney and other organs, including pancreas, retina, liver, and spleen.[125] Small arteries in diabetes also show an increased frequency of PAS-positive staining of the media without hyaline material being seen by light microscopy.[131] The significance of this finding is not known.

Microangiopathy

Diabetic microangiopathy[132–135] refers to widespread lesions that occur in the capillaries, small arterioles, and venules and are characterized by basement membrane thickening (Fig. 16-6) and microaneurysms (Fig. 16-7). The latter develop in thin-walled vessels, possibly because of loss of pericytes or smooth muscle cells or both.

Basement membrane thickening may be seen to some extent in aged nondiabetics[133] and in patients with other conditions including myopathies,[136] collagen disease,[137] myxedema,[138] chronic venous congestion[139] and, in some studies, hemochromatosis.[140, 141] However, the changes in diabetics are prominent, widespread, and associated with specific organ malfunction. The thickened basement membrane in either instance appears as a PAS-positive thickening by light microscopy. Ultrastructurally, a thickened basement membrane in either a diabetic or a nondiabetic

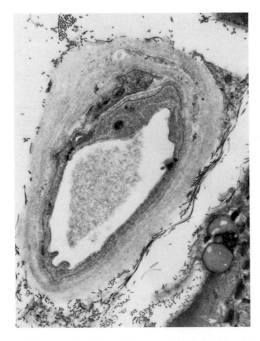

Figure 16-6 • Capillary from skeletal muscle biopsy in a patient with diabetes, showing a severely thickened basement membrane with a well-defined outer boundary. (Courtesy of J. Bilbao, MD, Toronto, Ontario.)

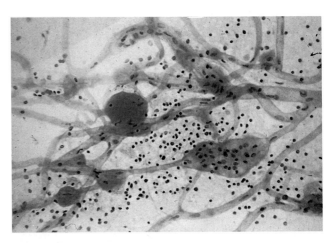

Figure 16-7 • Capillary microaneurysms in retina from a diabetic patient after tryptic digestion. (Courtesy of M.D. Silver, MD, Toronto, Ontario.)

patient is somewhat variable[142, 143] and is either homogenous or has a concentric lamellar pattern composed of both distinct and incomplete layers of basement membrane with cellular material and debris trapped between the layers (see Fig. 16-6). The lamellar pattern is most common in capillaries of the skin and peripheral nerves[120] and has been described in skeletal muscle[132] and the heart.[138]

Assessment of basement membrane thickness should be done cautiously. The capillaries of the renal glomerulus and skeletal muscle are most suitable for careful quantitative electron microscopic studies. Because the thickening is not uniformly concentric, several points must be measured around a capillary's circumference.[143] Although some researchers have found that the type of fixation is important when assessing membrane thickness,[144] others have not.[143, 145] In addition, nondiabetics show a variation in basement membrane thickness among samples of different skeletal muscles from the same individual.[142, 145, 146] There is also significant variation in capillary basement membrane thickness at different sites within the same muscle.[147] A skin biopsy is not a very suitable site for study because there is variability in basement membrane thickening in adjacent vessels,[148] the concentric lamellar membrane is characterized by numerous thickened complete and incomplete layers, and it is often difficult to define the external border.

Diabetic Glomerulosclerosis

Diabetic microangiopathy as described in the previous section is not typical of early diabetic glomerular disease. In its early stages, the kidney size and glomerular volume increase, and capillary wall surface area parallels the increase in glomerular filtration rate. The extent of endothelial injury and dysfunction during these early changes is not well understood. Disease progression is marked by extracellular matrix expansion that leads to obliteration of glomerular capillaries. Previously it was believed that capillary microaneurysms exist in the kidney and that, although they may not be related initially to Kimmelstiel-Wilson nodules, large nodules are formed by their organization.[118] Now, possible roles for platelet-derived growth factor (PDGF)[149] and transforming growth factor-β (TGF-β)[150] in the pathogenesis of progressive diabetic glomerulosclerosis have been presented. Microaneurysmal dilation of intrarenal arteries has also been described[151] in association with advanced arteriolar hyalinosis. They are much less common than glomerulocapillary microaneurysms.

Diabetic Retinopathy

The basement membranes of retinal capillaries and of very small vessels from diabetics show diffuse thickening, reduplication, and a specific vacuolization, referred to as a "Swiss cheese appearance," which may also affect the retinal vessels of nondiabetics older than 30 years of age.[152] In diabetics, changes are found more commonly around mural cells, whereas in nondiabetics there is no specific location.[153] Dilation and tortuosity of the veins is also an early change in diabetes. There may be focal or complete loss of endothelial cells and/or pericytes from single capillaries or groups of capillaries.[152, 119] Pericyte

loss may weaken the vessel wall and lead to microaneurysm formation; this is best seen by using tryptic digestion[154] (see Fig. 16-7).

Retinal microaneurysms are found on both the arterial and venous sides of capillaries, may have an associated thickened basement membrane, and may be either thin- or thick-walled. Although such aneurysms are very closely associated with diabetes, they occur occasionally in nondiabetics with retinoblastoma,[155] glaucoma,[156] sickle cell anemia,[157] or other conditions including hyperviscosity syndrome and malignant hypertension.[156] In these nondiabetic conditions, there are fewer aneurysms, and they are located less frequently in the posterior pole of the retina. It has been suggested that limbs of adjacent varicosed parts of a capillary wall may fuse and thereby form an aneurysm. Thick-walled aneurysms have a very thickened, laminated basement membrane and contain remnants of platelets, red blood cells, and fibrinoid material. The aneurysms may slowly regress and thrombose, or leak, or rupture. Well-defined yellowish-white, waxy exudates are prominent on funduscopy; less sharply outlined fluffy retinal exudates, related to microinfarcts, may also be present.

Proliferative retinopathy may be a complication; it is characterized by neovascularization in the retina, first as naked vessels and followed by an associated fibrous proliferation. In the retina, it is likely that pericytes regulate endothelial cell function. Tissue culture studies using cocultures show that pericytes inhibit endothelial cell migration[158] and proliferation,[159] features important in new vessel growth. These studies demonstrate that TGF-β, generated when both cell types are in contact or very close to each other, mediates migration and proliferation. The new retinal vessels have increased permeability, which may be related to changes in the vitreous leading to a severe vision deterioration.[160] Other parts of the eye[161] also show microangiopathic changes. Visual acuity decreases slowly in affected patients, but the ensuing proliferative retinopathy is more often the cause of marked deterioration and eventual blindness.

Pathogenesis of Diabetic Microangiopathy

The pathogenesis of diabetic microangiopathy is not known. Evidence exists of an increased capillary permeability to small ions and albumin in diabetes,[119, 162] and it is possible, although not proven, that substances leaking from the vessels interfere with basement membrane metabolism.[163] Quantitative vitreous fluorophotometry indicates that retinal vessels in diabetes have an increased permeability to fluorescein even before clinical evidence of a retinopathy is detected.[164] The basement membranes from glomeruli of long-term diabetics with glomerular lesions have a different composition from those of nondiabetic controls.[165] Vracko suggested that basement membrane thickening may be related to an accelerated rate of cell death in the vessel wall, with each new generation of endothelial cells depositing a new layer of basement membrane.[146, 166] Glycosylation of basement membrane proteins, such as collagen type IV and laminin, has also been implicated.[167, 168]

Several changes in the blood of diabetics could affect

the microvasculature. They have a two to three times higher level of glycosylated hemoglobin A_{1c} than do non-diabetics. Because this compound has a high affinity for oxygen,[169] the ability of erythrocytes to release oxygen may be impaired.[170, 171] Ditzel proposed that the venous end of the capillaries dilates because of local hypoxia induced by the increased affinity of hemoglobin for oxygen.[172] Recurrent local hypoxic injuries may increase vessel permeability and cause mild damage. Two studies reported no correlation between single measurements of glycosylated hemoglobins and either basement membrane thickening[173] or vitreous leakage as assessed by fluorescein angiography.[174] Because glycosylated hemoglobin measurements reflect control of diabetes in the previous 6 to 10 weeks, long-term prospective studies are required to correlate diabetic complications and glycosylated hemoglobin levels.

McMillan suggested that changes in the plasma proteins in diabetics cause an elevation in plasma viscosity and promote an increased affinity of erythrocytes for each other, affecting the microcirculation and promoting microangiopathy.[175]

Platelets from diabetics showed accelerated aggregation when studied in vitro.[176] Glycosylated hemoglobin levels were also positively correlated with fibrinogen concentration and increased platelet aggregation.[147] Diabetics have increased fibrinogen levels and fibrinolytic dysfunction, especially related to decreased plasminogen activator inhibitor type I.[177] However, it is not clear whether these changes are related to diabetes per se or are secondary to underlying vascular disease.[125, 178]

Control of Microangiopathy

Most studies indicate a positive correlation between angiopathy and the duration of diabetes.[133, 179–185] However, Siperstein and colleagues found no such correlation in a group of mainly elderly diabetics. He suggested that the thickening is part of the genetic syndrome of diabetes.[186]

Several risk factors have been identified in retinopathy.[187] The most significant appears to be the degree and duration of hyperglycemia.[188, 189] The Diabetes Control and Complications Trial studied 1441 patients between 13 and 39 years old with insulin-dependent diabetes mellitus and showed that intensive treatment reduced the incidence of retinopathy, nephropathy, and neuropathy.[190] The mechanisms by which hyperglycemia induces vascular damage is unknown. It is reasonable to hypothesize that it causes toxic injury as well as endothelial cell dysfunction resulting in permeability changes and/or synthesis and release of cytokines and reactive oxygen species, vasoactive agents, and other substances that promote further endothelial and medial smooth muscle cell injury and dysfunction. Several other factors besides hyperglycemia may injure the endothelial cell, including hemodynamic shear stress factors,[191] aberrant metabolic pathways (e.g., polyol pathway), glycosylation,[192] insulin,[193] oxidative stress,[194] and others.

High glucose concentration, independent of its hyperosmolar effects, does affect microvascular endothelial cells. Retinal capillary endothelial cells so treated accumulate sorbitol, while inositol phospholipids are unaltered and protein kinase C (PKC) is activated.[195, 196] In studies of human large vessel endothelium, some authors report that high glucose levels are toxic to endothelial cells.[197, 198] High glucose concentration results in an abnormal glutathione redox cycle in human umbilical vein endothelial cells, with cytotoxicity by hydrogen peroxide.[194] This impaired radical scavenger function may be very important, because there is an increased production of oxygen free radicals and increased lipid peroxidation.[199, 200] A high blood glucose level also enhances matrix production by endothelial cells.[201, 202]

Because abnormal vasomotor responses are a feature of diabetes, studies have been done on the effect of high glucose levels on endothelium-dependent vasomotor responses. Aortas from diabetic rabbits and rats and those from normal rabbits exposed to elevated concentrations of glucose in vitro demonstrate impaired endothelium-dependent relaxation in response to acetylcholine, enhanced contractile response to norepinephrine, and augmented generation of vasoconstrictor prostanoids.[203] The inhibition of angiotensin-converting enzyme (ACE) slows the progression of diabetic nephropathy by affecting the angiotensin system and reducing blood pressure.[204] ACE inhibition causes a further lowering of efferent arteriolar resistance and reduces intraglomerular pressure.

High glucose levels may stimulate the release of endothelin-1 (ET-1), a potent vasoactive protein, from endothelial cells in vitro. However, circulating ET-1 is not elevated in most diabetics with or without vascular complications.[205] High glucose inhibits,[206] whereas insulin stimulates, ET-1 gene expression in endothelial cells.[207]

High glucose concentration in the culture medium of bovine endothelial cells increases the permeability of the monolayer by activating PKC.[208] PKC activation may result from enhanced de novo synthesis of diacylglycerol from glucose, which subsequently stimulates sustained PKC activation. An oral PKC inhibitor ameliorated the glomerular filtration rate, albumin excretion rate, and retinal circulation in diabetic rats in a dose-responsive manner in parallel with its inhibition of PKC activities.[209] Further study of the role of PKC in signaling mechanisms leading to mesangial matrix accumulation in high-glucose conditions is required.

Proliferative Changes

Proliferative lesions[210] characterized by endothelial cell swelling and proliferation, basement membrane thickening, and the presence of a reticulated network of PAS-positive fibrils interspersed between endothelial cells, with the vessel lumen often narrowed by bridges of proliferating endothelial cells that eventually completely obliterate the lumen, have been reported to occur in smaller arteries and arterioles of many organs. They were twice as common in diabetics but were found in 20 to 35% of nondiabetics as well. The frequency of the lesions correlated more closely with patient age than with duration of diabetes. In amputated lower limbs, the lesion was described frequently adjacent to areas of gangrene in both diabetics and nondiabetics.[211] Sunni and coworkers suggested that such lesions are an artifact of vessel collapse[212]; the authors did not observe these lesions in pressure perfusion–fixed diabetic hearts. We agree with this viewpoint.

Large Vessel Disease

Atherosclerosis

Insulin-dependent and non–insulin-dependent diabetes mellitus are risk factors for atherosclerosis. Diabetics develop more extensive disease at an earlier age than do nondiabetics,[213] and they have increased plaque fissuring. Premenopausal women lose their protection against atherosclerosis when diabetic, and their prevalence rates for the vascular disease are similar to those of diabetic men. Hypertension is a major factor contributing to the vascular complications of diabetes, including atherosclerosis.[214] Atherosclerotic lesions tend to be more diffusely distributed in diabetics, and a larger number of coronary arteries are involved.[215] In addition, insulin promotes vascular smooth muscle cell proliferation, an important feature of atherogenesis. Both experimental and clinical support exists for the hypothesis that advanced glycosylation end products (AGE) contribute to atherogenesis in diabetic mellitus. With the use of immunofluorescent microscopy techniques, AGE reactivity was localized to diabetic coronary atheromas.[216] The most intense staining was in the fibrous areas of the plaques.[217] Receptors for AGE have been identified in macrophages and endothelial cells. AGE are thought to act within the vascular wall to cross-link and trap plasma proteins, including lipoproteins; to inactivate nitric oxide vasodilatory and antiproliferative activity; to activate cells to synthesize and release cytokines and growth factors; to cross-link matrix proteins[168, 218]; and to generate reactive oxygen species.[218]

Coronary Atherosclerosis

Diabetes mellitus accelerates coronary atherosclerosis,[213] with the initial severity of diabetes an important determinant of long-term survival in those undergoing coronary bypass surgery.[219] Diabetes is also a risk factor for poor outcome after myocardial infarction.[220] Because epicardial coronary artery disease is most often present,[131] it is difficult to attribute myocardial cell damage specifically to small-vessel pathology. However, an increased capillary basement membrane thickness and microaneurysms[221] are present in diabetic myocardial tissue.[138, 222]

Studies suggest that myocardial dysfunction occurs in diabetics beyond that resulting from ischemic heart disease.[223] Therefore, the term *diabetic cardiomyopathy* appeared in the literature[224–226] to describe the myocardial disease that develops in diabetics without significant epicardial coronary artery disease.[126, 227, 228] Disease of small vessels is assumed to be the cause. In a carefully controlled study, Sunni and coworkers failed to show any specific anatomic alteration in the intramyocardial arteries of diabetics.[212] An alternate point of view was presented by Siperstein and colleagues.[186]

Although self-limited edema is a recognized complication of insulin therapy, insulin-induced cardiac failure is rare.[229]

DIGEORGE SYNDROME/ VELOCARDIOFACIAL SYNDROME/ CATCH 22

Both the DiGeorge syndrome and the velocardiofacial syndrome are associated with deletions of the chromosome region 22q11.[230] The term CATCH 22 was proposed for the clinical defects associated with these deletions (*C*ardiac, *A*bnormal facies, *T*hymic hypoplasia, *C*left palate, and *H*ypocalcemia).[231] The DiGeorge or third and fourth pharyngeal pouch syndrome is characterized by hypoplastic or absent thymus and parathyroid glands and conotruncal defects, most often type B interrupted aortic arch, which features aortic interruption between carotid and subclavian artery origins, right-sided aortic arch, and persistent truncus arteriosus. Most patients with DiGeorge syndrome also have deletions in 22q11 when fluorescence in situ hybridization (FISH) technology is used.[230]

The velocardiofacial syndrome phenotype includes cleft palate, characteristic facies, learning disabilities, and cardiovascular defects, most often ventricular septal defect, right aortic arch, aberrant subclavian arteries, and tetralogy of Fallot. Some patients have a severe form of tetralogy manifested by pulmonary atresia with hypoplastic pulmonary arteries.[232] Some develop hypocalcemia. This disorder has also been labeled the conotruncal anomaly face syndrome.[233] Deletions of 22q11 are found in most patients.[234]

DISSEMINATED INTRAVASCULAR COAGULATION

Disseminated intravascular coagulation (DIC) is a systemic thrombohemorrhagic disorder that is associated with particular clinical situations and in which there is laboratory evidence of (1) procoagulant activation, (2) activation of fibrinolysis, (3) consumption of inhibitors, and (4) biochemical features of end-organ damage or failure.[235] DIC occurs in association with obstetric accidents, hemolysis, sepsis, uremias, malignancy, burns, trauma, prosthetic devices (e.g., LeVeen shunts, intra-aortic balloon pumps), giant hemangiomata, and acute liver disease. Saffitz and associates described five patients who developed DIC after undergoing aortic operations with deep hypothermic circulatory arrest and receiving high-dose aprotinin to decrease blood loss.[236]

Fibrin platelet thrombi are found within capillaries in various organs, including the heart, and may be associated with microinfarcts and hemorrhages. A blood smear may contain schistocytes.

EHLERS-DANLOS SYNDROMES

There are at least 10 types of Ehlers-Danlos syndrome, and many patients are unclassifiable. Generally, the features of these syndromes encompass laxity of joints, bruising, "cigarette paper" scars, and hyperextensible skin.[237]

Type I (gravis) is autosomal dominant and features prominent skin involvement. The molecular defect is not known. Skin collagen fibrils are enlarged, show increased variation in fiber diameter, and may form irregular clusters,[238] sometimes termed cauliflower collagen fibrils.[239] Cardiovascular abnormalities include (1) tricuspid valve prolapse, (2) mitral valve prolapse, (3) aortic root dilation, (4) aortic dissection, (5) pulmonary artery dilation, (6) conduction defects (PR interval prolongation, right bundle branch block), and (7) varicose veins.[240]

Type II (mitis) is autosomal dominant and clinically less severe than type I. Mitral valve prolapse has been reported.[241]

Type III is autosomal dominant. Increased joint mobility is the major feature.[238] Mitral valve prolapse and conduction defects occur in these patients.[240, 242]

Type IV Ehlers-Danlos syndrome (usually autosomal dominant) is caused by mutations in the gene for type III collagen at chromosome 2q. This results in an abnormal structure or synthesis of type III procollagen. Type III collagen is abundant in blood vessels, skin, and hollow viscera. The skin is thin and easily bruised, but joint mobility and skin extensibility may not be increased and scars are usually normal.[238] Some patients have a particular facies with prominent eyes, thin nose and lips, and absent earlobes.[243] In the skin, collagen fibrils are small or vary greatly in diameter; dermal fibroblasts have a dilated endoplasmic reticulum containing abnormal type III collagen in patients with some of the mutations.[244] Individuals with type IV syndrome may experience rupture of the colon or the pregnant uterus, pneumothorax, or stroke. Cardiovascular features include (1) arterial rupture, (2) arterial dissections, (3) arterial aneurysms, and (4) mitral valve prolapse.[243, 241, 245]

Microscopically, arterial aneurysms in type IV Ehlers-Danlos syndrome have thin fibrous walls. There may be elastic fiber clumping in the arterial wall and increased glycosaminoglycan within the media. Collagen fibers are loose and delicate.[246, 247] Accordion pleating of the internal elastic lamina of non–pressure-fixed arteries has been reported.[248] The lack of type III collagen in skin and arteries can be demonstrated by immunohistochemistry.[247] Ultrastructural study of blood vessels revealed significant variation in collagen fibril diameter and a decrease in the average collagen fibril cross-sectional area in arteries.[249]

Type V Ehlers-Danlos syndrome is X-linked recessive and may be associated with mitral valve prolapse.[241]

Type VI Ehlers-Danlos syndrome (autosomal recessive) features skin, joint, and ocular problems, as well as kyphoscoliosis. Most cases are caused by lysyl hydroxylase deficiency, which interferes with the generation of hydroxylysine for collagen cross-linking. Arterial rupture is reported.[238, 250]

Type VII. There are autosomal dominant and autosomal recessive subtypes of this form of the disease. Cardiovascular abnormalities do not appear to be a feature.

Type VIII Ehlers-Danlos syndrome is autosomal dominant. Periodontal disease is the prominent feature, but aortic and mitral regurgitation and mitral valve prolapse have been reported.[241]

Type IX. This defect is sometimes called X-linked cutis laxa, but it features defective copper transport, similar to Menkes syndrome.[238]

Type X disease (autosomal recessive) may be caused by a fibronectin deficiency. Mitral valve prolapse can occur in this condition.[241]

See the discussion in Chapter 5.

EMERY-DREIFUSS MUSCULAR DYSTROPHY

Emery-Dreifuss muscular dystrophy is a late-onset disease in which there is muscle wasting and weakness initially involving humeroperoneal muscles, causing contractures of the elbows, Achilles tendons, and postcervical muscles, as well as cardiac involvement. It differs from other muscular dystrophies in that there is a lack of pseudohypertrophy, the distribution of affected muscles is different, and the contractures develop before there is much muscle weakness. Most cases are X-linked recessive, but some may be autosomal dominant or autosomal recessive. X-linked cases are caused by mutations in a gene on distal chromosome Xq28, which encodes for the protein emerin. It resembles other proteins involved in vesicular transport and is absent from cardiac and skeletal muscle in patients with the disease.[251]

Sudden death is well documented in Emery-Dreifuss dystrophy. Patients, and female carriers, may develop third-degree AV block and atrial paralysis, usually in adulthood. Pacing of the atrium may be impossible in these patients.[252] Examination of the heart at autopsy reveals fibroadipose tissue replacement of atrial muscle. There is no change or a minimal increase in SA node fibrous tissue.[253] A patient with marked luminal narrowing of the AV node artery has been reported.[253] Some patients develop features of a dilated cardiomyopathy and have ventricular interstitial fibrosis and myocyte hypertrophy on biopsy or at autopsy.[253, 254]

FABRY DISEASE

Fabry disease is an X-linked disorder caused by deficiency of the lysosomal hydrolase α-galactosidase. This causes accumulation of trihexosylceramide (globotriaosylceramide) within endothelial and smooth muscle cells, cardiac myocytes, valve interstitial cells, glomerular cells, and renal tubular cells. The signs and symptoms include cutaneous angiokeratoma corporis diffusum, acroparesthesias, anhidrosis, and renal failure as well as symptoms of cardiac disease. There is a variant of Fabry disease in which disease is limited to the heart.[255, 256] Some heterozygous females are symptomatic, depending on random cellular X chromosome inactivation. Evaluation of 130

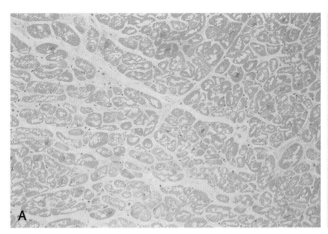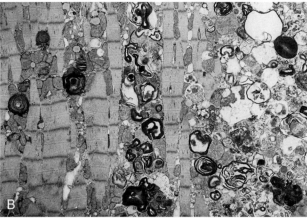

Figure 16-8 • Fabry disease. *A,* Lace-like appearance of cardiac myocytes. (H&E stain.) *B,* Electron micrograph reveals lamellar bodies.

unrelated Fabry disease families disclosed six different gene rearrangements and an exonic point mutation.[257]

Accumulation of trihexosylceramide in the myocardium causes left ventricular hypertrophy. The clinical features may mimic hypertrophic, restrictive, or dilated cardiomyopathy.[256, 258] Electrocardiographic changes include a short P-R interval,[259] ST- and T-wave changes, or AV block. Trihexosylceramide has been demonstrated within the conduction system.[260] Deposition of trihexosylceramide within valves can cause mitral stenosis,[261] aortic stenosis, or mitral regurgitation. The regurgitant mitral valve has been described as thickened with hooding,[262] and mitral valve prolapse is frequently found echocardiographically.[263] Involvement of the aorta, coronary arteries, or other arteries occurs, Fabry disease being a rare cause of coronary artery disease in younger patients.[264] Necrotizing vasculitis involving the gastrointestinal tract has also been reported.[265]

Histologically, involved cells are vacuolated with cardiac myocytes having a lace-like appearance (Fig. 16-8A). The deposits stain positively with toluidine blue, PAS stain, or Sudan black B and are birefringent. Transmission electron microscopy reveals lamellar bodies (Fig. 16-8B).[266] This finding is not specific, and confirmatory diagnosis requires biochemical assay for α-galactosidase. Recently a specific monoclonal antibody has been used to make the diagnosis on heart biopsies using immunofluorescence.[267]

FACIOSCAPULOHUMERAL DYSTROPHY

This autosomal dominant disorder is caused by mutations in a gene on chromosome 4q35.[268] It occurs in 3 to 10 of every 1 million people. Weakness and atrophy of facial and shoulder girdle muscles are characteristic. Some reported cases of cardiac involvement may actually represent cases of Emery-Dreifuss muscular dystrophy.[269] An electrophysiologic study of 30 patients with facioscapulohumeral dystrophy revealed sinus node dysfunction and susceptibility to atrial fibrillation.[269]

FARBER DISEASE

Farber disease (disseminated lipogranulomatosis) is an autosomal recessive sphingolipid storage disorder caused by a deficiency of the lysosomal enzyme acid ceramidase.[270] Lipogranulomas are found in the skin, joints, central nervous system, and larynx. They have also been reported within the endocardium and cardiac valves, where they appear as yellow plaques and nodules.[271] Ultrastructurally, the foam cells contain curvilinear structures and "banana" bodies.[272]

FRAGILE X SYNDROME

Fragile X syndrome, the most common type of hereditary mental retardation, is usually worse in affected males than in females (X-linked). The former have macroorchidism and large ears, face, and jaw. The X chromosome has a fragile site at position Xq27.3, which is induced by culturing cells in media lacking folic acid and thymidine.[273] The gene involved is called FMR1 and contains a CGG repeat. Although carrier males and some carrier females have few CGG amplifications, affected individuals have more than 200 repeats of CGG. The CGG repeat and promoter region are hypermethylated in affected subjects, inhibiting transcription of FMR1.

An echocardiographic study of 23 affected adult men revealed aortic root dilation in 52% and mitral valve prolapse in 22%.[274] However, another echocardiographic study of 16 affected boys 13 years old or younger disclosed mitral valve prolapse in only one and aortic root dilation in none, suggesting that cardiac abnormalities in fragile X syndrome develop with increasing age.[275] Little evidence is available on the pathology of the cardiovascular changes. A male with fragile X syndrome who died suddenly with pneumonia and myocarditis had hypoplasia of the descending thoracic and abdominal aorta and a coarctation just distal to the left subclavian artery origin. Histologically, there was a loss of elastic fibers in the aorta, with fragmentation of the remaining ones, and a decrease in medial glycosaminoglycans. There was no valve prolapse. Mitral valve elastic fibers were thickened and fragmented; collagen in the valve was increased and glycosaminoglycans decreased.[276]

FUCOSIDOSIS

This autosomal recessive lysosomal storage disease is caused by α-fucosidase deficiency. The affected gene is on chromosome 1p. Subjects are mentally retarded, have motor defects, and develop angiokeratomas and visceromegaly.[277] Left ventricular hypertrophy with storage of weakly PAS-positive material within cardiac myocytes has been reported.[278]

GANGLIOSIDOSES

GM$_1$ Gangliosidosis

This autosomal recessive condition is caused by a deficiency of GM$_1$ β-galactosidase and manifests in infantile, juvenile, and adult forms.[279] Cardiomegaly and cardiac valve involvement occur in the infantile form.[280] Mitral valve thickening and nodularity with histologic demonstration of foamy cells containing PAS-positive granules, as well as narrowing of a coronary artery by intimal thickening, were described in a 15-month-old patient.[281]

GM$_2$ Gangliosidoses

These are produced by impaired degradation of GM$_2$ ganglioside. A deficiency of the α subunit of N-acetyl-β-hexosaminidase causes *Tay-Sachs disease.*[279] Electrocardiographic abnormalities and GM$_2$ ganglioside storage in the heart have been reported.[282]

Sandhoff disease is a result of a deficiency of the β subunit of N-acetyl-β-hexosaminidase.[279] GM$_2$ ganglioside, asialo-GM$_2$-ganglioside, and globoside accumulate in tissues. Patients with Sandhoff disease may have endocardial fibroelastosis, valve thickening, left ventricular hypertrophy, and intimal proliferation in coronary arteries. Ultrastructurally, cells contain lamellar structures.[283]

GAUCHER DISEASE

Gaucher disease is an autosomal recessive lysosomal storage disease caused by deficiency of the enzyme glucocerebrosidase (glucosylceramidase). It results from many different mutations in the gene, located on chromosome 1. Accumulation of glucocerebroside (glucosylceramide) occurs within macrophages and in the nervous system in the neuropathic forms. Clinical expression varies, even in homozygous patients from the same family.[284]

The Gaucher cell is a lipid-laden macrophage with striated cytoplasm resembling crinkled tissue paper. Ultrastructurally, the appearance derives from tubular structures 20 to 60 nm in diameter.[285] The histologic appearance is not specific; similar cells are found in chronic myelogenous leukemia, for example. Diagnosis of Gaucher disease is made by measuring the activity of the leukocyte enzyme.

Cardiovascular complications are rare. Pulmonary hypertension, either caused by Gaucher cell infiltration or featuring the pathology of primary pulmonary hypertension, has been reported.[286, 287] When Gaucher cells are located in the lung, they are found within the interstitium, capillaries, or alveolar spaces.[287] Pericardial disease may manifest as acute or constrictive pericarditis or as cardiac tamponade. It is probably caused by hemorrhage secondary to thrombocytopenia, because Gaucher cells are not found in the pericardium.[288] There has been one report of Gaucher cell infiltration of the myocardial interstitium at autopsy; the cells were not identified in conduction tissue in that case.[289] Gaucher cells were demonstrated in a right ventricular heart biopsy.[290] Echocardiographic study of two teenage siblings with Gaucher disease disclosed aortic and mitral valve thickening and stenosis.[291] Young patients with Gaucher disease and calcification of the aortic and mitral valves and of the ascending aorta have the D409H mutation in the gene for glucocerebrosidase.[292, 293] However, Gaucher cells have not been found in calcified aortic valve tissue when it has been available for study.[292]

GLYCOGEN STORAGE DISEASES

Type I Glycogen Storage Disease

Type Ia glycogen storage disease, known as *von Gierke disease,* is caused by a deficiency of the enzyme glucose-6-phosphatase, whereas type Ib is caused by defective transport of glucose-6-phosphatase. The gene for glucose-6-phosphatase is on chromosome 17.[294] Primary cardiac involvement is not a feature, but right-sided heart failure may occur secondary to pulmonary hypertension and has been reported in four patients.[295]

Type II Glycogen Storage Disease

Type II glycogen storage disease (autosomal recessive) results from a deficiency of lysosomal acid α-glucosidase, also known as acid maltase. The gene for this enzyme is on chromosome 17q21-q23.[296] There is a fatal infantile form called *Pompe disease,* as well as juvenile and adult onset forms in which muscle weakness is the major problem and respiratory failure causes death. Infants with Pompe disease have characteristic electrocardiographic changes including short P-R interval, left ventricular hypertrophy with or without right ventricular hypertrophy, and large Q waves in precordial leads. Echocardiography reveals hypertrophy and may show outflow tract obstruction resembling hypertrophic cardiomyopathy.[297] At autopsy, cardiac hypertrophy is found, and some patients have endocardial fibroelastosis.[298] Histologically, the myocardium reveals vacuolization because of storage of structurally normal glycogen in myocytes. Ultrastructurally, the increased glycogen is both free in the cytoplasm and membrane bound within lysosomes.[299] Histologic examination of the conduction system reveals glycogen storage in these cells as well, and it is hypothesized that the short P-R interval may be caused by enhanced conduction through the enlarged conduction fibers.[300]

A single patient has been reported with adult-onset acid maltase deficiency and cardiac symptoms. Autopsy study of two patients with adult-onset disease revealed no gross cardiac abnormality, but membrane-bound glycogen was found in one heart and not in the other.[301]

Danon Disease

In Danon disease, glycogen is stored in lysosomes but acid maltase levels are normal. Heredity is either X-linked or autosomal dominant.[302] Patients have childhood-onset mental retardation, cardiomyopathy featuring cardiac hypertrophy, and muscle weakness. Cardiac involvement is first detected either in childhood or adulthood and may cause cardiac failure and sudden death. There has been a case report of a patient presenting with complete heart block.[303] Some patients have elevated serum muscle enzymes without skeletal muscle weakness or atrophy and echocardiographic left ventricular hypertrophy. Skeletal muscle biopsy may be positive.[304] Heart biopsy reveals mild interstitial fibrosis and vacuolated cardiac myocytes containing glycogen. Ultrastructural examination reveals free and membrane-bound lysosomal glycogen.[303, 304] At autopsy the heart demonstrates ventricular dilation and hypertrophy.

Type III Glycogen Storage Disease

Type III glycogen storage disease, or *Cori disease*, is an autosomal recessive disorder that results from deficiency of the glycogen-debranching enzyme, amylo-1,6-glucosidase. This impairs glucose release from stored glycogen, with the accumulated glycogen having an abnormal structure, resembling limit dextrin. Some patients have liver and skeletal muscle involvement; others have liver involvement only. The gene is located on chromosome 1p.[305] Patients with debranching enzyme deficiency in the liver but normal enzyme levels in skeletal muscle may not develop myopathy or cardiomyopathy.[306] Symptomatic cardiac involvement is uncommon, but electrocardiographic abnormalities such as those of ventricular hypertrophy and echocardiographic evidence of left ventricular hypertrophy are common.[307] Some patients have echocardiographic features resembling hypertrophic cardiomyopathy.[308] A patient with glycogen storage disease type III and recurrent ventricular tachycardia has been reported.[309] Heart biopsy in one patient with type III glycogen storage disease and pulmonary edema revealed increased glycogen content, the tissue being fixed in absolute ethanol to prevent glycogen dissolution, and debrancher enzyme deficiency was demonstrated in fresh frozen cardiac muscle samples.[310] The glycogen deposits are ultrastructurally normal.

Type IV Glycogen Storage Disease

Type IV glycogen storage disease, also called *Andersen disease* or amylopectinosis, is autosomal recessive and caused by branching enzyme deficiency. The gene is found on chromosome 3.[311] The structure of the stored glycogen in these patients is abnormal. Hepatic and skeletal muscle dysfunction cause the clinical abnormalities in most patients but occasionally cardiomyopathy is the major feature. At autopsy, cardiomegaly may or may not be found; if it occurs, it is of dilated form. On light microscopic examination and hematoxylin and eosin staining, cardiac myocytes contain colorless[312] or basophilic[313] deposits that are spherical to irregular.[313] These stain with PAS and at least their central portions are diastase resistant.[314] They also stain with toluidine blue or sulfated Alcian blue and are negative with Meyer mucicarmine.[314] Ultrastructurally, cardiac myocytes contain glycogen particles and rosettes, as well as 6-nm wide filaments separated from myofilaments by electron-lucent areas.[312–314] These deposits are not membrane bound. When patients with type IV glycogen storage disease receive a liver transplant, cardiac deposits of abnormal glycogen may decrease,[315] but one patient who developed cardiac failure after liver transplantation has been reported.[316] There has also been a patient with dilated cardiomyopathy and the pathology of type IV glycogen storage disease but normal levels of branching enzyme.[317]

Other Glycogen Storage Diseases

Cardiomyopathy does not occur in the remaining glycogen storage diseases except type IX, which is induced by a cardiac phosphorylase kinase deficiency.[318] Three patients with this disorder all died at less than 5 months of age.[319] This rare condition causes striking cardiac hypertrophy. Light microscopic examination shows a lace-like appearance, with myocyte cytoplasm pushed to the cell periphery by glycogen. The latter is PAS positive and is digested completely by diastase. It is free in the cytoplasm ultrastructurally.[319]

GOUT

The association between gout, atherosclerosis, and coronary heart disease is well known.[320] Increased serum lipoprotein Lp(a) has been reported in gouty patients.[321] Those with gout can develop tophi in the heart. These have been observed in the myocardium, conduction system, valves, coronary arteries, and pericardium.[322] If grossly evident, tophi are chalky white. Histologically, the urate crystals appear amorphous in formalin-fixed material but are preserved by fixation in absolute ethanol. The deposits are ringed by macrophages and foreign body giant cells.[323]

HEMOCHROMATOSIS

Iron overload can be primary and caused by hereditary hemochromatosis, or secondary to a number of conditions, such as ineffective erythropoiesis, chronic liver disease, or excessive iron intake, as occurs in some regions of Africa.[324] Hereditary hemochromatosis is caused by a mutation in a gene linked to the HLA class I region on chromosome 6. Complications occur in homozygotes,[325] who make up 0.5 to 0.8% of the white population. Measurement of transferrin saturation and serum ferritin serve as screening tests.[326]

Clinical manifestations of cardiac iron overload include (1) heart failure with congestive or restrictive physiology (see Chapter 10), (2) atrial and ventricular arrhythmias, and (3) AV block. Echocardiographic study of patients with thalassemia and secondary iron overload discloses abnormalities of left ventricular diastolic function, which precede any systolic dysfunction,[327] and increased myocardial reflectivity.[328] Iron deposition produces a characteristic signal attenuation on magnetic resonance imaging.[329]

The diagnosis of cardiac iron overload is made by demonstrating hemosiderin in cardiac biopsy material.[330] Minor interstitial fibrosis can be found in such biopsies. At autopsy, the heart may appear rusty brown. Its weight may be increased, and the chambers may be dilated. Hemosiderin deposition is greatest in the subepicardial myocardium[331] and can be absent from the right ventricular septal subendocardium despite involvement elsewhere. This can be a source of sampling error in the cardiac biopsy diagnosis of iron overload.[332] The hemosiderin is located in the perinuclear zones of cardiac myocytes and is well demonstrated by the Prussian blue stain (Fig. 16-9).[333] Hemosiderin is also found in the conduction system but is uncommon in the sinus node.[334, 332] Myocardial fibrosis is, at most, mild.[332] An autopsy study of patients with hemochromatosis and multiorgan hemosiderosis disclosed a low prevalence of atherosclerotic coronary artery disease.[335] Because iron catalyzes the generation of the hydroxyl radical, there is a hypothetic risk that iron storage may increase the risk of ischemic myocardial injury.[336] This point is controversial.

Hereditary hemochromatosis is treated by phlebotomy with or without chelation therapy, whereas chelation therapy alone is used in the secondary iron overload disorders (e.g., thalassemia). Cardiac function usually improves with treatment,[337, 338] and hemosiderin deposits diminish.

Combined liver and heart transplantation has been performed in patients with genetic hemochromatosis.[339]

HOLT-ORAM SYNDROME

The Holt-Oram syndrome is the most common heart-hand syndrome. It is autosomal dominant in inheritance and occurs in 1 of every 100,000 live births. The condition is produced by a mutation on chromosome 12q2.[340, 341] The upper limb abnormalities may be unilateral or bilateral. They include triphalangeal or digitalized thumb, absent or hypoplastic thumb, foreshortened arms, and phocomelia. Associated cardiac abnormalities include atrial secundum and ventricular septal defects, sinus bradycardia, and AV block.

Other Heart-Hand Syndromes

The genetic defects in some other heart-hand syndromes, such as heart-hand syndrome type III and familial atrial septal defect with conduction disease, do not map to chromosome 12q2.[342]

HOMOCYSTINURIA AND HYPERHOMOCYSTEINEMIA

Homocysteine is a sulfur-containing amino acid derived from methionine by demethylation. In the serum, homocysteine occurs as homocysteine-homocysteine, called homocystine, or as homocysteine-cysteine. Homocysteine can be metabolized to cystathionine by the enzyme cystathionine synthase with vitamin B$_6$ as a cofactor. Alternatively, homocysteine can be transformed back into methionine by a pathway requiring the enzyme methionine synthase, vitamin B$_{12}$, and folic acid. The enzyme methylene tetrahydrofolate reductase generates 5-methyl tetrahydrofolate to serve as a carbon donor in this pathway.[343]

Homozygous deficiencies of cystathionine synthase (the gene for which is located on chromosome 21), of methylene tetrahydrofolate reductase, or of cobalamin (vitamin B$_{12}$) cause homocystinuria. Patients with this disorder have elevated serum concentrations of both homocysteine and methionine. Patients are characteristically mentally retarded, with ectopia lentis and skeletal abnormalities resembling those of Marfan syndrome. Venous and arterial thrombosis occurs, often before 30 years of age, and is a common cause of death. Arteries in children show fibrous intimal thickening, which may induce severe stenosis, and splitting of the internal elastic lamina. Small, medium-sized, and large arteries are involved.[344] The occlusive vascular lesions produce infarcts and other pathology comparable to that seen with atherosclerosis. Cystic medial necrosis of the aorta occurs.[345]

Elevated plasma homocysteine concentrations are now considered to be a risk factor for premature arterial occlusive disease,[346] myocardial infarction in young women,[347] and mortality in subjects with angiographic coronary artery disease.[348] (See Chapter 4 also.) Only a minority of

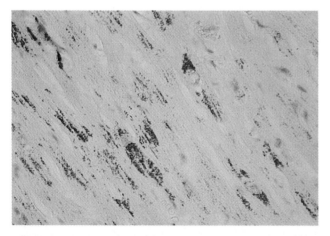

Figure 16-9 • Hemochromatosis. Hemosiderin deposition within cardiac myocytes demonstrated by Prussian blue stain. (Courtesy of M.D. Silver, MD, Toronto, Ontario.)

such patients have homocystinuria resulting from homozygous gene defects; some have heterozygous defects. Apart from gene defects, increased homocysteine levels are associated with increased age; male gender; renal failure; deficiencies of vitamin B_{12}, folate, and possibly vitamin B_6; psoriasis; cancer; and some medications. Possible mechanisms for the deleterious effects of homocysteine on vascular function and pathology include effects on endothelium, platelets, lipids, and clotting factors.[346]

HYPERTENSION

Systemic hypertension is a risk factor for atherosclerosis (see Chapter 4); it is also associated with systemic vascular changes (see Chapter 6). Systemic hypertension also causes left ventricular hypertrophy and heart failure. Echocardiography is about ten times as sensitive as electrocardiography in detecting left ventricular hypertrophy. The left ventricular hypertrophy in systemic hypertension is typically concentric, but 10 to 20% of elderly hypertensives have disproportionate ventricular septal thickening.[349] Left ventricular hypertrophy is associated with impaired diastolic function, increased myocardial oxygen demand, arrhythmias, and sudden death.[349] The risk of complications may be reduced if the left ventricular hypertrophy can be induced to regress by the pharmacologic treatment of hypertension.[350]

KESHAN DISEASE

This condition was first observed in the Keshan district of China, where soil is deficient in selenium. Children and young women present with acute or chronic heart failure. At autopsy, the heart has an increased weight and the ventricles are dilated. Coronary arteries are normal. Mural thrombi may be present in atrial appendages and in the left ventricle. The ventricular walls are not thickened. Areas of myocardial necrosis and fibrosis may be apparent grossly. The left ventricle is damaged before the right, and subendocardial damage precedes that to the outer ventricular wall. Affected areas may follow the course of intramyocardial arteries. The conduction system is also damaged, especially bundle branches. Atrial lesions are common. Histologically, contraction-band necrosis and myocytolysis are found. The necrosis may be focal or infarct-like, and inflammation is not prominent. Replacement fibrosis develops. Lesions of different ages can be found in the same heart.[351, 352] The cause of the disorder is thought to be nutritional, probably a result of selenium deficiency, which also produces "white muscle disease" in cattle.

Patients with poor selenium intake, such as those receiving long-term parenteral nutrition, also develop heart failure which responds to selenium administration.[353] Selenium is a component of glutathione peroxidase. Decreased antioxidant activity may result from its deficiency and may be responsible for myocardial damage.[354] Selenium is also a component of enzymes that convert thyroxine to the active form of thyroid hormone, tri-iodothyronine (T_3).[355]

KUGELBERG-WELANDER SYNDROME

Kugelberg-Welander syndrome is a chronic, juvenile-onset form of spinal muscular atrophy. The disorder is autosomal recessive, and the involved gene is on chromosome 5q.[356] Atrial arrhythmias, AV block, and congestive heart failure may occur.[357] Fibrosis in right atrial and right ventricular biopsies has been reported.[358]

LEOPARD SYNDROME

LEOPARD syndrome is an autosomal dominant complex that may encompass *L*entigines, *E*lectrocardiographic changes, *O*cular hypertelorism, *P*ulmonary stenosis, *A*bnormal genitals, *R*etardation of growth, and *D*eafness. The lentigines are brown-black macules that do not involve mucous membranes and are found on both sun-exposed and non–sun-exposed skin. Typical electrocardiographic abnormalities are axis deviation and conduction defects.[359] Patients may have clinical features of hypertrophic cardiomyopathy. Pulmonary valve stenosis is typical, but a case of primary pulmonary hypertension associated with the syndrome has been reported.[360] Aortic valve or mitral valve stenosis has also been described.[361] (See Chapter 13.)

Other familial syndromes in which lentigenes are associated with cardiac abnormalities include the familial cardiac myxoma syndrome,[14] hypertrophic cardiomyopathy,[362] and arterial dissections.[363]

LIGHT CHAIN DEPOSITION DISEASE

About 70% of cases of nonamyloid deposition of light chains are associated with multiple myeloma, and another 15% with monoclonal gammopathy. Occasionally, a patient has light chain deposition with a malignant lymphoplasmacytic disease other than myeloma.[364] Those affected usually present with proteinuria and renal failure. Cardiac involvement was found in 28% of patients with light chain deposition renal disease in one series.[365] This was manifested by heart failure and arrhythmias. Restrictive cardiomyopathy is typical.[366] A unique sudden death victim who had thick deposits of gelatinous material on the intimal surface of the aorta (causing coronary ostial stenosis), along the intimal surface of the pulmonary artery, and on cardiac valves and endocardium was found to have κ light chains in these deposits.[367] Another patient had myocardial infarcts secondary to the occlusion of intramyocardial blood vessels by light chain deposits within their walls.[368]

Histologically, eosinophilic amorphous material can be found along basement membranes, sometimes forming nodules (Fig. 16-10A). This material may be difficult to see and is better demonstrated on toluidine blue–stained 1-μm sections.[366] The light chain deposits are often PAS

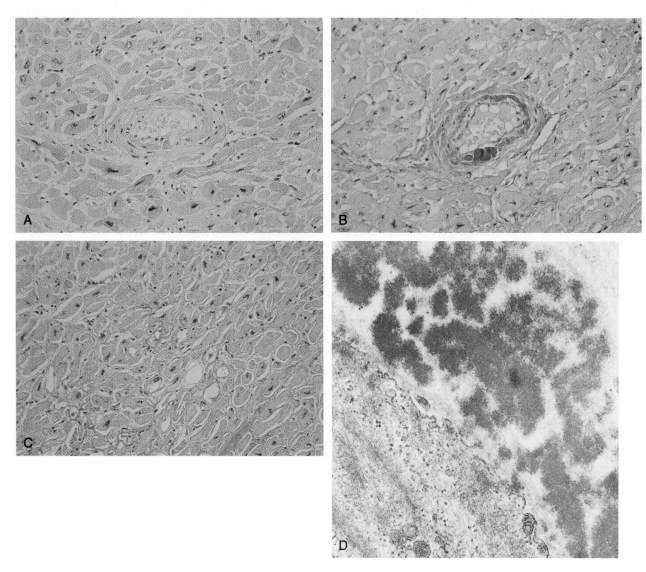

Figure 16-10 • Myocardial light chain deposition disease. Eosinophilic deposits within a vessel wall *(A)* (H&E stain) are periodic acid–Schiff (PAS)–positive *(B)* (PAS diastase). Deposits also surround cardiac myocytes *(C)* (PAS diastase). *D,* Electron micrograph of a renal capillary in the same patient reveals dark granular deposits to right of cell.

positive (Fig. 16-10*B, C*). They are Congo red negative. Immunofluorescence is diagnostic. Eighty percent of cases are κ light chain positive, the remainder being λ light chain positive. Ultrastructurally, deposits are granular and electron-dense (Fig. 16-10*D*).[369]

MALNUTRITION

Marasmus is a state of malnutrition caused by protein and calorie deficiency. *Kwashiorkor* is the result of a deficiency of protein relative to calories. Loss of weight and of adipose tissue without edema is typical of marasmus, whereas subjects with kwashiorkor may develop reddish hair discoloration, edema, and fatty liver. Subjects with the eating disorder *anorexia nervosa* are also malnourished. They tend to maintain protein intake while

decreasing fat and carbohydrate consumption.[370] *Cachexia* refers to ill health and malnutrition.

Marasmus and Kwashiorkor

One echocardiographic study of children with kwashiorkor showed decreased left ventricular end-diastolic and end-systolic dimensions, posterior ventricular wall thickness, and shortening fraction.[371] Another echocardiographic study of malnourished children revealed decreased left ventricular mass but also an increased ratio of left ventricular mass to body weight, suggesting relative cardiac sparing. Ejection fraction did not differ from normal, but stroke volume and cardiac output were reduced in proportion to the decreased body size. However, 20% of the malnourished patients did have a decreased ejection fraction and a reduced left ventricular mass/body weight ratio.[372] QRS amplitude was decreased.[371] Electrocardiography may also reveal bradycardia, T-wave changes, and a prolonged Q-T interval.[373] When subjects with kwashiorkor are refed, there is a risk of precipitating heart failure. Sudden death occurs in subjects with kwashiorkor.

Autopsies of children with marasmus or kwashiorkor reveal an absence of fat on the external surface of the heart and an absence of aortic fatty streaks. In 22.5% of kwashiorkor cases there is a decreased heart weight/body weight ratio, but 43% of cases of marasmus show an increased ratio. Histologically, atrophy and vacuolization of myocytes have been found.[374, 375] Atrophy of conduction tissue is reported.[373]

Cachexia

Patients with malignancies, end-stage disease of other organs, or severe malabsorption syndrome may become cachectic. Serial electrocardiograms reveal decreasing voltage of the QRS complex and T waves, and heart size may decrease on serial chest radiographs. At autopsy, heart weight is diminished with loss of epicardial fat. The heart may be particularly brown. The loss of adipose tissue from its usual sites on the atria and both atrioventricular and interventricular grooves may give the epicardial surface a gelatinous appearance. Marantic or nonbacterial thrombotic endocarditis may be found. Histologically, myocytes are atrophied and lipofuscin is prominent.[376] Patients with severe cardiac disease may also develop cachexia. The pathology of the original cardiac disease must be distinguished from that of secondary cachexia.[377]

Low-Calorie Diets

Sudden death has been reported in subjects who have used very-low-calorie diets to lose weight.[378] This was associated with electrocardiographic Q-T interval prolongation during life. At autopsy, the heart weight was found to be decreased in proportion to the decreased body weight. Myocytes were atrophied and contained increased lipofuscin in most patients. Myocarditis was present in 1 of 16 hearts. Sudden death also occurs in those who have had gastric stapling.

Clinical studies of patients who lost weight on very-low-calorie diets show decreased left ventricular mass and left ventricular wall thickness by echocardiography, and bradycardia, Q-Tc interval prolongation, and low voltage by electrocardiography. Although hypokalemia, hypocalcemia, or hypomagnesemia can precipitate Q-T interval prolongation and ventricular arrhythmias, these electrolyte abnormalities are absent in many of the cases of sudden death.[379]

Eating Disorders

The eating disorders are associated with altered cardiovascular function. There is overlap between the clinical features of anorexia nervosa and *bulimia,* but vomiting and laxative abuse are typical of bulimia and body weight is better preserved in bulimia than in anorexia nervosa. Dehydration and electrolyte abnormalities are seen in bulimics. Their misuse of ipecac may be associated with electrocardiographic abnormalities.[380]

Anorexia nervosa is associated with Q-T interval prolongation and sudden death.[370] Echocardiographic studies of patients revealed decreased left ventricular mass, abnormalities of left ventricular diastolic and systolic function, and a 62% incidence of mitral valve motion abnormalities.[381] Mitral valve prolapse in most of these patients is attributed to decreased left ventricular cavity size. During refeeding, anorexics risk developing heart failure.[370]

MARFAN SYNDROME

This autosomal dominant condition affects about 1 in every 10,000 persons. Approximately 30% of cases represent de novo mutations. Patients have a combination of physical defects such as tall stature, arachnodactyly, pectus excavatum or carinatum, high arched palate, kyphoscoliosis, ectopia lentis, myopia, and cardiovascular abnormalities.[243] Marfan syndrome is caused by mutations in the fibrillin-1 gene on chromosome 15.[382] This protein is a major component of connective tissue microfibrils, which form the scaffolding on which tropoelastin is deposited to create elastic fibers. However, microfibrils are also found in nonelastic tissues, such as the suspensory ligaments of the lens.[383] So far, more than 50 different mutations in the fibrillin-1 gene on chromosome 15 have been discovered in subjects with Marfan syndrome.[383] There can be considerable clinical variability even among family members who all carry the same fibrillin-1 mutation.[384] Conversely, mutations of the fibrillin-1 gene are apparently found in patients who do not satisfy the clinical criteria for Marfan syndrome.[385] For example, mutations in the fibrillin-1 gene are found in patients with aneurysms of the thoracic aorta but no other stigmata of Marfan syndrome.[386]

The cardiovascular abnormalities associated with Marfan syndrome are (1) ascending aortic aneurysm with secondary aortic regurgitation, (2) aortic dissection, (3) floppy mitral valve, (4) mitral annular dilation, and (5) mitral annular calcification.[387] (See Chapter 5 also.)

Patients with Marfan syndrome and aneurysm of the ductus arteriosus,[388] atrial septal aneurysm,[389] or pulmonary artery root dilation or tricuspid valve prolapse[390] have also been reported. Healed intimal and medial tears may be found in the aortic root aneurysms.[389] Although aortic dissection and rupture is an important cause of death in adolescent and adult patients, young children with Marfan syndrome have relatively greater morbidity from mitral valve prolapse.[390, 391]

Patients with Marfan syndrome are urged to undergo serial echocardiographic study of the aortic root, with prophylactic surgery when an aneurysm measures 6 cm in diameter.[392] Treatment with β-blockers has a beneficial effect on aortic root dilation and complications in some patients.[393] One echocardiographic study suggested that

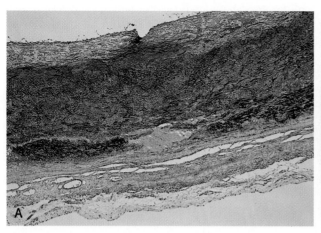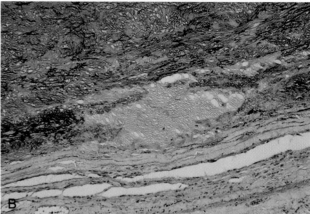

Figure 16-11 • Marfan syndrome. *A,* Section of aorta revealing loss of elastic laminas and accumulation of glycosaminoglycan in cyst-like spaces, so-called cystic medial necrosis. *B,* Higher magnification of the cyst-like spaces containing glycosaminoglycan. (Both, Movat stain.)

complications occur less often in patients with aortic root dilation confined to the sinuses of Valsalva than in those in whom dilation involves the sinuses of Valsalva, the supra-aortic ridge, and the proximal ascending aorta.[394] However, there is much variability in the rate of aortic dilation among patients. An echocardiographic study used the maximum diameter of the sinus of Valsalva region of the aorta, compared with a predicted dimension determined on the basis of body surface area and age, to attempt to establish a low-risk subgroup of patients with Marfan syndrome.[395]

Microscopic evaluation of the aorta in these patients may reveal "cystic medial necrosis" (Fig. 16-11; and see Figs. 5-8 to 5-10), which is characterized by loss of elastic fibers and smooth muscle cells and deposition of pools of glycosaminoglycan and collagen.[396] This histologic change is by no means specific to Marfan syndrome and can be seen with normal aging.[397] The gross pathology and complications of aortic dissection in patients with Marfan syndrome do not differ from aortic dissections caused by other conditions[391] (see Chapter 5). The prolapsing mitral valve in patients with Marfan syndrome demonstrates typical pathologic features of a myxomatous valve.[387]

MENINGOCOCCEMIA

Bacteremic infection with *Neisseria meningitidis* is associated with DIC. Myocarditis has been observed in 27 to 78% of autopsied cases[398, 399]; pericarditis is less common and classically purulent.[398]

MENKES DISEASE

In this X-linked disorder of copper transport, the element cannot be absorbed from intestinal cells. The resulting severe deficiency causes kinky hair, neurologic degeneration, and connective tissue defects.[400] It is usually fatal in infancy, but an experimental treatment with copper histidine is now available.[401] The cause of Menkes dis-

ease is a mutation in the gene for a copper-transporting adenosine triphosphatase (ATPase).

Abnormal arteries are found in these patients. Arterial dilations, arterial wall thinning, internal elastic lamina fragmentation, and intimal thickening occur.[402] The deficiency of elastic lamellas and irregular clumping of elastin are confirmed ultrastructurally.[403] Defects in vascular innervation have also been reported.[404]

MUCOLIPIDOSES

The mucolipidoses are hereditary disorders with some phenotypic similarities to the mucopolysaccharidoses but lacking urinary excretion of glycosaminoglycans. There is storage of mucopolysaccharides, sphingolipids, and glycolipids.

Mucolipidosis I

Here, a deficiency of α-N-acetylneuraminidase causes sialic acid–containing compounds to accumulate. The physical features resemble Hurler syndrome, and there is a severe neurologic disorder. Cardiomegaly, mitral valve abnormality, and pericardial effusion have been detected echocardiographically in some patients.[405]

Mucolipidosis II

Mucolipidosis II, or I-cell disease, is autosomal recessive and produced by a deficiency of N-acetylglucosamine-1-phosphotransferase. This results in a deficiency of lysosomal acid hydrolases. The term "I cell" refers to a fibroblast with inclusion bodies. The inclusions are 0.5 to 1 μ in diameter, contain lipid and mucopolysaccharide vacuoles, and stain positively with PAS and Sudan black stains. On electron microscopy, they contain lamellar and granular material.[406] Granular inclusions are also found in peripheral blood lymphocytes.

Affected subjects have physical similarities to those with Hurler syndrome. Cardiac dysfunction is a common cause of death. At autopsy, thickening of the endocardium, of the aortic and mitral valves and sometimes the tricuspid valve, and of chordae tendineae have been reported, as well as left ventricular hypertrophy.[406-409] Clear cells containing granules are found within the coronary artery intima and in the valves, and there is also mucopolysaccharide accumulation within valves. Vacuolated cardiac myocytes, which stain positively with Sudan black B and PAS, contain lamellar bodies and vacuoles ultrastructurally.[407]

Mucolipidosis III

Mucolipidosis III (pseudo-Hurler polydystrophy) is similar to mucolipidosis II biochemically.[410] Mitral valve prolapse and aortic regurgitation have been reported in some of these patients.[408, 411]

MUCOPOLYSACCHARIDOSES

The mucopolysaccharidoses are a group of hereditary disorders of proteoglycan metabolism[412, 413] (Table 16-1). Mucopolysaccharides are stored in tissue and excreted in urine. Cardiovascular disease occurs in some of these disorders. The frequency of cardiovascular disease may diminish when a mucopolysaccharidosis is treated by bone marrow transplantation.[414]

Hurler Syndrome

Echocardiographic study of patients with Hurler syndrome reveals thickened mitral valve leaflets. The left ventricle may be dilated or show features of a restrictive or hypertrophic cardiomyopathy.[415, 416] Angiography underestimates the extent of the diffuse coronary artery disease.[417] At autopsy, coronary arteries, endocardium, and all four cardiac valves are thickened, with worse involvement of left-sided chambers. There is no commissural fusion of valves. Chordae tendineae are shortened and thickened. Mitral annular and valvular calcification may

be found. Histologically, an accumulation of large clear cells and excessive collagen deposition account for valve and endocardial thickening. Focal fibrosis with clear cells is found in the myocardium. Severe intimal thickening of coronary arteries is caused by clear cells and collagen,[418] and similar changes are seen in aortic intimal plaques (pseudoatherosclerosis) (Fig. 16-12). Ultrastructurally, clear vacuoles and lamellar bodies may be found.[416]

Scheie Syndrome

Scheie syndrome is associated with mucopolysaccharide deposits in aortic and mitral valves. The aortic valve thickening can be nodular.[419] Valve replacement for aortic and mitral stenosis has been performed.[420] An excised stenotic aortic valve revealed calcification and fibrosis but no clear cells on histologic examination. However, when analyzed biochemically, it contained increased dermatan sulfate, chondroitin sulfate, and chondroitin with decreased hyaluronic acid.

Hunter Syndrome

Cardiovascular involvement in Hunter syndrome is similar to that in Hurler syndrome.[412, 415] In a series of 31 patients with mild Hunter syndrome, 91% had evidence of cardiac disease, often of aortic and mitral valves.[421] Involved heart valves contain vacuolated cells which stain positively with Alcian blue and PAS.[422]

Sanfilippo Syndrome

Echocardiographic study of patients with Sanfilippo syndrome reveals valve thickening in some patients.[415] Mitral valve replacement was performed for mitral regurgitation in one patient, and the excised valve had shortened chordae tendineae with a cartilaginous consistency and a thickened free edge. Histologic examination revealed dense fibrosis with increased metachromatic staining by toluidine blue.[423] Autopsy examination of a child with Sanfilippo B syndrome revealed nodules that con-

TABLE 16-1 • **The Mucopolysaccharidoses**

Eponym	Type	Enzyme Defect	Chromosome Location	Inheritance	MP Stored
Hurler	MPS-I-H	α-L-Iduronidase	4p 16.3	AR	DS, HS
Scheie	MPS-I-S	α-L-Iduronidase	4p 16.3	AR	DS, HS
Hunter	MPS-II	Iduronate sulfatase	Xq 27/Xq 28	XR	DS, HS
Sanfilippo A	MPS-III-A	Heparan N-sulfatase	17q 25[433]	AR	HS
Sanfilippo B	MPS-III-B	N-acetyl-α-D-glucosaminidase	17q 21[434]	AR	HS
Sanfilippo C	MPS-III-C	Lysosomal N-acetylase	?	AR	HS
Sanfilippo D	MPS-III-D	N-acetyl-α-D-glucosaminidine B sulfatase	12 q 14	AR	HS
Morquio A	MPS-IV-A	Galactose, N-acetyl galactosamine-6-sulfatase	16 q 24[432]	AR	KS
Morquio B	MPS-IV-B	β-Galactosidase	3	AR	KS
Maroteaux-Lamy	MPS-VI	(arylsulfatase B), N-acetyl galactosamine-4-sulfatase	5q 13.3	AR	DS
Sly-Neufeld	MPS-VII	β-Glucuronidase	7q 21.1-q22	AR	DS, HS

AR, autosomal recessive; DS, dermatan sulfate; XR, X-linked recessive; HS, heparan sulfate; KS, keratan sulfate; MPS, mucopolysaccharidosis.

Data from Fann JI, Dalman RL, Harris EJ Jr: Genetic and metabolic causes of arterial disease, Ann Vasc Surg 7:594, 1993; Fensom AH, Benson PF: Recent advances in the prenatal diagnosis of the mucopolysaccharidoses, Prenat Diagn 14:1, 1994; Morris CP, Guo X-H, Apostolou S, et al: Morquio A syndrome: Cloning, sequence, and structure of the human N-acetylgalactosamine 6-sulfatase (GALNS) gene, Genomics 22:652, 1994; Scott HS, Blanch L, Guo X-H, et al: Cloning of the sulphamidase gene and identification of mutations in the Sanfilippo A syndrome, Nat Genet 11:465, 1995; Zhao HG, Li HH, Bach G, et al: The molecular basis of Sanfilippo syndrome type B, Proc Natl Acad Sci USA 93:6101, 1996.

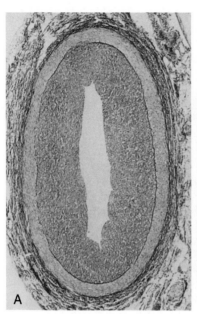
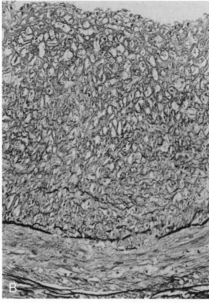

Figure 16-12 • Hurler syndrome (mucopolysaccharidosis I-H). *A,* Coronary artery showing marked intimal thickening and luminal narrowing. *B,* Higher magnification of part of the vessel shown in *A.* The intimal thickening is caused by proliferation of vacuolated intimal cells, which on electron microscopic study are smooth muscle cells. (Both, Movat stain.) (From Ferrans VJ: Metabolic and familial disease. In Silver MD [ed]: Cardiovascular Pathology. 2nd ed. New York, Churchill Livingstone, 1991, p 1080.)

tained vacuolated cells on aortic and mitral valves. Similar cells were found within the myocardium, endocardium, and coronary artery intima.[424]

Morquio Syndrome

Echocardiographic study in patients with Morquio syndrome may demonstrate aortic regurgitation and features of hypertrophic cardiomyopathy.[415] Autopsy examination has revealed endocardial and valvular thickening,[425] with mitral stenosis caused by leaflet and chordal thickening and chordal shortening reported in one patient.[426] Vacuolated cells are found within cardiac valves and coronary artery intima. Ultrastructurally, the vacuoles may be clear or contain lipid or finely granular material.[427]

Maroteaux-Lamy Syndrome

Endocardial fibroelastosis,[428] dilated cardiomyopathy,[429] and stenosis of aortic and mitral valves are reported in Maroteaux-Lamy syndrome. Aortic valve cusps are thick, calcified, and fused, while mitral valve leaflets and chordae are thickened. Light microscopy reveals foam cells within the valves[430] and myocardial interstitium.[429] The cells contain vacuoles and membranous bodies on ultrastructural examination.[430]

Sly-Neufeld syndrome

Autopsy of a patient with Sly-Neufeld disease revealed diffuse and nodular thickening of cardiac valves, calcification of aortic and mitral valves, coronary artery stenosis, and aortic plaques. Vacuolated cells were found microscopically, and ultrastructurally the material was lamellar and filamentous.[431]

NEMALINE MYOPATHY

Nemaline myopathies are characterized by rod-like bodies within skeletal muscle fibers. They contain α-actinin and actin. Nemaline myopathies may be congenital nonprogressive, congenital and quickly fatal, or of adult onset, and they may be either autosomal dominant or recessive. An autosomal recessive form is linked to a gene on chromosome 2q[435]; an autosomal dominant form is caused by a mutation in the α-tropomyosin gene, TPM3, on chromosome 1p.[436] Cardiomyopathy has been reported in the congenital rapidly fatal[437], congenital nonprogressive,[438] and adult-onset asymptomatic[439, 440] forms. The clinical and gross pathology of cardiac involvement is that of dilated cardiomyopathy. Sudden death has been reported.[440] Characteristic rods are found in cardiac myocytes and in the conduction system.[440] They can be demonstrated with a trichome stain and also stain positively with phosphotungstic acid hematoxylin (PTAH), elastic, or toluidine blue stains. The rods are weakly positive with PAS-diastase.[439] Electron microscopy may reveal rod-shaped bodies with the same electron density as Z bands, sometimes emerging from the Z bands, and consisting of thin filaments forming a crystalline-like lattice.[437] (See Chapter 10 also.)

NEUROFIBROMATOSIS

Neurofibromatosis (NF) is now divided into two types. Type I (NF1) is caused by defects in a gene on chromosome 17q that encodes a protein called neurofibromin.[441] This is the disorder that is associated with peripheral neurofibromas, pheochromocytoma, and vascular lesions.[243] NF1 is autosomal dominant, but 30 to 50% of patients represent new mutations.[441] It is associated with congenital valvular pulmonic stenosis.[442] Segmental tubular narrowing of the abdominal aorta and its branches, termed midaortic syndrome or coarctation of the abdominal aorta, has been reported in children with neurofibromatosis.[443] This usually manifests with hypertension. Adventitial neurofibromas may compress arteries, but there may be intrinsic lesions of the arteries themselves which consist of a proliferation of spindle and/or epithelioid cells within intima and/or media. Medial smooth muscle cells are lost, and elastic fibers fragment with aneurysm formation.[444] Aneurysms of renal, superior mesenteric, and popliteal arteries have been described.[445] The pathology of the renal artery in patients with NF1 features stenoses and dilations similar to those seen with intimal fibromuscular dysplasia, but it is typical that intrarenal arteries are also involved in neurofibromatosis. Histologic examination in a reported case[446] revealed intimal proliferation, breaks in the internal elastic lamina, and loss of medial tissue. Immunohistochemistry was consistent with a smooth muscle origin of proliferating cells.[446]

Neurofibromatosis type II (NF2) is autosomal dominant and is related to a mutation on chromosome 22 that encodes a protein called merlin. The major clinical manifestation is bilateral acoustic neuromas, but other central nervous system tumors also occur (e.g., meningioma, glioma). Hence, the findings in NF2 are primarily neurologic.

NIEMANN-PICK DISEASE

The five types of Niemann-Pick disease are all autosomal recessive conditions. Types A and B are caused by sphingomyelinase deficiency, with sphingomyelin accumulating within foam cells in the bone marrow, liver, spleen, lungs, and brain. Type C Niemann-Pick disease is caused by defective intracellular cholesterol metabolism which leads to accumulation of LDL-derived cholesterol in lysosomes. The gene for type C1 disease is on chromosome 18.[447] Cardiovascular involvement in Niemann-Pick disease is uncommon. Single cases of cor pulmonale secondary to pulmonary involvement in a patient with probable type B disease,[448] of endocardial fibroelastosis in a patient with type A disease[9, 449] of epicardial foam cell nodules,[450] and of echocardiographically mild mitral regurgitation[451] have all been reported.

NOONAN SYNDROME

Noonan syndrome is an autosomal dominant or sporadic condition occurring in 1 of every 1000 to 2500 live births. The diagnosis is made on clinical grounds. The NF1 gene on chromosome 17 and a locus near the DiGeorge syndrome locus on chromosome 22q have been excluded as sites for the Noonan syndrome. Some cases are linked to a gene on chromosome 12q.[452] Subjects with Noonan syndrome have a physical appearance similar to that of individuals with Turner syndrome (e.g., webbed neck, short stature). About 50% of patients have cardiac abnormalities, most commonly congenital pulmonary valve stenosis, often caused by valvular dysplasia; atrial septal defect, peripheral pulmonary artery stenosis, patent ductus arteriosus, aortic stenosis, and coarctation of the aorta also have been reported. Hypertrophic cardiomyopathy is found in 20 to 30% of patients. Particular electrocardiographic features include left-axis deviation and a prominent S wave; they are found in many patients.[453] An echocardiographic study of 145 affected individuals disclosed pulmonary valve dysplasia in 7%, pulmonary valve stenosis without dysplasia in 20%, and left ventricular hypertrophy in 25% of those without pulmonary stenosis. Ten percent of patients had a secundum atrial septal defect. Forty-one percent of those with left ventricular hypertrophy had localized hypertrophy involving the anterior septum, sometimes forming a discrete bulge in the upper septum.[454] Histologic examination of hearts from patients with Noonan syndrome showed myocyte disarray.[455] Patients with restrictive cardiomyopathy have been reported.[456] (See Chapter 10 also.)

OBESITY

There is no standard definition of obesity. It may be diagnosed by measuring body weight or skinfold thicknesses, by determining body-mass index, or by quantifying total body fat and lean tissue mass using techniques such as dual-energy x-ray absorptiometry.[457] In some studies, obesity was defined as 20% or more over ideal body weight[458] or as a body mass index (BMI) greater than 27.8 in men and 27.3 in women,[459] in which BMI is equal to the weight (in kilograms) divided by the square of the height (in meters).

Obesity is clearly associated with systemic hypertension. Studies show increases of 2 to 3 mm Hg in systolic and diastolic blood pressure for every 10 kg increase in body weight. Lipid profiles are often abnormal in the obese, with lower HDL cholesterol, normal or elevated total and LDL cholesterol, and higher triglyceride levels. The risk of diabetes mellitus increases 2 to 10 times with increasing degrees of obesity.[459]

The role of obesity in coronary atherosclerotic heart disease is controversial. Some difficulties in this area stem from confounding factors such as cigarette smoking, which tends to lower body weight but is itself a risk factor; short-term follow-up; the undetermined role of weight fluctuations over time; the association of obesity with other risk factors such as non–insulin-dependent diabetes mellitus; and the possibly varying influence of obesity at different ages. Central or upper body fat distribution (android pattern) increases risk. Fat distribution can be determined by skinfold measurements or hip-to-waist circumference ratios or by more sophisticated techniques.[457, 460] Possible mechanisms by which central obesity increases the risk of coronary disease include the association of central adiposity with unfavorable lipid profiles and insulin resistance.[457, 460] Autopsy studies in which obesity was defined as a body weight greater than 99 kg[461] or greater than 136 kg[462] have not demonstrated an excessive amount of coronary atherosclerosis.

The electrocardiogram in severely obese persons may show low voltage owing to increased chest wall fat or increased voltage resulting from increased heart mass. Left- or right-axis deviation reflecting left or right ventricular hypertrophy may be observed.[458, 463] Atrial and ventricular ectopy is frequent.[464] Sinus node dysfunction may be detected in Pickwickian patients.[458] Obesity is associated with echocardiographic left ventricular hypertrophy even after controlling for age and blood pressure. There is increased left ventricular wall thickness and chamber size: the eccentric hypertrophy pattern.[465] The increased left ventricular mass may cause left ventricular diastolic dysfunction.[466] Weight reduction leads to regression of increased left ventricular mass regardless of blood pressure levels.[467] Cardiac output in the obese is increased in proportion to the increased body weight. Right and left ventricular systolic function can be depressed in severely obese persons, and congestive heart failure is common at death. About 5% of severely obese persons have a sleep apnea syndrome (*Pickwickian syndrome*) and develop chronic pulmonary hypertension.[458]

An autopsy study of 136 obese patients (obesity defined as a body weight at least 13% higher than in standard actuarial charts) revealed increased epicardial fat in 95%. The heart weight rose roughly in proportion to increased body weight until about 105 kg, falling off thereafter.[468] Increased left and right ventricular wall thicknesses and dilation of right and left ventricular cavities have been found in autopsied obese persons,[462] and myocyte hypertrophy has been observed histologically.[461] A study of the conduction systems of obese young patients who died suddenly revealed fatty infiltration in some of them.[469]

An autopsy study of 10 patients with obesity and sleep apnea hypoventilation syndrome revealed right ventricular hypertrophy, evidence of biventricular failure, and pulmonary hypertensive changes with prominent pulmonary hemosiderosis. Some patients had prominent pulmonary capillary proliferation.[470]

OSLER-WEBER-RENDU DISEASE

Osler-Weber-Rendu disease, or *hereditary hemorrhagic telangiectasia,* encompasses a group of autosomal dominant conditions characterized by telangiectases of the nose, skin, and gastrointestinal system that cause hemorrhage. In some forms, arteriovenous malformations are present in lung and brain. Pulmonary lesions cause cyanosis, dyspnea, and fatigue and are most often found in the lower lobes or in the right middle lobe.[471] Arteriovenous malformations in the liver can cause high-output cardiac failure.[472] The gene for one form of Osler-Weber-Rendu disease is on chromosome 9q3 and encodes endoglin, an endothelial cell–binding protein for TGF-β.[473] The gene for another form is on chromosome 12q.[474]

OSTEOGENESIS IMPERFECTA

Osteogenesis imperfecta affects 1/10,000 of the population. There are four types. Types I, II, and IV are autosomal dominant; type III may be either autosomal dominant or recessive. Type II is lethal in the perinatal period. Parental mosaicism for osteogenesis imperfecta is an important factor in genetic counseling.[475] Bone fragility is present in all types. Scleral color, frequency of hearing loss, and frequency of dentinogenesis imperfecta vary among the types. The molecular deficit in all types causes abnormalities of type I collagen, which is found in bone, ligaments, sclerae, and blood vessels. Type I and type III collagen are found in about equal amounts in blood vessel walls, but type III provides more tensile strength.[243] There is a decreased quantity of type I collagen in most patients with type I osteogenesis imperfecta, whereas most of those with other forms of the disease have qualitative deficits in type I collagen. Ultrastructurally, collagen fibers in skin and osteoid have decreased diameter.[476]

Cardiovascular findings at autopsy of infants with type II osteogenesis imperfecta include deficiency of collagen in valves and blood vessels.[477] In the other types, chest deformity resulting from bone disease can cause secondary cor pulmonale.[478] Aortic regurgitation secondary to aortic root dilation and mitral regurgitation due to mitral valve prolapse also occur.[114, 479, 480] An echocardiographic study of 109 patients from 66 families with osteogenesis imperfecta revealed aortic root dilation in 12%, but the frequency of mitral valve prolapse was not clearly different from that in a normal adult population.[480]

Histologic examination of the aorta reveals thinning of its wall and cystic medial necrosis.[479] Mitral valve prolapse is caused by myxomatous degeneration. There have been case reports of atrial rupture in osteogenesis imperfecta.[481, 482] Patients who undergo cardiac surgery are said to be at increased risk because of tissue fragility[483] and bleeding complications.

OXALOSIS

The three types of primary hyperoxaluria or oxalosis are all autosomal recessive in inheritance. Type I results from a deficiency of hepatic peroxisome alanine:glyoxylate aminotransferase, and type II is caused by glyoxylate reductase deficiency. In both, glyoxylate accumulates proximal to the enzymatic block and is metabolized to oxalate. Type III hyperoxaluria is caused by increased oxalate absorption in the gastrointestinal tract.[484] Secondary oxalosis is usually induced by chronic renal failure but can follow ingestion of oxalates or ethylene glycol, xylitol infusion, methoxyflurane anesthesia, or gastrointestinal disease.[485] Cardiovascular manifestations of primary oxalosis or secondary uremic oxalosis are similar, with congestive heart failure and heart block occurring. The heart may take up ^{99m}Tc-methylene diphosphonate on bone scan.[486] Arterial involvement can cause peripheral ischemia (e.g., gangrene).[487] There have been reports of patients with type I hyperoxaluria in whom successful liver-kidney transplantation reversed cardiac dysfunction.[486]

Deposition of calcium oxalate crystals occurs in the heart and arterial media. The crystals are positively bire-

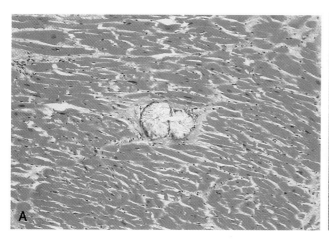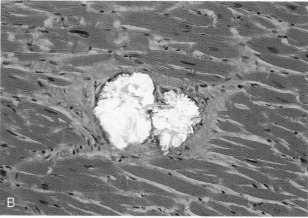

Figure 16-13 • Oxalosis. *A,* Crystals deposited within the myocardium. *B,* Crystals at higher magnification and partly polarized. (Both, H&E stain.)

fringent and form rosettes, dipyramids, diamond shapes, or plate-like structures (Fig. 16-13). They are deposited within cardiac myocytes, in conduction tissue, or in the interstitium.[488] There may be associated necrosis, fibrosis, and a mononuclear and foreign body giant cell reaction.[485]

PARATHYROID DISORDERS

Hyperparathyroidism, whether primary and caused by parathyroid adenoma or hyperplasia, or secondary to chronic renal failure, induces hypercalcemia. Electrocardiographic changes produced in the condition include prolongation of the PR and QRS intervals and shortening of ST and Q-T intervals.[489] Echocardiographic study of a series of 54 patients undergoing surgery for primary hyperparathyroidism revealed aortic valve calcification in 63%, mitral valve calcification in 49%, myocardial calcifications in 69%, and left ventricular hypertrophy in 68%. One year after parathyroid surgery, the left ventricular hypertrophy had regressed, but cardiac calcifications had not altered.[490] Similarly, autopsy study of hypercalcemic patients reveals valvular and myocardial calcifications. Some hypercalcemic patients have tricuspid annular calcification and calcification within pulmonary valve cusps, findings rare in other settings. Medial calcification occurs in coronary and peripheral arteries.[491] Hypercalcemia can also cause calcification that impinges on the AV node.[492] Calcific occlusion of intramyocardial coronary arteries fosters ischemia,[493] while small vessel calcification in the skin causes necrosis and ulceration.[494]

Hypoparathyroidism due to absent parathyroid glands is a component of the DiGeorge syndrome discussed previously. Hypoparathyroidism causes hypocalcemia that is associated with a prolonged Q-T interval on the electrocardiogram. There are many case reports of congestive heart failure related to chronic hypocalcemia that responds to calcium repletion. A Doppler echocardiographic study of eight chronically hypocalcemic subjects lacking cardiovascular symptoms disclosed normal left ventricular function.[495]

PITUITARY DISORDERS

Acromegaly

Hypertension occurs in 13 to 50% of patients with acromegaly,[496] and diabetes is found in 15%.[497] Echocardiography reveals left ventricular hypertrophy in more than 50% of acromegalics in some series; it occurs even in nonhypertensive acromegalics. Asymmetric septal hypertrophy is described in a minority. Decreased left ventricular function sometimes develops, but overt heart failure in the absence of ischemic or hypertensive heart disease is uncommon.[496] Studies examining regression of left ventricular hypertrophy after treatment led to conflicting results.[496] An autopsy study revealed left ventricular hypertrophy in more than 80% of acromegalic patients, with cardiac enlargement disproportionate to enlargement of other organs in some. Histologically, myocyte hypertrophy and interstitial fibrosis were found.[498]

Growth Hormone Deficiency

Subjects with growth hormone deficiency often have carbohydrate intolerance and hypertriglyceridemia and may have hypercholesterolemia.[499] They have a low incidence of atherosclerosis[500] but may have impaired cardiac function.[501] Autopsy study of individuals with hypopituitarism reveals decreased heart weight and basophilic degeneration of myocytes.[502] Treatment with growth hormone increases levels of Lp(a) and HDL cholesterol[499] and seems to normalize cardiac function. There have been trials of growth hormone in the treatment of dilated cardiomyopathy.[501]

A patient with a prolactin-producing pituitary tumor and congestive heart failure has been reported.[503]

POLYCYSTIC KIDNEY DISEASE

Autosomal dominant polycystic kidney disease is produced by a mutation in the polycystic kidney disease 1

(PKD1) gene on chromosome 16, or a mutation in a gene on chromosome 4, or a mutation in a yet unidentified gene. Polycystin, the PKD1 product, is involved in cell-matrix interactions.[504]

The association of autosomal dominant polycystic kidney disease with intracranial arterial aneurysms is well known.[505] Aortic root dilation with aortic regurgitation and pathologically confirmed floppy mitral valve have also been reported.[506] An echocardiographic study revealed a significantly increased (26%) prevalence of mitral valve prolapse.[507] A single patient with coronary artery aneurysms and autosomal dominant polycystic kidney disease[508] and a family with clustering of aortic dissection and cystic kidneys[509] have been described. Because hypertension is common in these patients, secondary left ventricular hypertrophy is to be expected.

POLYMYOSITIS/DERMATOMYOSITIS

These inflammatory myopathies occur in about 1 per 100,000 population and may be associated with other connective tissue diseases. Up to 40% of patients with polymyositis/dermatomyositis develop cardiac abnormalities, specifically arrhythmias and heart failure.[510] Patients may have various autoantibodies. An antibody directed against histidyl transfer RNA or Jo-1 is associated with interstitial lung disease[511] but was also positive in a patient reported to have polymyositis and cardiomyopathy on heart biopsy.[512] Pericardial effusion and pericarditis are less frequently associated with polymyositis and dermatomyositis than with other collagen vascular disorders[513] but do occur, and cardiac tamponade has been reported.[514] Myocarditis was found in 6 of 20 autopsied patients with polymyositis in one series[515]; 4 of them also had myocardial fibrosis and medial thickening of small intramyocardial arteries. Four patients with myocarditis at autopsy had heart failure during life. Fibrosis, with or without chronic inflammation and not considered an infarct, was found in 3 individuals with dermatomyositis in an autopsy series of 16 patients with polymyositis/dermatomyositis.[516]

Electrocardiographic study may reveal different degrees of AV block, bundle branch block, and nonspecific ST-T changes. Atrial fibrillation and atrial and ventricular arrhythmias occur but are not common.[513] Lymphocytic infiltration and fibrosis of the SA node and contraction-band necrosis with lymphocytes involving the left bundle branch were found in one dermatomyositis patient who had left bundle branch block during life.[516] Fibrosis of bundle branches[517] in a polymyositis patient with complete heart block, and fibrosis with mononuclear inflammation in the right bundle branch with additional fibrosis in the SA node and AV node in a dermatomyositis patient with right bundle branch block[518] have been reported.

Echocardiographic mitral valve prolapse occurred in 65% of polymyositis patients in a 1978 study.[519] Floppy mitral valve was found at autopsy in 1 of 16 dermatomyositis patients in another autopsy series[516] but was not described in any of 10 autopsied polymyositis patients in

a third study.[515] Vasculitis is associated with childhood dermatomyositis.[520]

POTASSIUM DISORDERS

Hyperkalemia

Hyperkalemia is associated with the following electrocardiographic changes: tall thin T waves, PR interval prolongation, ST depression, QRS prolongation, loss of P waves, and development of ventricular fibrillation.[489]

Hypokalemia

Hypokalemia can be caused by gastrointestinal losses, treatment of diabetic ketoacidosis, or excessive steroid or aldosterone. Electrocardiographic features of hypokalemia include ST depression, diminution of the T wave, increased height of the U wave, P wave enlargement, and QRS widening.[489] Hypokalemia predisposes to torsades de pointes ventricular tachycardia. Myocyte necrosis has been described at autopsy.[521, 522] Renal tubular vacuolization is usually prominent.

PREGNANCY

Beginning at the fifth to sixth weeks, blood volume and cardiac output rise in pregnancy, with the blood volume increase exceeding increased red cell mass so that a relative anemia develops. Elevated stroke volume accounts for an increased cardiac output in early pregnancy, whereas increased heart rate is responsible subsequently. Systemic vascular resistance falls because of vasodilation and shunting through the placenta. Caval compression by the gravid uterus can significantly depress cardiac output when a pregnant woman is supine. Cardiac output increases further during labor.[523] Serial echocardiographic studies in normal pregnant women show left ventricular hypertrophy and atrophy temporally coupled with changes in hemodynamic load.[524]

Because of the physiologic changes of pregnancy, women with underlying cardiovascular disease have increased morbidity and mortality with pregnancy and delivery, depending on the specific nature of the cardiovascular lesions.[525, 526] Women with left-sided obstruction, pulmonary hypertension, abnormal aorta, impaired ventricular function, prosthetic valves, or cyanosis are at especially high risk.[527] If a pregnant patient must undergo surgery with cardiopulmonary bypass, normothermia[528] and fetal and uterine monitoring are advised.[529]

Gestational diabetes develops in 2 to 4% of pregnant women. About 5% have pre-eclampsia (hypertension, edema, and proteinuria after 20 weeks of gestation in a previously normotensive subject), and 0.2% have eclampsia (pre-eclampsia plus seizures).[523] Reduced organ perfusion is an important feature of pre-eclampsia. Some patients develop a potentially lethal disorder featuring hemolysis, liver dysfunction, and coagulation defects—the HELLP syndrome (*H*emolysis, *E*levated *L*iver enzymes, *Low Platelets*).[530] Possible causes of pre-eclampsia include prostaglandin deficiency, endothelial cell dysfunction,[530] and sympathetic overactivity.[531] The condition resolves with delivery. One study revealed an association between a history of pre-eclampsia and subsequent development of hypertension, ischemic heart disease, and venous thrombosis.[532]

Acute myocardial infarction occurs in about 1 per 10,000 pregnant women. A review of 125 such cases showed that the infarct usually occurs in the third trimester and in women older than 33 years of age. Autopsy or coronary angiography was performed in 68 of the 125 patients and revealed coronary atherosclerosis with or without thrombus in 29 and probable or definite coronary thrombus without atherosclerosis in 14. Sixteen percent had coronary artery dissection, and 29% had normal coronary arteries.[533] It has been suggested that hormonal changes associated with pregnancy may predispose to arterial dissection. The aortic media of pregnant women was found to have decreased glycosaminoglycans, fragmentation of reticulin and elastic fibers, and loss of corrugations of elastic fibers,[534] but this was not confirmed in a subsequent study.[535] Coronary artery dissection is also discussed in Chapter 8.

Venous thromboembolism occurs in 0.1 to 0.2% of pregnancies, the risk being increased five-fold by the pregnancy. Venous stasis due to compression by the uterus and venous relaxation is the major cause, but bed rest, sepsis, and cesarean delivery may also be factors.[536] Pregnancy may hasten the development of varicose veins.

The topic of peripartum cardiomyopathy is addressed in Chapter 10.

PSEUDOXANTHOMA ELASTICUM

Both autosomal dominant and autosomal recessive forms of pseudoxanthoma elasticum occur.[243] Classification is controversial and genetic heterogeneity likely. In this condition elastic fibers in the skin, eyes, and cardiovascular system undergo fragmentation, clumping, and calcification.[537] Skin lesions manifest as yellow-orange papules similar to xanthomas, typically found in the axillae, sides of the neck, and groin. Angioid streaks are found in the ocular fundi. Medium-sized arteries may develop stenoses or aneurysms. Histologically, they show elastic fiber fragmentation and calcification as well as intimal thickening[538] (Fig. 16-14). Calcification involves the elastic lamina, intima, and media. The aorta usually is not involved.[243] Arterial intimal changes resemble the usual forms of atherosclerosis but can differ clinically in being symptomatic at an early age and affecting upper extremity arteries. Involvement of gastric arteries may be associated with fatal hemorrhage, and renovascular involvement can cause hypertension. A group of patients with early-onset coronary artery disease, absent skin lesions, but with angioid streaks and histologic features of pseudoxanthoma elasticum on skin biopsy were described, and their condition was labeled "occult pseudoxanthoma elasticum."[539] The authors suggested that this entity should be considered in subjects who have early-onset

coronary disease in the absence of other risk factors and raised the possibility that arterial grafts to the coronary arteries might be inadvisable because of possible calcification. However, this has not been proven. The atrial endocardium may be thickened with white-yellow plaques. Histologically, these reveal degeneration and calcification of elastic fibers.[537] Sometimes, the endocardial plaques involve mitral or tricuspid valve leaflets[114] or encase the bundle branches.[540] Rarely, involvement of the left ventricular endocardium causes a clinical condition resembling restrictive cardiomyopathy.[541]

REFSUM DISEASE

Adult Refsum disease is an autosomal recessive disorder that features retinitis pigmentosa, peripheral neuropathy, and ataxia. It is caused by a defect in the catabolism of phytanic acid.[542] Conduction defects and left ventricular dysfunction occur.[543] Left ventricular hypertrophy and interstitial fibrosis with myocyte hypertrophy and vacuolization have been described at autopsy.[544]

RHEUMATOID ARTHRITIS

Patients with rheumatoid arthritis have a shortened life-span. In a population-based study about 40% of the excess mortality in women with rheumatoid arthritis was attributable to cardiovascular disease.[545] An echocardiographic survey of 35 patients who lacked cardiac symptoms revealed pericardial effusion in 57%, aortic root enlargement in 34%, mitral valve thickening and/or calcification in 23%, and aortic valve thickening and/or calcification in 20%.[546]

Rheumatoid nodules are typically found in patients who have high serum titers of rheumatoid factor. Microscopically, the nodule has a central zone of necrosis, a surrounding zone of palisaded histiocytes and fibroblasts, and an outer zone of perivascular mononuclear inflammatory cells.[547] Rheumatoid nodules are found in the pericardium, myocardium, conduction tissue, cardiac skeleton and valves, and aorta. Treatment of rheumatoid arthritis with methotrexate may cause "accelerated nodulosis," with a dramatic increase in the size of extra-articular rheumatoid nodules,[548] even while synovial disease improves. Some patients have developed cardiac tamponade[549] and heart failure or sudden death[550] while receiving methotrexate therapy.

Pericarditis is found in about one third of autopsied patients with rheumatoid arthritis, and in almost half of patients on echocardiographic surveys. However symptomatic pericarditis is uncommon. Acute pericarditis is more common than tamponade or constriction. If pericardiocentesis is performed, the pericardial fluid typically has increased leukocytes, protein, and lactate dehydrogenase with decreased glucose. It may contain rheumatoid factor.[551] Histologic examination of resected pericardium from patients with constrictive pericarditis revealed fibrosis and chronic inflammation with or without rheumatoid nodules.[552] See Chapter 12 for further discussion.

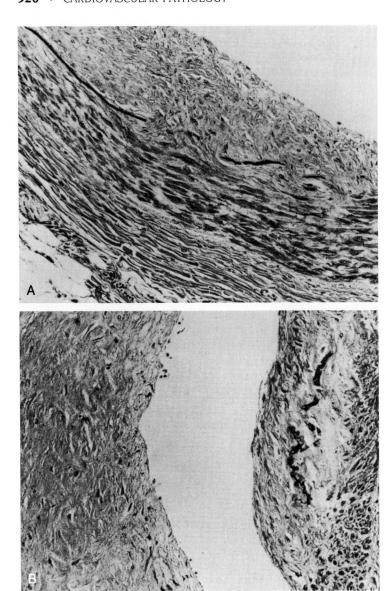

Figure 16-14 • Pseudoxanthoma elasticum. *A* and *B*, Two views of coronary arteries, showing dark areas of calcification and fragmentation of the internal elastic lamina (H&E stain). (From Ferrans VJ: Metabolic and familial diseases. In: Silver MD [ed]: Cardiovascular Pathology. 2nd ed. New York, Churchill Livingstone, 1991, p 1100.)

Rheumatoid nodules are also found within the endocardium, affecting any of the cardiac valves, or in the myocardium.[553] When valves are involved, the nodules are located within the leaflet surrounded by valve tissue. They may cause no valve dysfunction, or, by thickening and distorting the valve, they may lead to regurgitation. Valve stiffening due to the inflammation can cause stenosis. The mitral valve is more often involved than the aortic or right-sided valves.[553] A left atrial rheumatoid nodule mimicking a left atrial myxoma, with a pedunculated lesion prolapsing into the mitral valve, has been reported.[554]

Aortitis was found in 10 of a series of 188 autopsied patients.[555] (See also Chapter 5.) Two had aneurysms of the ascending aorta and/or aortic root, and 1 had aortitis as well as an abdominal aortic aneurysm. Intimal plaques and adventitial nodules were found on gross examination. Four patients with aortitis had grossly abnormal aortic valves, including three with rheumatoid nodules in the aortic root extending into the base of the valve cusps and

1 with a mononuclear inflammation and necrosis in the aortic valve cusps. Histologic examination of the aorta revealed inflammatory infiltrates consisting of lymphocytes, plasma cells, and occasional histiocytes and polymorphonuclear cells, involving all three aortic tunica in 3 of the 10 cases, or else just medial and adventitial involvement. There was inflammation around vasa vasorum but no luminal obliteration. Necrosis of aortic medial smooth muscle cells and/or elastic fiber disruption were present in 8 of 10 cases. Intimal necrosis and fibrosis occurred in those with intimal inflammation. Five patients had rheumatoid nodules in their aortic adventitia, and 3 had them in the media as well. Four had vasculitis involving branches of the aorta, with this vasculitis a cause of myocardial, gut, or kidney infarcts in some patients.[555] (Fig. 5-26 presents histologic findings in the aorta.)

Patients with rheumatoid arthritis can develop small-vessel vasculitis involving the skin or vasculitis of small and medium-sized arteries, typically causing mononeuritis multiplex or gangrene.[556, 557]

RUBELLA

Intrauterine rubella infection induces deafness, cataracts, microcephaly, and cardiac defects.[558] The typical cardiac lesions are patent ductus arteriosus, peripheral pulmonary artery stenoses, and ventricular septal defect.[559] Intimal thickening in the aorta and systemic arteries have also been described.[560] Widespread vaccination against rubella has not completely eliminated this problem.[561]

SCLERODERMA

Scleroderma, a *progressive systemic sclerosis,* is a systemic disorder in which there is fibrosis of skin and viscera, microcirculatory abnormalities, and the production of antinuclear antibodies. Patients may have diffuse or limited skin involvement, the latter termed CREST (for *C*alcinosis, *R*aynaud phenomenon, *E*sophagus, *S*clerodactyly, *T*elangiectasia). Cardiac involvement is not common.[562] Its clinical features are (1) congestive heart failure, (2) typical or atypical chest pain, (3) pericarditis, and (4) arrhythmias.

Pericardial effusion, myocardial fibrosis, myocarditis, right ventricular hypertrophy secondary to pulmonary disease, left ventricular hypertrophy secondary to systemic hypertension, and valvular lesions have been described. Pericardial effusion and acute pericarditis may affect patients with scleroderma.[563] Cardiac tamponade has been reported in those with either systemic scleroderma or CREST.[564] A patient with CREST and pericardial calcification in the absence of peripheral calcinosis has also been described.[565] Pneumopericardium due to esophagopericardial fistula can occur.[566]

Conduction defects, supraventricular tachycardia, and ventricular arrhythmias develop in patients with scleroderma.[567, 568] Scarring is found within the conduction system but overall seems less extensive than that within the ventricular myocardium.[569] Some large autopsy series[570, 571] failed to show that cardiac valvular abnormali-

ties were increased in scleroderma patients compared with controls.

Scleroderma involving myocardium causes a patchy fibrosis that is randomly located in the ventricular walls[572] (Fig. 16-15) and not related to perfusion territories of epicardial coronary arteries. The areas of fibrosis can be large enough to mimic an infarct. There may be associated contraction-band necrosis. It is unusual to find histologic disease of intramyocardial coronary arteries,[573] although there is evidence for such disease on thallium scans and coronary flow reserve measurements. Myocardial inflammation is not common. Heart biopsies showing fibrosis have been reported,[574, 575] as well as others with lymphocytic inflammation.[576] Increased numbers of myocardial mast cells were described in 3 scleroderma patients who came to autopsy.[577] Associations between myositis and myocardial dysfunction have been reported.[578]

Digital arteries in patients with scleroderma and Raynaud phenomenon demonstrate intimal fibrosis with, sometimes, severe luminal stenosis, internal elastic lamina breaks and reduplication, normal medial thickness, and, occasionally, adventitial fibrosis. Digital artery thrombi may sometimes be found but not vasculitis.[579] The typical vascular lesions of scleroderma in organs such as the kidney consist of intimal proliferation in small arteries and arterioles.[580] Cases of vasculitis involving skin and peripheral nerves in patients with CREST plus Sjögren syndrome have been reported.[581]

SCURVY

Vitamin C (ascorbic acid) is an antioxidant. It improves iron absorption and serves as a cofactor for collagen synthesis. In scurvy, the perivascular connective tissue degenerates; therefore, hemorrhages occur.[582] Scurvy may be mistaken for vasculitis.[583] Sudden death,[584] right ventricular hypertrophy,[585] and cardiomegaly have also been described. Peripheral edema may rapidly respond to replacement therapy,[586] and so may ST and T-wave changes.[587]

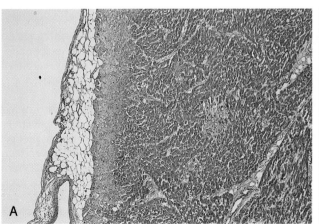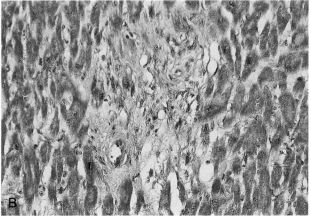

Figure 16-15 • Scleroderma. *A,* Patchy myocyte loss in the subepicardial zone. *B,* Higher magnification reveals fibroblasts and glycosaminoglycan accumulation. No scleroderma vascular lesions were found within this heart. (Both, Movat stain.)

Because vitamin C is an antioxidant, its role in coronary atherosclerosis has been examined. Investigations of the effects of vitamin C supplements on coronary events have had inconsistent results, but in one recent study there was an association between vitamin C deficiency and myocardial infarction.[588]

SEPSIS

Sepsis is a clinical syndrome in which altered organ perfusion is caused by systemic responses to infection. Mortality is 20 to 50%, with sepsis the most common cause of death in adult noncoronary intensive care units.[589] Precise criteria for the diagnosis of systemic inflammatory response syndrome, sepsis, severe sepsis, and septic shock have been established for use in trials of innovative therapies.[589] These incorporate determinations of temperature, respiratory rate, heart rate, arterial blood gases, urine output, blood pressure, systemic vascular resistance, coagulation parameters, and mental status. Mediators thought to be involved in the development of sepsis syndromes include tumor necrosis factor-α; interleukins 1, 6, and 8; interferon-α; arachidonic acid metabolites; platelet activating factor; histamine; bradykinin; angiotensin; complement components; vasoactive intestinal peptide; and nitric oxide. Endothelial injury is important in pathogenesis. Septic shock typically features hypotension, decreased systemic vascular resistance, and normal or increased cardiac output.[590] The right and left cardiac ventricles have impaired function and dilate if fluid-loaded.[591] Both depressed myocardial contractility and impaired peripheral vascular response to vasoactive drugs may be partly mediated by nitric oxide.[590]

SICKLE CELL DISEASE

The sickle cell diseases are hereditary disorders of hemoglobin structure and consist of homozygous sickle cell anemia (HbSS), HbSC disease, and HbS-thalassemia.

Sickle cell anemia is characterized by a chronic hemolytic anemia and vaso-occlusion. It is caused by a valine substitution for glutamic acid in the sixth position of the β globin chain.[592] Vascular occlusion results from sickling (see Fig. 8-44C and D), intimal thickening, or thrombosis.[593] Clinically, cardiac output is increased as in other anemias. Patients may complain of dyspnea and palpitations.[594] An echocardiographic study of clinically stable patients revealed cardiac chamber dilation, increased ventricular septal thickness, and normal contractility.[595]

At autopsy, in chronic cases, cardiomegaly, chamber dilation, and hypertrophy are found.[596] Hemosiderosis may be seen in patients with HbS-thalassemia. Scarring of left ventricular papillary muscles is common,[597] and degenerative changes in the conduction system have been reported.[598] (See also Chapter 8.)

Pulmonary vascular occlusion occurs in patients with HbSS, HbSC, and HbS-thalassemia. This is most often a result of in situ sickling and thrombosis, although fat and bone marrow emboli have also been reported. Patients may develop chronic pulmonary hypertensive disease. Those with the "acute chest syndrome"—an acute illness with a new pulmonary infiltrate on chest radiographs—may have pulmonary infection, pulmonary infarction, or both.[592, 599]

Stroke is a common cause of death in affected children. It is usually a result of vascular occlusion. Hemorrhagic stroke tends to occur in older patients.[592, 600]

The median age of death in patients with HbSS is 42 years for males and 48 years for females; for those with HbSC, it is 60 years for males and 68 years for females.[601]

Sickle cell trait (HbSA) may be a risk factor for exercise-related sudden death.[602]

SJÖGREN SYNDROME

Sjögren syndrome is characterized by lymphocytic destruction of lacrimal and salivary glands. Associations with pericarditis,[603] leukocytoclastic vasculitis,[604] and pulmonary hypertension[605] have been described. A Sjögren syndrome patient with a clinically noninfected vegetation of the mitral valve has been reported.[606] Individuals with Sjögren syndrome may have antibodies to SSA/Ro antigens,[607] and the fetus of a mother with such antibodies risks heart block.[608]

SYSTEMIC LUPUS ERYTHEMATOSUS

Systemic lupus erythematosus (SLE), an autoimmune disease, affects women more frequently than men. Cardiovascular disease is an important cause of death.[609] The heart may also be affected secondarily by systemic or pulmonary hypertension. Systemic hypertension occurs in 25 to 49% of SLA patients,[610] and sensitive Doppler echocardiographic techniques demonstrated mild pulmonary hypertension in 43% in one study.[611]

Pericarditis and/or pericardial effusion develop in more than 30% of affected individuals. Cardiac tamponade occurs occasionally, but constriction is rare.[612, 613]

Indium-111–antimyosin Fab imaging has been used to demonstrate myocardial involvement in patients with SLE.[614] Clinical features of myocarditis may correlate with myositis.[615] Myocardial mononuclear inflammation was found in 3 of 36 autopsied patients in one series[616] (Fig. 16-16). However, cases described as myocarditis in the literature do not always satisfy the Dallas criteria for diagnosis. (See also Chapter 9.)

The mortality rate from ischemic heart disease in SLE patients is estimated to be nine times higher than expected. Risk factors such as hypertension and hyperlipidemia are common in these patients.[617] Their coronary artery disease may correlate with the duration of steroid use,[618] and it has been proposed that corticosteroids accelerate atherosclerosis in SLE patients.[616] An autopsy series of 21 women with SLE who were between 16 and 37 years of age revealed >75% cross-sectional area narrowing by atherosclerosis of one or more coronary arteries in 10 of them.[619] Myocardial infarcts occur in young pa-

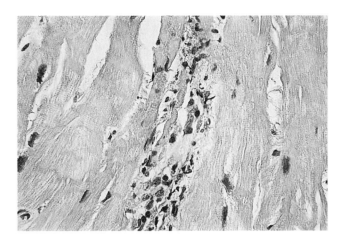

Figure 16-16 • Systemic lupus erythematosus. Myocarditis found in a right ventricular heart biopsy (H&E stain).

tients,[620] most caused by atherosclerotic coronary disease. However, occasional cases are the result of coronary vasculitis,[621] and some are embolic or related to the antiphospholipid antibody syndrome. Several cases of coronary artery aneurysm have been reported[620]; the cause of at least some of them was thought to be vasculitis.

Cardiac conduction tissue may show scarring or inflammation. Luminal narrowing of the SA and AV node arteries is common.[616]

An echocardiographic study revealed abnormalities of the cardiac valves in more than 50% of patients.[622] This was most often a diffuse thickening of aortic and/or mitral valves, often associated with decreased mobility. Fewer than 10% of the subjects had valvular calcification. More than one third had valve vegetations, usually on the atrial side of the mitral valve or the aortic side of the aortic valve. Overall, about 25% of patients had valvular regurgitation, and 3% had stenosis. On follow-up evaluation, the valve disease was an important cause of morbidity and mortality due to stroke, heart failure, or infective endocarditis.

Libman and Sacks reported endocardial lesions at au-topsy in four patients with SLE. They consisted of thrombotic vegetations involving any of the four cardiac valves plus the atrial and ventricular endocardium.[623] They were often found along the lines of closure of valves but were not restricted to this zone and were also present on either side of the line of closure (Fig. 16-17). Vegetations were also common on the ventricular surface of the posterior mitral leaflet, extending from there to the left ventricular endocardium, toward the papillary muscles. Some valves were also thickened with fibrous tissue. Histologically, vegetations were formed of fibrin and platelets and the underlying valve or endocardium showed neovascularization, active fibroblasts, and mononuclear inflammation. Hematoxylin bodies could be found. Cultures and special stains for organisms were negative. It has been suggested that, with modern therapy for SLE, the valve lesions (of nonbacterial thrombotic endocarditis [NBTE] type) seen at autopsy now show more evidence of healing, with fibrosis, calcification, and valvular distortion resulting in regurgitation.[616] There has been a report of tricuspid stenosis and regurgitation in one patient with SLE.[624] Mitral valve chordal rupture, apparently in the absence of myxomatous degeneration or infection, can occur.[625] Systemic emboli may derive from the endocardial vegetations. It is not always possible to determine whether ischemic lesions in body organs were caused by in situ thrombosis or by emboli from valves. NBTE is discussed in Chapter 14.

Small-vessel vasculitis in SLE is especially common in the kidneys.[626] Noninflammatory vascular thromboses are associated with the antiphospholipid antibody syndrome (see next paragraph). Atherosclerosis of peripheral arteries occurs in SLE patients and causes the usual range of complications.[627] There have been rare reports of aortitis in patients with SLE.[628, 629]

Antiphospholipid Antibody Syndrome

The lupus anticoagulant and antibodies to cardiolipin are autoantibodies to phospholipid and are demonstrated in patients with SLE and other disorders. The antibodies prolong phospholipid-dependent coagulation tests in vitro; in vivo, they are not usually associated with bleeding[630]

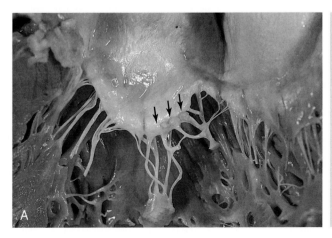
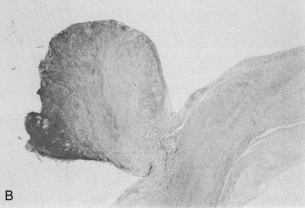

Figure 16-17 • Systemic lupus erythematosus—Libman-Sacks endocarditis. *A*, Note three thrombotic vegetations on the anterior leaflet of the mitral valve, near its line of closure (arrows). *B*, Histologic section revealing a partly organized vegetation on the mitral valve (H&E stain).

but with thrombus formation in arteries and veins. They may also cause thrombocytopenia and recurrent fetal loss due to placental thrombosis.[631] Because a number of assays have been used to detect these antibodies historically, there is variability in the data regarding their prevalence. Between 28 and 44% of SLE patients have a lupus anticoagulant. Steroid treatment can decrease its level. Correlation exists between the presence of anticardiolipin and lupus anticoagulant, but they are separate entities. Antiphospholipid antibodies are also found in other autoimmune disorders, with malignancy, and in HIV infection and can be induced by drugs that produce lupus-like syndromes. (See Chapter 17.) Anticardiolipin antibodies also occur in patients with syphilis, in those with acute infection, and even in the healthy elderly. At least half of the patients with the antiphospholipid antibody syndrome do not have SLE.[632] The prevalence of lupus anticoagulant in the general population has been estimated at 2%, and that of anticardiolipin at 0 to 7.5%. The clinical features of the antiphospholipid antibody syndrome include neurologic deficits, obstetric complications, cardiac valvular disease, and skin lesions.[633]

Thrombi (NBTE) are common on cardiac valves in affected patients, and their organization produces thickened, deformed, fibrotic valves. Echocardiographic studies reveal valvular abnormalities in approximately one third of patients with the syndrome.[633] Some echocardiographic studies indicate a higher prevalence of valve defects in SLE patients with antiphospholipid antibodies than in those without the antibodies, but other investigators have demonstrated no such difference. The valve abnormalities detected by echocardiography have consisted of verrucous or diffuse thickening of aortic and mitral valves and regurgitation.[633] (See further discussion in Chapter 14.)

The role of antiphospholipid antibodies in the pathogenesis of coronary artery disease is controversial. Certainly, acute coronary occlusion in young patients with SLE is well recognized. There have been several reports of thrombosis of intramyocardial arteries in patients with SLE and in those with the antiphospholipid antibody syndrome. Thrombotic occlusion occurs in large and small peripheral arteries, causing complications such as gangrene and livedo reticularis.[634] Aortic occlusion[635] and frequent occlusion of hemodialysis grafts[636] have also been reported in SLE patients with antiphospholipid antibodies. Histologic examination reveals fresh or organizing thrombi within small arteries. Vasculitis is not a feature. Concentric cellular and fibrous intimal thickening similar to hypertensive arteriolosclerosis may also be found.[637] Venous thrombosis and pulmonary emboli are part of the syndrome.[634] Thrombi within the right or left atrium can mimic cardiac myxoma.

Congenital Heart Block

Isolated congenital heart block occurs in 1 of every 15,000 to 22,000 live births and can cause fetal death.[638] Even if a permanent pacemaker is not required in infancy, it may be necessary later.[639] About 90% of cases are the result of neonatal lupus.[639] The cause is the transplacental passage of maternal antibodies to Ro/SS-A and La/SS-B ribonucleoproteins. Neonatal lupus features skin and hepatic involvement as well as heart block, but only the heart block is permanent. More than 40% of mothers of affected infants are asymptomatic at the time of the birth, whereas others have SLE or Sjögren syndrome. The mothers may develop SLE subsequently.[640]

Examination of the conduction system reveals fibrofatty replacement of the AV node and adjacent atrial septal tissue, sometimes with calcification and rarely with leukocyte infiltration. A case report describes an infant with congenital heart block and maternal anti-Ro antibodies[641] who also had mitral and tricuspid regurgitation due to fibrosis and calcification of chordae tendineae with a chordal rupture near the papillary muscles.[642]

THALASSEMIA

Cardiovascular complications of thalassemia include heart failure, arrhythmias, and pericarditis. Apart from the effect of chronic anemia on the heart, hemosiderin deposition in the myocardium causes dysfunction[643] (see earlier discussion of hemochromatosis). Histologic myocarditis has been reported[644] in patients with β-thalassemia major.

THIAMINE DEFICIENCY (CAUSES BERIBERI)

Thiamine (vitamin B_1) deficiency causes *Wernicke-Korsakoff syndrome* and *beriberi*. Thiamine diphosphate is a coenzyme for the oxidative decarboxylation of α-keto acids and for transketolase in the hexose monophosphate shunt. Thiamine deficiency was first described in subjects who ate a polished rice diet in the Orient. In the West, where flour is supplemented with thiamine, deficiency now occurs mostly in alcoholics and food faddists.[645] Deficiency may also occur with hyperthyroidism, diuresis, dialysis, diarrhea,[646] and total parenteral nutrition.[647] Diagnosis of this vitamin deficiency can be made by measuring transketolase activity in red blood cells or by a direct measurement of thiamine levels in blood by high-performance liquid chromatography.[648] *Dry beriberi* refers to the associated neuropathy. *Wet beriberi* refers to congestive heart failure, which, when fulminant, is called *Shoshin disease.* A possible role for thiamine deficiency in the sudden death of young expatriate Asian workers is controversial.[649, 650] Thiamine-deficient alcoholics may manifest acute lactic acidosis[651] because lack of thiamine affects pyruvate and lactate metabolism.[652] A report of six patients with acute beriberi emphasized the triad of heart failure and lactic acidosis without hypoxemia.[652] The heart failure is characterized by high cardiac output, low peripheral vascular resistance, and chiefly signs and symptoms of right-sided heart failure.[653] The response to thiamine is dramatic in some patients.

At autopsy, myocardial hypertrophy and chamber dilation, hydropic degeneration of myocytes, and interstitial edema and fibrosis have been described.[654, 655] These changes are nonspecific. Right ventricular hypertrophy and dilation have been emphasized by some authors.[656]

THROMBOTIC THROMBOCYTOPENIC PURPURA

A thrombotic microangiopathy is the characteristic pathologic feature of thrombotic thrombocytopenic purpura (TTP) and of the *hemolytic-uremic syndrome.* The clinical pentad of these disorders is thrombocytopenia, nonimmune hemolytic anemia, neurologic defects, renal disease, and fever.[657] Some cases of hemolytic-uremic syndrome are related to infection with *Escherichia coli* 0157:H7.[658] Others have been reported in patients with adenocarcinoma treated with mitomycin C,[659] after bone marrow transplantation,[660] and in cyclosporine-treated patients who have undergone kidney and pancreas transplantation.[661]

Patients with TTP may have thrombi in capillaries and arterioles and hemorrhages in the heart (Fig. 16-18), including the conduction system.[662] Such involvement can cause heart failure, arrhythmias, or sudden death. Heart biopsy in one patient revealed myocarditis as well as vascular thrombosis.[663] (See discussion in Chapter 8.)

THYROID DISORDERS

Hyperthyroidism

Hyperthyroidism, or *Graves disease,* has characteristic effects on cardiovascular physiology, namely (1) resting tachycardia, (2) increased cardiac index, (3) decreased systemic vascular resistance, (4) increased left ventricular contractility,[664] and (5) risk for developing atrial fibrillation.[665]

It is associated with echocardiographic left ventricular hypertrophy,[666] although only a minority of patients have an increased heart weight at autopsy once coexisting factors such as hypertension are excluded.[667] In some studies,[668] mitral valve prolapse had an increased incidence in patients with Graves disease. Angina pectoris was reported in patients with hyperthyroidism and normal coronary arteries.[669] It was presumed to be a result of coronary artery spasm and responded to treatment of the thyroid disorder.

Hypothyroidism

Hypothyroidism causes (1) a low cardiac index, (2) decreased intravascular volume, (3) increased systemic vascular resistance, (4) sometimes hypertension,[664] and (5) pericardial effusion in about one third of patients.[670]

A long-standing pericardial effusion may contain cholesterol crystals, giving it the appearance of gold paint, but this finding is not specific for hypothyroidism. Fatal cardiac tamponade has been reported in hypothyroidism.[671] (See also Chapter 12.) Some patients develop reversible asymmetric septal hypertrophy.[672] Basophilic degeneration of cardiac myocytes may be found (see Chapter 3). Chronic lymphocytic thyroiditis is associated

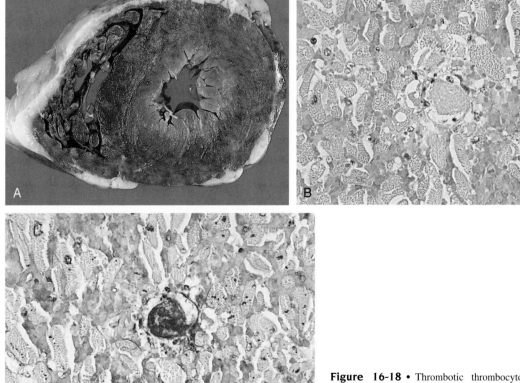

Figure 16-18 • Thrombotic thrombocytopenic purpura. *A,* Gross photograph of heart reveals multiple myocardial hemorrhages. *B,* Histologic section demonstrates myocardial hemorrhage surrounding a capillary thrombus (H&E stain). *C,* The latter is strongly periodic acid–Schiff–positive (PAS diatase).

with an increased incidence of mitral valve prolapse[673] and with giant cell myocarditis.[674] Whether hypothyroidism predisposes to coronary artery disease is uncertain.[675] However, its treatment may worsen symptoms of ischemic heart disease because of increased cardiac oxygen demand. Increased creatine kinase and creatine kinase MB in the absence of myocardial infarction may occur in hypothyroid patients because of altered metabolism.[676] Myocardial capillary basement membranes may be thickened, but this is neither a uniform nor a specific change.[138, 677]

Cardiopulmonary bypass causes a euthyroid sick state with drops in T_3 levels of 50 to 75% that last for 1 to 4 days. T_3 administration immediately after bypass is associated with increased cardiac output and decreased systemic vascular resistance.[664]

TRISOMY SYNDROMES

Patau Syndrome

Trisomy 13 occurs in 1 of 5000 births. Typical features are holoprosencephaly, polydactyly, growth retardation, omphalocele, and cystic renal dysplasia.[678]

Cardiac defects include (1) infundibular ventricular septal defect, (2) double-outlet right ventricle,[676] (3) patent ductus arteriosus, (4) atrial septal defect,[679] and (5) calcification of papillary muscle.[681]

Edwards Syndrome

The incidence of trisomy 18 or Edwards syndrome is about 1 in 3000 at birth.[676] Survival beyond 1 year of age is rare. Characteristic features include polyhydramnios, growth retardation, diaphragmatic hernia, rocker bottom feet, and omphalocele.[676] Associated cardiac anomalies are (1) ventricular septal defect, (2) complete atrioventricular canal, (3) double-outlet right ventricle,[676] (4) atrial septal defect, (5) dysplasia of pulmonic and tricuspid valves,[679, 680] (6) tetralogy of Fallot, (7) bicuspid aortic valve, (8) coarctation of aorta, and (9) rapid development of pulmonary hypertensive disease. Transposition of the great arteries and inversions of the heart or viscera are not found.[681]

Down Syndrome

Down syndrome occurs in 1 of 600 births and is usually caused by trisomy 21. The congenital heart defects seen are (1) complete or partial atrioventricular canal, (2) ventricular septal defect, (3) tetralogy of Fallot, (4) atrial septal defect, and (5) patent ductus arteriosus.[682]

Calcification of papillary muscle and epicardial lymphocytic infiltration are reported in fetuses with the syndrome.[680] Children with Down syndrome and complete atrioventricular canal develop pulmonary hypertensive changes more rapidly than those without Down syndrome who have the same cardiac defect.[683] An echocardiographic study of adults with the syndrome and no cardiac symptoms disclosed mitral valve prolapse in 57% and

mild aortic regurgitation in 11%.[684] The molecular mechanisms of meiotic nondisjunction causing Down syndrome associated with AV canal defects have been reported.[685]

TUBEROUS SCLEROSIS

Tuberous sclerosis is an autosomal dominant disease in which benign tumors develop in many organ systems (e.g., facial angiofibromas, renal angiomyolipomas, subependymal nodules).[686] Two genetic loci, on chromosomes 9q34 and 16p13.3, are linked to the disease.[687] Cardiac rhabdomyomas are common (see Chapter 19 for further discussion).[688] Right ventricular hypertrophy may occur secondary to pulmonary lymphangiomyomatosis. Hemangiomas, intracranial aneurysms, and eight cases of thoracic or abdominal aortic aneurysms have been reported. Histologic examination of one such aneurysm revealed cystic medial necrosis,[689] a nonspecific change.

TURNER SYNDROME

Turner syndrome occurs in 1 of every 1500 to 2500 live-born female infants. The karyotype can be monosomy X (45,X) or mosaic monosomy X (45,X/46,XX), or one X chromosome may be structurally abnormal. In two thirds of patients, it is the maternal X chromosome that is retained. More than 50% of Turner syndrome patients are mosaics. The use of FISH technology increases the ability to detect mosaicism.[690]

Typical clinical features are (1) webbed neck, (2) cystic hygroma, (3) horseshoe kidney, (4) short stature, (5) amenorrhea, (6) low hairline, (7) shield chest, (8) deformed ears, and (9) cardiovascular abnormalities. Poor development of the lymphatic system in these patients is a proposed mechanism for many of the anomalies.[690]

A bicuspid aortic valve can be found in up to 34% of Turner syndrome patients but was present in only 14% of cases in one series.[691] A congenitally bicuspid aortic valve increases the risk for aortic root dilation. Coarctation of the aorta, usually postductal, occurs in fewer than 20% of patients.[690] Pulmonary valve abnormalities are uncommon.[691] Pulmonary stenosis is usual and is apparently found only in patients with mosaic monosomy. Associations of Turner syndrome with hypoplastic left heart syndrome[692] and with partial anomalous pulmonary venous return[693] have also been noted. Patients with Turner syndrome have an increased risk of aortic dissection, even in the absence of aortic coarctation or a bicuspid aortic valve. Cystic medial necrosis, which is nonspecific, has been found in dissected aortas.[694] Associations between specific karyotypes and particular cardiovascular abnormalities in Turner syndrome are under active investigation.[692]

UREMIA

Death due to cardiovascular disease is common in uremic subjects, occurring 20 times more frequently than in the general population.[695] Congestive heart failure in these patients may be related to hypertension, fluid overload, pericardial disease, and the increased cardiac output necessitated by arteriovenous fistulas, anemia, and/or pericardial disease.[696] Left ventricular hypertrophy occurs and may not be completely explained by hypertension and increased cardiac output.[695] Interstitial myocardial fibrosis is more prominent in uremic subjects than in those with hypertension or diabetes mellitus.[695] A study of iliac vein histology revealed increased medial thickness in hypertensive uremic patients.[697] The effect of hypercalcemia on the heart is discussed in the section on parathyroid disorders. The specific topic of mitral annular calcification is addressed in Chapter 3. Uremic pericardial disease is discussed in Chapter 12.

WHIPPLE DISEASE

Typical clinical features of Whipple disease include fever, weight loss, abdominal pain, arthritis, and lymphadenopathy. Cardiovascular involvement includes (1) pericarditis, (2) myocarditis, (3) endocarditis, and (4) coronary arteritis. Valvular disease may cause mitral stenosis or aortic regurgitation, and involvement of a bioprosthetic valve has been reported.[698] Myocardial involvement may cause heart failure or sudden death.[699]

Traditionally the diagnosis was made by the histologic identification of foam cells containing PAS-positive material. Because a similar light microscopic appearance is found in AIDS patients with *Mycobacterium avium-intracellulare* infection, acid-fast staining must be performed to exclude mycobacterial infection. Ultrastructurally, rod-shaped organisms 0.25 × 1.1 to 1.5 μm are present within macrophages,[700] and the electron microscopic appearances are quite typical.[701] Molecular biology techniques are used to identify an organism called *Tropheryma whippelii*, a gram-positive actinomycete.[702]

At autopsy, typical foam cells may be seen in pericardium, myocardium, and valves, associated with chronic inflammation and fibrosis.[703] Heart biopsy may reveal lymphocytic infiltration and interstitial fibrosis without identifiable organisms.[704] A sarcoid-like histologic appearance, with granulomas and multinucleated giant cells, has also been described.[704] An involved mitral valve may grossly resemble one affected by rheumatic disease, with thickening and fibrosis of leaflets and chordae tendineae.[703] Platelet-fibrin vegetations containing characteristic macrophages may be found.[705] Involved aortic valves demonstrate thickening and fibrosis of cusps with the microscopic features of Whipple disease.[706] Whipple disease involving a bioprosthetic valve was responsible for erosions and vegetations[707] of the leaflets.

WILLIAMS SYNDROME

Williams syndrome encompasses abnormal ("elfin") facies, mental retardation, infantile hypercalcemia, connective tissue abnormalities, and cardiovascular defects, most often supravalvular aortic stenosis.[708] It is caused by a deletion in the elastin gene at 7q11.23.[709] Most cases are sporadic. It should be noted that supravalvular aortic stenosis can also occur as an isolated autosomal dominant condition.[710]

Apart from supravalvular aortic stenosis, patients with Williams syndrome may have stenosis of peripheral pulmonary,[708] renal, celiac, or mesenteric arteries; stenosis of the aortic arch branches; or a more diffuse stenosis of the aorta,[711] sometimes termed midaortic syndrome.[443] Because coronary arteries arise proximal to the aortic stenosis, they are exposed to elevated blood pressure and may develop tortuosity, intimal thickening, and histologically disorganized medial fibroelastic tissue.[712] The coronary disease can cause myocardial ischemia and infarction.[712] An aortic valve cusp may adhere to the area of supravalvular stenosis, excluding a coronary artery from blood flow. Such nonperfused coronary arteries are thin-walled.[713]

Supravalvular aortic stenosis consists of three types: membranous, diffuse, and hourglass. Patients with Williams syndrome may have any of these. Sections of the narrowed portion of aorta in hourglass or diffuse lesions reveal a disorganized arrangement of thick elastic fibers, increased fibrous tissue, and hypertrophied smooth muscle cells. The membranous type of stenosis contains fibroelastic tissue and glysosaminoglycans.[714] (See also Chapter 13.)

WILSON DISEASE

This autosomal recessive disorder of copper transport occurs in about 1 of every 30,000 people. The defect affects incorporation of copper from liver into ceruloplasmin and excretion of copper into bile.[715] Wilson disease is caused by mutations in the gene for a copper-transporting ATPase that is expressed in the liver. The gene is on chromosome 13q. More than 50 different mutations have been discovered so far, and there appear to be correlations between the type of mutation and clinical features of the disease.[400] The accumulated copper has toxic effects, especially on liver and brain. In most patients the diagnosis is made by the findings of Kayser-Fleischer rings on slit-lamp examination and hypoceruloplasminemia.[716] Treatment is with the chelating agents penicillamine or trientene, occasionally with zinc, or with liver transplantation.[716]

Cardiovascular involvement is rarely reported, but the disease may be associated with arrhythmias and heart failure.[717] An autopsy study of nine patients revealed cardiac hypertrophy, interstitial fibrosis, and fibrous thickening of the walls of intramural small vessels. Rubeanic acid and rhodamine stains for copper were negative despite a greatly increased myocardial copper content demonstrated by spectrophotometry. Cardiac changes did not seem to correlate with penicillamine therapy or with cirrhosis in these patients.[718]

REFERENCES

1. Oelkers W: Adrenal insufficiency. N Engl J Med 335:1206, 1996
2. Hartog M, Joplin GF: Effects of cortisol deficiency on the electrocardiogram. BMJ 2:275, 1968

3. Baker NW: The pathologic anatomy in 28 cases of Addison's disease. Arch Pathol Lab Med 8:432, 1929

4. Bravo EL: Primary aldosteronism. Cardiol Clin 6:509, 1988

5. Denolle T, Chatellier G, Julien E, et al: Left ventricular mass and geometry before and after etiologic treatment in renovascular hypertension, aldosterone-producing adenoma, and pheochromocytoma. Am J Hypertens 6:907, 1993

6. Rossi GP, Sacchetto A, Pavan E, et al: Remodeling of the left ventricle in primary aldosteronism due to Conn's adenoma. Circulation 95:1471, 1997

7. Geist M, Dorian P, Davies T, et al: Hyperaldosteronism and sudden cardiac death. Am J Cardiol 78:605, 1996

8. Biglieri EG: Rare causes of adrenocortical hypertension. Cardiology 72(suppl 1):70, 1985

9. Howlett TA, Rees LH, Besser GM: Cushing's syndrome. Clin Endocrinol Metab 14:911, 1985

10. Sugihara N, Shimizu M, Ino H, et al: Cardiac characteristics and postoperative courses in Cushing's syndrome. Am J Cardiol 69:1475, 1992

11. Younge PA, Shmidt D, Wiles PG: Cushing's syndrome: Still a potential killing disease. J R Soc Med 88:174, 1995

12. Nashel DJ: Is atherosclerosis a complication of long-term corticosteroid treatment? Am J Med 80:925, 1986

13. Carney JA: Psammomatous melanotic schwannoma: A distinctive, heritable tumor with special associations, including cardiac myxoma and the Cushing syndrome. Am J Surg Pathol 14:206, 1990

14. Carney JA, Hruska LS, Beauchamp GD, Gordon H: Dominant inheritance of the complex of myxomas, spotty pigmentation, and endocrine overactivity. Mayo Clin Proc 61:165, 1986

15. Bravo EL, Gifford RW Jr: Pheochromocytoma: Diagnosis, localization and management. N Engl J Med 311:1298, 1984

16. Moriguchi A, Otsuka A, Kohara K, et al: Evaluation of orthostatic hypotension using power spectral analysis. Am J Hypertens 6:198, 1993

17. Van Vliet PD, Burchell HB, Titus JL: Focal myocarditis associated with pheochromocytoma. N Engl J Med 274:1102, 1966

18. Huddle KR, Kalliatakis B, Skoularigis J: Pheochromocytoma associated with clinical and echocardiographic features simulating hypertrophic obstructive cardiomyopathy. Chest 109:1394, 1996

19. Quigg RJ, Om A: Reversal of severe cardiac systolic dysfunction caused by pheochromocytoma in a heart transplant candidate. J Heart Lung Transplant 13:525, 1994

20. Jessurun CR, Adam K, Moisek J Jr, Wilansky S: Pheochromocytoma-induced myocardial infarction in pregnancy. Tex Heart Inst J 20:120, 1993

21. Pickard JL, Ross G Jr, Silver D: Coexisting extraadrenal pheochromocytoma and renal artery stenosis: A case report and review of the pathophysiology. J Pediatr Surg 30:1613, 1995

22. Morris K, McDevitt B: Phaeochromocytoma presenting as a case of mesenteric vascular occlusion. Ir Med J 78:356, 1985

23. Gulliford MC, Hawkins CP, Murphy RP: Spontaneous dissection of the carotid artery and phaeochromocytoma. Br J Hosp Med 35:416, 1986

24. DeSouza TG, Berlad L, Shapiro K, et al: Pheochromocytoma and multiple intracerebral aneurysms. J Pediatr 108:947, 1986

25. Kulp-Shorten CL, Rhodes RH, Peterson H, Cullen JP: Cutaneous vasculitis associated with pheochromocytoma. Arthritis Rheum 33:1852, 1990

26. Rote AR, Flint LD, Ellis FH Jr: Intracaval recurrence of pheochromocytoma extending into right atrium: Surgical management using extracorporeal circulation. N Engl J Med 296:1269, 1977

27. De la Monte S, Hutchins GM, Moore GW: Peripheral neuroblastic tumors and congenital heart disease. Am J Pediatr Hematol Oncol 7:109, 1985

28. Jougasaki M, Wei C-M, McKinley LJ, Burnett JC Jr: Elevation of circulatory and ventricular adrenomedullin in human congestive heart failure. Circulation 92:286, 1995

29. Scriver CR: Alkaptonuria: Such a long journey. Nat Genet 14:5, 1996

30. Gaines JJ Jr: The pathology of alkaptonuric ochronosis. Hum Pathol 20:40, 1989

31. Albers SE, Brozena SJ, Glass LF, Fenske NA: Alkaptonuria and ochronosis: Case report and review. J Am Acad Dermatol 27:609, 1992

32. Gaines JJ Jr, Pai GM: Cardiovascular ochronosis. Arch Pathol Lab Med 111:991, 1987

33. Schievink WI, Björnsson J, Parisi JE, Prakash UBS: Arterial fibromuscular dysplasia associated with severe α_1-antitrypsin deficiency. Mayo Clin Proc 69:1040, 1994

34. Schievink WI, Prakash UBS, Piepgras DG, Mokri B: α_1-Antitrypsin deficiency in intracranial aneurysms and cervical artery dissection. Lancet 343:452, 1994

35. Cox DW: α_1-Antitrypsin: A guardian of vascular tissue. Mayo Clin Proc 69:1123, 1994

36. Gertz MA, Skinner M, Connors LH, et al: Selective binding of nifedipine to amyloid fibrils. Am J Cardiol 55:1646, 1985

37. Kyle RA: Amyloidosis. Circulation 91:1269, 1995

38. Pomerance A, Slavin G, McWatt J: Experience with the sodium sulphate–Alcian blue stain for amyloid in cardiac pathology. J Clin Pathol 29:22, 1976

39. Ferrans VJ, Butany JW: Ultrastructural pathology of the heart. In: Trump BF, Jones RT (eds): Diagnostic Electron Microscopy. Vol 4. New York, John Wiley & Sons, 1983, p 391

40. Factor SM, Menegus MA, Kress Y, et al: Microfibrillar cardiomyopathy: An infiltrative heart disease resembling but distinct from cardiac amyloidosis. Cardiovasc Pathol 1:307, 1992

41. Walley VM, Kisilevsky R, Young ID: Amyloid and the cardiovascular system: A review of pathogenesis and pathology with clinical correlations. Cardiovasc Pathol 4:79, 1995

42. Kyle RA, Gertz MA, Greipp PR, et al: A trial of three regimens for primary amyloidosis: Colchicine alone, melphalan and prednisone, and melphalan, prednisone, and colchicine. N Engl J Med 336:1202, 1997

43. Saffitz JE, Sazama K, Roberts WC: Amyloidosis limited to small arteries causing angina pectoris and sudden death. Am J Cardiol 52:1234, 1983

44. Navarro JF, Rivera M, Ortuño J: Cardiac tamponade as presentation of systemic amyloidosis. Int J Cardiol 36:107, 1992

45. Carroll JD, Gaasch WH, McAdam KPWJ: Amyloid cardiomyopathy: Characterization by a distinctive voltage/mass relation. Am J Cardiol 49:9, 1982

46. Falk RH, Plehn JF, Deering T, et al: Sensitivity and specificity of the echocardiographic features of cardiac amyloidosis. Am J Cardiol 59:418, 1987

47. Klein AL, Hatle LK, Burstow DJ, et al: Doppler characterization of left ventricular diastolic function in cardiac amyloidosis. J Am Coll Cardiol 13:1017, 1989

48. Falk RH, Lee VW, Rubinow A, et al: Cardiac technetium-99m pyrophosphate scintigraphy in familial amyloidosis. Am J Cardiol 54:1150, 1984

49. Simons M, Isner JM: Assessment of relative sensitivities of noninvasive tests for cardiac amyloidosis in documented cardiac amyloidosis. Am J Cardiol 69:425, 1992

50. Hachulla E, Maulin L, Deveaux M, et al: Prospective and serial study of primary amyloidosis with serum amyloid P component scintigraphy: From diagnosis to prognosis. Am J Med 101:77, 1996

51. Valantine HA, Billingham ME: Recurrence of amyloid in a cardiac allograft four months after transplantation. J Heart Transplant 8:337, 1989

52. Dubrey S, Mendes L, Skinner M, Falk RH: Resolution of heart failure in patients with AL amyloidosis. Ann Intern Med 125:481, 1996

53. van Buren M, Hené RJ, Verdonck LF, et al: Clinical remission after syngeneic bone marrow transplantation in a patient with AL amyloidosis. Ann Intern Med 122:508, 1995

54. Crotty TB, Li C-Y, Edwards WD, Suman VJ: Amyloidosis and endomyocardial biopsy: Correlation of extent and pattern of deposition with amyloid immunophenotype in 100 cases. Cardiovasc Pathol 4:39, 1995

55. Roberts WC, Waller BF: Cardiac amyloidosis causing cardiac dysfunction: Analysis of 54 necropsy patients. Am J Cardiol 52:137, 1983

56. Smith RRL, Hutchins GM: Ischemic heart disease secondary to amyloidosis of intramyocardial arteries. Am J Cardiol 44:413, 1979

57. Kaiserling E, Kröber S: Lymphatic amyloidosis, a previously unrecognized form of amyloid deposition in generalized amyloidosis. Histopathology 24:215, 1994

58. Ridolfi RL, Bulkley BH, Hutchins GM: The conduction system in cardiac amyloidosis: Clinical and pathologic features of 23 patients. Am J Med 62:677, 1977

59. Booth DR, Tan S-Y, Booth SE, et al: Hereditary hepatic and systemic amyloidosis caused by a new deletion/insertion mutation in the apolipoprotein A I gene. J Clin Invest 97:2714, 1996
60. Jacobson DR, Pastore RD, Yaghoubian R, et al: Variant-sequence transthyretin (isoleucine 122) in late-onset cardiac amyloidosis in black Americans. N Engl J Med 336:466, 1997
61. Gertz MA, Kyle RA, Thibodeau SN: Familial amyloidosis: A study of 52 North American–born patients examined during a 30-year period. Mayo Clin Proc 67:428, 1992
62. Booth DR, Tan SY, Hawkins PN, et al: A novel variant of transthyretin, 59 Thr→Lys, associated with autosomal dominant cardiac amyloidosis in an Italian family. Circulation 91:962, 1995
63. Hongo M, Ikeda S-I: Echocardiographic assessment of the evolution of amyloid heart disease: A study with familial amyloid polyneuropathy. Circulation 73:249, 1986
64. Eriksson A, Eriksson P, Olofsson B-O, Thornell L-E: The sinoatrial node in familial amyloidosis with polyneuropathy: A clinicopathological study of nine cases from Northern Sweden. Virchows Arch [Path Anat] 402:239, 1984
65. Holmgren G, Ericzon B-G, Groth C-G, et al: Clinical improvement and amyloid regression after liver transplantation in hereditary transthyretin amyloidosis. Lancet 341:1113, 1993
66. Goffin YA: Microscopic amyloid deposits in the heart valves: A common local complication of chronic damage and scarring. J Clin Pathol 33:262, 1980
67. Ladefoged C, Rohr N: Amyloid deposits in aortic and mitral valves: A clinicopathological investigation of material from 100 consecutive heart valve operations. Virchows Archiv [Path Anat] 404:301, 1984
68. Goffin YA, Gruys E, Sorenson GD, Wellens F: Amyloid deposits in bioprosthetic cardiac valves after long-term implantation in man: A new localization of amyloidosis. Am J Pathol 114:431, 1984
69. Gal R, Korzets A, Schwartz A, et al: Systemic distribution of β_2-microglobulin derived amyloidosis in patients who undergo long-term hemodialysis: Report of seven cases and review of the literature. Arch Pathol Lab Med 118:718, 1994
70. Barrett-Connor E, Khaw K-T, Yen SSC: A prospective study of dehydroepiandrosterone sulfate, mortality, and cardiovascular disease. N Engl J Med 315:1519, 1986
71. Mitchell LE, Sprecher DL, Borecki IB, et al: Evidence for an association between dehydroepiandrosterone sulfate and nonfatal premature myocardial infarction in males. Circulation 89:89, 1994
72. Pratico D, Fitzgerald GA: Testosterone and thromboxane: Of muscles, mice, and men. Circulation 91:2694, 1995
73. Herrington DM, Nanjee N, Achuff SC, et al: Dehydroepiandrosterone and cardiac allograft vasculopathy. J Heart Lung Transplant 15:88, 1996
74. Zgliczynski S, Ossowski M, Slowinska-Srzednicka J, et al: Effect of testosterone replacement therapy on lipids and lipoproteins in hypogonadal and elderly men. Atherosclerosis 121:35, 1996
75. Kalin MF, Zumoff B: Sex hormones and coronary disease: A review of the clinical studies. Steroids 55:330, 1990
76. Phillips GB: Relationship of serum sex hormones to coronary heart disease. Steroids 58:286, 1993
77. Phillips GB: Evidence of hyperoestrogenemia as a risk factor for myocardial infarction in man. Lancet 2:14, 1976
78. Guzick DS, Talbott EO, Sutton-Tyrrell K, et al: Carotid atherosclerosis in women with polycystic ovary syndrome: Initial results from a case-control study. Am J Obstet Gynecol 174:1224, 1996
79. Birdsall MA, Farquhar CM, White HD: Association between polycystic ovaries and extent of coronary artery disease in women having cardiac catheterization. Ann Intern Med 126:32, 1997
80. Bagatell CJ, Bremner WJ: Androgens in men: Uses and abuses. N Engl J Med 334:707, 1996
81. Strauss RH, Yesalis CE: Anabolic steroids in the athlete. Annu Rev Med 42:449, 1991
82. McNutt RA, Ferenchick GS, Kirlin PC, Hamlin NJ: Acute myocardial infarction in a 22 year old world class weight lifter using anabolic steroids. Am J Cardiol 62:164, 1988
83. DePiccoli B, Giada F, Benettin A, et al: Anabolic steroid use in body builders: An echocardiographic study of left ventricle morphology and function. Int J Sports Med 12:408, 1991
84. Thompson PD, Sadaniantz A, Cullinane EM, et al: Left ventricular function is not impaired in weight lifters who use anabolic steroids. J Am Coll Cardiol 19:278, 1992
85. Varat MA, Adolph RJ, Fowler NO: Cardiovascular effects of anemia. Am Heart J 83:415, 1972
86. Yu DT, Choo SY, Schaack T: Molecular mimicry in HLA-B27 related arthritis. Ann Intern Med 111:581, 1989
87. Lehtinen K: Mortality and causes of death in 398 patients admitted to hospital with ankylosing spondylitis. Ann Rheum Dis 52:174, 1993
88. O'Neill TW: The heart in ankylosing spondylitis. Ann Rheum Dis 51:705, 1992
89. Haverman F, Van Albada-Kuipers GA, Dohmen HJM, Dijkmans BAC: Atrioventricular conduction disturbance as an early feature of Reiter's syndrome. Ann Rheum Dis 47:1017, 1988
90. Misukiewicz P, Carlson RW, Rowan L, et al: Acute aortic insufficiency in a patient with presumed Reiter's syndrome. Ann Rheum Dis 51:686, 1992
91. Labresh KA, Lally EV, Sharma SC, Ho G Jr: Two-dimensional echocardiographic detection of preclinical aortic root abnormalities in rheumatoid variant diseases. Am J Med 78:908, 1985
92. Bulkley BH, Roberts WC: Ankylosing spondylitis and aortic regurgitation: Description of the characteristic cardiovascular lesion from study of eight necropsy patients. Circulation 48:1014, 1973
93. Brewerton DA, Gibson DG, Goddard DH, et al: The myocardium in ankylosing spondylitis: A clinical, echocardiographic, and histopathological study. Lancet 1:995, 1987
94. Cohen PR, Kurzrock R: Miscellaneous genodermatoses: Beckwith-Wiedemann syndrome, Birt-Hogg-Dubé syndrome, familial atypical multiple mole melanoma syndrome, hereditary tylosis, incontinentia pigmentii, and supernumerary nipples. Dermatol Clin 13: 211, 1995
95. Greenwood, RD, Sommer A, Rosenthal A, et al: Cardiovascular abnormalities in the Beckwith-Wiedemann syndrome. Am J Dis Child 131:293, 1977
96. Stanley CA: Carnitine disorders. Adv Pediatr 42:209, 1995
97. Vockley J: The changing face of disorders of fatty acid oxidation. Mayo Clin Proc 69:249, 1994
98. Tripp ME, Katcher ML, Peters HA, et al: Systemic carnitine deficiency presenting as familial endocardial fibroelastosis. N Engl J Med 305:385, 1981
99. Bennett MJ, Hale DE, Pollitt RJ, et al: Endocardial fibroelastosis and primary carnitine deficiency due to a defect in the plasma membrane carnitine transporter. Clin Cardiol 19:243, 1996
100. Abrahamsson K, Mellander M, Eriksson BO, et al: Transient reduction of human left ventricular mass in carnitine depletion induced by antibiotics containing pivalic acid. Br Heart J 74:656, 1995
101. Servidei S, Bertini E, DiMauro S: Hereditary metabolic cardiomyopathies. Adv Pediatr 41:1, 1994
102. Hug G, Bovek E, Soukup S: Lethal neonatal multiorgan deficiency of carnitine palmitoyl transferase II. N Engl J Med 325:1862, 1991
103. Sewell AC, Bender SW, Wirth S, et al: Long-chain 3-hydroxyacyl-CoA dehydrogenase deficiency: A severe fatty acid oxidation disorder. Eur J Pediatr 153:745, 1994
104. Ino T, Sherwood G, Benson LN, et al: Cardiac manifestations in disorders of fat and carnitine metabolism in infancy. J Am Coll Cardiol 11:1301, 1988
105. Amirkhan RH, Timmons CF, Brown KO, et al: Clinical, biochemical, and morphological investigations of a case of long-chain 3-hydroxyacl-CoA dehydrogenase deficiency. Arch Pathol Lab Med 121:730, 1997
106. Kelly DP, Strauss AW: Inherited cardiomyopathies. N Engl J Med 330:913, 1994
107. Winter S, Jue K, Prochazka J, et al: The role of l-carnitine in pediatric cardiomyopathy. J Child Neurol 10(suppl 2):S45, 1995
108. Bodensteiner J: Congenital myopathies. Muscle Nerve 17:131, 1994
109. Gospe SM Jr, Armstrong DL, Gresik MV, Hawkins HK: Life-threatening congestive heart failure as the presentation of centronuclear myopathy. Pediatr Neurol 3:117, 1987
110. Verhiest W, Brucher JM, Goddeeris P, et al: Familial centronuclear myopathy associated with cardiomyopathy. Br Heart J 38: 504, 1976
111. Wilkins LE, Brown JA, Nance WE, Wolf B: Clinical heterogeneity in 80 home-reared children with cri du chat syndrome. J Pediatr 102:528, 1983
112. Imaizumi K, Kurosawa K, Makita Y, et al: Male with type II autosomal recessive cutis laxa. Clin Genet 45:40, 1994

113. Weir EK, Joffe HS, Blaufuss AH, Beighton P: Cardiovascular abnormalities in cutis laxa. Eur J Cardiol 5:255, 1977

114. Pyeritz RE: Cardiovascular manifestations of heritable disorders of connective tissue. Prog Med Genet 5:191, 1983

115. Hashimoto K, Kanzaki T: Cutis laxa: Ultrastructural and biochemical studies. Arch Dermatol 111:861, 1975

116. Tsuji A, Yanai J, Miura T, et al: Vascular abnormalities in congenital cutis laxa: Report of two cases. Acta Paediatr Jap 32:155, 1990

117. Edelman M, Silverstein D, Strom J, Factor SM: Cardiomyopathy in a male with cystinosis. Cardiovasc Pathol 6:43, 1997

118. Bloodworth JMB Jr: A re-evaluation of diabetic glomerulosclerosis 50 years after the discovery of insulin. Hum Pathol 9:439, 1978

119. De Oliveira F: Pericytes in diabetic retinopathy: Evolution of the retinal lesions. Br J Opthalmol 50:134, 1966

120. Behse F, Buchthal F, Carlsen F: Nerve biopsy and conduction studies in diabetic neuropathy. J Neurol Neurosurg Psychiatry 40:1072, 1977

121. Stary HC: Disease of small blood vessels in diabetes mellitus. Am J Med Sci 252:357, 1966

122. Neubauer B: A quantitative study of peripheral arterial calcification and glucose tolerance in elderly diabetics and non diabetics. Diabetologia 7:409, 1971

123. Lester WM, Roberts WC: Diabetes mellitus for 25 years or more: Analysis of cardiovascular findings in seven patients studied at necropsy. Am J Med 81:275, 1986

124. Dybdahl H, Ledet T: Diabetic macroangiopathy. Diabetologia 30:882, 1987

125. Berkman J, Rafkin H: Newer aspects of diabetic microangiopathy. Annu Rev Med 17:83, 1966

126. Fein FS, Sonnenblick EH: Diabetic cardiomyopathy. Prog Cardiovasc Dis 27:255, 1985

127. Smith JP: Hyaline arteriosclerosis in the kidney. J Pathol Bacteriol 69:147, 1955

128. Sinclair RA, Antonovych TT, Mostofi FK: Renal proliferative arteriopathies and associated glomerular change: A light and electron microscopic study. Hum Pathol 7:565, 1976

129. McKluskey ET, Hall CL, Colvin RB: Immune complex mediated disease. Hum Pathol 9:71, 1978

130. Gamble CN: The pathogenesis of hyaline arteriosclerosis. Am J Pathol 122:410, 1986

131. Crall FV, Robarts WC: The extramural and intramural coronary arteries in juvenile diabetes mellitus. Am J Med 64:221, 1978

132. Bencosme SA, West RO, Kerr JW, Wilson DL: Diabetic capillary angiography in human skeletal muscle. Am J Med 40:67, 1966

133. Kilo C, Vogler N, Williamson JR: Muscle capillary basement membrane changes related to aging and to diabetes cellitus. Diabetes 21:881, 1972

134. Camerubu-Davakis RA, Velasco C, Glasser M, Bloodworth KMB Jr: Drug induced reversal of early diabetic microangiopathy. N Engl J Med 309:1551, 1983

135. Dyck PJ, Hansen S, Karnes J, et al: Capillary number and percentage closed in human diabetic sural nerve. Proc Natl Acad Sci USA 82:2513, 1985

136. Danowski TS, Khurana RC, Gonzalcz AR, Fisher ER: Capillary basement membrane thickness and pseudodiabetes of myopathy. Am J Med 51:757, 1971

137. Norton WL: Comparison of the microangiopathy of systemic lupus erythematosus, dermatomyositis, scleroderma, and diabetes mellitus. Lab Invest 22:301, 1970

138. Silver MD, Huckel VF, Lorber M: Basement membranes of small cardiac vessels in patients with diabetes and myxoedema: Preliminary observations. Pathology 9:213, 1977

139. Pardo V, Perez-Stable E, Allozamora DB, Cleveland WW: Incidence and significance of muscle capillary basal lamina thickness in juvenile diabetes. Am J Pathol 68:67, 1972

140. Becker D, Miller M: Presence of diabetic glomerulosclerosis in patients with hemochromatosis. N Engl J Med 263:367, 1960

141. Kerines K, Kim O, Knowles HC: Glomerulosclerosis, hemochromatosis and diabetes cellulitis. Am J Clin Pathol 54:47, 1970

142. Siperstein MD, Unger RH, Madison LL: Studies of muscle capillary basement membranes in normal subjects, diabetics, and prediabetic patients. J Clin Invest 47:1973, 1968

143. Yodaiken RE, Pardo V: Diabetic capillaropathy. Hum Pathol 6:455, 1975

144. Siperstein MD, Raskin P, Burns H: Electron microscopic quantification of diabetic microangiopathy. Diabetes 22:514, 1973

145. Williamson JR, Rowold E, Hoffman P, Kilo C: Regional variations in the width of the basement membrane of muscle capillaries in man and giraffe. Am J Pathol 63:359, 1971

146. Vracko R: Basal lamina scaffold. Front Matrix Biol 7:78, 1979

147. Peterson GE, Forsham PH: Variation in thickness of the capillary basement membrane in single muscles of diabetic subjects. Diabetes 28:548, 1979

148. Cream JJ, Brycesson ADM, Ryder G: Disappearance of immunoglobin and complement from the Arthus reaction and its relevance to the studies of vasculitis in man. Br J Dermatol 84:106, 1971

149. Abboud HE: Role of platelet derived growth factor in renal injury. Annu Rev Physiol 57:297, 1995

150. Ketteler M, Noble NA, Border WA: Transforming growth factor-β and angiotensin II: The missing link from glomerular hyperfiltration to glomerulosclerosis? Annu Rev Physiol 57:279, 1995

151. Nakamoto Y, Takazakura E, Hayakawa H, et al: Intrarenal microaneurysms in diabetic nephropathy. Lab Invest 42:433, 1980

152. Bloodworth JMB Jr: Diabetic retinopathy. Diabetes 11:1, 1962

153. Cogan DG: Vascular complications of diabetes mellitus. In: Kimura SJ, Caygill WM (eds): Vascular Complications of Diabetes Mellitus with Special Emphasis on Microangiopathy of the Eye. St. Louis, Mosby, 1967

154. Kuwabara T, Cogan DG: Studies of retinal vascular patterns. I. Normal architecture. Arch Opthalmol 64:904, 1960

155. Wolter JR: The blood vessels of retinoblastomas. Arch Opthalmol 66:545, 1961

156. Kuwabara T, Carroll JM, Cogan DG: Retinal vascular patterns. III. Age, hypertension, absolute glaucoma, injury. Arch Opthalmol 65:708, 1961

157. Neetens A: Microcirculation in the diabetic eye. In: Davis E (ed): The Microcirculation in Diabetes. Basel, S Karger, 1979

158. Sato Y, Rifkin DB: Inhibition of EC movement by pericytes and smooth muscle cells: Activation of a latent transforming growth factor $\beta 1$-like molecule by plasmin during co-culture. J Cell Biol 109:309, 1989

159. Antonelli-Orlidge A, Saunders KB, Smith SR, D'Amore PA: An activated form of transforming growth factor β is produced by cocultures of endothelial cells and pericytes. Proc Natl Acad Sci USA 86:4544, 1989

160. McMeel JW: Diabetic retinopathy: Fibrotic proliferation and retinal detachment. Trans Am Opthalmol Soc 69:440, 1971

161. Landau J, Davis E: The small blood vessels of the conjunctiva and nailbed in diabetes mellitus. Lancet 2:731, 1960

162. Trap-Jensen J, Lassen NA: Increased capillary diffusion capacity for small ions in skeletal muscle in long term diabetes. Scand J Clin Lab Invest 21:116, 1968

163. Williamson JR, Kilo C: Basement-membrane thickening and diabetic microangiopathy. Diabetes 25:925, 1976

164. Krupin T, Waltman ST, Oestrich C, et al: Vitreous fluorophotometry in juvenile-onset diabetes mellitus. Arch Ophthalmol 96:812, 1978

165. Beisswenger PJ, Spiro RG: Studies on the human glomerular basement membrane: Composition, nature of the carbohydrate units and chemical changes in diabetes mellitus. Diabetes 22:180, 1973

166. Vracko R, Benditt EP: Capillary basal lamina thickening: Its relationship to endothelial cell death and replacement. J Cell Biol 47:281, 1970

167. Raskin P: Diabetic regulation and its relationship to microangiopathy. Metabolism 27:235, 1978

168. Brownlee M: Glycation and diabetic complications. Diabetes 43:836, 1994

169. Trivelli LA, Ranney HM, Lai HT: Hemoglobin components in patients with diabetes mellitus. N Engl J Med 284:353, 1971

170. Bunn HF, Gabbay KH, Gallop PM: The glycosylation of hemoglobin: Relevance to diabetes mellitus. Science 200:21, 1978

171. Ditzel J: Oxygen transport impairment in diabetes. Diabetes 25:832, 1976

172. Ditzel J: Diabetic vascular disease: The importance of insulin deficiency, hyperglycemia, hypophosphatemia on red cell oxygen unloading. Acta Paediatr Scand Suppl 270:112, 1977

173. Koenig RJ, Peterson CM, Kilo C, et al: Hemoglobin A1c as an indicator of the degree of glucose tolerance in diabetes. Diabetes 25:230, 1976

174. Malone JI, Simons CA, van Cade TC: Correlation of HbAI and diabetic microvascular disease (MVD) (abstract). Diabetes 27:434, 1978

175. McMillan DE: Plasma protein changes, blood viscosity, and diabetic microangiopathy. Diabetes 25:858, 1976

176. Halushka PV, Lurie D, Colwell JA: Increased synthesis of prostaglandin-E-like material by platelets from patients with diabetes mellitus. N Engl J Med 297:1306, 1977

177. Ganda OP, ArkinCF: Hyperfibrinogenemia: An important risk factor for vascular complications in diabetes. Diabetes Care 15:1245, 1992

178. Mustard JF, Packham MA: Platelets and diabetes mellitus. N Engl J Med 311:665, 1984

179. Mauer SM, Barbosa J, Vernier RL, et al: Development of diabetic vascular lesions in normal kidneys transplanted into patients with diabetes mellitus. N Engl J Med 295:916, 1976

180. Lazarow A: Glomerular basement membrane thickening in diabetes. In: Ostaman J, Miller RD (ed): Proceedings of the 6th Congress of the International Diabetes Federation, Stockholm. Amsterdam, Experpta Medica, 1967, p 302

181. Osterby Hansen R: A quantitative estimate of the peripheral glomerular basement membrane in recent juvenile diabetes. Diabetologia 1:97, 1965

182. Osterby Hansen R: Morphometric studies of the peripheral glomerular basement membrane in early juvenile diabetes. I. Development of initial basement membrane thickening. Diabetologia 8:84, 1972

183. Osterby Hansen R: Early phases in the development of diabetic glomerulopathy: A quantitative electron microscopic study. Acta Med Scand Suppl 574:3, 1974

184. Otto H, Thermann H, Wagner H: Qualitative and quantitative elekronenmikroskopische Untersuchungen an Hauptcapillaren jugendlicher Diabetiker. Klin Wochschr 45:299, 1967

185. Hanssen KF, Dahl-Jorgensen K, Lauritzen T, et al: Diabetic control and microvascular complications: The near-normoglycaemic experience. Diabetologia 29:677, 1986

186. Siperstein MD, Foster DW, Knowles HC, et al: Control of blood glucose and diabetic vascular disease. N Engl J Med 296:1060, 1977

187. Rand LI, Krolewski SA, Aiello LM, et al: Multiple factors in the prediction of risk of proliferative diabetic retinopathy. N Engl J Med 313:1433, 1985

188. Williamson JR, Kilo C: Vascular complications in diabetes mellitus. N Engl J Med 302:399, 1980

189. Bilous RW, Mauer SM, Sutherland DER, et al: The effects of pancreas transplantation on the glomerular structure of renal allografts in patients with insulin-dependent diabetes. N Engl J Med 321:80, 1989

190. The Diabetes Control and Complications Trial Research Group. The effect of intensive treatment of diabetes on the development and progression of long-term complications in insulin-dependent diabetes mellitus. N Engl J Med 329:977, 1993

191. Abboud HE, Pinzani M, Knauss T, et al: Actions of platelet derived growth factor isoforms in mesangial cells. J Cell Physiol 158:140, 1994

192. Doi T, Vlassara H, Kirstein M, et al: Receptor-specific increase in extracellular matrix production in mouse mesangial cells by advanced glycosylation end products is mediated via platelet-derived growth factor. Proc Natl Acad Sci U S A 89:2873, 1992

193. Eshraghi S, Gotlieb AI: Insulin does not disrupt actin microfilaments, microtubules, and in vitro aortic endothelial wound repair. Biochem Cell Biol 73:507, 1995

194. Kashiwagi, Asahina T, Ikebuchi M, et al: Abnormal glutathione metabolism and increased cytotoxicity caused by H_2O_2 in human umbilical vein EC cultured in high-glucose medium. Diabetologia 37:300, 1994

195. Lee TS, MacGregor LC, Fluharty SJ, King GL: Differential regulation of protein kinase C and (Na,K)-adenosine triphosphatase activities by elevated glucose levels in retinal capillary endothelial cells. J Clin Invest 83:90, 1989

196. Lee TS, Saltsman KA, Ohashi H, King GL: Activation of protein kinase C by elevation of glucose concentration: Proposal for a mechanism in the development of diabetic vascular complications. Proc Natl Acad Sci USA 86:5141, 1989

197. Lorenzi M, Cagliero E, Toleda S: Glucose toxicity for human EC in culture: Delayed replication, disturbed cell cycle and accelerated death. Diabetes 34:621, 1985

198. Lorenzi M, Cagliero E: Perspectives in diabetes: Pathobiology of endothelial and other vascular cells in diabetes mellitus. Diabetes 40:653, 1991

199. Morel DW, Chisolm GM: Antioxidant treatment of diabetic rats inhibits lipoprotein oxidation and cytotoxicity. J Lipid Res 30: 1827, 1989

200. Jain SK: Hyperglycemia can cause membrane lipid peroxidation and osmotic fragility in human red blood cells. J Biol Chem 264: 21340, 1989

201. Cagliero E, Roth T, Roy S, Lorenzi M: Characteristics and mechanisms of high-glucose-induced overexpression of basement membrane components in cultured human EC. Diabetes 40:102, 1991

202. Ziyadeh FN, Sharma K, Wolf G: Stimulation of collagen gene expression and protein synthesis in murine mesangial cells by high glucose is mediated by autocrine activation of transforming growth factor β. J Clin Invest 93:536, 1994

203. Weisbrod RM, et al: Effect of elevated glucose on cyclic GMP and eicosanoids produced by porcine aortic endothelium. Arterioscler Throm Vasc Biol 13:915, 1993

204. Taguma Y, Kitamoto Y, Futaki G, et al: Effect of captopril on heavy proteinuria in azotemic diabetics. N Engl J Med 313:1617, 1985

205. Kanno K, Hirata Y, Shichiri M, et al: Plasma endothelin-1 levels in patients with diabetes mellitus with or without vascular complication. J Cardiovasc Pharmacol 17(suppl 7):S475, 1991

206. Oliver FJ, de la Rubia G, Feener EP, et al: Stimulation of endothelin-1 gene expression by insulin in EC. J Biol Chem 266: 23251, 1991

207. Hattori Y, Kasai K, Nakamura T, et al: Effect of glucose and insulin on immunoreactive endothelin-1 release from cultured porcine EC. Metabolism 40:165, 1991

208. Mandarino LJ: Current hypotheses for the biochemical basis of diabetic retinopathy. Diabetes Care 15:1892, 1992

209. Ishii H, Jirousek MR, Koya D, et al: Amelioration of vascular dysfunctions in diabetic rats by an oral PKC β inhibitor. Science 272:728, 1996

210. Blumenthal HT: The relation of microangiopathies to arteriosclerosis with special reference to diabetes. Ann N Y Acad Sci 149:834, 1968

211. Goldberg S, Alex M, Joshi RA, Blumenthal HT: Nonatheromatous peripheral vascular disease of the lower extremity in diabetes mellitus. Diabetes 8:261, 1959

212. Sunni S, Bishop SP, Kent SP, Geer JC: Diabetic cardiomyopathy: A morphological study of intramyocardial arteries. Arch Pathol Lab Med 110:375, 1986

213. Garcia MJ, McNamara PM, Gordon T, Kannell WD: Morbidity and mortality in diabetics in the Framingham population. Diabetes 23:105, 1974

214. Hsueh WA, Andderson PW: Systemic hypertension and the renin-angiotensin system in diabetic vascular complications. Am J Cardiol 72(suppl):14, 1993

215. Waller BF, Palumbo PJ, Lie JT, Roberts WC: Status of the coronary arteries at necropsy in diabetes mellitus with onset after age 30 years: Analysis of 229 diabetic patients with and without clinical evidence of coronary heart disease and comparison to 183 control subjects. Am J Med 69:498, 1980

216. Palinski W, Koschinsky T, Butler SW, et al: Immunological evidence for the presence of advanced glycosylation end products in atherosclerotic lesions of euglycemic rabbits. Arterioscler Thromb Vasc Biol 15:571, 1995

217. Nakamura Y, Horii Y, Nishino T, et al: Immunohistochemical localization of advanced glycosylation endproducts in coronary atheroma and cardiac tissue in diabetes mellitus. Am J Pathol 143: 1649, 1993

218. Schmidt AM, Hori O, Brett J, et al: Cellular receptors for advanced glycation end products: Implications of induction of oxidant stress and cellular dysfunction in the pathogenesis of vascular lesions. Arterioscler Throm Vasc Biol Thromb 14:1521, 1994

219. Lawrie GM, Morris GC, Glaeser DH: Influence of diabetes mellitus on the results of coronary bypass surgery. JAMA 256:2967, 1986

220. Singer DE, Moulton AW, Nathan DM: Diabetic myocardial infarction. Diabetes 38:350, 1989

221. Factor SM, Okun EM, Minase T: Capillary microaneurysms in the human diabetic heart. N Engl J Med 302:384, 1980

222. Fischer VW, Barner HB, Leskiw ML: Capillary basal laminar thickness in diabetic human myocardium. Diabetes 28:713, 1979

223. Mildenberger RR, Bar-Shlomo B, Druck MN, et al: Clinically unrecognized ventricular dysfunction in young diabetic patients. J Am Coll Cardiol 4:234, 1984

224. Hamby RI, Zoneraich S, Sherman L: Diabetic cardiomyopathy. JAMA 229:1749, 1974

225. Rubler S, Dlugash J, Yuceogly YZ, et al: New type of cardiomyopathy associated with diabetic glomerulosclerosis. Am J Cardiol 30:595, 1972

226. Regan TJ: Congestive heart failure in the diabetic. Annu Rev Med 34:161, 1983

227. Opie LH, Tansey MJ, Kennelly BM: The heart in diabetes mellitus. I. Biochemical basis for myocardial dysfunction. S Afr Med J 56:207, 1979

228. Vered Z, Battler A, Segal P, et al: Exercise-induced left ventricular dysfunction in young men with asymptomatic diabetes mellitus (diabetic cardiomyopathy). Am J Cardiol 54:633, 1984

229. Sheehan JP, Sisam DA, Schumacher PO: Insulin-induced cardiac failure. Am J Med 79:147, 1985

230. Greenberg F: DiGeorge syndrome: An historical review of clinical and cytogenetic features. J Med Genet 30:803, 1993

231. Hall JG: CATCH 22. J Med Genet 30:801, 1993

232. Jedele KB, Michels VV, Puga FJ, Feldt RH: Velo-cardio-facial syndrome associated with ventricular septal defect, pulmonary atresia, and hypoplastic pulmonary arteries. Pediatrics 89:915, 1992

233. Momma K, Kondo C, Matsuoka R, Takao A: Cardiac anomalies associated with a chromosome 22q 11 deletion in patients with the conotruncal anomaly face syndrome. Am J Cardiol 78:591, 1996

234. Driscoll DA: Genetic basis of DiGeorge and velocardiofacial syndromes. Curr Opin Pediatr 6:702, 1994

235. Bick RL: Disseminated intravascular coagulation: Objective clinical and laboratory diagnosis, treatment, and assessment of therapeutic response. Semin Thromb Hemost 22:69, 1996

236. Saffitz JE, Stahl DJ, Sundt TM, et al: Disseminated intravascular coagulation after administration of aprotinin in combination with deep hypothermic circulatory arrest. Am J Cardiol 72:1080, 1993

237. Byers PH: Ehlers-Danlos syndrome: Recent advances and current understanding of the clinical and genetic heterogeneity. J Invest Dermatol 103(suppl):S47, 1994

238. Yeowell HN, Pinnell SR: The Ehlers-Danlos syndromes. Semin Dermatol 12:229, 1993

239. Piérard GE, Lê T, Piérard-Franchimont C, Lapière CM: Morphometric study of cauliflower collagen fibrils in Ehlers-Danlos syndrome type I. Coll Relat Res 8:453, 1988

240. Leier CV, Call TD, Fulkerson PK, Wooley CF: The spectrum of cardiac defects in the Ehlers-Danlos syndrome types I and III. Ann Intern Med 92:171, 1980

241. Adés LC, Waltham RD, Chiodo AA, Bateman JF: Myocardial infarction resulting from coronary artery dissection in an adolescent with Ehlers-Danlos syndrome type IV due to a type III collagen mutation. Br Heart J 74:112, 1995

242. Cabeen WR Jr, Reza MJ, Kovick RB, Stern MS: Mitral valve prolapse and conduction defects in Ehlers-Danlos syndrome. Arch Intern Med 137:1227, 1977

243. Schievink WI, Michels VV, Piepgras DG: Neurovascular manifestations of heritable connective tissue disorders: A review. Stroke 25:889, 1994

244. Byers PH, Holbrook KA, McGillivray B, et al: Clinical and ultrastructural heterogeneity of type IV Ehlers-Danlos syndrome. Hum Genet 47:141, 1979

245. Jaffe AS, Geltman EM, Rodey GE, Uitto J: Mitral valve prolapse, a consistent manifestation of type IV Ehlers-Danlos syndrome: The pathogenetic role of the abnormal production of type III collagen. Circulation 64:121, 1981

246. Imahori S, Bannerman RM, Graf CJ, Brennan JC: Ehlers-Danlos syndrome with multiple arterial lesions. Am J Med 47:967, 1969

247. Nishiyama Y, Manabe N, Ooshima A, et al: A sporadic case of Ehlers-Danlos syndrome type IV: Diagnosed by a morphometric study of collagen content. Pathol Int 45:524, 1995

248. Dunmore PJ, Roach MR: The effects of age, vessel size, and Ehlers-Danlos type IV syndrome on the waviness index of arteries. Clin Invest Med 13:67, 1990

249. Crowther MA, Lach B, Dunmore PJ, Roach MR: Vascular collagen fibril morphology in type IV Ehlers-Danlos syndrome. Connect Tissue Res 25:209, 1991

250. Wenstrup RJ, Murad S, Pinnell SR: Ehlers-Danlos syndrome type VI: Clinical manifestations of collagen lysyl hydroxylase deficiency. J Pediatr 115:405, 1989

251. Bione S, Small K, Aksmanovic VMA, et al: Identification of new mutations in the Emery-Dreifuss muscular dystrophy gene and evidence for genetic heterogeneity of the disease. Hum Mol Genet 4:1859, 1995

252. Marshall TM, Huckell VF: Atrial paralysis in a patient with Emery-Dreifuss muscular dystrophy. Pacing Clin Electrophysiol 15:135, 1992

253. Fishbein MC, Siegel RJ, Thompson CE, Hopkins LC: Sudden death of a carrier of X-linked Emery-Dreifuss muscular dystrophy. Ann Intern Med 119:900, 1993

254. Voit T, Krogmann O, Lenard HG, et al: Emery-Dreifuss muscular dystrophy: Disease spectrum and differential diagnosis. Neuropediatrics 19:62, 1988

255. Nakao S, Takenaka T, Maeda M, et al: An atypical variant of Fabry's disease in men with left ventricular hypertrophy. N Engl J Med 333:288, 1995

256. von Scheidt W, Eng CM, Fitzmaurice TF, et al: An atypical variant of Fabry's disease with manifestations confined to the myocardium. N Engl J Med 324:395, 1991

257. Bernstein HS, Bishop DF, Astrin KH, et al: Fabry disease: Six gene rearrangements and an exonic point mutation in the α-galactosidase gene. J Clin Invest 83:1390, 1989

258. Hillsley RE, Hernandez E, Steenbergen C, et al: Inherited restrictive cardiomyopathy in a 74 year old woman: A case of Fabry's disease. Am Heart J 129:199, 1995

259. Roudebush CP, Foerster JM, Bing OHL: The abbreviated PR interval of Fabry's disease. N Engl J Med 289:357, 1973

260. Ikari Y, Kuwako K, Yamaguchi T: Fabry's disease with complete atrioventricular block: Histological evidence of involvement of the conduction system. Br Heart J 68:323, 1992

261. Leder AA, Bosworth WC: Angiokeratoma corporis diffusum universale (Fabry's disease) with mitral stenosis. Am J Med 38:814, 1965

262. Desnick RJ, Blieden LC, Sharp HL, et al: Cardiac valvular anomalies in Fabry disease: Clinical, morphologic, and biochemical studies. Circulation 54:818, 1976

263. Goldman ME, Cantor R, Schwartz MF, et al: Echocardiographic abnormalities and disease severity in Fabry's disease. J Am Coll Cardiol 7:1157, 1986

264. Fisher EA, Desnick RJ, Gordon RE, et al: Fabry disease: An unusual cause of severe coronary disease in a young man. Ann Intern Med 117:221, 1992

265. Drachenberg CB, Schweitzer EJ, Bartlett ST, et al: Polyarteritis nodosa-like necrotizing vasculitis in Fabry disease. J Inher Metab Dis 16:901, 1993

266. Ferrans VJ, Hibbs RG: The heart in Fabry's disease: A histochemical and electron microscopic study. Am J Cardiol 24:95, 1969

267. Itoh K, Takenaka T, Nakao S, et al: Immunofluorescence analysis of trihexosylceramide accumulated in the hearts of variant hemizygotes and heterozygotes with Fabry disease. Am J Cardiol 78:116, 1996

268. Deidda G, Cacurri S, Piazzo N, Felicetti L: Direct detection of 4q 35 rearrangements implicated in facioscapulohumeral muscular dystrophy. J Med Genet 33:361, 1996

269. Stevenson WG, Perloff JK, Weiss JN, Anderson TL: Facioscapulohumeral muscular dystrophy: Evidence for selective, genetic electrophysiologic cardiac involvement. J Am Coll Cardiol 15:292, 1990

270. Bernardo K, Hurwitz R, Zenk T, et al: Purification, characterization, and biosynthesis of human acid ceramidase. J Biol Chem 270:11098, 1995

271. Abul-Haj SK, Martz DG, Douglas WF, Geppert LJ: Farber's disease: Report of a case with observations on its histogenesis and notes on the nature of the stored material. J Pediatr 61:221, 1962

272. Abenoza P, Sibley RK: Farber's disease: A fine structural study. Ultrastruct Pathol 11:397, 1987

273. Tsongalis GJ, Silverman LM: Molecular pathology of the fragile X syndrome. Arch Pathol Lab Med 117:1121, 1993

274. Sreeram N, Wren C, Bhate M, et al: Cardiac abnormalities in the fragile X syndrome. Br Heart J 61:289, 1989

275. Crabbe LS, Bensky AS, Hornstein L, Schwartz DC: Cardiovascular abnormalities in children with fragile X syndrome. Pediatrics 91:714, 1993

276. Waldstein G, Hagerman R: Aortic hypoplasia and cardiac valvular abnormalities in a boy with fragile X syndrome. Am J Med Genet 30:83, 1988

277. Willems PJ, Gatti R, Darby JK, et al: Fucosidosis revisited: A review of 77 patients. Am J Med Genet 38:111, 1991
278. Durand P, Borsone C, Cella CD: Fucosidosis. J Pediatr 75:665, 1969
279. Rapola J: Lysosomal storage diseases in adults. Pathol Res Pract 190:759, 1994
280. Rosenberg H, Frewen TC, Li MD, et al: Cardiac involvement in diseases characterized by β-galactosidase deficiency. J Pediatr 106:78, 1985
281. Hadley RN, Hagstrom JWC: Cardiac lesions in a patient with familial neurovisceral lipidosis (generalized gangliosidosis). Am J Clin Pathol 55:237, 1971
282. Rodriguez-Torres R, Schneck L, Kleinberg W: Electrocardiographic and biochemical abnormalities in Tay-Sachs disease. Bull N Y Acad Med 47:717, 1971
283. Blieden LC, Desnick RJ, Carter JB, et al: Cardiac involvement in Sandhoff's disease: Inborn error of glycosphingolipid metabolism. Am J Cardiol 34:83, 1974
284. Balicki D, Beutler E: Gaucher disease. Medicine (Baltimore) 74:305, 1995
285. Naito M, Takahashi K, Hojo H: An ultrastructural and experimental study on the development of tubular structures in the lysosomes of Gaucher cells. Lab Invest 58:590, 1988
286. Roberts WC, Fredrickson DS: Gaucher's disease of the lung causing severe pulmonary hypertension with associated acute recurrent pericarditis. Circulation 35:783, 1967
287. Dawson A, Elias DJ, Rubenson D, et al: Pulmonary hypertension developing after alglucerase therapy in two patients with type I Gaucher disease complicated by the hepatopulmonary syndrome. Ann Intern Med 125:901, 1996
288. Mester SW, Weston MW: Cardiac tamponade in a patient with Gaucher's disease. Clin Cardiol 15:766, 1992
289. Smith RRL, Hutchins GM, Sack GH Jr, Ridolfi RL: Unusual cardiac, renal, and pulmonary involvement in Gaucher's disease: Interstitial glucocerebroside accumulation, pulmonary hypertension, and fatal bone marrow embolization. Am J Med 65:352, 1978
290. Edwards WD, Hurley HP III, Partin JR: Cardiac involvement by Gaucher's disease documented by right ventricular endomyocardial biopsy. Am J Cardiol 52:654, 1983
291. Saraçlar M, Atalay S, Koçak N, Özkutlu S: Gaucher's disease with mitral and aortic involvement: Echocardiographic findings. Pediatr Cardiol 13:56, 1991
292. Abrahamov A, Elstein D, Gross-Tsur V, et al: Gaucher's disease variant characterized by progressive calcification of heart valves and unique genotype. Lancet 346:1000, 1995
293. Chabás A, Cormand B, Grinberg D, et al: Unusual expression of Gaucher's disease: Cardiovascular calcification in three sibs homozygous for the D409H mutation. J Med Genet 32:740, 1995
294. Lei K-J, Pan C-J, Shelly LL, et al: Identification of mutations in the gene for glucose-6-phosphatase the enzyme deficient in glycogen storage disease type 1A. J Clin Invest 93:1994, 1994
295. Ohura T, Inoue CN, Abukawa D, et al: Progressive pulmonary hypertension: A fatal complication of type I glycogen storage disease. J Inherit Metab Dis 18:361, 1995
296. Raben N, Nichols RC, Boerkoel C, Plotz P: Genetic defects in patients with glycogenesis type II (acid maltase deficiency). Muscle Nerve 3(suppl):S70, 1995
297. Hwang B, Meng L, Lin C-Y, Hsu H-C: Clinical analysis of five infants with glycogen storage disease of the heart—Pompe's disease. Jpn Heart J 27:25, 1986
298. Dincsoy MY, Dincsoy HP, Kessler AD, et al: Generalized glycogenesis and associated endocardial fibroelastosis. J Pediatr 67:728, 1965
299. Hug G, Schubert WK: Glycogenesis type II: Glycogen distribution in tissues. Arch Pathol 84:141, 1967
300. Bharati S, Serrato M, DuBrow I, et al: The conduction system in Pompe's disease. Pediatr Cardiol 2:25, 1982
301. Felice KJ, Alessi AG, Grunnet ML: Clinical variability in adult-onset acid maltase deficiency: Report of affected sibs and review of the literature. Medicine (Baltimore) 74:131, 1995
302. Byrne E, Dennett X, Crotty B, et al: Dominantly inherited cardioskeletal myopathy with lysosomal glycogen storage and normal acid maltase levels. Brain 109:523, 1986
303. Tripathy D, Coleman RA, Vidaillet HJ Jr, et al: Complete heart block with myocardial membrane–bound glycogen and normal peripheral α glucosidase activity. Ann Intern Med 109:985, 1988
304. Tachi N, Tachi M, Sasaki K, et al: Glycogen storage disease with normal acid maltase: Skeletal and cardiac muscles. Pediatr Neurol 5:60, 1989
305. Shen J, Bao Y, Liu H-M, et al: Mutations in exon 3 of the glycogen debranching enzyme gene are associated with glycogen storage disease type III that is differentially expressed in liver and muscle. J Clin Invest 98:352, 1996
306. Coleman RA, Winter HS, Wolf B, et al: Glycogen storage disease type III (glycogen debranching enzyme deficiency): Correlation of biochemical defects with myopathy and cardiomyopathy. Ann Intern Med 116:896, 1992
307. Moses SW, Wanderman KL, Myroz A, Frydman M: Cardiac involvement in glycogen storage disease type III. Eur J Pediatr 148:764, 1989
308. Carvalho JS, Matthews EE, Leonard JV, Deanfield J: Cardiomyopathy of glycogen storage disease type III. Heart Vessels 8:155, 1993
309. Tada H, Kurita T, Ohe T, et al: Glycogen storage disease type III associated with ventricular tachycardia. Am Heart J 130:911, 1995
310. Olson LJ, Reeder GS, Noller KL, et al: Cardiac involvement in glycogen storage disease III: Morphologic and biochemical characterization with endomyocardial biopsy. Am J Cardiol 53:980, 1984
311. Thon VJ, Khalil M, Cannon JF: Isolation of human glycogen branching enzyme cDNAs by screening complementation in yeast. J Biol Chem 268:7509, 1993
312. Reed GB Jr, Dixon JFP, Neustein HB, et al: Type IV glycogenesis: Patient with absence of a branching enzyme α-1,4-glucan: α-1,4-Glucan 6-glycosyl transferase. Lab Invest 19:546, 1968
313. Schochet SS, McCormick WF, Zellweger H: Type IV glycogenesis (amylopectinosis). Arch Pathol 90:354, 1970
314. Ishihara T, Uchino F, Adachi H, et al: Type IV glycogenesis: A study of two cases. Acta Pathol Jpn 25:613, 1975
315. Starzl TE, Demetris AJ, Trucco M, et al: Chimerism after liver transplantation for type IV glycogen storage disease and type I Gaucher's disease. N Engl J Med 328:745, 1993
316. Sokal EM, Van Hoof F, Alberti D, et al: Progressive cardiac failure following orthotopic liver transplantation for type IV glycogenesis. Eur J Pediatr 151:200, 1992
317. Greene GM, Weldon DC, Ferrans VJ, et al: Juvenile polysaccharidosis with cardioskeletal myopathy. Arch Pathol Lab Med 111:977, 1987
318. Schwartz ML, Cox GF, Lin AE, et al: Clinical approach to genetic cardiomyopathy in children. Circulation 94:2021, 1996
319. Elleder M, Shin YS, Zuntová A, et al: Fatal infantile hypertrophic cardiomyopathy secondary to deficiency of heart specific phosphorylase b kinase. Virchows Archiv [Path Anat] 423:303, 1993
320. Abbott RD, Brand FN, Kannel WB, Castelli WP: Gout and coronary heart disease: The Framingham study. J Clin Epidemiol 41:237, 1988
321. Takahashi S, Yamamoto T, Moriwaki Y, et al: Increased concentrations of serum Lp(a) lipoprotein in patients with primary gout. Ann Rheum Dis 54:90, 1995
322. Pund EE Jr, Hawley RL, McGee HJ, Blount SG Jr: Gouty heart. N Engl J Med 263:835, 1960
323. Lichtenstein L, Scott HW, Levin MH: Pathologic changes in gout: Survey of 11 necropsied cases. Am J Pathol 32:871, 1956
324. Bacon BR: Causes of iron overload. N Engl J Med 326:126, 1992
325. Bulaj ZJ, Griffen LM, Jorde LB, et al: Clinical and biochemical abnormalities in people heterozygous for hemochromatosis. N Engl J Med 335:1799, 1996
326. Edwards CQ, Kushner JP: Screening for hemochromatosis. N Engl J Med 328:1616, 1993
327. Spirito P, Lupi G, Melevendi C, Vecchio C: Restrictive diastolic abnormalities identified by Doppler echocardiography in patients with thalassemia major. Circulation 82:88, 1990
328. Lattanzi F, Bellotti P, Picano E, et al: Quantitative ultrasonic analysis of myocardium in patients with thalassemia major and iron overload. Circulation 87:748, 1993
329. Waxman S, Eustace S, Hartnell GG: Myocardial involvement in primary hemochromatosis demonstrated by magnetic resonance imaging. Am Heart J 128:1047, 1994
330. Olson LJ, Edwards WD, Holmes DR Jr, et al: Endomyocardial biopsy in hemochromatosis: Clinicopathologic correlates in 6 cases. J Am Coll Cardiol 13:116, 1989
331. Buja LM, Roberts WC: Iron in the heart: Etiology and clinical significance. Am J Med 51:209, 1971

332. Olson LJ, Edwards WD, McCall JT, et al: Cardiac iron deposition in idiopathic hemochromatosis: Histologic and analytic assessment of 14 hearts from autopsy. J Am Coll Cardiol 10:1239, 1987

333. Brown GG: Pigments and minerals. I. Hematogenous pigments. J Histotechnol 11:109, 1988

334. James TN: Pathology of the cardiac conduction system in hemochromatosis. N Engl J Med 271:92, 1964

335. Miller M, Hutchins GM: Hemochromatosis, multiorgan hemosiderosis, and coronary artery disease. JAMA 272:231, 1994

336. McCord JM: Is non-sufficiency a risk factor in ischemic heart disease? Circulation 83:1112, 1991

337. Dabestani A, Child JS, Henze E, et al: Primary hemochromatosis: Anatomic and physiologic characteristics of the cardiac ventricles and their response to phlebotomy. Am J Cardiol 54:153, 1984

338. Brittenham GM, Griffith PM, Nienhuis AW, et al: Efficacy of deferoxamine in preventing complications of iron overload in patients with thalassemia major. N Engl J Med 331:567, 1994

339. Surakomol S, Olson LJ, Rastogi A, et al: Combined orthotopic heart and liver transplantation for genetic hemochromatosis. J Heart Lung Transplant 16:573, 1997

340. Basson CT, Cowley GS, Solomon SD, et al: The clinical and genetic spectrum of the Holt-Oram syndrome (heart-hand syndrome). N Engl J Med 330:885, 1994

341. Terrett JA, Newbury-Ecob R, Cross GS, et al: Holt-Oram syndrome is a genetically heterogeneous disease with one locus mapping to human chromosome 12q. Nat Genet 6:401, 1994

342. Basson CT, Solomon SD, Weissman B, et al: Genetic heterogeneity of heart-hand syndromes. Circulation 91:1326, 1995

343. Meleady RA, Mulcahy DA, Graham IM: Genes, greens, and homocysteine. Heart 76:103, 1996

344. McCully KS: Vascular pathology of hyperhomocysteinemia: Implications for the pathogenesis of arteriosclerosis. Am J Pathol 56:111, 1969

345. Gibson JB, Carson NAJ, Neill DW: Pathological findings in homocystinuria. J Clin Pathol 17:427, 1964

346. Mayer EL, Jacobsen DW, Robinson K: Homocysteine and coronary atherosclerosis. J Am Coll Cardiol 27:517, 1996

347. Schwartz SM, Siscovick DS, Malinow R, et al: Myocardial infarction in young women in relation to plasma total homocysteine, folate, and a common variant in the methylenetetrahydrofolate reductase gene. Circulation 96:412, 1997

348. Nygård O, Nordrehaug JE, Refsum H, et al: Plasma homocysteine levels and mortality in patients with coronary artery disease. N Engl J Med 337:230, 1997

349. Frohlich ED, Apstein C, Chobanian AV, et al: The heart in hypertension. N Engl J Med 327:998, 1992

350. Devereux RB: Do antihypertensive drugs differ in their ability to regress left ventricular hypertrophy? Circulation 95:1983, 1997

351. Ge K, Xue A, Bai J, Wang S: Keshan disease: An endemic cardiomyopathy in China. Virchows Archiv [Path Anat] 401:1, 1983

352. Li G, Wang F, Kang D, Li C: Keshan disease: An endemic cardiomyopathy in China. Hum Pathol 16:602, 1985

353. Reeves WC, Marcuard SP, Willis SE, Movahed A: Reversible cardiomyopathy due to selenium deficiency. J Parenter Enter Nutr 13:663, 1989

354. Hensrud DD, Heimburger DC, Chen J, Parpia B: Antioxidant status, erythrocyte fatty acids, and mortality from cardiovascular disease and Keshan disease in China. Eur J Clin Nutr 48:455, 1994

355. Rayman MP: Dietary selenium: Time to act. BMJ 314:387, 1997

356. Brzustowicz LM, Lehner T, Castilla LH, et al: Genetic mapping of chronic childhood-onset spinal muscular atrophy to chromosome 5q 11.2–13.3. Nature 344:540, 1990

357. Tanaka H, Uemura N, Toyama Y, et al: Cardiac involvement in the Kugelberg-Welander syndrome. Am J Cardiol 38:528, 1976

358. Tanaka H, Nishi S, Nuruki K, Tanaka N: Myocardial ultrastructural changes in Kugelberg-Welander syndrome. Br Heart J 39:1390, 1977

359. Józwiak S, Schwartz RA, Janniger CK: LEOPARD syndrome (cardiocutaneous lentiginosis syndrome). Cutis 57:208, 1996

360. Blieden LC, Schneeweiss A, Neufeld HN: Primary pulmonary hypertension in leopard syndrome. Br Heart J 46:458, 1981

361. Seuanez H, Mañe-Garzon F, Kolski R: Cardiocutaneous syndrome (the "LEOPARD" syndrome): Review of the literature and a new family. Clin Genet 9:266, 1976

362. St. John Sutton MG, Tajik AJ, Giuliani ER, et al: Hypertrophic obstructive cardiomyopathy and lentiginosis: A little known neural ectodermal syndrome. Am J Cardiol 47:214, 1981

363. Schievink WI, Michels VV, Mokri B, et al: Brief report: A familial syndrome of arterial dissections with lentiginosis. N Engl J Med 332:576, 1995

364. Feiner HD: Pathology of dysproteinemia: Light chain amyloidosis, non-amyloid immunoglobulin deposition disease, cryoglobulinemia syndromes, and macroglobulinemia of Waldenstrom. Hum Pathol 19:1255, 1988

365. Ganeval D, Noël L-H, Preud'homme J-L, et al: Light-chain deposition disease: Its relation with AL-type amyloidosis. Kidney Int 26:1, 1984

366. McAllister HA Jr, Seger J, Bossart M, Ferrans VJ: Restrictive cardiomyopathy with κ light chain deposits in myocardium as a complication of multiple myeloma: Histochemical and electron microscopic observations. Arch Pathol Lab Med 112:1151, 1988

367. Walley VM, Silver MD: Unusual cardiovascular localization of nonamyloid immunoglobulin deposition disease causing sudden death. Mod Pathol 5:89, 1992

368. Peng S-K, French WJ, Cohen AH, Fausel RE: Light chain cardiomyopathy associated with small-vessel disease. Arch Pathol Lab Med 112:844, 1988

369. Gallo G, Goñi F, Boctor F, et al: Light chain cardiomyopathy: Structural analysis of the light chain tissue deposits. Am J Pathol 148:1397, 1996

370. Cooke RA, Chambers JB: Anorexia nervosa and the heart. Br J Hosp Med 54:313, 1995

371. Olowonyo MT, Ogunkunle OO, Akinbami FO, Jaiyesimi F: The echocardiographic findings in kwashiorkor. J Trop Pediatr 41:74, 1995

372. Kothari SS, Patel TM, Shetalwad AN, Patel TK: Left ventricular mass and function in children with severe protein energy malnutrition. Int J Cardiol 35:19, 1992

373. Sims BA: Conducting tissue of the heart in kwashiorkor. Br Heart J 34:828, 1972

374. Piza J, Troper L, Cespedes R, Miller JH, Berenson GS: Myocardial lesions and heart failure in infantile malnutrition. Am J Trop Med Hyg 20:343, 1971

375. Wharton BA, Balmer SE, Somers K, Templeton AC: The myocardium in kwashiorkor. Q J Med 38:107, 1969

376. Ansari A: Syndromes of cardiac cachexia and the cachectic heart: Current perspective. Prog Cardiovasc Dis 30:45, 1987

377. Webb JG, Kiess MC, Chan-Yan CC: Malnutrition and the heart. Can Med Assoc J 135:753, 1986

378. Isner JM, Sours HE, Paris AL, et al: Sudden, unexpected death in avid dieters using the liquid-protein-modified-fast diet: Observations in 17 patients and the role of the prolonged QT interval. Circulation 60:1401, 1979

379. Fisler JS: Cardiac effects of starvation and semistarvation diets: Safety and mechanisms of action. Am J Clin Nutr 56(suppl):S230, 1992

380. Mitchell JE, Seim HC, Colon E, Pomeroy C: Medical complications and medical management of bulimia. Ann Intern Med 107:71, 1987

381. de Simone G, Scalfi L, Galderisi M, et al: Cardiac abnormalities in young women with anorexia nervosa. Br Heart J 71:287, 1994

382. Tsipouras P, Del Mastro R, Sarfarazi M, et al: Genetic linkage of the Marfan syndrome, ectopia lentis, and congenital contractual arachnodactyly to the fibrillin genes on chromosomes 15 and 5. N Engl J Med 326:905, 1992

383. Dietz HC, Pyeritz RE: Mutations in the human gene for fibrillin-1 (FBN1) in the Marfan syndrome and related disorders. Hum Mol Genet 4:1799, 1995

384. Pereira L, Levran O, Ramirez F, et al: A molecular approach to the stratification of cardiovascular risk in families with Marfan's syndrome. N Engl J Med 331:148, 1994

385. Francke U, Furthmayer H: Marfan's syndrome and other disorders of fibrillin. N Engl J Med 330:1384, 1994

386. Milewicz DM, Michael K, Fisher N, et al: Fibrillin-1 (FBN1) mutations in patients with thoracic aortic aneurysms. Circulation 94:2708, 1996

387. Roberts WC, Honig HS: The spectrum of cardiovascular disease in the Marfan syndrome: A clinicomorphologic study of 18 necropsy patients and comparison to 151 previously reported necropsy patients. Am Heart J 104:115, 1982

388. Crisfield RJ: Spontaneous aneurysm of the ductus arteriosus in a patient with Marfan's syndrome. J Thorac Cardiovasc Surg 62:243, 1971

389. Magherini A, Margiotta C, Bandini F, et al: Atrial septal aneurysm, ectasia of a sinus of Valsalva, and mitral valve prolapse in Marfan's syndrome. Am J Cardiol 58:172, 1986

390. Geva T, Sanders SP, Diogenes MS, et al: Two-dimensional and Doppler echocardiographic and pathologic characteristics of the infantile Marfan syndrome. Am J Cardiol 65:1230, 1990

391. Roberts WC: Aortic dissection: Anatomy, consequences, and causes. Am Heart J 101:195, 1981

392. Gott VL, Pyeritz RE, Magovern GJ Jr, et al: Surgical treatment of aneurysms of the ascending aorta in the Marfan syndrome: Results of composite—graft repair in 50 patients. N Engl J Med 314:1070, 1986

393. Shores J, Berger KR, Murphy EA, Pyeritz RE: Progression of aortic dilatation and the benefit of long-term β adrenergic blockade in Marfan's syndrome. N Engl J Med 330:1335, 1994

394. Roman MJ, Rosen SE, Kramer-Fox R, Devereux RB: Prognostic significance of the pattern of aortic root dilation in the Marfan syndrome. J Am Coll Cardiol 22:1470, 1993

395. Legett ME, Unger TA, O'Sullivan CK, et al: Aortic root complications in Marfan's syndrome: Identification of a lower risk group. Heart 75:389, 1996

396. Schlatmann TJM, Becker AE: Pathogenesis of dissecting aneurysm of aorta: Comparative histopathologic study of significance of medial changes. Am J Cardiol 39:21, 1977

397. Schlatmann TJM, Becker AE: Histologic changes in the normal aging aorta: Implications for dissecting aortic aneurysm. Am J Cardiol 39:13, 1977

398. Pierce HI, Cooper EB: Meningococcal pericarditis: Clinical features and therapy in five patients. Arch Intern Med 129:918, 1972

399. Neveling U, Kaschula ROC: Fatal meningococcal disease in childhood: An autopsy study of 86 cases. Ann Trop Paediatr 13:147, 1993

400. Cox DW: Genes of the copper pathway. Am J Hum Genet 56:828, 1995

401. Kaler SG: Menkes' disease mutations and response to early copper histidine treatment. Nat Genet 13:21, 1996

402. Danks DM, Campbell PE, Stevens BJ, et al: Menkes' kinky hair syndrome: An inherited defect in copper absorption with widespread effects. Pediatrics 50:188, 1972

403. Oakes BW, Danks DM, Campbell PE: Human copper deficiency: Ultrastructural studies of the aorta and skin in a child with Menkes' syndrome. Exp Mol Pathol 25:82, 1976

404. Uno H, Arya S, Laxova R, Gilbert EF: Menkes' syndrome with vascular and adrenergic nerve abnormalities. Arch Pathol Lab Med 107:286, 1983

405. Kelly TE, Bartoshesky L, Harris DJ, et al: Mucolipidosis I (acid neuraminidase deficiency). Am J Dis Child 135:703, 1981

406. Blank E, Linder D: I-cell disease (mucolipidosis II): a lysosomopathy. Pediatrics 54:797, 1974

407. Patriquin HB, Kaplan P, Kind HP, Giedion A: Neonatal mucolipidosis II (I-cell disease): Clinical and radiologic features in three cases. AJR Am J Roentgenol 129:37, 1977

408. Satoh Y, Sakamoto K, Fujibayashi Y, et al: Cardiac involvement in mucolipidosis: Importance of non-invasive studies for detection of cardiac abnormalities. Jpn Heart J 24:149, 1983

409. Nagashima K, Sakakibara K, Endo H, et al: I-cell disease (mucolipidosis II): Pathological and biochemical studies of an autopsy case. Acta Pathol Jpn 27:251, 1977

410. Kelly TE, Thomas GH, Taylor HA Jr, et al: Mucolipidosis III (pseudo-Hurler polydystrophy): Clinical and laboratory studies in a series of 12 patients. Johns Hopkins Med J 137:156, 1975

411. Sensenbrenner JA: Pseudo-Hurler polydystrophy (mucolipidosis III) with aortic regurgitation. Birth Defects 8:295, 1972

412. Fann JI, Dalman RL, Harris EJ Jr: Genetic and metabolic causes of arterial disease. Ann Vasc Surg 7:594, 1993

413. Fensom AH, Benson PF: Recent advances in the prenatal diagnosis of the mucopolysaccharidoses. Prenat Diagn 14:1, 1994

414. Gatzoulis MA, Vellodi A, Redington AN: Cardiac involvement in mucopolysaccharidoses: Effects of allogeneic bone marrow transplantation. Arch Dis Child 73:259, 1995

415. Gross DM, Williams JC, Caprioli C, et al: Echocardiographic abnormalities in the mucopolysaccharide storage diseases. Am J Cardiol 61:170, 1988

416. Rentería VC, Ferrans VJ, Roberts WC: The heart in Hurler syndrome: Gross, histologic and ultrastructural observations in five necropsy cases. Am J Cardiol 38:487, 1976

417. Braunlin EA, Hunter DW, Krivit W, et al: Evaluation of coronary artery disease in the Hurler syndrome by angiography. Am J Cardiol 69:1487, 1992

418. Ferrans VJ: Metabolic and familial disease. In: Silver MD (ed): Cardiovascular Pathology. 2nd ed. New York, Churchill Livingstone, 1991, p 1080

419. Butman SM, Karl L, Copeland JG: Combined aortic and mitral valve replacement in an adult with Scheie's disease. Chest 96:209, 1989

420. Masuda H, Morishita Y, Taira A, Kuriyama M: Aortic stenosis associated with Scheie's syndrome: Report of successful valve replacement. Chest 103:968, 1993

421. Young ID, Harper PS: Mild form of Hunter's syndrome: Clinical delineation based on 31 cases. Arch Dis Child 57:828, 1982

422. Nagashima K, Endo H, Sakakibara K, et al: Morphological and biochemical studies of a case of mucopolysaccharidosis II (Hunter's syndrome). Acta Pathol Jpn 26:115, 1976

423. Herd JK, Subramanian S, Robinson H: Type III mucopolysaccharidosis: Report of a case with severe mitral valve involvement. J Pediatr 82:101, 1973

424. Shimamura K, Hakozaki H, Takahashi K, et al: Sanfilippo B syndrome: A case report. Acta Pathol Jpn 26:739, 1976

425. Schenk EA, Haggerty J: Morquio's disease: A radiologic and morphologic study. Pediatrics 34:839, 1964

426. Ireland MA, Rowlands DB: Mucopolysaccharidosis type IV as a cause of mitral stenosis in an adult. Br Heart J 46:113, 1981

427. Factor SM, Biempica L, Goldfischer S: Coronary intimal sclerosis in Morquio's syndrome. Vircho Arch [Path Anat] 379:1, 1978

428. Fong LV, Menahem S, Wraith JE, Chow CW: Endocardial fibroelastosis in mucopolysaccharidosis type VI. Clin Cardiol 10:362, 1987

429. Hayflick S, Rowe S, Kavanaugh-McHugh A, et al: Acute infantile cardiomyopathy as a presenting feature of mucopolysaccharidosis VI. J Pediatr 120:269, 1992

430. Tan CTT, Schaff HV, Miller FA Jr, et al: Valvular heart disease in four patients with Maroteaux-Lamy syndrome. Circulation 85:188, 1992

431. Vogler C, Levy B, Kyle JW, et al: Mucopolysaccharidosis VII: Postmortem biochemical and pathological findings in a young adult with β glucuronidase deficiency. Mod Pathol 7:132, 1994

432. Morris CP, Guo X-H, Apostolou S, et al: Morquio A syndrome: Cloning, sequence, and structure of the human N-acetylgalactosamine 6-sulfatase (GALNS) gene. Genomics 22:652, 1994

433. Scott HS, Blanch L, Guo X-H, et al: Cloning of the sulphamidase gene and identification of mutations in the Sanfilippo A syndrome. Nat Genet 11:465, 1995

434. Zhao HG, Li HH, Bach G, et al: The molecular basis of Sanfilippo syndrome type B. Proc Natl Acad Sci U S A 93:6101, 1996

435. Wallgren-Pettersson C, Avela K, Marchand S, et al: A gene for autosomal recessive nemaline myopathy assigned to chromosome 2q by linkage analysis. Neuromuscul Disord 5:441, 1995

436. Laing NG, Wilton SD, Akkari PA, et al: A mutation in the α tropomyosin gene TPM3 associated with autosomal dominant nemaline myopathy. Nat Genet 9:75, 1995

437. Ishibashi-Ueda H, Imakita M, Yutani C, et al: Congenital nemaline myopathy with dilated cardiomyopathy: An autopsy study. Hum Pathol 21:77, 1990

438. Rosenson RS, Mudge GH Jr, St. John Sutton MG: Nemaline cardiomyopathy. Am J Cardiol 58:175, 1986

439. Jones JG, Factor SM: Familial congestive cardiomyopathy with nemaline rods in heart and skeletal muscle. Virchows Arch [Path Anat] 408:307, 1985

440. Meier C, Voellmy W, Gertsch M, et al: Nemaline myopathy appearing in adults as cardiomyopathy: A clinicopathologic study. Arch Neurol 41:443, 1984

441. von Deimling A, Krone W, Menon AG: Neurofibromatosis type 1: Pathology, clinical features and molecular genetics. Brain Pathol 5:153, 1995

442. Kaufman RL, Hartmann AF, McAlister WH: Family studies in congenital heart disease associated with neurofibromatosis. Birth Defects 8:92, 1972

443. Panayiotopoulos YP, Tyrrell MR, Koffman G, et al: Mid-aortic syndrome presenting in childhood. Br J Surg 83:235, 1996

444. Salyer WR, Salyer DC: The vascular lesions of neurofibromatosis. Angiology 25:510, 1974

445. Huffman JL, Gahtan V, Bowers VD, Mills JL: Neurofibromatosis and arterial aneurysms. Am Surg 62:311, 1996

446. Westenend PJ, Smedts F, de Jong MCJW, et al: A 4-year-old boy with neurofibromatosis and severe renovascular hypertension due to renal arterial dysplasia. Am J Surg Pathol 18:512, 1994

447. Carstea ED, Morris JA, Coleman KG, et al: Niemann-Pick C1 disease gene: Homology to mediators of cholesterol homeostasis. Science 277:228, 1997

448. Lever AML, Ryder JB: Cor pulmonale in an adult secondary to Niemann-Pick disease. Thorax 38:873, 1983

449. Westwood M: Endocardial fibroelastosis and Niemann-Pick disease. Br Heart J 39:1394, 1977

450. Chan WC, Lai KS, Todd D: Adult Niemann-Pick disease: A case report. J Pathol 121:177, 1977

451. Şenocak F, Sarçlar M, Ozkutlu S: Echocardiographic findings in some metabolic storage diseases. Jpn Heart J 35:635, 1994

452. Jamieson CR, van der Burgt I, Brady AF, et al: Mapping a gene for Noonan syndrome to the long arm of chromosome 12. Nat Genet 8:357, 1994

453. Noonan JA: Noonan syndrome: An update and review for the primary pediatrician. Clin Pediatr 33:548, 1994

454. Burch M, Sharland M, Shinebourne E, et al: Cardiologic abnormalities in Noonan syndrome: Phenotypic diagnosis and echocardiographic assessment of 118 patients. J Am Coll Cardiol 22:1189, 1993

455. Burch M, Mann JM, Sharland M, et al: Myocardial disarray in Noonan syndrome. Br Heart J 68:586, 1992

456. Wilmshurst PT, Katritsis D: Restrictive and hypertrophic cardiomyopathies in Noonan syndrome: The overlap syndromes. Heart 75:94, 1996

457. Walton C, Lees B, Crook D, et al: Body fat distribution, rather than overall adiposity, influences serum lipids and lipoproteins in healthy men independently of age. Am J Med 99:459, 1995

458. Alpert MA, Hashimi MW: Obesity and the heart. Am J Med Sci 306:117, 1993

459. Pi-Sunyer FX: Medical hazards of obesity. Ann Intern Med 119:655, 1993

460. Freedman DS: The importance of body fat distribution in early life. Am J Med Sci 310(suppl):S72, 1995

461. Amad KH, Brennan JC, Alexander JK: The cardiac pathology of chronic exogenous obesity. Circulation 32:740, 1965

462. Warnes CA, Roberts WC: The heart in massive (more than 300 pounds or 130 kilograms) obesity: Analysis of 12 patients studied at necropsy. Am J Cardiol 54:1087, 1984

463. Frank S, Colliver JA, Frank A: The electrocardiogram in obesity: Statistical analysis of 1,029 patients. J Am Coll Cardiol 7:295, 1986

464. Messerli FH, Nunez BD, Ventura HO, Snyder DW: Overweight and sudden death: Increased ventricular ectopy in the cardiopathy of obesity. Arch Intern Med 147:1725, 1987

465. Lauer MS, Anderson KM, Kannel WB, Levy D: The impact of obesity on left ventricular mass and geometry: The Framingham heart study. JAMA 266:231, 1991

466. Lavie CJ, Amodeo C, Ventura HO, Messerli FH: Left atrial abnormalities indicating diastolic ventricular dysfunction in cardiopathy of obesity. Chest 92:1042, 1987

467. Himeno E, Nishino K, Nakashima Y, et al: Weight reduction regresses left ventricular mass regardless of blood pressure level in obese subjects. Am Heart J 131:313, 1996

468. Smith HL, Willius FA: Adiposity of the heart: A clinical and pathological study of 136 obese patients. Arch Intern Med 52:911, 1933

469. Bharati S, Lev M: Cardiac conduction system involvement in sudden death of obese young people. Am Heart J 129:273, 1995

470. Ahmed Q, Chung-Park M, Tomashefski JF Jr: Cardiopulmonary pathology in patients with sleep apnea/obesity hypoventilation syndrome. Hum Pathol 28:264, 1997

471. Smalling RW, Soohoo W, Chen P: A 25-year-old white woman with a cerebrovascular accident and a right to left shunt. Circulation 90:2540, 1994

472. Guttmacher AE, Marchuk DA, White RI Jr: Hereditary hemorrhagic telangiectasia. N Engl J Med 333:918, 1995

473. McAllister KA, Grogg KM, Johnson DW, et al: Endoglin, a TGF-β binding protein of endothelial cells, is the gene for hereditary hemorrhagic telangiectasia type I. Nat Genet 8:345, 1994

474. Vincent P, Planchu H, Hazan J, et al: A third locus for hereditary haemorrhagic telangiectasia maps to chromosome 12q. Hum Mol Genet 4:945, 1995

475. Marini JC, Gerber NL: Osteogenesis imperfecta: Rehabilitation and prospects for gene therapy. JAMA 277:746, 1997

476. Stöss H, Freisinger P: Collagen fibrils of osteoid in osteogenesis imperfecta: Morphometrical analysis of the fibril diameter. Am J Med Genet 45:257, 1993

477. Wheeler VR, Cooley NR Jr, Blackburn WR: Cardiovascular pathology in osteogenesis imperfecta type II A with a review of the literature. Pediatr Pathol 8:55, 1988

478. McAllion SJ, Paterson CR: Causes of death in osteogenesis imperfecta. J Clin Pathol 49:627, 1996

479. Criscitiello MG, Ronan JA Jr, Besterman EMM, Schoenwetter W: Cardiovascular abnormalities in osteogenesis imperfecta. Circulation 31:255, 1965

480. Hortop J, Tsipouras P, Hanley JA, et al: Cardiovascular involvement in osteogenesis imperfecta. Circulation 73:54, 1986

481. Rogerson ME, Buchanan JD, Morgans CM: Left atrial rupture in osteogenesis imperfecta. Br Heart J 56:187, 1986

482. Wong JSK, O'Neill DM, Cunningham NE: Atrial rupture in osteogenesis imperfecta. Br J Hosp Med 38:139, 1987

483. Wong RS, Follis FM, Shively BK, Wernly JA: Osteogenesis imperfecta and cardiovascular diseases. Ann Thorac Surg 60:1439, 1995

484. Watts RWE: Primary hyperoxaluria type I. Q J Med 87:593, 1994

485. Chaplin AJ: Histopathological occurrence and characterization of calcium oxalate: A review. J Clin Pathol 30:800, 1977

486. Fyfe BS, Israel DH, Quish A, et al: Reversal of primary hyperoxaluria cardiomyopathy after combined liver and renal transplantation. Am J Cardiol 75:210, 1995

487. Arbus GS, Sniderman S: Oxalosis with peripheral gangrene. Arch Pathol 97:107, 1974

488. Salyer WR, Hutchins GM: Cardiac lesions in secondary oxalosis. Arch Intern Med 134:250, 1974

489. Surawicz B: Relationship between electrocardiogram and electrolytes. Am Heart J 73:814, 1967

490. Stefenelli T, Mayr H, Bergler-Klein J, Globits S, et al: Primary hyperparathyroidism: Incidence of cardiac abnormalities and partial reversibility after successful parathyroidectomy. Am J Med 95:197, 1993

491. Roberts WC, Waller BF: Effect of chronic hypercalcemia on the heart: An analysis of 18 necropsy patients. Am J Med 71:371, 1981

492. King M, Huang J-M, Glassman E: Paget's disease with cardiac calcification and complete heart block. Am J Med 46:302, 1969

493. Katz JH, Dias SM, Ferguson RP: Fatal cardiac calcifications secondary to primary hyperparathyroidism. Am J Med 85:122, 1988

494. Pulitzer DR, Martin PC, Collins PC, Reitmeyer WJ: Cutaneous vascular calcification with ulceration in hyperparathyroidism. Arch Pathol Lab Med 114:482, 1990

495. Vered I, Vered Z, Perez JE, et al: Normal left ventricular performance documented by Doppler echocardiography in patients with long-standing hypocalcemia. Am J Med 86:413, 1989

496. Terzolo M, Avonto L, Matrella C, et al: Doppler echocardiographic patterns in patients with acromegaly. J Endocrinol Invest 18:613, 1995

497. Coggeshall C, Root HF: Acromegaly and diabetes mellitus. Endocrinology 26:1, 1940

498. Lie JT, Grossman SJ: Pathology of the heart in acromegaly: Anatomic findings in 27 autopsied patients. Am Heart J 100:41, 1980

499. Edén S, Wiklund O, Oscarsson J, et al: Growth hormone treatment of growth hormone-deficient adults results in a marked increase in Lp(a) and HDL cholesterol concentrations. Arterioscler Thromb Vasc Biol 13:296, 1993

500. Merimee TJ, Fineberg SE, Hollander W: Vascular disease in the chronic HGH-deficient state. Diabetes 22:813, 1973

501. Fazio S, Sabatini D, Capaldo B, et al: A preliminary study of growth hormone in the treatment of dilated cardiomyopathy. N Engl J Med 334:809, 1996

502. Sheehan HL, Summers VK: The syndrome of hypopituitarism. Q J Med 18:319, 1949

503. Curtarelli G, Ferrari C: Cardiomegaly and heart failure in a patient with prolactin-secreting pituitary tumor. Thorax 34:328, 1979

504. Peters DJM, Spruit L, Klingel R, et al: Adult, fetal, and polycystic kidney expression of polycystin, the polycystic kidney disease-1 gene product. Lab Invest 75:221, 1996

505. Gabow PA: Autosomal dominant polycystic kidney disease. N Engl J Med 329:332, 1993

506. Leier CV, Baker PB, Kilman JW, Wooley CF: Cardiovascular abnormalities associated with adult polycystic kidney disease. Ann Intern Med 100:683, 1984

507. Hossack KF, Leddy CL, Johnson AM, et al: Echocardiographic findings in autosomal dominant polycystic kidney disease. N Engl J Med 319:907, 1988

508. Adubofour K, Sidaway L, Glatter T: Coronary artery aneurysms in association with adult polycystic kidney disease. Am Heart J 127:1411, 1994

509. Biagini A, Maffei S, Baroni M, et al: Familial clustering of aortic dissection in polycystic kidney disease. Am J Cardiol 72:741, 1993

510. Lie JT: Cardiac manifestations in polymyositis/dermatomyositis: How to get to the heart of the matter. J Rheumatol 22:809, 1995

511. Dalakas MC: Polymyositis, dermatomyositis, and inclusion-body myositis. N Engl J Med 325:1487, 1991

512. Gómez FP, Merino JL, Maté I, et al: Polymyositis associated with anti-Jo1 antibodies: Severe cardiac involvement as initial manifestation. Am J Med 94:110, 1993

513. Askari AD, Huettner TL: Cardiac abnormalities in polymyositis/dermatomyositis. Semin Arthritis Rheum 12:208, 1982

514. Yale SH, Adlakha A, Stanton MS: Dermatomyositis with pericardial tamponade and polymyositis with pericardial effusion. Am Heart J 126:997, 1993

515. Denbow CE, Lie JT, Tancredi RG, Bunch TW: Cardiac involvement in polymyositis: A clinicopathologic study of 20 autopsied patients. Arthritis Rheum 22:1088, 1979

516. Haupt HM, Hutchins GM: The heart and conduction system in polymyositis/dermatomyositis: A clinicopathologic study of 16 autopsied patients. Am J Cardiol 50:998, 1982

517. Lynch PG: Cardiac involvement in chronic polymyositis. Br Heart J 33:416, 1971

518. Behan WMH, Aitchison M, Behan PO: Pathogenesis of heart block in a fatal case of dermatomyositis. Br Heart J 56:479, 1986

519. Gottdiener JS, Sherber HS, Hawley RJ, Engel WK: Cardiac manifestations in polymyositis. Am J Cardiol 41:1141, 1978

520. Jimenez C, Rowe PC, Keene D: Cardiac and central nervous system vasculitis in a child with dermatomyositis. J Child Neurol 9:297, 1994

521. Perkins JG, Petersen AB, Riley JA: Renal and cardiac lesions in potassium deficiency due to chronic diarrhea. Am J Med 8:115, 1950

522. Keye JD: Death in potassium deficiency: Report of a case including morphologic findings. Circulation 5:766, 1953

523. Rizk NW, Kalassian KG, Gilligan T, et al: Obstetric complications in pulmonary and critical care medicine. Chest 110:791, 1996

524. Mone SM, Sanders SP, Colan SD: Control mechanisms for physiological hypertrophy of pregnancy. Circulation 94:667, 1996

525. Gianopoulos JG: Cardiac disease in pregnancy. Med Clin North Am 73:639, 1989

526. Presbitero P, Somerville J, Stone S, et al: Pregnancy in cyanotic congenital heart disease: Outcome of mother and fetus. Circulation 89:2673, 1994

527. Oakley CM: Pregnancy and congenital heart disease. Heart 78:12, 1997

528. Pomini F, Mercogliano D, Cavalletti C, et al: Cardiopulmonary bypass in pregnancy. Ann Thorac Surg 61:259, 1996

529. Parry AJ, Westaby S: Cardiopulmonary bypass during pregnancy. Ann Thorac Surg 61:1865, 1996

530. Cunningham FG, Lindheimer MD: Hypertension in pregnancy. N Engl J Med 326:927, 1992

531. Schobel HP, Fischer T, Heuszer K, et al: Pre-eclampsia: A state of sympathetic overactivity. N Engl J Med 335:1480, 1996

532. Hannaford P, Ferry S, Hirsch S: Cardiovascular sequelae of toxaemia of pregnancy. Heart 77:154, 1997

533. Roth A, Elkayam U: Acute myocardial infarction associated with pregnancy. Ann Intern Med 125:751, 1996

534. Manalo-Estrella P, Barker AE: Histopathologic findings in human aortic media associated with pregnancy. Arch Pathol 83:336, 1967

535. Cavanzo FJ, Taylor HB: Effect of pregnancy on the human aorta and its relationship to dissecting aneurysms. Am J Obstet Gynecol 105:567, 1969

536. Toglia MR, Weg JG: Venous thromboembolism during pregnancy. N Engl J Med 335:108, 1996

537. Mendelsohn G, Bulkley BH, Hutchins GM: Cardiovascular manifestations of pseudoxanthoma elasticum. Arch Pathol Lab Med 102:298, 1978

538. Ferrans VJ: Metabolic and familial diseases. In: Silver MD (ed): Cardiovascular Pathology. 2nd ed. New York, Churchill Livingstone, 1991, p 1100

539. Lebwohl M, Halperin J, Phelps RG: Brief report: Occult pseudoxanthoma elasticum in patients with premature cardiovascular disease. N Engl J Med 329:1237, 1993

540. Huang S-N, Kumar G, Steele HD, Parker JO: Cardiac involvement in pseudoxanthoma elasticum. Am Heart J 74:680, 1967

541. Challenor VF, Conway N, Monro JL: The surgical treatment of restrictive cardiomyopathy in pseudoxanthoma elasticum. Br Heart J 59:266, 1988

542. Nadal N, Rolland M-O, Tranchant C, et al: Localization of Refsum disease with increased pipecolic acidaemia to chromosome 10p by homozygosity mapping and carrier testing in a single nuclear family. Hum Mol Genet 4:1963, 1995

543. Leys D, Petit H, Bonte-Adnet C, et al: Refsum's disease revealed by cardiac disorders. Lancet 1:621, 1989

544. Gordon N, Hudson REB: Refsum's syndrome: Heredopathia atactica polyneuritiformis. Brain 82:41, 1959

545. Myllykangas-Luosujärvi R, Aho K, Kautiainen H, Isomäki H: Shortening of life span and causes of excess mortality in a population-based series of subjects with rheumatoid arthritis. Clin Exp Rheumatol 13:149, 1995

546. Corrao S, Salli' L, Arnone S, et al: Cardiac involvement in rheumatoid arthritis: Evidence of silent heart disease. Eur Heart J 16:253, 1995

547. Veys EM, De Keyser F: Rheumatoid nodules: Differential diagnosis and immunohistological findings. Ann Rheum Dis 52:625, 1993

548. DiFrancesco L, Miller F, Greenwald RA: Detailed immunohistologic evaluation of a methotrexate-induced nodule. Arch Pathol Lab Med 118:1223, 1994

549. Abu-Shakra M, Nicol P, Urowitz MB: Accelerated nodulosis, pleural effusion, and pericardial tamponade during methotrexate therapy. J Rheumatol 21:934, 1994

550. Bruyn GAW, Essed CA, Houtman PM, Willemse FW: Fatal cardiac nodules in a patient with rheumatoid arthritis treated with low dose methotrexate. J Rheumatol 20:912, 1993

551. Hara KS, Ballard DJ, Ilstrup DM, et al: Rheumatoid pericarditis: Clinical features and survival. Medicine (Baltimore) 69:81, 1990

552. Thadani U, Iveson JM, Wright V: Cardiac tamponade, constrictive pericarditis, and pericardial resection in rheumatoid arthritis. Medicine (Baltimore) 54:261, 1975

553. Roberts WC, Kehoe JA, Carpenter DF, Golden A: Cardiac valvular lesions in rheumatoid arthritis. Arch Intern Med 122:141, 1968

554. Webber MD, Selsky EJ, Roper PA: Identification of a mobile intracardiac rheumatoid nodule mimicking an atrial myxoma. J Am Soc Echocardiogr 8:961, 1995

555. Gravallese EM, Corson JM, Coblyn JS, et al: Rheumatoid aortitis: A rarely recognized but clinically significant entity. Medicine (Baltimore) 68:95, 1989

556. Bacon PA, Kitas GD: The significance of vascular inflammation in rheumatoid arthritis. Ann Rheum Dis 53:621, 1994

557. Vollertsen RS, Conn DL, Ballard DJ, et al: Rheumatoid vasculitis: Survival and associated risk factors. Medicine (Baltimore) 65:365, 1986

558. Esterly JR, Oppenheimer EH: Congenital anomalies associated with intrauterine rubella infection. Birth Defects 8:75, 1972

559. Givens KT, Lee DA, Jones T, Ilstrup DM: Congenital rubella syndrome: Ophthalmic manifestations and associated systemic disorders. Br J Ophthalmol 77:358, 1993

560. Esterly JR, Oppenheimer EH: Vascular lesions in infants with congenital rubella. Circulation 36:544, 1967

561. Robinson J, Lemay M, Vaudry WL: Congenital rubella after anticipated maternal immunity: Two cases and a review of the literature. Pediatr Infect Dis J 13:812, 1994

562. Schumacher HR Jr, Klippel JH, Koopman WJ: Systemic sclerosis. In: Primer on the Rheumatic Diseases. Atlanta, Arthritis Foundation, 1993, p 118

563. McWhorter JE, LeRoy EC: Pericardial disease in scleroderma (systemic sclerosis). Am J Med 57:566, 1974

564. Sattar MA, Guindi RT, Vajcik J: Pericardial tamponade and limited cutaneous systemic sclerosis (CREST syndrome). Br J Rheumatol 29:306, 1990

565. Taylor HG, Sheldon P, McCance AJ, Skehan JD: CREST syndrome with pericardial but not peripheral calcinosis. Ann Rheum Dis 52:767, 1993

566. Sporn PHS, Albertson RD III, Orringer MB, Morganroth M: Fever and pneumopericardium in a patient with systemic sclerosis. Chest 90:117, 1986

567. Follansbee WP, Curtiss EI, Rahko PS, et al: The electrocardiogram in systemic sclerosis (scleroderma): Study of 102 consecutive cases with functional correlations and review of the literature. Am J Med 79:183, 1985

568. Ferri C, Bernini L, Bongiorni MG, et al: Noninvasive evaluation of cardiac dysrhythmias, and their relationship with multisystemic symptoms, in progressive systemic sclerosis patients. Arthritis Rheum 28:1259, 1985

569. Ridolfi RL, Bulkley BH, Hutchins GM: The cardiac conduction system in progressive systemic sclerosis: Clinical and pathologic features of 35 patients. Am J Med 61:361, 1976

570. Bulkley BH, Ridolfi RL, Salyer WR, Hutchins GM: Myocardial lesions of progressive systemic sclerosis: A cause of cardiac dysfunction. Circulation 53:483, 1976

571. D'Angelo WA, Fries JF, Masi AT, Shulman LE: Pathologic observations in systemic sclerosis (scleroderma): A study of 58 autopsy cases and 58 matched controls. Am J Med 46:428, 1969

572. Weiss S, Stead EA Jr, Warren JV, Bailey OT: Scleroderma heart disease with a consideration of other visceral manifestations of scleroderma. Arch Intern Med 71:749, 1943

573. Follansbee WP: The cardiovascular manifestations of systemic sclerosis (scleroderma). Curr Probl Cardiol 11:242, 1986

574. Winters GL, Costanzo-Nordin MR: Pathological findings in 2300 consecutive heart biopsies. Mod Pathol 4:441, 1991

575. Kahan A, Nitenberg A, Foult J-M, et al: Decreased coronary reserve in primary scleroderma myocardial disease. Arthritis Rheum 28:637, 1985

576. Clemson BS, Miller WR, Luck JC, Feriss JA: Acute myocarditis in fulminant systemic sclerosis. Chest 101:872, 1992

577. Lichtbroun AS, Sandhaus LM, Giorno RC, et al: Myocardial mast cells in systemic sclerosis: A report of 3 fatal cases. Am J Med 89:372, 1990

578. Follansbee WP, Zerbe TR, Medsger TA Jr: Cardiac and skeletal muscle disease in systemic sclerosis: A high risk association. Am Heart J 125:194, 1993

579. Rodnan GP, Myerowitz RL, Justh GO: Morphologic changes in the digital arteries of patients with progressive systemic sclerosis (scleroderma) and Raynaud phenomenon. Medicine (Baltimore) 59:393, 1980

580. Norton WL, Nardo JM: Vascular disease in progressive systemic sclerosis (scleroderma). Ann Intern Med 73:317, 1970

581. Oddis CV, Eisenbeis CH Jr, Reidbord HE, et al: Vasculitis in systemic sclerosis: Association with Sjögren's syndrome and the CREST syndrome variant. J Rheumatol 14:942, 1987

582. Reuler JB, Broudy VC, Cooney TG: Adult scurvy. JAMA 253:805, 1985

583. Adelman HM, Wallach PM, Gutierrez F, et al: Scurvy resembling cutaneous vasculitis. Cutis 54:111, 1994

584. Sament S: Cardiac disorders in scurvy. N Engl J Med 282:282, 1970

585. Follis RH: Sudden death in infants with scurvy. J Pediatr 20:347, 1942

586. Singh D, Chan W: Cardiomegaly and generalized edema due to vitamin C deficiency. Singapore Med J 15:60, 1974

587. Shafar J: Rapid reversion of electrocardiographic abnormalities after treatment in two cases of scurvy. Lancet 2:176, 1967

588. Nyyssönen K, Parviainen MT, Salonen R, et al: Vitamin C deficiency and risk of myocardial infarction: Prospective population study of men from eastern Finland. BMJ 314:634, 1997

589. Sands KE, Bates DW, Lanken PN, et al: Epidemiology of sepsis syndrome in 8 academic medical centers. JAMA 278:234, 1997

590. Pastores SM, Katz DP, Kvetan V: Splanchnic ischemia and gut mucosal injury in sepsis and the multiple organ dysfunction syndrome. Am J Gastroenterol 91:1697, 1996

591. Bunnell E, Parrillo JE: Cardiac dysfunction during septic shock. Clin Chest Med 17:237, 1996

592. Lane PA: Sickle cell disease. Pediatr Clin North Am 43:639, 1996

593. Francis RB Jr, Johnson CS: Vascular occlusion in sickle cell disease: Current concepts and unanswered questions. Blood 77:1405, 1991

594. Lindsay J Jr, Meshel JC, Patterson RH: The cardiovascular manifestations of sickle cell disease. Arch Intern Med 133:643, 1974

595. Covitz W, Espeland M, Gallagher D, et al: The heart in sickle cell anemia: The cooperative study of sickle cell disease. Chest 108:1214, 1995

596. Gerry JL Jr, Bulkley BH, Hutchins GM: Clinicopathologic analysis of cardiac dysfunction in 52 patients with sickle cell anemia. Am J Cardiol 42:211, 1978

597. Berezowski K, Mautner GC, Roberts WC: Scarring of the left ventricular papillary muscles in sickle-cell disease. Am J Cardiol 70:1368, 1992

598. James TN, Riddick L, Massing GK: Sickle cells and sudden death: Morphologic abnormalities of the cardiac conduction system. J Lab Clin Med 124:507, 1994

599. Bromberg PA: Pulmonary aspects of sickle cell disease. Arch Intern Med 133:652, 1974

600. Wood DH: Cerebrovascular complications of sickle cell anemia. Stroke 9:73, 1978

601. Platt OS, Brambilla DJ, Rosse WF, et al: Mortality in sickle cell disease: Life expectancy and risk factors for early death. N Engl J Med 330:1639, 1994

602. Kark JA, Posey DM, Schumacher HR, Ruehle CJ: Sickle-cell trait as a risk factor for sudden death in physical training. N Engl J Med 317:781, 1987

603. Rantapää-Dahlqvist S, Backman C, Sandgren H, Östberg Y: Echocardiographic findings in patients with primary Sjögren's syndrome. Clin Rheumatol 12:214, 1993

604. Markusse HM, Schoonbrood M, Oudkerk M, Henzman-Logmans SC: Leucocytoclastic vasculitis as presenting feature of primary Sjögren's syndrome. Clin Rheumatol 13:269, 1994

605. Sato T, Matsubara O, Tanaka Y, Kasuga T: Association of Sjögren's syndrome with pulmonary hypertension: Report of two cases and review of the literature. Hum Pathol 24:199, 1993

606. Staub HL, Capobianco KG, Rosa CH, Keiserman MW: Verrucous endocarditis and sicca syndrome. Scand J Rheumatol 22:202, 1993

607. Ben-Chetrit E: The molecular basis of the SSA/Ro antigens and the clinical significance of their autoantibodies. Br J Rheumatol 32:396, 1993

608. Veille JC, Sunderland C, Bennett RM: Complete heart block in a fetus associated with maternal Sjögren's syndrome. Am J Obstet Gynecol 151:660, 1985

609. Ward MM, Pyun E, Studenski S: Causes of death in systemic lupus erythematosus. Arthritis Rheum 38:1492, 1995

610. Schieppati A, Remuzzi G: Prevalence and significance of hypertension in systemic lupus erythematosus. Am J Kidney Dis 21:58, 1993

611. Winslow TM, Ossipov MA, Fazio GP, et al: Five-year follow-up study of the prevalence and progression of pulmonary hypertension in systemic lupus erythematosus. Am Heart J 129:510, 1995

612. Sturfelt G, Eskilsson J, Nived O, et al: Cardiovascular disease in systemic lupus erythematosus: A study of 75 patients from a defined population. Medicine (Baltimore) 71:216, 1992

613. Ansari A, Larson PH, Bates HD: Cardiovascular manifestations of systemic lupus erythematosus: Current perspective. Prog Cardiovasc Dis 27:421, 1985

614. Morguet AJ, Sandrock D, Stille-Siegener M, Figulla HR: Indium-111-antimyosin Fab imaging to demonstrate myocardial involvement in systemic lupus erythematosus. J Nucl Med 36:1432, 1995

615. Borenstein DG, Fye WB, Arnett FC, Stevens MB: The myocarditis of systemic lupus erythematosus: Association with myositis. Ann Intern Med 89:619, 1978

616. Bulkley BH, Roberts WC: The heart in systemic lupus erythematosus and the changes induced in it by corticosteroid therapy: A study of 36 necropsy patients. Am J Med 58:243, 1975

617. Boumpas DT, Austin HA III, Fessler BJ, et al: Systemic lupus erythematosus: Emerging concepts. Part I: Renal, neuropsychiatric, cardiovascular, pulmonary, and hematologic disease. Ann Intern Med 122:940, 1995

618. Petri M, Perez-Guttman S, Spence D, Hochberg MC: Risk factors for coronary artery disease in patients with systemic lupus erythematosus. Am J Med 93:513, 1992

619. Haider YS, Roberts WC: Coronary arterial disease in systemic lupus erythematosus: Quantification of degrees of narrowing in 22 necropsy patients (21 women) aged 16 to 37 years. Am J Med 70:775, 1981

620. Wilson VE, Eck SL, Bates ER: Evaluation and treatment of acute myocardial infarction complicating systemic lupus erythematosus. Chest 101:420, 1992

621. Bonfiglio TA, Botti RE, Hagstrom JWC: Coronary arteritis, occlusion, and myocardial infarction due to lupus erythematosus. Am Heart J 83:153, 1972
622. Roldan CA, Shively BK, Crawford MH: An echocardiographic study of valvular heart disease associated with systemic lupus erythematosus. N Engl J Med 335:1424, 1996
623. Libman E, Sacks B: A hitherto undescribed form of valvular and mural endocarditis. Arch Intern Med 33:701, 1924
624. Ames DE, Asherson RA, Coltart JD, et al: Systemic lupus erythematosus complicated by tricuspid stenosis and regurgitation: Successful treatment by valve transplantation. Ann Rheum Dis 51:120, 1992
625. Kinney EL, Wynn J, Ward S, et al: Ruptured chordae tendineae: Its association with systemic lupus erythematosus. Arch Pathol Lab Med 104:595, 1980
626. Belmont HM, Abramson SB, Lie JT: Pathology and pathogenesis of vascular injury in systemic lupus erythematosus. Arthritis Rheum 39:9, 1996
627. McDonald J, Stewart J, Urowitz MB, Gladman DD: Peripheral vascular disease in patients with systemic lupus erythematosus. Ann Rheum Dis 51:56, 1992
628. Guard RW, Gotis-Graham I, Edmonds JP, Thomas AC: Aortitis with dissection complicating systemic lupus erythematosus. Pathology 27:224, 1995
629. MacLeod CB, Johnson D, Frable WJ: "Tree-barking" of the ascending aorta: Syphilis or systemic lupus erythematosus. Am J Clin Pathol 97:58, 1992
630. Love PE, Santoro SA: Antiphospholipid antibodies: Anticardiolipin and the lupus anticoagulant in systemic lupus erythematosus (SLE) and in non-SLE disorders—prevalence and clinical significance. Ann Intern Med 112:682, 1990
631. Bick RL: The antiphospholipid-thrombosis syndromes: Fact, fiction, confusion, and controversy. Am J Clin Pathol 100:477, 1993
632. Lockshin MD: Answers to the antiphospholipid-antibody syndrome. N Engl J Med 332:1025, 1995
633. Hojnik M, George J, Ziporen L, Shoenfeld Y: Heart valve involvement (Libman-Sacks endocarditis) in the antiphospholipid syndrome. Circulation 93:1579, 1996
634. Ford SE, Ford PM: The cardiovascular pathology of phospholipid antibodies: An illustrative case and review of the literature. Cardiovasc Pathol 4:111, 1995
635. Drew P, Asherson RA, Zuk RJ, et al: Aortic occlusion in systemic lupus erythematosus associated with antiphospholipid antibodies. Ann Rheum Dis 46:612, 1987
636. Prieto LN, Suki WN: Frequent hemodialysis graft thrombosis: Association with antiphospholipid antibodies. Am J Kidney Dis 23:587, 1994
637. Hughson MD, McCarty GA, Brumback RA: Spectrum of vascular pathology affecting patients with the antiphospholipid syndrome. Hum Pathol 26:716, 1995
638. Groves AMM, Allan LD, Rosenthal E: Outcome of isolated congenital complete heart block diagnosed in utero. Heart 75:190, 1996
639. Silverman ED: Congenital heart block and neonatal lupus erythematosus: Prevention is the goal. J Rheumatol 20:1101, 1993
640. Buyon JP: Neonatal lupus syndromes. Curr Opinion Rheumatol 6:523, 1994
641. Ho SY, Esscher E, Anderson RH, Michaëlsson M: Anatomy of congenital complete heart block and relation to maternal anti-Ro antibodies. Am J Cardiol 58:291, 1986
642. Weber HS, Myers JL: Maternal collagen vascular disease associated with fetal heart block and degenerative changes of the atrioventricular valves. Pediatr Cardiol 15:204, 1994
643. Bartolini G, Italia F, Ferraro G, et al: Histopathology of thalassemic heart disease: An endomyocardial biopsy study. Cardiovasc Pathol 6:205, 1997
644. Kremastinos DT, Tiniakos G, Theodorakis GN, et al: Myocarditis in β-thalassemia major: A cause of heart failure. Circulation 91:66, 1995
645. Paul O: Background of the prevention of cardiovascular disease. I. Nutrition, infections, and alcoholic heart disease. Circulation 79:1361, 1989
646. Leslie D, Gheorghiade M: Is there a role for thiamine supplementation in the management of heart failure? Am Heart J 131:1248, 1996
647. Naidoo DP, Singh B, Haffejee A: Cardiovascular complications of parenteral nutrition. Postgrad Med J 68:629, 1992
648. Sinha S, Norell MS, Nanda BS: Cardiac and renal failure in a 38 year-old alcoholic. Postgrad Med J 71:293, 1995
649. Phua KH, Goh LG, Koh K, et al: Thiamine deficiency and sudden deaths: Lessons from the past. Lancet 335:1471, 1990
650. Thurnham DI: Thiamine and sudden death in South-East Asians. Lancet 335:1472, 1990
651. Campbell CH: The severe lactic acidosis of thiamine deficiency: Acute pernicious or fulminating beriberi. Lancet 2:446, 1984
652. ter Maaten JC, Hoorntje SJ, Hillen HFP: Acute pernicious or fulminating beriberi heart disease: A report of 6 patients. Neth J Med 46:217, 1995
653. Wagner PI: Beriberi heart disease: Physiologic data and difficulties in diagnosis. Am Heart J 69:200, 1965
654. Blankenhorn MA, Vilter CF, Scheinker IM, Austin RS: Occidental beriberi heart disease. JAMA 131:717, 1946
655. Wolf PL, Levin MB: Shoshin beriberi. N Engl J Med 262:1302, 1960
656. Vedder EB: The pathology of beriberi. JAMA 110:893, 1938
657. Bell W: Thrombotic thrombocytopenic purpura. JAMA 265:91, 1991
658. Boyce TG, Swerdlow DL, Griffin PM: *Escherichia coli* O157:H7 and the hemolytic-uremic syndrome. N Engl J Med 333:364, 1995
659. Sheldon R, Slaughter D: A syndrome of microangiopathic hemolytic anemia, renal impairment, and pulmonary edema in chemotherapy-treated patients with adenocarcinoma. Cancer 58:1428, 1986
660. Rabinowe SN, Soiffer RJ, Tarbell NJ, et al: Hemolytic-uremic syndrome following bone marrow transplantation in adults for hematologic malignancies. Blood 77:1837, 1991
661. Young BA, Marsh CL, Alpers CE, Davis CL: Cyclosporine-associated thrombotic microangiopathy/hemolytic uremic syndrome following kidney and kidney-pancreas transplantation. Am J Kidney Dis 28:561, 1996
662. Ridolfi RL, Hutchins GM, Bell WR: The heart and cardiac conduction system in thrombotic thrombocytopenic purpura: A clinico pathologic study of 17 autopsied patients. Ann Intern Med 91:357, 1979
663. Webb JG, Butany J, Langer G, et al: Myocarditis and myocardial hemorrhage associated with thrombotic thrombocytopenic purpura. Arch Intern Med 150:1535, 1990
664. Klemperer JD, Ojamaa K, Klein I: Thyroid hormone therapy in cardiovascular disease. Prog Cardiovasc Dis 38:329, 1996
665. Sawin CT, Geller A, Wolf PA, et al: Low serum thyrotropin concentrations as a risk factor for atrial fibrillation in older persons. N Engl J Med 331:1249, 1994
666. Ching GW, Franklyn JA, Stallard TJ, et al: Cardiac hypertrophy as a result of long-term thyroxine therapy and thyrotoxicosis. Heart 75:363, 1996
667. Friedberg CK, Sohval AR: The occurrence and the pathogenesis of cardiac hypertrophy in Graves' disease. Am Heart J 13:599, 1937
668. Brauman A, Algom M, Gilboa Y, et al: Mitral valve prolapse in hyperthyroidism of two different origins. Br Heart J 53:374, 1985
669. Moliterno D, DeBold CR, Robertson RM: Case report: Coronary vasospasm—relation to the hyperthyroid state. Am J Med Sci 304:38, 1992
670. Hardisty CA, Naik DR, Munro DS: Pericardial effusion in hypothyroidism. Clin Endocrinol 13:349, 1980
671. Kelly JK, Butt JC: Fatal myxedema pericarditis in a Christian Scientist. Am J Clin Pathol 86:113, 1986
672. Santos AD, Miller RP, Puthenpurakal KM, et al: Echocardiographic characterization of the reversible cardiomyopathy of hypothyroidism. Am J Med 68:675, 1980
673. Marks AD, Channick BJ, Adlin EV, et al: Chronic thyroiditis and mitral valve prolapse. Ann Intern Med 102:479, 1985
674. Davies MJ, Pomerance A, Teare RD: Idiopathic giant cell myocarditis: A distinctive clinicopathological entity. Br Heart J 37:192, 1975
675. Murkin JM: Anesthesia and hypothyroidism: A review of thyroxine physiology, pharmacology, and anesthetic implications. Anesth Analg 61:371, 1982
676. Pierce GF, Jaffe AS: Increased creatine kinase MB in the absence of acute myocardial infarction. Clin Chem 32:2044, 1986
676a. Wladimiroff JW, Stewart PA, Reuss A, Sachs ES: Cardiac and

extra-cardiac anomalies as indicators for trisomies 13 and 18: A prenatal ultrasound study. Prenat Diagn 9:515, 1989

677. Baker SM, Hamilton JD: Capillary changes in myxedema. Lab Invest 6:218, 1957

678. Moerman P, Fryns J-P, van der Steen K, et al: The pathology of trisomy 13 syndrome: A study of 12 cases. Hum Genet 80:349, 1988

679. Musewe MN, Alexander DJ, Teshima I, et al: Echocardiographic evaluation of the spectrum of cardiac anomalies associated with trisomy 13 and trisomy 18. J Am Coll Cardiol 15:673, 1990

680. Roberts DJ, Genest D: Cardiac histologic pathology characteristic of trisomies 13 and 21. Hum Pathol 23:1130, 1992

681. van Praagh S, Truman T, Firpo A, et al: Cardiac malformations in trisomy-18: A study of 41 postmortem cases. J Am Coll Cardiol 13:1586, 1989

682. Tandon R, Edwards JE: Cardiac malformations associated with Down's syndrome. Circulation 47:1349, 1973

683. Clapp S, Perry BL, Farooki ZQ, et al: Down's syndrome, complete atrioventricular canal, and pulmonary vascular obstructive disease. J Thorac Cardiovasc Surg 100:115, 1990

684. Goldhaber SZ, Brown WD, St. John Sutton MG: High frequency of mitral valve prolapse and aortic regurgitation among asymptomatic adults with Down's syndrome. JAMA 258:1793, 1987

685. Zittergruen MM, Murray JC, Lauer RM, et al: Molecular analysis of nondisjunction in Down syndrome patients with and without atrioventricular septal defects. Circulation 92:2803, 1995

686. Kwiatkowski DJ, Short P: Tuberous sclerosis. Arch Dermatol 130:348, 1994

687. Menchine M, Emelin JK, Mischel PS, et al: Tissue and cell-type specific expression of the tuberous sclerosis gene, TSC2, in human tissues. Mod Pathol 9:1071, 1996

688. Mühler EG, Turniski-Harder V, Engelhardt W, von Bernuth G: Cardiac involvement in tuberous sclerosis. Br Heart J 72:584, 1994

689. Lie JT: Cardiac, pulmonary, and vascular involvement in tuberous sclerosis. Ann N Y Acad Sci 615:58, 1991

690. Saenger P: Turner's syndrome. N Engl J Med 335:1749, 1996

691. Gøtzsche C-O, Krag-Olsen B, Nielson J, et al: Prevalence of cardiovascular malformations and association with karyotypes in Turner's syndrome. Arch Dis Child 71:433, 1994

692. Natowicz M, Kelley RI: Association of Turner syndrome with hypoplastic left-heart syndrome. Am J Dis Child 141:218, 1987

693. Moore JW, Kirby WC, Rogers WM, Poth MA: Partial anomalous pulmonary venous drainage associated with 45,X Turner's syndrome. Pediatrics 86:273, 1990

694. Lin AE, Lippe BM, Geffner ME, et al: Aortic dilation, dissection, and rupture in patients with Turner syndrome. J Pediatr 109:820, 1986

695. Amann K, Ritz E: Cardiac structure and function in renal disease. Curr Opin Nephrol Hypertens 5:102, 1996

696. Lazarus JM, Lowrie EG, Hampers CL, Merrill JP: Cardiovascular disease in uremic patients on hemodialysis. Kidney Int Suppl 2:S167, 1975

697. Kooman JP, Daemen MJAP, Wijnen R, et al: Morphological changes of the venous system in uremic patients: A histopathologic study. Nephron 69:454, 1995

698. Feldman M: Southern Internal Medicine Conference: Whipple's disease. Am J Med Sci 291:56, 1986

699. Khairy P, Graham AF: Whipple's disease and the heart. Can J Cardiol 12:831, 1996

700. Keren DF: "Whipple's disease": The causative agent defined. Its pathogenesis remains obscure. Medicine (Baltimore) 72:355, 1993

701. Dobbins WO III: The diagnosis of Whipple's disease. N Engl J Med 332:390, 1995

702. Relman DA: The identification of uncultured microbial pathogens. J Infect Dis 168:1, 1993

703. McAllister HA Jr, Fenoglio JJ Jr: Cardiac involvement in Whipple's disease. Circulation 52:152, 1975

704. Southern JF, Moscicki RA, Magro C, et al: Lymphedema, lymphocytic myocarditis, and sarcoidlike granulomatosis: Manifestations of Whipple's disease. JAMA 261:1467, 1989

705. Rose AG: Mitral stenosis in Whipple's disease. Thorax 33:500, 1978

706. Bostwick DG, Bensch KG, Burke JS, et al: Whipple's disease presenting as aortic insufficiency. N Engl J Med 305:995, 1981

707. Ratliff NB, McMahon JT, Naab TJ, Cosgrove DM: Whipple's disease in the porcine leaflets of a Carpentier-Edwards prosthetic mitral valve. N Engl J Med 311:902, 1984

708. Beuren AJ: Supravalvular aortic stenosis: A complex syndrome with and without mental retardation. Birth Defects 8:45, 1972

709. Brewer CM, Morrison N, Tolmie JL: Clinical and molecular cytogenetic (FISH) diagnosis of Williams syndrome. Arch Dis Child 74:59, 1996

710. Jalal SM, Crifasi PA, Karnes PS, Michels VV: Cytogenetic testing for Williams syndrome. Mayo Clin Proc 71:67, 1996

711. Ottesen OE, Antia AU, Rowe RD: Peripheral vascular anomalies associated with the supravalvular aortic stenosis syndrome. Radiology 86:430, 1966

712. van Son JAM, Edwards WD, Danielson GK: Pathology of coronary arteries, myocardium, and great arteries in supravalvular aortic stenosis. J Thorac Cardiovasc Surg 108:21, 1994

713. Peterson TA, Todd DB, Edwards JE: Supravalvular aortic stenosis. J Thorac Cardiovasc Surg 50:734, 1965

714. O'Connor WN, Davis JB Jr, Geissler R, et al: Supravalvular aortic stenosis: Clinical and pathologic observations in six patients. Arch Pathol Lab Med 109:179, 1985

715. Brewer GJ, Yuzbasiyan-Gurkan V: Wilson disease. Medicine (Baltimore) 71:139, 1992

716. Yarze JC, Martin P, Muñoz J: Wilson's disease: Current status. Am J Med 92:643, 1992

717. Kuan P: Cardiac Wilson's disease. Chest 91:579, 1987

718. Factor SM, Cho S, Sternlieb I, et al: The cardiomyopathy of Wilson's disease. Virchows Arch [Path Anat] 397:301, 1982

Chapter 17

Adverse Effects of Drugs on the Cardiovascular System

William Lewis • Malcolm D. Silver

Each year, an increasing number of therapeutic agents are licensed for use; also, many patients receive a combination of medications in treatment. Thus, a clinician's awareness of the potentially adverse effects of drugs and their interactions must be acute. Although the exact incidence is not known, it is estimated that 2 to 5% of medical hospital admissions are occasioned by adverse drug reactions and that 15 to 40% of hospitalized patients experience at least one such reaction.[1, 2] Overall, they may be secondary to the following:

- Hypersensitivity
- Pharmacologic idiosyncrasy caused by genetic differences that affect an individual's ability to metabolize a drug[3]
- Direct toxicity
- Overdose
- Interactions between drugs

The effects so induced may mimic systemic disease or manifest organ-specific signs and symptoms.

The heart's function can be adversely affected by many external agents. For example, radiotherapy and both hyper- and hypothermia do so (see Chapter 18), as do the venoms of certain scorpions,[4–7] wasps,[8, 9] snakes,[10–13] and jellyfish[14] acting through one of several different pathogenic mechanisms. Electrolyte disturbances produce electrocardiographic abnormalities and left ventricular dysfunction, with some disturbances associated with cardiac arrest. Metastatic calcification affecting the myocardium is discussed in Chapter 16.

Many drugs cause functional abnormalities. For example, clinicians are aware that some drugs induce chest pain or exacerbate angina pectoris; some cause arrhythmias or heart block; some promote fluid retention, edema, and congestive heart failure; and some stimulate either hypo- or hypertension, making a detailed history of a patient's drug use mandatory. Pathologists, too, must be aware of these effects when making clinical-pathologic correlations. None of the agents mentioned earlier or the drugs that cause functional disturbances are discussed in this chapter. The reader is referred to other texts for that information.[15–17] The untoward effects of inborn errors of metabolism, glandular hyper- or hypofunction, or tumors are presented in Chapter 16; interstitial fibrosis related to cyclosporine therapy is discussed in Chapter 23. Thus, this chapter is not a comprehensive review of *all* agents that may affect the cardiovascular system adversely. Rather, it emphasizes therapeutic drugs whose detrimental effects induce morphologically observable changes, which are discussed under hypersensitivity reactions, toxic effects, vascular changes (including thrombosis induced by oral contraceptives), and heart valve fibrosis. A final section deals with the effects of substances of abuse. Because a drug may incite several reactions, some overlap occurs.

The unambiguous attribution of morphologic changes to a given drug and its characterization as an etiologic agent may be problematic. Some of this difficulty relates to distinguishing drug-induced structural changes from those caused by naturally occurring cardiovascular diseases. Moreover, initial knowledge of a drug reaction is often derived from retrospective analysis of clinical signs and symptoms, whereas morphologic observations may be included in a single case report. In this setting, morphologic changes may be assumed on the basis of these previous but not necessarily proved reports. In other words, the association between a drug and an adverse tissue reaction may be based on presumptive evidence. Proof of the relationship rests on the weight of accumulated evidence that a particular morphologic change is associated with a specific drug. Here, use of endomyocardial biopsy or other investigative tools helps to clarify the situation. When a series of fatal cases is available for autopsy study or altered tissue is consistently recovered in surgical pathology, an association between drug and injury may be simpler to forge.

Linking a putative agent to observed morphologic changes also requires that the suspect drug be eligible temporally, with linkage established by one of several methods, such as exclusion, dechallenge, rechallenge, singularity of the agent, pattern of injury, and quantitative determination of the drug. The method has been defined by Irey, although it is not applied rigorously, especially in case reports.[18] A definite causative relationship is established either by reproducing the tissue reaction in an experimental animal model or by rechallenging the patient. The latter may be used to document adverse reactions but has limited applicability and may be contraindicated both medically and ethically.

HYPERSENSITIVITY REACTIONS

Clinically, the criteria for diagnosing drug hypersensitivity reactions are as follows:[19]

- Previous use of a drug without incident
- No relationship between hypersensitivity and drug dosage
- Not caused by the pharmacologic or toxic effect of the drug

- Classic hypersensitivity symptoms, symptoms of serum sickness, or syndromes suggesting infectious disease
- Immunologic confirmation
- Persistence of symptoms until the drug is discontinued

Hypersensitivity Myocarditis

In hypersensitivity myocarditis and in toxic myocarditis (discussed later), one finds at endomyocardial biopsy or at autopsy histologic features in the myocardium that fit the current pathologic definition of myocarditis. As the authors of the Dallas criteria have indicated, pathologists already distinguish ischemic myocardial damage and histologic malignant infiltrates from other myocarditic lesions.[20] It is time to broaden this diagnostic differentiation. In toxic myocarditis, the definition may cast a net wider than consideration of mechanistic processes allows. The prime question is whether the observed myocarditic reaction is the result of an inflammatory reaction leading to cell death or the result of cell death producing an associated inflammatory reaction; either mechanism, although each has a different trigger, is capable of presenting a comparable histology. This topic is also discussed in Chapter 9. In our view *toxic myocarditis* is the result of cell death inducing an inflammatory reaction after release of cytosolic molecules. Nishiura and colleagues provide insight into a possible mechanism.[21] The authors observed that covalent dimerization of a ribosomal protein, S19, generates a molecule that binds to the C5a receptor of both neutrophils and monocytes. This protein dimer also acts as a competitive antagonist of C5a binding to neutrophils, but it is a chemotactic agonist for monocytes. The generation of S19 dimers, formed when cytoplasmic ribosomes are exposed to cellular or extracellular transglutaminases, has the capacity to change a skin infiltrate elicited by C5a injection from neutrophil-rich to monocyte-rich. We believe that the current pathologic definition of myocarditis as morphologic rather than mechanistic prompts confusion, which is mirrored in the literature. Because such lesions are obvious by endomyocardial biopsy, there must be greater clarity of thought in relating pathologic mechanisms and diagnosis to better define and guide the most appropriate therapy. Nevertheless, in the subsequent discussion, we use the terms *hypersensitivity* and *toxic myocarditis* based on the current pathologic definitions.

Hypersensitivity myocarditis is also discussed in Chapter 9. Its exact incidence is not known, although it may represent the most prevalent form of morphologically observable, drug-induced heart disease. Formerly, the diagnosis of hypersensitivity myocarditis was established primarily by retrospective analyses of autopsy material and rested on historical data from the patient; it was rarely diagnosed solely on clinical information.[22–25] Nowadays, a suspected diagnosis is readily established by endomyocardial biopsy and ancillary studies.

Etiology and Pathogenic Mechanisms

Data from clinical and autopsy studies implicate a variety of pharmacologic agents as causal agents. For example, penicillin and its congener, sulfonamides, and methyldopa are the most common.[19, 22–28] Table 17-1 lists

TABLE 17-1 • Drugs Associated With a Hypersensitivity Myocarditis

Acetazolamide*	Furosemide	
Amitriptyline*	Heparin	Penicillin*
Amphotericin B*	Hydralazine	Phenindione*
Ampicillin*	Hydrochlorothiazide*	Phenylbutazone*
Azathioprine	Indomethacin*	Phenytoin*
Bumetanide	Interleukin-2	Spironolactone*
Captopril	Isoniazid*	Streptomycin*
Carbamazepine*	Isorbide dinitrate	Sulfadiazine*
Cefazolin	Methyldopa*	Sulfisoxazole*
Chloramphenicol*	Metolazone	Sulfonylureas*
Chlorthalidone*	Nitroprusside	Tetracyclines*
Cyclosporin	Oxyphenbutazone*	Triazolam
Dobutamide	Para-aminosalicylic acid*	

* A frequent cause.
Tetanus toxoid is also associated with a hypersensitivity myocarditis.

some drugs that are associated with hypersensitivity myocarditis.

Hypersensitivity drug reactions are not mediated directly through the drug but through chemically reactive metabolites. The latter, now acting as haptens, combine with endogenous macromolecules, especially proteins, with that combination being antigenic. The protein carrier is able to interact with T lymphocytes, initiating an immune response. Once T cells are activated, hapten-specific activation is induced in B lymphocytes, and antihapten antibodies are formed. The antigen must have multiple combining sites that permit the formation of a bridge between antibody molecules, to elicit symptoms of hypersensitivity. This allows soluble antibody molecules to react with complement and release cytokines which damage the cell. Bridging between cell-bound antibody molecules or antigen receptors on lymphocytes produces changes in cell membrane conformation required for mediator release or lymphocyte transformation. The requirement that multivalent haptens initiate antihapten antibodies is one explanation for the relative infrequency of hypersensitivity drug reactions, because most drugs and drug metabolites are univalent haptens. They compete with multivalent haptens for antibody and thus inhibit the response. Organ-specific allergic reactions may also be explained by this theory. Conjugation of hapten with an organ-specific protein can produce an immunologic response with specificity for the protein as well as the haptenic group.

Pathology

The pathologic features of a hypersensitivity myocarditis are fairly typical, irrespective of the cause. Grossly, the heart in a fatal case resembles one that has an inflammatory myocarditis with cardiomegaly, biventricular dilation, and pallor. There is patchy subendocardial erythema or mottling. An associated pericarditis may be seen.

Histology is characterized by all lesions having a similar morphology, suggesting a comparable age. The interstitial inflammatory reaction may be focal or diffuse. It is often of mixed cell type and contains eosinophils, lymphocytes, and plasma cells (Fig. 17-1A). Eosinophils may predominate in this exudate, whereas in other instances, histiocytes are the major cell type. Focal myocytolysis is always present (Fig. 17-1B) but is often obscured by the interstitial inflammatory cell infiltrate. Foci of extensive

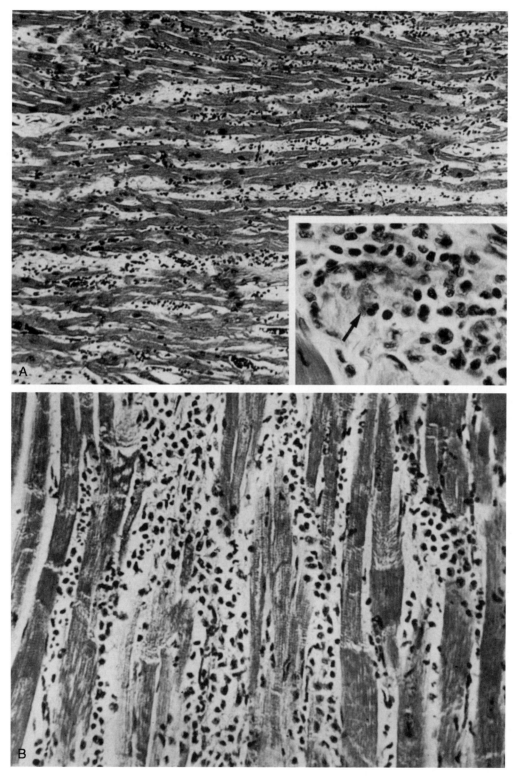

Figure 17-1 • *A,* Hypersensitivity myocarditis associated with penicillin. Inflammatory reaction is usually diffuse and interstitial, with separation of myocardial cells by edema. The inflammatory infiltrate (insert) is composed of lymphocytes, plasma cells, and prominent eosinophils (arrow). *B,* Hypersensitivity myocarditis associated with methyldopa. Foci of acute cell death are usually not observed, but contraction band necrosis and myocytolysis are always present. Extensive cellular necrosis is unusual. Foci of myocytolysis are usually most prominent in areas of extensive interstitial infiltrate. (Both H&E stain)

cellular necrosis are rare, which can help to distinguish hypersensitivity myocarditis from other types of myocarditis in which eosinophils predominate but extensive myocardial necrosis and replacement fibrosis are seen. Evidence of interstitial or replacement fibrosis is uniformly absent in hypersensitivity myocarditis. Nor are true granulomatous lesions a feature, although isolated giant cells, presumably derived from myocytes, are found occasionally. Rarely, the histology of a giant cell myocarditis results. Edema is frequently present. Vascular involvement is common in areas of extensive interstitial infiltrates and, like that found in drug-related vasculitis, has a bland histology. It affects small arteries, arterioles, and veins. Necrotizing vascular lesions are not associated with hypersensitivity myocarditis. (Fig. 9-11 also demonstrates a hypersensitivity myocarditis.)

The lack of extensive myocardial necrosis or interstitial fibrosis suggests that the drug-induced disease is self-limited. Once the offending agent is withdrawn, the myocarditis presumably resolves without serious residual cardiac damage. There are no reports of cardiac fibrosis or cardiomyopathy developing after drug-induced hypersensitivity myocarditis.

Hypersensitivity Myocarditis and Heart Transplantation

With the advent of heart transplantation, hypersensitivity myocarditis has become prevalent in a new clinical setting. In patients who underwent orthotopic heart transplantation, up to 22% of explanted hearts had histologic evidence of hypersensitivity myocarditis.[29-31] Although the responsible etiologic agents were not identified with certainty, the list of candidate agents included drugs commonly used in the aggressive treatment of congestive heart failure, hypertension and hypotension, and ischemic heart disease. Spear suggested that long-term intravenous dobutamine therapy may be responsible.[31] Alternatively, sodium nitrate used as a preservative in intravenous solutions may contribute pathogenetically to the myocarditis found in this unique population of patients. (See Chapter 23 also.)

Eosinophilia Myalgia Syndrome

Eosinophilia myalgia syndrome includes peripheral blood eosinophilia, generalized disabling myalgias, scleroderma-like skin manifestations, and arthralgias. In a series of 20 patients, one had myocarditis along with skeletal muscle changes. An endomyocardial biopsy in that case demonstrated lymphocytic myocarditis with focal necrosis and few eosinophils. Interstitial pneumonitis with eosinophils also was present.[32]

An epidemic of the syndrome occurred in New Mexico in 1989, affecting predominantly non-Hispanic white women,[33-35] 5 to 7% of whom developed pulmonary hypertension. An impurity in L-tryptophan taken as a nutritional supplement or therapuetic agent was believed to be the cause. The mechanism of injury was eosinophil activation and release of major basic protein and eosinophil-derived products into the extracellular space.

Lupus-like Syndromes

Syndromes indistinguishable from systemic lupus erythematosus (SLE) may appear after drug administration.[36] (See also Chapter 16.) They usually occur after months of therapy with large doses of a drug and affect only 1 to 2% of the population exposed to the agent. Most cases reverse completely within weeks to months of drug withdrawal.

Clinical Features

Unlike the situation in spontaneously occurring SLE, in which females are affected more often than males, in drug-associated SLE, the sexes are affected equally. This form of adverse reaction occurs among those who have so-called lupus diathesis, with patients exhibiting certain HLA and DR antigens of the major histocompatability complex—in the case of lupus, DR2, and DR3. Clinical complaints vary widely and include fever, skin lesions, and renal involvement, although the last is usually both less frequent and less severe than in spontaneouly occurring SLE. A high proportion of patients (75–100%) have antinuclear antibodies with a positive LE test. However, these antibodies may also be present in the absence of other signs of the disease, especially in individuals receiving procainamide.

Etiology and Pathogenic Mechanisms

Table 17-2 provides a list of drugs associated with lupus-like syndromes. The exact mechanism of their action is not known. The reaction may be a type 3 hypersensitivity, with the drug either modifying nucleoprotein antigenicity or reinforcing the antigenicity of circulating DNA normally present in small amounts with procainamide. The syndrome seems to occur more frequently and earlier in those who are "slow acetylators" of the drug, and the aromatic amine group in procainamide is important in inducing the syndrome.[37] The systemic injury is caused by deposition of autoantibodies in tissues, which triggers acute inflammation. The uncommon arteritis of major coronary arteries and the vasculitis of small coronary artery branches that induce a myocarditis-like histologic picture that is sometimes seen in spontaneously occuring SLE are not usually present when the syndrome is

TABLE 17-2 • **Drugs Associated With Lupus-like Syndromes**

Carbamazepine
Chlorpromazine
Diphenylhydantoin
D-penicillamine
Isoniazid
Mephenytoin
Methyldopa
Methylthiouracil
Para-aminosalicylate
Phenylbutazone
Procainamide
Propylthiouracil
Reserpine
Trimethadione

caused by a drug. The possibility of a type 2 hypersensitivity reaction having a role cannot be excluded, because cytotoxic antibodies develop against red and white blood cells and platelets.

TABLE 17-3 • **Drugs and Agents Associated With a Toxic Myocardial Damage**

Amphetamine	Doxorubicin (Adriamycin)
Amsacrine	Emetine hydrochloride
Anabolic steroids	Ethanol
Antimony compounds	5-fluorouracil
Antiviral agents (notably,	Interferon-alpha
antinitroural	Interleukin-2
mucilloid analogs)	Lead
Arsenicals	Lithium carbonate
Catecholamines	Mitomycin C
Chloroquine	Mitoxantrone
Cobalt	Phenothiazines
Cocaine	
Cyclophosphamide	
Daunorubicin (daunomycin)	

TOXIC EFFECTS

Etiology and Pathogenic Mechanisms

In addition to eliciting a hypersensitivity response, drugs may injure myocardial or other cells of the cardiovascular system by their direct toxic action. Table 17-3 lists drugs and agents known to have such effects.

The mechanisms of toxicity vary. For example, some drugs interfere with or inhibit cell metabolism, others block or alter cell transport, and still others induce hemodynamic alterations that prompt cell ischemia. Drug toxicity is dose related, and its effects are usually cumulative. The extent of cell damage depends on the toxicity of an individual drug, the total dose administered, and its absorption by a cell. The combination of these factors determines both the extent and the speed of cell death; therefore, drug toxicity produces a variable histologic picture and different clinical manifestations. For example, histologic findings may vary from acute cell death as the most prominent finding to cell death associated with an inflammatory reaction producing the morphology of a toxic myocarditis. Alternatively, if cellular damage or death

with loss of function has been subtle and insidious, the histologic findings may be those of a cardiomyopathy, usually a dilated type. Histologic findings may also evolve over the duration of the reaction after the onset of clinical symptoms. This must be remembered when endomyocardial biopsies are interpreted. Nevertheless, some individual drugs commonly produce only one pathologic or clinical presentation, whereas the toxicity of others induces more than one. Table 17-4 presents the main histologic effects of some of the drugs listed in Table 17-3. Clinical manifestation can vary too, from sudden death, to symptoms of an acute or chronic myocarditis that appear suddenly over a few days or evolve over weeks, to symptoms of a cardiomyopathy with progresssive and worsening congestive heart failure.

Histologic Presentations

Cell Death

Acute catecholamine-induced cardiovascular damage is a model. An excess of catecholamines may develop in the blood stream from endogenous sources, such as during stressful situations; in association with a functioning pheochromocytoma (see Chapter 8); or after a head injury (see Chapter 15).[38] Alternatively, the excess can arise from exogenous sources when these agents are used therapeutically. Catecholamines are present in many prescription and nonprescription medications commonly used for upper respiratory tract illnesses and other diseases.

Although specific sympathomimetic drugs vary in their action, there are two potential pathogenetic mechanisms by which they can induce cardiac injury: direct myocardial toxicity or effect on vascular tone. It is possible that constriction of large and small coronary arteries is a critical event. (See Chapter 8 for a contrary viewpoint.) Direct cardiac effects are determined largely by β_2-receptors, although β_2- and, to a lesser extent, α-receptors can be involved. β-receptor activation induces an increased calcium influx into cardiac cells, causing their hypercontraction. The potential role of catecholamines in various toxic and nontoxic heart muscle diseases has been explored on both theoretical and pathologic bases (see also Chapter 8).[38, 39]

The earliest myocardial lesions appear as subendocardial and intramyocardial hemorrhages found more fre-

TABLE 17-4 • **Drugs Having Toxic Effects on the Myocardium**

Associated With Myocardial Necrosis	Associated With Toxic Myocarditis	Associated With Cardiomyopathy
Catecholamines	Antimony compounds	Amphetamine
Interleukin-2	Arsenicals	Antiviral agents
	Catecholamines	Arsenicals
	Cyclophosphamide	Chloroquine
	Emetine hydrochloride	Cobalt
	Lithium carbonate	Doxorubicin
	Phenothiazines	Endogenous catecholamines
		Ephedrine
		Ethanol
		Lithium carbonate
		Mitomycin C

quently in the left ventricle. Histologically, catecholamine-induced lesions are similar, irrespective of the agonist used, its route of administration, or the species. For example, experimental studies in which isoproterenol hydrochloride was administered to many animals demonstrated cardiac myofilament fragmentation and contraction band necrosis. In humans, histopathologic features include intermyocyte hemorrhage, edema, and patchy (or more extensive) eosinophilic changes in myofibers, with granularity, focal myofibril degeneration, and prominent contraction bands. Ultrastructural correlates include hypercontraction of Z disks (contraction bands) and dilation of the sarcoplasmic reticulum (see Figs. 8-7 and 8-8). Mitochondrial changes are profound and include swelling, lysis, and calcification.[40, 41] Similar changes may occur in skeletal muscles.

With temporal evolution, this acute myocyte necrosis is followed by a mononuclear or, less fequently, a mixed inflammatory cell infiltrate, producing the histology of a toxic myocarditis. The reparative reaction involves lysis of cellular cortex with vacuolation of fibers; it finally produces small scars, which are the only late evidence of previous myocardial damage caused by catecholamines. At this stage, the finding is not specific. It has been postulated that repeated myocardial injury induced in this manner could produce sufficient myocardial fibrosis to affect cardiac function, and thus the term *stress cardiomyopathy* was coined.[42] Patients with a functioning pheochromocytoma have developed clinical manifestations of a cardiomyopathy that disappeared when the tumor was excised.[43]

Myocarditis

In this instance, arsenic poisoning provides a model. Gross examination of a heart with a toxic myocarditis often reveals chamber dilation without significant hypertrophy. The myocardium is usually pale and soft. Microscopically, the myocarditis is characterized by multifocal areas of cell death of different ages, accompanied by an extensive inflammatory infiltrate of lymphocytes, plasma cells, and polymorphonuclear leukocytes (Fig. 17-2A). Eosinophils are usually not a feature in this exudate but are present in rare cases, raising the possibility of a combined toxic and hypersensitivity effect. Coagulative necrosis may be present, suggesting ischemic changes. Healing areas of cell damage are marked by proliferating fibroblasts and a sparse infiltrate of macrophages (Fig. 17-2B), but patchy areas of fibrosis, indicating healed cellular damage, are uncommon in fatal cases or on endomyocardial biopsy (Fig. 17-2C). Frequently, there is moderate interstitial edema and a sparse, nonspecific, interstitial infiltrate of lymphocytes, plasma cells, and macrophages. The endocardium and heart valves are usually not affected. Endothelial damage and capillary microthrombosis may be prominent features, especially with cyclophosphamide cardiotoxicity (see later). Although microthrombosis is best appreciated by electron microscopy, small arterial thrombi are occasionally seen by light microscopy. Larger vessels are normal, and a true vasculitis is rarely present.

Mixed Cellular Reactions

Some cases of toxic myocarditis present mixed pathologic features. One case of severe, acute necrotizing eosinophilic myocarditis was reported as a manifestation of hypersensitivity myocarditis.[44] A possible toxic myocarditis may have been caused by hydroxychloroquine in this patient, who had SLE.

Table 17-5 provides some histologic pointers that may help to distinguish hypersensitivity from toxic myocarditis.

TABLE 17-5 • **Histologic Features That Help to Differentiate Hypersensitivity From Toxic Myocarditis**

Hypersensitivity Myocarditis	Toxic Myocarditis
Myocyte cell death presents as myolysis and may not be prominent	Myocyte death prominent; may mimic foci of myocardial infarction
Lesions of approximately comparable age	Areas of cell death of different age
Eosinophils likely a feature of mixed inflammatory exudate	Eosinophils usually not prominent in exudate, which may include polymorphonuclear leukocytes
Vascular involvement frequent, with features of hypersensitivity vasculitis	Endothelial damage and capillary microthrombi prominent in some instances of toxic myocarditis
Necrotizing vascular lesions not a feature	Large vessels usually normal, and true vasculitis rarely present
Interstitial or replacement fibrosis uniformly present	Healing marked by proliferating fibroblasts
	Healed cellular damage, marked by fibrosis, is not often seen in fatal cases or by endomyocardial biopsy

Cardiomyopathy

A patient with dilated cardiomyopathy has an enlarged heart and irreversible congestive heart failure (see Chapter 10). Drugs and substances of abuse can induce the condition through their toxic effects and produce nonspecific clinical and gross pathologic findings like those in dilated cardiomyopathy caused by many other agents. In one retrospective study, 6.5% of cases of dilated cardiomyopathy were attributed to the toxic effects of drugs.[45] In many insances, the pathogenetic mechanisms of the induced dilated cardiomyopathy are poorly understood, despite identification of the etiologic agent, pathologic features, and natural history of disease.

We now discuss in alphabetical order specific drugs associated with toxic myocardial injury.

Anthracyclines

In the past, antitumor agents were always associated with cardiotoxicity, but their use in clinical oncology raised awareness of this effect.[46, 47] The anthracyclines are a group of pigmented glycosidic antibiotics that possess potent antineoplastic activity. They are administered intra-

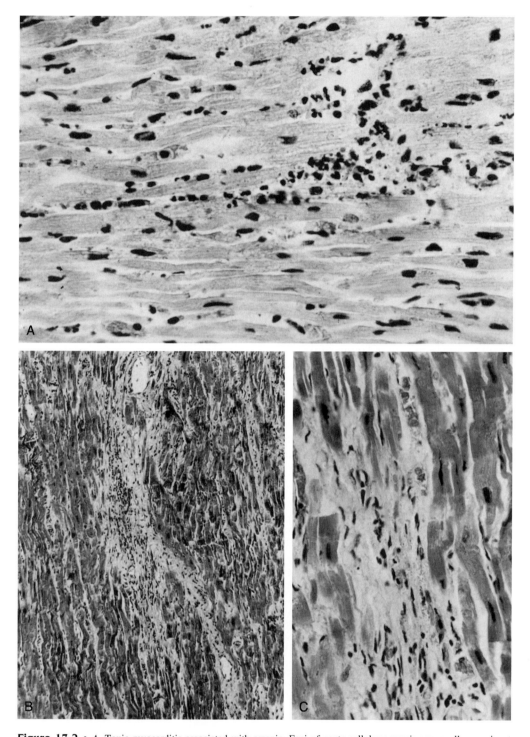

Figure 17-2 • *A,* Toxic myocarditis associated with arsenic. Foci of acute cellular necrosis are usually prominent and marked by an inflammatory infiltrate rich in polymorphonuclear leukocytes. *B,* Healing areas of myocardial damage imply chronicity. Note interstitial inflammatory infiltrate. *C,* Proliferation of fibroblasts and capillaries and scattered mononuclear cells and macrophages. (H&E stain)

venously and intercalate into DNA, interfering with both DNA and RNA synthesis and DNA strand scission through effects on topoisomerase II. They also bind to cell membranes, altering fluidity and ion transport and generate semiquinone free radicals and oxygen radicals through an enzyme-mediated reductive process. The two most common congeners, doxorubicin (Adriamycin) and

daunorubicin (Daunomycin), are used to treat solid tumors, leukemias, and lymphomas.

Clinical Features

Shan and colleagues described three distinct clinical types of anthracycline-induced cardiotoxicity.[48] First, up to 11% of patients developed acute cardiovascular effects within days of drug administration. They consisted of electrocardiographic changes, including sinus tachycardia, ST segment depression, T wave flattening, and premature atrial and ventricular contractions.[49] Left ventricular dysfunction and contractile abnormalities have also been reported but are usually transient and reverse after therapy is discontinued.[50, 51] Myocytes may show marked cytoplasmic vacuolation (Fig. 17-3). Clinically, it has not been determined that these acute changes are related to the dilated cardiomyopathy observed with long-term drug administration.[52, 53] A second form of anthracycline cardiotoxicity evolved with the aggressive treatment of neoplasms in pediatric and adult patients. This late-onset (delayed) toxicity was identified in children who were treated for malignancies and in women who survived breast cancer. Clinical features varied from minor abnormalities on echocardiogram to ventricular dysfunction and arrhythmias manifesting years after anthracycline treatment in breast cancer patients.[48] Irradiation appeared to increase the risk for myocardial damage. The delayed onset was a discriminator of this toxicity. Third, the dilated cardiomyopathy associated with doxorubicin therapy was cumulative, dose dependent, irreversible, and progressive, leading to congestive heart failure and death. Clinical manifestations included congestive heart failure with sinus tachycardia, tachypnea, cardiomegaly, peripheral and pulmonary edema, hepatomegaly, venous congestion, and pleural effusion.[52, 54] In initial clinical trials, the drug did not reveal significant evidence of cardiac toxic-

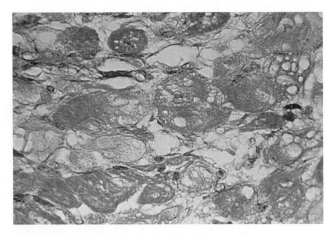

Figure 17-3 • Acute myocardial changes after Adriamycin therapy. Note myocyte vacuolation. (Verhoeff elastic stain) (Courtesy of F.J. Schoen, MD.)

ity. In fact, the cardiomyopathy may develop after the last drug administration.[54]

The overall incidence of severe congestive heart failure with anthracycline toxicity is between 2 and 3%.[49, 54, 55] Once apparent pathologic changes are evident, mortality may be as high as 70%.[49, 54]

Pathology

The pathologic features of the dilated cardiomyopathy induced in humans by doxorubicin treatment are similar to

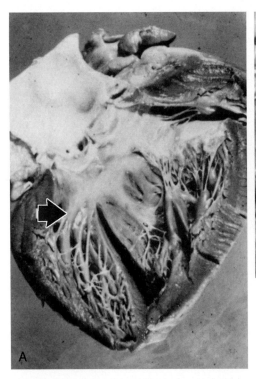

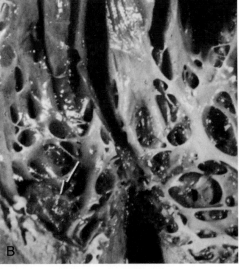

Figure 17-4 • *A,* Adriamycin-related dilated cardiomyopathy with dilated left ventricular chamber. The wall is not thickened, despite the heart's weight of 750 g. Mitral and aortic valves are normal, but endocardial sclerosis is obvious, especially in the outflow region (arrow). *B,* Mural thrombus formation between prominent trabeculae in the right ventricle. This type of formulation can be present in any cardiac chamber.

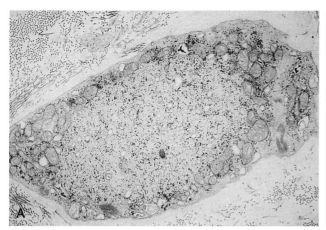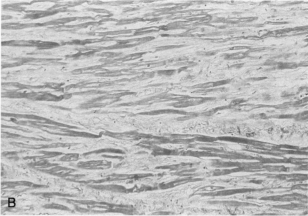

Figure 17-5 • *A*, Electron micrograph of Adria cell. *B*, Late-stage Adriamycin cardiomyopathy showing interstitial fibrosis. (H&E stain.) (*A*, Courtesy of J. Butany, M.D. *B*, Courtesy of F.J. Schoen, MD.)

those found in most species studied experimentally.[56, 57] Gross examination in patients reveals an enlarged, pale, flabby heart with ventricular dilation and hypertrophy (Fig. 17-4*A*). Mural thrombi are frequently present (Fig. 17-4*B*).[58] These changes are indistinguishable from those found in dilated cardiomyopathies from other causes.

Light microscopic and ultrastructural examination of the myocardium reveals focal and disseminated degeneration of cardiac myocytes characterized by myofibrillar loss and myocyte dropout, with or without marked cytoplasmic vacuolation (see Fig. 17-3).[56, 58] An early ultrastructural manifestation includes distention of the sarcoplasmic reticulum. It eventually swells and coalesces to form large membrane-bound clear spaces in the myocyte cytoplasm, producing the so-called Adria cell.[56] These lesions progress to ultrastructural features that include loss of some mitochondria and swelling of others with cristolysis, the presence of myelin figures and dense bodies, focal membrane thickening, myofibrillar loss, Z band remnants, and, finally, myocyte death[48, 57] (Fig. 17-5*A*). Nuclear and nucleolar changes have been described by some investigators and include clumped chromatin and nucleolar alterations,[59] with these changes obvious after a single injection of the drug. Such myocardial cell alterations have been noted to some degree not just at necropsy but in virtually all patients treated with doses of 240 mg/m² or greater.[56] There is a relative increase in interstitial connective tissue (Fig. 17-5*B*).[50] An inflammatory reaction, even in necrotic areas, is usually minimal or absent.[56]

These pathologic features have been analyzed semiquantitatively by a grading system that helps to determine the extent of cardiac myocyte damage and provides a prognostic indicator of the therapeutic limits to anthracycline cumulative dose.[56] The endomyocardial biopsy has added immeasurably to the effectiveness of clinical care in patients receiving anthracyclines.[56] Biopsy findings lead clinicians to modify its use and arrest or attenuate adverse effects before they become clinically obvious. Endomyocardial biopsy with histopathologic and ultrastructural findings is used for comparison studies when newer anthracycline antineoplastics are used.[60]

Factors That Affect the Risk of Doxorubicin Cardiomyopathy

An increased frequency of dilated cardiomyopathy resulting from anthracyclines occurs with cumulative doses above 550 mg/m². However, symptomatic congestive heart failure may develop in patients at lower cumulative doses when other risk factors are present. For example, it is believed that preexistent coronary artery disease, hypertention, or myocardial disease; extremes of age; high cumulative or peak serum levels of doxorubicin; and mediastinal radiation and coexistent chemotherapy with dactinomycin, dacarbazine, cyclophosphamide, or mitomycin can all increase the risk of cardiotoxicity.[48–50, 54, 55, 61] This suggests caution in administering doxorubicin to patients who are also receiving the other drugs.[62] In a dose-matched study, doxorubicin's effect was enhanced by previous mediastinal radiotherapy of varying doses and durations compared with biopsy findings in patients without that therapy.[61]

Mechanism of Cardiotoxicity

Doxorubicin and daunorubicin are the best-studied members of the anthracycline family, yet the mechanism of their cardiotoxicity is obscure.[63, 64] The free radical hypothesis is the one that has been most thoroughly investigated. As indicated earlier, anthracyclines generate free radicals and compromise the heart's ability to protect itself against the resulting injury by depleting glutathione or reducing glutathione peroxidase activity. Alternatively, free radical cardiac dysfunction may occur by affecting the sarcoplasmic reticulum and relate to alterations in release or sequestration of calcium. Mitochondrial injury may occur. Free radical scavengers such as vitamin E and *N*-acetylcysteine should decrease the severity of the cardiomyopathy and attenuate myocardial functional changes. However, although the free radical hypothesis is attractive, numerous experiments suggest that neither protection with antioxidants nor exacerbation can be uniformly created experimentally.

Calcium overload is associated with anthracycline treatment, but its causal relationship to cardiomyopathy is not certain. Mechanistically, excessive levels of intracellular calcium may occur. These levels could induce mitochondrial dysfunction and deplete adenosine triphosphate and creatine phosphate, with resulting contractile dysfunction and myocyte death.

Other suggested mechanisms of injury include (1) interference with the sarcolemmic sodium-potassium pump or with electron transplant in mitrochondria; (2) prostaglandin-induced damage, although direct evidence for cardiac injury resulting from products of arachidonic acid metabolism is not available; (3) histamine-induced cardiotoxicity, possibly involving free radical–mediated mechanisms (an attractive hypothesis, but clinical correlates are lacking); and (4) a direct effect on the expression of specific cardiac proteins, but these changes are likely secondary. Additionally, many metabolites of the anthracyclines could contribute to the dilated cardiomyopathy.

Antiviral Agents

Dilated cardiomyopathy is a complication of acquired immunodeficiency syndrome (AIDS).[65–67] (See Chapter 9 also.) Postulated causes include a direct human immunodeficiency virus (HIV)–1 infection of the heart (with or without myocarditis); the toxicity of therapeutic agents, particularly zidovudine (AZT) and related reverse transcriptase inhibitors; the effects of circulating or systemic toxins or cytokines; cardiac opportunistic infections; the toxicity of illicit or self-prescribed pharmaceuticals or home remedies; and nutritional disorders.[68, 69]

D'Amati and colleagues examined pathologic features of four cases of dilated cardiomyopathy associated with AZT treatment.[70] All patients had a documented HIV-1 infection, long-term AZT therapy, and intractable congestive cardiac failure. In each instance, myocarditis was absent. However, mitochondrial degeneration was present, with the organelles being swollen and showing vacuolation, fragmentation, and loss of cristae. Despite differences in patient ages and behavioral risk factors for AIDS, all four showed these pathologic changes in cardiac mitochondria.[70]

Clinical and experimental evidence links an altered mtDNA replication in various tissues to the mitochondrial toxicity of antiviral nucleoside agents in AIDS and other chronic viral infections such as hepatitis B.[71–76] However, controversy prevails regarding the prevalence and overall clinical impact of such toxicities. ATZ, zalcitabine (DDC), didanosine (DDI), and stavudine (d4T) provide models of mitochondrial DNA polymerase-*y* inhibition.[77, 78] This enzyme replicates mitochondrial DNA. Some of these agents have been implicated in causing a clinical dilated cardiomyopathy.

Other agents, such as fialuridine (FIAU), 1-2-deoxy-2-fluoro-B-D-arabinofuranosyl-5-iodouridine, and 3-TC, which showed promise in treating AIDS-related viral infections, proved extremely toxic to the liver, skeletal and cardiac muscle, and peripheral nerve tissues. Recently, fluorodideoxyadenosine has been used in clinical trials. Preclinical data in rats suggest that it has potentially acute cardiotoxicity, producing myocyte necrosis.

The DNA *poly* hypothesis is the pharmacologic theory that helps to explain the pathogenesis and pathophysiology of dilated cardiomyopathy induced by antiviral nucleoside agents. It is based on alterations of mitochondrial DNA replication occurring in target tissues.[79]

Arsenic

Accidental arsenic poisoning may be acute or chronic.[80] It is a problem in children. Frequently, the element is found at the workplace in metallurgy, textile, tanning, glass, and paint manufacture. It is also a component of various pesticides.

Grossly, the heart is not enlarged in this toxic myocarditis, which may develop with acute or chronic poisoning. Microscopically, perinuclear vacuolation of cardiac myocytes is found. Infiltrates of mixed inflammatory cells, including erythrocytes and polymorphonuclear leukocytes, and edema are present. They are often prevascular (see Fig. 17-2). Arsenic may act mechanistically through the inhibition of oxidative phosphorylation in cardiac mitochondria.

Cobalt

Dilated cardiomyopathy from cobalt exposure is uncommon in the general population; however, industrial exposure puts certain populations at risk.[81] Dilated cardiomyopathy among heavy beer drinkers was observed in Quebec City, Canada; Omaha, Nebraska; and Louvain, Belgium.[82] In each instance, it was related to the use of cobalt sulfate as an antifoaming agent. The "epidemics" disappeared when cobalt was removed from beer processing. Nevertheless, in these cases, the adverse reaction may have been an interactive one, because affected individuals also had thiamine and protein deficiencies, which enhance cobalt toxicity. Ethanol also produces sensitivity to cobalt toxicity.

Pathology

Pathologic changes included cardiomegaly and a flabby heart. Punctate hemorrhages of the epicardium were present. Focal acutely necrotic myocytes were surrounded by histiocytes. Interstitial fibrosis was common. Ultrastructural changes included myofilament loss, lysosomal accumulation, and mitochondrial changes, including matrix lysis.[81] Cobalt also induced a diffuse thyroid hypoplasia. This finding gave Quebec City pathologists a clue about the cause of the cardiomyopathy.

Chloroquine

Chloroquine and its congeners are effective agents in treating malaria and some immunologic and rheumatologic illnesses such as sarcoidosis and rheumatoid arthritis. Known side effects are relatively uncommon. They include retinopathy, skeletal myopathy, and neuromyopathy.[83] Both acute and chronic toxic effects on the heart have been reported.[84–86] The former include hypotension; conduction disturbances, including complete heart block; myocardial hypertrophy; and myocardial insufficiency.

Long-term therapy with chloroquine results in changes in patients' hearts, including cardiomegaly with ventricular enlargement.

Pathology

Grossly, myocardial fibrosis is absent, but the heart is said to cut with a gritty sensation. Microscopic examination reveals dark, hypertrophied, and vacuolated myocytes that exhibit positive staining with the periodic acid Schiff technique. Fine interstitial sclerosis is present. Ultrastructurally, myocytes contain accumulated lipid droplets with lamellae and membrane-enclosed aggregates that resemble curvilinear bodies present in distended lysosomes, with myelin figures and large secondary lysosomes. Glycogen granules may be found. In some cases, related changes are present in skeletal muscle samples.

Other antimalarial agents may also have cardiovascular side effects that could lead to dilated cardiomyopathy. In Southeast Asia, treatment with halofantrine induced consistent, dose-related increases in the PR and QT intervals that affected all treated patients.[87]

Cyclophosphamide

The alkylating agent cyclophosphamide, used for both immunosuppression and chemotherapy, can induce cardiomyopathy. In a study of patients undergoing bone marrow transplantation, 17% had signs and symptoms of cyclophosphamide cardiotoxicity within 10 days after initiation of therapy, and nearly half died with congestive heart failure. If the drug dosage exceeded 1.55 g/m per day, 25% of patients were affected. This group was older than those who had no apparent cardiac injury clinically. Cardiotoxicity was not fatal when it occurred in children, and adults who recovered exhibited no residual cardiac abnormalities.

Clinically, this drug's toxic effect is acute in onset and not the result of cumulative dosage. It is marked by diffuse voltage loss, cardiomegaly, pulmonary vascular congestion and pleural effusions, decreased fractional ventricular wall shortening, increased end-diastolic volume, and pericardial effusions.

The adverse effects of high doses of cyclophosphamide appear secondary to capillary endothelial damage.[88, 89] This leads to fibrin deposition, interstitial edema, blood extravasation, and foci of necrosis in the adjacent myocardium, characterized structurally by extensive contraction bands, myofibrillar lysis, and electron-dense intramitochondrial inclusions. These lesions heal by fibrosis. The drug may also cause a fibrinous pericarditis. Transmission electron microscopy reveals widespread myocardial necrosis and microvascular fibrin thrombi. In earlier reports, combined chemotherapy was used with cyclophosphamide, 6-thioguanine, bis-chloroethyl-nitrosourea, or 5-azacitidine.[88] Buja and colleagues indicated that such drug combinations could alter the nature of pathologic findings.[89]

Emetine

Emetine hydrochoride is employed to treat amebiasis. Toxic effects are usually associated with long-term use of the drug and are rarely fatal. It induces a toxic myocarditis (Fig. 17-6). The agent inhibits oxidative phosphorylation.[90] Structurally, the anatomic targets of its toxicity

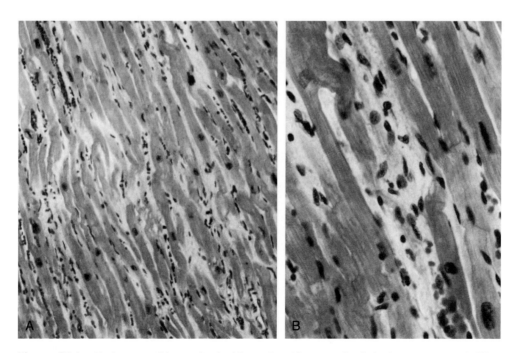

Figure 17-6 • Toxic myocarditis associated with emetine. All stages of cell death are present, and diffuse interstitial inflammation is usually prominent. *A,* Areas of recent cell damage are characterized by focal loss of myocytes and myocytolysis. *B,* Higher power shows areas of myocyte loss with cellular infiltrate consisting of lymphocytes, macrophages, and polymorphonuclear leukocytes. (H&E stain.)

are cardiac mitochondria. Pathologic features after 10 days of therapy include severe mitochondrial distortion with swelling and dissolution of cristae, leading to widespread cell death.[91]

Morphologically, there are similarities to the changes found in the cardiotoxicity resulting from antiretroviral agents. Accompanying clinical and electrophysiologic changes include nonspecific electrocardiographic changes and an absence of any effect on right- or left-sided heart pressures.

5-Fluorouracil

Although the point is controversial, 5-fluorouracil is believed to cause severe left ventricle dysfunction and reversible cardiogenic shock by inducing vaso-occlusive problems.[92] Acute myocardial infarction may develop. There is controversy because this agent is often used in combination with other antineoplastic drugs, making exact attribution difficult. Ischemic myocardial complications have also been reported after treatment with cisplatinum, bleomycin, and vinca alkaloids, with comparable reservations. Paclitaxel has been noted to cause arrhythmias and, possibly, ischemia.[93]

Interleukin-2

A relatively recent addition to the causes of toxic myocarditis is interleukin-2 therapy.[94–97] Although death from its administration is relatively rare, eight patients who received it died of cardiopulmonary causes within 4 days of its initiation. Noninfectious myocarditis was present in five autopsy heart samples. One additional case showed an eosinophilic myocarditis, perhaps indicating a hypersensitivity reaction secondary to this therapy.[98] The pathogenetic mechanism is obscure and may be related to decreased contractility through an altered adrenergic response of the heart, illustrated by the interaction of interleukin-1 and myocytes.[99, 100] Both interleukin-1 and -2 can induce a diffuse capillary leak syndrome, with resultant myocardial infarction.

Psychotropic Drugs

Several reports link acute cardiovascular changes with the administration of psychotropic drugs.[101] Echocardiographic changes have been reported in patients receiving imipramine or amitriptyline.[102] A group of patients who received the tricyclic antidepressant amitriptyline had an increased rate of sudden death.[102]

Acute poisoning with thioridazine and imipramine leads to arrhythmic death. Cardiac changes observed in individuals taking phenothiazines long term include electrocardiographic abnormalities and myocardial ultrastructural changes of increased lipochrome pigment, clusters of misshapen mitochondria, and dilated sarcoplasmic reticulum. Lithium also produces adverse cardiac effects.[103, 104] Lithium therapy is associated with ventricular arrhythmia and myocarditis. However, the latter association is considered tenuous because of intercurrent illnesses that could influence the observed changes.

VASCULAR CHANGES INDUCED BY DRUGS

Vascular changes may manifest as the main pathology causing a patient's symptoms or be part of the overall adverse response to an agent. Drugs can induce vascular spasm, hypersensitivity, non-necrotizing vasculitis, necrotizing vasculitis, endothelial damage with thrombosis, vascular thrombosis, or proliferative changes in the vessel wall. Any vascular change may promote intraluminal thrombus formation, aggravating distal effects.

Hypersensitivity Vasculitis

Drug hypersensitivity may account for approximately 10% of all cases of vasculitis, with most drug-related vasculitides being non-necrotizing and secondary to delayed hypersensitivity. The topic of hypersensitivity vasculitis is discussed in Chapter 6.

Here, we emphasize the following points: (1) Drug-induced hypersensitivity vasculitis is not dependent on dose and may occur at any time a drug is being administered. (2) Affected patients develop either a localized skin reaction without other clinical signs or symptoms or a systemic vasculitis, often with skin involvement. In the latter group, clinical findings may be confusing owing to specific organ involvement. Skin rash and eosinophilia are the most reliable clinical clues to the possibility of a systemic drug-related vasculitis, irrespective of the organs involved. (3) In this condition, drug history, clinical findings, and laboratory results, such as positive serologic tests, are important. (4) The diagnosis should not be made solely on the basis of morphologic findings. Nevertheless, the presence of a bland vasculitis (usually in a skin biopsy, although other organs such as heart, liver, and kidney may be affected) marked by a mainly mononuclear cell infiltrate with prominent eosinophils and rare polymorphonuclear leukocytes that affects arterioles, capillaries, venules, small veins, and occasional small arteries (if not affecting muscular or elastic arteries and larger veins), all in the absence of necrotizing vascular lesions, strongly suggests a drug-related hypersensitivity vasculitis (Fig. 17-7). The inflammatory infiltrate involves all tunics in the full thickness of the affected vessel.

Table 17-6 lists drugs that are associated with hypersensitivity vasculitis. Many also induce hypersensitivity myocarditis.

Toxic Vasculitis

This produces a necrotizing vasculitis that may be indistinguishable from classic panarteritis nodosa (see Chapter 6). As in that condition, medium and small arteries are usually affected, with capillaries, arterioles, and veins spared. Lesions are most often observed at vessel bifurcations and may be acute, healing, or healed. Acute lesions manifest fibrinoid necrosis affecting the full thickness of the wall, often in an arc of its circumference, with the associated inflammatory reaction comprised mainly of polymorphonuclear leukocytes, although eosinophils occasionally predominate. Older lesions show focal scarring of

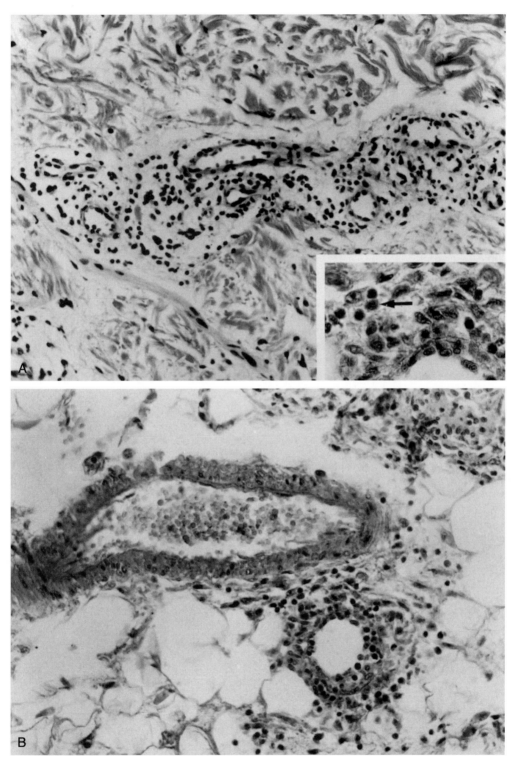

Figure 17-7 • *A,* Hypersensitivity vasculitis associated with ampicillin. The skin is a common site for vascular involvement in hypersensitivity drug reactions. The inflammatory infiltrate rings small vessels and extends through the vessel wall. Capillaries, arterioles, and small veins are all involved. The infiltrate (inset) consists of mononuclear cells and prominent eosinophils (arrow). *B,* Hypersensitivity vasculitis associated with allopurinol. Large vessels, arteries, and veins are characteristically spared in hypersensitivity vasculitis. The arteriole, adjacent to the larger vein, is involved, whereas the vein is spared. The inflammatory infiltrate extends through the entire thickness of the arteriole wall. (H&E stain.)

TABLE 17-6 • **Drugs Associated With Non-necrotizing Hypersensitivity Vasculitis**

Allopurinol	Indomethacin
Ampicillin	Isoniazid
Bromide	Levamisole
Carbamazepine	Methylthiouracil
Chloramphenicol	Oxyphenbutazone
Chlorothiazide	Penicillin
Chlorpropamide	Phenylbutazone
Chlortetracycline	Potassium iodine
Chlorthalidone	Procainamide
Colchicine	Propylthiouracil
Cromolyn sodium	Quinidine
Dextran	Spironolactone
Diphenhydramine	Sulfonamide
Diphenylhydantoin	Tetracycline
Griseofulvin	Trimethadione

the media, adventitial fibrosis, and marked intimal proliferation with luminal narrowing. Occlusive thrombi may be found in both acute and healing phases. In many instances, there is aneurysmal dilation of the affected area of the vessel wall. Only a few drugs are associated with necrotizing vasculitis (Table 17-7). The cause of this form of drug-related vasculitis is unclear. Precipitated drug, a foreign material, is occasionally found in the vessel wall in areas of necrosis. In these instances, a direct toxic effect is likely. However, in serum sickness, similar necrotizing vascular lesions can develop. In this circumstance, its cause appears to be an immediate hypersensitivity reaction.

Vascular Proliferative Conditions

Appetite Suppressant Agents

Aminorex

In the late 1960s and early 1970s, an outbreak of pulmonary hypertension in Western Europe resulted from use of the anorectic agent aminorex fumarate.[105, 106] Two percent of individuals taking the drug were affected, suggesting a genetic predisposition, and women were affected four times more often than men. Patients developed intimal proliferation in small muscular pulmonary arteries. The pulmonary hypertension often progressed after treatment ceased, but in other patients it regressed over many years. The drug was withdrawn from the market in 1972 (see also Chapter 7).

Fenfluramines

As Fishman[107] points out, the fenfluramines, like aminorex, are congeners of amphetamines and are related to phenylethylamines. They were used as appetite suppres-

TABLE 17-7 • **Drugs Associated With Necrotizing Vasculitis**

Arsenic
Bismuth
Gold
Methamphetamine
Sulfonamides

sants, with dexfenfluramine preferred. It induces increased serotoninergic activity by stimulating serotonin release from cellular stores, notably nerve endings and platelets; inhibits serotonin uptake from presynaptic neurons; and directly stimulates presynaptic serotonin receptors. The drug is metabolized to dexnorfenfluramine, which also releases serotonin into synapses and activates serotonin $5H_2$. Serotonin is an intense pulmonary vasoconstrictor that stimulates vascular smooth muscle proliferation by interacting synergistically with platelet-derived growth factor. Vessels draining the site of an actively secreting intestinal carcinoid often show intimal proliferation. The 1996 report of the International Primary Pulmonary Hypertension study related use of fenfluramine and its congener dexfenfluramine with cases of pulmonary hypertension.[108]

Fenfluramine/Phentermine

Weintraub and colleagues reported that the anorexigenic effects of fenfluramine could be duplicated and its side effects minimized if it were given in smaller doses combined with phentermine, an amphetamine-like agent.[109] Isolated reports of pulmonary hypertension had been reported when fenfluramine or phentermine alone was used.[110] Five of the 24 patients reported with valvular lesions following combined fenfluramine/phentermine (fen/phen) treatment developed pulmonary hypertension.[111] In this instance, the hypertension was attributed to a direct toxic effect of serotonin on small muscular arteries and arterioles in the lung and on the secondary hemodynamic effects of associated valvular insufficiency. Here, with combined drug therapy the need to satisfy Irey's postulates[18] is paramount in linking a drug or combination of drugs to pathological findings. Nevertheless, the combined therapy was withdrawn from the market in 1997. Experimental studies seeking mechanisms have been reported.[111a–c] It is noted that phentermine also induces phospholipidosis.

Ergot and Methysergide

Intimal fibroplasia and fibromuscular hyperplasia were also reported in association with ergotamine and methysergide therapy[112, 113] (Fig. 17-8). In patients treated with these agents, the intima was thickened by a proliferation of myofibroblasts in a loose myxomatous tissue. The internal elastic lamina was focally disrupted, but the media was not thickened. The adventitia also thickened. These vascular lesions were focal, with only selective vascular involvement. The intimal thickening produced focal luminal narrowing and symptoms of ischemic disease in distal organs.

Oral Contraceptives and Vascular Thrombosis

The introduction of oral contraceptives was thought to provide an ideal method of birth control. However, by the late 1960s, reports of cardiovascular complications began to appear. Premenopausal women taking high-dose estrogen oral contraceptives had an increased risk of hypertension, venous thromboembolism, stroke, and myocardial infarction. Connell noted that hypertension contributed to the morbidity and mortality resulting from stroke, myo-

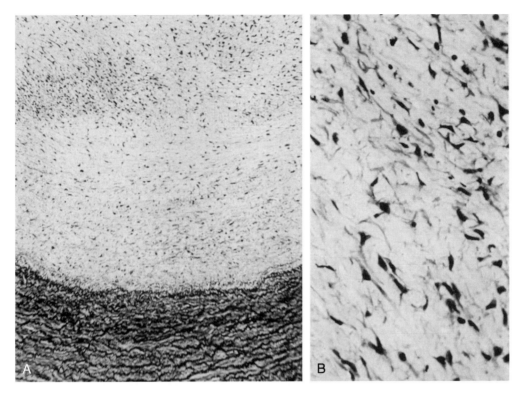

Figure 17-8 • *A* and *B,* Intimal fibroplasia of the common carotid artery associated with methysergide therapy. This process is focal, and the vessel lumen is usually compromised. *B,* At higher power the thickened intima is composed of fibroblasts and prominent myointimal cells in a matrix of glycosamine glycans. The myointimal cells are branching and contain abundant myofilaments, similar to smooth muscle cells, although they lack a well-defined basement membrane. (H&E stain.)

cardial infarction, and both cardiac and renal failure; the risk of a previously normal woman developing venous thromboembolism was increased, but the absolute risks varied considerably; the risk of stroke was greater, with that risk continuing after discontinuance; and there was an association between pill use and coronary heart disease, but heart attacks occurred mainly in women who had additional risk factors such as increasing age and smoking.[114]

Meanwhile, to overcome the risk of thrombotic disease, second-generation pills containing low-dose estrogens were succeeded by third-generation types containing the progestins desogestrel, gestodene, or norgestimate. Although the debate on oral contraceptives and thrombotic disease continues,[115, 116] second-generation oral contraceptives seem to confer a smaller increased risk of venous thrombosis and a higher risk of arterial thrombosis than third-generation pills. What is clear is that women with inherited or acquired thrombophilia have a greater risk for venous thromboembolism when they use either second- or third-generation oral contraceptives, because of the drugs' potential to activate clotting factors.[115, 117, 118]

HEART VALVE FIBROSIS

Carcinoid Heart Disease

Patients with carcinoid intestinal tumors and metastatic lesions in the liver may develop plaque-like deposits on the endocardium and right-sided heart valves. Much less often, left-sided heart valve lesions are seen if such a patient has a right or left heart shunt or if a patient has a pulmonary carcinoid (see Chapter 13 for further discussion). Here, an excess production of serotonin and other biologically active agents is the likely pathogenic mechanism.

Ergot and Methysergide

Ergot alkaloids are produced by *Claviceps purpurea,* a fungus that infects grains, especially rye, under damp growing or storage conditions. Epidemics of ergot poisoning caused by accidental ingestion can be traced back more than 2000 years.[119] The alkaloids act on several types of receptors. Their effects include agonist, partial agonist, and antagonist actions against α-adrenoreceptors and serotonin receptors and agonist action at central nervous system dopamine receptors.[16] Ergot derivatives, including methysergide, a derivative of the amine subgroup, are used to treat migraine. An uncommon side effect is a fibrotic disease of vessels and connective tissue deposition on cardiac valves. The latter leads to valve stenosis or incompetence (see Chapter 13 and Fig. 13-18*A*). Not all patients treated with the drug develop this valvular change, suggesting that there is a genetic predisposition. The lesion can regress if methysergide treatment ceases. Similar lesions are produced by ergot.

Fenfluramine/Phentermine

The similarity in pathology of valvular lesions seen in carcinoid heart disease, after methysergide therapy,[120] and associated with fen/phen is remarkable. (Fig. 13-18B demonstrates mitral valve lesions after fen/phen therapy.) However, the pathogenic mechanism is obscure and, as indicated earlier, with combined drug therapy the particular role of each drug and of any combined effect needs clarification. It is suggested that a common mechanism, possibly related to that of the vascular fibrotic lesion described earlier, prevails. Two mechanisms have been postulated to operate in most of these fibrotic syndromes: (1) an inherited susceptibility that predisposes individuals to vasoconstriction and obliterative lesions confined predominantly to the pulmonary precapillary muscular arteries and arterioles, and (2) either a direct action on the right heart endocardium and valves (and on left-sided valves when their fibrosis is associated with a shunt or a pulmonary carcinoid) or an impaired clearance of biologically active substances such as serotonin and other agents by the lungs, enabling toxic concentrations to reach and damage left-sided heart valves and some larger vessels. Fitzgerald and colleagues report an experimental study seeking mechanisms.[121a]

EFFECTS OF SUBSTANCES OF ABUSE

Ethanol

Acute Clinical Effects

Some cardiovascular effects of ethanol consumption occur acutely, without the development of its more common and later effect—dilated cardiomyopathy. For example, a *holiday heart* is marked by a rhythm disturbance, usually a supraventricular tachyarrhythmia (atrial fibrillation being the most common), that manifests after weekend or holiday imbibition. Holiday heart is considered benign and generally does not require antiarrhythmic therapy.[122]

Dilated Cardiomyopathy

A dilated cardiomyopathy resulting from long-term, excessive ethanol consumption was described more than a century ago. In some early reports, it was considered a relatively common cause of heart failure, and that fact was rediscovered in the mid-20th century.[123–125]

In the Western world, alcoholic dilated cardiomyopathy is one of the most common causes of nonischemic heart muscle disease and may be the most frequent identifiable cause.[126] (See also Chapter 10.) Its incidence at autopsy is as high as 45% in urban medical centers. Commonly quoted data range from 20 to 30%.[127] In the United States, chronic ethanol consumption is the leading cause of heart muscle disease of known etiology, and 4.2% of cardiomyopathic deaths are related to it.[128] If abstinence from ethanol consumption is accomplished after a diagnosis of alcoholic dilated cardiomyopathy, a more favorable clinical course results.[129] Recent clinical evidence shows that patients admitted to the hospital for alcoholic cardiomyopathy have a higher prevalence of liver cirrhosis than unselected alcoholics without heart disease.[130]

Pathology

Pathologic changes resemble those of other dilated cardiomyopathies produced by a wide range of different agents.[127, 131] The heart is usually enlarged, dilated, flabby, and pale. Diffuse zones of fibrosis may be seen in the myocardium and on the ventricular and atrial endocardial surfaces. Endocardial fibrotic thickening is sometimes associated with mural thrombosis.[132, 133] Interstitial fibrosis is common and may be visible grossly.

Histopathologic changes are found in the endocardium, interstitium, and myocytes but are not considered specific. Microscopic features resemble those of other idiopathic dilated cardiomyopathies.[134] Fibrosis, increased lipid deposits, and lipofuscin staining are considered characteristic changes by some authors.[135–137] Histochemical staining is positive for mitochondrial cytochrome oxidase.[135, 138] In a study of endomyocardial biopsies from patients with alcoholic dilated cardiomyopathy, the most common findings included endocardial thickening and fibrosis, focal and diffuse interstitial fibrosis, and hypertrophic and myocytolytic changes.[139] In that study, the estimated total lifetime dose of ethanol correlated inversely with cardiac ejection fractions.

Various myocardial ultrastructural findings have been reported. Specific ones cannot be attributed unambiguously to ethanol. This relates to the confounding effects of coexistent malnutrition, vitamin deficiencies, and other disturbances that frequently coexist in alcoholic patients. In one early ultrastructural study,[140] the morphology of cardiac myocytes varied greatly. Scattered patches of fibrous connective tissue were prominent. Cardiac myocytes were enlarged, and few mitochondria were normal. Rather, they showed great variation within myocytes,[135, 140, 41] with many being swollen, having few or no cristae, and containing osmophilic inclusions. The sarcoplasmic reticulum was swollen in damaged myocytes—a change then considered an early one in alcoholic cardiomyopathy.[127] In another report on septal biopsy specimens, loss of contractile elements, dilation of the sarcoplasmic reticulum, and increased glycogen abundance were found. These features were common to both idiopathic and alcoholic cardiomyopathy and could not be used to discriminate between the entities diagnostically.[142]

Pathogenesis

From both pathophysiologic and pathogenetic perspectives, the effects of ethanol consumption in inducing and maintaining an alcoholic cardiomyopathy have not yet been determined although many hypotheses are supported by positive data.[143] One suggests that the deleterious effects of ethanol relate to perturbations of molecular organization in the cardiac myocyte membrane or ion channels in the membrane. Similarly, sarcoplasmic reticulum or mitochondrial membranes may serve as targets for ethanol toxicity. Decreased sarcoplasmic reticulum calcium binding and uptake, altered Na^+ and K^+ ATPase activity, and altered mitochondrial function with decreased oxidative enzyme activity have all been described in experimental models. Oxidative or free radical damage from products of ethanol metabolism, such as acetaldehyde, may be linked to membrane damage.[144–146] Decreased actin-myosin ATPase activity was demonstrated in vitro and may occur in vivo. Data concerning acute and chronic effects of ethanol on myocardial protein synthesis are less clear. Early in vitro studies suggest that relatively low doses of ethanol had no effect on myocardial protein synthesis. Other in vivo studies support the concept that ethanol dosage reduces the fractional synthesis rate in heart muscle.[144]

So-called cirrhotic cardiomyopathy occurs in patients with nutritional cirrhosis who are challenged by pharmacologic or physiologic stress.[147] It may occur in the absence of ethanol ingestion. Diminished myocardial adrenergic receptor signal transduction function is considered critical in this clinical entity.

Cocaine

Cocaine is an alkaloid extract of *Erythroxylon coca,* that has been used as a local anesthetic for more than a century. Its abuse and that of crack cocaine (made by adding ammonium and baking soda to an aqueous solution of cocaine hydrochloride to precipitate alkaloid cocaine, which is dried and smoked, producing high blood levels of the drug very quickly) is a major societal problem in many countries. For example, it is estimated that over 30 million Americans have used cocaine at least once.[148]

Clinical Effects

The drug has both direct and indirect clinical effects. Acute pulmonary edema, angina pectoris, myocardial infarction, coronary artery spasm, cardiac arrhythmias, and sudden death have all been reported, as well as dilated cardiomyopathy with congestive cardiac failure. Endocarditis is also a frequent complication among intravenous drug users (see Chapter 14). Ischemic bowel disease also occurs, and acute dissecting aneurysms have been reported among young black addicts.

Pathogenic Mechanisms

The cardiac consequences of cocaine abuse (1) are not unique to parenteral administration of the drug; (2) may occur in patients who do not necessarily have underlying heart disease; (3) may develop in those without seizure activity, a well-documented noncardiac complication of cocaine abuse; and (4) are not limited to massive doses of the drug. Most cases have been reported among patients 20 to 40 years old, with a greater frequency in males.

Although the mechanisms of cocaine cardiotoxicity are not fully elucidated, its primary pharmacologic properties can be related to the pathophysiology of disease. It acts as an anesthetic and blocks sodium and potassium channels in the heart and vasculature. It also has a powerful stimulant action that accentuates the effects of the sympathetic nervous system by blockading the presynaptic reuptake of norepinephrine and dopamine, the latter resulting in an excess of neurotransmitters at the postsynaptic receptor site.[149, 150] Cocaine may also enhance presynaptic catecholamine release.

Local anesthetic effects can impair conduction and foster arrhythmias. High doses of cocaine can depress contractile function by inhibiting sodium and potassium pumps. Adrenergic effects might be related to coronary artery spasm, ischemic events, increased contractile force, and arrhythmias.[149, 150] Nevertheless, cocaine-associated vascular events are not completely explained by adrenergic stimulation. Wilbert-Lampen and colleagues found that cocaine increases endothelin-1 release both in vitro and in vivo.[151] This may facilitate cocaine-induced vasoconstriction or vasospasm. Cocaine appears to be an exogenous stimulator of endothelial σ-receptors. The endogenous hazards of the antiopioid system may prove to play a role in vasospastic angina, acute myocardial infarction, and sudden cardiac death.

Cocaine hydrochloride is marketed on the street with many adulterants. Because of this, care must be observed in relating the drug to observed clinical events and morphologic findings.

Pathology

Sudden Death

As mentioned earlier, the effects of cocaine relate to both vascular and myocardial dysfunction. The most frequent cardiovascular complication temporally associated with cocaine abuse is acute myocardial infarction.[148, 152, 153] Pathologic changes in the infarct are similar to those found in atherosclerotic heart disease. Sudden death from cocaine abuse is associated with histopathologic evidence of increased contraction band change in the cardiac myocytes.[154] Karch and Billingham reviewed myocardial histology from 30 cases of sudden death associated with cocaine use, comparing the findings with histology from 20 patients who died of sedative-hypnotic drug overdose.[155] The later were used as controls for the effects of hypoxia and resuscitation, which are known to be associated with contraction band necrosis. The authors found that contraction band necrosis was significantly more prevalent ($P <$ .001) in the group taking cocaine and that the extent of their myocardial injury correlated well with urinary and blood levels of the drug. Fineschi and coworkers quantitated myocardial necrosis in 26 cocaine-associated deaths.[155a] (See also Chapter 8.)

Cocaine Myocarditis

Cocaine abuse may be associated with a myocarditis. The histology of a myocarditis must be carefully separated from the inflammatory reaction and myocel dropout that mark repair of contraction band necrosis. Perhaps because of this difficulty, conflicting data exist regarding its pathology and pathogenesis. Isner and colleagues reported an eosinophilic myocarditis in an endomyocardial biopsy from a man who had cocaine-related cardiac symptoms.[152] Virmani's group reported a 20% incidence of inflammatory myocarditis in hearts from cocaine abusers at postmortem examination.[156] The observed inflammatory infiltrates consisted of mixed mononuclear cells with lymphocytes and macrophages.

Although not clarified yet, the mechanism of myocardial damage from cocaine may relate to a hypersensitivity or a toxic myocarditis. However, inflammatory changes may not be attributable to drug abuse alone, because patients may have intercurrent conditions in which myocardial disease is an important factor. Microvascular spasm or changes that resemble those found in the myocardial catecholamine effect also occur.[157]

Cocaine Cardiomyopathy

Cocaine-induced dilated cardiomyopathy is not as prevalent as myocardial ischemia induced by cocaine. It is marked clinically by increased ventricular volumes and impaired systolic function.[158] Despite physiologic and clinical bases for its occurrence, strong pathologic correlation is lacking.[148, 155] Karch and Billingham described the features of three cases. Pathologically, they observed focal lymphocytic infiltrates, less hypertrophy, and fewer nuclear abnormalities than are usually seen in end-stage dilated cardiomyopathy.[155] Fibrosis in the hearts of those with cocaine cardiomyopathy was described as microfocal. This latter feature may be relatively distinctive but is not diagnostic. Microvascular disease, possibly through cocaine-induced vascular spasm, may cause patchy necrosis and replacement fibrosis. Baroldi, in Chapter 8, challenges this proposal. Equally, features in cocaine cardiotoxicity resemble those of catecholamine excess, in which contraction band changes in myocytes are a prominent feature. Their healing can also induce microfocal fibrosis.

Anabolic Steroids

Sholter and Armstrong review the adverse effects of corticosteroid therapy on the cardiovascular system.[158a]

During the 1990s, concern arose over the use of self-prescribed anabolic steroids employed by some athletes for nonmedicinal purposes. Their administration has dangerous cardiovascular side effects. However, the association between these self-administered steroids and death may be overemphasized in the lay press. The cardiovascular system, including heart muscle and vascular tissues, possesses androgen receptors that are specific and have a high affinity. Adverse cardiovascular effects of anabolic steroids include tachycardia, precordial pain, weakness, and edema.[159, 160] In many studies of healthy men and women some of whom were and some of whom were not "power" athletes, no clear changes in blood pressure were observed. Evidence of functional alterations in cardiac performance caused by anabolic steroids was reported, but data were conflicting in different animal experimental systems.[159, 160] Six studies of humans evaluated left ventricular dimension echocardiographically. Mild left ventricular diastolic function was reported in top-ranking competitive athletes who used self-administered steroids. This suggested that use of steroids during training caused mildly increased concentric left ventricular wall thickness. Other indices of left ventricular structure were similar to those found in body builders who did not use steroids.

An increased incidence of thrombosis may be associated with steroid abuse. A few documented cases exist in which acute myocardial infarction was associated with self-administration of steroids in male body builders and power lifters. Investigating competitive athletes for cardiovascular diseases, Maron and colleagues identified significant structural abnormalities in the hearts of conditioned athletes who died suddenly.[161] Many had left ventricular hypertrophy or hypertrophic cardiomyopathy. However, the impact of illicit medication was not the principal focus of this study.

Myocardial Injury From Polysubstance Abuse

It is reasonable to think that individuals who abuse one substance may abuse others. This creates a situation of polydrug abuse. The mixing of agents could potentially cause mixed, additive, or synergistic effects and alter pathologic features. One study demonstrated additive deleterious effects on the myocardium that resulted from mixed substance abuse. The observed effects included myocardial ischemia and infarction, cardiomyopathy and myocarditis, and ventricular arrhythmias.[162] Moreover, in some populations, other factors, such as AIDS and its related pathologic changes, may be critical additions to the pathologic picture.

We note that the adverse effects of bleomycin therapy and of paraquat poisoning are discussed in Chapter 7.

REFERENCES

1. Gotti EW: Adverse drug reactions and the autopsy. Arch Pathol 97:201, 1974
2. Rubin E, Farber JL: Environmental and nutritional pathology. In: Rubin E, Farber JL (eds): Pathology. Philadelphia, Lippincott 1988, p 288
3. La Du BN Jr: Genetic variations in humans and toxicokinetics. In: Welling PG, de la Inglesia FA (eds): Drug Toxicokinetics. New York, Marcel Dekker, 1993
4. Murthy KR, Zolfagharaina H, Medh JD, et al: Disseminated intravascular coagulation and disturbances in carbohydrate and fat metabolism in acute myocarditis produced by scorpion (Buthus tamulus) venom. Indian J Med Res 87:318, 1988
5. Sofer S, Shahak E, Slonim A, Gueron M: Myocardial injury without heart failure following envenomation by the scorpion Leiurus quinquestriatus in children. Toxicon 29:382, 1991
6. Amaral CF, Lopes JA, Magalhaes RA, de Rezende NA: Electrocardiographic, enzymatic and echocardiographic evidence of myocardial damage after Tityu serrulatus scorpion poisoning. Am J Cardiol 67:655, 1991
7. Cupo P, Jurca M, Azedo-Marques MM, et al: Severe scorpion envenomation in Brazil: Clinical, laboratory and anatomopathological aspects. Rev Inst Med Trop Sao Paulo 36:67, 1994
8. Levine HD: Acute myocardial infarction following wasp sting: Report of two cases and critical survey of the literature. Am Heart J 91:365, 1976
9. Wagdi P, Mehan VK, Burgi H, Salzmann C: Acute myocardial infarction after wasp stings in a patient with normal coronary arteries. Am Heart J 128:820, 1994
10. Than-Than FN, Tin-Nu-Swe M-L, Tun-Pe S-S, et al: Contribution of focal haemorrhage and microvascular fibrin deposition to fatal envenoming by Russell's viper (Vipera russelli siamensis). Burma Acta Trop 46:23, 1989
11. Gaynor B: An unusual snake bite story. Med J Aust 2:191, 1977
12. Tibballs J, Sutherland SK, Kerr S: Studies on Australian snake venoms. Part I. The hemodynamic effects of brown snake (Pseudonaja) species in the dog. Anaesth Intensive Care 17:466, 1991
13. Tibballs J, Sutherland SK, Kerr S: Studies on Australian snake venoms. Part II. The haematological effects of brown snake (Pseudonaja) species in the dog. Anaesth Intensive Care 19:338, 1991
14. Tibballs J, Williams D, Sutherland SK: The effects of antivenom and verapamil on the haemodynamic actions of Chironex fleckeri (box jellyfish) venom. Anaesth Intensive Care 26:40, 1998
15. Bristow MR (ed): Drug Induced Heart Disease. Amsterdam, Elsevier, 1980
16. Katzung BG (ed): Basic and Clinical Pharmacology. 6th ed. Norwalk, CT, Appleton & Lange, 1995

17. Wood AJ: Adverse reactions to drugs. In: Isselbacker KJ, Braunwald E, et al (eds): Harrison's Principles of Internal Medicine. 13th ed. New York, McGraw-Hill, 1994
18. Irey NS: Tissue reactions to drugs. Am J Pathol 1976:82, 617
19. Lilienfeld A, Hochstein E, Weiss W: Acute myocarditis with bundle branch block due to sulfonamide sensitivity. Circulation 1: 1060, 1950
20. Aretz HT, Billingham ME, Edwards WD, et al: Myocarditis: A histopathologic definition and classification. Am J Cardiovasc Pathol 1:3, 1987
21. Nishiura H, Shibuya Y, Yamamoto T: S19 ribosomal protein cross-linked dimer causes monocyte-predominant infiltration by means of molecular mimicry to complement C5a. Lab Invest 78: 1615, 1998
22. Burke AP, Saenger J, Mullick F, Virmani R: Hypersensitivity myocarditis. Arch Pathol Lab Med 115:764, 1991
23. Kounis NG, Zavras GM, Soufras GD, Kitrou MP: Hypersensitivity myocarditis. Ann Allergy 62:71, 1989
24. Taliercio CP, Olney BA, Lie JT: Myocarditis related to drug hypersensitivity. Mayo Clin Proc 60:463, 1985
25. Fenoglio JJ Jr, McAllister HA Jr, Mullick FG: Drug related myocarditis: Hypersensitivity myocarditis. Hum Pathol 12:900, 1981
26. Markus CK, Chow LH, Wycoff DM, McManus BM: Pet food–derived penicillin residue as a potential cause of hypersensitivity myocarditis and sudden death. Am J Cardiol 63:1154, 1989
27. Garty BZ, Offer I, Livini E, Danon YL: Erythema multiforme and hypersensitivity myocarditis caused by ampicillin. Ann Pharmacother 28:730, 1994
28. French AJ, Weller CD: Interstitial myocarditis following the clinical and experimental use of sulfonamide drugs. Am J Pathol 18: 109, 1942
29. Lewin D, d'Amati G, Lewis W: Hypersensitivity myocarditis: Findings in native and transplanted hearts. Cardiovasc Pathol 1: 225, 1992
30. Gravanis MB, Hertzler GL, Franch RH, et al: Hypersensitivity myocarditis in heart transplant candidates. J Heart Transplant 10: 688, 1991
31. Spear GS: Eosinophilic explant carditis with eosinophilia: Hypersensitivity to dobutamine infusion. J Heart Lung Transplant 14: 755, 1995
32. Martin RW, Duffy J, Engel AG, et al: The clinical spectrum of the eosinophilia-myalgia syndrome associated with L-tryptophan ingestion. Ann Inter Med 113:124, 1990
33. Clinical spectrum of eosinophilia-myalgia syndrome: California. MMWR Morb Mortal Wkly Rep 112:85, 1990
34. Varga J, Uitto J, Jimine S: The cause and pathogenesis of the eosinophilia-myalgia syndrome. Ann Intern Med 116:140, 1992
35. Silver RM, Heyes MP, Maize JC, et al: Scleroderma, fasciitis and eosinophilia associated with the ingestion of tryptophan. N Engl J Med 322:874, 1990
36. Harpy JP: Lupus-like syndromes induced by drugs. Ann Allergy 33:256, 1974
37. Adams LE, Balakrishnan K, Roberts SM, et al: Genetic, immunologic and biotransformation studies of patients on procainamide. Lupus 2:89, 1993
38. Samuels MA: Neurally induced cardiac damage: Definition of the problem. Neurol Clin 11:273, 1993
39. Reichenbach DD, Benditt EP: Catecholamines and cardiomyopathy: The pathogenesis and potential importance of myofibrillar degeneration. Hum Pathol 1:125, 1970
40. Csapo Z, Dusek J, Rona G: Early alterations of the cardiac muscle cell in isoproterenol-induced necrosis. Arch Pathol 93:363, 1972
41. Bloom S, Cancilla PA: Myocytolysis and mitochondrial calcification in rat myocardium after low dose isoproterenol. Am J Pathol 54:373, 1969
42. Cebelin MS, Hirsch, CS: Human stress cardiomyopathy. Hum Pathol 11:123, 1980
43. Scott J, Parker R, Cameron DP: Pheochromocytoma and cardiomyopathy. Med J Aust 14:894, 1988
44. Getz MA, Subramanian R, Logemann T, Ballantyne F: Acute necrotizing eosinophilic myocarditis as a manifestation of severe hypersensitivity myocarditis. Ann Intern Med 115:201, 1991
45. Kasper EK, Agema WRP, Hutchins GM, et al: The causes of dilated cardiomyopathy: A clinicopathological review of 673 consecutive patients. J Am Coll Cardiol 23:586, 1994
46. Kantrowitz NE, Bristow MR: Cardiotoxicity of antitumor agents. Prog Cardiovasc Dis 27:195, 1984
47. Frishman WH, Sung HM, Yee HCM, et al: Cardiovascular toxicity with cancer chemotherapy. Curr Probl Cardiol 21:226, 1996
48. Shan K, Lincoff AM, Young JB: Anthracycline-induced cardiotoxicity. Ann Intern Med 125:47, 1996
49. Lefrak EA, Pitha J, Rosenheim S, Gottlieb JA: A clinicopathologic analysis of Adriamycin cardiotoxicity. Cancer 32:302, 1973
50. Rinehart JJ, Lewis RP, Balcerzak SP: Adriamycin cardiotoxicity in man. Ann Intern Med 81:475, 1974
51. Borow KM, Henderson IC, Neuman A, et al: Assessment of left ventricular contractility in patients receiving doxorubicin. Ann Intern Med 99:750, 1983
52. Carter SK: Adriamycin, a review. J Natl Cancer Inst 55:1265, 1975
53. Singal PK, Deally CMR, Weinberg LE: Subcellular effects of Adriamycin in the heart: A concise review. J Mol Cell Cardiol 19: 817, 1987
54. Von Hoff DD, Layard MW, Basa P, et al: Risk factors for doxorubicin-induced congestive heart failure. Ann Intern Med 91:710, 1979
55. Saltiel E, McGuire W: Doxorubicin (Adriamycin) cardiomyopathy. West J Med 139:332, 1983
56. Billingham ME, Mason JW, Bristow MR, Daniels JR: Anthracycline cardiomyopathy monitored by morphologic changes. Cancer Treat Rep 62:865, 1978
57. Ferrans VJ: Overview of cardiac pathology in relation to anthracycline cardiotoxicity. Cancer Treat Rep 62:955, 1978
58. Kajihara H, Yokozaki H, Yamahara M, et al: Anthracycline induced myocardial damage. Pathol Res Pract 181:434, 1986
59. Unverferth BJ, Megorien RD, Balerzak SP, et al: Early changes in human myocardial nuclei after doxorubicin. Cancer 52:215, 1983
60. Torti FM, Bristow M, Lum BL, et al: Cardiotoxicity of epirubicin and doxorubicin: Assessment by endomyocardial biopsy. Cancer Res 46:3722, 1986
61. Billingham ME, Bristow MR, Glatstein E, et al: Adriamycin cardiotoxicity: Endomyocardial biopsy evidence of enhancement by irradiation. Am J Surg Pathol 1:17, 1977
62. Greene HL, Reich SD, Dalen JE: Drug therapy: How to minimize doxorubicin toxicity. J Cardiovasc Med 7:306, 1982
63. Speth PAJ, van Hoesel QCGM, Haanen C: Clinical pharmacokinetics of doxorubicin. Clin Pharmacokinet 15:15, 1988
64. Olson RD, Mushlin PS: Doxorubicin cardiotoxicity: Analysis of prevailing hypotheses. FASEB J 4:3076, 1990
65. Currie PF, Boon N: Cardiac involvement in human immunodeficiency virus infection. Q J Med 86:751, 1983
66. Hsia JA, McQuinn LB: AIDS cardiomyopathy. Res Staff Physician 39:21, 1993
67. Jacob AJ, Boon NA: HIV cardiomyopathy: A dark cloud with a silver lining. Br Heart J 66:1, 1991
68. Lewis W: AIDS: Cardiac findings from 115 autopsies. Prog Cardiovasc Dis 32:207, 1989
69. Lewis W, Grody WW: AIDS and the heart: Review and consideration of pathogenetic mechanisms. Cardiovasc Pathol 1:53, 1992
70. d'Amati G, Kwan W, Lewis W: Dilated cardiomyopathy in a zidovudine-treated AIDS patient. Cardiovasc Pathol 1:317, 1992
71. Swartz MN: Mitochondrial toxicity: New adverse drug effects. N Engl J Med 333:1146, 1995
72. Dalakas MC, Illa I, Pezeshkpour G, et al: Mitochondrial myopathy caused by long term zidovudine therapy. New Engl J Med 322: 1098, 1990
73. Lewis W, Papoian T, Gonzalez B, et al: Mitochondrial ultrastructural and molecular changes induced by zidovudine in rat hearts. Lab Invest 65:228, 1991
74. Lewis W, Chomyn A, Gonzalez B, et al: Zidovudine induces molecular, biochemical and ultrastructural changes in rat skeletal muscle mitochondria. J Clin Invest 89:1354, 1992
75. Lewis W, Simpson JF, Meyer RR: Cardiac mitochondrial DMA polymerase is inhibited competitively and non-competitively by phosphorylated zidovudine. Circ Res 74:344, 1994
76. Herskowitz A, Willoughby SB, Baughman KL, et al: Cardiomyopathy associated with antiretroviral therapy in patients with HIV infection: A report of 6 cases. Ann Intern Med 116:311, 1992
77. Lamperth L, Dalakas MC, Dagani F, et al: Abnormal skeletal and cardiac mitochondria induced by zidovudine (AZT) in human muscle in vitro and in an animal model. Lab Invest 65:742, 1991

78. Cocuera Pindado MT, Lopez Bravo A, Martinez-Rodriguez R, et al: Histochemical and ultrastructural changes induced by zidovudine in mitochondria of rat cardiac muscle. Eur J Histochem 38: 311, 1994

79. Lewis W, Dalakas MC: Mitochondrial toxicity of antiviral drugs. Nature Med 1:417, 1995

80. Hall JC, Harruff R: Fatal cardiac arrhythmia in a patient with interstitial myocarditis related to chronic arsenic poisoning. South Med J 82:1557, 1989

81. Jarvis JQ, Hammond E, Meier R, Robinson C: Cobalt cardiomyopathy: A report of two cases from mineral assay laboratories and a review of the literature. J Occup Med 34:620, 1992

82. Quebec beer-drinker's cardiomyopathy. Can Med Assoc J 97:881, 1967

83. Estes ML, Ewing-Wilson D, Chou SM, et al: Chloroquine neuromyotoxicity. Am J Med 82:447, 1987

84. Ratliff NB, Estes ML, Myles JL, et al: Diagnosis of chloroquine cardiomyopathy by endomyocardial biopsy. N Engl J Med 316: 191, 1987

85. McAllister HA, Ferrans VJ, Hall RJ, et al: Chloroquine-induced cardiomyopathy. Arch Pathol Lab Med 111:953, 1987

86. August C, Holzhausen H-J, Schmoldt A, et al: Histological and ultrastructural findings in chloroquine-induced cardiomyopathy. J Mol Pathol 73:73, 1995

87. Nosten F, ter Kuile FO, Luxemburger C, et al: Cardiac effects of antimalarial treatment with halofantrine. Lancet 341:1054, 1993

88. Slavin RE, Woodruff JM: The pathology of bone marrow transplantation. Pathol Annu 19:291, 1974

89. Buja LM, Ferrans VJ, Graw RG: Cardiac pathologic findings in patients treated with bone marrow transplantation. Hum Pathol 7: 17, 1976

90. Murphy ML, Bullock RT, Pearce MB: The correlation of metabolic and ultrastructural changes in emetine myocardial toxicity. Am Heart J 87:105, 1974

91. Pearce MB, Bullock RT, Murphy ML: Selective damage of myocardial mitochondria to emetine hydrochloride. Arch Pathol 91:8, 1971

92. Robben NC, Pippas AW, Moore JO: The syndrome of 5-fluorouracil cardiotoxicity. Cancer 71:493, 1993

93. Hochster H, Wasserheit C, Speyer J: Cardiotoxicity and cardioprotection during chemotherapy. Curr Opin Oncol 7:304, 1995

94. Kragel AH, Travis WD, Steis RG, et al: Pathologic findings associated with interleukin-2-based immunotherapy for cancer: A postmortem study of 19 patients. Hum Pathol 21:493, 1990

95. Kragel AH, Travis WD, Steis RG, et al: Myocarditis or acute myocardial infarction associated with interleukin-2 therapy for cancer. Cancer 66:1513, 1990

96. Samlowski WE, Ward JH, Craven CM, Freedman RA: Severe myocarditis following high dose interleukin-2 administration. Arch Pathol Lab Med 113:838, 1989

97. Nora R, Abrams JS, Tait NS, et al: Myocardial toxic effects during recombinant interleukin-2 therapy. J Natl Cancer Inst 81:59, 1989

98. Schuchter LM, Hendricks CB, Holland KH, et al: Eosinophilic myocarditis associated with high dose interleukin-2 therapy. Am J Med 88:439, 1990

99. Fink S, Finiasz M, Sterin-Borda L, et al: Interleukin-2 stimulates heart contractility in the presence of exogenous arachidonate or the calcium ionophor A23187. Immunol Lett 17:183, 1988

100. Gulick T, Chumg MK, Pieper SJ, et al: Interleukin-1 and tumor necrosis factor inhibit cardiac myocyte adrenergic responsiveness. Proc Natl Acad Sci U S A 86:6753, 1989

101. Alexander CS, Nini A: Cardiovascular complications in young patients taking psychotropic drugs. Am Heart J 78:757, 1969

102. Moir DC, Crooks J, Cornwell WB, et el: Cardiotoxicity of amitriptyline. Lancet 2:561, 1972

103. Tseng HL: Interstitial myocarditis probably related to lithium carbonate intoxication. Arch Pathol 92:444, 1971

104. Brady HR, Horgan JB: Lithium and the heart. Chest 93:166, 1988

105. Greiser R: Epidemiologische untersuchungen zum zusammenhang Swischen Appetitizueglere, Innahme Und Primaer Vasculaer Pulmonaler Hypertonie. Internist 14:437, 1973

106. Gurtner HP: Aminorex and pulmonary hypertension. In: Fishman AP (ed): The Pulmonary Circulation: Normal and Abnormal. Philadelphia, University of Pennsylvania Press, 1999, p 397

107. Fishman AP: Aminorex to fen/phen. Circulation 99:156, 1999

108. Abenhaim L, Moride Y, Brenot F, et al: Appetite suppressant drugs and the risk of primary pulmonary hypertension. N Engl J Med 335:609, 1996

109. Weintraub M, Hasday JD, Mushlin AI, et al: A double-blind clinical trial in weight control: Use of fenfluramine and phenterimine alone and in combination. Arch Intern Med 144:1143, 1984

110. Mark EJ, Patalas ED, Chang HT, et al: Fatal pulmonary hypertension associated with short-term use of fenfluramine and phentermine. N Engl J Med 337:602, 1997

111. Connolly HM, Crary JL, McGoon MD: Valvular heart disease associated with fenfluramine-phentermine. N Engl J Med 337:581, 1997

111a. Baumann HM, Schuster CR, Rothman RB: Effects of phentermine and cocaine on fenfluramine-induced depletion of serotonin in mouse brain. Drug Alcohol Depend 41:71, 2000

111b. Baumann HM, Ayestas MA, Dersch CM, et al: Effects of phentermine and fenfluramine on extracellular dopamine and serotonin in rat nucleus accumbens: Therapeutic implications. Synapse 36: 102, 2000

111c. Valodia P, Syce JA: The effect of fenfluramine on the pulmonary disposition of 5-hydroxytryptamine in the isolated perfused rat lung: A comparison with chlorphentermine. J Pharm Pharmacol 53:53, 2000

112. Young JR, Humphries AW: Severe arteriospasm after use of ergotamine tartrate suppositories. JAMA 175:114, 1961

113. Regan JF, Poletti BJ: Vascular adventitial fibrosis in a patient taking methysergide maleate. JAMA 203:1069, 1968

114. Connell EB: Oral contraceptives: The current risk-benefit ratio. J Reprod Med 29(suppl 7):513, 1984

115. Lidegaard O, Bygdeman M, Milsom I, et al: Oral contraceptives and thrombosis: From risk estimates to health impact. Acta Obstet Gynecol Scand 78:142, 1999

116. Lewis MA: Myocardial infarction and stroke in young women: what is the impact of oral contraceptives. Am J Obstet Gynecol 179(pt 2):S68, 1998

117. Waselenko JK, Nace MC, Alving B: Women with thrombophilia: Assessing the risks for thrombosis with oral contraceptives hormone replacement therapy. Semin Thromb Hemost 24(suppl 1):33, 1998

118. Rosing J, Tans G, Nicolaes GA, et al: Oral contraceptives and venous thrombosis: Different sensitivities to activated protein C in women using second and third generation oral contraceptives. Br J Haematol 97:223, 1997

119. Fuller JG: The Day of St. Anthony's Fire. London, Macmillan, 1968

120. Bana DS, MacNeal PS, LeComte PM, et al: Cardiac murmurs and endocardial fibrosis associated with methysergide therapy. Am Heart J 88:640, 1974

121. Cannistra L: Valvular heart disease associated with dexfenfluramine. N Engl J Med 337:635, 1997

121a. Fitzgerald LW, Burn TC, Brown BS, et al: Possible role of valvular serotonin 5-HT(2B) receptors in the cardiomyopathy associated with fenfluramine. Mol Pharmacol 57:75, 2000

122. Menz V, Grimm W, Hoffmann J, Maisch B: Alcohol and rhythm disturbance: The holiday heart syndrome. Herz 21:227, 1996

123. Steel G: Heart failure as a result of chronic alcoholism. Med Chron 18:1, 1893

124. Burch GE, Walsh JJ: Cardiac insufficiency in chronic alcoholism. Am J Cardiol 6:864, 1960

125. Brigden W, Robinson J: Alcoholic heart disease. BMJ 2:1283, 1964

126. Fabrizio L, Regan TJ: Alcoholic cardiomyopathy. Cardiovasc Drugs Ther 8:89, 1994

127. Regan TJ: Alcoholic cardiomyopathy. Prog Cardiovasc Dis 27:141, 1984

128. Piano MR, Schwertz DW: Alcoholic heart disease: A review. Heart Lung 23:3, 1994

129. Demakis JG, Proskey A, Rahimtoola SH, et al: The natural course of alcoholic cardiomyopathy. Ann Intern Med 80:293, 1974

130. Estruch R, Fernandez-Sol J, Sacanella E, et al: Relationship between cardiomyopathy and liver disease in chronic alcoholism. Hepatology 22:532, 1995

131. Olsen EGJ: The pathology of the cardiomyopathies. Am Heart J 98:385, 1979

132. Urbano-Marquez A, Rubin E: Alcoholic cardiomyopathy. Alcohol Clin Exp Res 18:111, 1994

133. Rubin E: Alcoholic myopathy in heart and skeletal muscle. N Engl J Med 301:28, 1979
134. Ursell PC, Fenoglio JJ: Spectrum of cardiac disease diagnosed by endomyocardial biopsy. Pathol Annu 19:197, 1984
135. Ferrans VJ, Hibbs RG, Weilbaecher DG, et al: Alcoholic cardiomyopathy: A histochemical study. Am Heart J 69:748, 1965
136. Ferrans VJ: Alcoholic cardiomyopathy. Am J Med Sci 252:89, 1966
137. Jaatinen P, Saukko P, Hervonen A: Chronic ethanol exposure increases lipopigment accumulation in human heart. Alcohol Alcohol 28:559, 1993
138. Tsiplenkova VG, Vikhert AM, Cherpachenko NM: Ultrastructural and histochemical observations in human and experimental alcoholic cardiomyopathy. J Am Coll Cardiol 8:22A, 1986
139. Urbano-Marquez A, Estruch R, Navarro-Lopez F, et al: The effects of alcoholism on skeletal and cardiac muscle. N Engl J Med 320:409, 1989
140. Hibbs RG, Ferrans VJ, Black WC, et al: Alcoholic cardiomyopathy: An electron microscopic study. Am Heart J 69:766, 1965
141. Alexander CS: Electron microscopic observations in alcoholic heart disease. Br Heart J 29:200, 1967
142. Bulloch RT, Pearce MB, Murphy ML, et al: Myocardial lesions in idiopathic and alcoholic cardiomyopathy: Study by ventricular septal biopsy. Am J Cardiol 29:15, 1972
143. Thomas AP, Rozanski DJ, Renard DC, Rubin E: Effects of ethanol on the contractile function of the heart: A review. Alcohol Clin Exp Res 18:121, 1994
144. Preedy VR, Atkinson LM, Richardson PJ, et al: Mechanisms of ethanol induced cardiac damage. Br Heart J 69:197, 1993
145. Preedy VR, Richardson PJ: Ethanol induced cardiovascular disease. Br Med Bull 50:152, 1994
146. Preedy VR, Siddiq T, Why H, Richardson PJ: The deleterious effects of alcohol on the heart: Involvement of protein turnover. Am Heart J 127:1432, 1994
147. Ma Z, Lee SS: Cirrhotic cardiomyopathy: Getting to the heart of the matter. Hepatology 24:451, 1996
148. Kloner RA, Hale S, Alker K, Rezkalla S: The effects of acute and chronic cocaine use on the heart. Circulation 85:407, 1992
149. Billman GE: Mechanisms responsible for the cardiotoxic effects of cocaine. FASEB J 4:2469, 1990
150. Billman GE: Cocaine: A review of its toxic actions on cardiac function. Crit Rev Toxicol 25:113, 1995
151. Wilbert-Lampen U, Seliger C, Zilker T, et al: Cocaine increases the endothelial release of immunoreactive endothelin and its concentration in human plasma and urine. Circulation 98:385, 1998
152. Isner JM, Estes MNA III, Thompson PD, et al: Acute cardiac events temporally related to cocaine abuse. N Engl J Med 315:1438, 1986
153. Rezkalla SH, Halle S, Kloner RA: Cocaine-induced heart diseases. Am Heart J 120:1403, 1990
154. Tazelaar H, Karch SB, Billingham ME, et al: Cocaine cardiotoxicity. Hum Pathol 18:195, 1987
155. Karch SB, Billingham ME: The pathology and etiology of cocaine-induced heart disease. Arch Pathol Lab Med 112:225, 1988
155a. Fineschi V, Welti CW, di Paulo M, Baroldi G: Myocardial necrosis and cocaine. A quantitative morphological study in 26 cocaine-associated deaths. Int J Legal Med 110:193, 1997
156. Virmani R, Robinowitz M, Smialek JE: Cardiovascular effects of cocaine: An autopsy study of 40 patients. Am Heart J 115:1068, 1988
157. Samuels MA: Neurally induced cardiac damage. Neurol Clin North Am 11:273, 1993
158. Willens H, Chakko SC, Kessler KM: Cardiovascular manifestations of cocaine abuse: A case of recurrent dilated cardiomyopathy. Chest 106:594, 1994
158a. Sholter DE, Armstrong PW: Adverse effects of corticosteroids on the cardiovascular system. Can J Cardiol 16:505, 2000
159. Melchert RB, Welder AA: Cardiovascular effects of androgenic-anabolic steroids. Med Sci Sports Exerc 27:1252, 1995
160. Rockhold RW: Cardiovascular toxicity of anabolic steroids. Annu Rev Pharmacol Toxicol 33:497, 1993
161. Maron BJ, Shirani J, Poliac LC, et al: Sudden death in young competitive athletes: Clinical, demographic and pathological profiles. JAMA 276:199, 1996
162. Lam D, Goldschlager N: Myocardial injury associated with polysubstance abuse. Am Heart J 115:675, 1988

Chapter 18

Cardiovascular Trauma

· · · · ·

Francesca V.O. Lobo • H. Alexander Heggtveit

Cardiovascular trauma ranks second only to craniocerebral injury as a major cause of morbidity and mortality in both civilian and military spheres. Mechanical injuries of the heart and blood vessels are increasingly a basis for accident insurance or workers' compensation claims. Wounds, including those of the heart and blood vessels, were among the earliest lesions depicted with their causative agents (Fig. 18-1). The spectrum of cardiovascular trauma has enlarged over the centuries, with respect to both penetrating and nonpenetrating injuries, including a widening array of iatrogenic trauma related to cardiac surgical and invasive cardiologic procedures. In addition, cardiovascular injury may result from exposure to radiation, electrical currents, hypothermia, or certain occupations. Rich and Spencer,[1] Symbas,[2–4] and DeSanctis[5] have addressed the clinical aspects and management of cardiovascular trauma. The pathologic features and older literature are assessed in books by Gould[6] and Hudson.[7] In this chapter, the basic types and mechanisms of heart and blood vessel injuries are reviewed. Although some consequences may be the same, it is convenient to consider the effects of penetrating and nonpenetrating injury separately.

PENETRATING INJURIES

Common in military casualties,[1] penetrating wounds of the heart and great vessels are becoming much more frequent in the civilian population as urban violence escalates.[8, 9] Penetrating wounds are usually the result of a bullet (Fig. 18-2) or knife (Figs. 18-3 and 18-4) wound to the chest or neck; less often, they are caused by puncture wounds from other sharp objects such as ice picks, metal shrapnel, pins, or arrows (Fig. 18-5). Multiple penetrating wounds of the heart can result from indriven fragments of fractured ribs in falls from great heights or other severe crushing injuries of the chest (Fig. 18-6). The nature of an injury inflicted on vascular structures is related to the physical properties of the missile as well as its velocity and force. High-velocity projectiles such as rivets or bullets possess great kinetic energy. Even a small-caliber bullet can inflict extensive injury, out of proportion to its size. More massive wounds result from larger caliber bullets or shotgun injuries (Figs. 18-7 and 18-8). Generally speaking, the closer the range, the greater the destructive force released; in the case of very close range or contact gunshot wounds, the destructive force is compounded by the effect of the muzzle blast of hot gases. Gunshot wounds tend not only to penetrate but also to perforate the heart or great vessels. Associated massive tissue destruction often leads to exsanguinating hemorrhage.

In contrast, knife wounds are of low velocity and are more likely to produce localized penetrating injuries, which, although transmural, do not necessarily perforate a chamber. Such wounds may seal or close spontaneously, especially when confined to the thicker left ventricle. Despite lower intracavity pressures in atria and right ventricle, these thin-walled chambers are more likely to bleed when punctured. Therefore, the site of a wound is important in determining the outcome of injury. Hemopericardium with cardiac tamponade is a common sequel of major penetrating wounds of the heart and aortic root. Rapid accumulation of 150 to 200 ml of blood in the pericardial sac increases intrapericardial pressure and decreases systolic ejection of the ventricles, leading to a decline in central aortic pressure and diminution of coronary blood flow with ultimate cessation of cardiac function. If the associated pericardial wound communicates with the pleural cavity, fatal hemothorax may result.

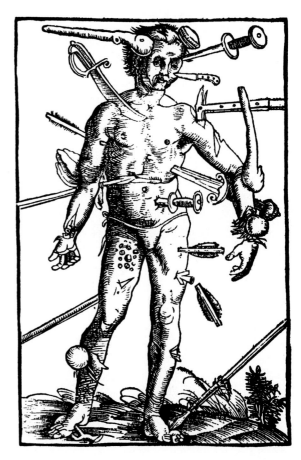

Figure 18-1 • The Wound Man. Plate from the Grosse Wundartzney by Paracelsus, 1536.

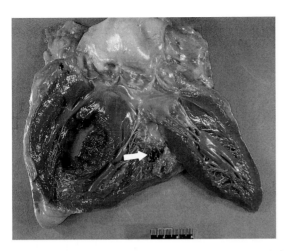

Figure 18-2 • Suicidal gunshot wound of heart (.22-caliber handgun). The bullet produced a small entry wound in the anterior free wall of the right ventricle (not shown), a large ventricular septal defect, and a small exit wound in the posterobasal wall of the left ventricle beneath the mitral valve (arrow).

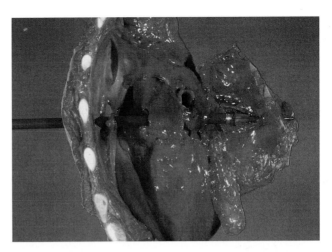

Figure 18-5 • Suicidal crossbow wound of aorta in a 21-year-old man. Thoracic structures are viewed from the left side. Bolt penetrated ascending aorta (behind pulmonary artery in the photograph) and passed through descending aorta before lodging in the thoracic spine. The hunting tip extended through 6.0 cm of bone. Death resulted from a massive left-sided hemothorax. (Courtesy of D.E.L. King, MD, Hamilton, Ontario.)

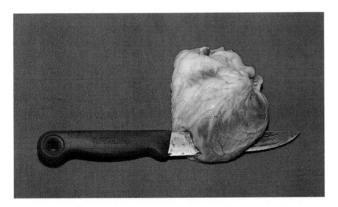

Figure 18-3 • Suicidal stab wound of heart in a 45-year-old depressed male. Knife perforated diaphragm, pericardium, and heart, entering the anteroapical aspect of the left ventricle and exiting higher on the posterior wall. Associated massive left hemothorax. (Courtesy of D.E.L. King, MD, Hamilton, Ontario.)

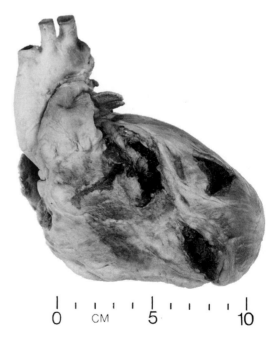

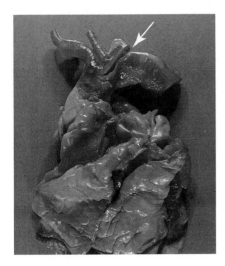

Figure 18-4 • Self-inflicted, sharply incised stab wound of aortic arch (arrow) resulting from a single downward thrust of a broad kitchen knife in the left supraclavicular region.

Figure 18-6 • Specimen from a 19-year-old youth who fell from the 22nd floor of an apartment block, sustaining multiple traumatic injuries. Several irregular penetrating wounds of the atria and ventricles resulted from indriven ends of broken ribs, most of which were fractured anteriorly and posteriorly. This is an example of nonpenetrating thoracic trauma causing penetrating cardiac wounds.

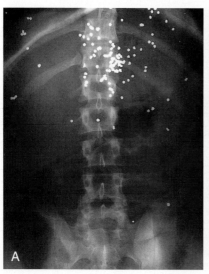
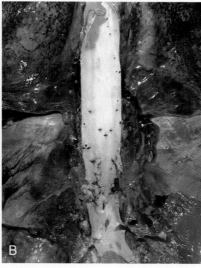

Figure 18-7 • Close-range homicidal shotgun wound (.20 gauge, no. 5 shot) in a young man. *A,* Radiograph showing lead pellets clustered in lower chest and upper abdomen. *B,* Aorta with multiple perforating wounds above level of celiac artery.

Table 18-1 lists the locations and types of lesions seen in penetrating wounds of the heart.[10] Arrhythmias and conduction defects may occur in addition to structural damage to any of the cardiac tissues. Intracardiac shunts[11, 12] or fistulas[13–15] develop, as do valvular[16] and coronary artery lacerations. Coronary artery injuries, depending on the size of the injured vessels, result in cardiac tamponade and varying degrees of myocardial ischemia or even infarction.[2]

The resorption of hematomas produced by penetrating wounds is slow; healing begins at the epicardial and endocardial portions of the wound and extends gradually

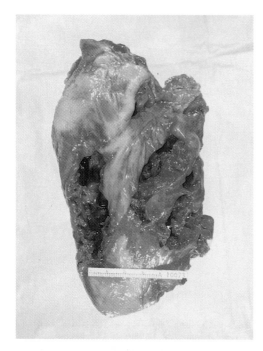

Figure 18-8 • Close-range homicidal shotgun (.410 gauge) wound of heart in a young man. The ventricular walls have been lacerated and portions carried away by the charge of shot at point-blank range.

TABLE 18-1 • Cardiac Lesions Produced by Penetrating Wounds

I. Pericardial injury
 A. Laceration
 B. Hemopericardium
  1. With cardiac tamponade
  2. Without cardiac tamponade
 C. Effusion with fibrinous pericarditis
 D. Recurrent pericarditis with effusion
 E. Pneumopericardium
 F. Suppurative pericarditis
 G. Constrictive pericarditis

II. Myocardial injury
 A. Laceration
 B. Penetration or perforation
 C. Rupture
 D. Retained foreign body
  1. Infected (abscess)
  2. Sterile
 E. Structural defects
  1. Aneurysm formation
  2. Septal defects
  3. Aortocardial fistula

III. Valvular injury
 A. Leaflet injury
 B. Papillary muscle or chordae tendineae laceration or rupture

IV. Coronary artery injury
 A. Thrombosis or laceration
  1. With myocardial infarction
  2. Without myocardial infarction
 B. Arteriovenous fistula
 C. Aneurysm

V. Embolism
 A. Foreign body
 B. Thrombus
  1. Septic
  2. Sterile

VI. Infective endocarditis

VII. Rhythm or conduction disturbances

Adapted from Parmley LF, Symbas PN: Traumatic heart disease. In: Hurst JW (ed): The Heart. Vol. 2. New York, McGraw-Hill, 1978, p 1683, with permission of The McGraw Hill Companies.

into the transmural segment.[6] The end result is focal endocardial fibrosis and localized fibrous pericardial adhesions with a connecting, often ill-defined path of myocardial scarring between. Constrictive pericarditis does not usually result unless there is organization of an associated hemopericardium. Post-traumatic aneurysm of the left ventricle may be an early or late consequence of penetrating or nonpenetrating wounds.[4, 17]

Infection, leading to suppurative pericarditis, myocardial abscess, or endocarditis, is always a risk with penetrating wounds of pericardium and heart. One of the unique features of missile injury to the heart and blood vessels is the possibility of intracardiac retention or embolization of a bullet or other foreign object.[4, 13, 18, 19] In persons surviving the acute injury, surgical treatment of penetrating wounds of the heart, aorta, and peripheral vessels generally produces good results.[1, 4, 8, 20, 21]

NONPENETRATING INJURIES

Nonpenetrating chest trauma with injury to the heart and aorta has become increasingly common, particularly as a result of rapid deceleration in high-speed vehicular accidents.[3, 22, 23] Airplane crashes, falls from great height, and other severe crushing injuries of the thorax and the lower body may lead to nonpenetrating cardioaortic injuries. Damage from blunt trauma is often masked by associated major visceral or musculoskeletal injury or by lack of external evidence of chest injury.[22] The effects are governed by the site and extent of injury and the phase of the respiratory and cardiac cycles during which trauma was sustained. Physical forces acting externally on the body to produce major cardiovascular lesions do so through one or more of the mechanisms listed in Table 18-2.[10] The major sequelae of nonpenetrating trauma to the heart and great vessels are listed in Table 18-3.

Pericardial Lesions

Pericardial tears from blunt trauma are usually transverse across the base of the heart near the reflection of visceral and parietal pericardium, at a site which represents an area of relative fixation or suspension.[22] Such rents carry a potential danger of herniation or luxation of the heart.[24] When myocardial tears coexist, the integrity of the parietal pericardium may prevent exsanguination by inducing tamponade to control bleeding long enough to permit surgical treatment. Larger pericardial defects

TABLE 18-2 • **Mechanisms of Blunt Force Injury Producing Cardiovascular Lesions**

Unidirectional force against chest
Bidirectional or compressive force against thorax
Indirect forces (i.e., compression of abdomen and lower extremities resulting in markedly increased intravascular pressure)
Decelerative forces, particularly when imparting differential deceleration to heart and great vessels
Blast forces of great magnitude
Concussive force, indicating jarring force that interferes with cardiac rhythm but not of magnitude to produce a significant lesion

TABLE 18-3 • **Nonpenetrating Trauma of Heart and Great Vessels**

I. Pericardial injury
   A. Hemopericardium
   B. Rupture or laceration
   C. Serofibrinous or suppurative pericarditis
   D. Constrictive pericarditis
   E. Recurrent pericarditis with effusion

II. Myocardial injury
   A. Concussion
   B. Contusion
     1. Anginal syndrome
     2. Myocardial necrosis with or without cardiac failure
     3. Myocardial fibrosis
     4. Aneurysm
     5. Delayed rupture
     6. Thromboembolism
   C. Laceration
   D. Rupture, including septal rupture

III. Coronary artery injury
   A. Laceration with or without myocardial infarction
   B. Thrombosis with or without myocardial infarction
   C. Arteriovenous fistula

IV. Valvular injury
   A. Laceration, rupture, contusion
   B. Papillary muscle or chordae tendineae injury

V. Disturbances of rhythm or conduction

VI. Great vessel injury
   A. Laceration, rupture
   B. Aneurysm formation
   C. Thrombotic occlusion

Modified from Parmley LF, Symbas PN: Traumatic heart disease. In: Hurst JW (ed): The Heart. Vol. 2. New York, McGraw-Hill, 1978, p 1683, with permission of The McGraw-Hill Companies.

can allow excessive bleeding from smaller myocardial lacerations that might otherwise seal, with some relative increase in intrapericardial pressure. Traumatic pericarditis is a common accompaniment of closed cardiac injuries and is usually characterized by simple serous or sanguinous effusions and fibrinous exudate. Such reactions are probably secondary to pericardial and underlying myocardial contusions. Delayed or recurrent pericarditis with effusion after trauma is a poorly understood clinical entity that may have an autoimmune basis. Chronic constrictive pericarditis with calcification may be a late sequela of recurrent post-traumatic pericarditis or result from organization of blood in the pericardial sac (see Chapter 12).

Cardiac Commotion

The spectrum of acute myocardial injury ranges from "concussion or commotion" to contusion, laceration, and rupture. Cardiac commotion (commotio cordis) or concussion is a term denoting a disturbance of cardiac function, induced by impact or agitation of the heart. It is out of proportion to the degree of observed anatomic alterations.[6] Nonfatal transient disturbances of cardiac activity may occur after chest trauma, but pathologic documentation of damage is obviously impossible in survivors. In cardiac concussion, however, despite the lack of myocardial cellular damage, patients can suffer a variety of arrhythmias, including ventricular tachycardia or fibrillation. Although rare, sudden death has been documented, typically after an abrupt blunt precordial blow, particularly during sporting activities.[25, 26] Rib fractures are characteristically absent and chest wall injuries insignificant.

Myocardial Contusions

Myocardial contusion falls within the spectrum of cardiac damage between cardiac rupture on the one hand and arrhythmias or heart failure without morphologic evidence of injury on the other.[23, 24] It has its own range of variable, often transient, clinical signs or functional consequences and is marked histologically by cellular injury. Myocardial contusion (Fig. 18-9) may occur with or without external signs of trauma or fractures of the bony structures of the chest wall. The most common cause of this injury is steering wheel impact, which compresses the heart between the sternum and vertebrae. Sudden accelerations or decelerations may cause the heart to be thrust against the sternum or vertebrae, injuring the myocardium. Also, a sudden increase in intrathoracic or intraabdominal pressure may result in subendocardial and myocardial hemorrhages.[2, 4]

Precordial pain, which clinically simulates angina pectoris or acute myocardial infarction,[27] is the most common symptom and may be associated with rhythm or conduction disturbances. When extensive damage is present throughout the myocardium, early death is the rule, although later deaths have been reported. Causes of death include ventricular fibrillation, prolonged cardiac standstill, myocardial rupture, and heart failure.[22] Pathologically, there may be subepicardial, intramyocardial, or

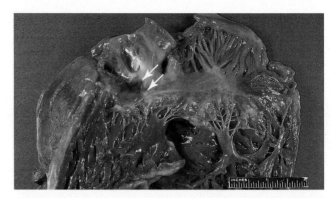

Figure 18-10 • Specimen from a patient involved in a motor vehicle accident, showing multiple injuries. Note focal subendocardial hemorrhage in the atrioventricular node region just proximal to the septal cusp of the tricuspid valve (small arrows). An incomplete transverse endomyocardial tear surrounded by hemorrhage is present in the right atrium immediately proximal to the posterior leaflet of the tricuspid valve.

subendocardial extravasation of blood with focal, microscopic fractures of the muscle bundles of the heart. Varying degrees of myocardial necrosis (often of the contraction-band type) may be present in contusions,[27] but this may be minimal, the dominant feature being interstitial hemorrhage. Healing takes place rapidly with infiltration of leukocytes and resorption of blood and necrotic tissue, followed by replacement fibrosis. Extensive transmural contusions may, with healing, give rise to true post-traumatic aneurysms of the ventricular wall,[22, 23, 28] in contrast to false aneurysms occurring after cardiac rupture (see later discussion).

Although subendocardial hemorrhages may be contusive in origin (Fig. 18-10), very similar (although usually smaller) extravasations are found in hypoxic or asphyxial states.[6] Larger subendocardial hemorrhages are often observed in patients with circulatory or hypovolemic shock or hemorrhagic diatheses. It is not as widely appreciated that subendocardial hemorrhage, myocytolysis, and myocardial necrosis develop in the left ventricular myocardium secondary to isolated spontaneous or traumatic intracranial hemorrhage (see Chapter 15).

Rupture of the Heart

Myocardial laceration and rupture may be produced by the same forces that cause contusion, and they are the lesions most often found at autopsy in fatalities attributable to nonpenetrating chest trauma.[4, 22] Rupture of the right ventricle occurs most frequently, followed in diminishing order by rupture of the left ventricle (see Fig. 18-9), right atrium, and left atrium (Fig. 18-11). Massive compression of the chest can cause explosive rupture of the roof of the atria and/or apex of the ventricles (Fig. 18-12). Rupture may occur immediately or within the first 2 weeks after injury, following softening and necrosis in a contused segment of the wall, before healing occurs. The heart is usually ruptured when the anterior chest wall is driven in by an external force or by forceful compression against the vertebral column.[4] The ventricles are most vulnerable in late diastole or early systole, when chambers are full and valves are closed. The atria are at

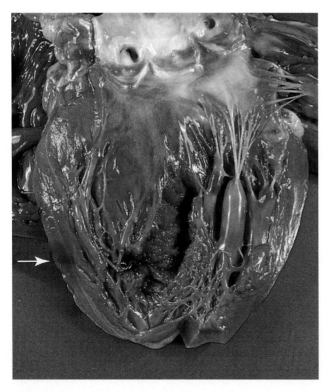

Figure 18-9 • Traumatic ventricular septal laceration caused by blunt thoracic injury in a young man struck by an automobile. The left ventricular free wall was contused (arrow) but not ruptured.

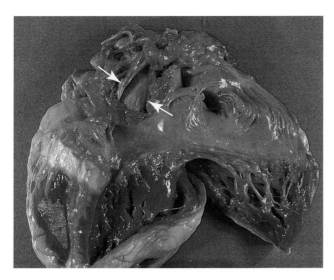

Figure 18-11 • Traumatic atrial septal defect (arrows) resulting from nonpenetrating thoracic trauma sustained in a motor vehicle accident.

risk during ventricular systole because of maximum venous return. A sudden increase in hydrostatic pressure within the heart chambers causes tearing of atrial or ventricular walls from within outward, beginning with the endocardium. As a result, partial or incomplete endomyocardial lacerations (see Fig. 18-10) or complete full-thickness tears (see Fig. 18-12) may be found. The size of a rupture tends to be larger on the endocardial aspect and smaller on the epicardial surface. Ventricular ruptures from blunt trauma usually have a vertical orientation, whereas those in the atria are most often horizontal. With larger ventricular free-wall lacerations, death from cardiac tamponade is commonly a swift sequela. Smaller tears may be compatible with survival long enough to permit surgical correction.[4, 22] Rarely, a false or pseudoaneurysm of the left ventricle develops when bleeding from a rupture is contained by pericardial adhesions and an organizing blood clot (see Chapter 12).[4, 17, 22] The interventricular septum appears to be acutely susceptible to injury secondary to nonpenetrating chest trauma (see Fig. 18-9). Isolated traumatic ventricular septal defects may occur as the

major cardiac lesion,[22, 29] or they may be associated with valvular damage[30] or ventricular aneurysm.[31] Although small ventricular defects may close spontaneously, the treatment of choice is surgical closure, particularly in the presence of cardiac failure.[22] Other, less common types of intracardiac or cardiothoracic shunt may develop secondary to nonpenetrating chest trauma.[32]

Coronary and Valvular Injuries

The question of whether nonpenetrating chest trauma can cause direct injury to coronary arteries has been hotly debated in the literature.[22, 23, 27] Cumulative evidence from clinical cases with angiographic documentation supports such a relationship,[33–37] although documented pathologic observations are few (Fig. 18-13). Most often, the left anterior descending coronary artery is the traumatized vessel, and myocardial infarction the result. Intimomedial tears and intramural dissections with superimposed thrombosis appear to be the major mechanisms involved. Rupture of a coronary artery is a rare occurrence (Fig. 18-14), and coronary artery fistulas have occasionally been described.[32, 38]

Nonpenetrating traumatic injuries of the atrioventricular or semilunar valves may induce clinically significant valvular incompetence.[4, 6, 22, 23] The aortic valve is most commonly involved, followed by the mitral and the tricuspid. The bodies of aortic cusps may be torn or the cusps avulsed along their basal attachments.[39] Injuries of the mitral valve may result in tears of the anterior or posterior leaflets but more commonly cause rupture of chordae tendineae or papillary muscles. Underdiagnosis of traumatic tricuspid insufficiency is possible,[40] and reports of pulmonary valve injury are rare (Fig. 18-15). Early operation with prosthetic valve replacement affords the best chance of survival.[22, 23, 28] Instances of bioprosthetic valve dysfunction and rupture after blunt chest trauma have also been described.[4, 41] Infective endocarditis may develop on traumatically ruptured valves.[7, 10, 42]

Laceration and Rupture of Aorta

An unusual occurrence until well into this century, traumatic laceration and rupture of the aorta now occurs

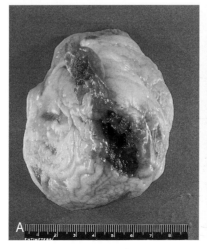
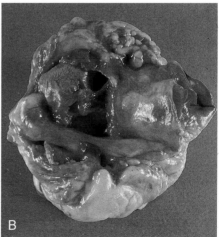

Figure 18-12 • *A,* Blowout lacerations of apex of right ventricle; *B,* dome of right atrium. The victim had been run over, the wheels of an automobile traversing his chest.

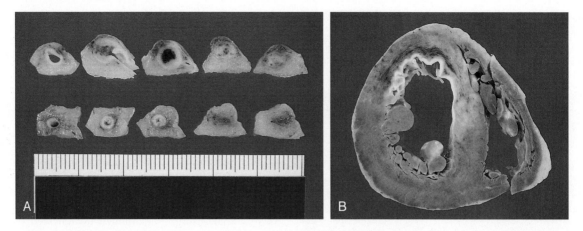

Figure 18-13 • Post-traumatic coronary occlusion and myocardial infarction in a 17-year-old boy who sustained a severe concussion and bilateral fractured clavicles in a motorbike accident. An aortogram was normal, but cardiac investigations were not done. He died suddenly 3 months later while playing basketball. *A,* Serial sections of left main coronary artery and left anterior descending (LAD) branch clockwise from upper left. Slight aneurysmal dilation and recent retrograde extension of thrombus are seen at the LAD origin (sections 2 and 3), followed by organized luminal occlusion (sections 4 to 7) and, further along, distal prolapse and LAD occlusion caused by a torn intimomedial flap. *B,* Transverse midventricular slice of heart showing late healing anteroseptal infarct with richly vascularized scar and secondary endocardial fibrosis.

with alarming frequency and is seen in 1 of every 6 to 10 automobile fatalities.[3, 4] The types of injury leading to aortic rupture are similar to those causing rupture of the heart and include direct blunt force to the chest, vertical deceleration, horizontal deceleration with or without chest compression, and crushing injuries involving some flexion mechanism to the spine. More than 95% of traumatic aortic injuries involve the thoracic aorta, and the usual site of tearing is the aortic isthmus at the ligamentum arteriosum, 2 to 3 cm beyond the origin of the left sub-clavian artery (Fig. 18-16). This represents a point of relative fixation or suspension of the descending thoracic aorta by the ligamentum, intercostal arteries, and parietal pleura, rendering it relatively immobile compared with the aortic arch and heart. The different rates of deceleration of the mobile arch and the relatively fixed descending aorta place unusual stresses on the aortic isthmus in deceleration accidents. The second most frequent site of

rupture is in the ascending aorta proximal to the innominate artery (Fig. 18-17). This too is a point of relative fixation by the pericardial reflection and partial suspension of the heart by bronchi and mediastinal structures.[4]

Four main mechanical stresses (shearing, bending, torsion, and waterhammer) appear to contribute to acute traumatic rupture of the aorta (Fig. 18-18).[4] Shearing and bending stresses are more likely to cause rupture at the isthmus. Shearing stress is related to differential deceleration and relative fixation, whereas bending stress is caused by chest compression with flexion of the aortic arch over the left main stem bronchus and left pulmonary artery. During sudden compression or direct blunt force to the chest, the heart may be displaced into the left posterior chest and the aorta rotated. The ascending aorta bears the brunt of this torsion. In addition, horizontal linear impact trauma to the sternum produces an acute lengthening of the vessel, creating an intra-aortic pressure wave —

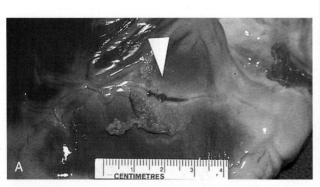
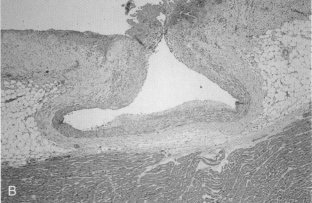

Figure 18-14 • This previously well 35-year-old man had a sudden onset of angina, collapsed, and died later the same day. He had no history of trauma apart from involvement in karate exercises the previous day. *A,* Focal hemorrhage and fibrinous exudate at site of rupture of posterior descending branch, right coronary artery. *B,* Photomicrograph of lacerated coronary artery branch sealed by fibrin platelet thrombus with associated inflammatory infiltrate. (H&E stain.) (Courtesy of D.E.L. King, MD, Hamilton, Ontario.)

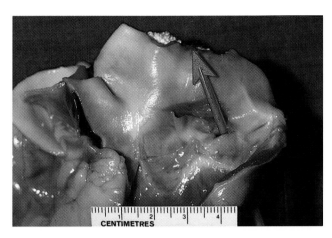

Figure 18-15 • Lacerated root of pulmonary artery with perforation of sinus of pulmonary valve (probe). This 38-year-old man, an automobile driver, was involved in a head-on collision. He died with hemopericardium and left hemothorax together with fractured sternum and ribs, left side. (Courtesy of D.E.L. King, MD, Hamilton, Ontario.)

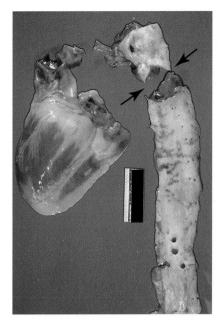

Figure 18-16 • Injuries sustained by 36-year-old male automobile driver in a head-on collision. There is complete transection of the aorta just beyond the attachment of the ligamentum arteriosum (arrows) with a number of transverse intimal tears and contusions in the descending thoracic aorta. There is coexistent partial avulsion of the heart through the atria. (Courtesy of D.E.L. King, MD, Hamilton, Ontario.)

or waterhammer stress—that is greatest in the ascending aorta.[4]

Traumatic rupture of the ascending aorta is often associated with other cardiac injuries. Combined rupture of the aortic valve and ascending aorta have been reported after blunt chest trauma,[43] including one patient with a prior aortic dissection.[44] Charles and colleagues[43] suggested that depression of a fractured sternum contacting the forward-moving heart in diastole resulted in injuries to the aortic root after a steering wheel injury in their case. Aronson[45] reported rupture of the ascending aorta after a minor fall in a patient with extreme cardiomegaly. It was postulated that the unusually heavy heart exerted a severe downward force as a result of its mass and the inertia concomitant with the fall. The aorta ripped at the proximal site of maximum stress. This type of rupture is usually seen in falls from great height or in air crash victims.

The aorta exhibits less tensile strength to longitudinal than to transverse stress; therefore, the majority of aortic lacerations are horizontal. Tears in the aorta range from small lacerations to circumferential transections with separation of proximal and distal aortic segments. As in the heart, aortic lacerations develop from within outward and may involve the intima only, the intima and a varying amount of media, or the full thickness of the aorta. In the latter situation, the parietal pleura tears and fatal hemothorax ensues. Nevertheless, a patient may survive complete transection of the aorta. The adventitia may remain intact because it is the toughest layer of the aortic wall and has the greatest tensile strength. Patients retaining a largely intact adventitia and pleura may survive initial injury with bleeding limited to the mediastinal tissues. Such cases are amenable to successful surgery if a diagnosis can be established.[46] Major aortic rupture may be accompanied by multiple intimal contusions and minor intimomedial lacerations (see Fig. 18-16). When minor lacerations alone are produced by chest trauma, they can give rise to post-traumatic aneurysm but the majority are likely to be of no great consequence and will probably

resolve, leaving small fibrous intimal plaques. However, if an accident victim survives, serious lacerations will require graft replacement of the lacerated aorta.

Major dissection is not a feature of traumatic rupture of the aorta because there is usually no underlying medial disease. However, limited "dissection" or undermining of the torn edges may lift an intimal or intimomedial flap,[47] and this can cause obstruction by prolapse or thrombosis or simulate coarctation in the thoracic[48] or abdominal[49, 50] aorta (Fig. 18-19). Although abdominal aortic injury is more commonly caused by penetrating wounds,[51] when

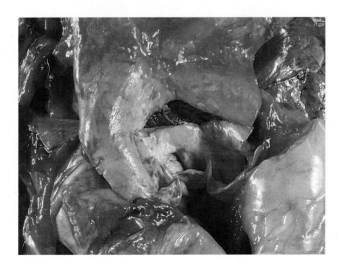

Figure 18-17 • Transverse laceration of ascending aorta just distal to the aortic valve. This middle-aged woman was driving a snowmobile on a country road and was struck by a car. Death was caused by hemopericardium with cardiac tamponade.

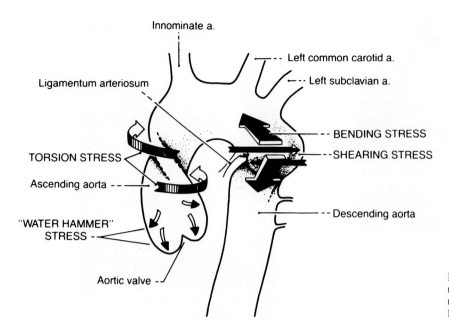

Innominate a.

Left common carotid a.

Left subclavian a.

Ligamentum arteriosum

BENDING STRESS

SHEARING STRESS

TORSION STRESS

Ascending aorta

Descending aorta

"WATER HAMMER" STRESS

Aortic valve

Figure 18-18 • Diagram of the stresses contributing to rupture of the aorta from blunt trauma. (Symbas PN: Cardiothoracic Trauma. Philadelphia, WB Saunders, 1989.)

lacerations from blunt force do occur, they are often associated with intimal flap prolapse and luminal stenosis.[6, 49, 50] Occlusive thrombi, frank rupture, intramural hematomas, simple contusions, false aneurysms, and atheroemboli also result from blunt trauma to the abdominal aorta.[52, 52a] Most cases of abdominal aortic injury manifest with signs of leg ischemia, an "acute abdomen," or both.[52]

Post-traumatic Aortic Aneurysm

Because of the ability of the adventitia to withstand great mechanical forces and remain intact, partial tears involving the inner layers of the aortic wall can result in post-traumatic aneurysms.

With full-thickness tears, the parietal pleura and organization of periaortic mediastinal hematoma may limit bleeding until healing occurs. Such aneurysms are usually found in the upper thoracic aorta some time after the injury (Fig. 18-20). They may be discovered by chance, or, since they continue to expand, they may cause pressure on an adjacent structure or rupture well after the trauma. Swanson and Gaffey reported a case of traumatically induced false aneurysm with secondary bacterial aortitis of the descending aorta and fistula formation between aorta and esophagus.[53] When diagnosed, the af-

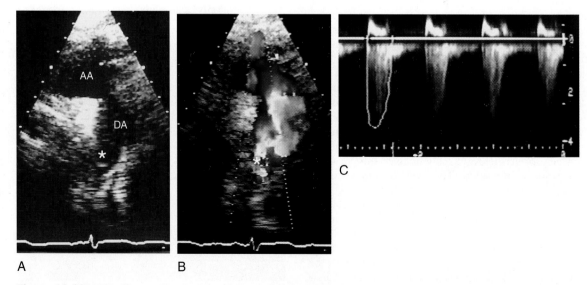

A

B

C

Figure 18-19 • This 25-year-old male driver (without seatbelt) was involved in a motor vehicle accident. A, Suprasternal two-dimensional echocardiogram of the thoracic aorta showing an intimal flap (below*) in the descending thoracic aorta. AA, aortic arch; DA, descending aorta. B, Color Doppler echocardiogram showing turbulent flow (mosaic of color*) at level of intimal flap. C, Continuous-wave Doppler echocardiogram showing significant gradient of 46 mm Hg (velocity of 3.4 m/sec) consistent with pseudocoarctation. (Courtesy of A. Mulji, MD, and Ms. H. Burley, Hamilton, Ontario.)

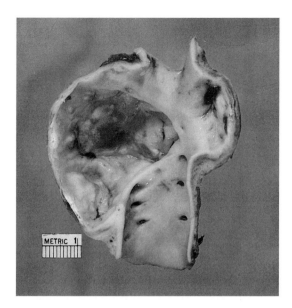

Figure 18-20 • Surgically resected post-traumatic aneurysm of descending thoracic aorta in a 23-year-old automobile driver involved in a head-on collision 9 months previously. The aortic injury escaped notice at the time of the accident. A mediastinal mass was detected on routine chest radiography when the patient returned for treatment of a nonunited fracture of the tibia and fibula. The specimen has been hemisected in the coronal plane. This is a true aneurysm, with the adventitia holding intact almost after complete circumferential laceration of the full thickness of intima and media.

fected patient requires early operation; surgical results are good.[54] The inner margins of post-traumatic aneurysms are formed by the edges of the original aortic laceration. The undermined edges may produce an intimal flap or rolled-in cuff of intima and media, which can manifest as a coarctation.[55] False aneurysm of the abdominal aorta

due to total rupture and periaortic hematoma formation has been reported after a fall causing blunt abdominal trauma.[56]

Blunt Injuries to Branches of the Aortic Arch

Nonpenetrating chest trauma may involve branches of the aortic arch, causing early laceration or avulsion of the innominate, common carotid, or subclavian arteries with resultant massive mediastinal hemorrhage.[4] Incomplete lacerations result in post-traumatic aneurysms, which most often involve the innominate artery.[57, 58] Heggtveit and colleagues[57] reported two cases of innominate arterial aneurysm after steering wheel injuries in young men (Fig. 18-21). One also involved the proximal portions of the right subclavian and common carotid arteries. Both were associated with partially obstructing intimomedial flap or shelf-like stenoses caused by limited dissection with lifting of the torn edges; in both cases, the adventitia remained intact, containing major bleeding. Resection and graft replacement of the aneurysms were performed 4 and 11 months, respectively, after the injuries were sustained and produced excellent long-term results.

Blunt Injuries of Peripheral Vessels

Although less frequent than penetrating injuries, blunt trauma to peripheral vessels may produce lacerations, transections, avulsions, contusions, secondary thrombosis, and arteriovenous fistulas.[9, 21] The intimal flap mechanism may play an important role in arterial stenosis[47]; occasionally, false aneurysms develop.[1] The development of post-traumatic pseudoaneurysm of the superficial temporal artery is a hazard of ice hockey puck injuries sustained in the absence of protective head gear.[59] We are also aware

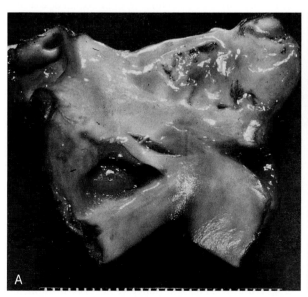

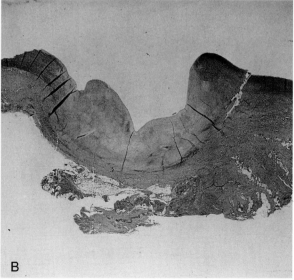

Figure 18-21 • *A,* Post-traumatic innominate arterial aneurysm associated with transverse intimomedial tears resulting from steering wheel injury of chest 10 months previously. *B,* Longitudinal histologic section through aneurysm showing intact adventitia and myointimal repair tissue partially filling the defect. (Hematoxylin, phloxine, and saffron stains.)

Illustration continued on next page

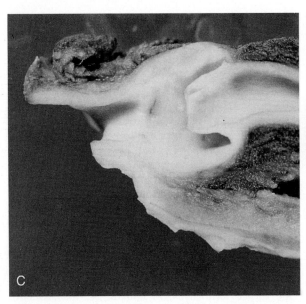

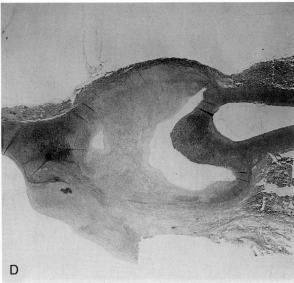

Figure 18-21 • *Continued. C,* Post-traumatic aneurysm involving innominate bifurcation and proximal common carotid artery discovered 4 months after steering wheel injury. The projecting intimal flap or shelf, caused by limited dissection, may result in obstruction to blood flow and secondary thrombosis. *D,* Low-power histologic section of aneurysm showing the dark intimomedial flap of the original vessel wall and the lightly textured myointimal repair tissue partially filling the sac. (Verhoeff–van Gieson.) (From Heggtveit HA, Campbell JS, Hooper GD: Innominate arterial aneurysms occurring after blunt trauma. Am J Clin Pathol 42:69, 1964.)

of occurrence of this injury in kick boxers (personal communication, Dr. J. Butany). Nonpenetrating or crush injuries of the abdomen may damage mesenteric arteries and veins. Instead of severe bleeding, the vessels may thrombose, resulting in infarction and subsequent perforation of the bowel.[60] Thrombosis of veins in the axilla or upper arm as a result of pressure, for example of one person's head against another's axilla during sleep (Fig. 18-22), or in alcoholics after a "bender" has been recognized.[61]

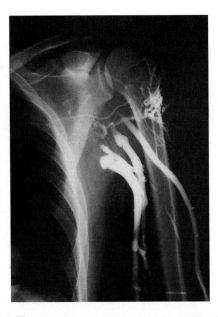

Figure 18-22 • Venogram from a previously healthy 23-year-old man who slept with his girlfriend's head on his left shoulder and awoke the next morning with marked swelling of that arm. Note extensive thrombotic occlusion of vessels in left upper arm. (From Silver MD: Man-made cardiovascular disease. Ann R Coll Phys Surg Can 16:533, 1983.)

IATROGENIC INJURY

Operative Injury

Operative injury to blood vessels, although uncommon during general surgical and orthopedic procedures, must be recognized and treated if permanent sequelae are to be avoided.[62] They may occur during a variety of procedures but are more often encountered during particularly difficult or complicated operations (Fig. 18-23). Cardiovascular surgery carries an inherent risk of damage when the heart and vascular structures are approached and manipulated directly. Penetrating wounds or vascular cross-clamp injuries may manifest as early or delayed bleeding or later as aneurysmal dilations. Black and colleagues[63] described 50 vascular injuries in 45 patients after cardiac valve replacement over a 10-year period. Lesions of the aorta were most common, and coronary and femoral arteries were damaged less frequently. The injuries included stenosis or occlusion (17 patients), laceration or perforation (16), dissecting aneurysm (13), and false aneurysm (4). Nine patients had injuries caused by surgical clamps, and 12 injuries were caused by sutures. Tearing of the aortic root from the base of the heart occurred in five patients. Inadvertent coronary ligation is apt to occur during emergency attempts to control major intraoperative bleeding, and the left circumflex coronary artery is at special risk during mitral valve replacement. Transverse lacerations, dissections, and small saccular aneurysms may develop in the proximal aorta at sites of cannulation (Fig. 18-24) or needle puncture or where aortic clamps were applied (see Fig. 18-23). Coronary ostial obstruction, resulting from intimal proliferation, may be a late result of coronary cannulation[64] or high-perfusion pressures that distend the proximal coronary arteries during

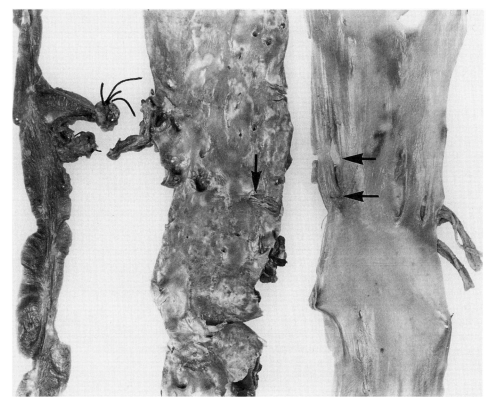

Figure 18-23 • Operative vascular injuries in a 64-year-old woman undergoing left nephrectomy for a large renal cell carcinoma. Massive hemorrhage occurred during the operation, and the patient died 2 days later from continued bleeding and ischemic infarction of liver, spleen, and stomach. The celiac artery was clipped and ligated (at left, with silk ligature); several small transverse intimomedial cross-clamp tears were present in the aorta (center, arrow); and a vertical, partially sutured 2-cm laceration was found in the inferior vena cava (right, arrows).

surgery.[65] Vascular grafts, particularly those used for vascular access,[66, 67] may be damaged or become infected, resulting in thrombosis, aneurysm, or rupture (Fig. 18-25).

Ventriculotomy sites represent penetrating wounds with the additional factor of ischemic necrosis at their margins as a consequence of incision or suture obliteration of subtending blood vessels.[68] False aneurysms develop at such points of injury.[69] Damage to components of the cardiac conduction system is a special hazard in surgical correction of congenital heart defects (see Chapter 20).[68] As increasing numbers of patients undergo a second or third cardiac operation, it is apparent that repeat median sternotomy is an especially hazardous procedure.[70, 71] If the pericardial sac has been left open after

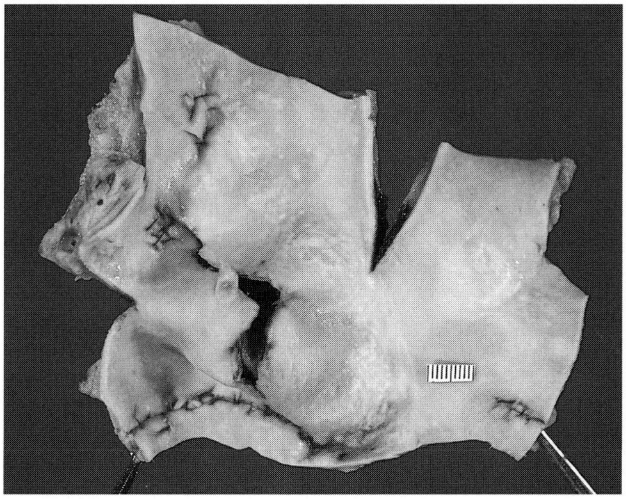

Figure 18-24 • Intimomedial tear and dissection of ascending aorta beginning at cannulation site. Proximally, the dissection stopped at the sutured aortotomy wound and ruptured externally into the pericardial sac, causing massive hemopericardium 10 days after aortic valve replacement. Histologically, there was mild cystic medionecrosis of the aorta.

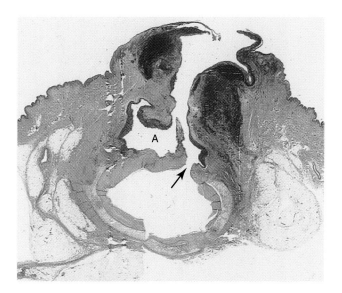

Figure 18-25 • This 30-year-old woman with end-stage diabetic renal disease was receiving hemodialysis. Exsanguination was caused by perforation of the vascular access graft of her left arm. There was recent infection of the graft, for which she had been treated and discharged from the hospital. Note site of graft disruption (arrow) with false aneurysm (A), hemorrhage around rupture tract (H), and external rupture through skin. (Masson trichrome stain.) (Courtesy of D.E.L. King, MD, Hamilton, Ontario.)

surgery, the heart becomes closely bound to the posterior surface of the sternum. Penetrating wounds of the great vessels, right atrium, or right ventricle may occur on reopening of the sternum or on subsequent blunt dissection to free the heart from encasing adhesions. Although the closed pericardial sac may become largely obliterated by fibrous adhesions, it serves as a cleavage plane that facilitates separation from the sternum. Therefore, the complications of pericardial tamponade or constriction from postoperative closure of the pericardium are probably less than the risks of repeat sternotomy when the pericardium has been left open at initial operation.[71]

Cardiac Massage

A wide range of cardiac injuries occur secondary to open- or closed-chest cardiac massage. Adelson documented the anatomic changes in the hearts of 60 patients who died during or after open-chest cardiac massage.[72] Manual massage can injure any or all cardiac tissues and gross laceration of the heart may occur in 10% of cases (Fig. 18-26). Closed-chest resuscitation may produce, in addition to cardiac contusions, traumatic rupture of the aorta or right ventricular structures from sternal compression.[73-75]

In a series of 705 autopsies on persons undergoing prehospital cardiac resuscitation, 42.7% were found to have thoracic complications (rib and sternal fractures, mediastinal hematomas); 30.8% had abdominal visceral complications; 13% had pulmonary complications; and only 0.5% displayed heart and great vessel trauma.[76] Among 130 hospitalized patients who died after cardiopulmonary resuscitation, 21% had major complications, including 8%

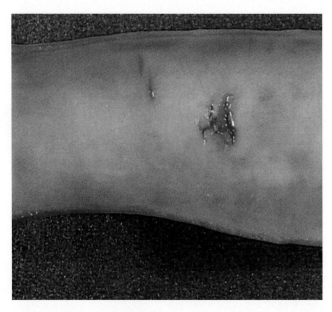

Figure 18-27 • Carotid angiogram puncture site in a young adult. Note two small, nonperforating intimal tears on opposite wall just above point of entry.

with cardiac laceration or hemorrhage[77]; all of the latter group had pericardiocentesis or placement of a transvenous pacemaker during attempted cardiopulmonary resuscitation. Subepicardial contraction-band necrosis of myocytes in the anterior or posterior myocardial wall is a common postmortem finding in patients who underwent cardiac massage before death.

Catheters and Cannulas

The use of a wide range of intravascular catheters, cannulas, and other invasive instruments for diagnosis and therapy is routine in medical and surgical wards. All vascular cannulations involve a penetrating wound of the vessel at the point of insertion (Fig. 18-27) and the possibility of further trauma as the catheter is advanced within the lumen (Table 18-4).

Polyethylene Catheters

Catheter embolization to the heart or pulmonary arteries is a well-recognized complication of intravenous fluid therapy using polyethylene tubing. This may result from disengagement of the catheter from the needle during administration of fluid or from severing of the tubing

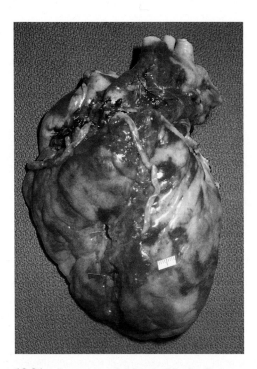

Figure 18-26 • Lacerations of right ventricle, focally transmural (arrowheads), in a 68-year-old patient, sustained during resuscitation attempts. Patient had had recent aortocoronary saphenous vein bypass grafting. The chest was reopened because of bleeding from the site of a slipped ligature on a branch of the venous graft.

TABLE 18-4 • **Complications of Catheterization and Cannulation**

Local bleeding
Mural tears or contusion
Intimal flaps
Thrombi, mural or occlusive
Emboli—thrombotic, atheromatous, foreign body
Intramural dissection
Aneurysms
Infection—local, systemic, endocarditis
Entrapment or entanglement
Damage to remote structures—contusion, laceration, perforation

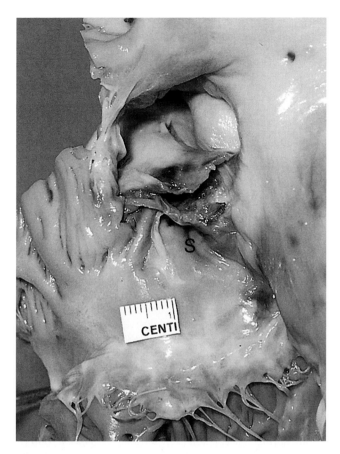

Figure 18-28 • Cannulation tip injury sustained by a 77-year-old woman who had recently undergone cardiac surgery with repeat sternotomy and evacuation of right pleural hematoma. There is an irregular endomyocardial tear in the right atrium, just superior to the ostium of the coronary sinus (S). The site corresponds to injury sustained from the tip of a right atrial cannula inserted for cardiopulmonary bypass.

by the needle through which the catheter was introduced.[78] Although much less common with current methods, catheter loss into the venous circulation sometimes occurs as a result of faulty bonding of the catheter shaft to the hub.[79] Embolization of polyethylene catheter fragments[80] or silicone rubber ventriculoatrial shunt tubing[81] has caused myocardial perforation and cardiac tamponade. Even intact indwelling polyethylene catheters of various types can perforate the right atrium (Fig. 18-28) or ventricle, causing fatal cardiac tamponade from hemopericardium[82-84] or intrapericardial infusion of intravenous fluid.[85-87]

Central Venous Lines

The ubiquitous insertion of central venous pressure (CVP) lines via subclavian and internal jugular veins is fraught with hazards ranging from simple knotting[88] and thrombosis to perforation of the heart and lethal tamponade.[82, 84, 86] Catheter-associated infections remain an important cause of nosocomial infection.[89] In a prospective study of 141 autopsies on patients with indwelling right-sided heart catheters,[90] 3 deaths were attributable to catheter use, 2 to perforation. Twelve (29%) of 42 patients with central venous catheters exhibited mural thrombi in the right side of the heart. Perforation of the dome of the

right pleural cavity with resultant hemothorax or hydrothorax has been seen on a number of occasions. It is not generally appreciated that the large veins of the neck are thin-walled, delicate structures with a network of venous valves at the junction of subclavian and jugular veins. These may snare or misdirect a CVP line or guide, leading to perforation of the vessel wall (Fig. 18-29).

Swan-Ganz Catheters

Balloon-tipped, flow-directed, Swan-Ganz catheters have been associated with cardiac arrhythmias[91, 92] and may become snared or entangled in the heart.[93] Tricuspid and pulmonary valve injury with insufficiency have been reported,[94, 95] as well as perforation of the pulmonary artery[96, 97]; however, minor pulmonary valve contusion is more frequent (Fig. 18-30). Other complications of these commonly employed devices include pulmonary thromboembolism and infarction, balloon rupture, catheter knotting, and infection.[92, 98] In one study, 33% of 99 patients with indwelling pulmonary arterial catheters had mural thrombi in the right side of the heart at autopsy.[90] We find a high incidence of mural or occlusive thrombi due to endothelial damage along the course of veins traversed by these catheters (Fig. 18-31). The incidence and severity of such venous thrombosis are directly proportional to the number of catheters passed, the degree of right-sided heart failure, and the duration of catheterization. The inferior vena cava virtually always exhibits mural thrombi

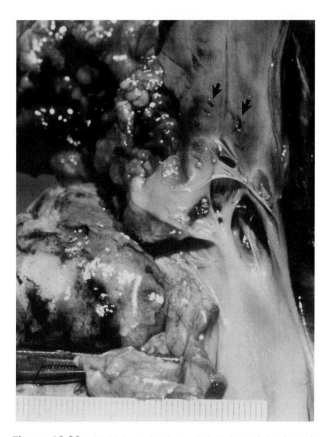

Figure 18-29 • Multiple perforations of right internal jugular vein (arrows) induced during insertion of central venous pressure line. The subclavian artery and the dome of the pleural cavity were also perforated, resulting in fatal hemothorax.

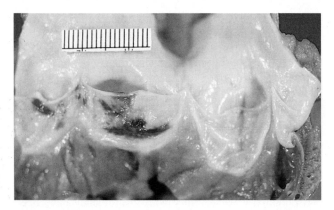

Figure 18-30 • Contusions and superficial thrombus on pulmonary valve after passage of a Swan-Ganz catheter.

when catheters have been inserted via the femoral veins in patients with congestive cardiac failure. Intimal injury and stasis both play a major role in their pathogenesis. In a critical assessment of the procedure, Robin[99] suggested that as many as 8% of patients with acute myocardial infarction die as a result of complications from pulmonary arterial catheterization; he called for a moratorium on their use. He expressed the belief that the information gained from the procedure does not justify the associated high morbidity and mortality.

Aortography and Angiography

Arterial trauma secondary to diagnostic procedures frequently involves a vessel at the point of vascular invasion or cannulation.[20, 100] Lacerations, stenoses, thromboses, false aneurysms, and arteriovenous fistulas occur locally and are usually amenable to surgical correction.[20, 100] Aortographic injection of contrast material may produce vasospasm with depression of renal function,[101] and intramural aortic dissection is a hazard of transfemoral or translumbar aortography.[102] Complications of peripheral angiography have been described by Nunn (Table 18-5).[103]

TABLE 18-5 • Complications of Peripheral Angiography

Reactions to contrast media (much less likely with nonionic media)
Vasovagal response to arterial puncture
Local hemorrhage
Local vein and nerve injuries
Subintimal injection of contrast material
Arterial thromboembolism
Intravascular injection of foreign material
Catheter and guidewire breakage, knots, kinks, and creation of false channels
Infection, localized or generalized

Intra-aortic Balloons

Intra-aortic balloon counterpulsation employed to treat cardiogenic shock may be associated with a higher frequency of complications than that predicted from purely clinical studies.[104] Most necropsy patients with counterpulsation devices inserted exhibit major or minor vascular injury. Damage ranges from small aortic intimal contusions, tears, and mural thrombi to extensive aortoiliac lacerations, dissections, and occlusive thrombi in iliac or femoral arteries (Figs. 18-32 and 18-33). Intramural dissection begins in the common iliac artery as it curves over the pelvic brim. Usually, the balloon catheter re-enters the aortic true lumen before reaching the upper abdominal segment. Soft atheromatous plaques also serve to divert the balloon intramurally and initiate dissection. Such retrograde re-entry dissections are more likely to occur during intraoperative insertion of balloon pumps without fluoroscopic guidance. Secondary ischemic changes in the lower extremities and spinal cord are not uncommon. Dissections have been encountered with both surgically installed and percutaneously inserted devices. Intraoperative insertion of balloon pumps through the ascending aorta has led to balloon-tip occlusion of the superior mesenteric artery with ischemic necrosis of the bowel or to stroke caused by occlusion of carotid arteries.

Coronary Angiography

The complication rate of coronary angiography is generally low in institutions where a large volume of case

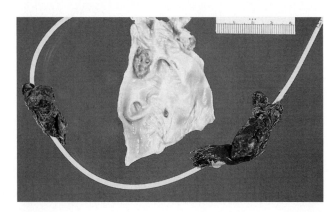

Figure 18-31 • Mural thrombi in the right internal jugular vein and on Swan-Ganz catheter in a patient who died after aortic valve replacement.

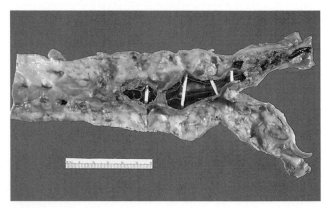

Figure 18-32 • Laceration and disruption of lower abdominal aorta and right common iliac artery by intra-aortic balloon inserted via right femoral artery in a patient with left ventricular failure at the end of coronary bypass surgery.

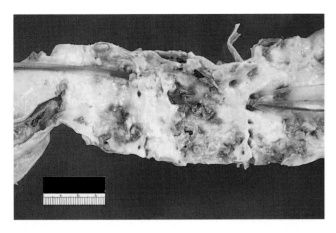

Figure 18-33 • Re-entry dissection of the abdominal aorta after placement of an intra-aortic balloon pump when the patient could not be weaned from cardiopulmonary bypass. The balloon tip burrowed into an atheromatous plaque and re-emerged in the true lumen at the ostium of the superior mesenteric artery. Ischemic bowel was found at autopsy.

material is studied[105-107] and higher in those where smaller groups of patients are investigated.[106, 108-110] As is the case with other angioinvasive procedures, thrombosis and distal thromboembolism may result from injury at entry sites.[1, 106] Sones,[107] reviewing his vast experience, found 39 deaths (0.07%). The most common complications were brachial artery occlusion, which occurred in 2.8%, and ventricular arrhythmias, which were seen in 0.82%. Other, less common sequelae included acute myocardial infarction, coronary artery dissection, coronary or cerebral emboli, and left ventricular perforation. Guss and coworkers[105] found 12 coronary dissections or embolizations among 2981 patients. There were significantly fewer coronary occlusions after the Sones brachial artery approach (0.19%), compared with the Judkins transfemoral technique (0.88%). In a study of 3044 coronary angiograms from 19 cooperating hospitals, Takaro and colleagues[108] reported 66 deaths (2.1%), the greater proportion when the transfemoral route was used. In a small series of patients, de la Torre and coworkers[111] found a relatively high incidence of coronary thromboemboli (4%) after switching from the transbrachial to the transfemoral approach; their six cases involved the left main coronary artery or one of its branches. It has been suggested that the left coronary system is the site of predilection for coronary thromboemboli occurring during transfemoral coronary arteriography.[112] Also, thrombus forming on a catheter may be wiped off on the vessel wall during removal and picked up on the tip of a second catheter when it is inserted over the retained guidewire.[108] We believe that there is a greater risk of picking up fragments of damaged endothelium, atheromatous debris, or mural thrombi from the aorta or iliofemoral vessels when catheters are introduced from below. Skeletal muscle coronary embolism is a less common complication of coronary angiography.[113] Coronary ostial stenosis due to intimal proliferation and atherosclerosis has been reported as a long-term complication of coronary angiography[114]; presumably, it represents a reparative response to endothelial injury induced during the procedure.

Angiocardiography

The passage of catheters through the left and right sides of the heart during angiocardiography may also induce perforating wounds[86, 115, 116] that may, in turn, cause hemopericardium or transmyocardial extravasation of contrast material, with resultant cardiac tamponade.[117] Exploration of the heart with semirigid catheters is more likely to cause intracardiac perforation, particularly in infants and children.[115] When this procedure was instituted in the 1960s, one of us (H.A.H.) observed three instances of fatal cardiac tamponade caused by right atrial perforation during angiocardiography in newborns. Atrial perforations are more serious because there is a tendency to tear the chamber wall, as opposed to a "clean" ventricular penetration.[116] Where myocardium is sparse or virtually absent, such as between pectinate muscles of the right atrium, in areas of fatty infiltration of the right ventricular wall, or wherever the chamber is abnormally thin, there is a greater tendency for continued bleeding with tamponade. The heart is probably perforated more frequently than is generally recognized, but seldom does this cause serious complication.[116] Infective endocarditis is a rare complication of right- and left-sided heart catheterization.[118] Morton and associates[119] reported an overall mortality rate of 0.1% in a series of 30,838 patients undergoing left- and right-sided cardiac catheterization and coronary angiography. Of 32 deaths, 6 were related to vascular complications of the procedure—coronary artery dissection (1), CVP-related hemothorax (1), and local femoral artery–related complications (4). The remaining deaths were attributable to high-grade left main or triple-vessel coronary artery disease.

MISCELLANEOUS FORMS OF INJURY

Variable degrees of damage to the heart and/or blood vessels result from radiation, electrical injury, lightning, burns and hyperthermia, hypothermia, carbon monoxide poisoning, barotrauma, and occupational injury of repetitive nature.

Radiation

Despite refinements in the radiotherapeutic management of lymphoma and other neoplasms, inadvertent damage to heart and blood vessels has been reported. Pericarditis is most commonly observed, but pancarditis may occur. Pericardial injury may manifest as acute nonspecific pericarditis during the course of radiation. It resolves rapidly but, more often months or years later, a delayed pericarditis (acute or chronic with effusion) with or without tamponade develops. There is pericardial fibrosis with fibrinous exudate (Fig. 18-34) and, in some cases, late constrictive pericarditis.[120, 121] Radiation-induced myocardial fibrosis is thought to result from injury to capillary endothelial cells that causes destruction or obstruction of capillaries and compromised microcirculation.[120] Such fibrosis may produce a cardiomyopathy. Focal endocardial fibrosis occurs, and cardiac valves may exhibit fibrous thickenings of leaflet or chordae.[120, 122] Radiation-induced

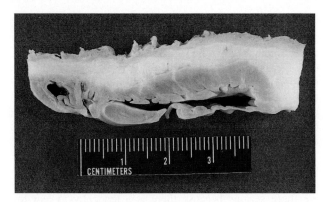

Figure 18-34 • Organizing fibrinous pericarditis and pericardial fibrosis in an elderly man who received radiotherapy for carcinoma of the esophagus.

coronary artery disease has been associated with myocardial infarction. Coronary lesions include the induction of bizarre fibroblasts, myointimal hyperplasia with luminal narrowing, encroachment on media, and fibrosis of media and adventitia.[123] Stewart and associates,[120] however, consider the morphology of radiation-induced coronary artery disease to be similar to that of spontaneous, albeit accelerated, atherosclerosis.

In the acute phase of vascular injury, radiation causes endothelial damage, with increased permeability of arterioles, venules, and capillaries. Medial necrosis, which may be fibrinoid, occurs in small arteries, and there are rare cases of necrotizing aortitis and rupture of major vessels.[124] Thrombosis may occur. In the chronic phase, there is intimal hyperplasia; larger vessels may exhibit mural and adventitial fibrosis, occasionally with complete fibrous occlusion. The aorta, in fields of radiation, may loose all nuclear structures and its wall may then condense, showing fibrous tissue and elastic lamellae only (M. D. Silver, personal communication). Amyloid deposition has been noted.[125] There is a predisposition to accelerated atherosclerosis and periarterial fibrosis as a late complication.[126] Vascular changes are the main site of injury in radiation bowel disease.[127]

Lightning

Death caused by lightning is rare, but when it does occur, it is usually immediate, with ventricular asystole resulting from depolarization of the myocardium due to very-high-voltage direct current. In some cases, other cardiac arrhythmias such as ventricular fibrillation occur.[128] Microscopic changes, with widespread contraction bands and disruption of myocytes, have been reported (Fig. 18-35). In survivors, myocardial injury resembling that of ischemia or infarction can occur. It is suggested that true vascular occlusion (possibly spasm) may be precipitated by "stress" in patients with coronary artery disease or by contusion of the myocardium secondary to lightning shock.[129] Wetli[130] documented gross and histologic features of myocardial contusion in three deaths that occurred 10.5 hours to 3 days after lightning strike. He also

noted aortic abnormalities in three patients with hemoglobin staining of aortic intima and horizontally arranged "creases," which apparently represented medial defects. Two other patients had microscopic separation of intima from media.

Other Forms of Electrical Injury

In cases of accidental electrocution, widespread focal necrosis involving the myocardium and the sinus and atrioventricular nodes, as well as contraction band necrosis of smooth muscle cells in the media of coronary arteries, has been noted.[131] High-voltage electrical injury produces manifestations similar to lightning, and myocardial injury resembling infarction or reperfusion-type injury has been documented.[132] Low-voltage alternating current is more dangerous than the corresponding direct current and causes death by ventricular fibrillation or respiratory arrest. Echocardiographic observations suggest that left ventricular dysfunction of variable degree persists in survivors of electrical injury.[133]

Vascular thromboses, mainly but not exclusively venous, may be seen in the vicinity of electrical burns. They are induced thermally or, in some cases, may be voltage dependent. There is necrosis of the intima and media of blood vessels with occasional rupture, focal hemorrhage or thrombosis, and subsequent reactive inflammatory response.[134, 135]

Attempts at cardioversion, where there is transthoracic administration of direct current with cardiac defibrillators, have produced small, sharply localized foci of myocyte necrosis in experimental animals. These have subsequently progressed to fibrous scar.[136] Similarly, catheter ablation (whether by direct current or radio frequency) used to treat arrhythmia produces variably sized foci of myocardial necrosis in the region of the conduction system.[137] (See Chapter 20 also.)

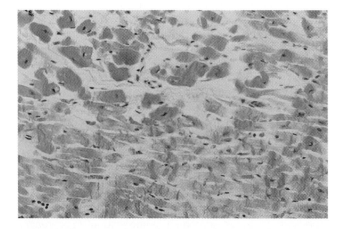

Figure 18-35 • Photomicrograph of section of left ventricle of a 19-year-old baseball player who was struck by lightning and was unresponsive to immediate cardiopulmonary resuscitation. Note prominent disruption of cardiac myocytes and contraction bands. (H&E stain.) (Courtesy of D.E.L. King, MD, Hamilton, Ontario.)

Burns and Hyperthermia

In cases of burn, although the seriousness of injury depends on the extent of burn and other associated factors, there is endothelial injury leading to vascular dilation and proteinaceous fluid exudation with an associated inflammatory reaction. Edema and petechial hemorrhages in various organs are frequently present in those who die rapidly[138]; congestive heart failure occurs in those who survive for longer periods (up to 91 days).[139] In the latter group, moderate cardiomegaly with microscopic foci of myocardial necrosis and inflammation (predominantly mononuclear) have been documented.[139] Sudden death associated with generalized microcirculatory thrombosis has been reported 3 days after adequately treated moderate burns in a 3-year-old child.[140] In burn cases, particularly those associated with shock, venous thrombosis and, less often, arterial thrombosis may occur. Coronary thrombosis with associated myocardial infarct has been described.[141] In a few cases, mural thrombus, endocardial thickening, or focal interstitial fibrosis has been found.[139]

Systemic hyperthermia or heat stroke, associated with an excessive rise of the temperature of circulating blood (to more than 40°C), results in generalized vascular and cardiac dilation.[142] Although autopsy findings in fatal cases are nonspecific, disseminated intravascular coagulation and contraction-band necrosis of myocardium have been recorded.[61]

Hypothermia

Depending on the severity and rapidity of the hypothermic insult, direct tissue injury as well as vasoconstriction may occur, in association with sludging, thrombosis, and resultant ischemic necrosis of tissues. This may be observed in the local freezing hypothermia of frostbite.[142, 142a] Likewise, in severe systemic hypothermia with whole body exposure, sludging of blood in peripheral and central vessels, partly from cold agglutinins, contributes to skin edema and necrosis and to microinfarcts in many organs. Deep vein thrombosis has been found on occasion.[143] Edematous changes are typical in slowly developing, non-freezing hypothermia, such as occurs in "trench foot" or in the phase of rewarming.[142] Frost-bitten skin exhibits markedly dilated and blood-filled capillaries in the superficial dermis, often associated with edema.[144] The late effects of local hypothermia are variable, but organization of the edema fluid could result in atrophy and fibrosis.[142] Death in severe hypothermia is attributable to central and peripheral circulatory failure. Although necropsy findings may be scarce, foci of cardiac myocyte fragmentation and degenerative change have been documented in fatal cases.[145]

Drowning

Although there is frequently a paucity of findings in immersed bodies, Lunt and Rose[146] noted smooth muscle contraction bands in the media of major coronary arteries, as well as increased eosinophilia and contraction-band necrosis of cardiac myocytes, in a significant proportion of cases, suggesting association with a "sympathetic storm" producing both coronary arterial spasm and myocyte injury. Diatoms, if present in the water, may be found in small intramyocardial vessels.

Carbon Monoxide Poisoning and Barotrauma

Foci of myocardial necrosis have been noted in both acute and delayed deaths resulting from carbon monoxide poisoning.[147] They can progress to myocardial fibrosis in survivors.

Barotrauma (decompression sickness, caisson disease) may be associated with air/gas or fat/bone marrow emboli that can involve the myocardium. The cardiac chambers, particularly on the right side, may be distended with air. Small foci of myocardial necrosis and disseminated intravascular coagulation have been observed.[148]

Repetitive Occupational Injury

Vibrating tool disease (vibration white finger or Raynaud phenomenon of occupational origin), first recognized in the early 1950s, may well depend not only on mechanical factors related to the vibrating tool in use but also on individual sensitivity and susceptibility.[149] Manifested by periodic ischemic attacks of the fingers, it can also affect neurologic, musculoskeletal, and osseous systems. There is controversy as to whether the initial injury is that of a vasospasm and subsequent medial muscular hypertrophy[150] or whether there is primary arterial endothelial injury with intimal thickening and thrombosis in addition to medial hypertrophy and fibrosis.[151] The affect is cumulative and can ultimately lead to necrosis/gangrene of the fingertips. The single objective test is that of cold provocation. In advanced stages, because the effects are cumulative, the changes are irreversible even if the patient is withdrawn from exposure. If exposed to vibration, similar changes can occur in the lower limbs.[149]

Chronic repetitive vascular injuries can result in thrombosis with embolism and aneurysm of the axillary and brachial arteries, for example, with prolonged use of crutches, cervical ribs, anomalous fibrous bands, compression of the axillary artery by the head of the humerus, or compression of the thoracic outlet while pitching ball. Axillary artery tears and thrombosis (in baseball pitchers), thrombosis of digital arteries (in the catching hand of baseball and handball participants), and thrombosis and aneurysm of the ulnar artery (in the dominant hand used as a mallet or with jackhammer use) have been documented.[149, 152] Similarly, popliteal artery thrombosis may result from repeated minor injuries. Incidentally, myointimal hyperplasia has been reported in the external iliac arteries of bicycle racers.[153] The so-called "effort or stress thrombosis" refers to thrombosis of axillary or subclavian vein resulting from occupational trauma or unusual exercise, although it may also occur in thoracic outlet or costoclavicular syndrome.[154] In some instances, organization of such thrombi may be associated with an exuberant intravascular papillary endothelial hyperplasia which should not be mistaken for a neoplasm.

REFERENCES

1. Rich NM, Spencer FC: Vascular Trauma. Philadelphia, WB Saunders, 1978
2. Symbas PN: Cardiac trauma. Am Heart J 92:387, 1976
3. Symbas PN: Great vessels injury. Am Heart J 93:518, 1977
4. Symbas PN: Cardiothoracic Trauma. Philadelphia, WB Saunders, 1989
5. De Sanctis RW: Trauma of the heart and great vessels. Sci Am Med 16:1, 1993
6. Gould SE (ed): Pathology of the Heart and Blood Vessels. 3rd ed. Springfield, IL, Charles C Thomas, 1968, p 834
7. Hudson RE: Cardiovascular Pathology. Vol 2. London, Edward Arnold, 1965, p 1604
8. Asfaw I, Arbulu A: Penetrating wounds of the pericardium and heart. Surg Clin North Am 57:37, 1977
9. Rich NM: Vascular trauma. Surg Clin North Am 53:1367, 1973
10. Parmley LF, Symbas PN: Traumatic heart disease. In: Hurst JW (ed): The Heart. Vol 2. New York, McGraw-Hill, 1978, p 1683
11. Rayner AV, Fulton RL, Hess PJ, Daicoff GR: Post-traumatic intracardiac shunts: Report of two cases and review of the literature. J Thorac Cardiovasc Surg 73:728, 1977
12. Thandroyen FT, Matisonn RE: Penetrating thoracic trauma producing cardiac shunts. J Thorac Cardiovasc Surg 81:569, 1981
13. Alter BR, Whelling JR, Martin HA, et al: Traumatic right coronary artery-right ventricular fistula with retained intramyocardial bullet. Am J Cardiol 40:815, 1977
14. Orlick AE, Hultgren HN, Stoner JD, et al: Traumatic pulmonary artery–left atrial fistula: An unusual case of cyanosis in an adult. Am Heart J 98:366, 1979
15. Hermoni Y, Engel PJ, Gallant TE: Sequelae of injury to the heart caused by multiple needles. J Am Coll Cardiol 8:1226, 1986
16. Pate JW, Richarson RL: Penetrating wounds of cardiac valves. JAMA 207:309, 1969
17. Killen DA, Gobbel WG, France R, Vix VA: Post-traumatic aneurysm of the left ventricle. Circulation 39:101, 1969
18. Ward PA, Suzuki A: Gunshot wound of the heart with peripheral embolization. J Thorac Cardiovasc Surg 68:440, 1974
19. Silverman EM, Littler ER: Bullet in the left ventricle from a remote gunshot wound to the heart. Chest 71:234, 1977
20. Rich NM, Hobson RW, Fedde CW: Vascular trauma secondary to diagnostic and therapeutic procedures. Am J Surg 128:715, 1974
21. Burnett HF, Parnell CL, Williams GD, Campbell GJ: Peripheral arterial injuries: A reassessment. Ann Surg 183:701, 1976
22. Liedtke AJ, DeMuth WE: Nonpenetrating cardiac injuries: A collective review. Am Heart J 86:687, 1973
23. Tenzer ML: The spectrum of myocardial contusion: A review. J Trauma 25;620, 1985
24. Rubio-Alvarez J, Fuster-Siebert F, Calzadilla-Martin G, et al: Traumatic rupture of the pericardium: Report of two cases with unusual features. Tex Heart Inst J 10:77, 1983
25. Abrunzo TJ: Commotio cordis: The single, most common cause of traumatic death in youth baseball. Am J Dis Child 145:1279, 1991
26. Maron BJ, Poliac LC, Kaplan JA, Mueller FO: Blunt impact to the chest leading to sudden death from cardiac arrest during sports activities. N Engl J Med 333:337, 1995
27. Jones FL: Transmural myocardial necrosis after nonpenetrating cardiac trauma. Am J Cardiol 26:419, 1970
28. Long WA, Willis IV PW, Henry GW: Childhood traumatic infarction causing left ventricular aneurysm: Diagnosis by two-dimensional echocardiography. J Am Coll Cardiol 5:1478, 1985
29. Bloch B, Meir J: Isolated traumatic tears of the intraventricular septum. Forensic Sci 9:81, 1977
30. Stephenson LW, MacVaugh H, Kastor JA: Tricuspid valvular incompetence and rupture of the ventricular septum caused by nonpenetrating trauma. J Thorac Cardiovasc Surg 77:768, 1979
31. Stinson EB, Rowles DF, Shumway NE: Repair of right ventricular aneurysm and ventricular septal defect caused by nonpenetrating cardiac trauma. Surgery 64:1022, 1968
32. DeSa'Neto A, Padnick MB, Desser KB, Steinhoff NG: Right sinus

of Valsalva-right atrial fistula secondary to nonpenetrating chest trauma: A case report with description of noninvasive diagnostic features. Circulation 60:205, 1979
33. Kohli S, Saperia GM, Waksmonski CA, et al: Coronary artery dissection secondary to blunt chest trauma. Cathet Cardiovasc Diagn 15:179, 1988
34. Pifarre R, Grieco J, Garibaldi A, et al: Acute coronary artery occlusion secondary to blunt chest trauma. J Thorac Cardiovasc Surg 83:122, 1982
35. Jessurun GAJ, den Heijer P, May JF, Lie KI: Coronary angioscopy confirms the presence of red thrombus in acute myocardial infarction after blunt chest trauma. Am Heart J 131:1216, 1996
36. Heyndrickx G, Vermeire P, Goffin Y, Van den Bogaert P: Rupture of the right coronary artery due to nonpenetrating chest trauma. Chest 65:577, 1974
37. Dueholm S, Fabrin J: Isolated coronary artery rupture following blunt chest trauma: A case report. Scand J Thorac Cardiovasc Surg 20:183, 1986
38. Sareli P, Goldman AP, Pocock WA, et al: Coronary artery–right ventricular fistula and organic tricuspid regurgitation due to blunt chest trauma. Am J Cardiol 54:697, 1984
39. German DS, Shapiro MJ, Willman VL: Acute aortic valvular incompetence following blunt thoracic deceleration injury: Case report. J Trauma 30:1411, 1990
40. Gayet C, Pierre B, Delahaye JP, et al: Traumatic tricuspid insufficiency: An underdiagnosed disease. Chest 92:429, 1987
41. Reinfeld HB, Agatston AS, Robinson MJ, Hildner FJ: Bioprosthetic mitral valve dysfunction following blunt chest trauma. Am Heart J 111:800, 1986
42. Morgan MG, Glasser SP, Sanusi ID: Bacterial endocarditis: Occurrence on a traumatically ruptured aortic valve. JAMA 233:810, 1975
43. Charles KP, Davidson KG, Miller H, Caves PK: Traumatic rupture of the ascending aorta and aortic valve following blunt chest trauma. J Thorac Cardiovasc Surg 73:208, 1977
44. Cleveland JC, Cleveland RJ: Successful repair of aortic root and aortic valve injury caused by blunt chest trauma in a patient with prior aortic dissection. Chest 66:447, 1974
45. Aronson W: Aortic rupture after a minor fall in a patient with extreme cardiomegaly. JAMA 186:729, 1963
46. Allmendinger PD, Low HB, Takata H, et al: Deceleration injury: Laceration of the thoracic aorta. Am J Surg 133:490, 1977
47. Hare RR, Gaspar MR: The intimal flap. Arch Surg 102:552, 1971
48. Koroxenidis GT, Moschos CB, Landy ED, et al: Traumatic rupture of the thoracic aorta simulating coarctation. Am J Cardiol 16:605, 1965
49. Sloop RD, Robertson KA: Nonpenetrating trauma of the abdominal aorta with partial vessel occlusion: Report of two cases. Am Surg 41:555, 1975
50. Dajee H, Richardson IW, Iype MO: Seat belt aorta: Acute dissection and thrombosis of the abdominal aorta. Surgery 85:263, 1979
51. Myles RA, Yellin AE: Traumatic injuries of the abdominal aorta. Am J Surg 138:273, 1979
52. Nizzero A, Miles JT: Blunt trauma to the abdominal aorta. Can Med Assoc J 135:219, 1986
52a. Bunai Y, Nagai A, Nakamura I, Ohya I: Traumatic rupture of an abdominal aortic aneurysm associated with the use of a seatbelt. J Forensic Sci 44:1304, 1999
53. Swanson SA, Gaffey MA: Traumatic false aneurysm of descending aorta with aortoesophageal fistula. J Forensic Sci 33:816, 1988
54. McCollum CH, Graham JM, Noon GP, DeBakey ME: Chronic traumatic aneurysms of the thoracic aorta: An analysis of 50 patients. J Trauma 19:248, 1979
55. Kinley CE, Chandler BM. Traumatic aneurysm of thoracic aorta: A case presenting as a coarctation. Can Med Assoc J 96:279, 1967
56. Sethi GK, Scott SM, Takaro T: False aneurysm of the abdominal aorta due to blunt trauma. Ann Surg 182:33, 1975
57. Heggtveit HA, Campbell JS, Hooper GD: Innominate arterial aneurysms occurring after blunt trauma. Am J Clin Pathol 42:69, 1964
58. Castagna J, Nelson RJ: Blunt injuries to branches of the aortic arch. J Thorac Cardiovasc Surg 69:521, 1975
59. Campbell JJ, Fournier P, Hill DP: Puck aneurysm. Can Med Assoc J 81:922, 1959

60. Knight B: Chest and abdominal injuries. In: Forensic Pathology. 2nd ed. New York, Oxford University Press, 1996, p 217

61. Silver MD: Man-made cardiovascular disease. Ann R Coll Phys Surg Can 16:533, 1983

62. Rich NM, Hobson II, RW, Fedde CW: Vascular trauma secondary to diagnostic and therapeutic procedures. Am J Surg 128:715, 1974

63. Black LL, McComb RJ, Silver MD: Vascular injury following heart valve replacement. Ann Thorac Surg 16:19, 1973

64. Chawla SK, Najafi H, Javid H, Serry C: Coronary obstruction secondary to direct cannulation. Ann Thorac Surg 23:135, 1977

65. Silver MD, Wigle ED, Trimble AJ, Bigelow WG: Iatrogenic coronary ostial stenosis. Arch Pathol 88:73, 1969

66. Raju S: PTFE grafts for hemodialysis access. Ann Surg 206:666, 1987

67. Eid A, Lyass S: Acute perigraft seroma simulating anastomotic bleeding of a PTFE graft applied as an arteriovenous shunt for hemodialysis. Ann Vasc Surg 10:290, 1996

68. Korns ME, Schwartz CJ, Edwards JE, Lillehei CW: Pathologic sequelae and complications of ventriculotomy. I. With special reference to the myocardium. Arch Pathol 88:269, 1969

69. Rittenhouse EA, Sauvage LR, Mansfield PB, et al: False aneurysm of the left ventricle: Report of four cases and review of surgical management. Ann Surg 189:409, 1979

70. Macmanus Q, Okies JE, Phillips SJ, Starr A: Surgical considerations in patients undergoing repeat median sternotomy. J Thorac Cardiovasc Surg 69:138, 1975

71. Asanza L, Rao G, Voleti C, et al: Should the pericardium be closed after an open-heart operation? Ann Thorac Surg 22:532, 1976

72. Adelson L: A clinicopathological study of the anatomic changes in the heart resulting from cardiac massage. Surg Gynecol Obstet 104:513, 1957

73. Nelson DA, Ashley PF: Rupture of the aorta during closed-chest cardiac massage. JAMA 193:681, 1965

74. Gerry JL Jr, Bulkley BH, Hutchins GM: Rupture of the papillary muscle of the tricuspid valve: A complication of cardiopulmonary resuscitation and a rare cause of tricuspid insufficiency. Am J Cardiol 40:825, 1977

75. Bodily K, Fischer RP: Aortic rupture and right ventricular rupture induced by closed chest cardiac massage. Minn Med 62:225, 1979

76. Krischer JP, Fine EG, Davis JH, Nagel EL: Complications of cardiac resuscitation. Chest 92:287, 1987

77. Bedell SE, Fulton EJ: Unexpected findings and complications at autopsy after cardiopulmonary resuscitation (CPR). Arch Intern Med 146:1725, 1986

78. Steiner ML, Bartley TD, Byers FM, Krovetz LJ: Polyethylene catheter in the heart: Report of a case with successful removal. JAMA 193:1054, 1965

79. Sprague DH, Sarwar H: Catheter embolization due to faulty bonding of catheter shaft to hub. Anaesthesiology 49:285, 1978

80. Johnson CE: Perforation of right atrium by a polyethylene catheter. JAMA 195:584, 1966

81. Dzenitis AJ, Mealey J, Waddell JR: Myocardial perforation by ventriculoatrial-shunt tubing. JAMA 194:1251, 1965

82. Dane TEB, King EG: Fatal cardiac tamponade and other mechanical complications of central venous catheters. Br J Surg 62:6, 1975

83. Iglesias A, Rufilanchas JJ, Maronas JM, Figuera D: Perforation of the right ventricle and cardiac tamponade caused by a venous catheter. Postgrad Med J 53:225, 1977

84. Collier PE, Goodman GB: Cardiac tamponade caused by central venous catheter perforation of the heart: A preventable complication. J Am Coll Surg 181:459, 1995

85. Friedman BA, Jurgelett HC: Perforation of atrium by polyethylene CV catheter (letter). JAMA 203:1141, 1968

86. Thomas CS, Carter JW, Lowder SC: Pericardial tamponade from central venous catheters. Arch Surg 98:217, 1969

87. Lamberti JJ: Serious complication of intracardiac catheters (letter). JAMA 231:463, 1975

88. McMichan JC, Michel L: Knotting of central venous catheters: Nonsurgical correction. Chest 74:572, 1978

89. Adal KA: Central venous catheter-related infections: A review. Nutrition 12:208, 1996

90. Ducatman BS, McMichan JC, Edwards WD: Catheter-induced lesions of the right side of the heart: A one-year prospective study of 141 autopsies. JAMA 253:791, 1985

91. Luck JC, Engel TR: Transient right bundle branch block with "Swan-Ganz" catheterization. Am Heart J 92:263, 1976

92. Nichols WW, Nichols MA, Barbour H: Complications associated with balloon-tipped, flow-directed catheters. Heart Lung 8:503, 1979

93. Block PC: Snaring of a Swan-Ganz catheter. J Thorac Cardiovasc Surg 71:917, 1976

94. Smith WR, Glauser FL, Jemison P: Ruptured chordae of the tricuspid valve: The consequences of flow-directed Swan-Ganz catheterization. Chest 70:790, 1976

95. Lindgren KM, McShane K, Roberts WC: Acute rupture of the pulmonic valve by a balloon-tipped catheter producing a musical diastolic murmur. Chest 81:251, 1982

96. Fraser RS: Catheter-induced pulmonary artery perforation. Hum Pathol 18:1246, 1987

97. Sekkal S, Cornu E, Christidès C, et al: Swan-Ganz catheter induced pulmonary artery perforation during cardiac surgery concerning two cases. J Cardiovasc Surg 37:313, 1996

98. Mermel LA, Maki DG: Infectious complications of Swan-Ganz pulmonary artery catheters. Am J Respir Crit Care Med 149:1020, 1994

99. Robin ED: Death by pulmonary artery flow-directed catheter: Time for a moratorium? (editorial). Chest 92:727, 1987

100. Bergentz SE, Bergqvist D: Injuries caused by diagnostic arterial catheterization or puncture. In: Iatrogenic Vascular Injuries. New York, Springer-Verlag, 1989, p 8

101. Beall AC, Crawford ES, Couves CM, et al: Complications of aortography. Surgery 43:364, 1958

102. Wolfman EF, Boblitt DE: Intramural aortic dissection as a complication of translumbar aortography. Arch Surg 78:629, 1959

103. Nunn DB: Complications of peripheral arteriography. Am J Surg 44:664, 1978

104. Isner JM, Cohen SR, Virmani R, et al: Complications of the intraaortic balloon counterpulsation device: Clinical and morphologic observations in 45 necropsy patients. Am J Cardiol 45:260, 1980

105. Guss SB, Zir LM, Garrison HB, et al: Coronary occlusion during coronary angiography. Circulation 52:1063, 1975

106. Bourassa MB, Noble J: Complication rate of coronary arteriography: A review of 5250 cases studied by a percutaneous femoral technique. Circulation 53:106, 1976

107. Sones FM Jr: Complications of coronary arteriography and left heart catheterization. Cleve Clin Q 45:21, 1978

108. Takaro T, Hultgren HN, Littman D, Wright EC: An analysis of deaths occurring in association with coronary angiography. Am Heart J 86:587, 1973

109. Nitter-Hauge S, Enge I: Complication rates of selective percutaneous transfemoral coronary arteriography: A review of 1094 consecutive examinations. Acta Med Scand 200:123, 1976

110. Morton BC, Beanlands DS: Complications of cardiac catheterization: One centre's experience. Can Med Assoc J 131:889, 1984

111. de la Torre A, Jacobs D, Aleman J, Anderson GA: Embolic coronary artery occlusion in percutaneous transfemoral coronary arteriography. Am Heart J 86:467, 1973

112. Hartveit F, Andersen KS, Maehle BO, Kalager T: Fatal coronary embolism due to thrombus detached from a coronary catheter: A case report. Acta Pathol Microbiol Immunol Scand [A] 248(suppl):95, 1974

113. McHenry MM, Lee J: Skeletal muscle coronary embolism: A complication of coronary angiography. Circulation 59:189, 1979

114. Knutson EL, Smith JC: Coronary ostial stenosis complicating coronary arteriography. Arch Pathol Lab Med 100:113, 1976

115. Krovetz LJ, Shanklin DR, Schiebler GL: Serious and fatal complications of catheterization and angiocardiography in infants and children. Am Heart J 76:39, 1968

116. Lawton RL, Rossi NP, Funk DC: Intracardiac perforation. Arch Surg 98:213, 1969

117. Nadimi M, Anagnostopoulos LD, Frank MJ: Cardiac tamponade after transmyocardial extravasation of contrast material. Am Heart J 72:369, 1966

118. Mason JW, Rossen RM, Colby T, Harrison DC: Bacterial endocarditis after cardiac catheterization. Chest 70:293, 1976

119. Morton BC, Higginson LAJ, Beanlands DS: Deaths in a catheterization laboratory. Can Med Assoc J 149:165, 1993
120. Stewart JR, Fajardo LF, Gillette SM, Constine LS: Radiation injury to the heart. Int J Radiat Oncol Biol Physiol 31:1205, 1995
121. Veinot JP, Edwards WD: Pathology of radiation-induced heart disease: A surgical and autopsy study of 27 cases. Hum Pathol 27:766, 1996
122. Arsenian MA: Cardiovascular sequelae of therapeutic thoracic radiation. Prog Cardiovasc Dis 33:299, 1991
123. Om A, Ellahham S, Vetrovec GW: Radiation-induced coronary artery disease. Am Heart J 124:1598, 1992
124. Fajardo LF, Lee A: Rupture of major vessels after radiation. Cancer 36:904, 1975
125. Stehbens WE: Thrombosis and Vascular Trauma. In: Stehbens WE, Lie JT (eds): Vascular Pathology. 1st ed. London, Chapman & Hall Medical, 1995, p 63
126. Butler MJ, Lane RHS, Webster JHH: Irradiation injury to large arteries. Br J Surg 67:341, 1980
127. Hasleton PS, Carr N, Schofield PF: Vascular changes in radiation bowel disease. Histopathology 9:517, 1985
128. King DEL: Deaths due to lightning strike: Case report and discussion of a well documented fatality. Can Soc Forens Sci J 29:213, 1996
129. Sinha AK: Lightning-induced myocardial injury: A case report with management. Angiology 36:327, 1985
130. Wetli CV: Keraunopathology. Am J Forensic Med Pathol 17:89, 1996
131. James TN, Riddick L, Embry JH: Cardiac abnormalities demonstrated postmortem in four cases of accidental electrocution and their potential significance relative to nonfatal electrical injuries of the heart. Am Heart J 120:143, 1990
132. Xenopoulos N, Movahed A, Hudson P, Reeves WC: Myocardial injury in electrocution. Am Heart J 122:1481, 1991
133. Homma S, Gillam LD, Weyman AE: Echocardiographic observations in survivors of acute electrical injury. Chest 97:103, 1990
134. Perper JA: Electrical injuries. In: Wecht C (ed): Legal Medicine Annual. New York, Appleton Century Crofts, 1977, p 135
135. Xuewei W, Wanrhong Z: Vascular injuries in electrical burns: The pathologic basis for mechanism of injury. Burns 9:335, 1983
136. Warner ED, Dahl C, Ewy GA: Myocardial injury from transthoracic defibrillator countershock. Arch Pathol 99:55, 1975
137. Huang SKS, Graham AR, Lee MA, et al: Comparison of catheter ablation using radiofrequency versus direct current energy: Biophysical, electrophysiologic and pathologic observations. J Am Coll Cardiol 18:1091, 1991
138. Argamaso RV: Pathology, mortality and prognosis of burns: A review of 54 critical and fatal cases. Can Med Assoc J 97:445, 1967
139. Joshi VV: Effects of burns on the heart: A clinicopathological study in children. JAMA 211:2130, 1970
140. Halleraker B: Microcirculatory thrombosis as a cause of death in thermal burns. Acta Chir Scand 138:731, 1972
141. Cole FM: Myocardial infarction after burns. Br Med J 2:1575, 1963
142. Hirsch CS, Zumwalt RE: Forensic pathology. In: Damjanov I, Linder J (eds): Anderson's Pathology. 10th ed. St. Louis, Mosby, 1996, p 80
142a. Thoma A, Rao J, Heggtveit HA: Treatment of the ischemic hand in frostbite by revascularization with interpositional vein graft and digital palmar sympathectomy: A case report. Can J Plast Surg 7:195, 1999
143. Knight B: Neglect, starvation and hypothermia. In: Forensic Pathology. 2nd ed. New York, Oxford University Press, 1996, p 407
144. Schoning P: Frozen cadaver: Antemortem versus postmortem. Am J Forensic Med Pathol 13:18, 1992
145. Hirvonen J: Necropsy findings in fatal hypothermia cases. Forensic Sci 8:155, 1976
146. Lunt DWR, Rose AG: Pathology of the human heart in drowning. Arch Pathol Lab Med 111:939, 1987
147. Knight B: Carbon monoxide poisoning. In: Forensic Pathology. 2nd ed. New York, Oxford University Press, 1996, p 551
148. Knight B: Dysbarism and barotrauma. In: Forensic Pathology. 2nd ed. New York, Oxford University Press, 1996, p 483
149. Stehbens WE: Thrombosis and vascular trauma. In: Stehbens WE, Lie JT (eds): Vascular Pathology. 1st ed. London, Chapman & Hall Medical, 1995, p 63
150. Takeuchi T, Futatsuka M, Imanishi H, Yamada S: Pathological changes observed in the finger biopsy of patients with vibration-induced white finger. Scand J Work Environ Health 12:280, 1986
151. Walton KW: The pathology of Raynaud's phenomenon of occupational origin. In: Taylor W (ed): The Vibration Syndrome. London, Academic Press, 1974, p 109
152. Von Kuster L, Abt AB: Traumatic aneurysms of the ulnar artery. Arch Pathol Lab Med 104:75, 1980
153. Chevalier JM, Enon B, Walder J, et al: Endofibrosis of the external iliac artery in bicycle racers: An unrecognized pathological state Ann Vasc Surg 1:297, 1986
154. Leu HJ, Lie JT: Diseases of the veins and lymphatic vessels, including angiodysplasias. In: Stehbens WE, Lie JT (eds): Vascular Pathology. 1st ed. London, Chapman & Hall Medical, 1995, p 489

Chapter 19

Tumors and Tumor-Like Conditions of the Heart

· · · · ·

Allen P. Burke • Renu Virmani

INCIDENCE AND CLASSIFICATION

Primary cardiac tumors are rare. They are found in only 0.01% of autopsies,[1] metastatic tumors being nearly 100 times more common. However, surgical resections of cardiac tumors are usually performed for primary lesions, so that the surgical pathologist, who must make a histologic diagnosis on the cardiac mass, must be familiar with the spectrum of primary tumors of the heart. The most common is the cardiac myxoma, which constitutes nearly 80% of surgically excised masses, and which is the only cardiac tumor well known to most physicians. It is unique to the heart, possessing several histologic and immunohistochemical features that clearly separate it from soft tissue myxomas. Other tumors that are found exclusively in the heart include cardiac rhabdomyoma, Purkinje cell hamartoma, cystic tumor of the atrioventricular node, and lipomatous hypertrophy of the atrial septum. The remaining lesions have extracardiac counterparts that are similar, if not identical, histologically.

Tumors of the heart may be classified broadly into five types: pseudotumors, ectopias and tumors arising from ectopic tissue, tumors of mesenchymal tissue, lymphoid neoplasms, and metastatic lesions (Table 19-1). Tumors of mesenchymal tissue are the most diverse, are further subdivided by tissue type, and may be benign or malignant. In this chapter, pseudotumors are discussed first, followed by benign and malignant lesions in turn. Tumors of mesothelial origin (malignant mesothelioma) are discussed in Chapter 12. The relative frequency of cardiac tumors that are surgically removed and the patients' mean ages at presentation are provided in Table 19-2.

REACTIVE CARDIAC MASSES AND PSEUDOTUMORS

Mural Thrombi

Although they are not strictly cardiac tumors, mural thrombi are occasionally removed surgically and may be clinically and pathologically misdiagnosed as myxomas. For these reasons, it is important for a pathologist to be familiar with the histologic and clinical features of cardiac thrombi. The majority of mural thrombi occur in association with underlying heart disease.[2] Left atrial thrombi are frequently associated with mitral valvular disease, especially mitral stenosis, and thrombi occur in either atrium in patients with atrial fibrillation. Ventricular thrombi likewise form with decreased or abnormal ventricular contractility, particularly in patients with cardiomyopathy or ischemic heart disease and especially at sites of transmural infarction or ventricular aneurysms. In patients with known cardiac disease, mural thrombi are readily diagnosed by imaging studies, and biopsies or resections are only rarely performed.

Mural thrombi in the absence of heart disease occur in any chamber, but they are most commonly found in the right atrium. In the majority of patients, a coagulation defect is either suspected or documented. One of the more common coagulopathies diagnosed in patients with mural thrombi is the antiphospholipid syndrome,[3] but a wide variety of conditions may be predisposing factors, including essential thrombocytosis (Fig. 19-1) and Behçet disease.[4] In some patients, the nature of the coagulopathy is not appreciated, and the preoperative diagnosis is cardiac myxoma.[4, 5] If venous emboli are dislodged into the right ventricle, a mistaken preoperative diagnosis of right ventricular tumor may be made.[6]

Histologically, organized thrombi are characterized by layers of degenerated blood cells with a margin of granulation tissue and, eventually, fibrosis (Fig. 19-2). The endocardium demonstrates thickening and elastosis. It is worthwhile to evaluate the underlying myocardium to make a specific diagnosis. Numerous eosinophils and extracellular eosinophil breakdown products may suggest hypereosinophilic syndrome (eosinophilic endocardial disease), and intramural arterioles are often thrombosed. Obliteration of intramural arterioles with fibrointimal proliferation raises the diagnostic possibility of essential thrombocytosis or embolic disease resulting in myocardial infarction and mural thrombus. In most cases, however, the diagnosis is simply mural thrombus, and the clinician must attempt to explain the mass on the basis of heart disease or a coagulation defect.

The pathologic differential diagnosis of mural thrombus includes cardiac myxoma. Before the histologic appearance is even considered, the site of attachment helps to make this distinction. Mural thrombi typically occur in the atrial appendages or posterior walls of the atrium, whereas myxomas almost exclusively occur at the fossa ovalis. Histologically, myxomas are heterogeneous proliferations of myxoma cells, capillaries, and inflammatory cells, which in the majority of cases allow the pathologist to make a straightforward diagnosis. Luckily, those rare myxomas that do not attach to the fossa ovalis are almost always of the highly myxoid type with a classic histologic appearance.

TABLE 19-1 • **Types of Cardiac Tumors**

Pseudotumors
　Mural thrombi
　Inflammatory masses (rare)
　Mesothelial/monocyte incidental cardiac excrescence (MICE)

Heterotopias and tumors of ectopic tissue
　Tumors of the atrioventricular nodal region
　Teratoma
　Ectopic thyroid

Tumors of mesenchymal tissue
　Hamartoma of endocardial tissue
　　Papillary fibroelastoma*
　Hamartomas of cardiac muscle
　　Rhabdomyoma
　　Histiocytoid cardiomyopathy (Purkinje cell hamartoma)
　Tumors and neoplasms of fat
　　Lipomatous hypertrophy, interarterial septum
　　Lipoma
　　Liposarcoma (rare)†
　Tumors and neoplasms of fibrous and myofibroblastic tissue
　　Fibroma
　　Inflammatory pseudotumor (inflammatory myofibroblastic tumor)
　　Sarcomas (malignant fibrous histiocytoma, fibrosarcoma, leiomyosarcoma)†
　Vascular tumors and neoplasms
　　Hemangioma
　　Epithelioid hemangioendothelioma (rare)
　　Angiosarcoma†
　Neoplasm of uncertain histogenesis
　　Myxoma
　Neoplasms of neural tissue
　　Granular cell tumor
　　Schwannoma/neurofibroma (rare)
　　Paraganglioma
　　Malignant schwannoma/neurofibrosarcoma (rare)†

Malignant lymphoma

Metastatic tumors to the heart

* Considered by some as a reactive endocardial lesion.
† In the text, sarcomas are discussed as a group after benign lesions.

TABLE 19-2 • **Primary Cardiac Tumors: Frequency and Mean Age at Presentation***

Tumor Type	(%)†	Mean Age at Presentation
Teratoma	<1	16 weeks
Rhabdomyoma	2	33 weeks
Fibroma	3	13 years
Rhabdomyosarcoma	2	15 years
Hemangioma	2	31 years
Atrioventricular (AV) nodal tumor	<1‡	33 years
Sarcoma (all)	10	41 years
Myxoma	77	50 years
Papillary fibroelastoma	1	59 years
Lipomatous hypertrophy	3	64 years

* Adapted from reference[1].
† Percentage of primary cardiac tumors removed surgically.
‡ AV nodal tumor has been anecdotally reported as a surgical specimen; most are autopsy findings.

Calcifying Amorphous Pseudotumor

Calcification within a mural thrombus often leads to the erroneous clinical diagnosis of cardiac myxoma.[3, 7] In some mural thrombi, the calcification may be diffuse, resulting in a rock-hard mass that must be subjected to days of decalcification before histologic sectioning is possible (Fig. 19-3). Calcified mural thrombi may occur in any cardiac chamber, but they are most common in the right atrium, are often associated with antiphospholipid syndrome or renal failure, and have been fancifully designated cardiac CAT, or calcifying amorphous tumor.[8] Histologically, there are abundant microcalcifications in a hyalin stroma (Fig. 19-4).

Inflammatory Masses

Reactive inflammatory masses in the myocardium are rare. The so-called inflammatory pseudotumor is currently considered a benign myofibroblastic neoplasm. In parts of the world where parasitic diseases are endemic, echinococcal cysts in the myocardium may produce a tumor.

Mesothelial Pseudotumors

Collections of macrophages, mesothelial cells, and fat globules are occasionally encountered in surgical biopsies of the heart and pericardium (Fig. 19-5). They are not true tumors at all and are incidental findings at surgery. These structures are histologically identified by their total lack of stroma or vascularity and by their characteristic cellular constituents. Most are thought to be artifacts of open heart surgery.[9] Originally considered a form of hemangioma,[10] they are currently designated mesothelial/monocytic incidental cardiac excrescences, or cardiac MICE.[11]

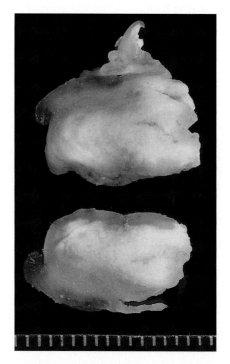

Figure 19-1 • Cardiac thrombus. A 37-year-old woman with essential thrombocytosis developed cerebral ischemia. An echocardiogram demonstrated a left ventricular mural mass that was resected and transected. Note appearance of layered thrombus.

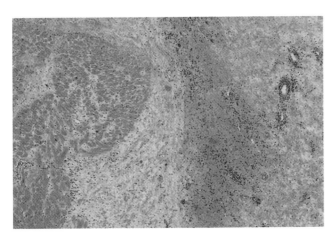

Figure 19-2 • Cardiac thrombus. The ventricular myocardium (left) is contrasted with the organized fibrin clot (right) (H&E stain).

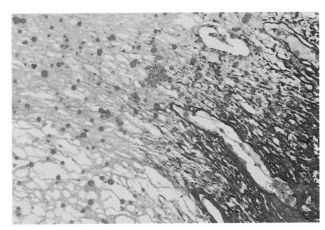

Figure 19-4 • Calcified mural thrombus (pseudotumor). Histologic section demonstrates microcalcifications and amorphous hyaline stroma (H&E stain).

ECTOPIAS

Cystic Tumor of the Atrioventricular Node

Although once considered of mesothelial[12] or even endothelial origin, these curious inclusions are almost certainly of endodermal derivation.[13–15] The majority of patients have congenital heart block, and almost three of four are female. Most tumors occur sporadically, but there is an association with cysts of endocrine organs and other midline defects, such as ventricular septal defect, nasal septal defect, encephalocele, thyroglossal duct cysts, and absent septum pellucidum.

Most tumors are diagnosed first at autopsy, although these lesions should be considered in the differential diagnosis of congenital heart block, especially in girls. Death is usually sudden and unexpected. Ventricular arrhythmias are somewhat more frequent in patients with heart block from any cause than in patients without heart disease.

The mean age at death is in the fourth decade, although there is a wide range, from birth to the eighth decade. There have been reports of biopsy diagnosis of atrioventricular (AV) nodal tumors.[16]

In almost one in two hearts with AV nodal tumors, cysts are grossly evident to the naked eye in the atrial approaches to the AV node; in the remainder of cases, the tumor is first noted on histologic examination of the conduction system (Fig. 19-6A). Histologically, there are multiple cysts that occur in the area of the AV node and the nearby atrial tissues, without involvement of the central fibrous body or penetrating bundle (Fig. 19-6B). The cysts are lined by cuboidal, transitional, or squamous epithelium, and there is often a combination of epithelial elements (Fig. 19-6C). Intervening stroma is generally composed of dense fibrous connective tissue. Many cysts are collapsed, forming nests of cells with an infiltrative appearance. There are no mitotic figures or atypical features of the nuclei. Immunohistochemically, the lining cells are positive for cytokeratin, carcinoembry-

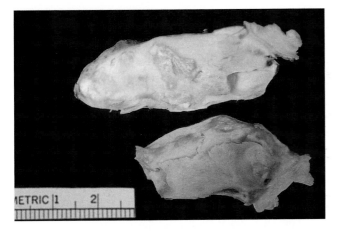

Figure 19-3 • Calcified mural thrombus (pseudotumor). This right atrial mass was removed from a patient with antiphospholipid syndrome. There was dense calcification resulting in rock-hard tumor that could be sectioned only after days of decalcification. The cut section is yellow tan.

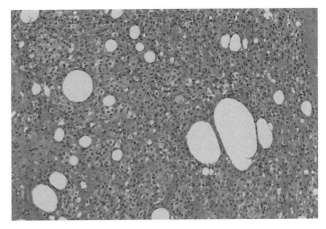

Figure 19-5 • Mesothelial/monocytic incidental cardiac excrescence. There is a collection of mononuclear cells and fat globules resembling a cytologic preparation. Note absence of stroma (H&E stain).

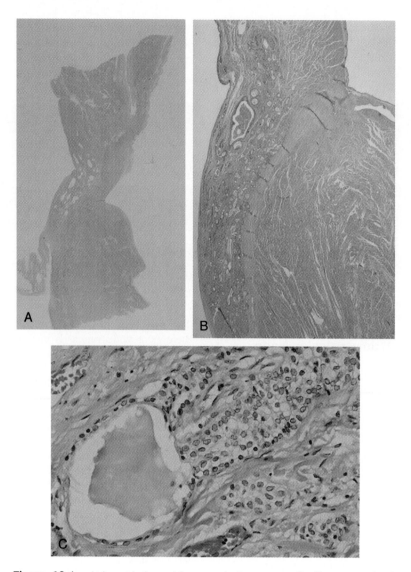

Figure 19-6 • Atrioventricular nodal tumor. *A,* Low power. Small cysts are barely perceptible superior to the tricuspid valve (left) and central fibrous body. *B,* A higher magnification demonstrates the cysts in the region of the atrioventricular node. They do not affect the central fibrous body. *C,* The cysts are lined by epithelium composed of a mixture of transitional and cuboidal cells (H&E stain).

onic antigen, B72.3 antigen, and, occasionally, chromogranin.[13, 14, 17–19] This tumor is also discussed in Chapters 11 and 20 (see Figs. 11-37 and 20-8).

There are few entities in the differential diagnosis. Rarely, teratomas may occur in the AV node region.[20] The diagnosis of teratoma rests on the identification of endodermal, ectodermal, and mesenchymal elements.

Germ Cell Tumors of the Heart

Almost all germ cell tumors of the heart are teratomas, but rare yolk sac tumors have also been described within the pericardium.[20–23] The majority of cardiac teratomas are located in the pericardial sac in fetuses, newborns, infants, or children. Rarely, they may occur within the

myocardium in the ventricular septum or in the area of the AV node. Histologically, they resemble testicular teratomas and are usually benign. The clinical diagnosis may be made in utero,[24] and symptoms include tamponade, hydrops fetalis, and sudden death.[23, 25, 26]

Thyroid Heterotopia

Ectopic thyroid that occurs in the myocardium is called "struma cordis." The right ventricular outflow is generally involved. The condition is believed to occur early in embryogenesis, when part or all of the functioning thyroid tissue becomes lodged in the ventricular outflow region.[27] Although pulmonary stenosis with right ventricular hypertrophy may occur, most patients

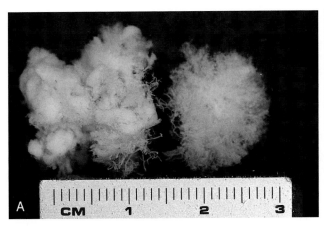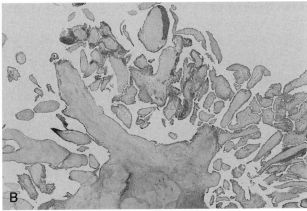

Figure 19-7 • Papillary fibroelastoma. *A,* The gross papillary appearance is often heightened by placing the specimen under water, as illustrated. *B,* Microscopically, the tumor is composed of avascular fronds lined by endothelial cells (H&E stain.)

are asymptomatic.[28, 29] Histologically, there are follicular structures containing colloid; if there is any difficulty in diagnosis, immunohistochemical stains for thyroglobulin may be performed. The differential diagnosis includes metastatic carcinoma of various origins and metastatic thyroid carcinoma. The latter distinction may be difficult to make on purely histologic grounds and is made clinically by exclusion of a dominant mass in the thyroid.

HAMARTOMAS AND BENIGN NEOPLASMS

Papillary Fibroelastoma

Also known as fibroelastic papilloma, this unusual lesion occurs exclusively on endocardial surfaces, most commonly on valve leaflets. A papillary fibroelastoma is probably an exaggerated form of Lambl excrescence,[30] which is a reactive filiform growth that occurs at sites of greatest hemodynamic stress, usually at the nodules of Aranti of the semilunar valves. Like Lambl excrescences, they occasionally occur in areas of previous endocardial damage or in patients with preexisting heart disease. We have seen them in patients with prosthetic heart valves and in those who have had previous radiation therapy. Unlike Lambl excrescences, papillary fibroelastomas can become quite large, and they may occur on any valve surface or any area of the endocardium. The pathogenesis of papillary fibroelastoma is unknown, and it is unclear whether it is a reactive or hamartomatous process. Thrombi may occur on the surface of the proliferation, and dislodged clots are responsible for embolic symptoms. However, we have not noted incipient thrombi lesions and doubt that thrombosis is the inciting event, a theory corroborated by established immunohistochemical differences between papillary fibroelastoma and organizing thrombus.[31]

The majority of cardiac papillary fibroelastomas are incidental findings at autopsy. However, left-sided lesions may cause symptoms by embolization of attached fibrin clots or prolapse into the coronary orifices.[32, 33] The most common symptoms are transient neurologic defects and myocardial ischemia, although sudden death has also been reported.[33]

Grossly, the papillary fibroelastoma has been compared to a "sea anemone," an appearance heightened by placing the tumor in a bowl of water (Fig. 19-7*A*). Their most common location is in the aortic valve, followed by the mitral and tricuspid valves, the pulmonary valve, and other endocardial surfaces. Histologically, they are avascular papillary structures lined by endothelial cells (Fig. 19-7*B*). The papillary cores contain a proteoglycan-rich stroma, and layers of elastic fibers and collagen are prominent near the base of the lesion. The cells covering the surface express vimentin, factor-VIII–related antigen, and CD34, and the stroma is rich in collagen type IV.[31]

The major differential diagnosis is cardiac myxoma. Most reported "myxomas" of cardiac valves are, in fact, papillary fibroelastomas. Myxomas are highly vascular lesions that rarely occur on the valve surfaces and contain stellate "myxoma" cells not seen in papillary fibroelastoma.

HAMARTOMAS OF CARDIAC MUSCLE

Rhabdomyoma

A rhabdomyoma is a hamartoma of cardiac myocytes that is intimately associated with the tuberous sclerosis syndrome. In infancy, most, if not all, patients with tuberous sclerosis demonstrate on echocardiography multiple cardiac masses that are presumed to be rhabdomyomas.[34] Conversely, 50% of patients with rhabdomyomas have other manifestations of the syndrome, such as intracranial hamartomas, facial angiofibromas, subungual fibromas, linear epidermal nevi, renal angiomyolipomas, and other hamartomas.[35, 36]

Rhabdomyomas in patients with tuberous sclerosis are usually multiple masses that with extensive cardiac involvement may result in intrauterine hydrops.[35, 37] In many patients, however, the tumors regress, and there are often no cardiac symptoms if the patient survives the first month of life. Sporadic rhabdomyomas are more likely to be solitary endocardial-based lesions that may cause ventricular outflow tract obstruction requiring surgical excision or that may induce cardiac arrhythmias. However, there is an overlap between the morphologic findings in patients with and without tuberous sclerosis.[37]

Most patients are diagnosed in the first few months of life, and the mean age at diagnosis is 2 months. However, cardiac rhabdomyomas may be detected in children and teenagers, and should, especially when multiple, prompt the pathologist to search for other manifestations of tuberous sclerosis.[38]

Grossly, rhabdomyomas are well-demarcated, yellow-tan nodules that occur within the myocardium or on the endocardial surface. Incidental rhabdomyomas are often endocardial lesions near the atrioventricular valves (Fig. 19-8A). Histologically, the characteristic cell is the vacuolated "spider cell," which possess strands of cytoplasm emanating from the nucleus (Fig. 19-8B). The apparent spaces within the cell contain large amounts of glycogen. Ultrastructurally, there are glycogen granules, myofibers, dispersed Z-band material, and intercalated disks along the cell periphery.[36]

There are few entities in the differential diagnosis. Vacuolated cells may occur in storage diseases in a diffuse, nondiscrete distribution. Purkinje cell hamartomas are usually smaller lesions with abundant mitochondria (see next section).

Histiocytoid/Oncocytic Cardiomyopathy, or Purkinje Cell Hamartoma

Often designated as simply "hamartoma," Purkinje cell hamartoma comprises a small percentage of surgical resections of heart tumors[39-41] in infants and children. The histogenesis of the lesion is debated, and it is unclear whether the cell of origin is the Purkinje cell or the cardiac myocyte.[42] The abundance of mitochondria revealed by ultrastructural study and their histologic appearance have led to the use of the term "oncocytic cardiomyopathy" (see Chapter 10 and Fig. 10-27 also).

At the time of diagnosis, most patients are younger than 3 years, and there is female predominance of four to one. The most common initial features are arrhythmias, followed by seizures, heart failure, cyanosis, dyspnea, and sudden death.[43] Associated cardiac and extracardiac anomalies, such as ventricular septal defect and midline defects of the central nervous system, affect approximately 25% of patients.

The nodules of histiocytoid cardiomyopathy are raised and yellowish, ranging from 1 mm to 1.5 cm in diameter, and usually measure less than 2 mm. They occur anywhere in the heart and are not limited to the endocardium. Histologically, there are clusters of foamy cells that are well demarcated from adjacent normal myocardium (Fig. 19-9). The abnormal cells are large, pale, rounded or oval, and often surrounded by thin collagen fibers. They stain faintly with periodic acid-Schiff. In contrast to a rhabdomyoma, large vacuoles and cytoplasmic streaming are absent. By immunohistochemical techniques, the cells are negative for lysozyme and α-1 antitrypsin and weakly positive for myoglobin, desmin, and myosin. Ultrastructurally, there is marked mitochondriosis, occasional leptomeric fibers, and few desmosomes. T tubules are absent, and intercalated discs are rarely seen.

BENIGN FATTY TUMORS

Lipomatous Hypertrophy of the Atrial Septum

A deposit of fat in the atrial septum resulting in a thickness greater than 2 cm has been termed lipomatous hypertrophy.[44] There are no precise criteria for the autopsy diagnosis, because the condition is an exaggeration of the normal components, and septal thickness may vary depending on the area measured. In general, the fat deposit is measured above the fossa ovalis, where it forms a triangular mass roofed by the epicardial surface of the

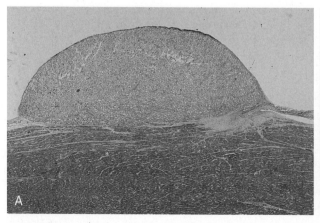
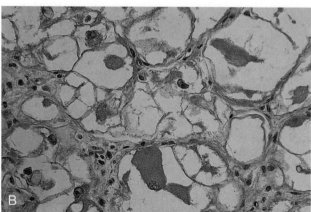

Figure 19-8 • Rhabdomyoma. A, The tumor is well circumscribed, composed of clear cells, and, in this case, is endocardial in location. This tumor was an incidental finding in the right ventricular inflow area in a 9-year-old boy. B, The clear cells contain retracted dark pink cytoplasm that may form fine strands resembling spider legs (H&E stain.)

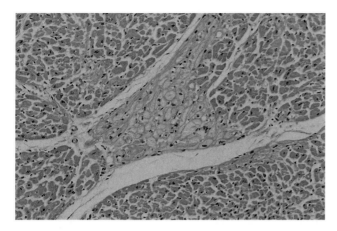

Figure 19-9 • Purkinje cell hamartoma (oncocytic/histiocytoid cardiomyopathy). There is a nest of clear microvesicular cells in the center of an otherwise unremarkable myocardium (H&E stain).

atria. Lipomatous hypertrophy occurs almost exclusively in adults, and there is an association with obesity, although not all patients are overweight.[45, 46] The true nature of lipomatous hypertrophy has been debated; it may be either a metabolic disturbance or a form of hamartoma.[47]

Lipomatous hypertrophy of the atrial septum is usually an incidental finding at autopsy. However, an association between interatrial fat deposits and arrhythmias, particularly atrial and supraventricular tachycardias, has been well established.[45, 48, 49] In the absence of other findings, lipomatous hypertrophy has even been blamed for sudden cardiac death.[45]

Recently, imaging techniques have allowed antemortem diagnosis.[46, 50, 51] The surgical pathologist now performs the diagnostic process in the rapid diagnosis suite, either because the surgeon has removed the mass incidentally during open heart surgery for relief of cardiac symptoms, such as congestive heart failure or vena caval obstruction,[46, 53] or for other causes.[52]

The preoperative diagnosis is usually right atrial myxoma, because the mass bulges into the right atrial cavity,[46] or, if tissue density has been ascertained, the correct diagnosis may be made before surgery is performed.[51]

Grossly, the tumor is not encapsulated and is bright yellow (Fig. 19-10A). Histologically, there is a mixture of mature and brown fat, which ultrastructurally contains abundant mitochondria.[46] Entrapped, enlarged myocytes are common and may lead to the false diagnosis of sarcoma, or the brown fat clusters may be mistaken for lipoblasts (Fig. 19-10B). The pathologist must remember that fatty masses of the atria, even if large and causing symptoms, are far more likely to be benign than malignant, because liposarcomas of the heart are extremely rare.

Cardiac Lipoma

Encapsulated lipomatous neoplasms occur in the heart but are very rare. Most are epicardial tumors, although any site of the heart may be affected. Occasionally, they are multiple.[54] If small, they are usually incidental findings at autopsy; larger lesions may result in pericardial constriction, heart failure, and sudden death. Histologically, they resemble lipomas of soft tissue, although entrapped cardiomyocytes may be seen.[54]

BENIGN TUMORS OF FIBROUS TISSUE

Cardiac Fibroma

After rhabdomyoma, cardiac fibroma is the second most common tumor of the heart in children. Unlike rhabdomyoma, it may also be first diagnosed in adults or elderly patients.[55] Because of their intramural location, cardiac fibromas often cause cardiac arrhythmias that may be life-threatening. There is an association with Gorlin-Goltz syndrome or basal cell nevus syndrome,[56] although

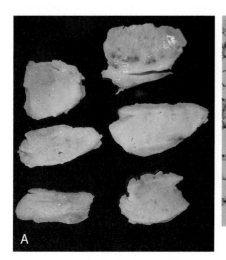
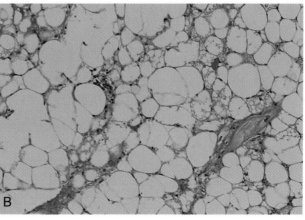

Figure 19-10 • Lipomatous hypertrophy, atrial septum. A, Although usually diagnosed incidentally at autopsy, this fatty specimen was removed surgically. B, Histologically, the lesion is composed of vesicular brown fat, enlarged cardiac myocytes, and normal fat cells (H&E stain.)

most patients with cardiac fibroma do not have the full expression of that genetic disorder.

Grossly, a cardiac fibroma is a firm, white, bulging mass that appears circumscribed.[57] It may occur anywhere in the heart but usually involves the ventricles, with a predilection for the ventricular septum. The tumor may attain massive size in proportion to the heart itself[58, 59] (Fig. 19-11A). Calcification is common, and, if seen on chest radiogram, is a helpful feature in distinguishing the tumor from a rhabdomyoma. Cardiac fibromas are virtually always single, although multiple tumors have been reported. Microscopically, one sees fibroblasts in a collagenous background, with variable numbers of elastic fibers. Despite the gross impression, the borders of the lesion are infiltrating (Fig. 19-11B). In young patients, the tumor may be markedly cellular (Fig. 19-11C). As the tumor matures, the degree of collagen increases so that in elderly patients it resembles scar (Fig. 19-11D).

The differential diagnosis in infants is fibrosarcoma. This distinction can be extremely difficult because fibromas may be markedly cellular in young patients. In general, sarcomas in children are quite rare, and a fibrous tumor in a young child should be considered benign if it occurs in the heart. In adults, the differential diagnosis is healed myocardial infarct, which is easily excluded because of the lack of a bulging mass in that condition and the presence of coronary artery disease.

There is no indication that cardiac fibromas are as aggressive as some of the soft tissue fibromatoses that they resemble histologically. Long-term survival after partial excision has been reported.[57, 60, 61] Fatal lesions usually result in cardiac arrhythmias, or, if massive, heart failure.

Miscellaneous Benign Fibrous Tumors

Inflammatory pseudotumors have been rarely reported in the heart.[62–64] Currently, these lesions are considered benign myofibroblastic neoplasms. In contrast to a fibroma, lesions are often endocardially based and contain a mixture of inflammatory cells and stellate plump myofibroblastic cells. Benign fibrous histiocytoma is another rare tumor of the heart that differs from fibroma by the presence of histiocytic-like mesenchymal cells.[65] In contrast to inflammatory myofibroblastic tumor, significant inflammation is absent. Like a fibroma, both inflammatory myofibroblastic tumor and fibrous histiocytoma lack cellular pleomorphism, atypia, and frequent mitotic figures, differentiating them from cardiac sarcomas.

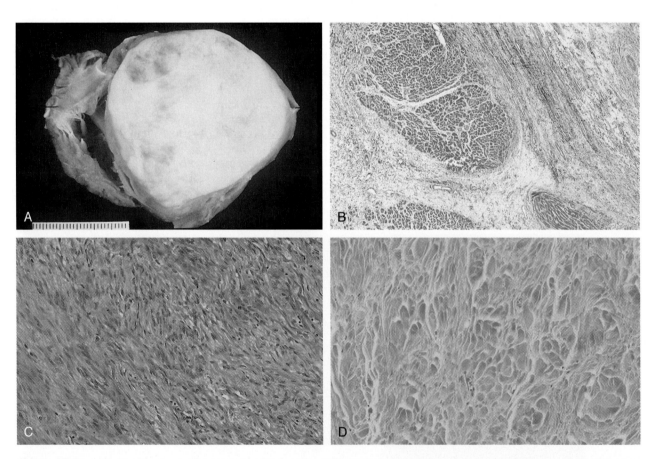

Figure 19-11 • Cardiac fibroma. *A,* The tumor is a bulging, firm white mass that often distorts the surrounding myocardium. This tumor obliterated the left ventricle and ventricular septum; note the tricuspid valve between the right atrium and the ventricle. *B,* A trichrome stain demonstrates infiltration of the collagenous tumor into cardiac muscle (Masson-trichrome). *C,* In children, cardiac fibromas may be markedly cellular, similar in appearance to fibrosarcoma. *D,* In adults, the tumors are composed almost entirely of nearly acellular collagen (*C & D,* H&E stain.)

CARDIAC HEMANGIOMA

Hemangiomas occur infrequently in the heart. Clinically, they may be incidental lesions discovered by chest radiogram or surgery for other purposes, or they may cause arrhythmias, pericardial effusions, congestive heart failure, or outflow tract obstruction.[66] They tend to occur in adults but may be found at any age. Although usually sporadic, they may be associated with hemangiomas of the gastrointestinal tract or skin[67] and result in a consumptive coagulopathy—Kasabach-Merritt syndrome—if they are large.[68]

Cardiac hemangiomas are of two basic pathologic types. Circumscribed ones are histologically uniform and composed of cavernous vascular spaces (Fig. 19-12A), often with a myxoid background (Fig. 19-12B). They may be easily shelled out at surgery, are often endocardially based masses that project into the lumen, but they may occur in the pericardium.[69] The lesions are occasionally misdiagnosed pathologically as myxomas because of their vascularity and myxoid stroma. Infiltrating cardiac hemangiomas are more likely to cause symptoms than circumscribed hemangiomas, and these often induce cardiac arrhythmias because of their intramural location.[66] In contrast to circumscribed cardiac hemangiomas, dysplastic arteries infiltrate the myocardium. In addition, there are often areas of capillary hemangioma and fat infiltrates, resulting in considerable histologic heterogeneity (Fig. 19-12C). These hemangiomas bear many histologic similarities to intramuscular hemangiomas of skeletal muscle. Occasionally, there may be areas of intravascular papillary endothelial hyperplasia that mimic angiosarcoma.[70] However, the presence of large vessels and areas of clearly benign vascular proliferation help the pathologist to distinguish cardiac hemangioma from angiosarcoma.

CARDIAC MYXOMA

Cardiac myxoma is a distinctive neoplasm that arises exclusively in the cardiac endocardium, usually near the fossa ovalis.[71–75] Although surface thrombus is common and may contribute to tumor growth, the idea that a cardiac myxoma is a form of thrombus is now antiquated[76] because there are several key differences between thrombus and myxoma (Table 19-3). The cell of origin of cardiac myxomas is unknown, but myxomas demonstrate remarkable pluripotentiality, expressing a variety of antigens and, occasionally, glandular structures.[77] Cardiac myxomas are composed of a variety of cellular elements, including stromal and inflammatory cells that secrete interleukins and coagulation factors.[78, 79] The diverse clinical symptoms experienced by patients with cardiac myxomas can likely be attributed, in part, to humoral factors expressed by the tumor.[71, 75]

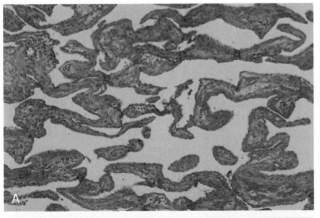

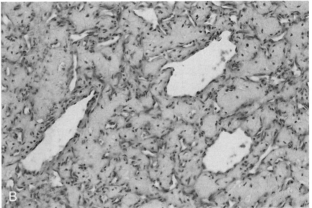

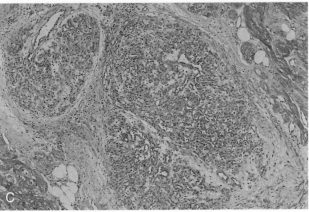

Figure 19-12 • Cardiac hemangioma. *A,* This tumor was easily shelled out of the atrium. It demonstrated the uniform histologic appearance of cavernous hemangioma. *B,* Endocardially based lesions may have a prominent myxoid stroma. Unlike myxoma, abundant hemosiderin and myxoma cells are absent. *C,* This cardiac hemangioma tumor is composed primarily of nodules of capillary hemangioma with occasional fat cells. Intramural cardiac hemangiomas are histologically similar to those arising in skeletal muscle. (*A–C,* H&E stain.)

TABLE 19-3 • **Cardiac Myxoma vs. Mural Thrombus: Differentiating Features**

	Mural Thrombus	Myxoma
Gross		
Common attachment site	Atrial appendage Ventricular endocardium	Fossa ovalis
Typical appearance of cut surface	Layered, with light and dark bands	Variegated, myxoid
Microscopic		
Cellular composition	Fibrin, red cells and leukocytes Endothelial cells Scattered fibroblasts Hemosiderin-laden macrophages (few)	Myxoma cells Hemosiderin-laden macrophages (numerous) Dendritic cells Capillaries
Immunohistochemical features	Actin + fibroblasts Endothelial cells expressing endothelial markers	S-100 + myxoma cells CD31 + myxoma cells Factor XIII + dendritic cells Endothelial cells expressing endothelial markers

Clinical Findings

Cardiac myxomas cause a multitude of symptoms related to obstruction of the mitral orifice, embolization, and elaboration of humoral substances (constitutional symptoms). Patients, on average, are 50 years of age at the time of diagnosis (Table 19-4), and there is a slight female predominance. Embolic myxoma may cause cerebral ischemia, claudication of the extremities, renal failure, coronary obstruction, and sudden death[80] (see Fig. 11-20). Before echocardiography was readily available as a diagnostic tool, patients often went for long periods without a diagnosis. In more recent series, a high proportion of tumors are found incidentally, representing approximately 15% of cases (Table 19-5). Constitutional symptoms associated with myxomas are believed to be secondary to elaboration of interleukin-1, a polyfunctional cytokine that stimulates B-cell differentiation in plasma cells and may result in polyclonal hypergammaglobulinemia.[81, 82] Furthermore, tumor size has been correlated with serum interleukin-1 activity.[83] In vitro studies have shown suppression of interleukin production of tumor cells with dexamethasone.[84] Tumor necrosis factor-α and interleukin-1 may also be elaborated by myxomas but are not thought to be responsible for constitutional symptoms.[85] Interleukin-8 and interleukin-6 have both been demonstrated immunohistochemically in three patients with cardiac myxoma and myocardial ischemia.[86]

The diagnosis of a cardiac myxoma is generally made

TABLE 19-4 • **Cardiac Myxoma: Sites of Endocardial Attachment and Mean Age***

Site	(%) Total	Mean Age (yr)
Single atrial tumors	89	53 ± 17
Left atrium at interatrial septum	64	
Right atrium at interatrial septum	15	
Left atrium at other sites†	5	
Right atrium at other sites	5	
Multiple or ventricular tumors	11	30 ± 11‡
Multiple sites, right atrium	2	
Multiple sites, left atrium	2	
Multiple chambers	5	
Left ventricle	1	
Right ventricle	1	

* Data derived from 128 cardiac myxomas (surgical and autopsy materials) reviewed by the authors.

† Some of these cases involved the mitral valve annulus or leaflets.

‡ Difference significant, p < 0.0001.

TABLE 19-5 • **Cardiac Myxoma: Initial Symptoms***

Symptom or Initial Manifestation	N		
	Left-Sided	Right-Sided	Total
Embolism	24	2	26
To central nervous system	18	—	18
To lower extremities	5	—	5
To kidneys (hematuria)	1	—	1
Lungs (pulmonary embolism)	—	2	2
Pulmonary congestion/heart failure	20	3	23
Shortness of breath/orthopnea	11	0	11
Dyspnea on exertion	7	1	8
Ankle edema	0	2	2
Hemoptysis	2	0	2
Arrhythmia/syncope	15	5	20
Syncope	3	3	6
Sudden death	5	0	5
Palpitation	3	0	3
Supraventricular tachycardia	3	0	3
Atrial fibrillation/flutter	1	1	2
Sick sinus syndrome	0	1	1
Incidental finding/no symptom	7	8	15
Detected at auscultation	4	5	9
Detected at chest X-ray	2	3	5
Detected at angiography for ischemic heart disease	1	0	1
Constitutional symptoms	0	6	6
Weakness	0	2	2
Fatigue	0	2	2
Weight loss	0	1	1
Fever of unknown origin	0	1	1
Other	7	3	10
Chest pain	5	1	6
Found in evaluation for syndrome	1	1	2
Fever/bacterial endocarditis	1	1	2
Total	73	27	100

* Data derived from 100 cardiac myxomas reviewed by the authors, excluding incidental myxomas found at autopsy.

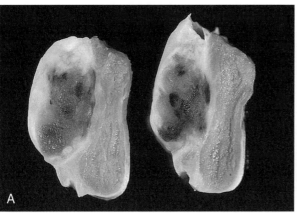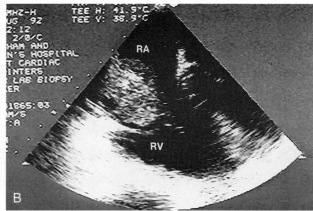

Figure 19-13 • Cardiac myxoma. *A,* Approximately 50% of cardiac myxomas are friable and prone to embolization. The photograph depicts the heart of a young woman who died suddenly. *A,* These cardiac myxomas are smooth-surfaced lesions. On section, the tumors are variegated with areas of hemorrhage. This tumor was an incidental left atrial mass discovered at autopsy in a young man who died of trauma. *B,* Echocardiogram demonstrates a right atrial mass in a patient with atrial myxoma. (RA = right atrium; RV = right ventricle.)

at echocardiography. Angiography is performed in elderly patients to evaluate the coronary arteries and often demonstrates a moderate degree of pulmonary hypertension in individuals with left atrial tumors. Transesophageal echocardiograms, computed tomography, and magnetic resonance imaging may be superior to transthoracic echocardiography in demonstrating precise tumor attachment and differentiating the lesion from a mural thrombus or atrial sarcoma. Over three fourths of tumors are located in the left atrium, and the majority of the remainder arise in the right atrium. Multiple tumors and tumors located in sites other than the fossa ovalis are rare and occur more frequently in patients with myxoma syndrome.

Surgically, tumors with a narrow stalk may be resected without removing atrial septal tissue. In many patients, however, a portion of atrial septum including the fossa is excised, and a synthetic or pericardial patch is placed in the defect. If the site of attachment is multifocal or in the atrial free wall, either myxoma syndrome should be suspected or the lesion is likely to be a myxoid sarcoma.

The postoperative prognosis of cardiac myxoma is excellent. The recurrence rate in combined series is less than 2%.[87] In the majority of patients with true recurrent myxomas, the tumor is part of an inherited syndrome. Many patients with so-called recurrent myxoma actually suffer from myxoid sarcomas, which may mimic myxoma clinically and pathologically.

Gross Pathologic Features

Cardiac myxoma are heterogeneous, variegated tumors that may have a smooth or irregular surface. Calcification is common, especially in right atrial tumors. Irregular tumors are more likely gelatinous, myxoid, and prone to embolization in contrast to smooth-surfaced lesions (Fig. 19-13), which often contain abundant collagen and are unlikely to fragment and dislodge into the circulation. Cardiac myxomas may be less than 1 cm and may be found incidentally at autopsy, or they may exceed 10 cm and distend the atria. As noted earlier, more than 90%

occur in the region of the fossa ovalis. Cardiac myxomas arising on cardiac valves are distinctly rare, and those reported are often papillary fibroelastomas misdiagnosed as myxomas.

Histologic Features

Cardiac myxomas demonstrate extensive cellular heterogeneity and frequent scarring and thrombosis. Characteristic histologic features are best seen close to the endocardial surface, where secondary changes are uncommon. The diagnostic element is the myxoma cell, which is a polygonal or stellate syncytial cell. It frequently forms cords or small nests. Toward the surface of the tumor, myxoma cells are closely associated with capillaries, often forming rings (Fig. 19-14*A*). It has been hypothesized that the myxoma cell differentiates into endothelial elements, which also line the surface of the tumor. Two percent of cardiac myxomas contain glands, usually near the atrial stalk; these glands are histologically, histochemically, and immunohistochemically identical to intestinal glands (Fig. 19-14*B*). The diagnosis of myxoma is apparent in areas of the tumor containing typical myxoma cells, which tend to merge imperceptibly with glandular elements. There is no clinical significant to the glands, which are not seen in excess in patients with the syndrome or in those with recurrent myxoma. The myxoid stroma contains dendritic cells that express factor XIII (Fig. 19-15*A*), KP-1 positive macrophages (many of which contain hemosiderin), and scattered lymphocytes. The typical proteoglycan-rich myxoid stroma is present throughout few cardiac myxomas because of degenerative changes. In over half of tumors, there is extensive scarring that replaces the myxoid areas, and calcification and metaplastic bone may be present in right atrial myxomas. Hemorrhage and organizing thrombus result in abundant hemosiderin-laden macrophages, which are virtually always present and a helpful diagnostic feature. In 10% of tumors, elastic tissue and calcification surround the hemosiderin, resulting in gamna bodies.

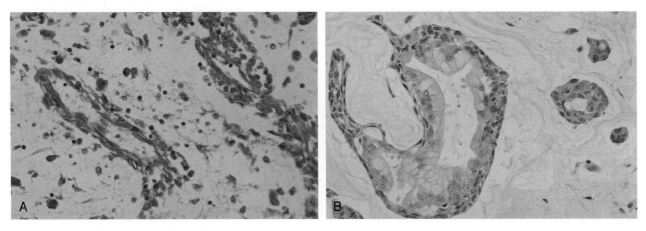

Figure 19-14 • Cardiac myxoma. *A,* Histologically, the tumor is composed of syncytia, many of which surround blood vessels. The stroma is rich in proteoglycans, inflammatory cells, and hemosiderin). *B,* In 1 to 2% of tumors, glandular structures are evident, which merge imperceptibly with typical myxoma cells (*A* and *B,* H&E stain.)

Immunohistochemical Features

The immunohistochemical findings of cardiac myxoma are as varied as their histologic appearance. The myxoma cell is variably positive for S-100 protein (Fig. 19-15*B*), muscle-specific actin, CD31, and vimentin.[87] A variety of other antigens have been demonstrated in the myxoma cell, including cytokeratin, desmin, myoglobin, factor VIII-related antigen, and CD34.[31, 88–90] The dendritic cells express factor XIII,[79] and the endothelial cells express CD34 and factor–VIII-related antigen.

The wide variation in the reported immunohistochemical profile of cardiac myxoma is hard to explain. In our experience, the myxoma cell expresses CD31 (Fig. 19-15*C*), Ulex europaeus lectin binding (focally), vimentin, S-100 protein (focally), and smooth muscle actin (focally). It only weakly expresses CD34 and factor–VIII-related antigen, which are found only in the capillaries

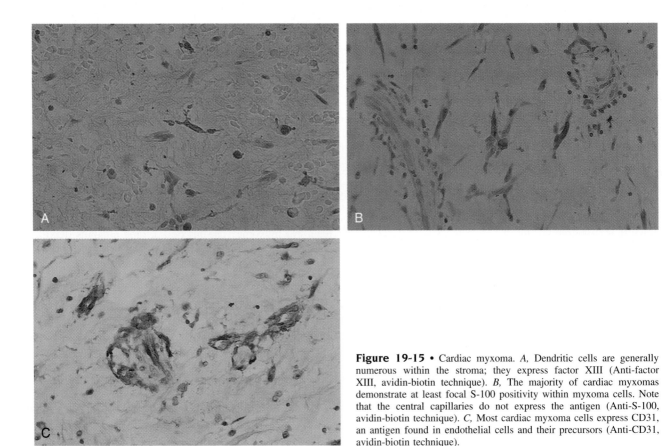

Figure 19-15 • Cardiac myxoma. *A,* Dendritic cells are generally numerous within the stroma; they express factor XIII (Anti-factor XIII, avidin-biotin technique). *B,* The majority of cardiac myxomas demonstrate at least focal S-100 positivity within myxoma cells. Note that the central capillaries do not express the antigen (Anti-S-100, avidin-biotin technique). *C,* Most cardiac myxoma cells express CD31, an antigen found in endothelial cells and their precursors (Anti-CD31, avidin-biotin technique).

TABLE 19-6 • **Myxoma Syndrome**

Skin lesions (eyes, ears, nipples, face, lips, trunk, limbs)
    Myxoma
    Lentigines
    Blue nevi
    Ephelides

Endocrine
    Cushing syndrome
    Acromegaly
    Calcifying Sertoli cell tumor

Schwannomas
    Melanocytic/psammomatous

and surface lining cells, and epithelial markers are seen only in the rare glandular structures. In general, immunohistochemical testing is not particularly helpful in diagnosis, which is almost always made on the identification of myxoma cell structures. However, the presence of S-100 protein may help to exclude the diagnosis of myxoid sarcoma, which rarely expresses this marker.

Differential Diagnosis

The histologic differential diagnosis of cardiac myxoma includes papillary fibroelastoma, myxoid sarcoma, organized thrombus, and hemangioma. Papillary fibroelastomas usually occur on valves, unlike myxomas, and do not contain capillaries or inflammatory cells within their stroma. Myxoid sarcomas do not possess myxoma cell structures and abundant hemosiderin and generally demonstrate cellular spindle cell areas with mitotic figures and nuclear atypia. Organized thrombi lack myxoma cells and are composed of granulation tissue with areas of scar and hyalinization. Cardiac hemangioma is rare and lacks myxoma cells and abundant hemosiderin.

Myxoma Syndrome

Approximately 1% of patients with cardiac myxoma have an autosomal dominant syndrome characterized by lentigines, blue nevi, myxoid tumors of the skin, schwannomas, endocrine overactivity, calcifying Sertoli cell tumors of the testis, and other lesions[91-96] (Table 19-6). Most patients with the syndrome do not have all of its features, and those who do are much younger than those with sporadic cardiac myxoma. Syndrome myxomas are often multiple, frequently recur or embolize, and do not necessarily occur at the fossa ovalis.

BENIGN NEURAL NEOPLASMS

Paraganglioma

Paraganglial cells are normally found within the atrial walls, and neoplasms arising from them are rare. Paragangliomas of the heart have been termed pheochromocytomas (when functioning)[97-99] and chemodectomas. The majority develop within the atria, are benign, and are functional, resulting in systemic hypertension. Most patients are young or middle-aged adults.[98, 100] Functional tumors have been successfully removed from patients, with subsequent remission of symptoms. Rare malignant cardiac paragangliomas have been reported.[101] Complete surgical excision is recommended for all cardiac paragangliomas, and often an atrial graft is used to repair the portion of atrium or atrial septum removed.

Grossly, paragangliomas are large, poorly circumscribed masses between 5 and 15 cm in greatest dimension. On section, they are often hemorrhagic and variegated. Pathologically, paragangliomas of the heart are similar histologically and immunohistochemically to extracardiac paragangliomas.[102] Without knowledge of the entity, the tumor may be mistaken for hemangiopericytoma (with a branching vascular pattern) (Fig. 19-16A) or metastatic carcinoma. The diagnosis is readily made by immunohistochemical stains and recognition of the endocrine or "Zellballen" appearance of tumor nests. The body cells are positive for chromogranin, neuron-specific enolase, and, commonly, met-enkephalin; the sustentacular cells are positive for S-100 protein (Fig. 19-16B).

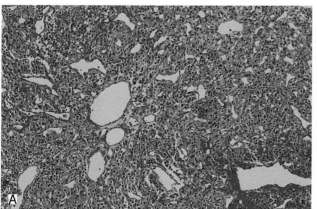
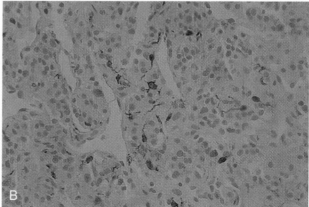

Figure 19-16 • Cardiac paraganglioma. *A,* There is a hemangiopericytoma-like vascular pattern at low magnification. This tumor was resected from a young man with hypertension, a cardiac murmur, and an atrial mass demonstrated by echocardiogram (H&E stain). *B,* A higher magnification demonstrates S-100 positive sustentacular cells (Anti-S-100 protein, avidin-biotin technique).

TABLE 19-7 • **Cardiac Sarcomas***

Histologic Type/Subtype	Number/%	Mean Age (Yrs)	Men %	Most Frequent Site(s) (%)
Myofibroblastic	58/34	41	45	Left atrium (68)
				Right atrium (14)
				Ventricles (12)
MFH (27)		42		Left atrium (70)
Osteosarcoma (15)		38		Left atrium (100)
Fibrosarcoma (8)		38		Left atrium (38)
Myxoid sarcoma		44		Left atrium (50)
Angiosarcoma	45/26	41	74	Right atrium (72)
				Pericardium (11)
				Left atrium (7)
Undifferentiated sarcoma	38/22	48	55	Left atrium (47)
				Ventricles (25)
				Right atrium (11)
Leiomyosarcoma	15/9	30	60	Left atrium (67)
Rhabdomyosarcoma	6/3	23	33	Left atrium (33)
				Left ventricle (33)
Synovial sarcoma	6/3	38	80	Pericardium (33)
				Right ventricle (33)
Neurofibrosarcoma	2/1	52	100	Pericardium (50)
				Right atrium (50)
Liposarcoma	2/1	67	50	Right atrium (100)
Epithelioid hemangio-endothelioma	1/1	71	0	Left atrium (100)
Totals	173/100	41	57	Left atrium (44)
				Right atrium (31)

* Data derived from 173 cardiac sarcomas reviewed by the authors. MFH = malignant fibrous histiocytoma.

Neurofibromas and Schwannomas

Nerve sheath tumors of the heart are extremely rare. They generally occur on epicardial surfaces and rarely cause outflow obstruction.[103–105] They have been described in patients with neurofibromatosis and in those who have had radiation therapy. Histologically, they resemble the nerve sheath minors of soft tissue.[106]

Granular Cell Tumor

Incidental granular cell tumors are occasionally found on the epicardial surface of the base of the heart at autopsy, usually near an epicardial artery. Grossly, they are circumscribed nodules that are homogeneously tan-yellow on section and that rarely exceed 1.5 cm in diameter. Histologically, they are identical to extracardiac granular cell tumors and contain nests of cells with PAS-positive granules that express S-100 protein immunohistochemically.

PRIMARY CARDIAC SARCOMAS

Classification and Prognosis

Primary sarcomas of the heart are similar histologically to those arising in extracardiac soft tissue. Almost all types have been reported as primary lesions in the myo-cardium, although certain subtypes have yet to be described in the heart. For this chapter, a simplified classification scheme has been followed (Table 19-7). Sarcomas of myofibroblastic differentiation, including those with malignant osteoid or chondrosarcoma, are considered as a group, because these tend to demonstrate considerable histologic and clinical overlap. Angiosarcomas and rhabdomyosarcomas are considered separately because their clinical and pathologic features are distinct from one another and from cardiac sarcomas with myofibroblastic differentiation. Because a high proportion of cardiac sarcomas defy classification, there is a separate discussion of undifferentiated lesions, and, for completeness, rare cardiac sarcomas that do not fit into any of these categories are addressed finally.

The prognosis of cardiac sarcoma is poor and is generally measured in months. Occasional patients live 2 to 3 years after diagnosis. The histologic type does not appear to affect prognosis. However, tumors with necrosis and numerous mitotic figures tend to behave more aggressively than those without these features. Patients with left-sided tumors and tumors without metastatic deposits at the time of diagnosis may survive longer than those with right-sided tumors or those without metastatic disease.[107] Heart transplantation has been used in treatment.

The most common sites of metastases are the lungs, accounting for nearly 50% of lesions, followed by the skeleton, the chest wall, the skin, lymph nodes, the pleura, and a variety of others.[107]

Myofibroblastic Sarcomas: Subtypes and Gross Findings

The largest group of primary cardiac sarcomas demonstrate fibroblastic or myofibroblastic differentiation that express intermediate filaments, vimentin, and smooth-muscle–cell actin.[39, 107] Classically, these are divided into malignant fibrous histiocytoma (comprising more than 50% of this group),[108–110] fibrosarcoma,[111, 112] and myxosarcoma or fibromyxosarcoma. When occurring in the heart, these three sarcomas share histologic and clinical features and are often difficult to distinguish one from the other both clinically and even pathologically.

The majority of cardiac myofibroblastic sarcomas are endocardially based, with a bulky tumor within a heart cavity. It is tempting to speculate that they originate from myofibroblastic cells that normally occur in the intima and that are analogous to intimal sarcomas of the great vessels.

A large proportion of malignant fibrous histiocytomas and fibrosarcomas of the heart demonstrate extensive myxoid changes in the stroma,[113, 114] perhaps because of their luminal location. The term "myxosarcoma" is often used in the surgical literature for these tumors, although it is probably best to avoid this designation, because it may give the erroneous impression that the tumor arises from a benign myxoma. In fact, there is very little evidence that cardiac myxomas undergo progressive malignant "transformation."[115]

Approximately 80% of cardiac sarcomas with myofibroblastic differentiation occur in the left atrium,[39, 107] for reasons that are unknown, and most of the remainder occur in the right atrium or the pericardium. Five to ten percent demonstrate areas of osteosarcoma, chondrosarcoma, or malignant giant cell tumor.[116] Generally, only a small proportion of the sarcoma shows one of these three histologic types of sarcoma, which occur exclusively in the left atrium.

Myofibroblastic Sarcomas: Clinical Findings

The majority of patients with primary cardiac sarcomas are adults. The mean age of about 40 at presentation is slightly younger than that of a patient with cardiac myxoma (50 years of age).[107] Sarcomas of the heart in children are quite rare. There is no sex predilection. The most common clinical symptom of myofibroblastic sarcomas is dyspnea related to obstruction of the mitral valve,[117] because sarcomas most often occur in the left atrium. There may be a host of other symptoms, including malaise, fever, chest pain, weight loss, palpitations, syncope, and stroke.[107] The most common clinical diagnosis is a cardiac myxoma. Imaging studies may demonstrate multiple attachment sites, mitral valve involvement, or infiltration into atrial or ventricular walls, none of which occurs with cardiac myxoma. Occasionally, complete tumor resection is impossible, and a palliative procedure is performed. It is best for the pathologist to attempt to determine completeness of excision if atrial

masses are removed surgically. Although there is no evidence that a patient with an incompletely excised myxoma may experience recurrence more frequently than one whose myxoma was a completely removed, it is likely that complete excision may lengthen survival in patients with a cardiac sarcoma.

As in all cardiac sarcomas, the prognosis for myofibroblastic cardiac sarcoma is poor and is generally measured in months.[107, 118–123] There is no evidence that one histologic type imparts a worse prognosis than any other.[119] It has been shown that high-grade tumors—those with numerous mitoses or necrosis—are more clinically aggressive than those with few mitoses and no necrosis.

Myofibroblastic Sarcomas: Histologic Findings and Differential Diagnosis

The histologic features of these cardiac sarcomas are identical to those of their extracardiac counterparts. In general, malignant fibrous histiocytoma denotes a pleomorphic tumor, which is typically myxoid in areas (Fig. 19-17), and often demonstrates prominent vascularity. Immunohistochemical studies are not particularly useful in helping the pathologist differentiate these tumors, although desmin expression is sometimes considered specific for leiomyosarcoma. Smooth-muscle actin, on the other hand, is not a specific marker for tumor differentiation. Epithelial markers are often helpful in excluding a mesothelioma or metastatic spindle cell carcinoma, although focal cytokeratin positivity may be seen in a small percentage of cardiac malignant fibrous histiocytomas. Malignant mesotheliomas are clinically quite different from myofibroblastic sarcomas because they encase the heart, obliterate the pericardial space, and rarely project into the cardiac chambers.

The primary differential diagnosis for myofibroblastic sarcomas is a cardiac myxoma (Table 19-8). A surprisingly high proportion of myxoid cardiac sarcomas are initially misdiagnosed histopathologically as myxomas. In

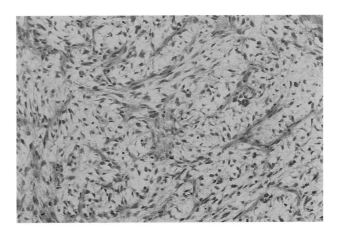

Figure 19-17 • Myxoid malignant fibrous histiocytoma, left atrium. There is a myxoid spindle cell proliferation with a prominent vascular pattern. In contrast to a myxoma, myxoma cell structures and abundant hemosiderin are absent (H&E stain).

TABLE 19-8 • **Differential Features, Cardiac Myxoma and Cardiac Sarcoma**

Feature	Myxoma	Sarcoma
Diagnostically helpful		
Myxoma cell rings, cords	++−+++	0
Hemosiderin-laden macrophages	++−+++	0−+
Factor XIII + dendritic cells	+−+++	0
Mitotic figures	0−+	+−+++
Cellular atypia	0−+	+−+++
Compact spindle cells	0	+−+++
Not diagnostically helpful		
Myxoid stroma	+−+++	0−+++
Fibrosis	+−+++	+−+++
Calcification	0−++	0−+

general, the distinction is easily made, provided that myxoma cells, hemosiderin-laden macrophages, and factor–XIII-positive dendritic cells are absent.

Angiosarcoma: Clinical and Gross Features

If the subtypes of myofibroblastic sarcomas are considered separately, angiosarcoma is the most common type of cardiac sarcoma,[124] accounting for approximately 37%.[116, 118–123]

The age range is 9 to 80 years, with a mean of 40 years.[125] In contrast to other cardiac sarcomas, there is a marked right-sided predominance, with nearly 90% of myofibroblastic sarcomas occurring in the right atrium.[118–123, 125] Initial clinical symptoms are most often related to hemopericardium or pericardial constriction and are rarely caused by distant metastases.[126] Because of the propensity for pericardial involvement, cardiac tamponade occurs more frequently than it does with other types of cardiac sarcomas. Metastases occur in 66 to 89% of patients, most often in the lungs.

Cardiac angiosarcoma is typically a multicentric mass that replaces the right atrial wall and either protrudes into or fills the chamber. The mass or masses are typically dark red or brown. Invasion of the vena cava and tricuspid valve is common, but the atrial septum and pulmonary artery are usually spared. The pericardium is frequently involved, and may be the only site of tumor.

Angiosarcoma: Histologic Features and Differential Diagnosis

Cardiac angiosarcomas are histologically similar to extracardiac angiosarcoma, and are composed of malignant endothelial cells that form vascular channels (Fig. 19-18A) or papillary structures (Fig. 19-18B). There may be areas of anaplastic or spindle cells with poorly formed vascular channels that resemble leiomyosarcoma or fibrosarcoma, but large numbers of extravascular erythrocytes and identification of vacuoles containing red blood cells may help diagnosis. Reticulin stains may be useful in highlighting vascular lumina. Extensive sampling is important for detecting endothelial vacuoles or diagnostic papillary structures in cardiac angiosarcomas with spindle cell areas.

Immunohistochemical studies indicate that factor–VIII-related antigen, although a specific marker, is not particularly sensitive.[39, 127] Angiosarcomas of the pericardium can be quite difficult to diagnose in pericardial biopsies and may be mistaken for mesothelioma or reactive mesothelial hyperplasia.[128] Nests of reactive mesothelial cells may become incorporated into the sarcoma and be mistaken for malignant cells. In these cases, immunohistochemical stains for cytokeratin and endothelial markers (factor–VIII-related antigen, CD31, and CD34) may help to delineate the two populations of cells.

Epithelioid angiosarcomas have not been reported in the heart. However, epithelioid hemangioendothelioma, a related low-grade tumor of vascular origin, may rarely arise in the atrium.[129]

Leiomyosarcoma

Approximately 10% of cardiac sarcomas demonstrate smooth muscle cell differentiation.[130–133] Leiomyosarcomas are composed of fascicles of spindle cells that intersect one another at right angles. Intracellular glycogen is

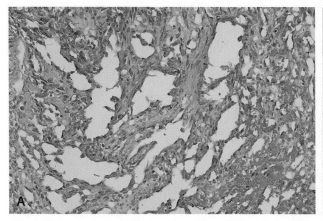
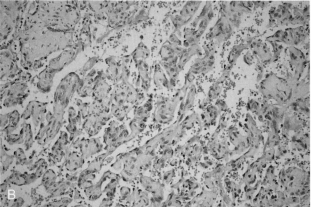

Figure 19-18 • Angiosarcoma. *A,* Histologically, irregular vascular channels are lined by typical endothelial cells. *B,* Another typical histologic pattern is that of anastomosing papillary structures lined by atypical endothelial cells. (*A* and *B,* H&E stain.)

present and more than 50% of tumors show focal desmin expression.

The mean age of patients with cardiac leiomyosarcoma is 30 years, approximately 15 years younger than those with most other cardiac sarcomas. As with myofibroblastic sarcomas, most tumors arise in the left atrium. A certain proportion of atrial leiomyosarcomas may derive from veins emptying the heart,[134] either the venae cavae on the right or pulmonary veins on the left.

The differential diagnosis includes myofibroblastic sarcoma, angiosarcoma, and myxoma. Compared with myofibroblastic sarcomas, leiomyosarcomas have more uniform cells and may demonstrate perinuclear vacuoles, abundant fuchsinophilic cytoplasm, and intracellular glycogen. Spindled areas of angiosarcoma may mimic leiomyosarcoma, but, with adequate sampling, the vascular nature of the former becomes apparent. Also, angiosarcomas rarely occur in the left atrium. A myxoid stroma is a characteristic feature of about 25% of leiomyosarcomas, but the dense cellular fascicles of leiomyosarcoma easily distinguish this tumor from cardiac myxoma.

Rhabdomyosarcoma

Rhabdomyosarcomas constitute approximately 5% of cardiac sarcomas.[39, 107, 119, 122, 123] Unlike a cardiac sarcoma, with fibrous or smooth muscle differentiation, cardiac rhabdomyosarcoma does not show any predilection for the left atrium; either atrium or ventricle may be the primary site. Cardiac rhabdomyosarcoma is slightly more common in males than females, at a ratio of 1.4 to 1.[135] The mean age of patients at first appearance of rhabdomyosarcoma is younger than that of patients who have other cardiac sarcomas (the second to third decade). These are bulky, invasive tumors that may exceed 10 cm at their greatest diameter. The majority are of the embryonal type and may be well differentiated, with numerous tadpole-shaped rhabdomyoblasts. Round cell tumors, by contrast, may show very few rhabdomyoblasts, which are identified only after extensive search. Rhabdomyoblasts contain abundant glycogen and express desmin and myoglobin, which prove helpful immunohistochemical markers. The alveolar subtype of embryonal rhabdomyosarcoma has been described in the heart as a metastatic lesion,[136] and cardiac sarcoma botryoides, another form of embryonal rhabdomyosarcoma, has also been reported.[137]

Undifferentiated Sarcoma

Depending on the criteria used for diagnosis of sarcomas with myofibroblastic differentiation, undifferentiated sarcomas make up either one fourth,[107] or less than 10%, of cardiac sarcomas.[39, 118–123] Like myofibroblastic sarcomas, the majority occur in the atria. Prognosis is poor, generally less than 2 years, but is not worse, on average, than prognosis in other types of cardiac sarcoma.[138] The major differential diagnosis of undifferentiated sarcoma, especially of right-sided lesions, is metastatic tumor. Malignant melanoma, metastatic carcinoma, and malignant mesothelioma should always be excluded if a pleomorphic tumor of the heart is encountered. In cases of small-cell tumors, a primary round cell liposarcoma should be considered if the typical vascular pattern is identified and embryonal rhabdomyosarcoma is excluded by absence of rhabdomyoblasts. A primitive neuroectodermal tumor has been described in the heart, which is a small round cell neoplasm that expresses CD99 (Ewing sarcoma marker).[139]

Miscellaneous Sarcomas

Sarcomas that may rarely arise within the myocardium include liposarcoma,[140] malignant peripheral nerve sheath tumor,[138] synovial sarcoma,[141, 142] and malignant mesenchymoma.[138] They are histologically similar to their extracardiac counterparts and often arise at the base of the heart on the epicardial surface.

CARDIAC LYMPHOMA

Incidence and Clinical Associations

Primary cardiac lymphomas, that manifest cardiac symptoms and are largely intrapericardial, are rare and generally diagnosed at autopsy.[143–146] Although there are occasional reports of cardiac lymphomas diagnosed at surgery,[144, 147] many series of surgically excised cardiac tumors do not include examples of lymphoma.[39, 119–121, 123]

The incidence of cardiac lymphoma is increasing because of Epstein-Barr–related lymphoproliferative disorders in acquired immunodeficiency syndrome (AIDS) patients[148] and in post-transplant patients.[149, 150] Post-transplant lymphoproliferative disease may develop in patients within months or many years after transplantation.[151] The incidence of post-transplant lymphomas at any site is greater in patients with heart and lung transplants (approximately 6%) than in those with renal transplants (less than 1%[152]). However, cardiac lymphomas comprise less than 5% of all lymphomas occurring in patients with AIDS and in those with organ transplants,[152–154] and location of the tumor in the donor heart is the exception rather than the rule in heart transplant patients.[149] Therefore, despite the increased prevalence of Epstein-Barr–related lymphomas, a considerable proportion of cardiac lymphomas still occur in immunocompetent patients. There is no evidence that cardiac lymphomas in immunocompetent patients contain genomic Epstein-Barr virus DNA.[145]

Patients with cardiac lymphomas may complain of a variety of symptoms, including cardiac tamponade,[155] heart failure,[146, 148, 149] exertional dyspnea, atrial fibrillation or flutter,[156, 157] and right-sided heart obstruction.[144, 158]

Pathologic Findings

Grossly, any portion of the heart may be involved by lymphoma, although there is a slight predilection for the right atrium.[143] Generally, the heart demonstrates multiple,

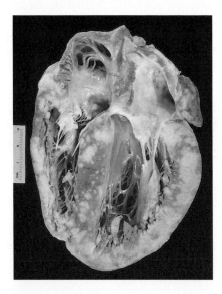

Figure 19-19 • Acquired immunodeficiency syndrome (AIDS)-associated lymphoproliferative disorder. A very small proportion of immunocompromised patients develop lymphomas of the heart that are associated with Epstein-Barr virus infection and that progress through a polyclonal phase. This patient died with multiple lymphomatous masses scattered throughout the myocardium.

firm, whitish-yellow nodules (Fig. 19-19). Extension into the epicardial fat is typical, epicardial arteries may be constricted by tumor, and gross hemorrhage and necrosis are usually minimal. Histologically, cardiac lymphomas span the spectrum of B cell proliferations and include follicle center-cell lymphomas, immunoblastic lymphomas, diffuse large-cell lymphomas, and Burkitt lymphoma. The differential diagnosis in low-grade lymphoma is post-transplant lymphoproliferative disorder, which is a heterogeneous infiltrate of reactive lymphocytes. Occasionally, cardiac lymphoma may clinically mimic cardiac rejection, and the histologic distinction between lymphoma and rejection may be difficult to establish by endomyocardial biopsy.[149]

METASTATIC TUMORS

Incidence and Pathways of Spread

Malignancies that involve the heart secondarily are, in order of frequency, carcinomas of the lung, lymphomas, carcinomas of the breast, leukemia, malignant melanoma, hepatocellular carcinoma, and carcinomas of the colon.[159] The following tumors have an especially high rate of cardiac metastasis if the incidence of the primary tumor is considered: leukemia, melanoma, thyroid carcinoma, extracardiac sarcoma, lymphoma, renal cell carcinoma, carcinoma of the lung, and carcinoma of the breast.[160, 161]

Malignancies spread to the heart by four paths: direct extension, usually from mediastinal tumor; hematogenous spread; lymphatic spread; and intracavitary extension from the inferior vena cava, or, rarely, the pulmonary veins. Although there are exceptions, epithelial malignancies typically spread to the heart by lymphatics. Mela-

noma, sarcoma, leukemia, and renal cell carcinoma metastasize to the heart by a hematogenous route, replacing large areas of myocardium not confined by vascular spaces (Fig. 19-20A). Lymphomas may involve the heart by virtually any path, including direct extension, hematogenous seeding, or lymphatic spread. Melanomas, renal tumors, including Wilms tumor and renal cell carcinoma, adrenal tumors, liver tumors, and uterine tumors are the most frequent intracavitary tumors. Renal cell carcinoma and hepatocellular carcinomas may extend into the vena cava and into the right atrium.[162]

Clinical Manifestations

The clinical manifestations of cardiac metastasis are, on the whole, similar to those of primary cardiac sarcomas, with the site of tumor within the heart greatly affecting the symptoms that a patient develops. Metastatic cardiac tumors affect the right side of the heart in 20 to 30% of cases and the left side in 10 to 33%; they are bilateral or diffuse in approximately 30 to 35% of cases, and they affect endocardium or chamber cavities in 5% of cases.[160] It is extremely uncommon for cardiac metastases to be isolated lesions.[163] Clinical manifestations include pericardial effusions, arrhythmias, congestive heart failure, syncope, and right-sided heart failure from ventricular outflow obstruction (Fig. 19-20B).[164–166]

Metastases From Epithelial Tumors

The frequency of cardiac metastasis in patients with metastatic epithelial malignancies ranges from 4.2 to approximately 30%.[159] It depends in part on the primary neoplasm; lung, breast, thyroid, and kidney cancers have the highest rates of spread to the heart. Ovarian carcinoma involves the pericardium in 2.4% of patients, and in 6% of those with stage IV disease. Cardiac metastases from the gastrointestinal and genitourinary tract tumors, especially prostatic cancer, are relatively rare.

Metastases From Nonepithelial Tumors

Sarcomas metastatic to the heart involve the myocardium (50%), pericardium (33%), or both myocardium and pericardium (17% of cases). Valvular metastases are uncommon.[167] Osteosarcoma, liposarcoma, leiomyosarcoma, unclassifiable sarcomas, rhabdomyosarcoma, neurofibrosarcoma, synovial sarcoma, sarcomatoid renal cell carcinoma, and malignant fibrous histiocytoma have been reported to involve the heart secondarily.[164, 168–173]

Malignant melanoma secondary tumors typically produce bulky, large lesions that are present throughout the cardiac chambers.[166, 174] Occasionally, isolated metastases occur; these may be removed surgically and have been reported in endomyocardial biopsy.[175, 176] Leukemic infiltrates are typically widespread, involving the pericardium in 61% of cases, the left ventricle in 55%, and the right atrium in 54%.[177] Lymphomatous involvement in the heart typically involves the epicardium and the myocardium and occurs in approximately 20% of autopsies.

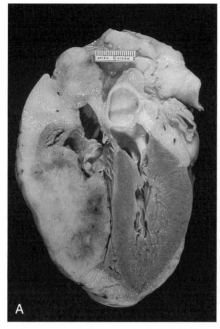
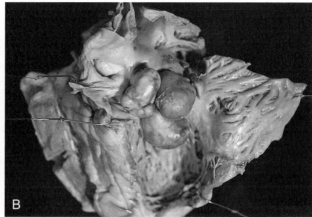

Figure 19-20 • Metastatic carcinoma. *A,* Primary, in the large bowel. Cardiac metastases arising from colonic tumors are relatively uncommon. Note the firm white mass replacing the right ventricular wall. *B,* Metastatic carcinoma with right ventricular outflow tract obstruction. Note bulky tumor in the region of the tricuspid valve. This patient developed symptoms of right ventricular outflow tract obstruction, and biopsy demonstrated high-grade metastatic endocrine carcinoma.

Pathologic Features and Surgical Biopsy

Establishing the autopsy diagnosis of metastatic cardiac tumor is not difficult, although small deposits may be missed on cursory examination. In surgical resections of cardiac tumors, a metastatic lesion should always be considered in the differential diagnosis, especially of right-sided lesions. The histologic appearance of primary and metastatic sarcomas of the heart may be identical; for this reason, a cardiac sarcoma may be considered primary only in the absence of a primary tumor elsewhere. If there is no history of other primary sarcomas, the majority of sarcomas that present as cardiac masses are primary in the heart. Spindle cell carcinomas and metastatic melanomas may histologically resemble a primary cardiac sarcoma; for this reason, immunohistochemical stains for epithelial and melanoma-specific antigens should be performed routinely on malignant cardiac lesions.

In a series of surgically resected cardiac tumors, about 20% were metastatic lesions.[120, 121] From a surgical standpoint, metastatic tumors are divided into invasive and intracavitary tumors and noninfiltrating tumors. Metastases that invade the myocardium and have been surgically removed are often sarcomas and nonepithelial neoplasms. Non-invasive intracavitary cardiac tumors that are surgically resected are often renal cell carcinomas that extend into the right atrium. Other neoplasms that grow into the right atrium without myocardial infiltration and that are amenable to surgical excision are Wilms tumor, hepatocellular carcinoma, adrenal pheochromocytoma, and uterine leiomyosarcomas. Rarely, lung carcinomas are resected after invading the pulmonary veins. Although long-term prognosis is poor in these patients, it is possible to temporarily improve cardiac function and quality of life by surgical excision.[164] Patients typically survive less than 10 months, but some, especially those with unusual tumor types, may live for extended periods. These tumors include metastatic teratoma,[178] breast carcinoma,[164] choriocarcinoma,[179] and pelvic leiomyosarcoma[173]; postoperative survival ranged from 1 to 5 years in these patients.

Acknowledgments

The opinions or assertions contained herein are the private views of the authors and are not to be construed as official or reflecting the views of the Department of the Army, the Department of the Air Force, or the Department of Defense.

REFERENCES

1. Burke A, Virmani R: Classification and incidence of cardiac tumors. In: Atlas of Tumor Pathology: Tumors of the Cardiovascular System. Washington, DC, Armed Forces Institute of Pathology, 1996
2. Waller B, Grider L, Rohr T, et al: Intracardiac thrombi: Frequency, location, etiology, and complications: A morphologic review. Part I. Clin Cardiol 18:477–479, 1995
3. Gertner E, Leatherman J: Intracardiac mural thrombus mimicking atrial myxoma in the antiphospholipid syndrome. J Rheumatol 19:1293–1298, 1992
4. Sayin A, Vural F, Bozkurt A, et al: Right atrial thrombus mimicking myxoma and bilateral pulmonary artery aneurysms in a patient with Behçet's disease—a case report. Angiology 44:915–918, 1993

5. Kmetzo J, Peters R, Plotnick G, et al: Left atrial mass. Thrombus mimicking myxoma. Chest 88:906–907, 1985

6. Shiu M, Abrams L: Echocardiographic features of free floating thrombus mimicking right ventricular myxoma. Br Heart J 49: 612–614, 1983

7. Zur-Binenboim C, Ammar R, Grenadier E, et al: Detection of round floating left atrial thrombus simulating left atrial myxoma by two-dimensional echocardiography. Am Heart J 110:492–493, 1985

8. Reynolds C, Tazelaar HD, Edwards WD: Calcified amorphous tumor of the heart (cardiac CAT). Hum Pathol 28:601–606, 1997

9. Courtice R, Stinson W, Walley V: Tissue fragments recovered at cardiac surgery masquerading as tumoural proliferations: Evidence suggesting iatrogenic or artefactual origin and common occurrence. Am J Surg Pathol 18:167–174, 1994

10. Luthringer D, Virmani R, Weiss S, Rosai J: A distinctive cardiovascular lesion resembling histiocytoid (epithelioid) hemangioma. Am J Surg Pathol 14:993–1000, 1990

11. Veinot J, Tazelaar H, Edwards W, et al: Mesothelial/monocytic incidental cardiac excrescences (cardiac MICE). Mod Pathol 7:9–16, 1994

12. Fenoglio J, Jacobs D, McAllister H: Ultrastructure of the mesothelioma of the atrioventricular node. Cancer 40:721–727, 1977

13. Monma N, Satodate R, Tashiro A, Segawa I: Origin of so-called mesothelioma of the atrioventricular node. An immunohistochemical study. Arch Pathol Lab Med 115:1026–1029, 1991

14. Burke AP, Anderson PG, Virmani R, et al: Tumor of the atrioventricular nodal region. A clinical and immunohistochemical study. Arch Pathol Lab Med 114:1057–1062, 1990

15. Fine G, Raju U: Congenital polycystic tumor of the atrioventricular node (endodermal heterotopia, mesothelioma): A histogenetic appraisal with evidence for its endodermal origin. Hum Pathol 18: 791–795, 1987

16. Balasundaram S, Halees SA, Duran C: Mesothelioma of the atrioventricular node: First successful follow-up after excision. Eur Heart J 13:718–719, 1992

17. Robertson AL Jr: The origin of primary tumors of the atrioventricular node. Resolving an old controversy (editorial). Arch Pathol Lab Med 114:1198, 1990

18. Yamazaki H, Hata J, Tamaoki N: "So-called mesothelioma" of the atrioventricular node—immunohistochemical study. Tokai J Exp Clin Med 10:589–593, 1985

19. Duray PH, Mark EJ, Barwick KW, et al: Congenital polycystic tumor of the atrioventricular node. Autopsy study with immunohistochemical findings suggesting endodermal derivation. Arch Pathol Lab Med 109:30–34, 1985

20. Ali SZ, Susin M, Kahn E, Hajdu SI: Intracardiac teratoma in a child simulating an atrioventricular nodal tumor. Pediatr Pathol 14: 913–917, 1994

21. John LC, Kingston J, Edmondson SJ: Teratoma associated with endodermal sinus tumor. Pediatr Hematol Oncol 10:49–54, 1993

22. Perez-Aytes A, Sanchis N, Barbal A, et al: Non-immunological hydrops fetalis and intrapericardial teratoma: Case report and review. Prenat Diagn 15:859–863, 1995

23. Swalwell CI: Benign intracardiac teratoma. A case of sudden death. Arch Pathol Lab Med 117:739–742, 1993

24. Todros T, Gaglioti P, Presbitero P: Management of a fetus with intrapericardial teratoma diagnosed in utero. J Ultrasound Med 10: 287–290, 1991

25. Kulthe SG, Nadkarni UB, Singh A, et al: Recurrent cardiac tamponade: Intrapericardial teratoma. Indian Pediatr 32:88–91, 1995

26. Rheuban KS, McDaniel NL, Feldman PS, et al: Intrapericardial teratoma causing nonimmune hydrops fetalis and pericardial tamponade: A case report. Pediatr Cardiol 12:54–56, 1991

27. Porqueddu M, Antona C, Polvani G, et al: Ectopic thyroid tissue in the ventricular outflow tract: Embryologic implications. Cardiology 86:524–526, 1995

28. Fujioka S, Takatsu Y, Tankawa H, et al: Intracardiac ectopic thyroid mass. Chest 110:1366–1368, 1996

29. Maillette S, Paquet E, Carrier L, et al: Asymptomatic heterotopic thyroid tumour in the right ventricular infundibulum. Can J Cardiol 10:37–40, 1994

30. Boone S, Campagna M, Walley V: Lambl's excrescences and papillary fibroelastomas: Are they different? Can J Cardiol 8:372–376, 1992

31. Rubin MA, Snell JA, Tazelaar HD, et al: Cardiac papillary fibroelastoma: an immunohistochemical investigation and unusual clinical manifestations. Mod Pathol 1995;8:402–7. 1995

32. Mann J, Parker D: Papillary fibroelastoma of the mitral valve: A rare cause of transient neurological defects. Br Heart J 71:6, 1994

33. Valente M, Basso C, Thiene G, et al: Fibroelastic papilloma: A not-so-benign cardiac tumor. Cardiovasc Pathol 1:161–166, 1992

34. Watson GH: Cardiac rhabdomyomas in tuberous sclerosis. Ann N Y Acad Sci 615:50–57, 1991

35. Burke AP, Virmani R: Cardiac rhabdomyoma: A clinicopathologic study. Mod Pathol 4:70–74, 1991

36. Fenoglio JJJ, McAllister HA, Ferrans VJ: Cardiac rhabdomyoma: A clinicopathologic and electron microscopic study. Am J Cardiol 38:241–251, 1976

37. Groves AM, Fagg NL, Cook AC, Allan LD: Cardiac tumours in intrauterine life. Arch Dis Child 67:1189–1192, 1992

38. Byard RW, Smith NM, Bourne AJ: Incidental cardiac rhabdomyomas: A significant finding necessitating additional investigation at the time of autopsy. J Forensic Sci 36:1229–1233, 1991

39. Tazelaar HD, Locke TJ, McGregor CG: Pathology of surgically excised primary cardiac tumors. Mayo Clin Proc 67:957–965, 1992

40. Kearney DL, Titus JL, Hawkins EP, et al: Pathologic features of myocardial hamartomas causing childhood tachyarrhythmias. Circulation. 75:705–710, 1987

41. Garson A Jr, Smith RT Jr, Moak JP, et al: Incessant ventricular tachycardia in infants: Myocardial hamartomas and surgical cure. J Am Coll Cardiol 10:619–626, 1987

42. Malhotra V, Ferrans VJ, Virmani R: Infantile histiocytoid cardiomyopathy: Three cases and literature review. Am Heart J 128: 1009–1021, 1994

43. Koponen MA, Siegel RJ: Histiocytoid cardiomyopathy and sudden death. Hum Pathol 27:420–423, 1996

44. Page D: Lipomatous hypertrophy of the cardiac interatrial septum: Its development and probable clinical significance. Hum Pathol 1: 151–163, 1970

45. Shirani WC Jr: Clinical, electrocardiographic and morphologic features of massive fatty deposits ("lipomatous hypertrophy") in the atrial septum. J Am Coll Cardiol 22:226–238, 1993

46. Burke A, Litovsky S, Virmani R: Lipomatous hypertrophy of the atrial septum presenting as a right atrial mass. Am J Surg Pathol 20:678–685, 1996

47. Agbamu DA, McMahon RF: Lipomatous hamartoma of the interatrial septum. Am J Cardiovasc Pathol 4:371–373, 1993

48. Reyes CJ, Jablokow VR: Lipomatous hypertrophy of the cardiac interatrial septum. A report of 38 cases and review of the literature. Am J Clin Pathol 72:785–788, 1979

49. Hutter AM, Page DL: Atrial arrhythmias and lipomatous hypertrophy of the cardiac interatrial septum. Am Heart J 82:16–21, 1971

50. Isner JM, Swan CS II, Mikus JP, Carter BL: Lipomatous hypertrophy of the interatrial septum. In vivo diagnosis. Circulation 66: 470–473, 1982

51. Fisher MS, Edmonds PR: Lipomatous hypertrophy of interatrial septum. Diagnosis by magnetic resonance imaging. J Comput Tomogr 12:267–269, 1988

52. Bhattacharjee M, Neligan MC, Dervan P: Lipomatous hypertrophy of the interatrial septum: An unusual intraoperative finding. Br Heart J 65:49–50, 1991

53. Scully RE, Mark EJ, McNeely WF, et al: Case Records of the Massachusetts General Hospital. Weekly clinicopathological exercises. Case 10. N Engl J Med 320:652–660, 1989

54. Lia J, Ho SW, Becker AE, Jones H: Multiple cardiac lipomas and sudden death. A case report and review of the literature. (In press)

55. Kanemoto N, Usui K, Fusegawa Y: An adult case of cardiac fibroma. Intern Med 33:10–12, 1994

56. Coffin CM: Congenital cardiac fibroma associated with Gorlin syndrome. Pediatr Pathol 12:255–262, 1992

57. Burke AP, Rosado-de-Christenson M, Templeton PA, Virmani R: Cardiac fibroma: Clinicopathologic correlates and surgical treatment. J Thorac Cardiovasc Surg 108:862–870, 1994

58. Busch U, Kampmann C, Meyer R, et al: Removal of a giant cardiac fibroma from a 4-year-old child. Tex Heart Inst J 22:261–264, 1995

59. Beghetti M, Haney I, Williams WG, et al: Massive right ventricular fibroma treated with partial resection and a cavopulmonary shunt. Ann Thorac Surg 62:882–884, 1996

60. Ceithaml EL, Midgley FM, Perry LW, Dullum MK: Intramural

ventricular fibroma in infancy: Survival after partial excision in 2 patients: Ann Thorac Surg 50:471–472, 1990

61. Yamaguchi M, Hosokawa Y, Ohashi H, et al: Cardiac fibroma. Long-term fate after excision. J Thorac Cardiovasc Surg 103:140–145, 1992

62. Chou P, Gonzalez-Crussi F, Cole R, Reddy V: Plasma cell granuloma of the heart. Cancer 62:1409–1413, 1988

63. Pearson P, Smithson WA, Driscoll DJ, et al: Inoperable plasma cell granuloma of the heart: Spontaneous decrease in size during an 11-month period. Mayo Clin Proc 63:1022–1025, 1988

64. Stark P, Sandbank JC, Rudnicki C, Zahari I: Inflammatory pseudotumor of the heart with vasculitis and venous thrombosis. Chest 102:1884–1885, 1992

65. Rose A: Fibrous histiocytoma of the heart. Arch Pathol Lab Med 102:389, 1978

66. Burke A, Johns JP, Virmani R: Hemangiomas of the heart. A clinicopathologic study of ten cases. Am J Cardiovasc Pathol 3:283–290, 1990

67. Weston C, Hayward M, Seymour R, Stephens M: Cardiac hemangioma associated with a facial port-wine stain and recurrent atrial tachycardia. Eur Heart J 9:668–671, 1988

68. Gengenbach S, Ridker P: Left ventricular hemangioma in Kasabach-Merritt syndrome. Am Heart J 121:202–203, 1991

69. Brodwater B, Erasmus J, McAdams HP, Dodd L: Case report: Pericardial hemangioma. J Comput Assist Tomogr 20:954–956, 1996

70. Abad C, Campo E, Estruch R, et al: Cardiac hemangioma with papillary endothelial hyperplasia: Report of a resected case and review of the literature. Ann Thorac Surg 49:305–308, 1990

71. Burke A, Virmani R: Cardiac myxomas. Am J Clin Pathol 100:671–680, 1994

72. Hutchins G, Bulkley B: Atrial myxomas: A fifty year review. Am Heart J 97:639, 1979

73. Markel M, Waller B, Armstrong W: Cardiac myxoma. A review. Medicine 66:114–125, 1987

74. Larsson S, Lepore V, Kennergren C: Atrial myxomas: Results of 25 years' experience and review of the literature. Surgery 105:695–698, 1989

75. Reynen K: Cardiac myxomas. N Engl J Med 333:1610–1617, 1995

76. Lie J: The identity and histogenesis of cardiac myxomas. A controversy put to rest. Arch Pathol Lab Med 113:724–726, 1989

77. Goldman B, Frydman C, Harpaz N, et al: Glandular cardiac myxomas. Histologic, immunohistochemical, and ultrastructural evidence of epithelial differentiation. Cancer 15:1767–1775, 1987

78. Kanda T, Sakamoto H, McManus BM, et al: Interleukin-6 secreted from human myxoma reduces murine viral myocarditis. Life Sci 58:1705–1712, 1996

79. Berrutti L, Silverman JS: Cardiac myxoma is rich in factor XIIIa positive dendrophages: Immunohistochemical study of four cases. Histopathology 28:529–535, 1996

80. Vassiliadis N, Vassiliadis K, Karkavelas G: Sudden death due to cardiac myxoma. Med Sci Law 37:76–78, 1997

81. Kanda T, Umeyama S, Sasaki A, et al: Interleukin-6 and cardiac myxoma. Am J Cardiol 74:965–967, 1994

82. Seguin JR, Beigbeder JY, Hvass U, et al: Interleukin 6 production by cardiac myxomas may explain constitutional symptoms. J Thorac Cardiovasc Surg 103:599–600, 1992

83. Soeparwata R, Poeml P, Schmid C, et al: Interleukin-6 plasma levels and tumor size in cardiac myxoma. J Thorac Cardiovasc Surg 112:1675–1677, 1996

84. Sakamoto H, Sakamaki T, Wada A, et al: Dexamethasone inhibits production of interleukin-6 by cultured cardiac myxoma cells. Am Heart J 127:704–705, 1994

85. Wiedermann CJ, Reinisch N, Fischer-Colbrie R, et al: Proinflammatory cytokines in cardiac myxomas. J Intern Med 232:263–265, 1992

86. Isobe N, Kanda T, Sakamoto H, et al: Myocardial infarction in myxoma patients with normal coronary arteries. Case reports. Angiology 47:819–823, 1996

87. Burke A, Virmani R: Cardiac myxomas. Atlas of Tumor Pathology: Tumors of the Cardiovascular System. Washington, DC, Armed Forces Institute of Pathology, 1996

88. Silverman JS, Berrutti L: Cardiac myxoma immunohistochemistry: Value of CD34, CD31, and factor XIIIa staining. Diagn Cytopathol 15:455–456, 1996

89. Johansson L: Histogenesis of cardiac myxomas. An immunohistochemical study of 19 cases, including one with glandular structures, and review of the literature. Arch Pathol Lab Med 113:735–741, 1989

90. Deshpande A, Venugopal P, Kumar AS, Chopra P: Phenotypic characterization of cellular components of cardiac myxoma: A light microscopy and immunohistochemistry study. Hum Pathol 27:1056–1069, 1996

91. Atherton D, Pitcher D, Wells R, MacDonald D: A syndrome of various cutaneous pigmented lesions, myxoid neurofibromata and atrial myxoma: The NAME syndrome. Br J Dermatol 103:421–429, 1980

92. Carney JA, Ferreiro JA: The epithelioid blue nevus. A multicentric familial tumor with important associations, including cardiac myxoma and psammomatous melanotic schwannoma. Am J Surg Pathol 20:259–272, 1996

93. Singh SD, Lansing AM: Familial cardiac myxoma—a comprehensive review of reported cases. J Ky Med Assoc 94:96–104, 1996

94. Stratakis CA, Jenkins RB, Pras E, et al: Cytogenetic and microsatellite alterations in tumors from patients with the syndrome of myxomas, spotty skin pigmentation, and endocrine overactivity (Carney complex). J Clin Endocrinol Metab 81:3607–3614, 1996

95. Richkind KE, Wason D, Vidaillet HJ: Cardiac myxoma characterized by clonal telomeric association. Genes Chromosomes Cancer 9:68–71, 1994

96. Carney JA: Carney complex: The complex of myxomas, spotty pigmentation, endocrine overactivity, and schwannomas. Semin Dermatol 14:90–98, 1995

97. David T, Lenkei S, Marquez-Julio A: Pheochromocytoma of the heart. Ann Thorac Surg 41:98–100, 1986

98. Orringer M, Sisson J, Glazer G, et al: Surgical treatment of cardiac pheochromocytomas. J Thorac Cardiovasc Surg 89:753–775, 1985

99. Aravot D, Banner N, Cantor A, et al: Location, localization and surgical treatment of cardiac pheochromocytoma. Am J Cardiol 69:283–285, 1992

100. Abad C, Jimenez P, Santana C, et al: Primary cardiac paraganglioma. Case report and review of surgically treated cases. J Cardiovasc Surg 33:758–772, 1992

101. Cruz P, Mahidhara S, Ticzon A, Tobon H: Malignant cardiac paraganglioma: Follow-up of a case. J Thorac Cardiovasc Surg 87:942–945, 1984

102. Johnson T, Shapiro B, Beierwaltes W, et al: Cardiac paragangliomas. A clinicopathologic and immunohistochemical study of four cases. Am J Surg Pathol 11:827–834, 1985

103. Kodama M, Aoki M, Sakai K: Images in cardiovascular medicine. Primary cardiac neurilemoma. Circulation 92:274–275, 1995

104. Ewy MF, Demmy TL, Perry MC, et al: Massive phrenic perineurioma mimicking an unresectable cardiac tumor. Ann Thorac Surg 60:188–189, 1995

105. Forbes AD, Schmidt RA, Wood DE, et al: Schwannoma of the left atrium: Diagnostic evaluation and surgical resection. Ann Thorac Surg 57:743–746, 1994

106. Burke A, Virmani R: Benign tumors of neural or smooth muscle origin. In: Tumors of the Heart and Great Vessels. Washington, DC, Armed Forces Institute of Pathology, 1996 pp. 105–109

107. Burke AP, Cowan D, Virmani R: Primary sarcomas of the heart. Cancer 69:387–395, 1992

108. Fang CY, Fu M, Chang JP, et al: Malignant fibrous histiocytoma of the left ventricle: A case report. Chang Keng I Hsueh 19:187–190, 1996

109. Maruki C, Suzukawa K, Koike J, Sato K: Cardiac malignant fibrous histiocytoma metastasizing to the brain: Development of multiple neoplastic cerebral aneurysms. Surg Neurol 41:40–44, 1994

110. Ovcak Z, Masera A, Lamovec J: Malignant fibrous histiocytoma of the heart. Arch Pathol Lab Med 116:872–874, 1992

111. Basso C, Stefani A, Calabrese F, et al: Primary right atrial fibrosarcoma diagnosed by endocardial biopsy. Am Heart J 131:399–402, 1996

112. Knobel B, Rosman P, Kishon Y, Husar M: Intracardiac primary fibrosarcoma. Case report and literature review. Thorac Cardiovasc Surg 40:227–230, 1992

113. Pasquale M, Katz NM, Caruso AC, et al: Myxoid variant of malignant fibrous histiocytoma of the heart. Am Heart J 122:248–250, 1991

114. Pucci A, Gagliardotto P, Papandrea C, et al: An unusual myxoid leiomyosarcoma of the heart. Arch Pathol Lab Med 120:583–586, 1996

115. Kasugai T, Sakurai M, Yutani C, et al: Sequential malignant transformation of cardiac myxoma. Acta Pathol Jpn 40:687–692, 1990

116. Burke AP, Virmani R: Osteosarcomas of the heart. Am J Surg Pathol 15:289–295, 1991

117. Domanski MJ, Delaney TF, Kleiner DE Jr, et al: Primary sarcoma of the heart causing mitral stenosis. Am J Cardiol 66:893–895, 1990

118. Dein J, Frist W, Stinson E, et al: Primary cardiac neoplasms. Early and late results of surgical treatment in 42 patients. J Thorac Cardiovasc Surg 93:502–511, 1987

119. Bear P, Moodie D: Malignant primary cardiac tumors. The Cleveland Clinic experience, 1956 to 1986. Chest 92:860–862, 1987

120. Miralles A, Bracamonte L, Soncul H, et al: Cardiac tumors: Clinical experience and surgical results in 74 patients. Ann Thorac Surg 52:886–895, 1991

121. Murphy M, Sweeney M, Putnam JJ, et al: Surgical treatment of cardiac tumors: A 25 year experience. Ann Thorac Surg 49:612–617, 1990

122. Putnam JB Jr, Sweeney MS, Colon R, et al: Primary cardiac sarcomas. Ann Thorac Surg 51:906–910, 1991

123. Reece I, Cooley D, Frazier O, et al: Cardiac tumors: Clinical spectrum and prognosis of lesions other than classical benign myxoma in 20 patients. J Thorac Cardiovasc Surg 88:439–446, 1984

124. Ohtahara A, Hattori K, Fukuki M, et al: Cardiac angiosarcoma. Intern Med 35:795–798, 1996

125. Herrmann MA, Shankerman RA, Edwards WD, et al: Primary cardiac angiosarcoma: A clinicopathologic study of six cases. J Thorac Cardiovasc Surg 103:655–664, 1992

126. Makhoul N, Bode FR: Angiosarcoma of the heart: Review of the literature and report of two cases that illustrate the broad spectrum of the disease. Can J Cardiol 11:423–428, 1995

127. Marafioti T, Castorini F, Gula G: Cardiac angiosarcoma. Histological, immunohistochemical and ultrastructural study. Pathologica 85:103–111, 1993

128. Lin BT, Colby T, Gown AM, et al: Malignant vascular tumors of the serous membranes mimicking mesothelioma. A report of 14 cases. Am J Surg Pathol 20:1431–1439, 1996

129. Marchiano D, Fisher F, Hofstetter S: Epithelioid hemangioendothelioma of the heart with distant metastases. A case report and literature review. J Cardiovasc Surg (Torino) 34:529–5333, 1993

130. Fox JP, Freitas E, McGiffin DC, et al: Primary leiomyosarcoma of the heart: A rare cause of obstruction of the left ventricular outflow tract. Aust N Z J Med 21:881–883, 1991

131. Fyfe AI, Huckell VF, Burr LH, Stonier PM: Leiomyosarcoma of the left atrium: Case report and review of the literature. Can J Cardiol 7:193–196, 1991

132. Han P, Drachtman RA, Amenta P, Ettinger LJ: Successful treatment of a primary cardiac leiomyosarcoma with ifosfamide and etoposide. J Pediatr Hematol Oncol 18:314–17, 1996

133. Takamizawa S, Sugimoto K, Tanaka H, et al: A case of primary leiomyosarcoma of the heart. Intern Med 31:265–268, 1992

134. Gyhra AS, Santander CK, Alarcon EC, et al: Leiomyosarcoma of the pulmonary veins with extension to the left atrium. Ann Thorac Surg 61:1840–1841, 1996

135. Hui K, Green L, Schmidt W: Primary cardiac rhabdomyosarcoma: Definition of a rare entity. Am J Cardiovasc Pathol 2:19–29, 1988

136. Orsmond GS, Knight L, Dehner LP, et al: Alveolar rhabdomyosarcoma involving the heart: An echocardiographic, angiographic and pathologic study. Circulation 54:837–8543, 1976

137. Hajar R, Roberts W, Folger GJ: Embryonal botryoid rhabdomyosarcoma of the mitral valve. Am J Cardiol 57:376, 1986

138. Burke A, Virmani R: Primary cardiac sarcomas. Atlas of Tumor Pathology: Tumors of the Heart and Great Vessels. Vol. 16. Washington, DC, Armed Forces Institute of Pathology, 1996 pp. 127–170

139. Charney DA, Charney JM, Ghali VS, Teplitz C: Primitive neuroectodermal tumor of the myocardium: A case report, review of the literature, immunohistochemical, and ultrastructural study. Hum Pathol 27:1365–1369, 1996

140. Paraf F, Bruneval P, Balaton A, et al: Primary liposarcoma of the heart. Am J Cardiovasc Pathol 3:175–180, 1990

141. Karn CM, Socinski MA, Fletcher JA, et al: Cardiac synovial sarcoma with translocation (X;18) associated with asbestos exposure. Cancer 73:74–78, 1994

142. Iyengar V, Lineberger AS, Kerman S, Burton NA: Synovial sarcoma of the heart. Correlation with cytogenetic findings. Arch Pathol Lab Med 119:1080–1082, 1995

143. Burke A, Virmani R: Hematologic tumors of heart and pericardium. Atlas of Tumor Pathology: Tumors of the Heart and Great Vessels. Vol. 16. Washington, DC, Armed Forces Institute of Pathology, 1996 pp 171–180

144. Margolin DA, Fabian V, Mintz U, Botham MJ: Primary cardiac lymphoma. Ann Thorac Surg 61:1000–1001, 1996

145. Ito M, Nakagawa A, Tsuzuki T, et al: Primary cardiac lymphoma. No evidence for an etiologic association with Epstein-Barr virus. Arch Pathol Lab Med 120:555–559, 1996

146. Chim CS, Chan AC, Kwong YL, Liang R: Primary cardiac lymphoma. Am J Hematol 54:79–83, 1997

147. Sommers KE, Edmundowicz D, Katz WE, Hattler BG: Primary cardiac lymphoma: Echocardiographic characterization and successful resection. Ann Thorac Surg 61:1001–1003, 1996

148. Holladay AO, Siegel RJ, Schwartz DA: Cardiac malignant lymphoma in acquired immune deficiency syndrome. Cancer 70:2203–2207, 1992

149. Burtin P, Guerci A, Boman F, et al: Malignant lymphoma in the donor heart after heart transplantation. Eur Heart J 14:1143–1145, 1993

150. Abu-Farsakh H, Cagle P, Buffone G, et al: Heart allograft involvement with Epstein-Barr virus-associated posttransplant lymphoproliferative disorder. Arch Pathol Lab Med 116:93–95, 1992

151. Rodenburg CJ, Kluin P, Maes A, Paul LC: Malignant lymphoma confined to the heart, 13 years after a cadaver kidney transplant. N Engl J Med 313:122, 1985

152. Mihalov ML, Gattuso P, Abraham K, et al: Incidence of post-transplant malignancy among 674 solid-organ-transplant recipients at a single center. Clin Transplant 10:248–255, 1996

153. Kowal-Vern A, Swinnen L, Pyle J, et al: Characterization of post-cardiac transplant lymphomas. Histology, immunophenotyping, immunohistochemistry, and gene rearrangement. Arch Pathol Lab Med 120:41–48, 1996

154. Selleslag DL, Boogaerts MA, Daenen W, et al: Occurrence of lymphoproliferative disorders in heart transplant recipients. Acta Clin Belg 46:68–74, 1991

155. Aboulafia DM, Bush R, Picozzi VJ: Cardiac tamponade due to primary pericardial lymphoma in a patient with AIDS. Chest 106:1295–1299, 1994

156. Pousset F, Le Heuzey JY, Pialoux G, et al: Cardiac lymphoma presenting as atrial flutter in an AIDS patient. Eur Heart J 15:862–864, 1994

157. Chao TY, Han SC, Nieh S, et al: Diagnosis of primary cardiac lymphoma. Report of a case with cytologic examination of pericardial fluid and imprints of transvenously biopsied intracardiac tissue. Acta Cytol 39:955–959, 1995

158. Stein M, Zyssman I, Kantor A, et al: Malignant lymphoma with primary cardiac manifestations: A case report. Med Pediatr Oncol 22:292–295, 1994

159. Burke A, Virmani R: Tumors metastatic to the heart and pericardium. Atlas of Tumor Pathology: Tumors of the Heart and Great Vessels. Vol. 16. Washington, DC Armed Forces Institute of Pathology, 1996, pp 195–210

160. McAllister H, Fenoglio J: Tumors of the cardiovascular system. Fascicles of the Armed Forces Institute of Pathology. Washington DC, 1977

161. Abraham KP, Reddy V, Gattuso P: Neoplasms metastatic to the heart: Review of 3314 consecutive autopsies. Am J Cardiovasc Pathol 3:195–198, 1990

162. Tse HF, Lau CP, Lau YK, Lai CL: Transesophageal echocardiography in the detection of inferior vena cava and cardiac metastasis in hepatocellular carcinoma. Clin Cardiol 19:211–213, 1996

163. Riccioni L, Damiani S, Pasquinelli G, Scarani P: Solitary left ventricle metastasis by renal cell carcinoma with sarcomatoid features. Tumori 82:266–269, 1996

164. Labib SB, Schick EC Jr, Isner JM: Obstruction of right ventricular

outflow tract caused by intracavitary metastatic disease: Analysis of 14 cases. J Am Coll Cardiol 19:1664–1668, 1992

165. Kasprzak JD, Religa W, Krzeminska-Pakula M, et al: Right ventricular outflow tract obstruction by cardiac metastasis as the first manifestation of follicular thyroid carcinoma. J Am Soc Echocardiogr 9:733–735, 1996

166. Rusconi C, Faggiano P, Ghizzoni G, et al: Congestive heart failure due to rapid right ventricular obliteration by metastatic malignant melanoma. Minerva Cardioangiol 44:123–125, 1996

167. Hallahan D, Vogelzang N, Borow K, et al: Cardiac metastases from soft-tissue sarcomas. J Clin Oncol 4:1662–1669, 1986

168. Bartels P, O'Callaghan W, Peyton R: Metastatic liposarcoma of the right ventricle with outflow tract obstruction: Restrictive pathophysiology predicts poor surgical outcome. Am Heart J 114:696–698, 1988

169. Bird D, Semple J, Seiler M: Sarcomatoid renal cell carcinoma metastatic to the heart: report of a case. Ultrastruct Pathol 15:361–366, 1991

170. Kamlow FJ, Padaria SF, Wainwright RJ: Metastatic cardiac malignant fibrous histiocytoma presenting as right ventricular outflow tract obstruction. Clin Cardiol 14:173–175, 1991

171. Leonard J, Raftery R: Metastatic osteogenic sarcoma involving the left ventricle. Identification with gallium-67 citrate. Clin Nucl Med 10:440, 1985

172. Lestuzzi C, Biasi S, Nicolosi G, et al: Secondary neoplastic infiltration of the myocardium diagnosed by two-dimensional echocardiography in seven cases with anatomic confirmation. J Am Coll Cardiol 9:439–445, 1987

173. Mitchell D, Mitchell D, Davidson M, et al: Nongenital pelvic leiomyosarcoma metastatic to the heart. Gynecol Oncol 43:84–87, 1991

174. Waller B, Gottdiener J, Virmani R, Roberts W: The "charcoal heart." Melanoma of the cor. Chest 77:671–676, 1980

175. Chen RH, Gaos CM, Frazier OH: Complete resection of a right atrial intracavitary metastatic melanoma. Ann Thorac Surg 61:1255–1257, 1996

176. Hanley P, Shub C, Seward J, Wold L: Intracavitary cardiac melanoma diagnosed by endomyocardial left ventricular biopsy. Chest 84:195–198, 1983

177. Roberts W, Hecht S, Berger M, et al: The heart in acute leukemia. A study of 420 autopsy cases. Am J Cardiol 21:388–412, 1968

178. Parker M, Russo P, Reuter V, et al: Intracardiac teratoma 15 years after treatment of a nonseminomatous germ cell tumor. J Urol 150:478–80, 1993

179. Perroni D, Grecchi GL, La Ciura P, Landoni F: Right ventricular metastasis from choriocarcinoma: Report of a rare case and review of the literature. Eur J Surg Oncol 19:378–381, 1993

Chapter 20

Pathology of the Conduction System

. . . . .

Saroja Bharati

In a broad sense, the pathology of the conduction system includes the pathology of the entire heart.[1-3] Thus, any disease or any type of a congenital cardiac anomaly that may affect the atria or ventricles has the potential of affecting various parts of that system to a varying degree. To understand the pathology of the system, it is imperative that we understand the anatomy of the normal conduction system. This chapter first briefly discusses normal anatomy including aging changes and their relevance to arrhythmias.[1-22] This is followed by a consideration of the common or usual types of congenital and acquired conduction system lesions that may cause arrhythmias in adults, with emphasis on the pathology of atrioventricular (AV) block.[1-3, 23-41] In addition, the pathologic changes in the system in sudden death associated with a benign tumor of the AV node, prolonged QT syndrome, mitral valve prolapse, hypertrophic cardiomyopathy, arrhythmogenic right ventricular dysplasia/cardiomyopathy, and heart transplantation are addressed.[42-48] Finally, the findings in the conduction system in sudden death in young and healthy adults; postoperative heart block and other arrhythmias that may occur several years after cardiac surgery in adults with congenital heart disease[49-57]; as well as the pathologic findings in the heart after radiofrequency ablation for intractable cardiac arrhythmias are dealt with briefly.[58-60]

NORMAL ANATOMY OF THE CONDUCTION SYSTEM

Although in a broad sense the conduction system includes the entire heart, for practical purposes this discussion includes the sinoatrial (SA) node and its approaches; the atrial preferential pathways; the AV node and its approaches; the AV bundle, including its penetrating, branching, and bifurcating parts; the right and left bundle branches; and the peripheral Purkinje nets.[1-15]

Sinoatrial Node and its Approaches

The SA node is situated in the sulcus terminalis between the junction of the superior vena cava and the right atrial appendage, extending from the hump of the atrial appendage inferiorly to the region of the intercaval band. (Fig. 20-1A). The node is a sizable structure, and most of it is situated in the epicardium, although some fibers may extend deep intramyocardially. Its size varies from heart to heart, but, generally, in the adult it is 1 to 2 cm in length and 0.5 cm in width. This is not a uniform structure; it has a rounded broad base that tapers considerably as it extends inferiorly.

The SA node cannot be dissected at the gross level. At the base (roof of the atrium), the node is in continuity with the Bachmann bundle (see Fig. 20-1B), which is the surrounding atrial myocardium including the crista terminalis and the pectinate muscles of the parietal wall of the right atrium. The Bachmann bundle more or less connects the SA node to the left atrium, which in turn is connected or fuses with the superior and middle preferential pathways in the atrial septum. At the light microscopic level, the node is easily recognizable (see Fig. 20-1C). It consists of fusiform cells with a small diameter, smaller than the surrounding atrial myocardial cells, arranged to a considerable extent along the line of the sulcus terminalis but also serpiginously surrounding the ubiquitous SA nodal artery. The cytoplasm of the cells stains lighter than that of the surrounding atrial myocardial cells. Also, its myofibrils have a smaller diameter than surrounding atrial myocardial cells, with few striations, and there is increased collagen connective tissue. There are no intercalated discs at the light microscopic level. The SA nodal cells lie in a great amount of thick collagenous and thinner elastic fibers.

At the electron microscopic level, nodal cells have fewer myofibrils compared with those of atrial cells. Their myofibrils and mitochondria are fewer and are arranged in a disorganized pattern. The sarcoplasmic reticulum is poorly developed, and the transverse tubular system is absent. There are very few fasciae adherentes and scant gap junctions. One may consider those cells that are more or less centrally located as the P, or pacemaker, cells of the SA node. There are transitional cells found at the periphery, which finally ends with surrounding atrial cells.

Approaches to the Sinoatrial Node

These consist of the ordinary or contracting type of atrial myocardial cells. In addition, some cells are somewhat larger and resemble Purkinje cells and other intermediate cells. Therefore, the cells surrounding the SA node are of varying size, and the SA node gradually merges with the surrounding atrial myocardium.

Blood Supply

The blood supply to the SA node is by way of the ramus ostii cavae superioris, reinforced by other atrial branches and branches from the bronchial arteries. In addition, the Kugel artery, a branch from the left coronary artery, may also supply the SA node. The ramus ostii cavae superioris, or SA nodal artery, originates in about 55% of cases from the right coronary artery, and in about 45% from the left coronary artery.

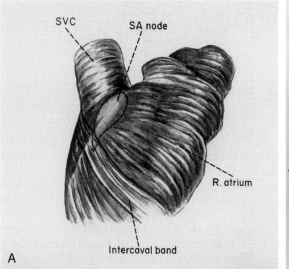

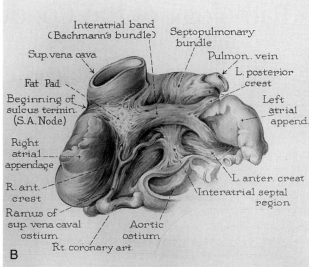

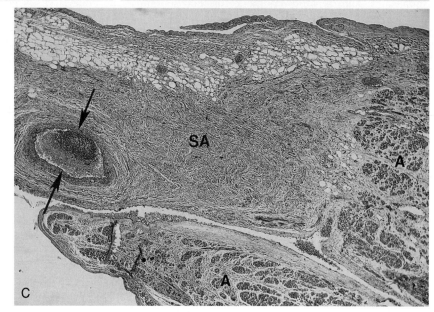

Figure 20-1 • *A,* Diagrammatic sketch of location of sinoatrial (SA) node. *B,* Diagrammatic sketch of the superior surface of the two atria showing the Bachmann bundle. *C,* Transverse section through the SA node and its approaches. Arrows define the SA nodal artery. A, atrial myocardium. (H&E stain.) (*A* and *C,* From Lev M: The conduction system. In: Gould SE (ed): Pathology of the Heart and Blood Vessels. 3rd ed. Springfield, IL, Charles C Thomas, 1968, p 180. Courtesy of Charles C. Thomas, Publisher, Springfield, IL. *B,* Lev M, Watne AL: Method for routine histopathologic study of human sinoatrial node. Arch Pathol 57:168–177, 1954. *B,* Copyrighted 1954, American Medical Association.)

Nerve Supply

There are nerve cells and fibers at the periphery of the SA node, and nerve fibers are present within it.

Atrial Preferential Pathways Including the Pectinate Muscles

The atrial preferential pathways (so-called internodal tracts or fibers) consist of regular, working-type, atrial myocardial fibers that proceed from the SA node to the AV node (Fig. 20-2). The anterior, superior, or upper preferential pathway is that part of the atrial myocardium that extends from the head of the SA node (superior part of the posterior crest) and the Bachmann bundle to the superior part of the atrial septum and that merges with the superior (anterior) approaches to the AV node. The middle preferential pathway is that part of the atrial myocardium that extends more or less from the middle part of the SA node along the proximal part of the right atrium

around the limbus fossae ovalis and that merges with or joins the anterior atrial septal approaches to the AV node. The inferior (posterior) or lower preferential pathway consists of that part of the atrial myocardium that extends from the tail end of the SA node along the inferior or posterior end of the sulcus terminalis (i.e., the crista terminalis) and proceeds along the lower part of the atrial septum adjacent to the mouth of the inferior vena cava to reach the coronary sinus area (see Fig. 20-2). Here, the myofibers are in continuity with the pectinate muscles. They then proceed to the posterior (inferior) approaches of the AV node.

These pathways consist of regular myocardial cells of a contractile type found elsewhere in the atrium. However, when cells near the approaches to the AV node are compared with cells within the atrial septum, or with the atrial approaches from the tricuspid valve and the approaches from the left atrial myocardium, the size, shape, and orientation of fibers are seen to vary considerably. Although these pathways are considered to be ordinary,

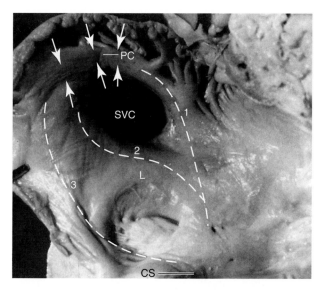

Figure 20-2 • Atrial preferential pathways from sinoatrial (SA) to atrioventricular (AV) node. 1, Anterior or superior preferential pathway; 2, middle preferential pathway; 3, posterior or inferior preferential pathway. Arrows depict the approximate location of the SA node. CS, coronary sinus; PC, porterior crest. (From Bharati S, Lev M: The anatomy and histology of the conduction system. In: Chang EK (ed): Artificial Cardiac Pacing: Practical Approaches. 2nd ed. Baltimore, MD, William and Wilkins, 1984, p 12.)

area. In general, the cells here are relatively loosely arranged and are smaller and somewhat lighter when stained. The arrangement of the myocardial fibers and both the size and shape of cells vary considerably from one approach to another in the vicinity of the AV node (Fig. 20-3).

The Atrioventricular Node

The AV node is situated between the coronary sinus and the medial (septal) leaflet of the tricuspid valve. In the majority of cases, it lies immediately deep to the endocardium of the right atrium, near the septal (medial) leaflet of the tricuspid valve (see Fig. 20-3). However, it may lie very close to the right ventricular aspect of the ventricular septum and the central fibrous body. Therefore, most of the AV node may be situated close to the summit of the right side of the ventricular septum. The node is a sizable structure; in an adult heart it is 5 to 7 mm long and 2 to 5 mm wide. Its size is not uniform, and both size and shape may vary considerably from heart to heart. The node can be dissected at the gross level. By light microscopy, it consists of a meshwork of cells that are about the size of atrial cells but are smaller than ventricular cells (see Fig. 20-3). The cyto-

working-type, atrial myocardial fibers, there are distinct variations; some cells resemble Purkinje cells, some are node-like, and some have an intermediate appearance. At the electron microscopic level, the cells in these pathways range from those with few myofibrils and mitochondria, resembling a conductive cell, to well-organized, working-type, myocardial cells.

The SA node is in continuity superiorly (anteriorly) in the parietal wall of the right atrium through the pectinate muscles, which in turn are in continuity with the posterior approaches to the AV node near the coronary sinus area. Myocardial fibers in these areas are not uniform and homogeneous but are characterized by small, relatively smooth, short fibers intermingled with scanty myocardial fibers. The intervening myocardium is quite thin and translucent, resulting in alternate thick and thin areas of atrial myocardium superiorly. It is again emphasized that the architecture of the right atrial myocardium varies considerably from one area to another.

The Atrioventricular Node and its Approaches

Approaches to the Atrioventricular Node

This vital part of the AV junction constitutes a wide area that includes the approaches from the coronary sinus (posterior or inferior), the septal leaflet of the tricuspid valve (approaches from the tricuspid valve), the atrial septal approaches, the left atrial approaches, the approaches from the mitral valve annulus, and the pectinate muscles from the superior wall. Therefore, the approaches to the AV node include the most distal fibers of the atrial preferential pathways as they merge toward the AV nodal

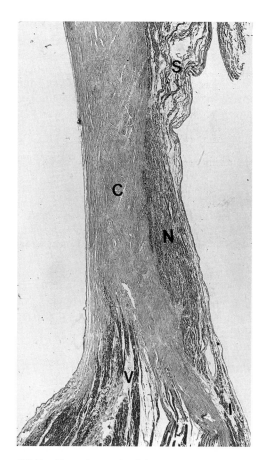

Figure 20-3 • Photomicrograph of the AV node with its approaches. N, AV node; S, superior approaches from the right atrium; I, inferior approaches; V, summit to the ventricular septum (H&E stain). (From Lev M, Widran J, Erickson EE: A method for the histopathological study of the atrioventricular node, bundle and branches. Arch Pathol 52:73, 1951. Copyrighted 1951, American Medical Association.)

plasm of the cells stains lightly and not as intensely as that of surrounding atrial or ventricular cells. Mesothelial-like cells and spaces are present between nodal cells. The elastic and collagenous tissue is more copious than that of the atria or the ventricles. Striations and intercalated disks are seen at the light microscopic level.

The AV node may be divided into three parts or layers: superficial, intermediate or middle, and deep (see Fig. 20-3). The structural variations in these layers may give rise to dual AV nodal pathways in a normal heart. The superficial layer is loosely arranged, with the smaller node-like cells oriented along the atrial cells, some intermingling with atrial cells; collagen, fat, elastic tissue, and nerve fibers are present. In the intermediate or middle layer, nodal cells tend to become compacted, but their orientation and arrangement vary considerably. The collagen and elastic tissue content is less than that found in the superficial layer, and there are fewer nerve fibers. In older persons, fat may be present in this area. In the deep layer of the AV node, nodal cells are tightly arranged and their orientation, again, varies considerably. Some amount of collagen and elastic tissue is present, but somewhat less than in the superficial and intermediate layers. Again, fat may be seen intermixed with the nodal cells in the older age group. Because the nodal fibers differ in their orientation and structure in these three layers, there are probably functional differences in the speed of conduction in these areas.

At the electron microscopic level, there are fewer mitochondria and myofibrils, with the latter arranged in a helter-skelter manner. The sarcoplasmic reticulum is poorly developed, and there is an absence of the transverse tubular system. It is unclear whether the node contains more glycogen than the surrounding atrial and ventricular myocardium. Gap junctions are scarce, but desmosomes are frequent. Fasciae adherentes are more copious than in SA nodal cells but not as frequent as in atrial or ventricular myocardial cells.

Blood Supply

In approximately 90% of hearts, the AV node is supplied by the ramus septi fibrosi, a branch from the right coronary artery, reinforced by branches from the left anterior descending coronary artery.

Nerve Supply

Copious nerve cells surround the AV node in the atrial septum and lie adjacent to the AV node and nerve fibers within the node.

Atrioventricular Bundle

Penetrating Portion

The AV node penetrates the central fibrous body to become the penetrating part of the AV bundle (Fig. 20-4). As it does so, the AV bundle assumes or undergoes different shapes and contours and the orientation of its fibers varies considerably. The so-called longitudinal orientation of the cells of the AV bundle is appreciated only from the branching part. However, even in the branching portion, there is some communication between cells. The penetrating part of the AV bundle measures 1.5 to 2 mm

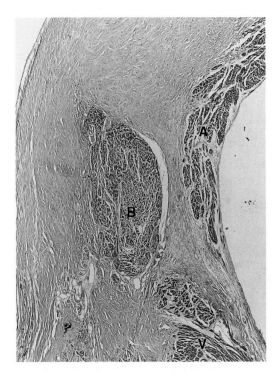

Figure 20-4 • Histology of penetrating portion of the AV bundle. B, penetrating AV bundle; A, superior approaches to the AV node; V, ventricular musculature (H&E stain). (From Lev M, Bharati S: Anatomic basis of impulse generation and atrioventricular transmission. In: Narula OS (ed): His Bundle Electrocardiology and Clinical Electrophysiology. Philadelphia, FA Davis, 1975, p 1.)

in greatest dimension and is surrounded by a space lined by mesothelial cells. The nature of the space is still unknown.

The diameter of the AV bundle cells is greater than those of the AV node but smaller than that of ventricular cells. Their cytoplasm, again, stains lighter than that of cells in the ventricles because there are fewer myofibrils. Intercalated disks and striations are present by light microscopy.

By electron microscopy, myofibrils and mitochondria are more plentiful than those in AV nodal cells but are not as numerous as those in ventricular cells. There are copious gap junctions, desmosomes, and fasciae adherentes.

The penetrating part of the AV bundle, as it enters the lower confines of the pars membranacea, may proceed some distance before it becomes the branching part of the AV bundle. This part of the AV bundle is usually situated on top of the ventricular septum.

Branching Portion

The branching part of the AV bundle gives rise to the fine fascicles of the posterior radiation of the left bundle branch in a wide manner (Fig. 20-5). In general, the left bundle branch fibers are quite superficial and subendocardial. However, more distally, some left bundle branch fibers may proceed intramyocardially and encircle groups of myocardial fibers. The branching AV bundle lies at the lower confines of the membranous part of the septum, at the summit of the ventricular septum, and below the non-

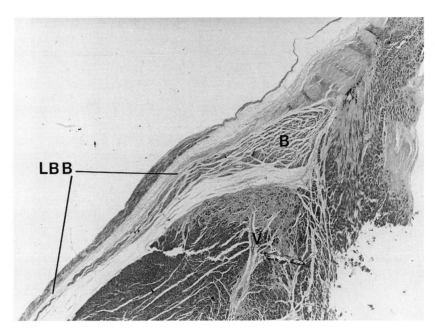

Figure 20-5 • Histology of branching portion of AV bundle from the normal heart of an older person. Note also the age changes in the summit of the septum. B, branching bundle; LBB, left bundle branch; V, ventricular septum (H&E stain). (From Lev M, Bharati S: Anatomic basis of impulse generation and atrioventricular transmission. In Narula OS [ed]: His Bundle Electrocardiology and Clinical Electrophysiology. Philadelphia, FA Davis, 1975, p 1.)

coronary, or posterior, aortic cusp. The entire bundle of His has a varying length, depending on the size of the pars membranacea. In general, in the adult, it is 1 to 3 mm wide and may vary from 6.5 to 20 mm in length.

Variations in Size, Location, and Course

The AV bundle may be located on the right or the left side of the ventricular septum or within the tricuspid valve annulus. The functional significance of these variations is not known.

Bifurcating Portion

The branching bundle, at the summit of the ventricular septum and as it proceeds to the junction beneath right

and posterior, or noncoronary, aortic cusps, becomes the bifurcating portion. This is also referred to as a pseudo-bifurcation. This is the region where the right bundle branch and the remaining fibers of the left bundle branch (anterior radiation) are given off (Fig. 20-6).

Left Bundle Branch

The main left bundle branch usually gives off a larger segment, forming the posterior radiation and a smaller segment of the anterior radiation (see Figs. 20-5 and 20-6). In general, the posterior and anterior radiations join together at the midseptal region to a varying degree, forming the septal arm of the left bundle branch. The functional significance of the midseptal fibers of the left bundle branch has not been documented, either electrocar-

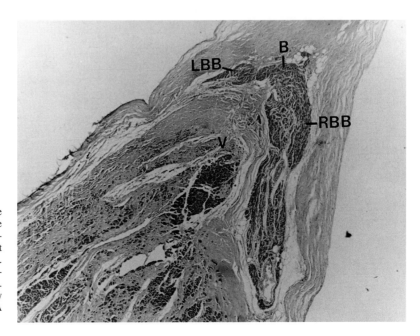

Figure 20-6 • Bifurcating part of the AV bundle from the normal heart of an older person. Note the age changes in the summit of the septum. B, bifurcating bundle; LBB, left bundle branch; RBB, right bundle branch; V, ventricular septum (H&E stain). (From Lev M, Bharati S: Anatomic basis of impulse generation and atrioventricular transmission. In: Narula OS [ed]: His Bundle Electrocardiology and Clinical Electrophysiology. Philadelphia, FA Davis, 1975, p 1.)

diographically or electrophysiologically. The posterior radiation proceeds along the posterior part of the ventricular septum toward the posterior group of papillary muscles. The anterior radiation of the left bundle branch fibers proceeds along the anteroseptal wall to the base of the anterolateral papillary muscle. The size and shape of the main left bundle branch and of the anterior, posterior, and midseptal fibers vary considerably from heart to heart. In an adult human, the main left bundle branch is approximately 1 cm wide at its origin and continues toward the apex for at least 1 to 3 cm before bifurcating into posterior and anterior radiations, respectively.

Right Bundle Branch

In contrast to the left bundle branch, this is a discrete, distinct structure in the majority of hearts and is given off distal to the insertion of the medial leaflet of the tricuspid valve on the pars membranacea, or the membranous part, of the ventricular septum. It passes along the lower septal band just distal to the muscle of Lancisi (Luschka, or the conal band) and reaches the moderator band. It then proceeds to the anterolateral papillary muscle of the right ventricle, where it divides into three segments, one supplying the anterolateral papillary muscle; one the parietal wall of the right ventricle; and the other, the distal septal surface of the right ventricle. The beginning of the right bundle branch and its third part are subendocardial (Fig. 20-7A); usually, the second part has an intramyocardial course (Fig. 20-7B). However, if the AV bundle is located on the left ventricular aspect, the entire right bundle branch may course intramyocardially. The right bundle branch measures approximately 50 mm in length and 1 mm in width.

At the light microscopic level, the cells of the first part of the right bundle branch are of the same size as AV bundle cells. Those of the second part are about the size

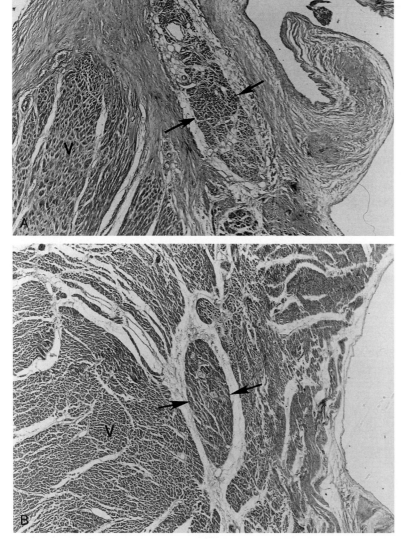

Figure 20-7 • Histology of right bundle branch from an older heart. *A,* First part; *B,* intramyocardial course of the second part (both defined by arrows). Note the fat in and around the first part of the right bundle branch. V, ventricular myocardium (H&E stain). (From Lev M, Bharati S: Anatomic basis of impulse generation and atrioventricular transmission. In: Narula OS (ed): His Bundle Electrocardiology and Clinical Electrophysiology. Philadelphia, FA Davis, 1975, p 1.)

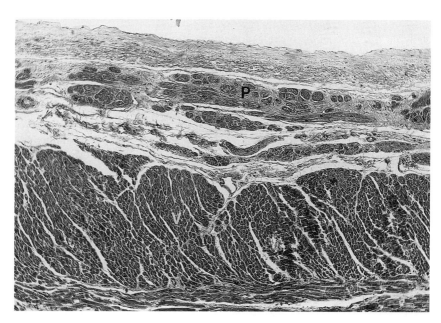

Figure 20-8 • Purkinje cells of left bundle branch lying deep to the endocardial layer of the left ventricle. P, Purkinje cells; V, ventricular myocardium (H&E stain). (From Lev M, Widran M, Erickson EE: A method for the histopathologic study of the atrioventricular node, bundle and branches. Arch Pathol 52:73, 1951. Copyright 1951–1955; American Medical Association.)

of surrounding myocardial fibers, and only the third part consists of typical Purkinje cells.

Purkinje Cells

The term *Purkinje cell* refers only to the large cells of the left bundle branch (Fig. 20-8) and those of the third part of the right bundle branch. These cells are larger than ventricular myocardial cells and are characterized by cross-striations and intercalated disks.

By electron microscopy, the myofibrils and mitochondria are few, with an irregular arrangement and an absent transverse tubular system. The connections, however, are well developed, with many desmosomes, gap junctions, and fasciae adherentes. Purkinje cells that are subendocardial become transitional cells as they penetrate the myocardium. The transitional cells eventually become regular, working myocardial cells.

Blood Supply

In approximately 90% of hearts, the right coronary artery supplies the AV bundle and is reinforced by branches from the left anterior descending coronary artery. The blood supply to the right bundle branch is by way of perforating branches from the anterior and posterior descending coronary arteries. In addition, a special large branch, the ramus limbi dextri, from the second anterior perforating artery, supplies the second or middle part of the right bundle branch. The blood supply to the main left bundle branch is by way of branches from the anterior and posterior perforating arteries; the supply to the anterior radiation is from anterior perforating branches. The posterior radiation is supplied by a posterior perforating artery in some hearts and in others by both anterior and posterior perforating branches.

Nerve Supply

Nerve fibers are present in both the AV node and AV bundle, but to a lesser extent in the beginning of the bundle branches. In general, very few nerves are observed in the areas distal to the AV sulcus.

Cardiac Innervation

In general, in the human, the cardiac plexus surrounding the arch of the aorta is responsible for cardiac innervation.[16] This is formed by sympathetic fibers originating from the upper thoracic spinal cord and parasympathetic ones originating from the medulla. The superior, middle, and inferior cardiac nerves from the superior, middle, and inferior cervical ganglia of the sympathetic nerves join the vagus nerve on both sides to form the cardiac plexus. It predominantly supplies the SA node and its approaches, the atrial septum, the approaches to the AV node, the AV node, and the AV bundle to a lesser degree. The cardiac plexus also supplies the right and left coronary arteries.

The exact distribution and destination of these nerves are unknown. However, the rich autonomic innervation of the SA and AV nodal areas noted in the canine heart indicates that in that species the SA node is especially responsive to parasympathetic adrenergic regulation, whereas the AV conduction is preferentially sensitive to sympathetic adrenergic regulation.[16]

Conductive Cells Versus Contractile Cells—Differentiating Features

The contracting cells of the ventricular myocardium are arranged in an organized manner, with tightly packed myofibrils, mitochondria, a well-developed sarcoplasmic reticulum, and a transverse tubular system with many gap junctions, desmosomes, and fasciae adherentes. (See Chapters 2 and 8.) On the other hand, mitochondria and myofibrils of atrial myocardial cells are not as well organized as those of ventricular myocardial cells, and some of these cells do not have a transverse tubular system.

In contrast to contracting cells, the conducting cells of

the myocardium have relatively few myofibrils and mitochondria that are poorly organized, with an absent transverse tubular system. The SA and AV nodes and the transitional cells peripheral to the Purkinje cells have scant gap junctions. Therefore, it may be said that the atrial myocardium is intermediate in nature and has the characteristics in part of conducting-type cells and in part of contractile ventricular myocardial cells.

Space Around the Atrioventricular Bundle and Bundle Branches

Endothelium-like cells, similar to those seen in and around the AV node, are also found within and around the AV bundle, where they form a distinct sheet lining a space. The sheet-lined space also surrounds the entire left and right bundle branches to the periphery. The nature and function of this space are unknown.

Paraspecific Fibers of Mahaim

Mahaim fibers are those myocardial fibers from the AV node, the AV bundle, and the left bundle branch that join the ventricular septum. They resemble the myocardial fibers of their origin and gradually become ventricular myocardial cells. Such connections are not normally present between the right bundle branch and the ventricular septum.

Accessory Bypass Pathways or Fibers of Kent

Accessory bypass pathways are seen in normal infants up to 6 months of age in the right or left AV rims between atrium and ventricle. The myocardial cells on the atrial side resemble atrial cells and those on the ventricular side resemble ventricular cells. These fibers are, in general, working myocardial fibers. It is not known whether such fibers exist in an adult heart without clinical evidence of Wolff-Parkinson-White syndrome.

Histochemical Features of the Conducting Cells

Histochemically, conductive cells have a well-developed anaerobic oxidative system and a poorly developed aerobic one. This is the opposite of a contracting myocardial cell. It has also been shown that the conduction system contains certain cholinesterases not found in working myocardium. There is a distinct increase in glycogen in the AV bundle and bundle branches. It is not clear whether there is more glycogen in the SA and AV nodes.

METHOD OF STUDY OF THE CONDUCTION SYSTEM

Blocks are taken from the SA node and its approaches, the atrial preferential pathways, the AV node and its approaches, the AV bundle (penetrating, branching, and bifurcating parts), and the bundle branches up to the region of the moderator band; all of these are serially sectioned (Fig. 20-9). If the block is large, it may be subdivided into two or three smaller ones. Every 20th section is retained, and alternate sections are stained with hematoxylin-eosin and Weigert-van Gieson stains. In addition, several sections are taken from the remainder of the heart. Depending on the size of the heart, approximately 1200 to 1600 sections are obtained for the study of the conduction system in an adult. The sections are then compared with those from an age-matched, control conduction system. This method of sectioning and sampling the entire heart yields a semiquantitative analysis of the conduction system.

Method of Study of the Conduction System and the Heart in Pre-excitation

Every attempt is made to retain the parietal walls of the atrioventricular rims without opening the coronary arteries. Blocks are taken from the parietal (superior) and posterior (inferior) walls of the AV rim, excluding the AV junction containing the conduction system, and are completely serially sectioned. The AV junctional block contains the summit of the ventricular septum, the central fibrous body, and the membranous septum. This block includes the approaches to the AV node, the AV node itself, the AV bundle, and the bundle branches. It is cut into several blocks and serially sectioned as previously described.

The Significance of Serial Section Examination of the Conduction System

In a limited sense, the conduction system is quite small and is situated in strategic parts of the heart in a curved manner, forming an arc. Therefore, a serial section examination, as described earlier, is mandatory to obtain information for meaningful interpretation that may be useful in correlation with electrocardiographic and/or electrophysiologic findings. Identification of the various parts of the conduction system through random single sections is impossible and a waste of time. The conduction system must be followed from beginning to end by means of serial sections. In pre-excitation, it is important to find the accessory pathways between the atria and ventricles that bypass the conventional conduction system.

When to Examine the Conduction System Studies

An examination of the conduction system is warranted in the following circumstances:

1. To correlate electrocardiographic and electrophysiologic findings and aid clinicians in their work
2. In postoperative congenital hearts, with or without arrhythmias, and/or sudden death

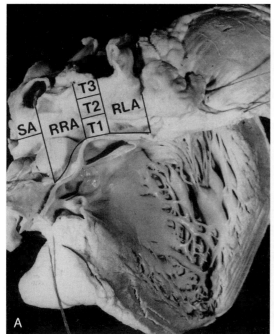

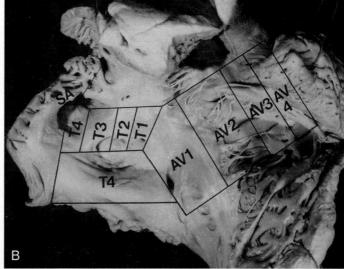

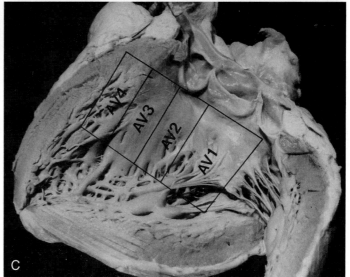

Figure 20-9 • *A* through *C,* Method of taking blocks from the heart for conduction system studies. SA, SA node; T_1 through T_4, atrial preferential pathways; RRA, roof of right atrium; RLA, roof of left atrium; AV_1 through AV_4, blocks containing atrioventricular (AV) node and its approaches, AV bundle, and bundle branches. (From Lev M, Bharati S: Lesions of the conduction system and their functional significance. In: Somers SC (ed): Pathology Annual 1974. New York, Appleton-Century-Crofts, 1974, pp 157–207.)

3. When death occurs either suddenly or otherwise after ablative procedures for varying types of arrhythmias
4. In pre-excitation (Wolff-Parkinson-White syndrome) with or without sudden death and/or arrhythmias
5. If death occurs suddenly and unexpectedly, especially in a young and apparently healthy person, including athletes

Transient cardiac arrhythmias may or may not have an anatomic or pathologic base. However, permanent cardiac arrhythmias almost always have an anatomic or pathologic substrate in the conduction system, including the surrounding myocardium.

NORMAL AGING CHANGES IN THE CONDUCTION SYSTEM AND THEIR RELEVANCE TO CARDIAC ARRHYTHMIAS

Normal aging changes generally take the form of fatty infiltration of the atria, including the atrial septum (atrial preferential pathways) and the approaches to the SA and AV nodes. Associated aging changes are loss of cells with space formation, atrophy, hypertrophy, fibroelastosis, calcification, and fibrotic and linear formation of all parts of the conduction fibers, with these changes occurring to a varying degree.[17-24]

Fatty infiltration as such may replace the SA node and its approaches, resulting in its isolation from the surrounding atrial myocardium. Senile amyloidosis, especially in patients older than 80 years of age, may affect the atria and small blood vessels with or without affecting the SA node and the SA nodal artery. Therefore, fat and/or amyloid of the atrial myocardium and the SA node and its approaches may give rise to atrial fibrillation, flutter, bradycardia-tachycardia, or sick sinus syndrome. Atrial fibrillation is the most common cardiac arrhythmia in the elderly, both men and women.

Similarly, fatty replacement of the AV node and its approaches, with or without fibroelastosis, may give rise to AV block (Fig. 20-10) or to varying types of junctional arrhythmias and a re-entrant type of arrhythmia at

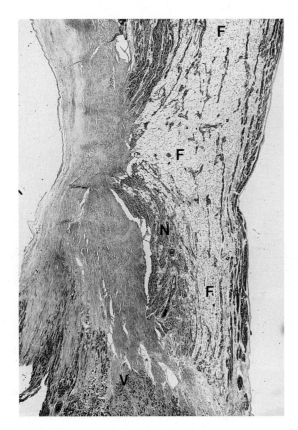

Figure 20-10 • Fatty metamorphosis in the approaches to the AV node and fat isolating the AV node from its approaches. The space to the left of AV node is an artifact. F, fat; N, AV node; V, summit of the ventricular septum (H&E stain). (From Lev M, Widran J, Erickson EE: Method for histological study of AV node, bundle and branches. Arch Pathol 52:73, 1951.)

the AV junction. The fat may involve the AV bundle and the bundle branches, especially the bifurcating part of the AV bundle.

Complete replacement of the main left bundle branch with fibrosis may produce complete left bundle branch block in the electrocardiogram. Marked fat and fibrosis of the beginning of the right bundle branch results in a complete right bundle branch block pattern. Similar changes in the bifurcating bundle may cause anterior fascicular block and right bundle branch block that can progress to complete AV block with time. The degree and extent of the fat and/or fibrosis and loss of conduction fibers in the AV conduction system form the anatomic base for arrhythmias in the elderly. Aging of the summit of the ventricular septum is discussed later.

PATHOLOGY OF THE CONDUCTION SYSTEM

Common Pathologic Causes of Arrhythmias

Coronary artery disease, hypertensive heart disease, collagen diseases, myocarditis, and infiltrative diseases such as sarcoidosis or amyloidosis may affect parts of the conduction system in varying degree and cause different types of AV block, bundle branch block, and ventricular and/or supraventricular arrhythmias.[1-3, 11, 13, 19, 22-41] Furthermore, their effect on various parts of the conduction system and the myocardium may cause different types of supraventricular, junctional, or ventricular arrhythmias at any given time in the same patient. More importantly, normal aging phenomena at the summit of the ventricular septum may affect the AV conduction system to a varying degree in a sclerodegenerative process associated with calcification and fat to induce AV block.[1-3, 11, 13, 17-24] A few examples of these conditions that affect the conduction system and in some instances cause sudden death are discussed.[49-52] Sudden death in tumor of the AV node, hypertrophic cardiomyopathy, mitral valve prolapse, arrhythmogenic right ventricular dysplasia/cardiomyopathy, Q-T prolongation syndrome, and heart transplantation are also dealt with briefly.[42-48] Cardiac conduction system pathology after heart surgery in congenital heart disease and the effects of ablative procedures using radiofrequency energy to treat intractable arrhythmias are discussed.[53-60]

No known definitive *common* congenital anomalies of the conduction system in the adult cause arrhythmia except for partial or complete absence of the AV node and/ or AV bundle, which result in heart block of varying degree.[27] However, varying types of congenital anomalies of the conduction system can cause arrhythmias and sudden death at any age, including sudden death in an otherwise "normal" adult or an athlete.[49-52]

Complete Atrioventricular Block

Any disease that affects the myocardium in either an acute or chronic stage may produce AV block. Such block may occur at the approaches to the AV node, at the AV node itself, at the penetrating part or branching part of the AV bundle, or at the level of the bundle branches. Pathologically, AV block may be classified as being caused by (1) a congenital condition, (2) coronary artery disease, (3) hypertensive heart disease, (4) sclerosis of the left side of the cardiac skeleton (idiopathic or primary AV block), (5) aortic valve disease, (6) collagen disease, (7) myocarditis, (8) infective endocarditis, (9) iatrogenic block, (10) neoplastic disease, or (11) miscellaneous diseases and altered physiologic states.[1-3, 11, 13, 21-41, 53-57]

Congenital Atrioventricular Block in the Adult

Congenital AV block in an otherwise normally developed heart is usually a benign condition. However, with advancing age, there may be further slowing of heart rate or congestive heart failure and an increase in mortality. Today, pacemakers are widely used to prevent symptoms such as syncopal episodes and congestive heart failure. In general, the pathologic substrate is a lack of connection between the atria and the peripheral conduction system, with total replacement by fat of the AV nodal approaches and AV node.[27] In addition, the AV bundle may show marked septation and/or fragmentation (Fig. 20-11). This may be associated with advanced sclerosis of the summit of the ventricular septum. Therefore, congenital AV block in the adult may be associated with premature aging of

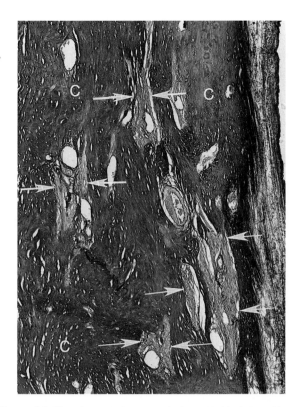

Figure 20-11 • Congenital atrioventricular (AV) block in a 42-year-old man. Fragments of the penetrating part of the AV bundle are defined by arrows in the central fibrous body (C) (Weigert-van Gieson stain). (From Bharati S, Rosen M, Strasberg B, et al: Anatomic substrate for atrioventricular block in middle aged adults. Pacing Clin Electrophysiol 5:860, 1982.)

the summit of the ventricular septum in the form of sclerosis affecting the branching bundle and the bundle branches.[27] The long-term hemodynamic stresses of chronic bradycardia most likely accelerate aging of the summit of the ventricular septum and may result in trifascicular involvement of the conduction system. This may

further worsen bradyarrhythmia by shifting the escape rhythm distally to lower foci, which are slower; this in turn may produce a further deterioration into a slower idioventricular escape rhythm and thereby worsen hemodynamics. The result is progressive conduction disease. Congenital AV block, especially in the young adult, may seemingly appear asymptomatic to start with and not require pacing. However, with advancing age, the hemodynamic effects of chronic bradycardia and progressive conduction system disease eventually prompt cardiac pacing.

Coronary Artery Disease

Pathologic changes may occur in the conduction system in coronary artery disease, either in its acute stage (i.e., acute myocardial infarction) or in chronic coronary insufficiency. It is important to differentiate these changes, because the mechanism of producing AV block differs in the two.[1-3, 11, 13, 24]

Acute Myocardial Infarction

When there is acute infarction of the posteroseptal wall, there may be infarction of part of the SA node and of the approaches to the AV node, with focal necrosis of the node (Fig. 20-12), the AV bundle, and the bundle branches. However, in some cases, there are no pathologic changes in the conduction system, and in still others there are no changes in the bundle branches. Clinically, these changes may manifest as complete AV block. Usually, if the patient recovers, the heart block disappears. On the other hand, in infarction of the anteroseptal wall, the branching bundle and bundle branches are usually affected by the necrotic process (Fig. 20-13), and the AV node and the penetrating portion of the AV bundle may be involved as well. In contrast to posteroseptal wall infarction with AV block, in which the mortality rate is 25%, anteroseptal wall infarction with AV block has a mortality rate of approximately 75%. The infarction is usually extensive in the latter instance. Usually, if a patient recovers, the heart block disappears; it is uncommon

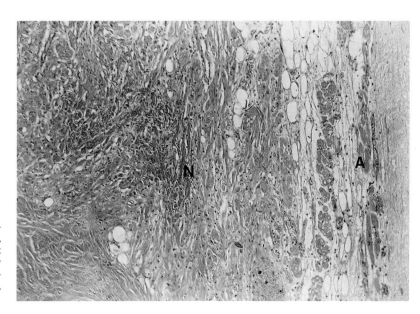

Figure 20-12 • Acute posterior wall myocardial infarction involving the AV node and its approaches, showing focal necrosis of the AV node (N) and recent infarct of the approaches (A) (H&E stain). (From Lev M, Kinare SG, Pick A: The pathogenesis of atrioventricular block in coronary disease. Circulation 42:409, 1970.)

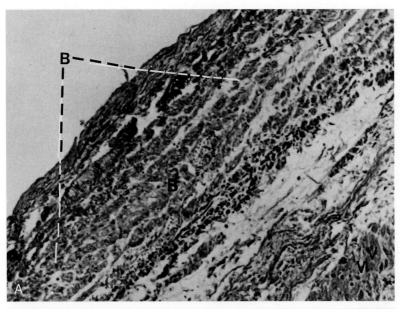

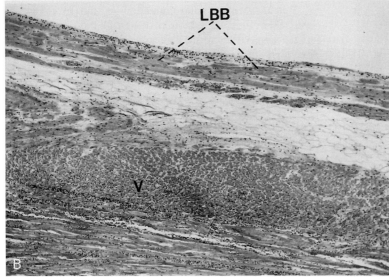

Figure 20-13 • *A,* Acute anteroseptal wall myocardial infarction. AV bundle showing necrosis and acute polymorphonuclear leukocytic exudate. *B,* Left bundle branch showing recent infarct. B, branching bundle; LBB, left bundle branch; V, ventricular septum (H&E stain). (From Lev M, Kinare SG, Pick A: The pathogenesis of atrioventricular block in coronary disease. Circulation 42:409, 1970.)

to develop chronic AV block after acute myocardial infarction. The site of infarction is more important than the site of coronary artery occlusion in producing lesions in the conduction system.

Chronic Coronary Insufficiency

When a patient has coronary insufficiency of long duration, with or without infarction, there may be involvement of varying parts of the conduction system, predominantly the bundle branches,[32] that may progress to complete AV block with time. However, the pathogenesis of AV block in chronic coronary insufficiency differs from that of acute infarction-induced block. In the former, in addition to the obvious ischemic factor, there are aging changes in the conduction system in the form of sclerosis of the left side of the cardiac skeleton and/or an abnormal formation of the AV bundle (e.g., right-sided AV bundle) and/or severe small vessel disease. Therefore, in chronic

coronary insufficiency it is a combination of several mechanisms that produces the pathologic changes in the conduction system. In these cases, the right bundle branch is destroyed by the chronic ischemic process and the left bundle branch by both the chronic ischemic process and other factors, such as a calcific mass in the summit of the ventricular septum that may impinge upon the branching bundle and the origin of the left bundle branch (Fig. 20-14A). The fibrosis of the main left bundle branch is probably mechanical and produced by calcific impingement, and that in the right bundle branch is caused by chronic coronary insufficiency (see Fig. 20-14B). Clinically, there may be chronic right bundle branch block or left bundle branch block progressing to chronic complete AV block. Arteriolosclerosis or disease of the small vessels may exacerbate the main coronary artery disease. In rare cases, arteriolosclerosis as such may be present without major coronary artery disease and may cause destruction of the

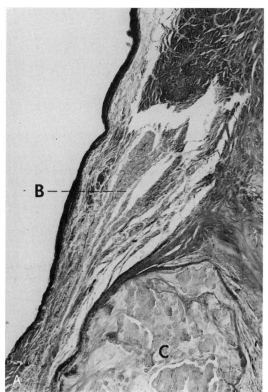
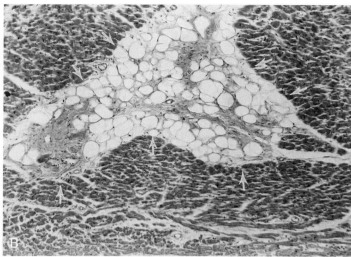

Figure 20-14 • *A,* Calcific mass (C) compressing the branching bundle (B) in chronic coronary insufficiency with chronic atrioventricular block (Weigert-van Gieson stain). *B,* Right bundle branch, second portion defined by arrows showing replacement by fibrous and fatty tissue (H&E stain). (From Lev M, Kinare SG, Pick A: The pathogenesis of atrioventricular block in coronary disease. Circulation 42:409, 1970.)

branching bundle and the bundle branches. Chronic coronary insufficiency is the most common cause of bilateral bundle branch block.[32]

Hypertensive Heart Disease

The pathologic effects of systemic hypertension on the conduction system are caused by mechanical forces as well as arteriolosclerosis.[1–3, 13, 19, 21–24] The injury to the beginning of the main left bundle branch occurs as a result of stress and strain on the fibrous skeleton of the heart and may be considered the mechanical factor. Arteriolosclerosis of the heart is frequently seen in hypertensive patients with conduction disturbances; there may be arteriolosclerosis of the SA node, the AV node, the AV bundle, and/or the bundle branches. Clinically, this may manifest as sick sinus syndrome, AV block, and/or right or left bundle branch block.

Age Changes at the Summit of the Ventricular Septum

In general, with advancing age degenerative changes occur at the summit of the ventricular septum and the contiguous aortic-mitral annulus, the mitral annulus, the central fibrous body, the membranous part of the ventricular septum, the aortic valve base, and the sinuses of Valsalva. The changes consist of fibrosis and hyalinization with or without associated calcification, fat deposition, and loss of conduction fibers. We have named this type of degenerative process "sclerosis of the left side of the cardiac skeleton." It occurs as a result of "stress and strain" in a high-pressure system, and the pathologic

changes may affect the adjacent AV bundle and bundle branches (Fig. 20-15). Often, the branching part of the AV bundle, the beginning of the right and left bundle branches, and the main left bundle branch are compressed by calcium or replaced by a fibroelastic process, such as linear fibroelastic strand formation, loss of cells, space formation, and/or fat. The left bundle branch may be totally disrupted from the main AV bundle; the second part of the right bundle branch may be completely replaced by a fibroelastic process, probably as a result of ischemia. These changes may induce complete AV block, left bundle branch block, or bilateral bundle branch block. Aging at the summit of the ventricular septum usually begins at 40 years and is accelerated by hypertensive heart disease, coronary artery disease, and diabetes mellitus. The branching and bifurcating part of the atrioventricular bundle and the beginning of the main left bundle branch are quite superficial subendocardial structures and, as such, are susceptible to degenerative changes caused by aging.[1–3, 13, 17, 19, 21–24, 28–33]

We believe that most cases of AV block seen in patients older than 55 years of age are a result of sclerosis of the left side of the cardiac skeleton. Some authors believe that chronic AV block in this age group is idiopathic in nature and follows a primary degenerative process that destroys the bundle branches.[29, 30] Others suggest that this destruction is related to interference with lymph drainage.[31] We have not encountered peripheral bundle branch disease as such producing AV block without involvement of the branching bundle and the main left bundle branch as reported in the literature.[32] We believe that sclerosis of the left side of the cardiac skeleton is fundamentally related to normal aging phenomena and

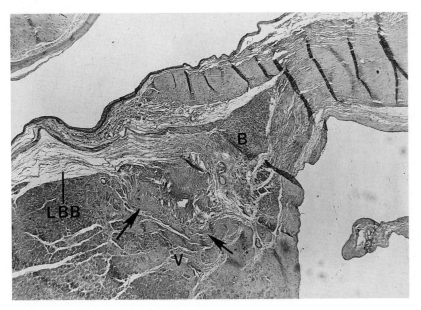

Figure 20-15 • Fibrocalcific degenerative changes in the summit of the ventricular septum pressing on the branching bundle and producing chronic atrioventricular block. Note the marked fibrosis of the branching bundle and marked linear formation of the left bundle branch. Arrows point to the calcific changes in the summit. B, fibrosis of the branching bundle; V, summit of the ventricular septum; LBB, left bundle branch fibers (Weigert–van Gieson stain). (From Lev M, Bharati S: Age-related changes in the cardiac conduction system. Internal Medicine for the Specialist 2:19, 1981.)

results in degenerative changes of the AV bundle and the beginning of the bundle branches. Likewise, mitral annular calcification as such may extend to the approaches to the AV node, the AV node, and the penetrating AV bundle to produce AV block.

Aortic Valve Disease

Normal aging changes of the aortic valve, with or without aortic stenosis and/or regurgitation, may cause fibrocalcific degenerative changes of the branching bundle and the main left bundle branch resulting in complete AV block.[2, 29, 31, 33, 35, 37]

Collagen Diseases

Since there is a considerable amount of collagen connective tissue in the conduction system, it is not surprising to find that collagen diseases such as lupus erythematosus, dermatomyositis, scleroderma, and other types affect the conduction system to varying degrees and may be associated with complete AV block or other arrhythmias.[1–3, 11, 34–36] Complete replacement of the AV node by granulation tissue in lupus (Fig. 20-16), fibrotic disruption of bundle branches to a varying extent in dermatomyositis, and granulomas in various parts of the conduction system in rheumatoid arthritis may be seen on histologic examination.[34–37]

Myocarditis

Myocarditis of any type, whether in an acute or chronic phase, may cause complete AV block and/or ventricular arrhythmias.[1–3, 11, 13, 25, 26] If the patient survives, the heart block usually disappears; it is uncommon for chronic AV block to develop after myocarditis. Pathologically, in the acute phase of the illness the inflammatory changes usually predominate in the ventricular myocardium, affecting the distal part of the conduction system such as the bundle branches (Fig. 20-17). Rarely is a part of the conduction system itself affected. Usually, the

myocardium surrounding the conduction system is involved by the inflammatory process, but in some cases, the conduction system is involved more than the surrounding myocardium. In myocarditis, there appears to be a predilection for the ventricular myocardium to be affected more than the atrial myocardium.

Infective Endocarditis

Infective endocarditis of the aortic and/or the mitral valve may extend to the aortic-mitral annulus, the central fibrous body, the membranous part of the ventricular septum, or the summit of the ventricular septum, thereby affecting the AV node and the AV bundle and producing AV block and/or bundle branch block.[1–3, 11, 38–41] (See also Chapter 14.)

Iatrogenic Atrioventricular Block

See discussion below.

Conditions Associated with Sudden Death

Sudden death is also discussed in Chapter 11.

Neoplastic Diseases

Any type of tumor that metastasizes to the heart has the potential to affect different parts of the conduction system to varying degrees and may produce AV block, junctional arrhythmias, atrial arrhythmias, or ventricular arrhythmias that can lead to sudden death.

There is one particular benign tumor, called mesothelioma or coelothelioma of the AV node, that has an affinity to involve only the AV node and its approaches.[2, 42] The tumor may replace the AV node and its approaches in the atrial septum (Fig. 20-18), producing complete AV block with narrow QRS complex in the electrocardiogram. Although this is a slow-growing tumor, it may manifest clinically as AV block from birth to old age. The tumor

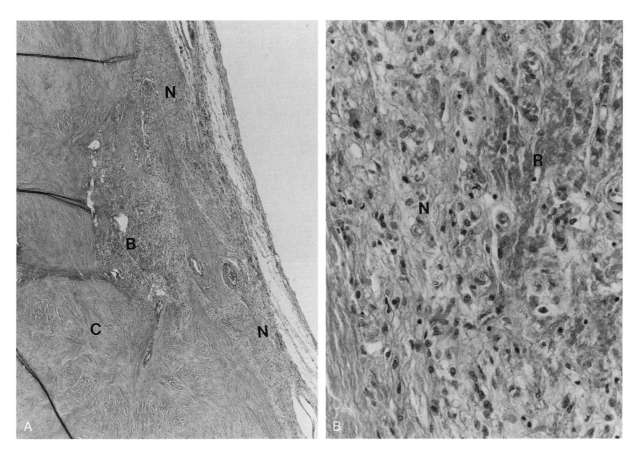

Figure 20-16 • Almost the entire AV node is replaced by granulation tissue in a 12-year-old girl with systemic lupus erythematosus and complete heart block. *A,* AV node (N) and beginning of penetrating portion of AV bundle (B). *B,* Higher power, AV node (N). R, remnants of nodal tissue (H&E stain). C, central fibrous body. (From Bharati S, de la Fuente DJ, Kallen RJ, et al: The conduction system in systemic lupus erythematosus with atrioventricular block. Am J Cardiol 35:299–304, 1975, with permission from Excerpta Medica Inc.)

consists of neoplastic cells of benign nature, with no anaplasia, and has a tendency to form cysts. The tumor is usually seen in young women who may remain totally asymptomatic. Sudden death may be the first manifestation.

Mesothelioma of the AV node, although a benign tumor, is a known cause of sudden death in otherwise young and healthy persons. This is surprising, because the tumor location produces a site of heart block proximal to the AV bundle with a narrow QRS complex in the elec-

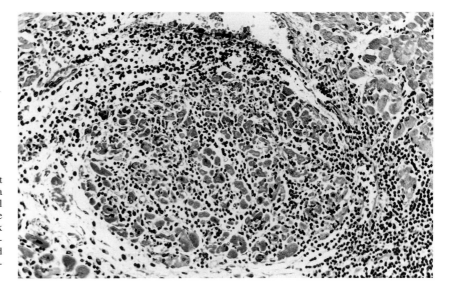

Figure 20-17 • Photomicrograph of right bundle branch in its midportion, showing a marked infiltration of lymphoid cells with focal necrosis, in a 30-year-old woman with acute myocarditis and complete atrioventricular block (H&E stain). (From Lev M, Unger PU: The pathology of the conduction system in acquired heart disease. Arch Pathol 60:502, 1955. Copyrighted 1955, American Medical Association.)

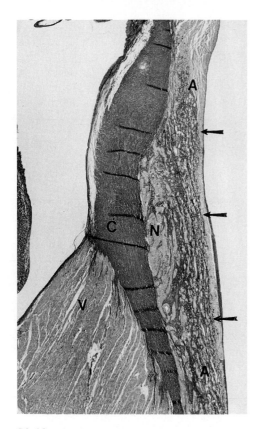

Figure 20-18 • A 16-year-old asymptomatic girl developed 2:1 AV block with intermittent complete AV block immediately after delivering a healthy full-term infant. Six weeks later, she developed complete AV block and died suddenly. Photomicrograph shows mesothelioma replacing the AV node (N) and its approaches (A). Arrows point to the tumor. C, central fibrous body; V, ventricular septum (Weigert-van Gieson stain). (From Bharati S, Lev M: The Cardiac Conduction System in Unexplained Sudden Death. Mt. Kisco, NY, Futura Publishing Co., 1992, pp 1–416.)

trocardiogram, which is consistent with a favorable clinical course. (See Figs. 11-37 and 19-6 also.)

Prolonged QT Interval

The only common finding in the conduction system in cases of prolonged QT interval with sudden death is marked fatty infiltration in the approaches to the AV node. The bundle is lobulated, with or without loop formation, with fibrosis of the summit of the ventricular septum predominately on the right side with arteriolosclerosis (Fig. 20-19). In addition, fibrotic changes are seen in the AV bundle and the bundle branches. The ventricular myocardium in all cases is chronically inflamed. In some, the AV node is partially embedded in the central fibrous body. Although it is not clear how these changes are related to the disturbance in the repolarization process and prolongation of the QT interval, it is notable that pathologic findings are, indeed, present in QT prolongation with sudden death.[43]

Several abnormal genes have been identified on several chromosomes in patients with prolonged QT interval syndrome. The familial QT syndrome is predominately an autosomal dominant disorder associated with syncopal ep-

isodes, ventricular tachycardia, and sudden death. Genetic heterogeneity has been documented through linkage studies with loci on chromosomes 3p21-24, 7q-35-36, 11p15.5, and 4q25-27. In addition, mutations in ionic channel genes, on chromosomes 3 and 7, have been demonstrated to be related to two other forms of long QT syndrome. More recently, a missense HERG mutation in affected members of a family with autosomal dominant long QT syndrome has been identified. (See discussion in Chapter 24.)

We hypothesize that the altered ion channel genes may create arrhythmias, which may remain silent for a long time. However, such "silent arrhythmias" may produce pathologic changes such as fat, fibrosis, and disruption of myocardial fibers, which in turn further affect the ion channel genes, creating a vicious cycle that leads to the development of arrhythmias and eventually, sudden death.

Mitral Valve Prolapse

In mitral valve prolapse with sudden death, the heart is usually hypertrophied and enlarged. The mitral valve, although redundant in all cases, shows considerable mor-

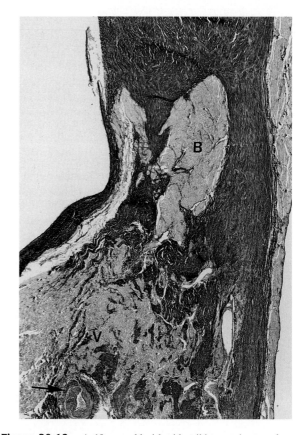

Figure 20-19 • A 19-year-old girl with mild to moderate pulmonary stenosis and prolonged QT interval had syncopal episodes for many years. During the last attack, she became unresponsive; immediately after cardiopulmonary resuscitation the electrocardiogram showed asystole, subsequently ventricular fibrillation, idioventricular rhythms, and then sinus tachycardia. She became comatose and died 10 days later. Note the lobulated atrioventricular bundle (B) with mild fibrosis and marked fibrosis of the summit of the ventricular septum (V) predominately on the right side. Arrow indicates thickened arteriole (Weigert–van Gieson stain).

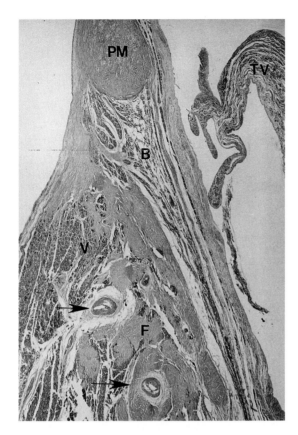

Figure 20-20 • A 45-year-old asymptomatic male physician died suddenly. Autopsy revealed marked mitral valve prolapse with calcification. Photomicrograph shows the beginning of the penetrating portion of the AV bundle (B) extending downward on the right side of the summit of the ventricular septum (V). Note the extensive fibrosis (F) of the ventricular septum on the right side with marked arteriolosclerosis. Arrow points to large arteriole. PM, pars membranacea; TV, tricuspid valve (H&E stain). (From Bharati S, Lev M, Granston A, et al: The conduction system in mitral valve prolapse syndrome with sudden death. Am Heart J 101:667–670, 1981.)

phologic variation. The conduction system in general shows fat, fibrosis, and degenerative changes to a varying extent in the SA node, AV node, AV bundle, and bundle branches. In addition, the AV node is in part situated within the central fibrous body or near the aortic-mitral annulus in some. In still others, the AV bundle is abnormal: there are connections between the atria and the AV bundle (atrio-Hisian connections), or the bundle forms loops within the central fibrous body, or the bundle remains on the right side of the ventricular septum. In addition, focal fibrotic scarring in the ventricular septum, predominately on the right side with arteriosclerosis, is noted in many cases (Fig. 20-20). In an occasional case, there is also calcification of the mitral valve.[44, 49]

Hypertrophic Cardiomyopathy

The heart is hypertrophied and enlarged in all cases. The AV node is almost always partly or mostly situated in the central fibrous body and occasionally partly embedded in the tricuspid valve annulus or at the aortic-mitral annulus. The AV nodal artery is frequently thickened and narrowed. The SA and the AV nodes are frequently infil-

trated with fat. The AV bundle is on the right side of the ventricular septum or is often loop-formed with fibrosis of the branching bundle (Fig. 20-21). Increase in fibrosis, disarray pattern, and arteriolosclerosis in the summit of the ventricular septum are observed.[45, 49]

Arrhythmogenic Right Ventricular Dysplasia/ Cardiomyopathy

The conduction system in this entity also presents remarkable changes in the form of fat, fibrosis, and infiltration of inflammatory cells to a varying extent. This is seen in all parts of the conduction system with partial or complete replacement of parts of the right ventricular wall with fat, inflammatory cells, and fibrosis in various proportions. The condition also affects the left ventricle. In addition, the AV bundle may present congenital abnormalities, including left-sided AV bundle, loop formation of the bundle, and atrio-Hisian connection[46, 47] (Fig. 20-22).

In all of the last three disease entities just described, there are distinct acquired pathologic changes as well as congenital anomalies of the conduction system that affect the SA node, AV node, and AV bundle. Although the

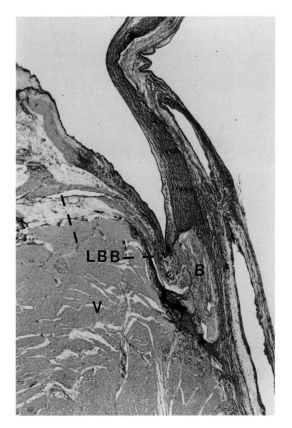

Figure 20-21 • A 25-year-old woman with hypertrophic cardiomyopathy died suddenly. Note the branching bundle (B) as it climbs over the hypertrophied ventricular septum (V) showing fibrosis, with marked disruption, fibrosis, and space formation of the left bundle branch fibers (LBB). Interrupted markers point to the disruption, fibrosis, and space formation of the LBB. PM, pars membranacea; V, ventricular septum (Weigert-van Gieson stain). (From Bharati S, Lev M, McAnutty J, et al: Idiopathic hypertrophic subaortic stenosis with split His bundle potential. Circulation 62:1373–1380, 1980.)

causes of the acquired pathologic changes in and around the conduction system remain unknown, it is conceivable that they may represent a previous myocarditis in some individuals, or they may be the end result of arrhythmias that patients had in the past. It is also of interest that in each of these three entities there is small vessel disease of the ventricular septum. The acquired pathologic changes in the myocardium can cause slowing of impulse conduction, thereby promoting a re-entry mechanism resulting in ventricular arrhythmias and sudden death.

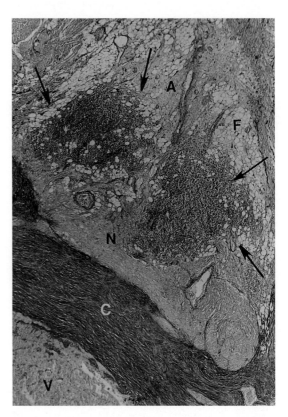

Figure 20-23 • A 55-year-old man died suddenly 2 years after heart transplantation. Photomicrograph of the AV nodal area demonstrates the AV node (N) and its approaches (A) with marked inflammatory cell infiltration (arrows), indicating acute rejection. Note also the fatty infiltration (F) of the AV node and its approaches. C, central fibrous body; V, ventricular septum (Weigert-van Gieson stain).

Several abnormal genes have been identified on several chromosomes in familial hypertrophic cardiomyopathy and arrhythmogenic right ventricular dysplasia/cardiomyopathy (see Chapter 10). Molecular genetic studies in all of the above disease entities will lead to a better understanding of the exact mechanisms responsible for associated arrhythmias and sudden death.

Sudden Death After Heart Transplantation

The transplanted heart is hypertrophied and enlarged in all cases studied.[48] There is also myocarditis to a varying degree, with arteriosclerosis and arteriolosclerosis. These findings are more dominant in the atria than in the ventricles. In the conduction system, myocarditis with fibrosis is seen in all the approaches to the SA node, SA node, atria, AV node (Fig. 20-23), AV bundle, and bundle branches to a varying degree. Compared with the previous endomyocardial biopsy findings, histologic examination at autopsy always reveals more myocarditis and fibrosis than that estimated in the biopsied specimen. In summary, in transplanted hearts there are fibrotic changes in the conduction system, with persistence of inflammatory phenomena in the conduction system and surrounding myocardium to a varying extent. This is associated with the ubiquitous coronary artery disease that affects not only large epicardial coronary arteries but also small vessels. (See Chapter 23 also.)

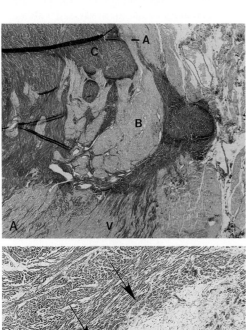

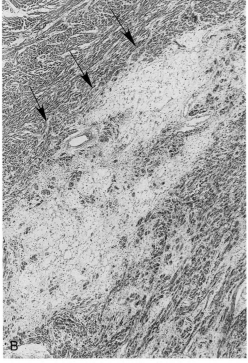

Figure 20-22 • A, A 22-year-old woman with a history of right ventricular tachycardia died suddenly. Autopsy revealed arrhythmogenic right ventricular dysplasia/cardiomyopathy. Photomicrograph of the penetrating AV bundle (B) shows loop formation and atrio-Hisian connection (A). C, central fibrous body; V, ventricular septum (Weigert-van Gieson stain). B, Photomicrograph of the middle part of the ventricular septum showing marked fatty infiltration and inflammatory cells with degeneration of myocardial fibers. Arrows point to fat, inflammatory cells, and degeneration of myocardial fibers (H&E stain). (A, From Bharati S, Lev M, Fold A, et al: Hypoplasia of the right ventricular myocardium with ventricular tachycardia. Arch Pathol Lab Med 107: 249–253, 1983.)

It is our belief that the pathologic changes in and around the conduction system are probably responsible for arrhythmias and sudden death in some cases of cardiac transplantation. Furthermore, the marked pathologic changes in the SA node and its approaches and in the atria are the pathologic substrate for the sinus node dysfunction seen clinically in many heart transplantation patients.

Iatrogenic Atrioventricular Block and Sudden Death After Correction of Congenital Cardiac Anomalies

Surgical injury to the conduction system may occur during closure of an isolated ventricular septal defect or repair of ventricular inversion associated with ventricular septal defect, also referred to as corrected transposition, which is one type of an atrioventricular discordant heart. Surgical AV block may also develop after surgical correction of an ostium primum atrial septal defect, repair in single ventricle, tricuspid valve replacement, or the Mustard procedure for complete transposition. The pathologic lesion is usually an interruption of the AV bundle in either the penetrating, branching, or bifurcating part, although other parts of the conduction system may be affected. The AV block or other arrhythmias may be temporary or permanent, and they can become manifest at any time after the operative procedure[53-57] (Fig. 20-24).

Today, complete AV block after corrective surgery for common congenital cardiac anomalies is rare. On the other hand, atrial and/or ventricular arrhythmias are frequently seen several years after surgical correction of such cardiac anomalies as atrial septal defect and tetralogy of Fallot and after the Mustard procedure for complete transposition, the Fontan procedure for tricuspid atresia or single ventricle, and various types of corrective procedures performed for double outlet right ventricle and other complicated congenital heart anomalies. In general, the arrhythmias are related to scar tissue adjacent to healthy myocardium that produces slowing of an impulse. This promotes a ventricular and/or atrial re-entry mechanism, imitating a premature ventricular or atrial contraction, which may eventually induce ventricular tachycardia and/or supraventricular tachycardia, that in turn degenerates into ventricular fibrillation and sudden death.[46-50]

Sudden Death in Young Persons, in Healthy Persons, and in Athletes

When to Study the Conduction System in Sudden Death

If, after a careful examination of the heart both grossly and microscopically, the cause of death cannot be determined, especially when death occurs suddenly and unexpectedly in the young and healthy individuals with or without a history of arrhythmias, it is then assumed that the death is caused by cardiac arrhythmias. Under these conditions, a thorough examination of the conduction system is warranted.

Findings in the Conduction System

In these so-called "normal" individuals who were living a normal life, the heart may not reveal any abnormalities on gross examination. However, it may be hypertro-

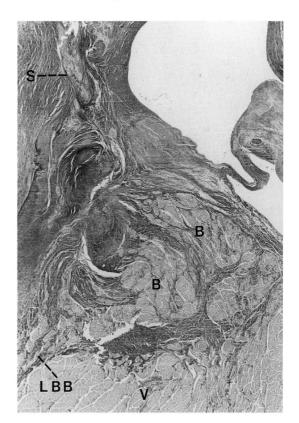

Figure 20-24 • Postoperative congenital heart. Sudden death in a 16-year-old boy 9 years after closure of both atrial and ventricular septal defects. Electrocardiograms demonstrated normal sinus rhythm before surgery, right bundle branch block after surgery, and much later atrial fibrillation with a ventricular rate of 70 to 80 beats/minute. Photomicrograph shows disruption of the branching bundle and marked fibrosis. B, marked fibrosis of the branching atrioventricular (AV) bundle; LBB, fibrotic disruption of left bundle branch; V, summit of the ventricular septum; S, sutures very close to the AV bundle with marked fibrosis of the membranous septum (Weigert-van Gieson stain). (From Bharati S, Lev M: Pathology of Congenital Heart Disease: A Personal Experience With More Than 6,300 Congenital Hearts. Vol 2. Armonk, NY, Futura Publishing Co, 1996, p 92.)

phied and enlarged.[49, 52] In general, the conduction system and surrounding myocardium show varying types of abnormalities that may be congenital or acquired. The congenital abnormalities may affect the SA node, the AV node, and/or the AV bundle. They may be in the form of a double SA (Fig. 20-25A) or AV node, or abnormal formation and location of the SA and/or AV nodes. The AV bundle may be markedly segmented or split into several components or abnormally located. Or, there may be accessory pathways that bypass the conventional conduction system and cause sudden death with or without a previous history of arrhythmias (Wolff-Parkinson-White syndrome, or pre-excitation).[49]

The acquired abnormalities may be in the form of fat, focal myocardial disarray, or fibrosis of varying severity disrupting or replacing different parts of the conduction system, with or without small vessel disease (arteriolosclerosis). Or, there may be a myocarditis of a chronic nature. Findings in the conduction system are usually accompanied by pathologic findings in the surrounding myocardium. In addition, there may be frequent association of mononuclear cell infiltration in the approaches to

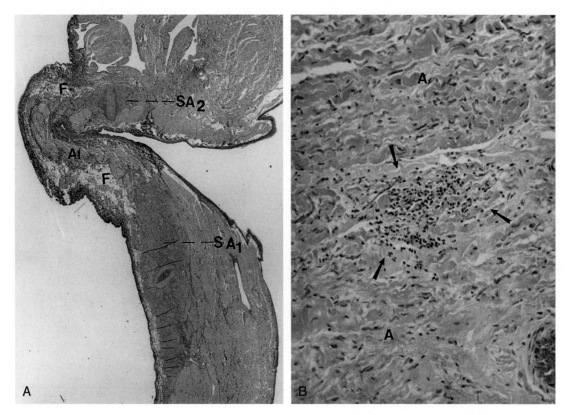

Figure 20-25 • *A,* Double SA node with two separate SA nodal arteries in a 22-year-old male football player who died suddenly. SA-1, body of the SA node; SA-2, head of the SA node; AT, atrial muscle; F, fat (Weigert-van Gieson stain). (Bharati S, Lev M: The Cardiac Conduction System in Unexplained Sudden Death. Mt. Kisco, NY, Futura Publishing Co, 1990, pp 1–416.) *B,* Accumulation of mononuclear cells in the approaches to the SA node, defined by arrows. A, approaches to the SA node (H&E stain.) (From Bharati S, Lev M: Sudden death in athletes—conduction system: Practical approach to dissection and pertinent pathology. Cardiovasc Pathol 3:117, 1994, with permission from Elsevier Science.)

the SA node (Fig. 20-25*B*) and in the SA node itself. Despite these findings in and around the conduction system, the patient can be totally "asymptomatic," with sudden death the first manifestation. We therefore hypothesize that the varying types of changes, whether congenital or acquired, found in different parts of the conduction system, although present for a long period, may form an anatomic substrate during an altered physiologic state and trigger an arrhythmia that progresses to ventricular tachycardia and degenerates into ventricular fibrillation and sudden death. A genetic tendency for abnormal formation of the conduction system and/or the surrounding myocardium may lead to sudden death in some cases.

The Conduction System and Myocardium After Radiofrequency Ablation Procedures

At present, radiofrequency energy is used to treat intractable AV nodal re-entrant tachycardia and atrial, as well as ventricular, arrhythmias.[58–60] All types of cardiac arrhythmias including pre-excitation syndrome, if not amenable to pharmaceutical management, are being ablated by radiofrequency energy with great success. However, death may occur suddenly in some patients several months after the procedure. Therefore, it is important to understand the pathologic findings of the ablated areas and surrounding structures in the heart.

At the gross level, a well-delineated scar is seen in the ablated area. Histologically, hemorrhage and coagulation necrosis are present in the acute stage and granulation tissue in the chronic stage. This may be accompanied by chronic inflammatory cells and fat.

Radiofrequency ablation is successfully used to cure fast and slow pathways, thereby modifying the AV nodal conduction selectively in selected patients. Selective ablation of the posterior and/or anterior approaches to the AV node can be accomplished without damaging the AV node or His bundle during abolishment of the slow or fast pathway in intractable AV nodal re-entrant tachycardias.

Uncommonly, perforations occur in the aortic, mitral, or tricuspid valve during the ablative procedure for Wolff-Parkinson-White syndrome, resulting in valvular insufficiency. Likewise, inadvertent damage to vital parts of the conduction system adjacent to the targeted area may result in incomplete or complete AV block. However selective the ablative procedure might be, the right ventricular side of the ventricular septum adjacent to the approaches to the AV node is almost always affected. This may result in focal scarred areas that could form a milieu for an arrhythmic event during an altered physiologic state at a later date and cause sudden death.

In summary, this chapter has briefly discussed the normal anatomy of the conduction system and the findings of the conduction system and surrounding myocardium in various types of cardiac diseases including sudden death in the young and healthy. The interested reader is encouraged to read the original works referred to in this chapter for further information.

REFERENCES

1. Bharati S, Lev M: The anatomy of the normal conduction system: Disease-related changes and their relationship to arrhythmogenesis. In: Podrid PJ, Kowey PR (eds): Cardiac Arrhythmias: Mechanism, Diagnosis and Management. Baltimore, MD, Williams & Wilkins, 1995, p 1
2. Lev M, Bharati S: Lesions of the conduction system and their functional significance. In: Sommers SC (ed): Pathology Annual 1974. New York, Appleton-Century-Crofts, 1974, p 157
3. Lev M: The conduction system. In: Gould SC (ed): Pathology of the Heart and Blood Vessels. 3rd ed. Springfield, IL, Charles C Thomas, 1968, p 180
4. Lev M, Bharati S: A method of study of the pathology of the conduction system for electrocardiographic and His bundle electrogram correlations. Anat Rec 201:43, 1981
5. Bharati S, Lev M: The anatomy and histology of the conduction system. In: Chung EK (ed): Artificial Cardiac Pacing: Practical Approach. 2nd ed. Baltimore, MD, Williams & Wilkins, 1984, p 12
6. Lev M, Bharati S: Anatomic basis for impulse generation and atrioventricular transmission. In: Narula OS (ed): His Bundle Electrocardiography and Clinical Electrophysiology. Philadelphia, FA Davis, 1975, p 1
7. Lev M, McMillan JB: A semiquantitative histopathologic method for the study of the entire heart for clinical and electrocardiographic correlations. Am Heart J 58:140, 1959
8. Wildran J, Lev M: The dissection of the human AV node, bundle and branches. Circulation 4:863, 1951
9. Truex RC, Smythe MO: Recent observations on the human cardiac conduction system with special considerations of the atrioventricular node and bundle. In: Taccardi B (ed): Electrophysiology of the Heart. New York, Pergamon Press, 1965, pp 177–198.
10. Lev M, Watne AL: Method for routine histopathologic study of the sinoatrial node. Arch Pathol 57:168, 1954
11. Bharati S, Lev M: The anatomy and pathology of the conduction system. In: Samet P, El-Sherif N (eds): Cardiac Pacing. 2nd ed. New York, Grune and Stratton, 1980, p 1
12. Truex RC, Bishof JK, Hoffman EL: Accessory atrioventricular muscle bundles of the developing human heart. Anat Rec 131:45, 1958
13. Lev M: The normal anatomy of the conduction system in man and its pathology in atrioventricular block. Ann N Y Acad Sci 111:817, 1964
14. Bharati S, Lev M: Morphology of the sinus and atrioventricular nodes and their innervation. In: Mazgalev T, Dreifus LS, Michelson El (eds): Progress in Clinical and Biological Research. Vol 275: Electrophysiology of the Sinoatrial and Atrioventricular Nodes. New York, Alan R. Liss, 1988, p 3
15. Bharati S, Lev M: The morphology of the AV junction and its significance in catheter ablation (editorial). Pacing Clin Electrophysiol 12:879, 1989
16. Randall WC: Differential autonomic control of SAN and AVN regions of the canine heart: Structure and function. In: Mazgalev T, Dreifus LS, Michelson EL (eds): Progress in Clinical and Biological Research. Vol. 275: Electrophysiology of the Sinoatrial and Atrioventricular Nodes. New York, Alan R. Liss, 1988, p 15
17. Erickson EE, Lev M: Aging changes in the human atrioventricular node, bundle, and bundle branches. J Gerontol 7:1, 1952
18. Lev M: Aging changes in the human sinoatrial node. J Gerontol 9: 1, 1954
19. Lev M, Bharati S: Age related changes in the cardiac conduction system. Internal Medicine for the Specialist 2:19, 1981
20. Bharati S, Lev M: Histologic abnormalities in atrial fibrillation: Histology of normal and diseased atrium. In: Falk RH, Podrid PJ (eds): Atrial Fibrillation: Mechanisms and Management. New York, Raven Press Ltd, 1992, p 15
21. Bharati S, Lev M: The pathologic changes in the conduction system beyond the age of ninety. Am Heart J 124:486, 1992
22. Bharati S, Lev M: Pathologic changes of the conduction system with aging. Cardiology in the Elderly 2:152, 1994
23. Lev M, Bharati S: Atrioventricular and intraventricular conduction disease. Arch Intern Med 135:405, 1975
24. Lev M, Bharati S: The conduction system in coronary artery disease. In: Donoso E (ed): Current Cardiovascular Topics. New York, Stratton Intercontinental Medical Book, 1978, p 1
25. Lev M, Bharati S: The pathologic base of supraventricular arrhythmias. In: Iwa T, Fontaine G (eds): Cardiac Arrhythmias: Recent Progress in Investigation and Management. Amsterdam, Elsevier, 1988, p 1
26. Bharati S, Lev M: The pathologic aspects of ventricular tachycardia. In: Iwa T, Fontaine G (eds): Cardiac Arrhythmias: Recent Investigation and Management. Amsterdam, Elsevier, 1988, p 15
27. Bharati S, Rosen KM, Strasberg B, et al: Anatomic substrate for congenital atrioventricular block in middle aged adults. Pacing Clin Electrophysiol 5:860, 1982
28. Rosenbaum MB, Elizari MV, Lazzari JO: The Hemiblocks. Oldsma, FL, Tampa Tracings, 1970
29. Davies MJ: Pathology of conducting tissue of the heart. New York, Appleton-Century Crofts, 1971
30. Lenegre J: Les block auriculoventriculaires complets chroniques: Étude des causes et des lésions à propose de 37 cas. Mal Cardiovasc 3:311, 1962
31. Rossi L: Histopathologic Features of Cardiac Arrhythmias. Milan, Ambrosiana, 1969
32. Lenegre J: Etiology and pathology of bilateral bundle branch block in relation to complete heart block. Prog Cardiovasc 6:409, 1963–1964
33. Davies MJ: Pathology of chronic AV block. Acta Cardiol 21(suppl): 19, 1976
34. Bharati S, de la Fuente DJ, Kallen RJ, et al: The conduction system in systemic lupus erythematosus with atrioventricular block. Am J Cardiol 35:299, 1975
35. Lightfoot PR, Bharati S, Lev M: Chronic dermatomyositis with intermittent trifascicular block: An electrophysiologic-conduction system correlation. Chest 71:413, 1977
36. Lev M, Landowne M, Matchar JC, et al: Systemic scleroderma with complete heart block: Report of case with comprehensive study of the conduction system. Am Heart J 72:13, 1966
37. Lev M, Bharati S, Hoffman FG, et al: The conduction system in rheumatoid arthritis with complete atrioventricular block. Am Heart J 90:78, 1975
38. Wang K, Gobel F, Gleason DF, et al: Complete heart block complicating bacterial endocarditis. Circulation 46:939, 1972
39. Kleid JJ, Kim ES, Brand B, et al: Heart block complicating acute bacterial endocarditis. Chest 61:301, 1972
40. Demoulin JC, Boniver J, Casters P, et al: Le bloc auriculo-ventriculaire complet dans l'endocardite bacterienne. Acta Cardiol 30:596, 1975
41. Théry C, Folliot JP, Gosselin B, et al: Les blocs auriculo-ventriculaires des endocardites bactériennes. Arch Mal Coeur 70:15, 1977
42. Bharati S, Lev M, Bicoff JP, et al: Sudden death caused by benign tumor of the atrioventricular node. Arch Intern Med 136:224–228, 1976
43. Bharati S, Lev M, Dreifus L, et al: The conduction system in patients with a prolonged QT interval. J Am Coll Cardiol 6:1110–1119, 1985
44. Bharati S, Lev M, Granston A, et al: The conduction system in mitral valve prolapse syndrome with sudden death. Am Heart J 101: 667–670, 1981
45. Bharati S, Lev M, McAnulty J, et al: Idiopathic hypertrophic subaortic stenosis with split His bundle potentials. Circulation 62: 1373–1380, 1980
46. Bharati S, Lev M, Ciraulo D, et al: Inexcitable right ventricle and bilateral bundle branch block in Uhl's disease. Circulation 57:636–644, 1978
47. Bharati S, Lev M, Feld A, et al: Hypoplasia of the right ventricular myocardium with ventricular tachycardia. Arch Pathol Lab Med 107:249–253, 1983
48. Bharati S, Billingham M, Lev M: The conduction system in transplanted hearts. Chest 102:1182–1188, 1992
49. Bharati S, Lev M: The Cardiac Conduction System in Unexplained

Sudden Death. Mt. Kisco, NY, Futura Publishing Co, 1990, pp 1–416

50. Bharati S, Bauernfiend R, Scheinman M, et al: Congenital abnormalities of the conduction system in two patients with tachyarrhythmias. Circulation 59:593, 1979
51. Bharati S, Moskowitz WB, Scheinman M, et al: Junctional tachycardias: Anatomic substrate and its significance in ablative procedures. J Am Coll Cardiol 18:179, 1991
52. Bharati S, Lev M: Sudden death in athletes—Conduction system: Practical approach to dissection and pertinent pathology. Cardiovasc Pathol 3:117, 1994
53. Bharati S, Lev M: Sequelae of atriotomy and ventriculotomy on the endocardium, conduction system and coronary arteries. Am J Cardiol 50:580, 1982
54. Bharati S, Molthan ME, Veasy LG, et al: Conduction system in two cases of sudden death two years after the Mustard procedure. J Thorac Cardiovasc Surg 77:101, 1979
55. Bharati S, Lev M: Conduction system in cases of sudden death in congenital heart disease many years after surgical correction. Chest 90:861, 1986
56. Bharati S, Lev M: Conduction system in sudden unexpected death a considerable time after repair of atrial septal defect. Chest 94:142, 1988
57. Bharati S, Lev M: The Pathology of Congenital Heart Disease: A Personal Experience with more than 6,300 Congenitally Malformed Hearts. Vol 2. Armonk, NY, Futura Publishing Co, 1996, p 1445
58. Huang SK, Bharati S, Graham AR, et al: Closed-chest catheter desiccation of the atrioventricular junction using radiofrequency energy: A new method of catheter ablation. J Am Coll Cardiol 9:349–358, 1987
59. Gamache C, Bharati S, Lev M, et al: Histopathologic study following catheter guided radio frequency current ablation of the slow pathway in a patient with AV nodal re-entrant tachycardia. Pacing Clin Electrophysiol 17:247–251, 1994
60. Bharati S, Lev M: Pathologic observation of radio frequency catheter ablation of cardiac tissue. In: Huang SKS (ed): Radio Frequency Catheter Ablation of Cardiac Arrhythmias: Basic Concepts and Clinical Applications. Armonk, NY, Futura Publishing Co, 1994, p 41

Chapter 21

Pathology of Heart Valve Substitution With Mechanical and Tissue Prostheses

· · · · ·

Frederick J. Schoen

First performed successfully in 1960,[1-3] cardiac valve replacement is now done frequently. Symptomatic patients with heart valve stenosis or regurgitation who are managed by replacement of the diseased valve with a synthetic or biologic substitute generally have increased survival, reduced symptoms, and an enhanced quality of life for extended intervals.[4-7] Nevertheless, the mechanical and tissue heart valve replacement devices that are available today remain imperfect. Prosthesis-associated complications occur frequently and have a considerable impact on patients' prognosis after valve replacement surgery.[8-13] Consequently, prosthetic valves are frequently encountered by pathologists when they are removed at reoperation or when a recipient comes to autopsy.

This chapter summarizes the pathologic anatomy and clinicopathologic considerations in patients who have had valve replacement surgery, encompassing pathology associated with the substitute valve as well as other pertinent cardiac and noncardiac pathology. Discussion of the following related areas provides additional context: (1) description of valve replacement devices, (2) clinical outcome, (3) ongoing research and development in this area, and (4) approach to evaluating substitute valves as pathologic specimens. We also recognize that a major (and increasing) fraction of contemporary valve surgery involves repairs and reconstructions.[14, 15]

GENERAL CONSIDERATIONS

Valvular disease causes marked secondary effects on the heart and other organs that vary with the valve involved and the nature, severity, and duration of the abnormality. (See Chapter 13.) In particular, the compensatory myocardial hyperfunction induced by the hemodynamic burden can eventually lead to muscle dysfunction, heart failure, and, occasionally, sudden death. Excessive delay in treatment can cause morbidity and mortality that might have been prevented by valve surgery. However, inappropriately early intervention may expose the patient to premature risk from the operation and any subsequent prosthetic valve-related pathology. Thus, in a patient with clinically overt valvular heart disease, surgery is usually deferred until the risks associated with continued medical therapy outweigh those of valve replacement and the subsequent postoperative course.[16] Optimally timed surgery balances the risk of complications with prolonged medical management against the dangers associated with both the surgical procedure and inserted device (Fig. 21-1).[17] Prognosis after surgery is determined by the quality of the myocar-

dium, other cardiac and systemic pathology, and the consequences of prosthesis-associated complications.

More specifically, and in each patient, the results of valve replacement and anticipated pathology depend on the (1) details of the procedure and both intraoperative and postoperative management; (2) extent of intraoperative myocardial injury (predominantly of ischemic origin); (3) overall functional status and irreversible and often chronic structural alterations in the heart and lungs secondary to the original valvular abnormality; (4) possibility of coexistent obstructive coronary artery disease and associated surgery, such as coronary artery bypass grafting; and (5) type of valve substitute used and its potential vulnerabilities, largely related to materials reliability and interactions of the device with natural tissues,[18, 19] as well as its relative benefit to cardiac structure and function.[20, 21]

Patients with valvular stenosis typically require operation sooner and have less operative risk than those with insufficiency; they recover better and obtain greater benefit from the operation. Moreover, in general, replacement of the aortic valve has a more favorable outcome than that of the mitral valve. These factors confound comparisons among published clinical data and may bear on the pathologist's understanding of a case under evaluation.

VALVE REPLACEMENT DEVICES

The characteristics of an ideal heart valve replacement were originally enumerated by Harken and colleagues in 1962[22] and have subsequently been modified (Table 21-1).[23] These criteria are difficult to achieve in any single fabricated valve; some have excelled in some respects only to fail miserably in others. No heart valve presently available satisfies them all.

Despite the development and investigation of countless models of substitute valves and progressive improvement in the techniques of their design and manufacture over the past four decades, only a small number have achieved wide clinical use. Heart valve prostheses fall into several general categories defined by design and materials of construction (Fig. 21-2). Prosthetic heart valves in current use either have all components manufactured of synthetic or naturally occurring but nonbiologic material (mechanical valves) or are constructed, at least in part, of either human or animal tissue (tissue valves).[24] The most commonly used valves (both past and present) and those most likely to be of interest to pathologists are listed in Table 21-2; several types are illustrated (see Figs. 21-3 to 21-5).

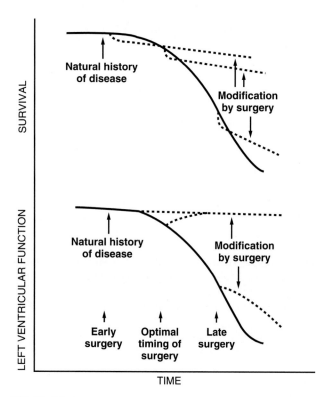

Figure 21-1 • Schematic representation of the concept of optimal timing of valve replacement surgery. Early surgery has a low operative mortality and preserves ventricular function. However, because of potential prosthesis-associated complications, postoperative risk exceeds that of pure medical treatment at this early phase of the disease. In contrast, if surgery is done too late, operative mortality is increased, and ventricular function may progressively deteriorate after surgery. Thus, postoperative survival is determined primarily by risks of prosthesis-associated complications and congestive heart failure. Optimal timing of surgery balances the risks of maintained medical management with the new risks associated with postoperative complications. With appropriate timing, operative mortality is relatively low, ventricular function is almost completely preserved, and postoperative risk is determined, as in early surgery, predominantly by the risk of prosthesis-associated complications. (From Schoen FJ, St. John Sutton M: Contemporary issues in the pathology of valvular disease. Hum Pathol 18:568, 1987.)

TABLE 21-1 • **Criteria for an Ideal Heart Valve Substitute**

Is chemically inert and does not damage blood elements
Offers no resistance to physiologic flow when open and, whenever possible, has central flow characteristics without a transvalvular gradient
Closes properly and remains closed during the appropriate phase of the cardiac cycle
Is nonthrombogenic (patient does not need anticoagulants)
Does not propagate emboli
Is resistant to infection
Does not induce a host reaction deleterious to the patient or the prosthesis
Has high durability
Is capable of permanent fixation
Is technically practical to insert in the appropriate anatomic site
Is not noisy or otherwise annoying to the patient
Is inexpensive

The terminology used to describe such devices is summarized in Table 21-3.

Available data suggest that each year 60,000 to 75,000 substitute valves are implanted in the United States and 170,000 to 250,000 worldwide, of which approximately 60 to 70% are mechanical and 30 to 40% are tissue.[25] Recent trends suggest that implant numbers are growing approximately 5 to 7% per year overall—approximately 8 to 11% for tissue valves and 3 to 5% for mechanical valves.

Substitute heart valves respond passively to hemodynamic stimuli manifested as pressure gradients and flow changes within the heart. The competency (i.e., ability to prevent backflow when closed) of a valve substitute generally derives from its intrinsic structure (either seating of mobile occluders or apposition of cuspal tissue). Moreover, except for a small percentage of tissue valves (discussed later), contemporary commercially manufactured mechanical and tissue valves have a fabric (usually Dacron mesh) sewing cuff that surrounds the base of the prosthesis. Sutures placed into this area by the surgeon are intended to anchor the device into the surgically prepared annulus. The sewing ring presents both inflow and outflow surfaces to the blood; its outer rim forms the peripheral margin of the prosthesis. Owing to the combi-

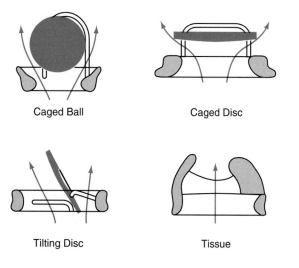

Caged Ball

Caged Disc

Tilting Disc

Tissue

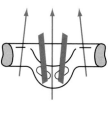

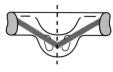

Bi-Leaflet
Tilting Disc

Figure 21-2 • Designs and flow patterns of the major categories of prosthetic heart valves: Caged-ball, caged disk, tilting disk, bileaflet tilting disk, and bioprosthetic (tissue) valves. Whereas flow in mechanical valves must course along both sides of the occluder, bioprostheses have a central flow pattern. (From Schoen FJ, Titus JL, Lawrie GM: Bioengineering aspects of heart valve replacement. Ann Biomed Eng 10:97, 1982; and from Schoen FJ: Pathology of cardiac valve replacement. In: Morse D, Steiner RM, Fernandez J [eds]: Guide to Prosthetic Cardiac Valves. New York, Springer-Verlag, 1985, p 209 [96123-2].)

TABLE 21-2 • **Prosthetic Heart Valve Types Likely to Be Encountered by Pathologists**

Type	Model
Mechanical	
Caged ball	Starr-Edwards*
	Braunwald-Cutter
Caged disk	Beall
Single tilting disk	Bjork-Shiley
	Bjork-Shiley Monostrut*
	Medtronic-Hall*
	Omniscience/Omnicarbon*
Bileaflet tilting disk	St. Jude Medical*
	Carbomedics*
	Edwards-Duromedics
Tissue	
Xenograft/hetero-graft	Carpentier-Edwards porcine aortic valve*
	Hancock standard porcine aortic valve*
	Hancock MO (modified orifice) porcine aortic valve*
	Hancock II porcine aortic valve
	Medtronic Freestyle stentless porcine aortic valve*
	Toronto SPV stentless porcine aortic valve*
	Ionescu-Shiley bovine pericardial valve
	Mitroflow bovine pericardial valve
	Carpentier-Edwards bovine pericardial valve*
Allograft/homograft*	

* Approved by the U.S. Food and Drug Administration as of mid-2000.

nation of passive function, rigid frame, and sewing ring, most mechanical and stented bioprosthetic valve types can be used to replace a diseased valve at any site. Nevertheless, sewing rings have different configurations in semilunar (i.e., mitral and tricuspid) and atrioventricular (i.e., aortic and pulmonary) prostheses, which are needed to conform to differences in annular anatomy, and there are more subtle differences to accommodate technical details of implantation within an anatomic region (e.g., aortic annular versus supra-annular).

The sewing ring is an important site of interaction between a prosthesis and its surrounding tissue, but little is known about its determinants.[26] In most cases, organized thrombus or fibrous tissue (pannus) derived from and contiguous with the adjacent myocardium or aortic wall ultimately covers the rough cloth surface. Small amounts of thrombus are probably beneficial initially to stimulate healing, but excessive deposits could potentiate thrombotic occlusion or emboli. Uncomplicated organization of thrombus and tissue overgrowth optimally yields a thin layer of largely endothelialized, mature collagen associated with minimal mononuclear inflammatory cells or giant cells. The gradual covering of heart valve prosthesis surfaces by endothelium may reduce thromboembolic episodes.

Heart valve substitutes are manufactured in a broad range of sizes, to match the size of the orifice remaining after the patient's diseased valve is excised. The sizes are expressed by diameter, typically 19 to 25 mm for aortic valves and 25 to 35 mm for mitral valves.

Mechanical Valves

In addition to the sewing cuff described earlier, mechanical heart valves have three essential components: (1) one or more rigid but mobile parts, each of which is called an occluder, usually a ball (a ball occluder is also called a *poppet*) or a hinged leaflet of circular or semicircular profile; (2) a cage-like superstructure or housing that guides and restricts occluder motion; and (3) a valve body or base that provides support for the housing or cage and provides the seat for the occluder.[27] The internal orifice of the valve housing defines the effective area through which blood can flow. In the closed phase, an occluder contacts the ring or seat and fills or overlies the prosthesis lumen. Mechanical valve prostheses can be separated into three major types, according to their flow characteristics (see Figs. 21-2 and 21-3): (1) those in which blood passing through the valve orifice impinges

TABLE 21-3 • **Substitute Heart Valve Terminology**

Term	Definition
Related to biomaterial, source, treatment, support	
Mechanical prosthesis	Valve in which the functional components are synthetic, composed of metals, polymers, ceramics, or carbon
Tissue (tissue-derived) valve	Any valve in which the functional components are derived from animal or human tissues, valvular or otherwise
Bioprosthesis	Valve composed of tissue, often chemically treated, usually but not always mounted on a prosthetic stent (e.g., porcine aortic valve or bovine pericardial bioprostheses, autologous fascia lata valve)
Heterograft/xenograft	Valve or tissue transplanted from an individual of one species to that of another (e.g., porcine aortic valve or bovine pericardium implanted into a human patient)
Homograft/allograft	Valve or tissue implanted in an individual of the same species (e.g., a valve from a human cadaver implanted into a human patient)
Autograft	Valve or tissue removed from one site to another in the same individual (e.g., a patient's own pericardium or fascia lata fashioned into valve cusps and mounted on a stent, or a pulmonic valve transplanted to the aortic root)
Stentless bioprosthesis	Bioprosthetic valve without prosthetic frame or sewing ring
Related to valve structure	
Occluder/poppet	Moving parts of a mechanical prosthesis that block reverse flow when valve is closed and partially move out of the flow stream when open
Cusps	Flexible, moving tissue components
Stent/struts	Prosthetic support structures of a mechanical or tissue valve
Sewing ring	Cloth that surrounds the base of a valve, through which sutures are placed to anchor it in the annulus

on a centrally placed occluder and must swirl around it (lateral flow prostheses exemplified by caged ball and disk valves); (2) those in which a single tilting occluder permits a semicentral flow; and (3) those of hinged, bileaflet tilting disk (double occluder) construction.

Widely used mechanical valves and those most likely to be encountered by pathologists include the Starr-Edwards (Edwards Life Sciences, Santa Ana, California) caged-ball valve[7, 28]; the Bjork-Shiley (previously manufactured by Shiley Co., Irvine, California)[29]; the Medtronic-Hall (Medtronic, Minneapolis, Minnesota)[30] tilting disk valve; and the St. Jude Medical (St. Jude Medical, St. Paul, Minnesota)[31, 32] and Carbomedics CPHV (Sulzer Carbomedics, Austin, Texas)[33] bileaflet tilting disk valve prostheses (see Fig. 21-3). Although slightly modified from its original form, the Starr-Edwards caged ball valve has been used longer than any other prosthesis type. Reported results using this prosthesis serve as a benchmark against which other valves can be measured. Presently, the most frequently implanted model, the St. Jude bileaflet tilting disk mechanical valve, accounts for approximately half of all valve replacements used worldwide. Owing to durability problems that became apparent only after extensive clinical use (discussed later), the previously popular Bjork-Shiley valve[34] with distinct inflow and outflow struts has been discontinued, but a more robust monostrut version is now available.[35] Moreover, several types of caged disk valves were used in the early decades of valve replacement, but intrinsic obstruction, poor durability, and tendency toward thromboembolism prompted their removal from the market.[36, 37]

The metallic cages of mechanical valves are composed of either cobalt-chromium alloy (e.g., Starr-Edwards and Bjork-Shiley valves) or nearly pure titanium (e.g., Medtronic-Hall valve). Although the Starr-Edwards valve has a silicone poppet, the occluders for single or bileaflet tilting disk valves available today are made of pyrolytic carbon. This material, originally developed as a coating for nuclear fuel particles in the 1960s, was and continues to be modified for medical applications. Pyrolytic carbon is rigid, strong, and highly resistant to wear, fatigue, and thrombus formation.[38, 39] In some designs, all rigid parts, including disks, housing, and superstructure, are composed of carbon (e.g., St. Jude or Carbomedics valve). The Carbomedics valve and OmniCarbon modification of the OmniScience valve also have a carbon-coated sewing cuff. A modification of the St. Jude valve was a silver-based coating intended to inhibit infection. However, the coating also seemed to impede healing (personal communication, J. Butany, Toronto), but this association has not been verified and the potential mechanism is not certain. Nevertheless, the particular model was withdrawn from the market in 2000.

Because the stream of blood flow through a mechanical valve prosthesis must separate, course around the occluder, and reconstitute distally (see Fig. 21-2), mechanical valves usually have areas of stasis, predominantly distal to the orifice. The combination of stasis and nonphysiologic surfaces potentiates thrombus formation.[40-42] Thus, virtually all patients with mechanical valves receive lifetime anticoagulation therapy to lessen the risk of thromboembolic complications.[43] However, as discussed later, anticoagulant therapy induces a significant risk of hemorrhage.

Tissue Valves

Tissue valves have a configuration that resembles natural anatomy and cusps composed of valvular or nonvalvular animal or human tissue. Tissue valves include *xenografts* (also called *heterografts* and include porcine aortic valves or bovine pericardial bioprostheses), *allografts* (also called *homografts* and include aortic or pulmonic valves primarily from human cadavers, with or without an associated aortic or pulmonary arterial sleeve as a conduit), or *autografts* (e.g., composed of pericardium or the patient's pulmonary valve transplanted to the aortic root). Fascia lata[44] and dura mater[45] have also been used. Clinically used xenografts are preserved by chemical cross-linking with aldehydes, and allografts and autografts have been used fresh, often treated with antibiotics, or otherwise preserved (see later).

The advantages of tissue valves include a central pattern of flow resembling that of native cardiac valves (see Fig. 21-2) and low thrombogenicity. Nevertheless, the original endothelium of porcine valves and allografts is denuded or damaged during preparation (and pericardium and other nonvalvular connective tissues are not naturally endothelialized). Most patients with bioprosthetic valves and virtually all those with allografts do not need long-term anticoagulation, and tissue valves are an attractive choice for patients in whom anticoagulation is either contraindicated or undesirable. However, durability limitations are the major impediment to the long-term success of commercially available, glutaraldehyde-pretreated porcine aortic valve–derived bioprostheses and most other tissue valve substitutes. This problem is discussed in detail later.

Chemical preservation allows a stable shelf-life of several years, enhances material stability, prevents autolysis, and permits the surgeon to have valves of various sizes readily available for implantation. These valves also minimize the theoretical potential of immunologic rejection while maintaining both the thromboresistance and antimicrobial sterility characteristic of the natural tissue.

The most frequently used chemical preservative for bioprosthetic tissue is glutaraldehyde (1,5 pentanedialdehyde; $CHO[CH2]_3CHO$), used historically for tanning leather and more recently as a fixative for electron microscopy.[46] This dialdehyde forms complex, degradation-resistant, Schiff base– and pyridinium salt–derived cross-links between protein molecules, especially collagen, the most abundant structural protein of natural valves and other tissue substitutes (such as pericardium). In contrast, formaldehyde-induced methylene-based protein cross-links are unstable. Thus, formaldehyde-pretreated bioprostheses used in the early days of tissue valve replacement frequently developed premature material failure.[47] Because the antibacterial and antifungal efficacy of low concentrations of glutaraldehyde is poor (especially against spores, as exemplified by a cohort of tissue valves over a decade ago that were contaminated with *Myobacterium chelonai*[48]), adjunctive solution sterilization procedures are

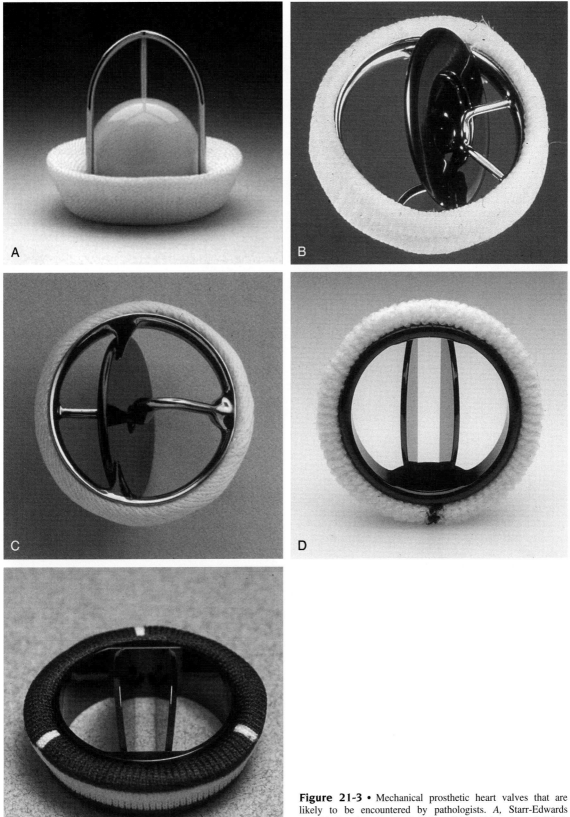

Figure 21-3 • Mechanical prosthetic heart valves that are likely to be encountered by pathologists. *A,* Starr-Edwards caged-ball valve. *B,* Bjork-Shiley tilting disk valve. *C,* Medtronic-Hall tilting disk valve. *D,* St. Jude Medical bileaflet tilting disk heart valve. *E,* Carbomedics bileaflet tilting disk heart valve.

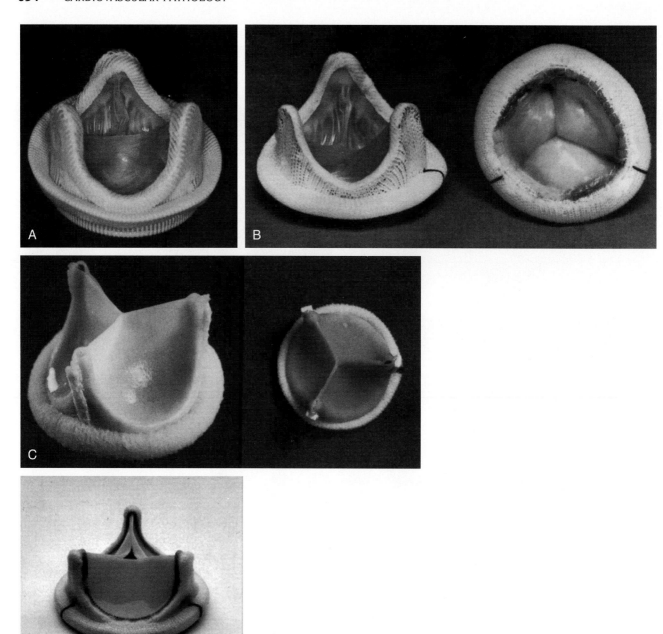

Figure 21-4 • Stented bioprosthetic heart valves that are likely to be encountered by pathologists. *A* and *B,* Porcine aortic valve bioprostheses. *A,* Hancock valve. *B,* Carpentier-Edwards valve. *C,* Ionescu-Shiley bovine pericardial valve. *D,* Carpentier-Edwards bovine pericardial valve.

necessary (e.g., transient treatment with alcoholic glutaraldehyde solutions).

Most commercially produced tissue valves are mounted on and supported by a metal or plastic *stent,* usually with three posts (called *struts*) to support their three cusps (Fig. 21-4). Stent mounting facilitates surgical implantation in either a semilunar or an atrioventricular valve site. Covered by Dacron or animal tissue (usually pericardium), the stents on which bioprosthetic tissue are mounted vary in structural design, flexibility, and composition among both manufacturers and models. In contrast, nonstented porcine valves (Fig. 21-5),[49, 50] semilunar valve allografts,[51] and pulmonary autografts[52] (see later) are usually sewn directly into the surgically prepared aor-

tic (or pulmonary) valve annulus; their configuration does not permit atrioventricular valve replacement. Thus, bioprostheses are hybrid structures, partly biologic (i.e., cuspal tissue) and partly synthetic (i.e., stent supports, fabric covering, and sewing ring). In general, the morphologic features before and after insertion, as well as the clinical success and specific failure modes of cardiac valvular tissue grafts, depend primarily on the type and source of the tissue, the preservation and handling before insertion, and the method of tissue attachment and support.

Historically, the most frequent type of tissue valve substitute used clinically, and still inserted in some patients, is a glutaraldehyde-preserved pig aortic valve mounted on a cloth-covered stent (porcine aortic bio-

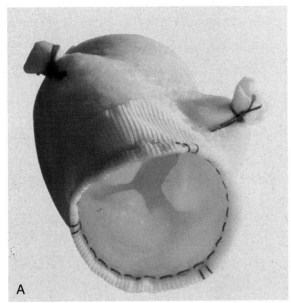

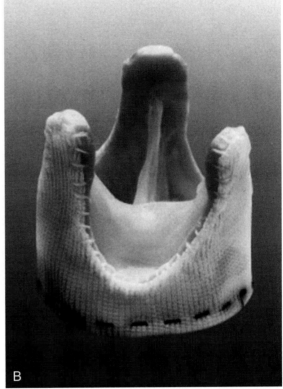

Figure 21-5 • Nonstented porcine bioprosthetic valves. *A,* Medtronic Freestyle valve. *B,* St. Jude Medical Toronto SPV valve.

prosthetic valve). Two commercially available products dominate: the Carpentier-Edwards valve (Edwards Life Sciences, Santa Ana, California) and the Hancock valve (Medtronic, Anaheim, California). Although much of the aortic wall is trimmed away in their fabrication, the aorta adjacent to the valve cusps and the intervening natural cuspal attachments are incorporated into each valve. These two commercial variants differ slightly in configuration, in the concentration of glutaraldehyde used in pretreatment (0.2% for the Hancock valve and 0.6% for the Carpentier-Edwards valve), and in stent composition (polyacetal [Delrin] in the Hancock valve, and Elgiloy metal alloy in the Carpentier-Edwards).

In contrast to human anatomy, in which there is no muscle in the aortic valve cusps, the right coronary cusp of the normal pig aortic valve has an extension of muscle from the ventricular septum. This "muscle shelf" within the right coronary cusp can cause delayed or incomplete opening of the cusp and ultimately become the site of calcific deposits. Its potential effect is inhibited by mounting valves on the stent with the minimum amount of muscle in the orifice and by discarding unsuitable valves. The Carpentier-Edwards porcine valve has a noncircular, contoured orifice to facilitate exclusion of the muscle portion of the right cusp. A modified orifice (MO) Hancock prosthesis for patients with small aortic roots substitutes the left cusp from another valve for the right coronary cusp as a means of widening the effective valve inlet area.[53]

Pericardial bioprosthetic valves have cusps composed of glutaraldehyde-treated parietal pericardium (usually of bovine origin) attached to a frame. The most frequently implanted first-generation bovine pericardial valves were the Ionescu-Shiley (Dacron-covered titanium frame) (see Fig. 21-4C) and the Mitroflow (Dacron-coated Delrin frame). Relative to porcine valves, pericardial bioprostheses generally have comparable or superior hemodynamic performance and low rates of thromboembolism, but problems associated with structural dysfunction dampened clinical enthusiasm for pericardial valves after failures in the original designs.[54–56] Nevertheless, a current model (the Carpentier-Edwards pericardial bioprosthesis [Edwards Life Sciences, Santa Ana, California]) has apparently improved durability (see later) and has become the most frequently implanted type of bioprosthetic heart valve. Without the inherent anatomic constraints of porcine valves, innovative design configurations are feasible, and both unicuspid and bicuspid pericardial valve designs have been investigated.[57, 58]

Detailed descriptions of porcine aortic valve and bovine pericardial bioprostheses are available.[59–61]

Structure-Function Correlations in Tissue Valve Substitutes

Aortic Valve and Pericardium

The natural aortic valve is remarkably well adapted to its function.[62–65] Aortic valve cusps open against the aortic wall during systole and close rapidly and completely under minimal reverse pressure, maintaining full competency throughout diastole. Although the pressure differential across the closed valve induces a large load on the cusps, cuspal prolapse does not normally occur, because the fibrous network effectively transfers the resultant

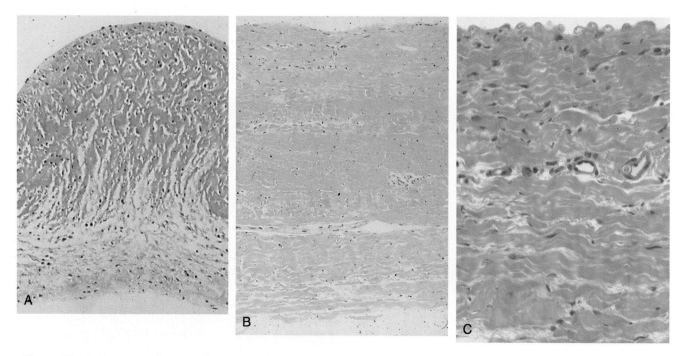

Figure 21-6 • Comparison of microscopic structures of porcine aortic valve and bovine pericardium. *A,* Cross section of porcine aortic valve cusp, showing layered architecture with diffusely distributed interstitial cells and endothelial cells at surface. The inflow surface is at the bottom. *B,* Cross section of bovine parietal pericardium, showing dense laminated fibrous tissue with diffusely distributed cells. *C,* Higher power photomicrograph of bovine pericardium showing collagen bundles and interstitial fibroblasts. In *B* and *C,* the former serosal surface is at the top. (All H & E stain).

stresses to the annulus. The structure of the aortic valve is discussed in detail and illustrated in Chapter 13. The structural details and functional motion of bioprosthetic valve cusps are altered by fixation, stent configuration, and tissue attachment (see later).

Bovine pericardium and porcine aortic valve cusps have different architectures (Fig. 21-6). Pericardial tissue is a relatively homogeneous sheet of laminated and compact collagen, but it is not as tightly arranged as porcine valve fibrosa. Although porcine valve contains a mixture of type I and type III collagens, bovine pericardial collagen is almost entirely type I.[66, 67] Parietal pericardium is composed of (1) a smooth serosal layer, originally covered by mesothelial cells; (2) fibrosa (accounting for almost the entire thickness), which contains collagen, elastic fibers, nerves, blood vessels, and lymphatics; and (3) rough epipericardial connective tissue, with loosely arranged collagen and elastic fibers.[68, 69] Thus parietal pericardium has two different surfaces—a smooth one previously facing the pericardial space, and a relatively rough external surface from which blood and fat are dissected

away. Most pericardial bioprostheses are fabricated with the smooth surface as the outflow aspect; thus, the inflow surface is rough. Pericardial bioprosthetic valve cusps are thicker than those of porcine valves, approximately 0.3 to 0.5 mm compared with 0.2 to 0.3 mm, respectively.

The complex, highly oriented array of connective tissue of a natural human valve (discussed earlier) ensures that excessive stress is not concentrated at the commissures, provided that normal coaptation is preserved. To a large extent, this feature is maintained in a porcine bioprosthesis. However, cuspal stresses at the valve commissures increase sharply with decreasing coaptation area, or with decreasing anisotropy of the cusp material (tending toward isotropy, or the same properties in all directions). The collagen fibrils in parietal pericardium are parallel to the surface and have a site-dependent and variable, although not random, orientation in the plane of the tissue.[70, 71] Pericardium lacks the functional adaptations of natural valves.

Thus, bioprostheses fabricated from bovine pericardium differ in several important respects from porcine bioprostheses (Table 21-4). As already indicated, pericardial tissue differs from aortic valve cusps in both architecture and mechanical properties. Moreover, in contrast to aortic valve cusps, whose natural attachments to the supporting aortic wall are preserved in a porcine bioprosthesis, pericardial bioprosthetic valve cusps are composed of individually obtained pieces of tissue that are artificially attached to stent supports. These features can contribute to untoward mechanical effects and tearing. For example, stresses in pericardial valves are directed toward commissural attachments, leading to stress concentrations

TABLE 21-4 • **Key Differences Between Porcine Aortic Valve (PAV) and Bovine Pericardial Valve (BPV) Bioprostheses**

Feature	PAV	BPV
Cusp structure	Layered	Uniform
Fibrosa	Oriented	Variable
Cuspal properties	Anisotropic	More isotropic
Cusp edges	Natural	Cut in manufacture
Wall stent attachments	Natural	Artificial

in the tissue at these sites. In addition, the cloth-covered inner support frame of some pericardial valves may induce abrasion on the inflow aspect of the tissue material, which can cause cusp tearing.[72] In the Ionescu-Shiley design, sutures placed in the tissue near its free edge at the stent post to maintain cuspal alignment, commissural apposition, and coaptation can exacerbate stress concentrations that occur during cusp flexure. Therefore, it is not surprising that cusp tearing beginning near the top of the stent post or along cuspal attachments is the most common mode of pericardial valve failure (see later). Finally, because new surfaces are generated during pericardial tissue procurement, dissection, and valve fabrication, the collagen bundles at the inflow surface and edges of pericardial cusps tend to splay during function, allowing host cells and fluid to enter cuspal tissue.

Tissue Changes Induced by Manufacture

Owing to changes in the tissue that are induced during various steps in the processes of valve treatment and further fabrication, a contemporary bioprosthesis differs structurally and functionally from a native valve in several important respects (summarized in Table 21-5 and discussed later). Typically, an interval of at least 24 to 36 hours transpires between harvest and glutaraldehyde treatment of bioprosthetic tissue. Moreover, the cells of bioprosthetic tissue are rendered nonviable and the extracellular matrix is altered by the current practice of fixation. Thus, the cells are incapable of repairing progressive damage and degenerative changes during function. Also, owing to fixation, the cuspal tissue is mechanically locked at a single point in the cardiac cycle, thereby hampering the dynamic microstructural alterations that accommodate normal valve function. Moreover, most porcine and pericardial valves are mounted on stents, further altering and providing constraints to cusp dynamics.

The tissue autolysis, chemical treatment, and physical changes induced by fabrication cause several histologic alterations that are revealed by pathologic examination of unimplanted bioprosthetic valves. These include, most prominently, loss of surface endothelium or mesothelium (aortic valve or pericardial bioprostheses, respectively); autolytic disruption of porcine or bovine interstitial cells; loosening of collagen bundles; loss of amorphous extracellular matrix (largely glycosaminoglycans [GAGs]); and, when there is backpressure during porcine valve fixation, flattening of the natural waviness (crimp) of collagen (Fig. 21-7).[13, 73] This emphasizes that in standard porcine

valves, the quality of structural preservation of valvular interstitial cells is especially poor, with loss of cytoplasmic membrane integrity, disruption of organelles, and vacuolation. With the endothelium denuded, the valve surfaces consist of subendothelial connective tissue. Occasionally, small textile fibers derived from materials used to pack the valves are noted adherent to and entangled in the superficial collagen bundles of bioprosthetic valve cusps.

The functional, mechanical, and morphologic characteristics of the porcine aortic valve and other tissues used in bioprostheses are also modified by glutaraldehyde cross-linking procedures, with the specific changes depending on the particular fixation techniques employed.[74–76] The collagenous skeleton becomes locked into a geometric configuration determined by the magnitude of the back pressure during pretreatment. When the aortic valve is preloaded by a back pressure during cross-linking, the collagen resembles that of a closed valve in diastole, causing flattened corrugations, straightened crimp waveform, and maximal cusp surface area. In first-generation porcine valves, fixation was done at a back pressure of 80 mm Hg, imparting a permanent diastolic configuration. When crimp and corrugations are preloaded in an elongated state, functional stresses must be absorbed by relatively noncompliant collagen fibers. Thus, porcine valve cusps fixed under load and bovine pericardial cusps are relatively stiff and inflexible; they do not open smoothly but rather bend in a series of kinks. During each subsequent cycle, the cusps bend sharply, thereby inducing substantial and repetitive mechanical stresses at the same site, buckling the fully stretched fibrosa and accentuating tissue fatigue.[77, 78]

To better preserve native cusp microstructure and anatomy, some bioprostheses are prepared using a low-pressure fixation technique in which there is a reduced gradient across the valve during fixation. However, fixation pressure as low as 2 to 4 mm Hg (relative to the full diastolic pressure of 80 mm Hg) is sufficient to straighten corrugations and crimp and reduce radial and circumferential compliance.[74, 76, 79] Some data suggest that the mechanical properties of cusps are improved when fixation occurs without any back pressure at all (i.e., zero pressure differential fixation), thereby retaining, at least initially, a histologically normal structure with full crimp and corrugation geometry. Valves so treated are under investigation.

Tissue Changes After Implantation

After implantation, additional pathologic changes occur to a variable degree in all types of bioprostheses. The most characteristic histologic changes are summarized in Table 21-6. Shortly after implantation, bioprostheses become variably covered on their cuspal surfaces with fibrin, platelets, and inflammatory cells, usually predominantly monocytes or macrophages and, occasionally, multinucleated giant cells. The presence of more than scattered monocytes or neutrophils deep within the cusp substance of porcine valves is unusual and suggests infection. Clusters of lymphocytes, macrophages, and a few plasma cells of host origin are sometimes found in the

TABLE 21-5 • **Changes in Bioprosthetic Tissue Induced by Fabrication**

Cross-linking of proteins
Loss of cell viability
Loss of endothelium (porcine valve) or mesothelium (pericardium)
Fragmentation of cuspal cell membranes
Flattening of the cusp and stretching and loosening of collagen bundles
Loss of amorphous extracellular matrix
Loss of tissue compliance, with resultant stiffening
Stress concentrations caused by mounting on a stent
Adherent textile fibers from packing

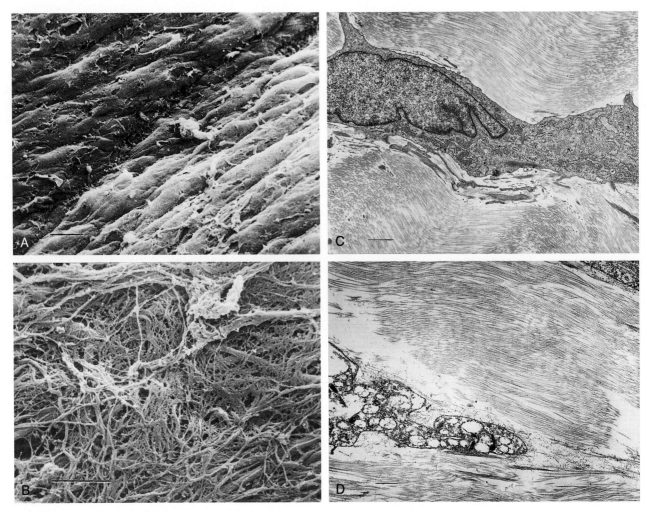

Figure 21-7 • Structural alterations induced by preservation and fabrication of a porcine aortic valve into a bioprosthesis. Scanning electron microscopy appearance of the surface of a fresh porcine valve (*A*) and a fabricated porcine bioprosthesis (*B*) before implantation. The confluent endothelial layer present in the fresh porcine aortic valve is entirely lost in the fabricated valve. A rough, fibrillar basement membrane forms the blood-contacting surface of the commercially produced valve shown in *B*. (*A*, ×1000; *B*, ×3800; bar in *A* = 10 μm; bar in *B* = 5 μm). *C* and *D*, Transmission electron microscopy of deep portions of the valve, illustrating degrees of cellular preservation and collagen waviness. In the freshly fixed porcine aortic valve (*C*) there is a morphologically normal cell, wavy collagen, and close apposition of cell to fibrillar and amorphous extracellular matrix. The fabricated valve (*D*, high-pressure-fixed) shows cellular autolysis and an empty space between cells and collagen. Moreover, the collagen is flat in the high-pressure-fixed valve illustrated in *D* but wavy in the fresh aortic valve shown in *C*. (*C* and *D*, ×8000; bars in *C* and *D*, = 1 μm). (From Flomenbaum MA, Schoen FJ: Effects of fixation back pressure and an antimineralization treatment on the morphology of porcine aortic bioprosthetic valves. J Thorac Cardiovasc Surg 105:154. 1993.)

connective tissue at the junction between valve tissue and sewing ring, particularly associated with the muscle shelf of the right coronary cusp of porcine valves and in pericordial valves. Foreign body giant cells may also be seen adjacent to suture materials traversing the base of a valve.

The basal regions of the cusps frequently become coated with a variably thick, fibrous sheath of host origin (*pannus*), which, when excessive, can lead to cusp immobilization or orifice obstruction (see later). Re-endothelialization of bioprosthetic valves is slow and limited to the basal attachments. It remains incomplete, even years after implantation.[80] Although it is reasonable to hypothesize that endothelialization of a bioprosthetic valve might decrease its propensity toward thrombosis, infection, insudation of fluid or blood, or calcific or noncalcific degeneration, no evidence exists that pre- or postimplantation endothelialization of a bioprosthesis is beneficial.

Focal superficial microthrombi are frequently noted along the surfaces of cusps, particularly at the cuspal attachments, and especially in pericardial valves. Owing to the absence of either a functional endothelium or other impermeable barrier, or to the sutures used in the manufacturing process piercing cuspal tissue, proteins, and other constituents of plasma penetrate into the cusps (*fluid insudation*). Erythrocytes are commonly noted deep in the cuspal tissue of removed porcine valve bioprostheses and occasionally in bovine pericardial valves (*cuspal hematoma*), probably for reasons similar to those that cause fluid insudation. Large accumulations of blood may yield grossly visible hematomas that can stiffen cusps or possibly provide sites for mineralization.[81]

TABLE 21-6 • **Postimplantation Changes in Bioprosthetic Tissue**

Deposition of platelets and fibrin
Superficial or deep mononuclear inflammatory cells
Endothelialization
Pannus overgrowth
Fluid insudation
Superficial collagen fragmentation
Generalized architectural homogenization and loss of staining
Delamination
Mechanical fatigue damage
Abrasion
Calcification
Cuspal sagging
Intracuspal hematomas
Infiltration of lipid and amyloid
Involvement with systemic disease (e.g., Whipple disease, carcinoid heart disease)
Colonization by infectious organisms
Cusp destruction by infection

Valve function in vivo also gradually results in generalized architectural homogenization with connective tissue disruption, mineralization (discussed later), and, in some cases, lipid accumulation (sometimes with cholesterol crystals)[82] or amyloid deposition.[83] With all types of bioprostheses, the intrinsic cuspal architecture is often disrupted with large collagen bundles appearing separated, distorted, indistinct, and hyalinized. After several months of function, there is loss of definition of virtually all basophilic (hematoxylinophilic) staining components, including cell nuclei. Thus, the valve structure becomes homogeneously eosinophilic. The pathologic changes that occur in bioprosthetic valves after implantation are to a large extent rationalized on the basis of the alterations in native valve tissue that occur during fabrication:

• The cusp-blood interface is not a natural blood-contacting biologic surface. Thus, with endothelial cells lost from the cusp-blood interface and exposure of subendothelial connective tissue plasma, erythrocytes, and inflammatory cells can penetrate into the cusp.
• Following cross-linking, the interstitial cells are nonviable. Thus, bioprostheses have no mechanism to remodel and replace collagen and other matrix components that are progressively degraded during valve function.
• Cellular debris, collagen, and elastin can serve as foci for calcification.
• Collagen is the most important structural element that confers the mechanical properties of a valve. It becomes locked in an altered and static geometry, yielding decreased tissue compliance. Thus, the cyclic rearrangements of the microstructure that accommodate normal valve function cannot occur, leading to abnormal motion of the cusps.

Bioprostheses can also be affected by systemic diseases. Whipple disease involving the cusps of a porcine bioprosthesis,[84] and plaque characteristic of carcinoid heart disease occurring on bioprosthetic tricuspid valves have been reported.[85, 86]

POSTOPERATIVE CLINICOPATHOLOGIC CORRELATIONS

Clinical Outcome: Mortality and Morbidity

Both early and late mortality and morbidity after cardiac valve replacement have decreased substantially in recent years, owing to improvements in the natural history of disease, timing of surgery, patient selection, surgical technique, and postoperative care.[87] The causes of patient problems are varied (Table 21-7).

Operative or Early

Operative (hospital) mortality is best defined as death from any cause during or after operation—within 30 days if the patient has been discharged from the hospital, or any interval if the patient has not. This classification is preferable to the traditional approach to analyses of valve replacement—"early" (<30 days) versus "late" (>30 days).

Contemporary operative mortality rates for otherwise uncomplicated cases are 5 to 9% for mitral valve replacement[88] and 4 to 6% for aortic valve replacement.[89] However, individualized estimated operative risk depends on case-specific clinical and pathologic details.[90, 91] For example, simultaneous replacement of two valves (double valve replacement) increases operative mortality twofold, and advanced age increases aortic valve replacement risk to approximately 14%.[92] Risk is increased substantially in patients with poor preoperative cardiac function but only modestly in those needing a valve replacement combined with coronary artery bypass. In general, the risk for a repeat valve replacement is increased, particularly when it is prompted by endocarditis or some other emergent problem.[93] Patient variables such as gender, original valve pathology, functional defect, urgency of surgery, and follow-up care may also influence outcome.

TABLE 21-7 • **Major Causes of Death and Pathologic Findings Following Cardiac Valve Replacement**

Cardiovascular disease and operative problems
  Pump failure with low cardiac output (intra- or postoperative)
  Progressive myocardial deterioration with congestive heart failure
  Arrhythmias/sudden death
  Myocardial infarction/necrosis, with or without coronary artery disease or embolus
  Technical difficulties
  Aortic dissection/hemorrhage
  Uncorrected cardiac lesions
  Extracardiac pathology related or unrelated to valve disease (pulmonary, gastrointestinal, cerebrovascular, wound infection or sepsis)

Prosthesis-associated complications
  Thrombosis, thromboembolism, bleeding event (anticoagulation-related hemorrhage)
  Prosthetic valve infective endocarditis
  Structural valvular deterioration (intrinsic failure)
  Nonstructural dysfunction

Noncardiac pathology

Late

After valve replacement with either mechanical or tissue valves, the probability of 5-year survival is about 80%, and 10-year survival about 70%. Strong patient-related correlates of excessive late statistical mortality are preoperatively impaired left ventricular function, increased left ventricular and left atrial size, and coronary artery obstructive disease. Clinical investigations of individual valves and randomized studies comparing different valve types consistently show that one or more valve-related problems cause reoperation or death in approximately 60 to 70% of patients with substitute valves within 10 years postoperatively,[11, 94, 95] with similar *overall* rates of valve-related complications for mechanical prostheses and bioprostheses. However, the frequency and nature of *specific* valve-related complications are markedly dependent on the prosthesis type, model, size, site of implantation, and patient characteristics (e.g., ventricular function, arrhythmias).

Sources of Morbidity and Mortality

Anticipated pathology in a recipient of a valve substitute varies according to the postoperative interval (Table 21-8).[94-98] For example, only a small fraction of deaths in the early postoperative period are attributable to complications of the valve substitute; rather, preexisting cardiovascular disease and operative complications are the overwhelming source of mortality.[97, 98] In contrast, prosthesis-associated complications are common in valve recipients after the early postoperative interval.[94-98] Thromboembolic complications with mechanical valves are most common in the first year, whereas limitations due to bioprosthetic durability become prevalent beginning approximately 4 to 5 years postoperatively.[11, 94-96] Prosthesis-associated complications can be catastrophic and fatal, or develop slowly and permit reoperation, with its attendant risks.

Pathologic Considerations in Operative Mortality

Cardiac, vascular, and noncardiac complications of operation account for the majority of operative deaths. These include hemorrhage, aortic dissection or disruption associated with cannulation sites or the aortotomy done for suturing an aortic valve replacement, emboli from plaques, calcific masses or thrombus, pulmonary embolism or insufficiency, low cardiac output, arrhythmias, and sudden death (with myocardial necrosis present or absent). The pericardium may be closed or left open after the surgery, deep to the closed sternum and skin incision. Occasionally, because of ongoing bleeding or edema of thoracic structures, the sternotomy cannot be closed, and reclosure is instituted only when there is resolution of the operative problems. With "clean" elective sternotomies, wound infection may occur in up to 5% of patients. In an excision of the valve, there may be trauma to adjacent structures: for the aortic valve, the coronary ostia, membranous septum, and conducting system (atrioventricular node and adjacent left bundle); for the mitral valve, the membranous septum, conducting system, and circumflex coronary artery. Occasionally, complications of investigative procedures or treatment undertaken before surgery contribute to the cause of death. As stated earlier, device-related pathology is unusual soon after operation.

Vascular Injury

Aortic dissection can result if a perfusion cannula enters the media, either during insertion or through an atherosclerotic plaque while being passed along the vessel. Alternatively, an intimal tear at the site of a vascular wound or clamp site may permit blood to enter the media, with resultant hemorrhagic dissection. Although coronary ostial injury does not necessarily manifest in the early postoperative interval, late fibrous proliferation of the intima with ostial stenosis may occur, owing to damage caused during surgery, such as when coronary artery cannulas are used for myocardial perfusion during bypass. Intimal thickening in the ascending aorta due to turbulence distal to a prosthesis can also contribute to ostial stenosis. Sutures may impinge on a vessel and distort or stenose its lumen or act as a nidus for thrombus, which can occlude or be a source of distal emboli.

Myocardial Injury

Acute myocardial necrosis caused by intraoperative ischemic injury may be observed in patients who die soon after valve replacement, especially but not exclusively those with chronic atherosclerotic coronary arterial stenotic occlusive disease. The extent of myocardial injury in patients with a benign postoperative course is not known. Ischemic myocardial injury is related to inade-

TABLE 21-8 • **Causes of Death in 378 Valve Replacement Patients**

Cause	Number
Early deaths	279 total
Cardiovascular and operative	**263 (94%)**
No anatomic lesion	108
Myocardial necrosis	68
Technical	4
Other cardiovascular	41
Pulmonary	18
Other	23
Prosthesis associated	**17 (6%)**
Thromboembolism	7
Endocarditis	2
Dehiscence/paravalvular leak	5
Disproportion	3
Late deaths	97 total
Cardiovascular and operative	**44 (44%)**
Congestive heart failure	14
Myocardial infarction	8
Sudden death	6
Other	16
Prosthesis-associated	**46 (47%)**
Thrombosis	13
Thromboembolism	8
Hemorrhage	3
Endocarditis	14
Paravalvular leak	6
Structural dysfunction	2
Noncardiac	**9 (9%)**

Data from Schoen FJ, Titus JL, Lawrie GM: Autopsy-determined causes of death after cardiac valve replacement. JAMA 249:899, 1983.

quate myocardial preservation (the most frequent cause), iatrogenic damage to the coronary arteries, direct trauma to the myocardium itself at the site of operation, or embolic phenomena. Improved techniques of intraoperative myocardial protection, particularly the use of cold cardioplegia, have greatly reduced the incidence of extensive perioperative ischemic myocardial injury.

Most commonly occurring during surgery for aortic stenosis are circumferential hemorrhagic necrosis[100] and "stone heart."[101] These complications of global myocardial ischemia occur during cardiopulmonary bypass followed by the restoration of perfusion after surgery. In the gross, the full-blown lesion is a red, beefy, swollen zone of hemorrhagic muscle encircling the left ventricular lumen, usually involving at least the entire subendocardium; it is often partially transmural, may be extensive from apex to base in the left ventricle, and can affect the right ventricle. After reperfusion of a globally ischemic heart, foci of necrosis with contraction bands and hemorrhage may be noted histologically. Although full-blown cardiac failure is rarely encountered today, focal lesions, particularly in the subendocardium of the left ventricle, are common in the hearts of patients who die after prosthesis insertion and may induce myocardial dysfunction or arrhythmias. The foci of such injury usually promote minimal polymorphonuclear leukocyte infiltrate but have mononuclear cells at their periphery and may undergo dystrophic calcification as early as hours to a few days postoperatively.[102, 103]

Valve and papillary muscle excision and suture placement, particularly in the implantation of a mitral prosthesis, can also be associated with important acute pathology. Rarely, the myocardium is ruptured at the level of either the papillary muscles or the chordae or in an immediately subannular location, causing massive hemorrhage with death on the operating table. Alternatively, with a partial-thickness tear, a subannular false aneurysm may form, which can subsequently rupture. Moreover, deep dissection or a deep suture placed in the anteromedial mitral annulus can damage the bundle of His and cause complete heart block. Deep excision or suturing along the posterior leaflet can lead to dissecting hematoma of the atrioventricular groove, with hemorrhage and possibly external perforation. The left circumflex coronary artery, in the atrioventricular groove and only a few millimeters away from the attachment of the posterior mitral leaflet, can be injured or entrapped by a suture placed to anchor a mitral prosthesis. A deep anterior suture can tear or tether the left or noncoronary cusp of the aortic valve. These complications have been virtually eliminated, and postoperative cardiac function has generally been improved by contemporary surgical procedures that in many cases maintain intact rather than excise the entire mitral leaflets and submitral apparatus; however, this may induce other problems.[104]

Late Pathology

Late mortality and morbidity after cardiac valve replacement result predominantly from prosthesis-associated complications or cardiac failure. Valve-related complications (discussed in detail later) frequently require reopera-

tion; repeat procedures now constitute approximately 15% of all valve procedures. Autopsy studies and clinical analyses show that late deaths are device-related in 25 to 61% of patients.[96, 97, 105] Prosthesis-associated fatalities often occur suddenly.[106] Late outcome after cardiac valve replacement is also critically dependent on both irreversible cardiac pathology secondary to the original valvular disease (especially myocardial hypertrophy and subsequent degeneration caused by chronic pressure or volume overload and uncorrected valvular pathology, as well as pulmonary vascular disease) and superimposed coronary artery disease, whether or not valve replacement is combined with aortocoronary bypass graft surgery. Nonvalve-related cardiac conditions collectively account for nearly half of late deaths.

Myocardial Hypertrophy and Heart Failure

The process of myocardial hypertrophy was discussed in detail in Chapter 13. Removal of a diseased heart valve and replacement by a substitute relieve much of the pressure or volume overload induced by the original disease. However, all prostheses have some degree of obstruction relative to normal valves.[107] Moreover, although left ventricular hypertrophy resulting from systemic hypertension is reversible in many cases,[108] the extent to which hypertrophy associated with valvular disease is capable of regression and the factors regulating the extent of resolution are uncertain.[109] Hemodynamic adjustment is not always accompanied by a reversal of the myocardial changes, and progressive cardiac failure may ensue, despite valve replacement or repair. Indeed, many patients with adequately functional heart valve prostheses eventually die of or require transplantation for congestive heart failure due to myocardial decompensation (Fig. 21-8).

VALVE-RELATED COMPLICATIONS: CLINICAL IMPORTANCE, MORPHOLOGY, SECONDARY EFFECTS, AND PATHOGENESIS

This section discusses the relative occurrence, importance, and clinicopathologic features of the four most important categories of valve-related complications: (1) thromboembolic problems and those resulting from anticoagulant therapy used to prevent them, (2) infection, (3) structural deterioration (failure or degeneration of the biomaterials composing a prosthesis), and (4) nonstructural dysfunction (a heterogeneous group of complications and modes of failure not encompassed in the previous groups). These are summarized with their usual functional presentations in Table 21-9.[110]

The cumulative incidence of mechanical and bioprosthetic valve failure 10 years postoperatively is similar. Nevertheless, the nature, time dependence, and consequences of major modes of failure differ markedly between these valve types. Representative data from one study randomizing patients to mechanical or bioprosthetic valves are shown in Table 21-10.

Mechanical prostheses have the advantage of good du-

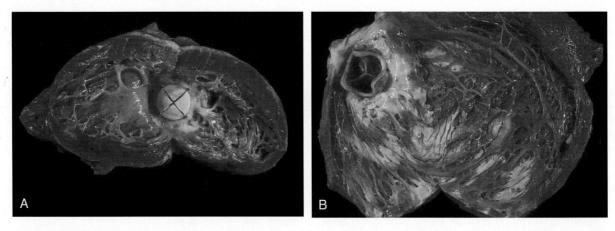

Figure 21-8 • Late postoperative cardiac failure after valve replacement prompting heart transplantation. *A,* Twenty-eight years after mitral valve replacement with a caged-disk valve for mitral stenosis. *B,* Four years after mitral valve replacement with a porcine bioprosthesis for congenital deformity causing mitral regurgitation. In neither case was the valve prosthesis dysfunctional. (From Schoen FJ: Pathologic considerations of the surgery of adult heart disease. In: Edmunds LH Jr [ed]: Cardiac Surgery in the Adult. New York, McGraw-Hill, 1997, p 85.)

rability but the disadvantage of a high risk of thrombosis, thromboembolism, and anticoagulation-related hemorrhage. These complications are frequently catastrophic and may be fatal. In contrast, bioprostheses have the advantage of relative low rates of thromboembolic complications, at least as low as those of mechanical prostheses, despite an absence of anticoagulation therapy (see Table 21-10).[8] However, bioprostheses have the disadvantage of limited durability, requiring more frequent reoperations for intrinsic structural deterioration. Tissue degradation leading to stenosis, regurgitation, or both is the predominant late valve-related complication of bioprostheses; calcification is contributory to most cases of porcine valve deterioration and to many cases of pericardial valve failure.[12, 13, 60, 61] Bioprosthetic structural dysfunction generally occurs 5 years or later postoperatively and generally induces slow patient deterioration; only approximately 5% of such failures require urgent reoperation.

The causes of prosthetic valve failure (see Tables 21-9 and 21-10) define indications for reoperation. They influence valve selection for individual patients (Table 21-11) and encompass the potential diagnoses rendered on recovered surgical pathology specimens and modes of valve-related death discovered at autopsy. Our experience with fatal valve-related complications and the most important causes of valve failure prompting reoperation are summarized in Figure 21-9. In that autopsy study, largely comprising mechanical valve recipients, 63 patients died of valve-related complications.[96] In particular, late death resulted from valve-related complications in 46% of 99 patients. Thrombosis, thromboembolism, and anticoagulant-associated hemorrhage caused 28, 17, and 7%, respectively, of these 46 late deaths. Thus, collectively, more than half (52%) of all valve-related deaths (and nearly one quarter of all postoperative valve replacement deaths) were related to the thrombogenicity of the mechanical prosthesis and its management.

Our surgical pathology study investigated the causes of dysfunction of 112 consecutive porcine bioprostheses and 45 mechanical valves surgically removed in a 5½-year interval during 1980 through 1985.[111, 112] The causes of failure included degenerative dysfunction (53%), endocarditis (16%), paravalvular leak (11%), thrombosis (9%), and tissue overgrowth (5%). Sterile paravalvular leak and prosthetic infective endocarditis were encountered with approximately equal frequency in mechanical and bioprosthetic valves. In agreement with the results of our

TABLE 21-9 • **Prosthetic Valve–Related Causes of Mortality and Morbidity and the Usual Functional Correlates**

Complication	Stenosis (S) or Insufficiency (I)
Thromboembolism (and its prevention)	
Thrombosis	S or I
Thromboembolism	—
Anticoagulant-related hemorrhage	—
Prosthetic valve infective endocarditis	I
Structural valvular deterioration (intrinsic failure)	
Wear	I
Fracture	I
Ball/disk variance	S or I
Poppet escape	I
Cuspal stretching	I
Root dilation*	I
Cusp tear	I
Calcification	S or I
Stent creep	S
Commissural dehiscence	I
Nonstructural dysfunction	—
Pannus	S or I
Suture/tissue entrapment	S or I
Paravalvular leak	I
Disproportion	S or I
Hemolytic anemia	—
Noise	—

*Primarily with nonstented substitutes such as allografts, pulmonary valve autografts, and *potentially* nonstented porcine valves.

Terminology modified from Edmunds LH, Clark RE, Cohn LH et al: Guidelines for reporting morbidity and mortality after cardiac valvular operations. J Thorac Cardiovasc Surg 112:708, 1996.

TABLE 21-10 • **Probability of Death or Valve-Related Complications 11 Years Postoperatively**

	Aortic Valve		Mitral Valve	
Event	*Mechanical Prosthesis*	*Bioprosthesis*	*Mechanical Prosthesis*	*Bioprosthesis*
Death from any cause	0.53	0.59	0.64	0.67
Any valve-related complication	0.62	0.64	0.71	0.79
Systemic embolism	0.16	0.15	0.18	0.15
Bleeding	0.43	0.24*	0.41	0.28*
Endocarditis	0.07	0.08	0.11	0.17
Valve thrombosis	0.02	0.01	0.01	0.01
Perivalvular leak	0.04	0.02	0.17	0.09
Reoperation	0.07	0.16	0.21	0.47
Structural valve failure	0.00	0.15*	0.00	0.36*

* $P < 0.05$ (difference in the probability of an event occurring in patients with mechanical prostheses and those with bioprostheses).

Modified with permission, from Hammermeister KE, Seth GK, Henderson WG et al: A comparison of outcomes in men 11 years after heart-valve replacement with a mechanical valve or bioprosthesis. N Engl J Med 328:1289, 1993. Copyright 1993 Massachusetts Medical Society. All rights reserved.

autopsy study,[97] thromboembolic complications were a frequent cause of mechanical valve dysfunction requiring reoperation (20% of failures), but they were infrequent with bioprostheses. Materials degradation causing dysfunction of mechanical valves was seen with a frequency similar to that of other complications. The valves recovered in that study were mostly older models not implanted in the current era. In contrast, primary tissue deterioration causing structural valve dysfunction was overwhelmingly the most frequent cause of bioprosthetic valve failure (74% of removals). Sterile paravalvular leak and device-associated infective endocarditis were encountered with approximately equal frequency in both mechanical and bioprosthetic valves, consistent with clinical observations that these problems are independent of prosthesis type. The morphology and clinicopathologic considerations germane to the various prosthesis-associated complications are discussed in greater detail next.

Thromboembolic Complications

Thromboembolic complications include thrombosis, manifest either by thrombotic deposits that spread across a valve orifice to stenose or occlude it or by inhibiting or preventing occluder movement or by thromboembolism to distal arterial beds. Moreover, systemic anticoagulation used to prevent thrombosis and thromboembolism can cause anticoagulation-related hemorrhage, which is also considered in this context. These complications are illustrated in Figure 21-10.

Thrombotic occlusion and thromboemboli occur with all currently available prostheses at rates of 1 to 4% per patient-year. Actuarial analyses of patient cohorts typically show 70 to 80% free of thrombosis or thromboembolism at 10 years.[11, 94-96] The complication rate is highest in the first postoperative year and then continues with a lesser but finite long-term risk. This trend is thought to be related in part to the early thrombogenicity of the sewing cuff and the decrease in this potentially thrombotic surface as healing by pannus progresses over it.

As discussed earlier, mechanical valves have a higher propensity for thromboembolic complications than tissue valves. Long-term therapy with warfarin (Coumadin) is required in all patients with mechanical prosthetic

valves but only in those tissue valve recipients who have specific indications for anticoagulation (e.g., atrial fibrillation). Interestingly (see Table 21-10), the risk of thromboembolism does not differ appreciably between patients with mechanical valves (on anticoagulation) and those with porcine bioprostheses (most not receiving anticoagulants).[8, 95, 113] Multiple factors beyond the type of valve substitute can affect the risk of systemic thromboembolism, including the adequacy of anticoagulation (risk is particularly high in poorly anticoagulated patients with mechanical valves), level of cardiac function (risk is increased with left ventricular dysfunction [ejection fraction <0.30]), whether cardiac rhythm is normal (risk is increased with atrial fibrillation), the anatomic site of valve replacement (mitral site has a higher risk than aortic).

As in the cardiovascular system in general, surface thrombogenicity, hypercoagulability, and locally static blood flow (Virchow's triad) contribute to predict the relative propensity toward thrombus formation and the location of thrombotic deposits. A high prevalence of

TABLE 21-11 • **Patient Factors Influencing Choice of Mechanical Versus Tissue Valve (Based on Known Failure Modes)**

Favoring a mechanical prosthesis
Long life expected
Mechanical prosthesis existing in a different position than the valve to be replaced
Renal failure, on hemodialysis or with hypercalcemia
Warfarin therapy required because of other risk factors for thromboembolism*
Age ≤65 years for AVR and ≤70 years for MVR
Previous thrombosis of a biologic valve
Child or adolescent with growth potential

Favoring a bioprosthesis
Contraindication to or expected noncompliance with warfarin therapy
Age ≥65 years; needs AVR and does not have risk factors for thromboembolism*
Age ≥70 years; needs MVR and does not have risk factors for thromboembolism*
Previous thrombosis of a mechanical valve

AVR, aortic valve replacement; MVR, mitral valve replacement
* Atrial fibrillation, severe left ventricular dysfunction, previous thromboembolism, and hypercoagulability.

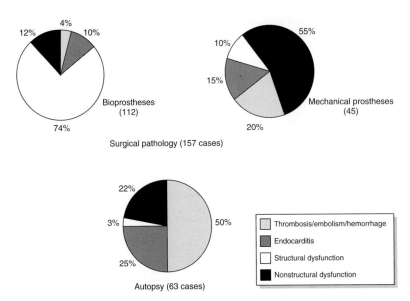

Figure 21-9 • Prosthesis-associated complications encountered at autopsy and surgical pathology. Half of all fatal problems are related to thromboembolism and anticoagulation therapy. Problems requiring reoperation on patients with mechanical valves are diverse, with a predominance of nonstructural dysfunction, including paravalvular leak and tissue overgrowth. In contrast, bioprosthetic valves fail most frequently by structural dysfunction consisting of calcific and noncalcific tissue degeneration. (Data from Schoen FJ, Titus JL, Lawrie GM, et al. Autopsy determined causes of death after cardiac valve replacement. JAMA 249:899, 1983; and Schoen FJ: Surgical pathology of removed natural and prosthetic heart valves. Hum Pathol 18:558, 1987.)

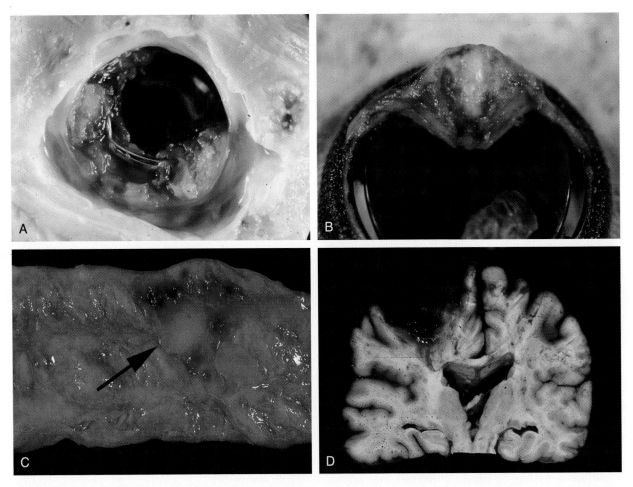

Figure 21-10 • Thrombosis, thromboembolism and complications of therapy used to prevent prosthesis-associated thrombotic and thromboembolic problems. *A,* Bjork-Shiley tilting aortic disk valve prosthesis, viewed from distal (outflow) aspect, demonstrating localization of thrombus to outflow strut near minor orifice, a site of flow stasis. *B,* Thrombus at pivot point of bileaflet tilting disk prosthesis. *C,* Thromboembolic infarct of the small bowel (arrow) secondary to embolus from valve prosthesis. *D,* Large fatal cerebral hemorrhage in a patient who had a mechanical valve prosthesis and received anticoagulant therapy. (*A,* From Schoen FJ, Levy RJ, Piehler HR: Pathological consideration in replacement cardiac valves. Cardiovasc Pathol 1:29, 1992, with permission from Elsevier Science.)

hypercoagulability states, including prothrombotic mutations has recently been reported in patients with recurrent thrombosis of mechanical valves.[114] Thus, patients with systemic hypercoagulability syndromes such as antiphospholipid (anticardiolipin) antibody syndrome, factor V Leiden (active protein C resistance), protein C or S deficiency, or antithrombin III deficiency may have increased risk.[115–117] Risk may also be increased when existing anticoagulation therapy is markedly and abruptly reduced. This may cause a transient rebound hypercoagulability.

Valve-associated regions where eddy currents or blood stasis persist are particularly vulnerable to thrombus formation. For example, with caged-ball prostheses, thrombi form at the cage apex distal to the ball, a location where flow is severely disrupted. Most thromboemboli are thought to arise from minute, often locally inconsequential thrombi at such sites. In contrast, thrombi on tilting disk prostheses are generally initiated at a region of critical flow disturbance, where stagnation occurs in the minor orifice at the outflow aspect. Thrombotic deposits on bileaflet tilting disk valves are generally localized predominantly on the outflow aspect of the valve superstructure, in the area of the pivot points (see Fig. 21-10). Indeed, one recently investigated novel design type (the Medtronic Parallel bileaflet tilting disk valve) suffered from frequent thrombotic occlusion in a clinical trial. Both pathologic examination and computerized flow dynamics strongly suggested that the thrombotic deposits were initiated at the depths of the hinge points of the hemidisks.[118, 119] Small thrombi may also be found in other crevices and junctions of mechanical valves, such as where the cage struts meet the inner portions of the housing or at the junction of the cloth sewing ring and the housing.

Thrombosis of tissue valves causing failure is less frequent than that of mechanical valves. When it occurs, it typically involves the bioprosthetic valve cusps, with large thrombotic deposits on the outflow aspect either partially or completely filling one or more prosthetic sinuses of Valsalva (Fig. 21-11). Although tissue overgrowth may be a contributing factor (see later), in most cases conventional pathologic examination is unable to demonstrate underlying cuspal pathology that can be considered causal.

Interpretation of the temporal progression of events from histologic examination of such thrombi must be done cautiously, as it is very difficult or impossible to assess the age of a thrombotic deposit on a valve substitute. The lack of vascularized tissue adjacent to prosthetic device thrombi in general, and to valves in particular, retards typical organization. It follows that valve-associated thrombi can be indefinitely friable, extending the risk of embolism. Moreover, the retarded organization of prosthetic valvular thrombi may permit restoration of valve function by thrombolytic therapy in some cases.[120] However, because thrombolytic therapy for a prosthetic valve obstructed by thrombus is ineffective in up to 18% of patients and has serious potential risks (e.g., thromboembolism, stroke, hemorrhage, recurrent thrombus), accounting for an acute mortality of 6%, thrombolytic therapy is generally reserved for those patients with high surgical risk or contraindications to surgery.

Platelet deposition dominates initial blood-surface interaction when valves and other cardiovascular devices are exposed to blood at high fluid shear stresses.[42, 121] Owing to an interaction of events mediated by platelet and coagulation proteins, valve and other device-associated thrombi are initially platelet rich and laminated (*white thrombus*), having formed in a high-flow. However, in the late stages of their formation there may be considerable fibrin and erythrocytes (*red thrombus*), indicating a static environment.

Warfarin decreases the activity of four vitamin K–dependent procoagulant factors (II, VII, IX, and X). The prothrombin time (PT) is sensitive to three of these factors and has previously been the most common test used for monitoring orally administered anticoagulant therapy. The International Normalized Ratio (INR) has supplanted the PT as a measure of intrinsic coagulation function in this context. The risk of thromboembolism is minimized when anticoagulation control is maximal, corresponding to an INR between 2.0 and 4.5.[122, 123] For most bileaflet mechanical valves, 2.0 to 3.0 is usually considered adequate; for patients or valves with enhanced risk, the INR is often increased to between 3.0 and 4.5, but the risk of bleeding is correspondingly worse. The INR system uses a PT methodology in which the local thromboplastin is compared with a World Health Organization standard.[124] Therefore, its use permits comparison of anticoagulation intensity among laboratories, clinical trials, and publications. Some centers also employ adjunctive antiplatelet agents such as aspirin, dipyridamole, or ticlopidine to reduce thromboembolic complications, with only a modestly increased risk of hemorrhage. However, antiplatelet therapy alone provides inadequate protection against thromboembolic complications with contemporary heart valve prostheses (except for short-term use after bioprosthesis implantation).[125, 126]

The risk of hemorrhage during long-term oral antico-

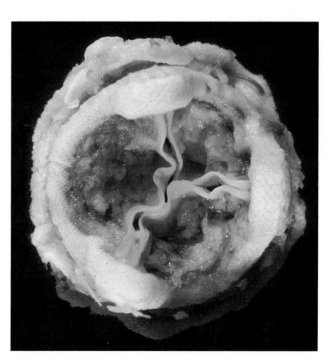

Figure 21-11 • Thrombosis of a porcine bioprosthesis with deposits localized to the prosthetic sinuses of Valsalva.

agulation therapy is 2 to 7% per patient-year overall, with cerebral, gastrointestinal, or retroperitoneal hemorrhage being most common in mechanical valve recipients on anticoagulation.[113, 127, 128] Major bleeding is often associated with a history of cerebrovascular disease, gastrointestinal bleeding, liver disease, and renal insufficiency.[129] Because only some recipients of tissue valves are anticoagulated, bleeding complications are less common in them than in those with mechanical valves (see Table 21-10).

Routine transesophageal echocardiographic (TEE) and transcranial Doppler (TCD) studies of patients with prosthetic heart valves frequently show the presence of high-intensity, high-velocity echoes (referred to as spontaneous echo contrasts, or "hits" [from High-Intensity Transcranial Doppler Signals]). With an appearance similar to that of saline contrast bubbles, they have been detected by TEE in approximately 28% of all patients with mechanical valves and are more frequently associated with mitral (41%) than aortic prostheses (15%).[130] They have been detected by TCD in 49 to 97% of patients with various valves.[131] Some investigators believe that these signals are microbubbles generated at valve closure when the leaflet or poppet strikes the valve housing, yielding microcavitation of dissolved gases in the plasma; others believe that they represent microemboli composed of formed blood elements.[132]

Prosthetic Valve Endocarditis

Infection associated with a valve substitute is termed *prosthetic valve endocarditis.* As an infrequent but serious complication, it affects 1 to 6% of valve replacement patients and has a poor outcome, with greater than 25 to 60% mortality.[133–135] Rates of infection are similar for mechanical and bioprosthetic valves, but patients whose original valve replacement surgery was prompted by endocarditis are at markedly greater risk. All patients with

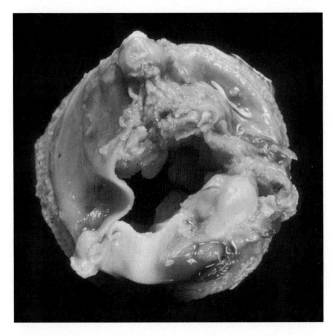

Figure 21-13 • Prosthetic valve endocarditis involving cusps of a bovine pericardial bioprosthesis.

mechanical prosthetic and bioprosthetic valves require antibiotic prophylaxis against prosthetic valve endocarditis during periods of vulnerability (see below).

Prosthetic valve endocarditis occurs most frequently in the first several months after surgery, with a preponderance of organisms constituting normal skin flora, such as staphylococci. In such cases, perioperative valve contamination or early postoperative bacteremia is the likely cause, whether or not there has been an overt wound infection. The infection rate is approximately linear thereafter, and infections are almost always caused by bacteremic seeding from the mouth or a breached mucosal surface, either iatrogenic (e.g., dental therapy or colonoscopy) or idiopathic. The high frequency of staphylococcal infection (especially *Staphylococcus epidermidis*) in prosthetic valve endocarditis contrasts with the relatively low frequency of such organisms in endocarditis occurring on natural valves. *Staphylococcus aureus,* streptococci, gram-negative bacilli, fungi, and unusual organisms can also cause prosthetic valve endocarditis.

As illustrated in Figure 21-12, infections of mechanical valves are almost always localized to the prosthesis-tissue interface at the sewing ring[136, 137] and often involve the periprosthetic tissues. This occurs because the synthetic biomaterials (polymers, metals, carbon) that make up mechanical prostheses and their sewing cuffs generally cannot support bacterial or fungal growth. Thus, tissues adjacent to the sewing cuff at the valve-tissue interface usually are infected and destroyed, causing a ring abscess. When a ring abscess is present, bioprosthetic valve endocarditis is similar to an infection of a mechanical valve. However, bioprosthetic valve infectious can also involve, or be limited to, the cusp tissue (Fig. 21-13), inducing its destruction with tearing, perforation, and valve incompetence.[138] In prosthetic valve endocarditis, deep clumps of bacterial or fungal organisms with sparse to exuberant

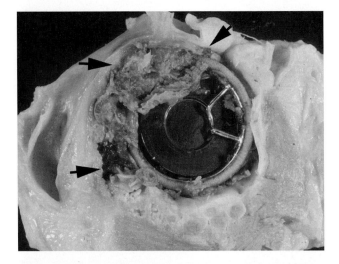

Figure 21-12 • Prosthetic valve endocarditis with large ring abscess (arrows), demonstrated from the ventricular surface of an aortic Bjork-Shiley tilting disk prosthesis. This patient died suddenly, owing to impingement of the abscess on the proximal atrioventricular conduction system. (From Schoen FJ: Cardiac valve prostheses: Pathological and bioengineering considerations. J Card Surg 2:65, 1987.)

inflammation may be demonstrated by histologic examination of periprosthetic tissue. In the case of infected bioprosthetic tissue valves, the cusps often contain organisms, with or without inflammation.

The complications of prosthetic valve endocarditis are potentially serious; they include embolization of vegetations, thrombi or, rarely, tissue valve fragments, heart failure secondary to obstruction or regurgitation caused by destructive bulky vegetations or secondary thrombi, and ring abscess–induced periprosthetic tissue destruction. Ring abscess may be further complicated either by separation (*dehiscence*) of the prosthesis from the annulus, causing regurgitation of blood around the device (*septic paravalvular leak*), which can induce cardiac failure or hemolysis, or by septic pericarditis, pseudoaneurysm, or atrioventricular conduction system block. (Fig. 14-13 demonstrates the possible pathways of spread for ring abscesses.) New cardiac murmurs or neurologic complications may appear. Blood cultures are usually positive if a patient has symptoms; the bacteremia associated with prosthetic valve endocarditis is often continuous. Echocardiography can demonstrate vegetations and helps to define complications such as valve dehiscence or annular abscess, but interference by echoes arising from the prosthesis may make interpretation difficult. Cinefluoroscopy may reveal valve instability resulting from dehiscence. Often owing to ring abscess and deep tissue involvement, prosthetic valve endocarditis is resistant to host defense mechanisms and antibiotics and is difficult to cure medically. Indications for reoperation during active infective

endocarditis on a heart valve prosthesis include severe heart failure, persistent sepsis, recurrent emboli, or a valve unstable in its annulus.

Structural Valve Deterioration

Biomaterials failure causing structural valve deterioration is an important cause of device dysfunction. Many valve models have been withdrawn from clinical use because of poor durability. Modes of degradation vary among valve types, models, and, in some cases, sites of implantation. Nevertheless, some patients with devices now considered obsolete have survived for extended periods without valve failure. This means that valves which are no longer inserted may be encountered by pathologists.

Mechanical Valves

The earliest substitute heart valves for either mitral or aortic implantation were of caged-ball type, with occluders fabricated from industrial-grade silicone elastomer. The most widely used models were the Starr-Edwards and Smeloff-Cutter prostheses. In many such valves, particularly in the aortic position, the poppets swelled, developed grooves, cracked, embolized fragments, and became distorted and immobile (a constellation of problems called *ball variance*) (Fig. 21-14). Mitral valves rarely suffered ball variance. Sudden death could occur when a swollen variant poppet impacted in the cage or obstructed an

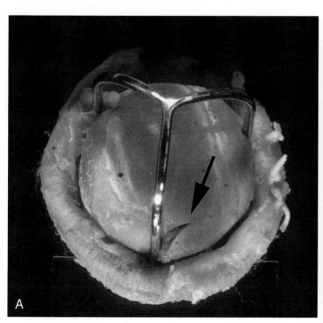
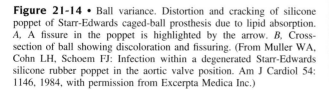
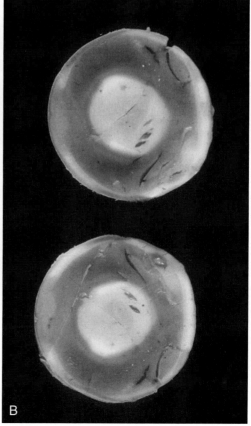

Figure 21-14 • Ball variance. Distortion and cracking of silicone poppet of Starr-Edwards caged-ball prosthesis due to lipid absorption. *A,* A fissure in the poppet is highlighted by the arrow. *B,* Cross-section of ball showing discoloration and fissuring. (From Muller WA, Cohn LH, Schoem FJ: Infection within a degenerated Starr-Edwards silicone rubber poppet in the aortic valve position. Am J Cardiol 54: 1146, 1984, with permission from Excerpta Medica Inc.)

orifice.[139] Ball variance was a consequence of lipid absorption (mainly cholesterol and cholesteryl esters, fatty acids, and triglycerides) by the silicone elastomeric poppet and embrittlement of the poppet, so that diameter was reduced sufficiently to permit escape from the cage.[140] Thrombi occasionally developed in crevices on the poppet surface. They could cause thromboemboli or become a nidus of infection.[141] This experience occasioned changes in elastomer fabrication in 1964 that have virtually eliminated lipid-related ball variance; caged-ball prostheses produced later rarely suffer such structural failure.[142]

Cloth-covered caged-ball valves were introduced to

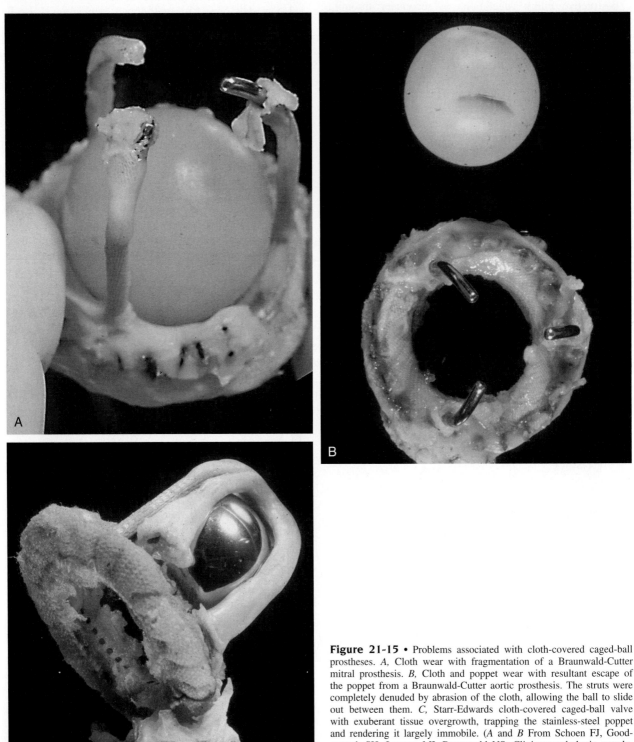

Figure 21-15 • Problems associated with cloth-covered caged-ball prostheses. *A,* Cloth wear with fragmentation of a Braunwald-Cutter mitral prosthesis. *B,* Cloth and poppet wear with resultant escape of the poppet from a Braunwald-Cutter aortic prosthesis. The struts were completely denuded by abrasion of the cloth, allowing the ball to slide out between them. *C,* Starr-Edwards cloth-covered caged-ball valve with exuberant tissue overgrowth, trapping the stainless-steel poppet and rendering it largely immobile. (*A* and *B* From Schoen FJ, Goodenough SH, Ionescu MI, Braunwald NS: Clinicomorphologic correlations following long-term implantation of cloth-covered prosthetic heart valves: Implications for device development. Trans Am Soc Artif Intern Organs 29:556, 1983.)

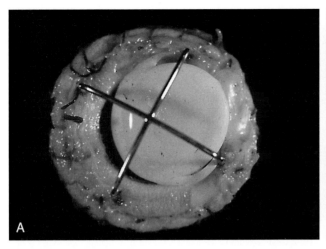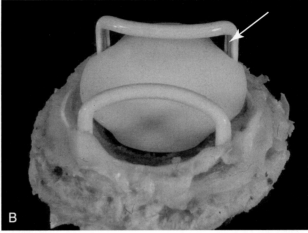

Figure 21-16 • Abrasive wear of disk valve prostheses. *A,* Silicone disk valve with disk damage as a result of abrasion on metallic struts. *B,* Beall valve with Teflon disk and Teflon-coated struts showing wear on both (strut wear highlighted by arrow).

lower the incidence of thromboembolism by encouraging tissue ingrowth into the fabric coating the struts, with the intention of yielding a favorable biologic surface. Two types were investigated and used: one with a hollow metal poppet and cage closed at its apex, and another with a silicone elastomeric poppet and a cage open at its apex. However, both suffered problems related to cloth abrasion and fragmentation by the occluder, with resultant cloth emboli and hemolysis; the metallic ball version (modified Starr-Edwards valve) also had frequent fibrous overgrowth, with ball entrapment and stenosis (Fig. 21-15).[143] In the type with a silicone ball and open cage (Braunwald-Cutter valve), cloth wear frequently denuded the struts; in addition, particularly in the aortic position, cloth loss coupled with a decrease in ball diameter due to wear occasionally permitted the occluder to escape between the bare metallic struts.[144, 145] One development to overcome cloth wear caused by a metal ball was the introduction of composite metal-cloth struts and metal studs in the seat so that a

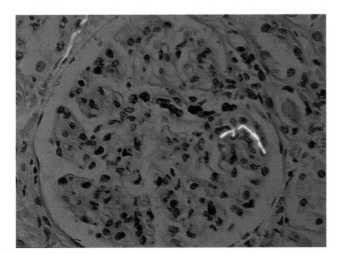

Figure 21-17 • Photomicrograph of renal glomerulus under partially polarized illumination showing fragment of Teflon from worn disk valve (H&E stain).

metal poppet could be in contact with metal rather than cloth during its excursion (further modified Starr-Edwards valve).[146] However, the metal studs also wore with time, eventually permitting the metal poppet to contact the cloth in the seat and, ultimately, to wear through it.

Patients with rheumatic mitral stenosis often have a small left ventricular chamber. In these patients, an introduced caged-ball prosthesis occupies a substantial fraction of left ventricular volume and could cause outflow tract obstruction or irritate or erode the septal wall. Caged-disk valves, designed with an increased orifice size and reduced cage height, helped overcome these problems. However, caged-disk valves at the mitral site had high-pressure gradients and disrupted flow across the prosthesis, leading to frequent thromboembolic complications. Disks composed of silicone or Teflon (polytetrafluoroethylene) frequently developed disk wear due to abrasion with the cage struts, with notching at their edges and a reduction in diameter, leading to slowly progressive valve incompetence[36, 37]; wear also occurred on polymer coated struts (Fig. 21-16).[19] A severely worn disk could lock in an abnormal orientation, inducing acute valvular dysfunction. Previously used tilting disk valves with polymeric disks formed of Delrin (polyacetal) or Teflon had limited durability due to abrasive wear, especially in those designs that did not permit free rotation of the disk.[34]

With abrasive wear or fracture of mechanical components of any prosthetic valve, fragments of nonphysiologic material can embolize to a distal organ bed (Fig. 21-17). Patients with degraded ball and disk valves frequently have foreign body granulomas or polymer fragments in random sections of various organs. Indeed, one study suggested that the presence of foreign body granulomas in a liver biopsy of a patient with a vulnerable valve prosthesis would aid the diagnosis of ball or disk deterioration.[147]

Contemporary single-leaflet or bileaflet tilting disk valves with pyrolytic carbon occluders and either metallic struts or carbon housing have generally favorable durability.[148] With the exception of two valve cohorts, fractures of either carbon or metallic components are rare. In one

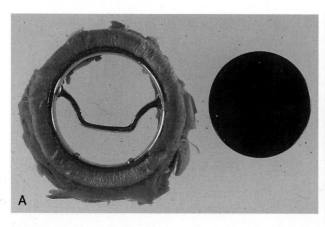

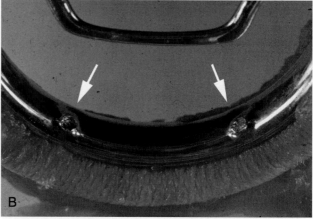

Figure 21-18 • Strut fracture of Bjork-Shiley valve. *A,* Valve housing with a single remaining strut and adjacent disk, which was found in the distal aorta. *B,* Close-up of fractured weld sites at strut bases (arrows). (*A* From Schoen FJ, Levy RJ, Piehler HR: Pathological consideration in replacement cardiac valves. Cardiovasc Pathol 1:29, 1992, with permission from Elsevier Science.)

instance, the Bjork-Shiley valve was redesigned with the intention of enhancing disk opening and relieving the obstruction and thromboembolic complications that occurred with the original and widely used model. The resultant Bjork-Shiley 60- and 70-degree convexoconcave tilting disk valves suffered fractures of the welded metallic outlet strut and separation from the valve, leading to frequently fatal disk escape (Fig. 21-18).[149, 150] As of August 1994, strut fracture had been reported in 557 of the 86,000 valves of this type implanted worldwide from 1979 to 1986; nearly 50,000 individuals are presently living with this valve. The underlying problem was due to the unanticipated consequence of the disk's moving at higher velocity and force during valve closure, causing its over-rotation and an excessively hard contact with the metallic outlet strut. The stress on the strut increases with elevated left ventricular contractile force, such as occurs with exercise, and many such failures occurred during physical exertion.[149–151] When the outlet strut suffers stresses that exceed its endurance limit, fatigue fracture may occur, especially in the region of the welds anchoring this strut to the housing. This occurs in part because welds are typically intrinsically brittle and thereby vulnerable regions of a metallic structure, owing to shrinkage porosity or inclusions. Valves are occasionally encountered with a unilateral outlet strut fracture, suggesting that one leg of the strut separates first, followed after some time by the second, thereby releasing the disk.[152] Prophylactic explantation has been recommended for some patients who are predicted to have an especially high fracture rate, dependent on gender, age, and valve position.

Fractures of carbon valve components (hemidisk or housing) occurred in at least 37 of an estimated 20,000 implanted Edwards (previously Hemex)-Duromedics bileaflet tilting disk valves (Fig. 21-19).[153] Studies of these explants suggest that valve fracture with leaflet escape resulted from variable combinations of five factors: (1) microporosity in the pyrolytic carbon coating in the leaflets, (2) cavitation bubbles impacting on the carbon surfaces during function, (3) unusual combinations of dimensional tolerances, (4) poor shock-absorbing qualities of the annular tissues in some patients (perhaps due to calcification-induced rigidity), and (5) structural defects in the valve prosthesis induced by fabrication or surgical mishandling.[154] Fractures of carbon components have been encountered only rarely with other carbon bileaflet tilting disk valves, such as the St. Jude Medical valve.[155, 156]

Figure 21-19 • Photograph of Edwards (previously Hemex)-Duromedics bileaflet tilting disk valve with fracture of hemileaflet and part of housing (arrow). (From Schoen FJ, et al: Pathological considerations in replacement cardiac valves. Cardiovasc Pathol 1:29, 1992, with permission from Elsevier Science.)

Bioprosthetic Valves

The major disadvantage of bioprosthetic valves is the substantial rate of time-dependent, progressive structural deterioration, particularly in younger recipients. Structural valve deterioration results from an intrinsic process of tissue degeneration that eventually results in stenosis or regurgitation.

Porcine Aortic Valves

The time-dependent rate of porcine valve structural deterioration has been established.[11, 157, 158] Fewer than 1% of porcine aortic valve bioprostheses implanted in adults suffer structural dysfunction after 5 years or less; however, 20 to 30% become dysfunctional within 10 years, and more than 50% fail due to degeneration within 15 years of implantation. Moreover, the risk of structural failure is strongly age dependent, with individuals younger than 35 years of age, and especially children, having the highest risk. Risk continues to be age dependent in older recipients. The rate of structural valve deterioration in patients older than 65 years is lower than in patients younger than 65 years. In patients older than 65 years, the rate of structural deterioration is relatively low, approximately 10% at 10 years. Failure rates are identical for the Hancock and Carpentier-Edwards types of porcine bioprosthetic valves.[159] The clinical presentation of bioprosthetic valve failure is heterogeneous; most patients develop cardiac dysfunction insidiously, permitting elective reoperation, but 5 to 10% of valves deteriorate rapidly and require urgent surgery.[160]

Two related but distinct processes dominate in bioprosthetic valve dysfunction owing to deterioration of the cuspal tissue: calcification within the substance of the cusps (*intrinsic mineralization*), and degradation with ultimate failure of the connective tissue matrix (*noncalcific mechanical failure*) (Fig. 21-20).[13, 161, 162] Approximately three fourths of degenerative failures manifest as regurgi-

tation through tears secondary to calcification.[163] Pure stenosis due to calcific cusp stiffening and cusp tears or perforations unrelated to either calcification or endocarditis occur less frequently (approximately 10 to 15% each) (Fig. 21-21). Tears may be spatially related to the underlying calcific deposits, which induce new and substantial sites of stress concentration at their junction with the surrounding tissue, potentiating the risk of cusp rupture. Rarely, calcific deposits in bioprosthetic valves fragment and embolize (Fig. 21-22). Calcific deposits are grossly visible, nodular gray or white masses that tend to be most apparent at the commissural tissue adjacent to the stent posts and in other areas of leaflet flexion where deformations are maximal (i.e., near the cusp commissures and basal attachment margins). Calcification can also occur at the surface of bioprosthetic valve cusps in thrombi or infective vegetations (*extrinsic mineralization*).

The extent of calcification of surgically removed failed bioprosthetic valves varies widely among patients after long-term implantation (Fig. 21-23). The calcium content of 32 excised porcine bioprostheses functioning for 36 to 156 months (mean, 87 months) and removed because of calcific failure was 113 ± 68 μm/mg; the maximal levels noted were 200 to 250 μg/mg calcium.[164] Calcification rarely causes dysfunction of valves implanted for less than 4 years in adults, and most failed valves removed after at least 4 years are mineralized. Nevertheless, some bioprostheses have minimal or no radiographically demonstrable calcific deposits after implantation for 10

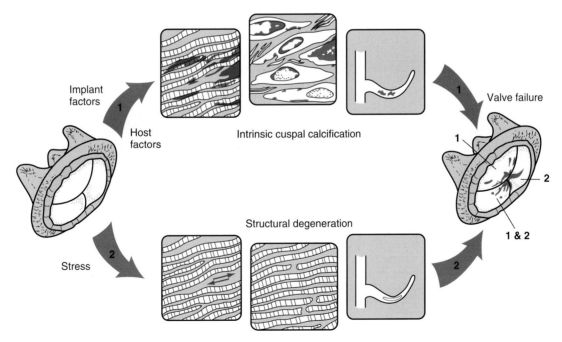

Figure 21-20 • Unified model for bioprosthetic heart valve failure relating isolated tissue processes of mineralization and collagen degeneration to gross clinical failures. These processes may occur independently, or be synergistic. Failures have calcification with cusp stiffening (pathway 1), cusp defects without calcific deposits (pathway 2), or cusp tears associated with mineralization (combination of pathways 1 and 2). Specifically, implant and host factors interact to induce the collagen-oriented and cell-oriented calcific deposits. These can be noted ultrastructurally. Calcific deposits predominate in the central portions of valve cusps, particularly at flexion points such as the commissures (pathway 1). Stress causes sheer between and fracture of collagen fibers, which may create gross cuspal defects (pathway 2). Also, although dynamic mechanical activity is not a prerequisite for calcification, stress may promote (i.e., accelerate) this process through unknown mechanisms. (From Schoen FJ, Levy RJ: Bioprosthetic heart valve failure: Pathology and pathogenesis. Cardiol Clin 2:717, 1984.)

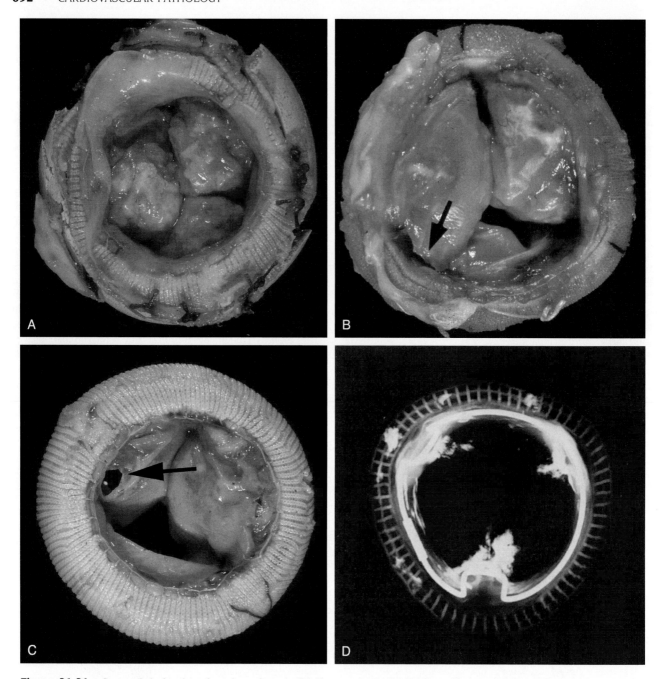

Figure 21-21 • Structural dysfunction of porcine valves. *A,* Calcific stenosis. *B,* Calcification with secondary tear (arrow) leading to severe regurgitation. *C,* Noncalcific cuspal defect (arrow) causing regurgitation of a porcine aortic valve. *D,* Radiograph of specimen shown in *B.* (*B* and *D,* from Schoen FJ, Hobson CE: Anatomic analysis of removed prosthetic heart valves: Causes of failure of 33 mechanical valves and 58 bioprostheses, 1980 to 1983. Hum Pathol 16:549, 1985. *C,* From Schoen FJ, Collins JJ Jr, Cohn LH: Long-term failure rate and morphologic correlations in porcine bioprosthetic heart valves. Am J Cardiol 51:957, 1983, with permission from Excerpta Medica Inc.)

years or longer. The underlying reasons for the considerable patient-to-patient and valve-to-valve variability in mineralization are poorly understood.

Percutaneous transluminal balloon dilation by catheter, used for stenosed natural mitral and aortic valves (see Chapter 13), has been employed to dilate calcified stenosed right-sided conduit-mounted valves and left-sided porcine bioprosthetic valves.[165] Balloon inflation induces commissural splitting, leaflet cracks, fractures, and tears. Although this procedure may be efficacious and safe in

some patients, breakage of friable calcific deposits poses a risk of calcific emboli.

Tears and other defects in bioprosthetic valves have several causes (Table 21-12). Factors in addition to calcification that contribute to cusp defects and tears are damage incurred during fabrication, implantation, or intravascular instrumentation such as catheterization; and patient-prosthesis interactions, such as infection, and factors related to otherwise uncomplicated function, such as progressive mechanically or chemically mediated degradation of the

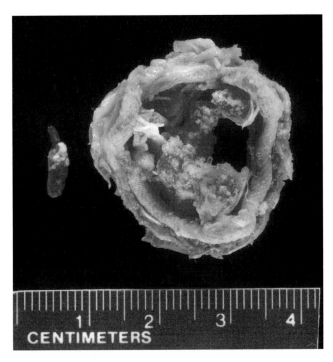

Figure 21-22 • Massive calcification of a porcine aortic valve bioprosthesis with secondary calcific embolus removed at surgery from the left anterior descending coronary artery (at left).

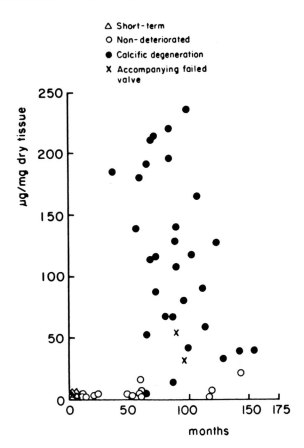

Figure 21-23 • Calcium concentration of removed porcine valves, measured by atomic absorption spectroscopy, plotted against duration of function. The accumulated valves were from very short-term implants, deteriorated valves removed at autopsy or cardiac transplantation, valves suffering structural deterioration, and those removed in tandem with a failed valve. Curiously, some valves seem to escape calcification. (From Schoen FJ, Kujovich JL, Webb CL, Levy RJ: Chemically determined mineral content of explanted porcine aortic valve bioprostheses: Correlation with radiographic assessment of calcification and clinical data. Circulation 76:1061, 1987.)

cuspal extracellular matrix (see later). In addition, buckling, abrasion, or fatigue may be potentiated by specific design features. Mechanical destruction of collagen architecture during cyclic and functional cuspal bending is revealed by scanning and transmission electron microscopy as fraying, disruption, and fracture of collagen fibers. Accelerated breakdown occurs at stress concentrations, particularly at cuspal attachment sites and foci of excessive leaflet stresses.

Valvular insufficiency may also be caused by commissural region dehiscence of transplanted aortic wall tissue from the luminal aspect of a porcine valve stent (Fig. 21-24).[166, 167] In such cases, the aortic wall and associated commissure collapse toward the center of the valve orifice. Although this complication has been reported primarily with Carpentier-Edwards porcine bioprostheses, we and others have noted this problem in several other models of porcine valves.

Bovine Pericardial Valves

Pericardial bioprostheses also fail by calcific and noncalcific deterioration (Fig. 21-25).[13, 54–56, 72] With first-generation pericardial bioprostheses, failure was most frequently caused by noncalcific cusp perforations and tears. The most common type of noncalcific pericardial valve structural defect is a large tear at the attachment margin of the cusp to a stent. However, pericardial bioprostheses also frequently suffer calcific degeneration leading to stiffening or secondary tearing, in both adults and children. The morphology of calcific deposits in pericardial valves is remarkably similar to that found in failed porcine valves.

TABLE 21-12 • **Factors Potentially Contributing to Cusp Defects or Tears in Bioprosthetic Valves**

Related to factors in design, manufacture, and implantation
Design flaws
Manufacturing defects

Related to interactions with the recipient
Infection
Inflammation
Calcification
Suture perforation
Tissue fatigue
Abrasion
Stress concentrations at commissures
Tissue delamination

Artifactual
Valve trauma during surgical removal

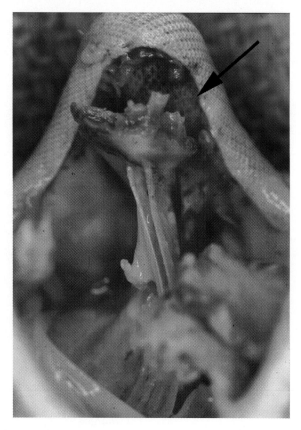

Figure 21-24 • Commissural dehiscence of aortic wall tissue from the inside of a strut of a porcine aortic valve bioprosthesis (arrow).

Tears in pericardial valves along the attachment points of cusps are frequently related to specific features of valve design and the resultant continuous trauma of tissue against bare Dacron cloth ("abrasion"), causing tissue fatigue along these repetitive flexure sites.[54–56, 72] Although the specific cause of a tear in a clinically retrieved valve often cannot be determined by gross or microscopic examination, a contribution by abrasion may be suggested by observing of a focal roughening or regional tapering of the tissue cross-section, with attrition of collagen bundles (Fig. 21-26). In the original Ionescu-Shiley design (see Fig. 21-4C), cusp perforations and tears were frequently associated with a commissural suture ("alignment stitch"), which held cusps in apposition near their free edge and adjacent to the stent post. Loss of commissural apposition may increase cusp excursion and potentiate fatigue or abrasion damage. In contemporary pericardial valve designs (e.g., Carpentier-Edwards Perimount, Edwards Life Sciences, Santa Ana, California; see Fig. 21-4D), the tissue is suspended from the inside of a flexible, low-profile stent, whereas the original pericardial valves had tissue mounted on the outside of the stent. Some studies suggest that such pericardial valves may have superior performance and durability,[168–71] but failures do occur that are morphologically identical to those of the previous generations of pericardial valves (personal communication, J. Butany, Toronto). A general comparison of the pathologic features observed with porcine valve and bovine pericardial bioprostheses is summarized in Table 21-13.

Pathobiology of Tissue Heart Valve Deterioration: Calcification and Structural Matrix Deterioration

Calcification

The pathophysiology and prevention of tissue calcification have been widely investigated using experimental circulatory models; orthotopic mitral and conduit-mounted valves in calves and sheep; and heterotopic implant models, including subcutaneous implantation, largely in rodents.[13, 67, 172, 173] Analogous to the accelerated rate of calcification in young patients discussed previously, these models use immature animals in which bioprosthetic tissue calcifies progressively and rapidly. Despite the markedly accelerated kinetics of calcification, the morphology is similar to that observed in clinical specimens. In the rat subcutaneous model using 3-week-old weanlings, clinically relevant calcification by amount and morphology is achieved in 3 weeks (80 to 120 μg/mg calcium), and maximal levels occur in approximately 8 weeks.[67, 172] In sheep mitral valve implants, a level of 109 to 118 μg/mg calcium is reached in 3 to 5 months.[173] Despite the absence of dynamic mechanical activity and blood contact characteristic of the circulatory environment, subcutaneous implants calcify with a morphology and extent analogous to those observed in clinical and experimental circulatory studies. In vitro models of calcification have been used, but none convincingly reproduced the in vivo environment or resultant pathology.[174, 175]

Calcification in chemically fixed or fresh bioprosthetic tissue or in the natural valves predominantly involves cells; however, extracellular matrix calcification can also occur (Fig. 21-27).[13, 67, 162, 172, 176–181] Recall that the residual cells in cross-linked bioprosthetic tissue are nonviable. The critical event in the nucleation of intrinsic cuspal mineralization is most likely the reaction of calcium derived from plasma with cell-associated (predominantly membrane-associated) organic phosphorus. This is hypothesized to occur as follows[13, 67]: Normal cells have an approximately 10,000-fold gradient of calcium from outside to inside, with the low intracellular calcium concentrations maintained by energy-dependent pumps at the cell membrane. In cells rendered nonviable or injured by glutaraldehyde fixation, autolysis, ischemia, or trauma, energy is unavailable, membranes are disrupted, and calcium exclusion is impaired. Thus, high concentrations of calcium in the fluid bathing the tissue can react with phosphorus (as cell membrane–based phospholipids or as intracellular organelles such as mitochondria) to nucleate calcific crystals. Considerable support for this hypothesis has recently been provided by an in vitro study of glutaraldehyde-treated porcine aortic valve fibroblasts.[177] Propagation of crystal formation depends on the concentration of Ca^{2+} and PO_4 and the balance of calcification inhibitors and accelerators in the extracellular space, such as the connective tissue matrix proteins. As demonstrated by analysis of clinical and experimental valve explants as well as experiments with purified proteins, calcification of collagen and elastin can also occur by independent but poorly understood mechanisms.[178, 179]

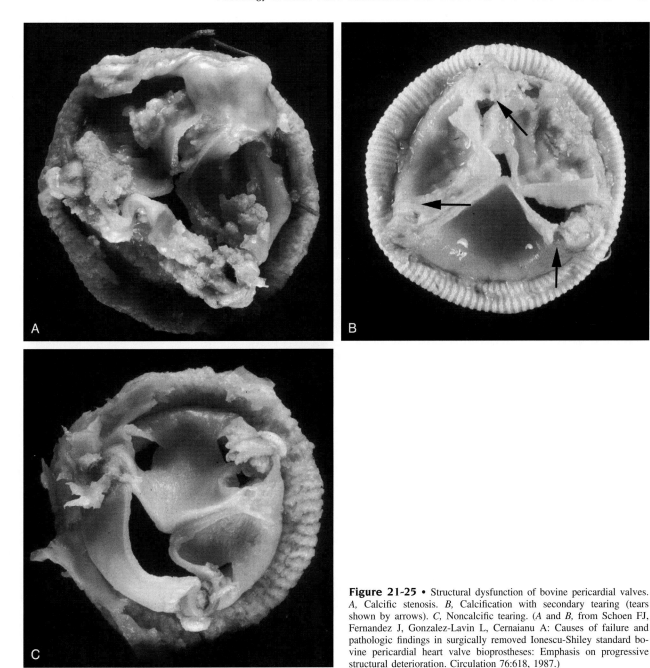

Figure 21-25 • Structural dysfunction of bovine pericardial valves. *A*, Calcific stenosis. *B*, Calcification with secondary tearing (tears shown by arrows). *C*, Noncalcific tearing. (*A* and *B*, from Schoen FJ, Fernandez J, Gonzalez-Lavin L, Cernaianu A: Causes of failure and pathologic findings in surgically removed Ionescu-Shiley standard bovine pericardial heart valve bioprostheses: Emphasis on progressive structural deterioration. Circulation 76:618, 1987.)

With increasing duration of implantation, cell-associated deposits propagate, progressively increasing in size and number, to obliterate cells and dissect among collagen bundles. Proliferation of nucleation sites and crystal growth in both porcine valve and bovine pericardium results in a progressive confluence of diffusely distributed microcrystals into macroscopic nodules. Analogous to those responsible for clinical valve failures, gross calcific nodules focally obliterate implant architecture and ulcerate through the cusp surface. This process is summarized schematically in Figure 21-28. In experimental models, the morphology, kinetics, and chemistry of calcification in porcine valve and bovine pericardial tissue are identical.

Mineralization of bioprosthetic valves has host, implant, and mechanical determinants.[13, 172, 180, 182] As indicated in Figure 21-28, the fundamental mechanisms of bioprosthetic tissue mineralization depend on implant microstructural components and their specific biochemical modifications induced by aldehyde pretreatment. In particular, glutaraldehyde cross-linking potentiates mineral deposition,[182] but the precise reasons are uncertain. The rate of clinical and experimental bioprosthetic tissue calcification also depends on host metabolic factors. For example, calcification is dramatically accelerated in younger patients; renal failure, hypercalcemia, and, possibly, dietary calcium supplementation also promote mineralization. The effect of mechanical factors is real but enigmatic. Clinical and experimental mineralization is accelerated and enhanced in areas of leaflet flexion where deformations are maximal, especially at cusp commissures and bases.[13]

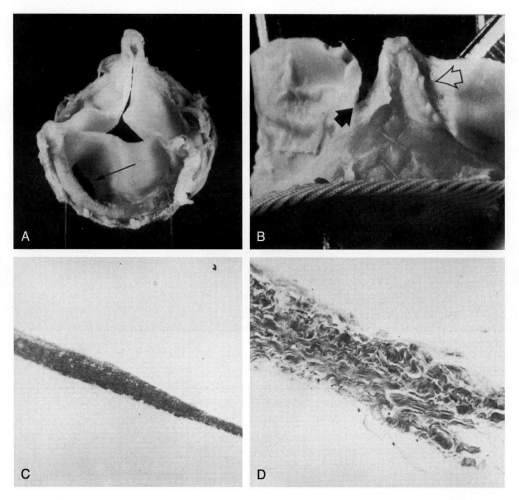

Figure 21-26 • Fatigue and abrasion causing tearing of pericardial valves. *A,* Basal cuspal tear in Ionescu-Shiley pericardial bioprosthesis (arrow). *B,* Tear at free edge (closed arrow) and abrasion causing thinning and incipient tear of pericardial bioprosthesis at commissural attachment (open arrow). *C* and *D,* Photomicrographs of valve in *B* through area shown by open arrow, indicating thinning and loss of pericardial tissue. (H & E stain.)

TABLE 21-13 • **Comparison of Pathologic Features: Porcine Aortic Valve Versus Bovine Pericardial Bioprosthesis**

Feature	Porcine Aortic Valve	Bovine Pericardial Bioprosthesis
Cusp calcification	+	+
Cusp tears	+	+
Tissue fatigue	+	+
Cusp abrasion	Minimal	+
Alignment or suture-related holes/tears	0	+
Cusp stretching/sagging	0	+
Tissue overgrowth	+	+
Endocarditis involving cusps	+	+
Endocarditis with ring abscess	+	+
Adherent macrophages	+	+
Deep inflammation (without infection)	Minimal	+
Deep fluid insudation	+	+
Inflow surface collagen fragmentation	0	+
Focal thrombi	+	+
Endothelialization	Minimal	0
Suture entrapment	Minimal	+
Suture perforation	+	Minimal

Nevertheless, in contrast to the prerequisite host and implant conditions, mechanical factors appear to be only contributory, as evidenced by the ability to achieve experimental calcification in the subcutaneous space. Moreover, the mechanism of calcification regulation by mechanical factors is uncertain.

Bioprosthetic tissue mineralization in particular and pathologic calcification in general resemble physiologic musculoskeletal mineralization.[176, 183] In cartilage and bone, the membrane fragments that initiate calcification are known as matrix vesicles; in pathologic calcification, a similar role is played by membranes and their fragments derived from degenerate, aging, injured, or dead cells. In both physiologic and pathologic calcification, the deposits are poorly crystalline calcium phosphate, chemically related to hydroxyapatite[180, 184]; in both, crystal formation is largely associated with cell membranes.

In normal bone calcification, the growth of apatite crystals is regulated by several noncollagenous matrix proteins, including *osteopontin,* an acidic calcium-binding phosphoprotein with high affinity to hydroxyapatite that is abundant in foci of dystrophic calcification;[185] *osteonectin,* also known as secreted protein acidic rich in cysteine (SPARC), which binds minerals and inhibits cell spreading and migration during new blood vessel formation or angiogenesis;[186] and *osteocalcin* and other γ-carboxyglutamic acid (GLA)–containing proteins, such as *matrix GLA protein* (Mgp).[187, 188] Mice lacking osteocalcin or Mgp exhibit inappropriate calcification of cartilage and die as a result of arterial calcification and blood vessel rupture.[189] These responses suggest that inhibition of calcification in arteries and cartilage requires Mgp and that this family of proteins may negatively regulate calcification. Noncollagenous matrix proteins have been demonstrated in calcific aortic stenosis, calcified atherosclerotic plaque, and calcified bioprosthetic heart valves. Additional evidence suggests that they serve a pathogenetic or regulatory role.[190, 191]

Noncalcific Deterioration

There is considerable evidence that degradation of the valvular structural matrix independent of calcification is a major mechanism of bioprosthetic valve structural degradation and potentially failure. Prosthesis failure has been reported to be due to localized cuspal damage at stressed regions, such as valvular commissures and points of maximal cuspal flexion. Ultrastructural disruption of bioprosthetic collagen fibrils has also been noted in clinical

retrievals. Chemical pretreatment not only renders cells nonviable and incapable of remodeling the matrix but also obviates the dynamic structural rearrangements that occur during natural valve function. This results in increased flexural compressive stresses that can induce delamination and fracture of the cuspal collagen fibers. Some aspects of the tissue degeneration can be reproduced by in vitro accelerated fatigue. In particular, in vitro accelerated testing yields a consistent pattern of collagen deterioration in regions located near the nodulus of Arantius and extending down toward the basal attachments.[192] In human explanted bioprosthetic heart valves, the regions of structural damage not corresponding to areas of calcification are also noted in a characteristic spatial distribution near the nodulus, with evidence of interlayer shearing in the damaged regions. Delaminations between the collagen fibers in the valve layers and fiber fractures are noted ultrastructurally. These structural changes are also accompanied by a dramatic loss of strength, flexural stiffness, collagen denaturation, and loss of GAGs.[193–195]

Molecular and biochemical changes in collagen may also contribute to progressive damage and the propensity

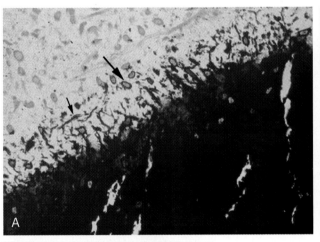

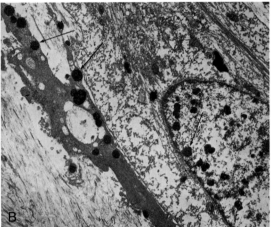

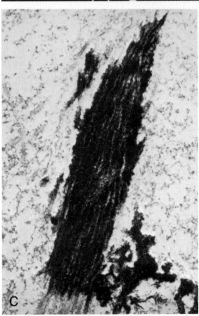

Figure 21-27 • Initiation of bioprosthetic valve calcification in structural tissue elements. *A,* Photomicrograph of the edge of a calcific deposit in an experimental porcine aortic valve bioprosthesis demonstrating both round and streak-like calcific densities, representing calcification initiated in cells (large arrow) and collagen (smaller arrow), respectively. (von Kossa stain: calcium phosphates black). *B,* Transmission electron microscopy photomicrograph of cell membrane–associated calcific deposits (arrows) (bar = 1 μm). *C,* Transmission electron microscopy photomicrograph of calcification in collagen (bar = 1 μm). (*B* and *C,* From Schoen FJ, Levy RJ, Nelson AC, et al: Onset and progression of experimental bioprosthetic heart valve calcification. Lab Invest 52: 523, 1985.)

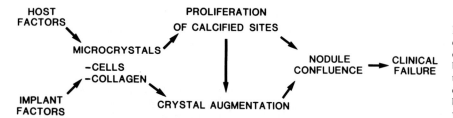

Figure 21-28 • Schematic sequence linking cellular and extracellular matrix–oriented events in the initiation of calcification responsible for clinical calcific failure of a bioprosthesis. (From Schoen FJ, Levy RJ, Nelson AC, et al: Onset and progression of experimental bioprosthetic heart valve calcification. Lab Invest 52:523, 1985.)

to calcify. Experimental in vitro accelerated cyclic fatigue of both type I collagen and porcine bioprosthetic heart valve cusps under conditions simulating actual aortic valve biomechanics causes a characteristic structural change in collagen fibers, which may indicate the creation of voids suitable for calcium phosphate nucleation; moreover, there is evidence for ongoing chemical degradation of the collagen framework and progressive loss of amorphous extracellular matrix (largely GAGs).[196-198] In particular, increased levels of extracellular matrix degrading activity—especially matrix metalloproteinases (MMPs), including MMP 9, beta glucuronidase, collagenase, and MMP 2—have been found clinically in explanted pericardial bioprostheses.[196]

Immunologic Processes

To what extent, if any, immunologic processes have a role in tissue valve deterioration is uncertain and highly controversial. Experimental animals can be sensitized to both fresh and cross-linked bioprosthetic valve tissues,[199, 200] antibodies to valve components can be detected in some patients following valve dysfunction,[201] and failed tissue valves often show a brisk mononuclear inflammation histologically. Thus, cross-linking reduces, but does not eliminate, the antigenicity of bioprosthetic material. Nevertheless, no causal immunologic basis has been demonstrated for clinical or experimental bioprosthetic valve failure. Moreover, neither nonspecific inflammation nor specific immunologic responses appear to mediate experimental bioprosthetic tissue calcification.[13, 180, 202]

Nonstructural Dysfunction

This group of complications is a heterogeneous collection of untoward outcomes that result predominantly from interactions of an otherwise structurally intact prosthesis with its environment. Prosthetic obstruction, paravalvular leak, extrinsic interference, and hemolysis are the most common problems.[19, 204-206]

Prosthetic Obstruction, Malposition, and Disproportion

Although normal native cardiac valves permit low-resistance central flow, all valve substitutes except non-stented tissue valves are to some degree obstructive to forward flow, largely a result of sewing cuff bulk, the housing and cage structures of a mechanical prosthesis or the struts of a bioprosthesis, and the poppet or tissue itself. Thus, the effective orifice area of all stented devices is considerably less than that of the normal annulus of the valve that it replaced. Functional prosthetic orifice areas and transvalvular gradients calculated at postoperative cardiac catheterization are often as high as those measured in nonoperated patients with mild to moderate valve stenosis. Hemodynamic obstruction is accentuated by smaller prosthesis size, even of the most efficient designs. Consequently, an otherwise normally functioning prosthesis occasionally requires removal because its size is insufficient for the needs of the patient. More typically, and important in many patients, myocardial pressure over-

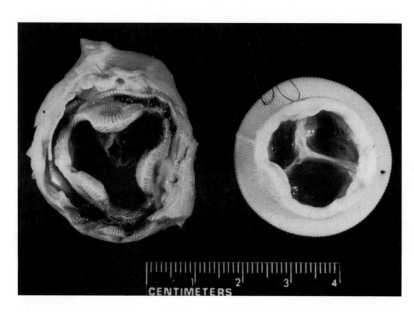

Figure 21-29 • Photograph demonstrating stent creep (left) of a 25-mm aortic prosthesis implanted for 36 months; an unimplanted 25-mm prosthesis is shown on the right for comparison. The compromise of the outflow orifice of the removed valve is apparent. (From Schoen FJ, Schulman LJ, Cohn LH: Quantitative anatomic analysis of "stent creep" of explanted Hancock standard porcine bioprostheses used for cardiac valve replacement. Am J Cardiol 56:110, 1985, with permission from Excerpta Medica Inc.)

work generally continues despite valve replacement with an entirely functional prosthesis. Bioprosthetic valves may show progressive obstruction as a result of subclinical cusp thickening, and stiffening and/or calcification. Moreover, inward deflection of stent posts (struts) during function of some porcine bioprostheses (*stent creep*) may contribute to progressive stenosis (Fig. 21-29).[203] Prosthetic valve function is generally accompanied by some degree of regurgitation, intentionally designed to enhance closing and provide washing of valve components, but it may continue during the completely closed phase of the cycle.

The effective orifice area of a valve prosthesis of a specific design increases with its diameter. Therefore, a surgeon generally implants the largest prosthesis possible into a fixed-size annulus. However, a valve disproportionately large for the anatomic site of implantation may have impeded movement of its components, cause damage to surrounding structures (such as septal irritation, erosion, or interference with left ventricular emptying for mitral valves), or be more severely obstructive than an appropriately sized valve. Prosthetic disproportion is most likely to occur with mitral replacements done for mitral stenosis and a small left ventricle; with aortic replacements when the aorta and aortic root are small; and in a double valve replacement for mitral and aortic stenosis, a situation generally associated with an extremely small, stiff left ventricle. Because chamber size and configuration are to some extent dynamic postoperatively, mitral disproportion may become apparent only after postoperative regression of preoperative left ventricular dilation.

Rarely, a heart valve prosthesis is not inserted in the proper position. Angulation or insertion proximal or distal to the ideal location may interfere with prosthesis function and cause low-output syndrome postoperatively. Malfunction often encourages thrombus formation. A malpositioned or poorly angled mitral prosthesis may cause left ventricular outflow tract obstruction, whereas an aortic prosthesis in an abnormal position can obstruct a coronary artery ostium.

Paravalvular Leak

A backward flow of blood passing between the prosthetic device and annular tissues when the device is closed is termed a paravalvular (also called a perivalvular or periprosthetic) leak (Fig. 21-30). An extreme and acute form is caused by dehiscence (i.e., separation) of a prosthesis from annular tissue that provides an unsatisfactory anchor for sutures. The most frequent conditions that potentiate paravalvular leak are inadequate suture placement, suture or knot failure, and a pathologic annulus due to infection, myxomatous valvular degeneration (floppy mitral valve), or degenerative calcification (calcific aortic stenosis or mitral annular calcification). Otherwise, tissue retraction from the sewing ring between sutures during healing is thought to be the cause. Paravalvular leak and dehiscence over a majority of the suture line were more frequent in the early days of valve replacement, when a continuous suture line was used to secure a prosthesis in situ and suture disruption caused a major separation. Currently, an interrupted suture line is used by most surgeons to anchor a substitute valve (approximately 16 to 18 individual ties). A small paravalvular leak may

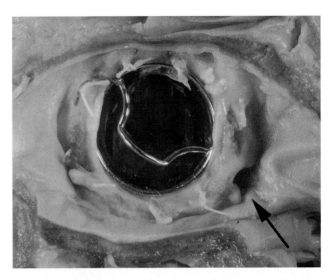

Figure 21-30 • Paravalvular leak with a defect at the edge of a healed sewing cuff of mechanical valve prosthesis (arrow). (From Schoen FJ: Pathologic considerations in replacement heart valves and other cardiovascular prosthetic devices. In: Schoen FJ, Gimbrone MA [eds]: Cardiovascular Pathology: Clinicopathologic Correlations and Pathogenetic Mechanisms. Baltimore, Williams & Wilkins, 1995, p 194.)

be clinically inconsequential, but a larger defect can aggravate hemolysis or cause heart failure.

Paravalvular defects can be difficult for a pathologist to demonstrate. Small defects may be overlooked at autopsy examination unless the perimeter of the prosthesis is carefully probed. Because a valve specimen received in surgical pathology has necessarily been removed from its tissue attachments, a prosthesis excised for an isolated paravalvular leak may appear normal. However, because most surgeons cut suture knots to excise a valve from the associated annular tissue at reoperation, residual intact suture loops with knots on an explant suggest that a paravalvular leak was present.

Extrinsic Interference, Occluder Entrapment, and Tissue Overgrowth

Prosthetic valve stenosis or regurgitation can also be promoted by factors extrinsic to a prosthesis, as illustrated in Figures 21-31 and 21-32. Occluder entrapment in mechanical heart valves is a serious and potentially fatal complication that can be related to both internal and external factors.[207]

The potential mechanisms of interference are diverse. Restriction of motion of a mechanical poppet or tissue cusps can occur by the looping of a suture around a portion of the superstructure (see Fig. 21-31A).[208] Sutures may be looped around mechanical valve struts of certain designs and bioprosthetic valve struts, particularly with pericardial bioprostheses, thereby restricting cusp motion; suture ends either unraveled or cut too long could perforate a bioprosthetic valve cusp.[209] Excursion of a tilting disk valve occluder can be inhibited by retained valve remnants such as chordae tendineae or leaflets, unraveled or excessively long ends of sutures,[210, 211] a large mitral annular calcific nodule, or septal hypertrophy (see Fig. 21-31B). Entrapment is more frequently reported after mi-

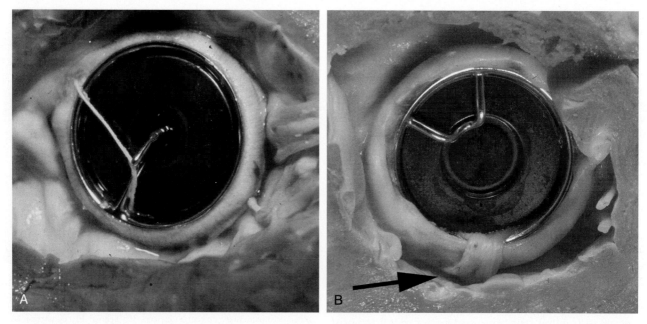

Figure 21-31 • Sutures and retained tissue affecting valve function. *A,* Early postoperative death due to suture looped around tilting disk valve strut, inhibiting free disk movement. *B,* Retained valvular tissue that spontaneously inserted between disk and housing (arrow), causing disk immobilization leading to sudden death 14 years postoperatively. (*A,* from Schoen FJ: Pathologic considerations in replacement heart valves and other cardiovascular prosthetic devices. In: Schoen FJ, Gimbrone MA [eds]: Cardiovascular Pathology: Clinicopathologic Correlations and Pathogenetic Mechanisms. Baltimore, Williams & Wilkins, 1995, p 194.)

tral than aortic valve replacement. Importantly, with mitral valves, the systolic valve closing pressure that may wedge foreign material can be as much as 10 times greater than the left atrial pressure. Thus, the latter may be insufficient to open the affected valve. The potential for valve malfunction exists whenever extraneous objects or anatomic structures migrate into the valve, but valve designs vary in their susceptibility to occluder entrapment and its consequences.[211] For example, suture, tissue, or other foreign material entrapment is less likely to occur in a bileaflet than a single-leaflet tilting disk valve, as a result of its design features. Moreover, a bileaflet valve with a single entrapped leaflet would be only partially stenotic, with the other leaflet being freely mobile.

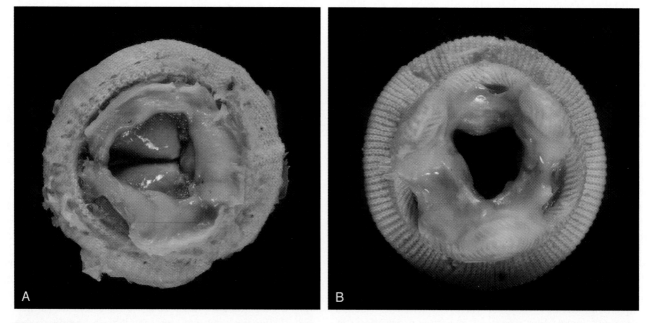

Figure 21-32 • Tissue overgrowth causing bioprosthetic valve dysfunction. *A,* Exuberant pannus overgrowth of the inflow side of a bioprosthesis extending over the cusps and reducing the effective orifice to approximately one third of its original size. This caused secondary thrombosis with massive thrombotic deposits in the prosthetic sinuses of Valsalva (not shown). *B,* Massive pannus overgrowth from outflow surface of porcine bioprosthesis, leading to retraction and immobilization of the cusps, with valvular regurgitation.

Exuberant overgrowth of fibrous tissue may obstruct the inflow orifice of any valve, prevent full mechanical valve occluder excursion, or cause stiffening or retraction with near obliteration of bioprosthetic valve cusps (*disappearing cusp syndrome*). Pannus extending from the tissue adjacent to the annulus can occur with any valve type at any site, and thrombosis may occur secondarily.

Intermittent sticking without an obvious anatomic cause following implantation of bileaflet tilting disk prostheses has been recognized.[212] Some such valves appear to function normally when removed. Specific details of valve orientation may contribute to the dysfunction, because reorientation of the valve at surgery resolves the problem in some cases.

Hemolysis

Hemolysis and occasionally hemolytic anemia were frequent complications of early mechanical valve prostheses.[213] Furthermore, certain models, exemplified by caged-ball valves with cloth-covered struts, had enhanced hemolysis by virtue of specific modes of degeneration superimposed on features of their intrinsic design. With contemporary substitute heart valves, the degree of red blood cell destruction is generally slight and well compensated by augmented hematopoietic function. However, when a high-velocity jet of blood is forced through a paravalvular leak or occurs in the presence of valvular dysfunction, severe hemolytic anemia can ensue. Pathologic markers for hemolysis include a blood smear with schistocytes or other evidence of erythrocyte fragmentation, renal tubular hemosiderosis, or pigment gallstones (Fig. 21-33).

OTHER TISSUE VALVE SUBSTITUTES

Stentless Porcine Aortic Valve Bioprostheses

Nonstented (stentless) porcine aortic valve bioprostheses are glutaraldehyde-pretreated pig aortic root and valve cusps without a supporting stent. Two such models were approved by the United States Food and Drug Administration (FDA) in 1997 for insertion into the aortic site: the St. Jude Medical Toronto SPV and the Medtronic Freestyle bioprosthesis (see Fig. 21-5).[214, 215] They differ slightly in overall configuration (particularly the amount of aortic wall included), details of glutaraldehyde pretreatment and overall fabrication, and whether anticalcification technology is used. Each has Dacron cloth covering at least the proximal edge of the prosthesis that contains the porcine right coronary cuspal muscle shelf (that area only in the Medtronic valve, and the entire aortic wall in the St. Jude). The Medtronic FreeStyle valve is treated with α-amino oleic acid, a compound shown to confer resistance to calcification in animal experiments (see later). Both have cusps fixed at zero-pressure differential. Both valves have performed well in limited clinical studies, showing low hemodynamic gradients and low rates of complications. Other variants of this concept are also in clinical trials.[216] It is expected that their use will increase and pathologists will begin to encounter them.

A stentless porcine aortic valve allows implantation of a larger bioprosthesis (than a stented one) in any given aortic root. As nearly as possible, such valves are designed to duplicate the nonobstructive configuration, mechanism of function and lack of sewing ring of a natural valve, while maintaining the full range of sizes and relative ease of implantation that typify fabricated bioprostheses. Such a bioprosthesis can be used as a valve, a root inclusion prosthesis (in which the graft is inserted as a cylinder inside the aorta), or as a total aortic root replacement (e.g., in cases of infective endocarditis or root dilation). Moreover, clinical and experimental evidence suggests that a biologic valve that is kept in its natural configuration and maintains the normal relationships of cusps, sinuses, and commissures not only performs better but also has a durability superior to that of a stent-mounted valve with its markedly altered geometry. Hemodynamic evidence suggests that the superior performance of stentless valves enhances ventricular remod-

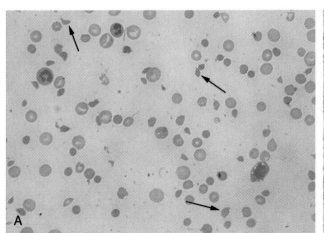
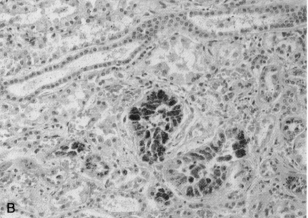

Figure 21-33 • Consequences of hemolysis. *A*, Blood smear of patient with paravalvular leak, showing abundant erythrocyte fragments (arrows) (Giemsa stain). *B*, Renal hemosiderosis, with pigment deposits in tubules (H&E stain.)

eling and recovery, and, thereby, patient survival.[21, 217] This makes the stentless porcine aortic valve a particularly attractive choice in elderly patients with aortic stenosis.[218]

Nevertheless, despite its superficial resemblance to the native aortic valve, a glutaraldehyde-fixed stentless porcine bioprosthesis differs considerably, in that the cusps and aortic wall are much less flexible, the collagen is altered by fixation, and the cells are not viable. The implantation of stentless valves also requires a longer period of intraoperative aortic cross-clamping, especially when the root replacement technique is used. Moreover, sizing and implantation technique overall are significantly more demanding than those associated with an equivalent stent-mounted valve.

The potential and observed complications with non-stented bioprostheses are comparable to those of stented valves, including thromboembolic complications, endocarditis, and structural dysfunction. However, root replacement has the potential for more xenograft tissue in contact with the recipient's tissue and possibly immunologic reactivity and adherence, leading to difficulty in reoperation as well as calcification of the aortic wall, and nonspecific inflammation. Although not yet observed clinically, calcification of the aortic wall may cause stiffening, ulceration, mural thrombosis or obstruction, and possible weakening and rupture. Moreover, host tissue overgrowth (pannus) beyond the suture lines, closer to the valve cusps than with stented valves, could be a more common problem. Nevertheless, the evaluation of results of explants in situ for an extended period suggests that such concerns have not been realized (Fig. 21-34).[219] Stentless porcine mitral valves are also being investigated.[220]

Valvular Allografts/Homografts

Used since 1962,[221, 222] aortic or pulmonary valves transplanted from one individual to another have exceptionally good hemodynamic profiles, a low incidence of thromboembolic complications without chronic anticoagulation, and a low infection rate.[223–226] Such valves are especially efficacious for replacing those excised because of endocarditis.[227] Nevertheless, the clinical outcome and reported pathologic features of allograft aortic valves vary greatly with the techniques used in valve preparation, particularly regarding sterilization and preservation procedures.[228] Recipients of allograft valves do not usually take immunosuppressive medications.

Allograft valves were initially collected by sterile technique and used fresh. However, logistic realities eventually required the antibiotic treatment or chemical or irradiation sterilization of valves obtained at autopsy. Valvular allografts sterilized or preserved with chemicals (using β-propiolactone or ethylene oxide), γ-irradiation, and freeze drying suffered failure rates of nearly 50% at 10 to 12 years and 50 to 90% at 15 to 20 years. Pathologic examination of retrieved valves revealed variable host fibrous tissue overgrowth and marked structural changes, including loss of architectural elements and cellularity, fibrosis, calcification, and often cusp ruptures.[229–233] Subsequent refinements in antibiotic sterilization and preservation techniques, including freezing, have produced a variety of improved fresh and the widely used cryopreserved allografts, with apparently enhanced longevity.

Human aortic valve allografts are usually derived from cadavers (in the past, they were occasionally obtained from diseased hearts removed at transplantation), cryopreserved without chemical cross-linking, stored, thawed for use, and then implanted directly into the aortic root without a stent as a valve or root inclusion prosthesis or as a full root replacement. In the most commonly applied cryopreservation method,[234] freezing is performed with protection from water crystallization by dimethyl sulfoxide, followed by storage at $-196°C$ in the vapor over liquid nitrogen. Cryopreservation permits a long shelf life and development of a banking system and the potential commercialization of processing. The quality of cryopreserved valvular tissue depends on details of freezing and thawing protocols, the interval from death to harvest, and additional warm and cold ischemic intervals.

Contemporary cryopreserved allograft valves are free of degeneration for periods equal to, or slightly better than, those of conventional porcine bioprosthetic valves (approximately 50 to 90% valve survival at 10 to 15

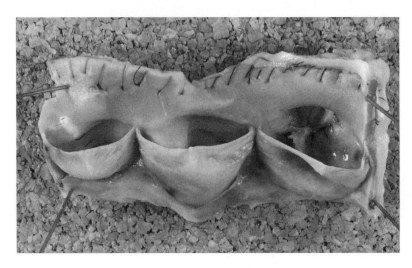

Figure 21-34 • Nonstented tissue valve implanted 48 months, demonstrating absence of calcification, tearing, or excessive pannus overgrowth. (From Fyfe B, Schoen FJ: Pathological analysis of nonstented Freestyle aortic root bioprostheses treated with amino oleic acid. Semin Thorac Cardiovasc Surg 11 [suppl]: 151, 1999.)

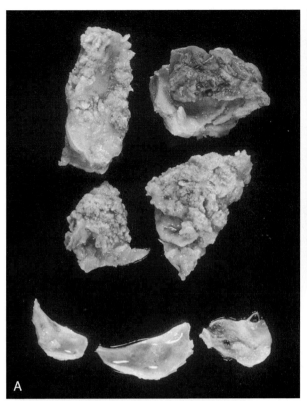

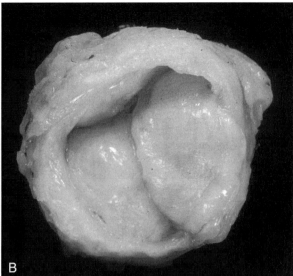

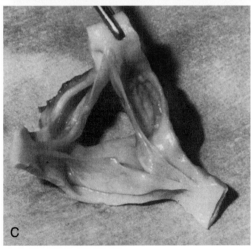

Figure 21-35 • Cryopreserved allograft heart valves: long-term explants and unimplanted valve. *A,* Pulmonary valve allograft and pulmonary artery conduit removed after 9 years for root stenosis in a child with repaired congenital heart disease. Despite diffuse nodular mineralization of the pulmonary artery conduit wall, the cusps (at bottom of photograph) were soft, pliable, and not calcified. *B,* Aortic valve allograft removed after 3 years for valvular insufficiency resulting from cusp prolapse. No calcification was noted. *C,* Unimplanted allograft aortic valve. (*A* and *B,* from Mitchell RN, Jonas RA, Schoen FJ: Pathology of explanted cryopreserved allograft heart valves: Comparison with aortic valves from orthotopic heart transplants. J Thorac Cardiovasc Surg 115:118, 1998.)

years for allografts). Nevertheless, progressive degeneration limits their long-term success (Fig. 21-35). The mode of failure of these valves when inserted on the left side of the heart is generally incompetence caused by cusp rupture, distortion with retraction, or perforations.[235] In contrast, right-sided valves in children who have right ventricle–to–pulmonary artery conduits usually stenose as a result of somatic growth of the recipient, with or without calcification of the cusps or distal aortic wall,[235] a mode of failure simulated experimentally in rapidly growing animals.[236] Stent-mounted aortic allografts can be used for mitral valve replacement, but failure by detachment of the allograft tissue from the supporting stent post limits their durability.[237]

The most critical and controversial issues in the pathology of valvular allografts relate to mechanisms of deterioration, cellular viability, extracellular matrix integrity, and the role of immune responses in causing dysfunction. The following description is based largely on our study of 33 cryopreserved human allograft heart valves explanted up to 9 years postoperatively, 14 nonimplanted cryopreserved allograft valves, and 16 aortic valves removed from transplanted allograft hearts in situ up to 4 years.[235] The results are summarized in Table 21-14.

Implanted cryopreserved allograft valves show a loss of normal structural complexity and cellularity of the cusps, including endothelium and deep connective tissue cells, and progressive collagen hyalinization (Fig. 21-36). The aortic or pulmonary artery wall associated with

TABLE 21-14 • **Morphology of Allograft Cardiac Values**

| | | Cryopreserved | | | Cardiac Transplant |
	Unimplanted	Implanted 0–8 Days	Implanted 2–11 Months	Implanted 1–9 Years	In Situ 0 Days–4 Years
Number of specimens	14	15	6	12	16
Trilaminar architecture	++	++	−	−	+++
Stainable connective tissue cells	++	+/++	−	− to +*	+++
Lymphocytic infiltrate (T cells)	− to +	−/+	− to +++†	− to +	+/++
Intact endothelium	−/+	−/+	−	−	+/++
Intimal hyperplasia/pannus	−	−	−	+/−	−
Cuspal hematoma/thrombus	−	−/+	+/++	− to ++	−
Calcification					
Cusps	−	−	−	− to +	−
Walls	−	−	−	− to +++	−/+

Cellularity and other morphologic measures of the explanted valves are semiquantified as −, not present; +, mild or minimal; ++, moderate; +++, severe or marked.

* Predominantly associated with pannus.

† Substantial only in those valves with endocarditis.

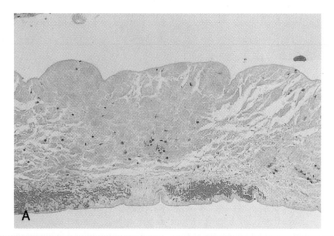

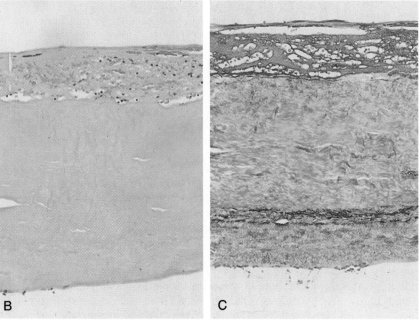

Figure 21-36 • Histology of allograft valve explants. *A,* Cross section of cusp from right-sided allograft explanted after 15 days. There is loss of endothelial cells and near complete loss of interstitial cells without inflammation. *B* and *C,* Cusp from allograft valve explanted after 7 years, showing flattening and loss of normal layered architecture. *B* highlights loss of endothelial and deep interstitial cells and absence of inflammation. *C* shows staining for connective tissue elements. (*A & B,* H&E stain, *C,* Elastin black stain.)

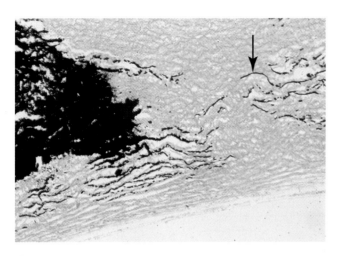

Figure 21-37 • Photomicrograph demonstrating nodular calcification in aortic wall portion of valvular allograft, largely involving elastic tissue (arrow) (von Kossa stain).

the valve becomes progressively and markedly scarred. Allografts have generally minimal or absent inflammatory cells at all postoperative intervals. Valves implanted for longer than 1 year have flattened and thinned cusps, with obliteration of the usual corrugations, indistinct layers, and no stainable interstitial or endothelial cells. Pannus overgrowth is generally mild and not clinically important. Lymphocytes and other inflammatory cells are occasionally present but sparse. Cusp calcification is usually absent or only focal, despite extensive wall calcification in some explants, especially in right ventricular–pulmonary artery conduits from children (Fig. 21-37). Transmission electron microscopy of long-term cryopreserved allograft valves reveals no viable cells, focal calcification centered around dead cell remnants, and distorted but preserved collagen. Thus, cryopreserved allografts are morphologically nonviable; their collagen is flattened but largely preserved. They are unlikely to grow, remodel, or exhibit active metabolic function, and their usual degeneration cannot be attributed to immunologic responses. Cryopreserved allograft valve durability must depend predominantly on the quality of the collagenous skeleton. Indeed, degeneration of the extracellular matrix likely accounts for the modest rate of progressive dysfunction (manifested predominantly as regurgitation) in the aortic site in adults. In contrast, aortic valves from transplanted hearts have remarkable structural preservation, including endothelium and abundant deep connective tissue cells; inflammatory infiltrates are generally mild and of no apparent deleterious consequence, including valves from patients who died of acute myocardial parenchymal rejection or graft coronary arteriosclerosis.

The lack of viable cells in cryopreserved human allograft valves, noted early after implantation, is most likely attributable to damage related to ischemia associated with harvest and that caused by cryopreservation and surgery. Nevertheless, some workers report long-term survival of certain cellular elements in both experimental systems and explanted allografts from human

recipients.[223, 238, 239] That fibroblasts cultured from one cryopreserved allograft after 9 years of implantation were found by chromosomal analysis to be donor derived is not surprising, because it is certainly possible that in some optimally preserved valves (i.e., minimal ischemic time and minimal death due to cryopreservation), a rare donor fibroblast may survive. However, an occasional viable cell cannot repopulate the entire valve or materially contribute to matrix remodeling.

Progressive loss of cusp cellular viability as well as cumulative changes in the cusp extracellular matrix occurred in the absence of significant mononuclear inflammatory cell infiltrates, although no patients were immunosuppressed and the valves were implanted without regard to HLA or blood group status. Because nonautologous endothelial cells, smooth muscle cells, and fibroblasts are all variably capable of eliciting an immune response,[240] preservation of these elements could theoretically have deleterious consequences by mediating immunologic reactivity. Other studies suggest that these processes elicit organ failure in children.[241]

Pulmonary Autograft Replacement of the Aortic Valve (Ross Procedure)

Since the original description by Ross in 1968, replacement of the aortic valve or root using the patient's own pulmonary valve (*pulmonary autograft*) has become widely accepted.[242, 243] The objective is to provide a hemodynamically superior and potentially "viable" valve that might grow with somatic growth of children in patients for whom there is no satisfactory alternative. The removed pulmonary valve is usually replaced by an allograft pulmonic valve.

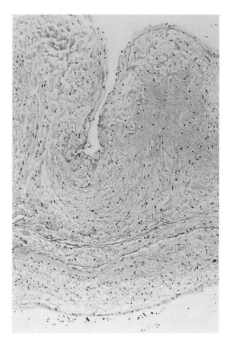

Figure 21-38 • Photomicrograph of largely intact cusp from an aortic valve autograft (Ross procedure) after 5 years (Movat stain).

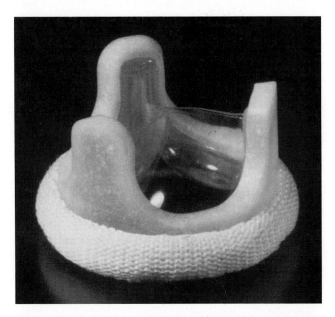

Figure 21-39 • Flexible trileaflet synthetic heart valve composed of thin polyurethane leaflets. (From Schoen FJ: Interventional and Surgical Cardiovascular Pathology: Clinical Correlations and Basic Principles. Philadelphia, WB Saunders, 1989.)

Although it is technically demanding, a pulmonary allograft valve transplant can be done with an operative risk not substantially greater than that for valve replacement using current prostheses (approximately 3%). The prevalence of perioperative complications ranges from 5 to 15%, with hemorrhage and difficulties of the requisite coronary arterial transfer being most prominent (e.g., damage to small blood vessels and leaks at the anastomoses of the buttons or kinking of the proximal coronary trunk). In some cases, progressive dilation of the aortic root occurs postoperatively.

Consistent with favorable clinical results yielding few late specimens, descriptive pathologic findings on pulmonary valve autografts to the aortic root have not been reported in detail. We have encountered several cases that span the perioperative period to long term. Following the procedure, the valve cusps of the autograft appear to retain the normal staining qualities of both cells and extracellular matrix. In valves examined up to 6 years postoperatively, the cuspal structure appeared essentially normal, with retention of corrugations, interstitial cellular staining, and collagen morphology, as well as endothelial cells lining the surface (Fig. 21-38). In contrast, the aortic wall seems to suffer ischemic necrosis after the procedure (probably due to the requisite transection of the vasa vasorum of the pulmonary artery during the procedure), leading to early inflammation and late scarring. For example, the aortic (previously pulmonary) wall of a valve implanted for 6 years had near-complete disruption of its structure by fibrosis, with only fragmented remnants of the elastic network of the original arterial media. The early injury to, and repair and remodeling of, the pulmonary arterial wall tissue most likely accounts for progressive luminal dilation following implantation into the systemic circulation.

NEW DEVELOPMENTS AND FUTURE CONSIDERATIONS

Pathologists may be called on to assist in studies of new and occasionally novel materials and design modifications and may encounter new valve types in clinical use. Therefore, some description of new technology is included here.

Novel rigid mechanical designs with two or three leaflets are currently in development,[244] and the concept of central flow trileaflet prostheses using three flexible synthetic polymeric leaflets in an anatomy that resembles the natural aortic valve is now being facilitated by major developments in the technology of polymeric materials, including polyurethanes (Fig. 21-39). Although such a valve has been used clinically in a cardiac assist device,[245] durability limitations remain the major concern with a flexible polymeric valve replacement; preclinical valve failures have been marked by tearing or calcification of the cusps.[246, 247] Most developmental activity is related to improving tissue valves.[13, 248, 249]

Major efforts are directed toward developing approaches to prevent calcification and tissue treatment technology to enhance durability of tissue valves.[13, 250, 251] The principal anticalcification approaches under investigation are summarized in Table 21-15. Strategies presently being investigated or used clinically include treatment with a detergent such as sodium dodecyl sulfate (SDS), two-amino oleic acid (used in the Medtronic Freestyle nonstented porcine valve discussed earlier),[252] aluminum salts,[253] ethanol,[254] a proprietary substance called No-React, epoxide compounds, extraction of nonviable cellular debris to yield a cell-free matrix,[255, 256] and a tissue preservation methodology that uses dye-mediated photo-oxidation instead of glutaraldehyde pretreatment.[257, 258] Toluidine blue has also been employed as an antimineralization agent in valves used in clinical trials; this approach is unique, in that the valve tissue takes on a blue color that slowly leaches after implantation. Explants of such valves may appear a discolored gray. Chemical neutralization of free aldehyde groups by amination after glutaraldehyde fixation has been reported to improve tissue biocompatibility and stimulate early valve re-endothelialization.[259] Although early porcine valves used a back-pressure of 80 mm during glutaraldehyde pretreatment,

TABLE 21-15 • **Current Approaches to Preventing Calcification of Tissue Heart Valves and the Mechanisms of Action of Agents Used**

Ethane hydroxybisphosphonate—inhibition of hydroxyapatite formation
Alpha-amino-oleic acid—inhibition of calcium uptake
Ferric/aluminum chloride exposure—inhibition of calcium phosphate crystal growth
Sodium dodecyl sulfate—phospholipid extraction
Ethanol exposure—phospholipid extraction and collagen conformation modification
Modification of (alternatives to) glutaraldehyde fixation—elimination of glutaraldehyde potentiation of calcification; amino acid neutralization of glutaraldehyde resides; polyepoxide (polyglycidal ether), acyl azide, carbodiimide, cyanimide, and glycerol cross-linking; dye-mediated photo-oxidation preservation

some newer valves use a zero-pressure gradient across the valve (termed *stress-free fixation*[260]), or even fixation while the valve is flexing (termed *dynamic fixation*), in an effort to eliminate preimplantation stretching and flattening of the cusp connective tissue.

Another approach uses autologous pericardium, excised and fixed in glutaraldehyde 5 to 15 minutes at the time of surgery. It is then cut by means of a specially designed die and subsequently mounted on a stent.[261] Short-term fixation stiffens the tissue and renders handling easier, but the effects on calcification and other biologic and physical properties are unknown. Nonstented aortic and mitral prostheses fabricated free-hand from similar lightly fixed autologous pericardium are also under investigation.

Exciting in concept but still early in practice is the approach to producing a nonobstructive, nonthrombogenic tissue valve substitute that will last the lifetime of the patient, provide ongoing remodeling and repair of cumulative injury, and potentially grow in maturing recipients (called *tissue engineering*). In this paradigm, an anatomically appropriate construct containing cells seeded on to a resorbable scaffold is fabricated in vitro in a bioreactor and then implanted.[13, 262, 263] Specific biologic signals may also be incorporated. Remodeling of the construct in vivo is intended to recapitulate normal functional architecture. Initial attempts to fabricate prototypes are encouraging.[264, 265]

A silver-coated polyethylene terephthalate polyester sewing ring fabric intended to inhibit prosthetic valve endocarditis associated with mechanical heart valves is under investigation, but an excessive incidence of paravalvular leaks have been reported.[265, 266] Other new concepts and configurations include those that will facilitate minimally invasive valve surgery[267] and, potentially, transluminal catheter implantation.[268]

PATHOLOGIC CONSIDERATIONS IN THE ANALYSIS OF HEART VALVE SUBSTITUTES

General Considerations

The goals of the surgical pathology or autopsy examination of artificial valves are generally restricted to documenting the specific valve type that either was removed at reoperation or that the patient had at death, and diagnosis of a clinical abnormality that requires therapeutic intervention. Detailed correlation of morphologic features with clinical signs, symptoms, and dysfunctional physiology is usually performed only by investigators specifically interested in this area. Nevertheless, pathologic examination of retrieved substitute heart valves can provide valuable information. Informed evaluation of failed (and nonfailed) substitute heart valves can contribute to the care of valve replacement patients; establish the rates, modes, morphology and mechanisms of prosthesis-associated complications; elucidate the structural basis of favorable valve performance; and predict the effects of developmental modifications on safety and efficacy.[25, 269]

For example, in an individual patient, determining a cause for valve failure can contribute to subsequent management. The diagnosis of infective endocarditis

---

TABLE 21-16 • **Surgical Pathology of Prosthetic Valves: Essential Processing Steps and Representative Diagnoses**

Processing Steps

1. Photograph from both proximal and distal aspects, at close range.
2. Radiograph all tissue valves.
3. Measure the external diameter of the sewing ring. Identify type of prosthesis by using structural or radiographic features.
4. Describe sewing ring tissue coverage; is it excessive, impairing either poppet or cuspal motion?
5. Describe thrombi or vegetations, including color, site (surface of valve, sewing ring), size, consistency (firm vs. friable), and any underlying material destruction.
6. For mechanical valves, describe any asymmetry, notches, or cracks in any of the components. Describe any impairment in poppet motion.
7. For tissue valves, describe size and condition of any tears or perforations of the cusps and/or any impairment of cusp motion. Describe any calcific deposits and their location; grade on a scale from 0 to 4, using the specimen radiograph.
8. Submit for histologic examination tissue adjacent to any valve prosthesis (or tissue loose in the specimen vial).
9. Submit a portion of bioprosthetic valve cusps for histologic examination, if clinical data suggest infection or if there is thrombus/vegetation, cusp destruction without calcification, or other questionably nondegenerative pathology.

Sample Diagnoses

Bioprosthetic mitral valve
    Hancock porcine mitral valve bioprosthesis (31 mm) with commissural calcification (2+/4+ by radiograph) and single cuspal tear near commissure, 4 mm long, involving cuspal free edge.
    Microscopic severe degeneration and mineralization, with focal mural thrombus.
    No evidence of endocarditis.

Mechanical mitral valve
    Bjork-Shiley tilting disk prosthesis (29 mm).
    Intact, without strut defects.
    Focal thrombus, at minor strut-housing junction (1 mm diameter), microscopically bland.

Mechanical aortic heart valve
    St. Jude bileaflet tilting disk prosthesis (21 mm); gross only.
    Intact, without thrombi, vegetations, or tissue overgrowth (consistent with paravalvular leak by clinical diagnosis).

From FJ Schoen: Approach to the analysis of cardiac valve prostheses as surgical pathology or autopsy specimens. Cardiovasc Pathol 4:241, 1995, with permission from Elsevier Science.

facilitates appropriate antibiotic therapy postoperatively. Intraoperative pathologic consultation that demonstrates accelerated degenerative calcification of a porcine bioprosthesis may stimulate replacement with a mechanical rather than a tissue valve for that patient. Demonstration of thrombosis on a removed valve prosthesis, despite adequate anticoagulation therapy, can be the initial indication of an identifiable and perhaps genetic predisposition to hypercoagulability (e.g., factor V Leiden, antithrombin III deficiency, or antiphospholipid antibody syndrome).

An appropriate surgical pathology or autopsy analysis requires knowledge of the established and potential failure modes of individual devices in particular situations, as well as pertinent clinical data on the patient. Moreover, although many of the different generic types and models of prosthetic heart valves used clinically in the past four decades have been discontinued because of design- or materials-related complications, pathologists may encounter some of these "obsolete" prosthesis types that are no longer implanted. Therefore, some access to historic treatments of prosthesis pathology may be helpful.[18, 19, 59, 270–272]

Pathologists also have an important regulatory role in recognizing clinical prosthesis-associated complications in their practices. This responsibility is a key element of the United States Federal Safe Medical Devices Act of 1990, the first major amendment to the Federal Food, Drug, and Cosmetic Act since the Medical Device Amendments of 1976.[273, 274] Under the "user reporting" requirements of this legislation, health care personnel and hospitals must report all device-related deaths, serious illnesses, and injuries to the FDA, the manufacturer, or both. Thus, a pathologist who initially discovers harm or death due to a malfunctioning cardiovascular device is required to initiate the reporting process (through his or her institution).

Explanted specimens requiring pathologic analysis include failed valves; nonfailed prostheses removed during operation on another valve, during coronary artery bypass grafting, or at cardiac transplantation prompted by ventricular failure despite a functional prosthesis; and prostheses obtained at autopsy. Generalized approaches to dissection of heart valve prostheses and documentation of their most important pathologic findings have been described in the literature.[25, 275] The anticipated pathology and the detailed protocol for analysis depend in large part on the type of prosthesis under consideration.

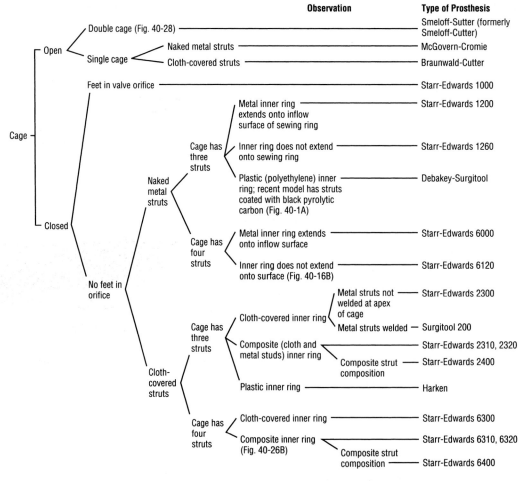

Figure 21-40 • Key to identify ball valve prostheses. (From Silver MD, Wilson GJ: Pathology of cardiovascular prostheses including coronary artery bypass and other vascular grafts. In: Silver MD [ed]: Cardiovascular Pathology. New York, Churchill Livingstone, 1983.)

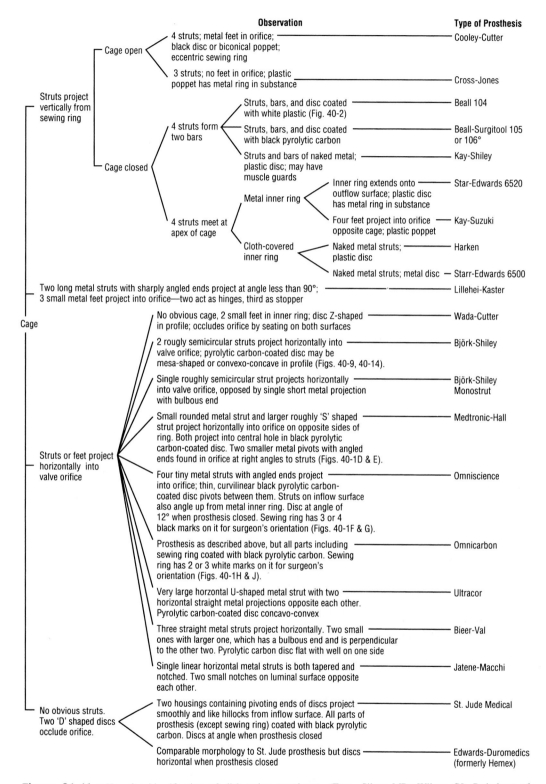

Figure 21-41 • Key for identification of disk valve prostheses. (From Silver MD, Wilson GJ: Pathology of cardiovascular prostheses including coronary artery bypass and other vascular grafts. In: Silver MD [ed]: Cardiovascular Pathology. New York, Churchill Livingstone, 1983.)

TABLE 21-17 • **Distinguishing Structural Features Among Various Contemporary Bileaflet Mechanical Valves**

Valve Type	Carbon Coating on Sewing Ring	Leaflet Shape	Housing Contours	Pivot Guard Protrusions	Radiopacity
CarboMedics CPHV	Yes	Flat	No	No obvious pivot guards	Leaflets radiopaque on edge; metal housing ring
Edwards-Duromedics (Tekna)	Some	Curved	No	Slight, outflow	Leaflets somewhat radiopaque; metal housing ring
Jyros	No	Curved	No	No pivot guards; leaflets can rotate	Metal housing ring
Medtronic Parallel	No	Flat	Inflow and outflow	Flat pivot guards	Leaflets radiopaque on edge; three metal housing rings
Sorin Bicarbon	Yes	Curved	No	No pivot guards	Metal housing ring
St. Jude Medical	No	Flat	Inflow	Large, inflow	Leaflets radiopaque on edge; no metal housing ring

From Schoen FJ: Approach to the analysis of cardiac valve prostheses as surgical pathology or autopsy specimens. Cardiovasc Pathol 4:241, 1995, with permission from Elsevier Science.

Prosthesis Evaluation

An overall summary of the pathologic analysis of valve substitutes obtained at either autopsy or following surgical removal, including sample diagnoses, is presented in Table 21-16. The specific type and model of a prosthesis are identified using radiographic and morphologic keys, as necessary (Figs. 21-40 and 21-41; Table 21-17).[59, 276] Models of tissue prostheses may be difficult to distinguish visually once they have been in situ for some time; radiography can be helpful (Fig. 21-42). A serial number placed by the manufacturer that uniquely identifies each valve is usually hidden under the sewing ring at the valve base. Photography should be done at close range from all pertinent aspects. Autopsy specimens are carefully probed for paravalvular leaks. The valve should be examined for thrombi, vegetations, exuberant tissue overgrowth, and structural defects. Mechanical heart valve prostheses are also checked for adequacy of poppet excursion and seating, defects and fractures of components,

asymmetries, sites of abrasive wear, and poppet swelling or distortion. Bioprostheses are gently palpated to assess cuspal excursion and are visually inspected for the presence of fenestrations, tears, cuspal hematomas, calcific nodules, commissural dehiscence, and central migration of struts. Morphologic analysis of bioprostheses should include radiography (we use the Faxitron, Hewlett Packard, McMinnville, OR, 0.8, 1 min × 35 KV), to aid both the identification of the prosthesis type and assessment of calcium deposits. Calcification is semiquantitatively graded,[164] and the locations of calcific deposits are noted (with respect to cusp bodies, commissures, basal attachment sites, and at the free cuspal edges) (Fig. 21-43).

Some investigators advocate describing cusp defects in bioprosthetic valves according to a schema developed primarily from observations of failed porcine valves but applicable to pericardial or other tissue valves (Fig. 21-44).[277] In this classification, type I tears involve the free edge of a cusp; type II lesions are linear perforations that extend along the cusp base, forming an arc parallel to the annular margin; type III lesions are large, round, or oval defects that occupy the central body of the cusp, often in association with severe cusp destruction owing to infection; and type IV lesions are small pinholes, often multiple, that appear in the central regions of the cusps.

Any thrombus attached to a heart valve prosthesis at autopsy or any thromboembolus removed surgically from a patient with a heart valve prosthesis should be regarded as infected until it is proved bland. Both microbiologic and histologic studies must be done. In the former, positive results are more likely if part of a vegetation is forwarded for culture rather than a swab of its surface. Gram and Gomori methenamine silver nitrate (GMS) stains are required histologically. After antibiotic treatment, some bacterial organisms may not stain or may stain in an aberrant fashion with Gram stain but may be obvious in the GMS stain.

Dissection of a bioprosthesis may be facilitated by removing the tissue from the stent and pinning it on a sheet of cork (Fig. 21-45). Specimens of cusp and adherent tissue are removed, specifically labeled, oriented in cross section, and embedded (some preferably in a hard medium such as glycol methacrylate) for histologic analy-

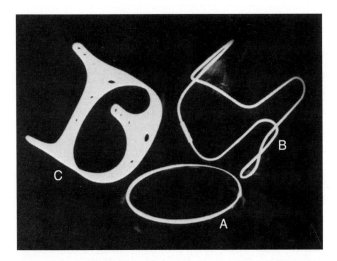

Figure 21-42 • Radiographs of Hancock (*A*), Carpentier-Edwards (*B*), and Ionescu-Shiley (*C*) xenograft tissue valve prostheses, showing distinctive characteristics. (From Schoen FJ: Interventional and Surgical Cardiovascular Pathology: Clinical Correlations and Basic Principles. Philadelphia, WB Saunders, 1989.)

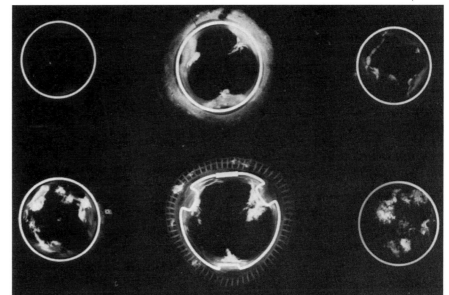

Figure 21-43 • Composite radiograph of calcified porcine aortic valve bioprostheses, demonstrating the various levels of mineralization and providing radiographic standards for examination. Uncalcified (0), 1+ and 2+ (top), 3+ and 4+ (bottom). (From Schoen FJ, Kujovich JL, Webb CL, Levy RJ: Chemically determined mineral content of explanted porcine aortic valve bioprostheses: Correlation with radiographic assessment of calcification and clinical data. Circulation 76: 101, 1987.)

TABLE 21-18 • **Pathologic Features to Be Reviewed in Examining Substitute Heart Valves**

Gross Examination	Radiography
Anatomic orientation of valve (at autopsy)	Valve type identification
Tissue overgrowth	Calcification: degree, morphology, location
Thrombus	Ring, stent, poppet fracture
Vegetations	**Histology**
Paravalvular leak	Cusp configuration/flattening
Cusp stiffness	Inflammation
Cusp hematomas	Thrombus
Calcification	Vegetations/organisms
Cusp fenestrations/tears	Host cell interactions
Cusp abrasion	Degenerative features
Cusp stretching	Abrasion
Strut relationships	Calcification
Mechanical dysfunction	Pannus overgrowth
Extrinsic interference or damage	Endothelialization
Commissural region dehiscence of tissue from stent	Cusp hematoma
	Adventitious material*

* Such as substances arising from an anticalcification treatment.

Modified from Schoen FJ, Levy RJ, Piehler HR: Pathological consideration in replacement cardiac valves. Cardiovasc Pathol 1:29, 1992, with permission from Elsevier Science.

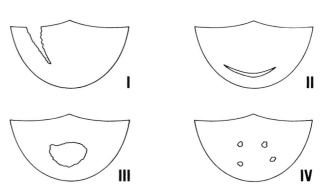

Figure 21-44 • Types of cusp tears and perforations that occur in cardiac valve bioprostheses. From Ishihara T, Ferrans VJ, Boyce SW, et al: Structure and classification of cuspal tears and perforations in porcine bioprosthetic cardiac valves implanted in patients. Am J Cardiol 48:665, 1981, with permission from Excerpta Medica Inc.)

TABLE 21-19 • **Studies Demonstrating the Value of and Approaches in Clinical Analysis of Retrieved Heart Valve Substitutes**

Prosthesis Type	Valve Problem	References
Braunwald-Cutter cloth-covered caged-ball valve	Cloth wear/ball escape	144, 145
Porcine aortic valve bioprostheses	Calcification	13, 111, 164, 181, 184
Bjork-Shiley 60/70 convexoconcave valve	Strut fracture	9, 152
Hemex-Duromedics bileaflet tilting disk valve	Disk, housing fracture	153
Medtronic Parallel bileaflet tilting disk valve	Thrombosis	119
Carbomedics PhotoFix-alpha bovine pericardial valve	Abrasion-related tears	258

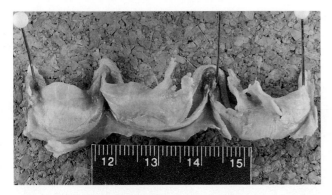

Figure 21-45 • Explanted porcine aortic valve bioprosthesis, pinned onto a sheet of cork. To open this valve, the commissure between the right and noncoronary cusps was incised. Cusp defects (in the right and left cusps) are clearly seen. This method of opening a valve facilitates the selection and excision of histologic sections.

sis. Embedding in glycol methacrylate is advantageous, because it allows sectioning of undecalcified bioprosthetic valve specimens or tissue-cloth composite specimens with good morphologic preservation. Paraffin-embedded sections, in contrast, permit staining for connective tissue elements using Masson trichrome, elastic-collagen or Movat pentachrome stains, von Kossa stains for calcium phosphate, and Gram stains for organisms. Histologic analysis is directed toward determining the morphology of tissue-prosthesis interactions, cuspal degeneration, and the degree and specific morphology of calcific deposits. The key morphologic findings sought in examination of a prosthesis are summarized in Table 21-18. Specialized approaches and analyses are used to answer specific questions regarding mechanisms of failure or other patient-prosthesis interactions.

When paravalvular leak is either present or reported by the surgeon, tissues submitted with the valve that were adjacent or adherent to the sewing ring should be examined histologically to assess the extent of healing and whether endocarditis was contributory. Indeed, it is good practice to sample adherent tissue, irrespective of accompanying data.

Table 21-19 exemplifies several situations in which studies of cohorts of clinically retrieved prosthetic valve specimens have had important impact. Table 21-20 lists

TABLE 21-20 • **Considerations in the Determination of Causal Factors in the Failure of a Heart Valve Prosthesis**

Related to the individual implant
Raw materials
Fabrication and assembly
Sterilization
Packaging, shipping, and storage
Patient-prosthesis interactions
Patient factors

Related to cohorts of patients with this type of prosthesis
Material properties
Design features
In vitro testing of prototypes
Preclinical animal testing
Clinical trials

important considerations in the analysis of cause of failure of a particular valve.

Acknowledgments

In the course of consultations on developmental or clinical research over approximately the past 5 years, the authors have received or may receive something of value from the following organizations that may be impacted by the work reviewed in this manuscript: Advanced Tissue Sciences; Allograft Heart Valve Tissue Bank Consortium; Autogenics, Inc.; Baxter, Inc.; BioMedical Design, Inc.; Bravo Cardiovascular, Inc.; CryoLife Cardiovascular, Inc.; Ethicon, Inc.; Medtronic, Inc.; Mitroflow Medical, Inc.; St. Jude Medical, Inc.; Sulzer Carbomedics, Inc.; and Tissue Engineering, Inc.

REFERENCES

1. Braunwald NS, Cooper T, Morrow AG: Complete replacement of the mitral valve: Successful clinical application of a flexible polyurethane prosthesis. J Thorac Cardiovasc Surg 40:1, 1960
2. Harken DE, Soroff HS, Taylor WJ, et al: Partial and complete prostheses in aortic insufficiency. J Thorac Cardiovasc Surg 40:744, 1960
3. Starr A, Edwards ML: Mitral replacement: Clinical experience with a ball valve prosthesis. Ann Surg 154:726, 1961
4. Rahimtoola SH: Perspective on valvular heart disease: An update. J Am Coll Cardiol 14:1, 1990
5. Emery RW, Arom KV, Nicoloff DM: Utilization of the St. Jude Medical prosthesis in the aortic position. Semin Thorac Cardiovasc Surg 8:231, 1996
6. Fann JI, Miller C, Moore KA, et al: Twenty-year clinical experience with porcine bioprostheses. Ann Thorac Surg 62:1301, 1996
7. Orszulak TA, Schaff HV, Puga FJ, et al: Event status of the Starr-Edwards aortic valve to 20 years: A benchmark for comparison. Ann Thorac Surg 63:620, 1997
8. Grunkemeier GL, Rahimtoola SH: Artificial heart valves. Annu Rev Med 41:251, 1990
9. Schoen FJ, Levy RJ, Piehler HR: Pathological considerations in replacement cardiac valves. Cardiovasc Pathol 1:29, 1992
10. Turina J, Hess OM, Turina M, Krayenbuehl HP: Cardiac bioprostheses in the 1990s. Circulation 88:775, 1993
11. Hammermeister K, Sethi GK, Henderson WG, et al: Outcomes 15 years after valve replacement with a mechanical versus a bioprosthetic valve: Final report of the Veterans Affairs Randomized Trial. J Am Coll Cardiol 36:1152, 2000
12. Vongpatanasin W, Hillis D, Lange RA: Prosthetic heart valves. N Engl J Med 335:407, 1996
13. Schoen FJ, Levy RJ: Tissue heart valves: Current challenges and future research perspectives. J Biomed Mater Res 47:439, 1999
14. Reul RM, Cohn LH: Mitral valve reconstruction for mitral insufficiency. Prog Cardiovasc Dis 39:567, 1997
15. Hammond GL, Franco KL: Mitral, tricuspid, and aortic valve repair or reconstruction. Curr Opin Cardiol 12:100, 1997
16. Carabello BA, Crawford FA Jr: Valvular heart disease. N Engl J Med 337:32, 1997
17. Schoen FJ, St. John Sutton M: Contemporary issues in the pathology of valvular heart disease. Hum Pathol 18:568, 1987
18. Roberts WC: Complications of cardiac valve replacement: Characteristic abnormalities of prostheses pertaining to any or specific site. Am Heart J 103:113, 1982
19. Schoen FJ: Interventional and Surgical Cardiovascular Pathology: Clinical Correlations and Basic Principles. Philadelphia, WB Saunders, 1989
20. Jin XY, Zhang Z-M, Gibson DG, et al: Effects on valve substitute on changes in left ventricular function and hypertrophy after aortic valve replacement. Ann Thorac Surg 62:683, 1996
21. Thompson HL, O'Brien MF, Almeida AA, et al: Hemodynamics

and left ventricular mass regression: A comparison of the stentless, stented and mechanical aortic valve replacement. Eur J Cardiothorac Surg 13:572, 1998

22. Harken DF, Taylor WJ, LeFemine AA, et al: Aortic valve replacement with a caged ball valve. Am J Cardiol 9:292, 1962
23. Roberts WC: Choosing a substitute cardiac valve: Type, size, surgeon. Am J Cardiol 38:633, 1976
24. Jamieson WR: Modern cardiac valve devices—bioprostheses and mechanical prostheses: State of the art. J Card Surg 8:89, 1993
25. Schoen FJ: Approach to the analysis of cardiac valve prostheses as surgical pathology or autopsy specimens. Cardiovasc Pathol 4:241, 1995
26. Berger K, Sauvage LR, Wood SJ, Wesolowski SA: Sewing ring healing of cardiac valve prostheses. Surgery 61:102, 1967
27. Silver MD, Wilson GJ: Pathology of mechanical heart valve prostheses and vascular grafts made of artificial material. In: Silver MD (ed): Cardiovascular Pathology. 2nd ed. New York, Churchill Livingstone, 1991, p 1487
28. Gödje OL, Fischlein T, Adelhard K, et al: Thirty-year results of Starr-Edwards prostheses in the aortic and mitral position. Ann Thorac Surg 63:613, 1997
29. Bjork VO, Henze A: Ten years' experience with the Bjork-Shiley tilting disk valve. J Thorac Cardiovasc Surg 78:331, 1979
30. Keenan RJ, Armitage JM, Trento A, et al: Clinical experience with the Medtronic-Hall valve prosthesis. Ann Thorac Surg 50:748, 1990
31. Debetaz LF, Ruchat P, Hurni M, et al: St. Jude Medical valve prosthesis: An analysis of long-term outcome and prognostic factors. J Thorac Cardiovasc Surg 113:134, 1997
32. Baudet EM, Puel V, McBride JT, et al: Long-term results of valve replacement with the St. Jude Medical prosthesis. J Thorac Cardiovasc Surg 109:858, 1995
33. Roedler SM, Moritz A, Schreiner W, et al: Five year follow-up after heart valve replacement with the CarboMedics bileaflet prosthesis. Ann Thorac Surg 63:1018, 1997
34. Roberts WC, Hammer WJ: Cardiac pathology after valve replacement with a tilting disc prosthesis (Bjork-Shiley type): A study of 46 necropsy patients and 49 Bjork-Shiley prostheses. Am J Cardiol 37:1024, 1976
35. Bjork VO, Lindblom D: The monostrut Bjork-Shiley heart valve. J Am Coll Cardiol 6:1142, 1985
36. Silver MD, Wilson GJ: The pathology of wear in the Beall Model 104 heart valve prosthesis. Circulation 56:617, 1977
37. Roberts WC, Fishbein MC, Golden A: Cardiac pathology after valve replacement by disc prosthesis: A study of 61 necropsy patients. Am J Cardiol 35:740, 1975
38. Haubold AD: On the durability of pyrolytic carbon in vivo. Med Prog Technol 20:201, 1994
39. Ely JL, Emken MR, Accuntius JA, et al: Pure pyrolytic carbon: Preparation and properties of a new material, On-X carbon for mechanical heart valve prostheses. J Heart Valve Dis 7:626, 1998
40. Yoganathan AP, Reamer HH, Corcoran WH, et al: The Starr-Edwards aortic ball valve: Flow characteristics, thrombus formation, and tissue overgrowth. Artif Organs 5:6, 1981
41. Yoganathan AP, Corcoran WH, Harrison EC, Carl JR: The Bjork-Shiley aortic valve prosthesis: Flow characteristics, thrombus formation and tissue overgrowth. Circulation 58:70, 1978
42. Anderson JM, Schoen FJ: Interactions of blood with artificial surfaces. In: Butchart EG, Bodnar E (eds): Thrombosis, Embolism, and Bleeding. London, ICR Publishers, 1992, p 60
43. Litin SC, Gastineau DA: Current concepts in anticoagulant therapy. Mayo Clin Proc 70:266, 1995
44. Senning A: Fascia lata replacement of aortic valves. J Thorac Cardiovasc Surg 54:465, 1967
45. Puig LB, Verginelli G, Iryia K, et al: Homologous dura mater cardiac valves. J Thorac Cardiovasc Surg 69:722, 1975
46. Jayakrishnan A, Jameela SR: Glutaraldehyde as a fixative in bioprostheses and drug delivery matrices. Biomaterials 17:471, 1996
47. Rose AG: Pathology of the formalin-treated heterograft porcine aortic valve in the mitral position. Thorax 27:401, 1972
48. Rumisek JD, Albus RA, Clarke JS: Late *Mycobacterium chelonai* bioprosthetic valve endocarditis: Activation of implanted contaminant? Ann Thorac Surg 39:277, 1985
49. Westaby S, Amarasena N, Long V, et al: Time-related hemodynamic changes after aortic replacement with the Freestyle stentless xenograft. Ann Thorac Surg 60:1633, 1995

50. Del Rizzo DF, Goldman BS, Christakis GT, David T: Hemodynamic benefits of the Toronto stentless valve. J Thorac Cardiovasc Surg 112:1431, 1996
51. Kirklin J, Smith D, Novick W, et al: Long-term function of cryopreserved aortic homografts: A ten-year study. J Thorac Cardiovasc Surg 106:154, 1993
52. Chambers JC, Somerville J, Stone S, Ross DN: Pulmonary autograft procedure for aortic valve disease: Long-term results of the pioneer series. Circulation 96:2206, 1997
53. Yun KL, Miller C, Moore KA, et al: Durability of the Hancock MO bioprosthesis compared with standard aortic valve bioprostheses. Ann Thorac Surg 60:S221, 1995
54. Walley VM, Keon WJ: Patterns of failure in Ionescu-Shiley bovine pericardial bioprosthetic valves. J Thorac Cardiovasc Surg 93:925, 1987
55. Schoen FJ, Fernandez J, Gonzalez-Lavin L, Cernaianu A: Causes of failure and pathologic findings in surgically removed Ionescu-Shiley standard bovine pericardial heart valve bioprostheses: Emphasis on progressive structural deterioration. Circulation 76:618, 1987
56. McGonagle-Wolff K, Schoen FJ: Morphologic findings in explanted Mitroflow pericardial bioprosthetic valves. Am J Cardiol 70:263, 1992
57. Shemin RJ, Schoen FJ, Hein R, et al: Hemodynamic and pathologic evaluation of a unileaflet pericardial bioprosthetic valve. J Thorac Cardiovasc Surg 95:912, 1988
58. Walker DK, Scotten LN, Hewgill DE, et al: Development and invitro assessment of a new two-leaflet replacement heart valve designed using computer-generated bubble surfaces. Med Biol Eng Comput 21:31, 1983
59. Morse D, Steiner RM: Cardiac valve identification atlas and guide. In: Morse D, Steiner RM, Fernandez J (eds): Guide to Prosthetic Cardiac Valves. New York, Springer Verlag, 1985, p 257
60. Schoen FJ: Pathology of bioprostheses and other tissue heart valve replacements. In: Silver MD (ed): Cardiovascular Pathology. 2nd ed. New York, Churchill Livingstone, 1991, p 1547
61. Ferrans VJ, Hilbert SL, Fujita S, et al: Abnormalities in explanted bioprosthetic cardiac valves. In: Virmani R, Atkinson JB, Fenoglio JJ (eds): Cardiovascular Pathology. Philadelphia, WB Saunders, 1993, p 373
62. Thubrikar M: The Aortic Valve. Boca Raton, CRC Press, 1990
63. Sutton JP, Yen S, Anderson RH: The forgotten interleaflet triangles: A review of the surgical anatomy of the aortic valve. Ann Thorac Surg 59:419, 1995
64. Schoen FJ: Aortic valve structure-function correlations: Role of elastic fibers no longer a stretch of the imagination. J Heart Valve Dis 6:1, 1997
65. Peskin CS, McQueen DM: Mechanical equilibrium determines the fractal fiber architecture of aortic heart valve leaflets. Am J Physiol 266:H319, 1994
66. Mannschott P, Herbage D, Weiss M, et al: Collagen heterogeneity in pig heart valves. Biochem Biophys Acta 434:177, 1976
67. Schoen FJ, Tsao JW, Levy RJ: Calcification of bovine pericardium used in cardiac valve bioprostheses: Implications for the mechanisms of bioprosthetic tissue mineralization. Am J Pathol 123:134, 1986
68. Ishihara T, Ferrans VJ, Jones M, et al: Histologic and ultrastructural features of normal human parietal pericardium. Am J Cardiol 46:744, 1980
69. Ishihara T, Ferrans VJ, Jones M, et al: Structure of bovine parietal pericardium and of unimplanted Ionescu-Shiley pericardial valvular bioprostheses. J Thorac Cardiovasc Surg 81:747, 1981
70. Hiester ED, Sacks MS: Optimal selection sites in the bovine pericardial sac. Part I. Measurement of fiber architecture and tissue thickness. J Biomed Mater Res 39:207, 1998
71. Hiester ED, Sacks MS: Optimal selection sites in the bovine pericardial sac. Part II. Cartographic analysis. J Biomed Mater Res 39:215, 1998
72. Hilbert SL, Ferrans VJ, McAllister HA, Cooley DA: Ionescu-Shiley bovine pericardial bioprostheses: Histologic and ultrastructural studies. Am J Pathol 140:1195, 1992
73. Ferrans VJ, Spray TL, Billingham ME, Roberts WC: Structural changes in glutaraldehyde-treated porcine heterografts used as substitute cardiac valves: Transmission and scanning electron microscopic observations in 12 patients. Am J Cardiol 41:1159, 1978

74. Flomenbaum MA, Schoen FJ: Effects of fixation back pressure and antimineralization treatment on the morphology of porcine aortic bioprosthetic valves. J Thorac Cardiovasc Surg 105:154, 1993

75. Broom ND, Thompson FJ: Influence of fixation conditions on the performance of glutaraldehyde-treated porcine aortic valves: Towards a more scientific basis. Thorax 34:166, 1979

76. Sacks MS, Smith DB, Hiester ED: The aortic valve microstructure: Effects of transvalvular pressure. J Biomed Mater Res 41:131, 1998

77. Gabbay S, Kadam P, Factor S, Cheung TK: Do heart valve bioprostheses degenerate for metabolic or mechanical reasons? J Thorac Cardiovasc Surg 55:208, 1988

78. Vesely I, Boughner D, Song T: Tissue buckling as a mechanism of bioprosthetic valve failure. Ann Thorac Surg 46:302, 1988

79. Hilbert SL, Barrick MK, Ferrans VJ: Porcine aortic valve bioprostheses: A morphologic comparison of the effects of fixation pressure. J Biomed Mater Res 24:773, 1990

80. Ishihara T, Ferrans VJ, Jones M, et al: Occurrence and significance of endothelial cells in implanted porcine bioprosthetic valves. Am J Cardiol 46:744, 1980

81. Ishihara T, Ferrans VJ, Barnhart GR, et al: Intracuspal hematomas in implanted porcine valvular bioprostheses. J Thorac Cardiovasc Surg 83:399, 1982

82. Ferrans VJ, Tomita Y, Hilbert SL, et al: Pathology of bioprosthetic cardiac valves. Hum Pathol 18:586, 1987

83. Goffin YA, Gruys E, Sorenson GD, Wellens F: Amyloid deposits in bioprosthetic cardiac valves after long-term implantation in man: A new localization of amyloidosis. Am J Pathol 114:431, 1984

84. Ratliff NB, McMahon JT, Naab TJ, Cosgrove DM: Whipple's disease in the porcine leaflets of a Carpentier-Edwards prosthetic mitral valve. N Engl J Med 311:902, 1984

85. Schoen FJ, Hausner RJ, Howell JF, et al: Porcine heterograft valve replacement in carcinoid heart disease. J Thorac Cardiovasc Surg 81:100, 1981

86. Ridker PM, Chertow GM, Karlson EW, et al: Bioprosthetic tricuspid valve stenosis associated with extensive plaque deposition in carcinoid heart disease. Am Heart J 121:1835, 1991

87. Bonow RO, Carabello B, de Leon AC Jr, et al: ACC/AHA guidelines for the management of patients with valvular heart disease: Executive summary. A report of the American College of Cardiology/American Heart Association Task Force on Practice Guidelines. Circulation 98:1949, 1998

88. Cohn LH: Mechanical and bioprosthetic mitral valve replacement. In: Edmunds LH (ed): Cardiac Surgery in the Adult. New York, McGraw-Hill, 1997, p 1025

89. Jamieson WRE: Mechanical and bioprosthetic aortic valve replacement. In: Edmunds LH (ed): Cardiac Surgery in the Adult. New York, McGraw-Hill, 1997, p 859

90. Jamieson WRE, Edwards FH, Schwartz M, et al: Risk stratification for cardiac valve replacement: National Cardiac Surgery Database. Ann Thorac Surg 67:943, 1999

91. Edwards FH, Peterson ED, Coombs LP, et al: Prediction of operative mortality after valve replacement surgery. J Am Coll Cardiol 37:885, 2001

92. Gehlot A, Mullany CJ, Ilstrup D, et al: Aortic valve replacement in patients aged eighty years and older: Early and long-term results. J Thorac Cardiovasc Surg 111:1026, 1996

93. Antunes MJ: Reoperations on cardiac valves. J Heart Valve Dis 1: 25, 1992

94. Bloomfield P, Wheatley DJ, Prescott RJ, Miller HC: Twelve-year comparison of a Bjork-Shiley mechanical heart valve with porcine bioprosthesis. N Engl J Med 324:573, 1991

95. Hammermeister KE, Sethi GK, Henderson WG, et al: A comparison of outcomes in men 11 years after heart-valve replacement with a mechanical valve or bioprosthesis. N Engl J Med 328:1289, 1993

96. Blackstone EH, Kirklin JW: Death and other time-related events after valve replacement. Circulation 72:753, 1985

97. Schoen FJ, Titus JL, Lawrie GM: Autopsy-determined causes of death after cardiac valve replacement. JAMA 249:899, 1983

98. Rose AG: Autopsy-determined causes of death following heart valve replacement. Am J Cardiovasc Pathol 1:30, 1987

99. Walley VM, Masters RG: Complications of cardiac valve surgery and their autopsy investigation. Cardiovasc Pathol 4:269, 1995

100. Gotlieb A, Masse S, Allard J, et al: Concentric hemorrhagic necro-

sis of the myocardium: A morphological and clinical study. Hum Pathol 8:27, 1977

101. Hutchins GM, Silverman KJ: Pathology of the stone heart syndrome. Am J Pathol 95:745, 1979

102. Cowan MJ, Reichenbach D, Turner P, Thostenson C: Cellular response of the evolving myocardial infarction after therapeutic coronary artery reperfusion. Hum Pathol 22:154, 1991

103. Reichenbach DD, Cowan MJ: Healing of myocardial infarction with and without reperfusion. Maj Probl Pathol 23:86, 1991

104. Esper E, Ferdinand FD, Aronson S, Karp RB: Prosthetic mitral valve replacement: Late complications after native valve preservation. Ann Thorac Surg 63:541, 1997

105. Hwang MH, Burchfiel CM, Sethi GK, et al: Comparison of the causes of late death following aortic and mitral valve replacement. J Heart Valve Dis 3:17, 1994

106. Burke AP, Farb A, Sessums L, Virmani R: Causes of sudden cardiac death in patients with replacement valves: An autopsy study. J Heart Valve Dis 3:310, 1994

107. Giddens DP, Yoganathan AP, Schoen FJ: Prosthetic cardiac valves. Cardiovasc Pathol 2:167S, 1993

108. Devereaux RB: Regression of left ventricular hypertrophy: How and why? (editorial). JAMA 275:1517, 1996

109. Roman MJ, Klein L, Devereaux RB, et al: Reversal of left ventricular dilatation, hypertrophy, and dysfunction by valve replacement in aortic regurgitation. Am Heart J 118:553, 1989

110. Edmunds LH, Clark RE, Cohn LH, et al: Guidelines for reporting morbidity and mortality after cardiac valvular operations. J Thorac Cardiovasc Surg 112:708, 1996

111. Schoen FJ, Hobson CE: Anatomic analysis of removed prosthetic heart valves: Cause of failure of 33 mechanical valves and 58 bioprostheses, 1980 to 1983. Hum Pathol 16:549, 1985

112. Schoen FJ: Surgical pathology of removed natural and prosthetic heart valves. Hum Pathol 18:558, 1987

113. Edmunds LH: Thrombotic and bleeding complications of prosthetic heart valves. Ann Thorac Surg 44:430, 1987

114. Gencbay M, Turan F, Degertekin M, et al: High prevalence of hypercoagulable states in patients with recurrent thrombosis of mechanical heart valves. J Heart Valve Dis 7:601, 1998

115. Bick RL, Ucar K: Hypercoagulability and thrombosis. Hematol Oncol Clin North Am 6:1421, 1992

116. Gonzalez-Lavin L: Thrombosis of an aortic porcine xenobioprosthesis associated with familial antithrombin III deficiency. J Thorac Cardiovasc Surg 88:631, 1984

117. Bick RL, Pegram M: Syndromes of hypercoagulability and thrombosis: A review. Semin Thromb Hemost 20:109, 1994

118. Ellis JT, Healy TM, Fontaine AA, et al: Velocity measurements and flow patterns within the hinge region of a Medtronic Parallel bileaflet mechanical valve with clear housing. J Heart Valve Dis 5: 591, 1996

119. Gross JM, Shu MC, Dai FF, et al: A microstructural flow analysis within a bileaflet mechanical heart valve hinge. J Heart Valve Dis 5:581, 1996

120. Hurrell DG, Schaff HV, Tajik AJ: Thrombolytic therapy for obstruction of mechanical prosthetic valves. Mayo Clin Proc 71:605, 1996

121. Anderson JM, Kottke-Marchant K: Platelet interactions with biomaterials and artificial devices. CRC Crit Rev Biocompat 1:111, 1985

122. Cannegieter SC, Rosendaal FR, Wintzen AR, et al: Optimal oral anticoagulant therapy in patients with mechanical heart valves. N Engl J Med 333:11, 1995

123. Huber KC, Gersh BJ, Bailey KR, et al: Variability in anticoagulation control predicts thromboembolism after mechanical cardiac valve replacement: A 23-year population-based study. Mayo Clin Proc 72:1103, 1997

124. Nichols WL, Bowie EJW: Standardization of the prothrombin time for monitoring orally administered anticoagulant therapy with use of the International Normalized Ratio system. Mayo Clin Proc 68: 897, 1993

125. Aramendi JL, Agredo J, Llorente A, et al: Prevention of thromboembolism with ticlopidine shortly after valve repair or replacement with a bioprosthesis. J Heart Valve Dis 7:610, 1998

126. Cannegieter SC, Rosendaal FR, Briët E: Thromboembolic and bleeding complications in patients with mechanical heart valve prostheses. Circulation 89:635, 1994

127. Levine MN, Raskob G, Landefeld S, Hirsch J: Hemorrhagic complications of anticoagulant treatment. Chest 108:276S, 1995

128. Koniaris LS, Goldhaber SZ: Anticoagulation in dilated cardiomyopathy. J Am Coll Cardiol 31:745, 1998
129. Landefield CS, Beyth RJ: Anticoagulant-related bleeding: Clinical epidemiology, prediction and prevention. Am J Med 95:315, 1993
130. Orsinelli DA, Pasierski TJ, Pearson AC: Spontaneously appearing microbubbles associated with prosthetic cardiac valves detected by transesophageal echocardiography. Am Heart J 128:990, 1994
131. Georgiadis D, Kaps M, Berg J, et al: Transcranial Doppler detection of microemboli in prosthetic heart valve patients: Dependency upon valve type. Eur J Cardiothorac Surg 10:253, 1996
132. Hwang NHC, Meltzer RS, Moehring MA, et al: Spontaneous echo contrast in patients with mechanical heart valve implants. ASAIO J 42:24, 1996
133. Calderwood SB, Swinski LA, Waternaux CM, et al: Risk factors for the development of prosthetic valve endocarditis. Circulation 72:31, 1985
134. Wilson WR, Danielson GK, Giuliani ER, Geraci JE: Prosthetic valve endocarditis. Mayo Clin Proc 57:155, 1982
135. Vlessis AA, Khaki A, Grunkemeier GL, et al: Risk, diagnosis and management of prosthetic valve endocarditis: A review. J Heart Valve Dis 6:443, 1997
136. Arnett EN, Roberts WC: Prosthetic valve endocarditis. Clinicopathologic analysis of 22 necropsy patients with active infective endocarditis involving natural left-sided cardiac valves. Am J Cardiol 38:281, 1976
137. Anderson DJ, Bulkley BH, Hutchins GM: A clinicopathologic study of prosthetic valve endocarditis in 22 patients: Morphologic basis for diagnosis and therapy. Am Heart J 94:324, 1977
138. Ferrans VJ, Boyce SW, Billingham ME, et al: Infection of glutaraldehyde-preserved porcine valve heterografts. Am J Cardiol 43:1123, 1979
139. Hylen JC, Kloster FE, Herr RH, et al: Phonocardiographic diagnosis of aortic ball variance. Circulation 38:90, 1968
140. Chin HP, Harrison EC, Blankenhorn DH, Moacanin J: Lipids in silicone rubber valve prostheses after human implantation. Circulation 43, 44 (suppl):I-51, 1971
141. Muller WA, Cohn LH, Schoen FJ: Infection within a degenerated Starr-Edwards silicone rubber poppet in the aortic valve position. Am J Cardiol 54:1146, 1984
142. Hylen JC, Hodam RP, Kloster FE: Changes in the durability of silicone rubber in ball-valve prostheses. Ann Thorac Surg 13:324, 1972.
143. Shah A, Dolgin M, Tice DA, Trehan N: Complications due to cloth wear in cloth-covered Starr-Edwards aortic and mitral valve prostheses—and their management. Am Heart J 96:407, 1978
144. Jonas RA, Garratt-Boyes BG, Kerr AR, Whitlock RM: Late follow-up of the Braunwald-Cutter valve. Ann Thorac Surg 33:554, 1982
145. Schoen FJ, Goodenough SH, Ionescu MI, Braunwald NS: Implications of late morphology of Braunwald-Cutter mitral heart valve prostheses. J Thorac Cardiovasc Surg 88:208, 1984
146. Macmanus Q, Grunkemeier G, Housman L, et al: Early results with composite strut caged ball prostheses. Am J Cardiol 46:566, 1980
147. Ridolfi RL, Hutchins GM: Detection of ball variance in prosthetic heart valves by liver biopsy. Johns Hopkins Med J 134:131, 1974
148. Silver MD: Wear in Bjork-Shiley heart valve prostheses recovered at necropsy or operation. J Thorac Cardiovasc Surg 79:693, 1980
149. Erichsen A, Lindblom D, Semb G, et al: Strut fracture with Bjork-Shiley 70° Convexo-Concave valve: An international multi-institutional follow-up study. Eur J Cardiothorac Surg 1992; 6:339
150. van der Graaf Y, de Waard F, van Herwerden LA, Defauw J: Risk of strut fracture of Bjork-Shiley valves. Lancet 339:257, 1992
151. Schreck S, Inderbitzen R, Wieting DW, et al: Dynamics of Bjork-Shiley convexo-concave mitral valves in sheep. J Heart Valve Dis 4(suppl I):S21, 1995
152. de Mol BA, Kallewaard M, McLellan RB, et al: Single-leg strut failures in explanted Bjork-Shiley valves. Lancet 343:9, 1994
153. Klepetko W, Moritz A, Mlczoch J, et al: Leaflet fracture in Edwards-Duramedics bileaflet valves. J Thorac Cardiovasc Surg 97:90, 1989
154. Hwang NHC (ed): Cavitation in mechanical heart valves. J Heart Dis 3(suppl I): S1, 1994
155. Odell JA, Durand J, Shama DM, Vythilingum S: Spontaneous embolization of a St. Jude Medical prosthesis. Ann Thorac Surg 39:569, 1985
156. Orsinelli DA, Becker RC, Cuenoud HF, Moran JM: Mechanical

157. Jamieson WR, Munro AI, Miyagishima RT, et al: Carpentier-Edwards standard porcine bioprosthesis: Clinical performance to seventeen years. Ann Thorac Surg 60:999, 1995
158. Cohn LH, Collins JJ, DiSesa VJ, et al: Fifteen-year experience with 1678 Hancock porcine bioprosthetic heart valve replacements. Ann Surg 210:435, 1989
159. Bolooki H, Kaiser GA, Mallon SM, Palatianos GM: Comparison of long-term results of Carpentier-Edwards and Hancock bioprosthetic valves. Ann Thorac Surg 42:494, 1986
160. Bortolotti U, Guerra F, Magni A, et al: Emergency reoperation for primary tissue failure of porcine bioprostheses. Am J Cardiol 60:920, 1987
161. Grunkemeier GL, Jamieson WRE, Miller DC, Starr A: Actuarial versus actual risk of porcine structural valve deterioration. J Thorac Cardiovasc Surg 108:709, 1994
162. Ferrans FJ, Boyce SW, Billingham ME, et al: Calcific deposits in porcine bioprostheses: Structure and pathogenesis. Am J Cardiol 46:721, 1980
163. Schoen FJ, Cohn LH: Explant analysis of porcine bioprosthetic heart valves: Mode of failure and stent creep. In: Bodnar E, Yacoub MH (eds): Biological and Bioprosthetic Valves. New York, Yorke, 1986, p 356
164. Schoen FJ, Kujovich JL, Webb CL, Levy RJ: Chemically determined mineral content of explanted porcine aortic valve bioprostheses: Correlation with radiographic assessment of calcification and clinical data. Circulation 76:1061, 1987
165. Waldman JD, Lamberti JJ, Schoen FJ, et al: Balloon dilatation of stenotic right ventricle-to-pulmonary artery conduits. J Card Surg 3:539, 1988
166. Butany J, Silver MD, Chiasson D, David TE: Tissue detachment in Carpentier-Edwards porcine bioprosthetic heart valves. Trans Soc Biomat 488, 1994
167. Allard MF, Thompson CR, MacNab JS, et al: Commissural region dehiscence from stent-posts of Carpentier-Edwards bioprosthetic cardiac valves. Cardiovasc Pathol 4:155, 1995
168. Aupart MR, Sirinelli AL, Diemont FF, et al: The last generation of pericardial valves in the aortic position: Ten-year follow-up in 589 patients. Ann Thorac Surg 61:615, 1996
169. Cosgrove DM: Carpentier pericardial valve. Semin Thorac Cardiovasc Surg 8:269, 1996
170. Grunkemeier GL, Bodnar E: Comparative assessment of bioprosthesis durability in the aortic position. J Heart Valve Dis 4:49, 1995
171. Jamieson WR, Marchand MA, Pelletier CL, et al: Structural valve deterioration in mitral replacement surgery: Comparison of Carpentier-Edwards supra-annular porcine and Perimount pericardial bioprostheses. J Thorac Cardiovasc Surg 118:297, 1999
172. Schoen FJ, Levy RJ, Nelson AC, et al: Onset and progression of experimental bioprosthetic heart valve calcification. Lab Invest 52:523, 1985
173. Schoen FJ, Hirsch D, Bianco RW, Levy RJ: Onset and progression of calcification in porcine aortic bioprosthetic valves implanted as orthotopic mitral valve replacements in juvenile sheep. J Thorac Cardiovasc Surg 108:880, 1994
174. Schoen FJ, Golomb G, Levy RJ: Calcification of bioprosthetic heart valves: A perspective on models. J Heart Valve Dis 1:110, 1992
175. Mako WJ, Vesely I: In-vivo and in-vitro models of calcification in porcine aortic valve cusps. J Heart Valve Dis 6:316, 1997
176. Majno G, Joris I: Cells, Tissues, and Disease: Principles of General Pathology. Cambridge, MA, Blackwell Science, 1996, p 229
177. Kim KM, Herrera GA, Battarbee HD: Role of glutaraldehyde in calcification of porcine aortic valve fibroblasts. Am J Pathol 154:671, 1999
178. Levy RJ, Schoen FJ, Sherman FS, et al: Calcification of subcutaneously implanted type 1 collagen sponges: Effects of formaldehyde and glutaraldehyde pretreatments. Am J Pathol 122:71, 1986
179. Vyavahare N, Ogle M, Schoen FJ, Levy RJ: Elastin calcification and its prevention with aluminum chloride pretreatment. Am J Pathol 155:973, 1999
180. Levy RJ, Schoen FJ, Levy JT, et al: Biologic determinants of dystrophic calcification and osteocalcin deposition in glutaraldehyde-preserved porcine aortic valve leaflets implanted subcutaneously in rats. Am J Pathol 113:143, 1983
181. Valente M, Bortolotti U, Thiene G: Ultrastructural substrates of

failure of a St. Jude Medical prosthesis. Am J Cardiol 67:906, 1991

dystrophic calcification in porcine bioprosthetic valve failure. Am J Pathol 119:12, 1985

182. Golomb G, Schoen FJ, Smith MS, et al: The role of glutaraldehyde-induced cross-links in calcification of bovine pericardium used in cardiac valve bioprostheses. Am J Pathol 127:122, 1987

183. Anderson HC: Molecular biology of matrix vesicles. Clin Orthop 314:266, 1995

184. Tomazic BB, Brown WE, Schoen FJ: Physicochemical properties of calcific deposits isolated from porcine bioprosthetic heart valves removed from patients following 2–13 years function. J Biomed Mater Res 38:35, 1994

185. McKee MD, Nanci A: Osteopontin: An interfacial extracellular matrix protein in mineralized tissues. Connect Tissue Res 35:197, 1996

186. Motamed K, Sage HE: Regulation of vascular morphogenesis by the matricellular protein SPARC. Kidney Int 51:1383, 1997

187. Boskey AL: Matrix proteins and mineralization: An overview. Connect Tissue Res 35:357, 1996

188. Ducy P, Desbois C, Boyce B, et al: Increased bone formation in osteocalcin-dependent mice. Nature 382:448, 1996

189. Srivatsa SS, Harrity PJ, Maerchlein PB, et al: Increased cellular expression of matrix proteins that regulate mineralization is associated with calcification of native human and porcine xenograft bioprosthetic heart valves. J Clin Invest 99:996, 1997

190. Parhami F, Bostrom K, Watson K, Demer LL: Role of molecular regulation in vascular calcification. J Atheroscler Thromb 3:90, 1996

191. Wada T, McKee MD, Steitz S, Giachelli CM: Calcification of vascular smooth muscle cell cultures: Inhibition by osteopontin. Circ Res 84:166, 1999

192. Sacks M, Schoen FJ: Calcification-independent damage in explanted clinical bioprosthetic heart valves. Transactions, Society For Biomaterials 1999, p 313

193. Gloeckner DC, Billiar KL, Sacks MS: Effects of mechanical fatigue on the bending properties of the porcine bioprosthetic heart valve. ASAIO J 45:59, 1999

194. Purinya B, Kasyanov V, Volkolakov J, et al: Biomechanical and structural properties of the explanted bioprosthetic valve leaflets. J Biomech 27:1, 1994

195. Vyavahare N, Ogle M, Schoen FJ, et al: Mechanisms of cardiac valve deterioration: Cyclic fatigue causes collagen structural alterations and loss of glycosaminoglycans. J Biomed Mater Res 46:44, 1999

196. Simionescu A, Simionescu D, Deac R: Biochemical pathways of tissue degeneration in bioprosthetic cardiac valves: The role of matrix metalloproteinases. ASAIO J 42:M561, 1996

197. Simionescu D, Simionescu A, Deac R: Detection of remnant proteolytic activities in unimplanted glutaraldehyde-treated bovine pericardium and explanted cardiac bioprostheses. J Biomed Mater Res 27:821, 1993

198. Mako JW, Calabro A, Ratliff NB, Vesely I: Loss of glycosaminoglycans from implanted bioprosthetic heart valves. Circulation 96:155, 1997

199. Salgaller ML, Bajpai PK: Immunogenicity of glutaraldehyde-treated bovine pericardial tissue xenografts in rabbits. J Biomed Mater Res 19:1, 1985

200. Dahm M, Lyman WD, Schwell AB, et al: Immunogenicity of glutaraldehyde-tanned bovine pericardium. J Thorac Cardiovasc Surg 99: 1082, 1990

201. Rocchini AP, Weesner KM, Heidelberger K, et al: Porcine xenograft valve failure in children: An immunologic response. Circulation 64:II-162, 1981

202. Levy RJ, Schoen FJ, Howard S: Mechanism of calcification of porcine aortic valve cusps: Role of T-lymphocytes. Am J Cardiol 52:629, 1983

203. Schoen FJ, Schulman LJ, Cohn LH: Quantitative anatomic analysis of "stent creep" of explanted Hancock standard porcine bioprostheses used for cardiac valve replacement. Am J Cardiol 56:110, 1985

204. Reddy SB, Pater JL, Pym J, Armstrong PW: Hemolytic anemia following insertion of Ionescu-Shiley mitral valve bioprostheses. Can Med J 131:1469, 1984

205. Roberts WC: Complications of cardiac valve replacement: Characteristic abnormalities of prostheses pertaining to any or specific site. Am Heart J 103:113, 1982

206. Roberts WC, Sullivan ME: Clinical and necropsy observations early after simultaneous replacement of the mitral and aortic valves. Am J Cardiol 58:1067, 1986

207. Williams DB, Pluth JR, Otszulak TA: Extrinsic obstruction of the Bjork-Shiley valve in the mitral position. Ann Thorac Surg 32:58, 1981

208. Kuo J, Rooney S, Breckenridge IM: Suture loop restriction of the Medtronic Hall valve: Late presentation of a rare complication. J Heart Valve Dis 5:117, 1996

209. Jones M, Rodriguez ER, Eidbo EE, Ferrans VJ: Cuspal perforations caused by long suture ends in implanted bioprosthetic valves. J Thorac Cardiovasc Surg 90:557, 1985

210. Waller BF, Jones M, Roberts WC: Postoperative aortic regurgitation from incomplete seating of tilting disc occluders due to overhanging knots or long sutures. Chest 78:565, 1980

211. Starek PJK: Immobilization of disc heart valves by unraveled sutures. Ann Thorac Surg 31:66, 1981

212. Ziemer G, Luhmer I, Oeler H, Borst HG: Malfunction of a St. Jude Medical heart valve in mitral position. Ann Thorac Surg 33: 391, 1982

213. Eyster E, Rothchild J, Mychajliw O: Chronic intravascular hemolysis after aortic valve replacement. Long-term study comparing different types of ball-valve prostheses. Circulation 44:657, 1971

214. David TE, Feindel CM, Scully HE, et al: Aortic valve replacement with stentless porcine aortic valves: A ten-year experience. J Heart Valve Dis 7:250, 1998

215. Westaby S, Jin XY, Katsuma T, et al: Valve replacement with a stentless bioprosthesis: Versatility of the porcine aortic root. J Thorac Cardiovasc Surg 116:477, 1998

216. Jin XY, Dhital K, Bhattacharya K, et al: Five-year hemodynamic performance of the prima stentless aortic valve. Ann Thorac Surg 66:805, 1998

217. David TE, Puschmann R, Ivanov J, et al: Aortic valve replacement with stentless and stented porcine valves: A case-match study. J Thorac Cardiovasc Surg 116:236, 1998

218. Westaby S, Huysmans HA, David TE: Stentless aortic bioprostheses: Compelling data from the Second International Symposium. Ann Thorac Surg 65:235, 1998

219. Fyfe B, Schoen FJ: Pathologic analysis of nonstented Freestyle aortic root bioprostheses treated with amino oleic acid. Semin Thorac Cardiovasc Surg 11(suppl):151, 1999

220. Vrandecic M, Gontijo B, Fantini FA, et al: Porcine mitral stentless valve mid-term clinical results. Eur J Cardiothorac Surg 12:56, 1997

221. Ross D: Homograft replacement of the aortic valve. Lancet 2:487, 1962

222. Barratt-Boyes B: Homograft aortic valve replacement in aortic incompetence and stenosis. Thorax 19:131, 1964

223. O'Brien M, Stafford E, Gardner M, et al: A comparison of aortic valve replacement with viable cryopreserved and fresh allograft valves with a note on chromosomal studies. J Thorac Cardiovasc Surg 94:812,1987

224. Barratt-Boyes BG, Roche AHG, Subramanyan R, et al: Long-term follow-up of patients with the antibiotic-sterilized aortic homograft valve inserted freehand in the aortic position. Circulation 75:768, 1987

225. Matsuki O, Robles A, Gibbs S, et al: Long-term performance of 555 aortic homografts in the aortic position. Ann Thorac Surg 46: 187, 1988

226. Kirklin JK, Smith D, Novick W, et al: Long-term function of cryopreserved aortic homografts. J Thorac Cardiovasc Surg 106: 154, 1993

227. Tuna IC, Orszulak TA, Schaff HV, Danielson GK: Results of homograft aortic valve replacement for active endocarditis. Ann Thorac Surg 49:619, 1990

228. Grunkemeier GL, Bodnar E: Comparison of structural valve failure among different "models" of homograft valves. J Heart Valve Dis 3:556, 1994

229. Smith JC: The pathology of human aortic valve homografts. Thorax 22:114, 1967

230. Davies H, Missen AK, Blandford G, et al: Homograft replacement of the aortic valve: A clinical and pathologic study. Am J Cardiol 22:195, 1968

231. Hudson REB: Pathology of the human aortic valve homograft. Br Heart J 28:291, 1966

232. Kosek JC, Iben AB, Shumway NE, Angell WW: Morphology of fresh heart valve homografts. Surgery 66:269, 1969
233. Gavin JB, Barratt-Boyes BG, Hitchcock GC, Herdson PB: Histopathology of "fresh" human aortic valve allografts. Thorax 28:482, 1973
234. O'Brien MF, Johnson N, Stafford G, et al: A study of the cells in the explanted viable cryopreserved allograft valve. J Card Surg 3:279, 1988
235. Mitchell RN, Jonas RA, Schoen FJ: Pathology of explanted cryopreserved allograft heart valves: Comparison with aortic valves from orthotopic heart transplants. J Thorac Cardiovasc Surg 115:118, 1998
236. Jonas RA, Ziemer G, Britton L, Armiger LC: Cryopreserved and fresh antibiotic-sterilized valved aortic homograft conduits in a long-term sheep model. J Thorac Cardiovasc Surg 96:746, 1988
237. Christie GW, Gavin JB, Barratt-Boyes BG: Graft detachment: A cause of incompetence in stent-mounted aortic valve allografts. J Thorac Cardiovasc Surg 90:901, 1985
238. Wheatley D, McGregor C: Post implantation viability in canine allograft heart valves. Cardiovasc Res 11:78, 1977
239. Angell W, Oury J, Lamberti J, Koziol J: Durability of the viable aortic allograft. J Thorac Cardiovasc Surg 98:48, 1989
240. Hogan P, Duplock L, Green M, et al: Human aortic valve allografts elicit a donor-specific immune response. J Thorac Cardiovasc Surg 112:1260, 1996
241. Rajani B, Mee RB, Ratliff NB: Evidence of rejection of homograft cardiac valves in infants. J Thorac Cardiovasc Surg 115:111, 1998
242. Kouchoukos NT, Davila-Roman VG, Spray TL et al: Replacement of the aortic root with a pulmonary autograft in children and young adults with aortic-valve disease. N Engl J Med 330:1, 1994
243. Elkins RC, Lane MM, McCue C: Pulmonary autograft reoperation: Incidence and management. Ann Thorac Surg 62:450, 1996
244. Lapeyre DM, Frazier OH, Conger JL, et al: In-vivo evaluation of a trileaflet mechanical heart valve. ASAIO J 40:M707, 1994
245. Leat ME, Fisher J: Comparative study of the function of the Abiomed polyurethane heart valve for use in left ventricular assist devices. J Biomed Eng 15:516, 1993
246. Braunwald NS, Morrow AG: A late evaluation of flexible Teflon prosthesis utilized for total aortic valve replacement: Postoperative clinical hemodynamic and pathological assessment. J Thorac Cardiovasc Surg 49:485, 1965
247. Fishbein MC, Roberts WC, Golden A, Hufnagel CA: Cardiac pathology after aortic valve replacement using Hufnagel trileaflet prostheses: A study of 20 necropsy patients. Am Heart J 89:443, 1975
248. Schoen FJ, Levy RJ: Pathology of substitute heart valves: New concepts and developments. J Cardiovasc Surg 9(suppl):222, 1994
249. Schoen FJ: Future directions in tissue heart valves: Impact of recent insights from biology and pathology. J Heart Valve Dis 8:350, 1999
250. Schoen FJ, Levy RJ, Hilbert SL, Bianco RW: Antimineralization treatments for bioprosthetic heart valves. J Thorac Cardiovasc Surg 104:1285, 1992
251. Vyavahare NR, Chen W, Joshi R, et al: Current progress in anticalcification for bioprosthetic and polymeric heart valves. Cardiovasc Pathol 6:219, 1997
252. Chen W, Schoen FJ, Levy RJ: Mechanism of efficacy of 2-amino oleic acid for inhibition of calcification of glutaraldehyde-pretreated porcine bioprosthetic valves. Circulation 90:323, 1994
253. Webb CL, Schoen FJ, Flowers WE, et al: Inhibition of mineralization of glutaraldehyde-pretreated bovine pericardium by AlCl3. Mechanisms and comparisons with FeCl3, LaCl3, and Ga(NO3)3 in rat subdermal model studies. Am J Pathol 138:971, 1991
254. Vyavahare N, Hirsch D, Lerner E, et al: Prevention of bioprosthetic heart valve calcification by ethanol preincubation: Efficacy and mechanism. Circulation 95:479, 1997
255. Courtman DW, Pereira CA, Omar S, et al: Biomechanical and ultrastructural comparison of cryopreservation and a novel cellular extraction of porcine aortic valve leaflets. J Biomed Mater Res 29:1507, 1995
256. Vesely I, Noseworthy R, Pringle G: The hybrid xenograft/autograft bioprosthetic heart valve: In-vivo evaluation of tissue extraction. Ann Thorac Surg 60:S359, 1995
257. Moore MA: Pericardial tissue stabilized by dye-mediated photooxidation: A review article. J Heart Valve Dis 6:521, 1979
258. Schoen FJ: Pathologic findings in explanted clinical bioprosthetic valves fabricated from photooxidized bovine pericardium. J Heart Valve Dis 7:174, 1998
259. Eybl E, Grimm M, Grabenwoger M, et al: Endothelial cell lining of bioprosthetic heart valve materials. J Thorac Cardiovasc Surg 104:763, 1992
260. Vesely I: Analysis of the Medtronic Intact bioprosthetic valve: Effects of "zero-pressure" fixation. J Thorac Cardiovasc Surg 101:90, 1991
261. Love JW, Schoen FJ, Breznock EM, et al: Experimental evaluation of an autologous tissue heart valve. J Heart Valve Dis 1:232, 1992
262. Langer R, Vacanti JP: Tissue engineering. Science 260:920, 1993
263. Mayer JE Jr, Shin'oka T, Shum-Tim D: Tissue engineering of cardiovascular structures. Curr Opin Cardiol 12:528, 1997
264. Hoerstrup SP, Sodian R, Daebritz S, et al: Functional living trileaflet heart valves grown in-vitro. Circulation 102:III-44, 2000
265. Tweden KS, Cameron JD, Razzouk AJ, et al: Biocompatibility of silver-modified polyester for antimicrobial protection of prosthetic valves. J Heart Valve Dis 6:553, 1997
266. Bodnar E: The Silzone dilemma—What did we learn? (Editorial) J Heart Valve Dis 9:170, 2000
267. Cosgrove DM, Sabik JF: Minimally invasive approach for aortic valve operations. Ann Thorac Surg 62:596, 1996
268. Knudsen LL, Andersen HR, Hasenkam JM: Catheter-implanted prosthetic heart valves. Int J Artif Organs 16:253, 1993
269. Schoen FJ: Role of device retrieval and analysis in the evaluation of substitute heart vales. In: Witkin KB (ed): Clinical Evaluation of Medical Devices. Totowa, New Jersey, Humana Press, 1998, p 209
270. Lefrak EA, Starr A: Cardiac Valve Prostheses. New York, Appleton-Century-Crofts, 1979
271. Roberts WC, Bulkley BH, Morrow AG: Pathologic anatomy of cardiac valve replacement: A study of 224 necropsy patients. Prog Cardiovasc Dis 15:539, 1973
272. Silver MD: Late complications of prosthetic heart valves. Arch Pathol Lab Med 102:281, 1978
273. Savage RA: New law to require medical device injury reports. CAP Today, July 1991, p 40
274. Kahan JS: The Safe Medical Devices Act of 1990. Med Dev Diagn Ind, January 1991, p 67
275. Silver MD, Butany J: Mechanical heart valves: Methods of examination, complications, and modes of failure. Hum Pathol 18:577, 1987
276. Morse D, Steiner RM: Cardiac valve identification atlas and guide. In: Morse D, Steiner RM, Fernandez J (eds): Guide to Prosthetic Cardiac Valves. New York, Springer Verlag, 1985, p 257
277. Mehlman DJ: A guide to the radiographic identification of prosthetic heart valves: An addendum. Circulation 69:102, 1984
278. Ishihara T, Ferrans VJ, Boyce SW, et al: Structure and classification of cuspal tears and perforations in porcine bioprosthetic cardiac valves implanted in patients. Am J Cardiol 48:665, 1981

Pathology of Cardiovascular Interventions, Including Endovascular Therapies, Revascularization, Vascular Replacement, Cardiac Assist/Replacement, Arrythmia Control, and Repaired Congenital Heart Disease

Frederick J. Schoen • William D. Edwards

The last several decades have witnessed a virtual explosion in the armamentarum of interventional and surgical procedures and medical devices available to manage cardiovascular diseases. For example, percutaneous treatment of coronary artery disease is one of the most widely done medical procedures, with greater than 1 million performed worldwide each year.[1] The total number of vascular and cardiac surgeries and procedures is over 5 million per year in the United States alone.[2] To a large extent, the use of these techniques and implants has created pathologic features that were not previously encountered. This chapter summarizes key morphologic, pathobiologic, and clinical considerations pertinent to the most important and widely used procedures and devices.

ENDOVASCULAR THERAPIES AND MYOCARDIAL REVASCULARIZATION

Thrombolysis

In his seminal paper of 1912, James Herrick attributed myocardial infarction (MI) to coronary artery thrombosis.[3] Controversy followed for many years as to whether the coronary thrombus was the cause or the consequence of the myocardial damage. However, DeWood and colleagues as well as many other investigators reported finding coronary thrombus by angiography in approximately 90% of patients shortly after MI.[4] Consequently, it is now well accepted that most instances of acute transmural MI are caused by intraluminal platelet-fibrin thrombus formation, generally related to underlying acute structural change in an atherosclerotic plaque.[5, 6] Although spontaneous lysis of the occluding thrombus occurs in some patients, persistent thrombotic occlusion is present in the majority during the progression of myocardial necrosis. Timely reperfusion of jeopardized myocardium by thrombolysis is the most effective means of restoring the balance between myocardial oxygen demand and supply, thereby alleviating ischemia and salvaging muscle.

The routine use of thrombolytic therapy in acute MI was established by the first Gruppo Italiano Per Lo Studio Della Streptochinasi Nell'Infarct Miocardico (GISSI) trial of over 11,000 patients. It showed that intravenous streptokinase significantly reduced mortality in patients treated within 6 hours of the onset of symptoms.[7] The benefits of thrombolysis are now well established; revascularization by thrombolysis in early acute MI limits infarct size, preserves left ventricular function, and improves survival.[8–14]

Early intravenous or intracoronary therapy with thrombolytic drugs yields an overall reduction in mortality of approximately 18%.[9–16] The clinical end points are largely determined by the time interval between the onset of symptoms and a successful intervention, adequacy of early coronary reflow, and the degree of residual stenosis of the infarct vessel. For both survival and improvement in left ventricular function, the greatest benefit accrues when the agents are administered as early as possible, particularly when this occurs less than 1 to 2 hours after symptoms begin.[17] The reduction in mortality can be dramatic; in one study, effective thrombolysis of the infarct-related artery within 90 minutes reduced 30-day mortality from 9 to 4% and enhanced parameters of left ventricular contraction.[18] Using the thrombolytic agents streptokinase, urokinase, or tissue-derived plasminogen activator (tPA), recanalization rates vary from 60 to 90%. No clear-cut benefit of any single agent has been confirmed,[19] but some studies favor tPA.[20] Despite reocclusion rates of the infarct-related artery as high as 10% in-hospital (corresponding to 5% reinfarction), half between the first and the second week,[21] and 30% in 3 months, the short-term survival benefit of thrombolytic therapy is maintained long term.

The clinical benefit of early thrombolysis in myocardial salvage is consistent with experimental studies of the progression of necrosis in acute MI, which show that in the dog approximately half of the jeopardized myocardium in the zone of perfusion becomes necrotic 3 to 4 hours after coronary occlusion.[22] However, studies also suggest that at least some benefit can occur after later reperfusion, usually within 12 hours of symptoms.[23] The mechanism of efficacy of late reperfusion is uncertain, but it is likely to be independent of myocardial salvage. Moreover, spontaneous recanalization, presumably due to intrinsic mechanisms of thrombolysis, can be beneficial to left ventricular function and has been well documented within 24 hours of infarct initiation. However, spontaneous thrombolysis with reperfusion probably occurs in fewer than 10% of patients within the critical 3 to 4 hours after symptom onset.

It is uncertain whether thrombolysis or primary percutaneous transluminal coronary angioplasty (PTCA) is superior treatment for acute MI.[24, 25] The largest trial showed that primary PTCA was beneficial in reducing the composite end point of death, recurrent MI, or stroke, but that this benefit was attenuated at 6 months. Thus, primary PTCA may ultimately achieve a higher patency rate, but thrombolytic therapy may actually open more arteries very early (before 60 minutes). However, the risk for reocclusion is nearly twofold higher for patients receiving thrombolysis than for patients receiving primary PTCA.

Pathologic Basis of Thrombolysis

The effectiveness of thrombolytic therapy depends on its ability to lyse infarct artery thrombi and achieve reperfusion of myocardium served by the infarct-related artery. The pathologic basis is as follows: (1) untreated thrombotic occlusion of a coronary artery usually causes transmural infarction; (2) the extent of necrosis during an evolving MI occurs progressively over time and becomes complete only 6 hours or more after coronary occlusion; (3) the progression of myocardial ischemic injury can be modified by *reperfusion* (restoration of flow) to an ischemic area; (4) early reperfusion prevents necrosis of some jeopardized myocardium; and (5) both early and long-term mortality after acute MI correlate strongly with the amount of residual functioning myocardium.[8]

There is heterogeneity in the responsiveness of the cardiac myocytes most vulnerable to ischemic injury.[26–28] As the time of ischemia is prolonged, more and more myocytes show irreversible injury in a "wavefront" of necrosis that begins in the subendocardial area and progressively involves more of the midmyocardial and subepicardial zones. The progression is probably slower in humans owing to collaterals. If reperfusion occurs before the onset of irreversible injury of any cells (approximately 20–30 minutes), then all myocytes survive. In contrast, if reperfusion is accomplished after some irreversible injury, then the already necrotic myocytes are lost but salvage of myocytes that are only reversibly injured is nearly complete.

However, despite the potential for myocardial salvage by reperfusion of ischemic myocardium, the process of reperfusion, per se, may damage some myocytes that were not already dead when reflow occurred; this is called *reperfusion injury*.[29] The most likely mechanism for reperfusion injury is cell injury mediated by toxic oxygen species that are overproduced on restoration of oxygen supply to the tissues. These may arise in the myocytes themselves or in the polymorphonuclear leukocytes entering areas of ischemic injury during reperfusion.

Although most of the viable myocardium existing at the time of reflow ultimately recovers after alleviation of ischemia, critical abnormalities in cellular biochemistry and function of myocytes salvaged by reperfusion may persist for several days (*prolonged postischemic ventricular dysfunction,* or *stunned myocardium*).[27, 28, 30–32] The mechanisms of stunning are poorly understood, but decreased intracellular Ca^{2+} and/or decreased Ca^{2+} sensitivity of the contractile machinery are the most likely. Moreover, free radicals also perturb Ca^{2+} homeostasis (i.e., exogenous radical generation leads to cellular calcium overload).

Morphology

The gross and histologic appearance of a reperfused infarct is illustrated in Fig. 22-1. Because some vasculature injured during the period of ischemia becomes leaky on restoration of flow, clinical or experimental reperfusion is often accompanied by hemorrhage, which can be

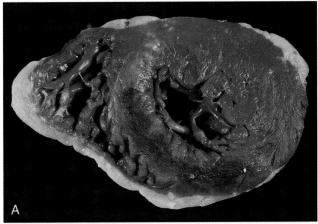

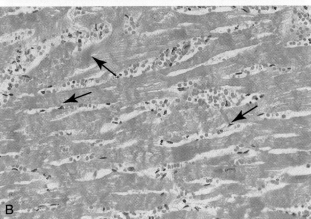

Figure 22-1 • Gross and microscopic appearance of myocardium modified by reperfusion. *A,* Large, densely hemorrhagic, anterior wall acute myocardial infarction from a patient with left anterior descending (LAD) artery thrombus treated with streptokinase intracoronary thrombolysis (triphenyl tetrazolium chloride [TTC]-stained heart slice making infarcted area is hemorrhagic and dark). *B,* Myocardial necrosis with hemorrhage and contraction bands, visible as dark bands spanning some myofibers (arrows). This is the characteristic appearance of markedly ischemic myocardium that has been reperfused (H & E stain). (Specimen in *A* oriented with posterior wall up.) (From Schoen FJ: The heart. In: Cotran RS, Kumar V, Collins T [eds]: Robbins Pathologic Basis of Disease, 6th ed. Philadelphia, WB Saunders, 1999, p 561)

apparent grossly, and patients with evolving infarction who receive thrombolysis often have massive hemorrhagic MI.[26–28, 33, 34] Injured myocytes show destruction of internal architecture with myofibril disruption and marked hypercontraction of some sarcomeres interspersed with sarcomeres that are torn apart (referred to as *necrosis with contraction bands* or *myofibrillar degeneration*[35]). Thus, reperfusion not only salvages reversibly injured cells but also alters the morphology of tissue with cells already lethally injured at the time of reflow. In animals, necrosis with contraction bands can be observed as early as 2 minutes of reperfusion after a prolonged period of ischemia (i.e., sufficient to cause irreversible injury).[36] The effects of reperfusion injury and hemorrhage on healing are largely unknown in humans.[37]

It is important to consider, however, that successful thrombolytic therapy reestablishes antegrade flow in the infarct-related coronary artery but does not reverse factors responsible for initiating the original thrombosis, such as advanced atherosclerotic plaque, acute intimal plaque rupture, superficial plaque erosion, enhanced platelet adhesiveness, or coronary spasm. Indeed, lysis of an offending thrombus at best restores the lesion to a condition of plaque disruption (most often). Thus, thrombolysis is not definitive therapy for chronic atherosclerosis or the acute plaque complication that initiated the infarct. A high-grade residual stenosis is likely to be associated with recurrent ischemic events, as evidenced by postinfarction angina or recurrent infarction. Thus, either balloon angioplasty or surgical revascularization during infarct evolution constitutes a more effective management of the underlying disease process than thrombolysis alone.

Complications

Failure to achieve successful pharmacologic thrombolysis may result from multiple anatomic factors related to the vascular pathophysiology that triggered the infarct. These include (1) geometric and compositional complexity of the culprit plaque, (2) intraplaque hemorrhage, (3) magnitude and accessibility of the thrombotic mass, (4) role in and proportion of platelets in the occluding thrombosis, (5) embolization of thrombotic and/or plaque fragments, (6) macro- and microvascular coronary spasm, and (7) coronary endothelial dysfunction.[8]

The most frequent and potentially the most serious complication of thrombolytic therapy is bleeding, with hemorrhage at sites of vascular puncture the most common (>70%) and intracranial hemorrhage (~1%) the most dreaded. The frequency varies with the clinical characteristics of the patient and the thrombolytic agent prescribed.[38] Hypotension occurs in approximately 10% and allergic reactions occur in approximately 2% of those receiving streptokinase.

Balloon Angioplasty

Catheter-based interventional techniques, of which PTCA is the prototype, represent a major therapeutic advance in the management of coronary artery disease. PTCA is widely used in patients with stable angina, un-

stable angina, or acute MI.[1, 24, 25, 39] According to the American Heart Association, over 400,000 of these procedures are presently done annually in the United States, at an average cost of approximately $20,000.[2]

The success rate for PTCA is currently greater than 90% with a complication rate of less than 5%.[39–41] Procedural failure rates have been reported at 4 to 8%.[42, 43]

Mechanisms of Luminal Expansion

The mechanisms of luminal expansion in coronary balloon angioplasty and its consequences have been characterized in animal models,[44] postmortem human hearts,[45] specimens obtained from patients who have undergone PTCA,[46] and by in vivo intravascular ultrasound.[47] Balloon dilation during angioplasty causes a radial force that induces an acute and complex arterial injury consisting of endothelial denudation, plaque fracture, intimal-medial separation accompanied by an intramural dissecting hematoma, and stretching of the media and adventitia.[48, 49] Waller postulated five possible mechanisms of luminal expansion: (1) plaque fracture, (2) medial dissection, (3) stretching of plaque-free arterial segments, (4) plaque stretching, and (5) plaque compression and redistribution (Table 22-1).[49]

In PTCA, the progressive and substantial expansile force induced by a balloon inflated at 8 to 12 atm of pressure causes the essentially nondistensible plaque to split at its weakest point. This site is not necessarily that most severely involved with atherosclerosis. The split extends at least to the intimal-medial border and often into the media, with consequent circumferential and longitudinal dissection of the media (Fig. 22-2).[48, 49] In essence, the plaque contents are redistributed. Dissimilar plaques respond differently to balloon dilation, and the composition and configuration of the original atherosclerotic lesion play a key role in the outcome of angioplasty.[50] Immediate success is probably enhanced in arteries having eccentric plaques with large lipid-rich necrotic cores and/or calcification, in contrast to concentric fibrotic lesions. For eccentric atheromas, balloon-induced splits most commonly involve the junction between the plaque and the disease-free portion of the arterial wall. Struc-

TABLE 22-1 • **Possible Mechanisms of Luminal Expansion in Balloon Angioplasty**

Mechanism	Clinicopathologic Correlation
Fracture of plaque	Major mechanism of expansion of lumen in complicated atherosclerotic plaque
Dissection into the media	Usually accompanies plaque fracture
Stretching of plaque-free segments	Largely reversible effect
Stretching of plaque	Most likely in eccentric lesions Minimal and largely reversible effect
Compression and redistribution of plaque	Does not usually account for significant long-term expansion of lumen

Modified from Schoen FJ: Interventional and Surgical Cardiovascular Pathology: Clinical Correlations and Basic Principles. Philadelphia, WB Saunders, 1989, p 74.

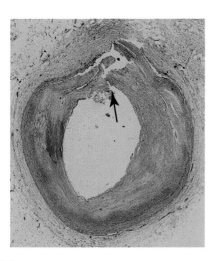

Figure 22-2 • Plaque fracture encompassing intima and media (arrow) and partial circumferential wall dissection induced by percutaneous coronary balloon angioplasty (PTCA). These features account for both the efficacy and potential complications of PTCA (Elastin stain). (From Schoen FJ: Blood vessels. In: Cotran RS, Kumar V, Collins T [eds]: Robbins Pathologic Basis of Disease, 6th ed. Philadelphia, WB Saunders, 1999, p 538)

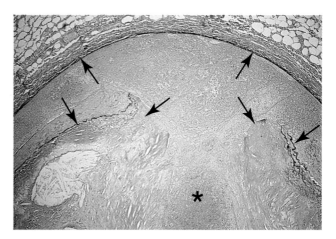

Figure 22-3 • Coronary lesion following angioplasty, demonstrating a plaque fracture region. New surfaces (arrows) have been generated by the process of angioplasty. They are highly thrombogenic and, indeed, have initiated early thrombosis in this case that involves both the original lumen (asterisk) and the new space created by the medial dissection (Elastin stain).

tural/stress analysis based on intravascular ultrasound imaging before balloon angioplasty can predict the location of plaque fracture that accompanies angioplasty.[51]

Thus, the key vascular consequences of angioplasty are plaque fracture, medial dissection, and stretching of the media beyond the dissection.[48, 49] These, in turn, are accompanied by local flow abnormalities and generation of new, thrombogenic blood-contacting surfaces (Fig. 22-3). This supports the concept that an atherosclerotic plaque after angioplasty has many features of a spontaneously disrupted plaque, namely those associated with the acute coronary syndromes. The immediate postangioplasty healing process in either arteries or bypass grafts is not well understood, but dissolution of soft atheromatous material, retraction of the split plaque, thrombus formation, and intimal healing with re-endothelialization likely contribute.

Complications

Major ischemic complications that prompt emergency bypass surgery occur in less than 1% of patients treated by PTCA.[52, 53] Features associated with increased risk for PTCA complications include advanced age, female gender, congestive heart failure or left ventricular dysfunction, recent thrombolytic therapy, and complex coronary lesional anatomy. Periprocedural myocardial infarction owing to side branch occlusion or embolization of thrombus, platelet aggregates, or plaque occurs in 5 to 20% of patients. The most important complications are abrupt closure (i.e., an early and sustained reduction of flow in the treated vessel) and restenosis (i.e., late loss of the acute luminal gain at the treated site).

Abrupt Closure

The incidence of abrupt closure after PTCA ranges from 4 to 9%, depending on precise definition and patient

risk factors, including unstable angina, diabetes, and chronic hemodialysis as well as target lesions that are long, angulated, calcified, or markedly (>80%) stenotic.[54, 55] The mechanisms of abrupt closure and therapeutic luminal expansion are related. For example, a dissection that involves a considerable portion of the circumference can generate a "flap" that may impinge on the lumen. Alternatively, a dissection that involves a substantial proximal-to-distal segment of the vessel, which traverses a large plaque-free wall segment, can induce compression of the vessel at a point of minimal disease (Fig. 22-4). Exposure of subendothelial vascular wall components (see Fig. 22-3), especially with the stasis engendered by medial flaps, induces platelet deposition and

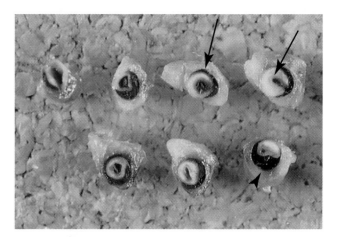

Figure 22-4 • Acute thrombotic occlusion of localized atherosclerotic coronary stenosis with extensive dissection extending both proximal and distal to plaque fracture of lesion (arrows), including and likely compressing a minimally stenotic distal vessel segment (arrowhead). (From Schoen FJ: Interventional and Surgical Cardiovascular Pathology: Clinical Correlations and Basic Principles. Philadelphia, WB Saunders, 1989, p 77)

activation with thrombin formation, often leading to obstructive thrombus. In a small number of patients, reduction in distal flow occurs without evidence of dissection or distal embolization. It is reversible with vasodilators, suggesting microvascular spasm as the cause.[56] Reduction in periprocedural adverse outcomes has occurred with the use of monoclonal antibody to the platelet glycoprotein IIb/IIIa receptor in some patients, but with increased risk of hemorrhage.[57, 58]

Late Restenosis

Restenosis accompanied by recurrent ischemic signs and symptoms limits the long-term success of angioplasty, particularly during the first year after PTCA, and dominates the late outcome. Proliferative restenosis is progressive, occurring over a period of months to years.[59, 60] Clinically significant restenosis occurs in approximately 30 to 40% of patients after coronary balloon angioplasty, most frequently within the first 4 to 6 months. Restenosis probably represents a fundamental but complex[61-63] vascular healing response that achieves clinical significance only in some patients. The risk of restenosis depends on definition used, patient population, and lesion complexity. For example, the long-term outcome is better among patients with single-vessel disease than those with multivessel disease. Many therapeutic approaches have been directed toward its prevention. Endovascular stents have reduced the frequency of this complication (see later). PTCA has also been used in coronary bypass grafts, but the late success rates are less than in native vessels.[64]

Although vessel wall recoil and organization of thrombus likely contribute, the major process leading to restenosis is excessive smooth muscle proliferation as a response to angioplasty-induced injury (Fig. 22-5). Medial smooth muscle cells migrate to the intima where, along with existing plaque smooth muscle cells, they proliferate and secrete abundant extracellular matrix, consisting predominantly of collagen and glycosaminoglycans. Early lesions have a loose myxoid matrix in which numerous stellate smooth muscle cells are haphazardly arranged

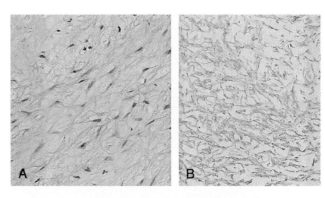

Figure 22-6 • Proliferative tissue causing occlusive restenosis several months after coronary balloon angioplasty and obtained by atherectomy. *A*, General morphology of the stellate mesenchymal cells haphazardly arranged in abundant loose myxoid matrix. *B*, Positive immunoperoxidase staining for α-smooth muscle cell actin demonstrating that these cells possess a smooth muscle cell phenotype (*A*, H&E stain; *B*, immunoperoxidase stain).

(Fig. 22-6). Over weeks to months, the extracellular matrix becomes more densely collagenous, and the neointima becomes less cellular, with scattered spindle-shaped cells in a more laminar arrangement. The process of restenosis has mechanistic similarities to both atherosclerosis and vascular graft healing described elsewhere (see later). Moreover, after prominent thrombus formation, or in a hyperlipidemic patient, the site of healing may also contain foam cells and lipid crystals, resembling a mature fibrofatty atheroma. There is considerable interest in locally delivered pharmacologic and molecular therapies to mitigate restenosis. However, despite there being efficacy of various approaches in animal models, success in humans has not yet been demonstrated.[65-68] In general, the largest acute luminal diameter safely possible provides better tolerance of subsequent intimal proliferation before hemodynamically significant renarrowing results at the treatment site.[69]

Atherectomy

In contrast to angioplasty, which effects a redistribution of atherosclerotic plaque constituents, atherectomy procedures, such as directional or rotational atherectomy, remove obstructive atherosclerotic tissue by excision or ablation.[70] The morphology of arterial vessel healing after transluminal plaque removal is similar to, but the rate of vascular complications is higher than, that after angioplasty.[71-73] Although restenosis is a limitation of directional atherectomy,[74] atherectomy techniques may permit a larger acute lumen than angioplasty, with potential benefit.[75] However, excisions deeper than an angiographically "normal" arterial lumen may occur.[76] Beyond therapeutic objectives, directional atherectomy obtains human tissue that may be used to investigate vascular pathobiology, including the mechanisms of restenosis and the effects of various pharmacologic or mechanical therapies or plaque ablation procedures.

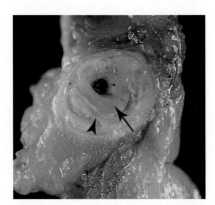

Figure 22-5 • Restenosis after balloon angioplasty. Gross photograph, demonstrating residual atherosclerotic plaque (arrowhead) and a new, glistening proliferative lesion (arrow). (From Schoen FJ: Blood vessels. In: Cotran RS, Kumar V, Collins T [eds]: Robbins Pathologic Basis of Disease, 6th ed. Philadelphia, WB Saunders, 1999, p 538)

Endoluminal Stents

As stated previously, balloon angioplasty alone is associated with rates of initial failure of 2 to 20%, early closure up to 15%, and restenosis of 40 to 50% (luminal diameter reduction of <50% compared with proximal reference segment) at 6 months. Recent studies suggest that as an adjunct to interventional procedures that manipulate plaque, metallic balloon-expandable and self-expanding intravascular stents may reverse the untoward effects of PTCA.[77–79] Intravascular stents could provide a larger and more regular lumen, initially acting as a scaffold to support the intimal flaps and dissections that occur in PTCA, limit elastic recoil, mechanically prevent vascular spasm, and increase blood flow, all of which could minimize thrombus formation and reduce the impact of postangioplasty restenosis.[80–82] Endoluminal stents also provide a means of delivering any localized therapy intended to reduce restenosis, such as a pharmacologic agent or radiation.

Stents are flexible endovascular prostheses usually fabricated from stainless steel alloys and designed as either coils or slotted tubes.[83] Stents are either expandable by a balloon or self-expanding. Mounted on a balloon catheter and with the aid of fluoroscopic screening and radiopaque markers, the stent is positioned across a stenotic lesion, which has usually been predilated with a balloon. Deployment involves expansion of the stent circumferentially in apposition to the endothelial surface of the coronary artery. Available stents range from 2.5 mm to 6 mm in diameter and from 8 mm to 50 mm in length. The proliferative restenosis that occurs after PTCA is not prevented by stenting, and the tissue between the stent and the blood *(neointima)* may progressively thicken. Important questions remain relative to determinants of healing and the potential for late complications of endovascular stents, such as migration, perforation, or infection.

Nevertheless, prospective randomized controlled trials comparing conventional coronary balloon angioplasty with stent implantation in patients with stable and unstable angina who had a single, de novo, focal stenosis in a large (>3 mm diameter) native coronary artery demonstrate clinical benefit to stenting. In one study, significantly fewer patients in the stent group than in the PTCA group—20% versus 30%, respectively—suffered the primary clinical end point (a composite of death, MI, cerebrovascular accident, coronary artery bypass grafting [CABG], or repeat PTCA).[84] In another study, the primary end point of angiographic restenosis at 6 months was significantly reduced in the stent group compared with the PTCA group—32% versus 42%.[85] Less impressive differences were found in patients with bypass graft disease.[86] Other studies also show superior rates of 6-month cardiac event–free survival (i.e., absence of death, reinfarction, or target vessel revascularization) for primary stenting compared with primary PTCA.[87, 88]

Complications

The complications and limitations of stenting include initial failure, early thrombosis (Fig. 22-7), and late restenosis. Subacute stent thrombosis occurs in 1 to 3% of patients, usually within 7 to 10 days of the procedure, and results in occlusion of the stented vessel with platelet-rich thrombus and associated MI or death. Antiplatelet treatment minimizes the risk of subacute stent thrombosis.[89] Attempts to reduce within-stent restenosis include evaluation of intracoronary radiotherapy using catheter-based γ radiation,[90] radioactive stents, the delivery of recombinant vascular endothelial growth factor with a balloon catheter to speed endothelialization of a stent,[91] gene therapy, and local drug delivery.[92, 93]

Pathologic Findings in Humans

The histologic changes induced in human atherosclerotic coronary arteries by a wide variety of commercial stents have been described.[94–98] In general, implantation is accompanied by damage to the endothelial lining and stretching of the vessel wall, stimulating early adherence and accumulation of platelets and leukocytes. Stent

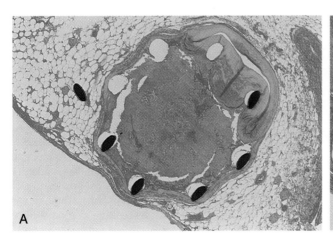
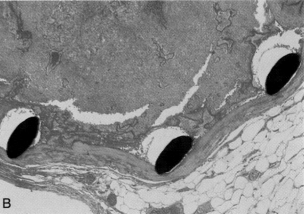

Figure 22-7 • Early thrombosis associated with a metallic coronary stent. *A,* Low-power view of occluded vessel and stent. *B,* Close-up showing interaction of stent wires with the atherosclerotic arterial wall and overlying thrombus, with several stent wire profiles (black), can be identified in both illustrations. (*A* and *B,* H&E stain.)

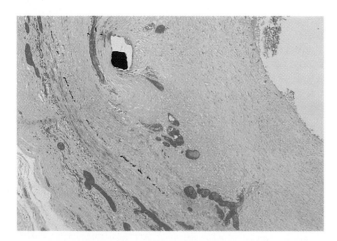

Figure 22-8 • Coronary arterial metallic stent implanted long term, demonstrating thickened proliferative neointima separating the stent wires (one shown as black structure) from the lumen (Movat stain).

wires are initially covered with a variable platelet-fibrin coating. They may eventually become completely covered by a neointima, whereby the wires are embedded in a layer of intimal thickening consisting of α-actin positive smooth muscle cells in a collagenous matrix, in some cases with foam cells, extracellular lipid and lipid crystals predominantly near the stent wires (Fig. 22-8).[92–101] Ultimately, there is a neointima lined by endothelium. Most stent struts are in direct contact with atherosclerotic plaque; in some cases, medial damage is associated with struts.

One study reported findings in 55 stents at a mean of 39 days after implantation, and in 10 patients later than 30 days.[98] Fibrin, platelets, and neutrophils were associated with stent struts early after deployment. In stents implanted 3 days or less, inflammatory cells were sparse when associated with struts in contact with fibrous plaque but were prominent with struts embedded in either lipid core or damaged media. Neointimal growth in stents implanted longer than 30 days was greatest at strut sites when medial laceration or rupture was present compared with struts in contact with plaque or with an intact media. Medial destruction and lipid core penetration increased inflammation, and neointimal growth increased as the ratio of stent area to reference lumen area increased. The presence of increased inflammation associated with stent struts in the vicinity of damaged media and increased neointimal thickness at struts associated with medial damage suggests that deployment strategies that reduce severe arterial injury during catheter-based interventions with stents may have a beneficial effect by lowering the frequency of in-stent restenosis.

Coronary Artery Bypass Graft Surgery

With 600,000 CABG operations per year in the United States, CABG remains one of the most frequently performed surgical procedures throughout the world and accounts for more resources expended in cardiovascular medicine than any other single procedure.[112] According to the American Heart Association, the average cost is approximately $45,000. The most frequent indication for CABG is chronic stable angina (48% of those undergoing bypass surgery in the United States and 61% of those in Canada), although many candidates have unstable angina or acute MI.

Operative mortality for CABG is approximately 3%.[112, 113] The most consistent predictors of mortality after coronary artery surgery are urgency of operation, age, prior heart surgery, female sex, left ventricular ejection fraction, percent stenosis of the left main coronary artery, and number of major coronary arteries with significant stenoses, with the first three factors of greatest importance. Additional variables augmenting short-term mortality risk include preceding coronary angioplasty during the admission in which surgery was done, recent MI, history of angina, ventricular arrhythmias, congestive heart failure, or mitral regurgitation, and comorbidities such as diabetes, cerebrovascular disease, peripheral vascular disease, chronic obstructive pulmonary disease, or renal dysfunction.

Major relief of angina pectoris occurs in more than 90% of appropriately selected patients after CABG.[114] Approximately three quarters of patients are free from ischemic events, sudden death, occurrence of MI, or return of angina for 5 years, nearly half for at least 10 years, and 15% by 15 years.[115] The reoperation rate for recurrence of symptoms is in the range of 6 to 8% per year. Symptomatic improvement is best maintained in patients with the most complete revascularization.

Meta-analyses have compared randomized trials of CABG versus medical therapy or balloon angioplasty.[113, 116] In one study, the CABG group had significantly lower mortality and morbidity than the medical group at 5 and 10 years (39% and 17% risk reductions, respectively[113]). In all comparisons, however, the benefit of surgery was greatest in the highest risk patients, that is, those with the most advanced disease, as defined by severity of ischemia, number of diseased vessels and presence of left ventricular dysfunction.[113, 116] For example, the risk reduction for patients with left main coronary artery disease was 68% and 33% at 5 and 10 years, respectively.[113] In contrast, in low and moderate risk patients, medical therapy or PTCA had results comparable to those of CABG.

Current clinical practice has been shaped by three major randomized trials into which patients were enrolled during the 1970s—The Veterans Administration (VA) study, European Cardiac Society Study (ECSS), and the National Institutes of Health–supported Coronary Artery Surgery Study (CASS)[117–124]—as well as several smaller trials. Relative to medical treatment, patients undergoing coronary bypass surgery had a significantly lower mortality at up to 10 years, but by that time 41% of the patients initially randomized to medical treatment had undergone CABG. The advantage for surgery was greatest in patients with left main coronary artery disease and stenosis of the proximal left anterior descending coronary artery, as well as the otherwise most ill patients (based on the severity of symptoms or ischemia, age, the number of vessels diseased, and the presence of left ventricular dysfunction).[120] Nevertheless, the likelihood of occurrence of

MI after 5 to 10 years of follow-up was similar in medically and surgically treated patients,[120–122] and congestive heart failure remains a powerful predictor of perioperative mortality and a poorer long-term outcome.[118, 123]

At least 10% of coronary artery procedures are now reoperations. The indications for reoperation include progression of atherosclerosis in native vessels, incomplete revascularization at the first operation, and both early and late graft failure. Operative mortality rates for reoperations are up to two to three times higher than that of the initial procedure and range from 2 to 10%.[124] The clinical results after reoperation are not as good as those after a primary procedure. By 5 years after reoperation surgery, approximately half of the patients have recurrent symptoms. However, late survival results are excellent, with 90% survival at 5 years and 75% at 10 years.

Mechanism of Efficacy

The mechanism of improved survival and left ventricular function after CABG is the reperfusion of viable but noncontractile or poorly contracting *hibernating* myocardium.[125, 126] Indeed, hypokinetic (and even akinetic) areas of the ventricular wall are composed entirely or in part of viable, hibernating myocardium or of a mixture of the latter and fibrous scar. Symptoms resulting from chronic left ventricular dysfunction may be inappropriately ascribed to myocardial necrosis and scarring when the symptoms may, in fact, be reversed when the chronic ischemia is relieved by coronary revascularization.

A major challenge in noninvasive diagnostic cardiology is the identification of viable but poorly contractile or noncontractile myocardium with potentially reversible dysfunction. Positron emission tomography has a positive predictive value of 78 to 85% and a negative predictive value of 78 to 92%.[127–129] Other useful techniques are thallium-201 scintigraphy, dobutamine echocardiography, myocardial contrast echocardiography, and contrast-enhanced MRI.[130]

In selected patients, PTCA is as effective as bypass surgery.[131] The early benefit of PTCA over medical treatment particularly applies to patients with severe angina and single-vessel coronary artery disease at baseline. This benefit, however, diminishes during long-term follow-up and in patients with multivessel coronary artery disease, partly because repeat revascularization is required for restenosis.[132, 133] Moreover, although the extent of revascularization achieved by bypass surgery is generally higher than with angioplasty, the outcomes for individuals who have had bypass surgery and medical therapy (including PTCA) converge after 10 to 12 years of follow-up, owing to progression of both native coronary disease and graft disease over time in surgical patients.

Complications

Overall mortality for elective first bypass procedures in the United States from 1980 to 1990 was 2.2% in 58,384 patients in the Society of Thoracic Surgeons database.[134] More recently, there may have been a slight overall increase in morbidity and mortality, reflecting the tendency to treat an older and sicker population of patients, in which a greater proportion have unstable angina, three-vessel disease, prior coronary revascularization with either coronary bypass surgery or PTCA, left ventricular dysfunction, and comorbid conditions, including hypertension, diabetes, and peripheral vascular disease. Many series have demonstrated a markedly higher perioperative morbidity (including MI, respiratory failure, and stroke) and mortality in coronary surgery in women than in men. Nevertheless, late survival is similar in men and women, but the relief of anginal symptoms confirmed by CABG appears to be less in women.[135–138] Coronary bypass surgery is now being carried out in increasing numbers of patients with multivessel coronary disease and either mild to moderate symptoms, left ventricular dysfunction, or poor exercise tolerance, because of the improved survival noted in these groups.

Approximately 6% of patients after bypass surgery have either major focal neurologic deficits, stupor or coma (seen particularly in patients with proximal aortic atherosclerosis, prior neurologic disease, intra-aortic balloon pump, diabetes, hypertension, unstable angina, and increased age), or perceptible deterioration in intellectual function. Deep sternal wound infection occurs in 1 to 4% of patients after bypass surgery and carries a mortality of approximately 25%. Predictors of this complication include obesity, reoperation, grafting using both internal mammary arteries (IMAs), duration and complexity of surgery, and diabetes. Postoperative renal dysfunction occurs in as many as 8% of patients; mortality among patients who develop postoperative renal dysfunction is 19%.

Pathologic Considerations

Myocardial Damage

Superior methods of myocardial preservation have been largely responsible for reducing the overall operative mortality rate of coronary bypass surgery. Clinically identifiable perioperative MI occurs in a few percent of patients undergoing aortocoronary bypass, although a somewhat larger number of patients have elevated creatine phosphokinase (CPK)-MB isoenzymes on the first postoperative day.

Acute cardiac failure is the most common mode of early death after CABG. In a combined Brigham and Women's Hospital/Massachusetts General Hospital autopsy study of 96 postoperative deaths less than 30 days after bypass operations, the causes of death included myocardial necrosis (57%), miscellaneous operative and systemic complications (25%), nonanatomic cause (10%), and technical factors (7%) (Table 22-2).[139] In 45 of the 55 patients dying 4 days or less postoperatively, the cause of death was clearly cardiac (either myocardial necrosis or cardiac decompensation without any demonstrable anatomic lesion sufficient to account for the profound cardiac failure). Fifty-three of all patients had myocardial necrosis histologically consistent with a perioperative onset; in 28, this lesion contributed heavily to the unfavorable outcome. Contraction bands were prominent in 25 patients, suggesting that ischemic injury with reperfusion was con-

TABLE 22-2 • **Causes of Early Death Following Aortocoronary Bypass**

	Number of Patients*		
Cause of Death	*0–4 Days Postoperative*	*5–30 Days Postoperative*	*Total No.*
No anatomic lesions†			
Pump failure in OR	4	NA	4
Low cardiac output	2	1	3
Sudden death	0	3	3
Myocardial necrosis†	39 (71%)	16 (39%)	55 (57%)
Technical mishap	4 (7%)	3 (7%)	7 (7%)
Pulmonary/renal/GI/CVA	3 (5%)	14 (34%)	17 (18%)
Other	3	4	7
Total	55	41	96

* Numbers in parentheses are percentage of all patients in group with specific cause of death.
† Mode of death was cardiac failure or arrhythmia.
OR, operating room; NA, not applicable; GI, gastrointestinal hemorrhage; CVA, cerebrovascular accident.
Modified from Schoen FJ: Interventional and Surgical Cardiovascular Pathology: Clinical Correlations and Basic Principles. Philadelphia, WB Saunders, 1989, p 83.

tributory. Thus, myocardial necrosis, most frequently perioperative, is associated with most early deaths after CABG, but necrosis is not always present in patients dying of low output failure.

Although *early cardiac failure* with low output or arrhythmias after uncomplicated CABG surgery occurs infrequently, the causes are unclear in many cases. Many such patients have no detectable myocardial necrosis, either clinically or at autopsy. In others, the extent of necrosis noted at autopsy seems insufficient to account for the profound ventricular dysfunction encountered clinically; possible explanations include (1) evolving myocardial necrosis either undetectable clinically or too recent to detect at autopsy,[140] (2) postischemic dysfunction of viable myocardium, for which no morphologic markers of the dysfunctional state are known, or (3) a metabolic cause, such as hypokalemia, for which there is no morphologic counterpart. Thus, although established myocardial necrosis causes cardiac dysfunction in many patients with postoperative failure, it may not be the predominant lesion or the cause or death. However, when such necrosis is detected at autopsy, it may be presumed that adjacent myocardium was biochemically and functionally (but not morphologically) deranged.

As in cardiac surgery in general, perioperative MI is more likely to occur in patients with cardiomegaly. Although perioperative infarction clearly adversely affects early prognosis, it probably has a minor role in the long-term prognosis of patients surviving the early postoperative interval.[141]

Most CABG surgery uses as grafts (1) saphenous veins excised from the patient's leg(s) (the vein segment is reversed [to obviate valves] and attached to both the proximal aorta and the coronary artery anastomosed to a site distal to an obstructive atherosclerotic lesion) and/or (2) the IMA, whose distal end is dissected free from the internal chest wall on a vascularized pedicle and is subsequently attached to the distal coronary artery. The proximal end retains its native attachment to the subclavian artery. IMA grafts have some advantages over saphenous vein grafts. (3) Recently the radial artery has been used more frequently as a conduit for coronary bypass surgery.

In general, graft patency deteriorates with time due to intrinsic and progressive pathologic changes, and acceler-

ated changes of atherosclerosis may develop in bypass vessels, especially saphenous veins.[142] The 5-year patency of coronary artery–vein bypass grafts is 74%, and at 10 years, just 41%; in contrast, patency of the IMA implanted into the left anterior descending coronary artery is as high as 83 to 90% at 10 years.

Saphenous Vein Grafts

The saphenous vein is used mainly for distal branches of the right and circumflex coronary arteries and for sequential grafts to these vessels and diagonal branches. Five-year patency appears to be in the range of 85%. The long-term patency of saphenous vein grafts is 75% at 5 years, 50 to 60% or less at 10 years, owing to pathologic changes, including thrombosis (early), intimal thickening (several months to several years postoperatively), and graft atherosclerosis (years).[143, 144] These may be associated with superimposed plaque rupture, thrombi, or aneurysms (usually more than 2 to 3 years postoperatively).

There are several phases of disease development in venous aortocoronary artery bypass grafts. Early occlusion (before hospital discharge) occurs in 8 to 12%, and by 1 year 15 to 30% of vein grafts have become occluded. The occlusion rate is high in the first year. After that period, the annual occlusion rate is 2% per year and rises to approximately 4% per year between years 6 and 10. Between 6 and 10 years after operation, the attrition rate for grafts increases again. At 10 years, approximately one third that were patent at 1 year have become occluded, one third demonstrate significant atherosclerosis, and one third appear to be unchanged.

Early thrombotic occlusion occurs in approximately 15% of grafts, and the clinical and autopsy incidences of early graft occlusion are not widely different (Fig. 22-9).[142] Graft thromboses account for only a minority of early cardiac deaths; most patients who die early have patent grafts.[145] Moreover, graft occlusions frequently do not account for early postoperative myocardial necrosis, which occurs most often in regions perfused by patent grafts. Perioperative infarction is usually caused by either hypotensive episodes during anesthesia induction or inadequate intraoperative regional preservation due to severe obstruction of the feeding artery and poor collaterals followed by reperfusion. Such necrosis usually predominates

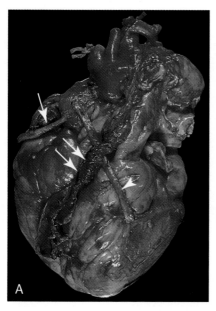

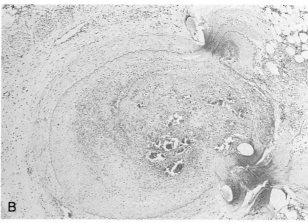

Figure 22-9 • Early thrombotic occlusion of saphenous vein coronary artery bypass graft. *A*, Gross photograph of heart. The graft to the posterior descending artery (arrow) in this frontal view is occluded. An internal mammary artery graft to the left anterior descending (double arrows) and a saphenous vein graft to the obtuse marginal branch of the left circumflex artery (arrowhead) are patent. *B*, Low-power histologic view of thrombosed distal anastomosis of coronary artery bypass graft, the location of most early graft thromboses. Several blue suture profiles can be identified. (H&E stain.)

in the subendocardium and often has the morphology of necrosis with contraction bands.

Factors in the acute occlusion of aortocoronary bypass grafts (with or without superimposed thrombus) include anastomotic compression by atherosclerosis, suboptimal insertion site, poor distal runoff, graft or native vessel mural dissection at the anastomotic site, and distortion of a graft that is too short or too long for the intended bypass. In some cases, thrombosis occurring early postoperatively involves only the distal portion of the graft, suggesting that early graft thrombosis is most frequently initiated at the distal anastomosis. Inadequate distal runoff in extremely small distal native coronaries, frequently further compromised by partial atherosclerotic occlusions, accounts for the major cause of early graft thrombosis.

Technical factors that may cause thrombotic closure at the proximal or distal anastomoses include kinking due to excessive length, tension due to insufficient length, poor graft flow, and inadequate distal runoff. Atheroma at the arteriotomy site may predispose to early thrombotic occlusion. Interruption of the nutrient blood flow to the vein wall may also be involved. Histologic studies of grafts that occlude within 1 year often show either substantial thrombosis with minimal intimal-medial changes or marked intimal hyperplasia or superimposed thrombus.[144, 146] Nearly all grafts examined after a year or more have at least some intimal hyperplasia (Fig. 22-10).

By 10 years, nearly one half of venous grafts patent at 5 years have occluded.[143, 147] Beyond the first year, particularly after 3 to 5 years, the histologic appearance of occluded or obstructed coronary bypass grafts is consistent with atherosclerosis analogous to disease in native coronary arteries, the plaques may rupture and precipitate thrombosis. Marked friability of the atherosclerotic lesions

may cause intermittent coronary embolization, which complicates revascularization procedures, such as reoperation or PTCA of vein grafts.[148] Disease progression, defined as a worsening of a preexisting lesion or appearance of a new diameter narrowing of 50% or greater, can occur at a rate of 20 to 40% over 5 to 10 years in nongrafted native vessels. Disease progression is also greater in arteries with patent grafts than in arteries with occluded grafts and usually occurs proximal to the site of graft insertion.[149-151]

Internal Mammary Artery

In contrast to saphenous veins, IMAs have a greater than 90% patency rate at 10 years.[152] Compared with

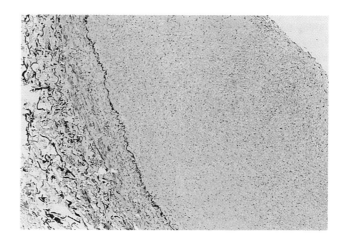

Figure 22-10 • Intimal hyperplasia of saphenous vein coronary artery bypass graft. Residual lumen is at upper right (Movat stain).

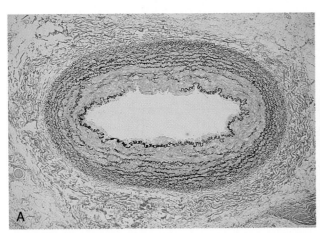
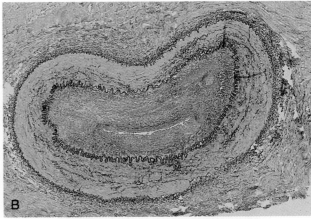

Figure 22-11 • Internal mammary arteries as coronary artery bypass grafts. *A,* Internal mammary graft after long-term implantation of 13 years, demonstrating nearly normal structure with preservation of the elastic arterial media. *B,* Internal mammary artery from another patient subsequent to long-term function, demonstrating marked stenosis by proliferative intimal hyperplasia (*A* and *B,* Elastin stain).

saphenous vein grafts, the pathology is markedly diminished, although occlusions occur owing to intimal proliferation or atherosclerosis (Fig. 22-11). Thus, routine use of the left IMA for left anterior descending coronary artery grafting with supplemental saphenous vein grafts to other coronary lesions is generally accepted as a standard grafting method. The use of bilateral IMAs appears to be safe and efficacious, although there is a higher rate of deep sternal wound infection when both IMAs are used.

Multiple factors likely contribute to the remarkably higher long-term patency of IMA grafts compared with vein grafts. During autotransplantation, free saphenous vein grafts sustain not only disruption of their vasa vasora but also endothelial damage, medial ischemia, and acutely increased internal pressure.[153] In contrast, the IMA generally has minimal preexisting atherosclerosis, requires minimal surgical manipulation, maintains its nutrient blood supply, is accustomed to arterial pressures, needs no proximal anastomosis, and has an artery-to-artery distal anastomosis. The sizes of graft and recipient vessel are comparable with the IMA but disparate (graft substantially larger) with a saphenous vein graft. As another distinguishing feature, the IMA is an elastic artery, whereas coronary arteries are muscular. The media of the artery may derive nourishment from the lumen as well as from the vasa vasorum, and the internal elastic lamina of the IMA is uniform. Moreover, the finding that the endothelium of the IMA produces significantly more prostacyclin than the saphenous vein may explain why endothelium-dependent relaxation is more pronounced, which may allow flow-dependent autoregulation to occur.[154] Patients receiving the IMA graft have a decreased risk of late death, MI, cardiac events, and reoperations, and this clinical advantage persists for up to 20 years.

Late Symptom Recurrence

Both progression of obstructive atherosclerosis in non-bypassed coronary artery segments and graft obstruction are major factors in *late symptom recurrence.* As in the coronary arteries, atherosclerosis in aortocoronary bypass grafts can cause myocardial ischemia through progressive luminal stenosis or plaque rupture with secondary throm-

botic obstruction. The potential for disruption and embolization of atherosclerotic lesions in vein grafts exceeds that for native coronary atherosclerotic lesions. Plaques in grafts generally involve dilated segments, often have poorly developed fibrous caps, have large necrotic cores, and develop secondary dystrophic calcific deposits that may be adjacent to the lumen rather than deep to the surface as in typical native arterial atherosclerosis (Fig. 22-12). Finally, because of the large size of the affected graft relative to the coronary artery to which it is anastomosed, atheroembolization is likely to be widespread, often with catastrophic results; balloon angioplasty or intraoperative manipulation of grafts may stimulate athero-

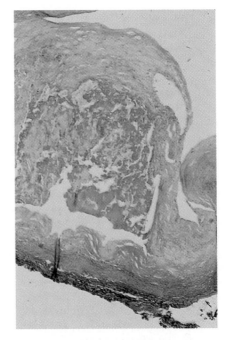

Figure 22-12 • Atherosclerotic plaque in a saphenous vein coronary artery bypass graft, demonstrating a poorly developed fibrous cap and large necrotic core, with calcification. Lumen is at upper right (Elastin stain).

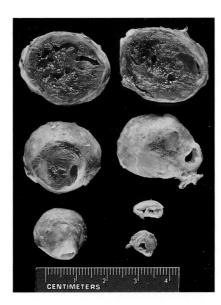

Figure 22-13 • Aneurysm in long-term atherosclerotic saphenous vein coronary artery bypass graft. (From Liang BT, Antman EM, Taus R, et al: Atherosclerotic aneurysms of aortocoronary vein grafts. Am J Cardiol 61:185, 1988)

embolism.[155] Aneurysms of saphenous vein grafts may also occur (Fig. 22-13).

Transmyocardial Revascularization

Transmyocardial revascularization (TMR) is a surgical procedure that uses a laser to create transmural channels through the myocardial wall to the left ventricular chamber intended to enhance intramyocardial perfusion. This therapy may be an attractive alternative for a subset of patients having coronary artery disease with intractable angina who are refractory to medical therapy but not candidates for direct revascularization procedures such as CABG or PTCA. Candidates often have diffuse or small vessel atherosclerosis or lack of distal targets, are poor surgical risks, and are unacceptable cardiac transplant candidates.

TMR is based on the hypothesis that myocardial sinusoids comprise a vascular network that could communicate between the ventricular chambers and the coronary arteries.[156] The concept of myocardial sinusoids is supported by extrapolation to more primitive vertebrate hearts such as the single-chambered hearts of hagfish and lampreys,[157] and reptilian hearts such as those of the crocodile, snake, and alligator.[158] In these reptiles, it has been postulated that the myocardium receives a substantial supply of blood directly via a meshwork of branching vessels that communicate with and are filled from the ventricular cavity and not from epicardial vessels. However, to what extent such a vascular network exists and is functional in the human heart is controversial. Nevertheless, in patients with pulmonary atresia and intact ventricular septum, proximal obstruction of the coronary arteries can result in a lumen-dependent perfusion of the myocardium.[159]

Clinical trials of TMR have showed encouraging results, although there is controversy about the mechanism of action.[160-166] Surgical studies using a CO_2 laser or holmium:yttrium-aluminum-garnet (YAG) laser have consistently demonstrated a marked reduction in anginal symptoms and, in most cases, an improvement in exercise tolerance and quality of life.[167]

Lasers Used in Transmyocardial Revascularization

Energy from a laser (an acronym for **l**ight **a**mplification by **s**timulated **e**mission of **r**adiation) differs from ordinary light in that all laser photons have the same wavelength and are coherent (spatially and temporally in phase). Early CO_2 lasers available for clinical use had only 80 watts of power and required at least one full cardiac cycle to complete creation of a transmyocardial channel. Therefore, the heart had to be stationary during channel creation. This limitation generally made it necessary to perform the procedure under conditions of ischemic arrest. Three types of lasers are currently used. The 1000-watt CO_2 laser (PLC Medical Systems, Franklin, MA), was recently approved by the US Food and Drug Administration for clinical use. Transmyocardial channels can be created in approximately 40 msec, fast enough to successfully make transmural channels in a beating heart. Introduced through a left anterolateral thoracotomy incision, the laser is placed against the epicardium and fired, with release triggered to the R wave of the electrocardiogram (ECG) to minimize arrhythmogenic activity.

The recently introduced holmium:YAG laser offers some advantages over the CO_2 laser; it is adaptable to a percutaneous approach using a fiberoptic system, uses a flexible probe, and can be manipulated along the ventricular contours. The energy is delivered as a pulsed triple burst of 350 μsec, at an output wavelength of 2.1 μm with an output of 2.0 joules. Like the CO_2 system it is also triggered by the ECG and water vaporization.[168]

CO_2 and holmium:YAG lasers emit infrared energy and rely on thermal ablation to produce intramyocardial channels. In contrast, excimer lasers operate in the deep ultraviolet spectrum and are therefore cold; they produce tissue ablation by dissociating molecular bonds (called photoablation), and incur less collateral damage. Nevertheless, to what extent thermal or more extensive tissue damage is detrimental or beneficial is unknown.

The wavelengths proposed for clinical TMR include the CO_2 laser (wavelength = 10.6 μm), holmium:YAG (wavelength = 2.1 μm), and excimer (wavelength = 193, 248 or 308 nm)[169] lasers. Percutaneous myocardial revascularization using a catheter-based holmium:YAG laser may be able to create nontransmural endocardial channels smaller in size but comparable in the tissue effect with surgical TMR.[170-173]

Pathologic Considerations

The histopathologic changes seen in TMR are similar for both CO_2 and holmium:YAG lasers, with minor quantitative differences in the size of the channel lumens and the amount of thermal injury to the adjacent myocytes.[174] Intramyocardial channels generated by TMR initially have a central region of vaporized myocardium surrounded by a thin rim of necrosis due to thermal damage.[175] Acute changes (within 24 hours) typically consist of circular to elliptic channels with a lumen filled to varying degrees

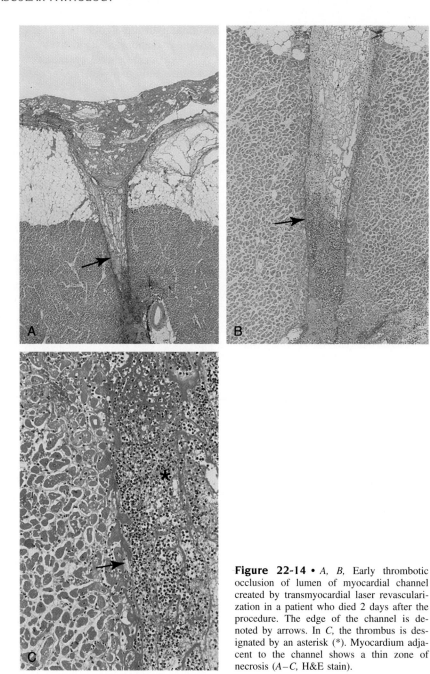

Figure 22-14 • *A, B,* Early thrombotic occlusion of lumen of myocardial channel created by transmyocardial laser revascularization in a patient who died 2 days after the procedure. The edge of the channel is denoted by arrows. In *C*, the thrombus is designated by an asterisk (*). Myocardium adjacent to the channel shows a thin zone of necrosis (*A–C*, H&E stain).

with thrombus composed of blood and fibrin (Fig. 22-14). This is surrounded by a zone of thermocoagulated myocytes with contraction bands, well demarcated from the adjacent normal myocytes.

It is perhaps not surprising that the new channels occlude in most cases. Thermal coagulation of muscle and exposure of interstitial connective tissue by channel-making creates a thrombogenic surface. In a patient who died 2 hours after treatment with a CO_2 laser, each of the 15 channels made were still open and no fibrin thrombi were seen.[176] However, we and most other observers have found that in the period from 1 to 10 days after treatment, the channels become occluded by a mixture of fibrin, platelets, polymorphonuclear leukocytes, macrophages, and foreign body giant cells.[177–180]

At 2 to 3 weeks, the epicardial lesions are difficult to identify macroscopically and often appear as pinpoint depressions on the epicardial surface. The channels usually are filled with loosely arranged granulation tissue rich in capillaries and small muscular arterioles embedded within the connective tissue matrix (Fig. 22-15). Well-formed scars are noted by 6 weeks, and both the scar size and its vascularity are reduced.

Mechanisms

The mechanism accounting for the clinical benefit of TMR remains unknown and is controversial.[181, 182] The initial hypothesis considered direct myocardial perfusion from the ventricular chamber through new penetrat-

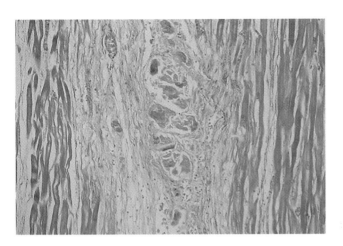

Figure 22-15 • Organizing thrombus in channel 18 days after transmyocardial laser revascularization (Masson trichrome stain).

ing and branching channels.[183, 184] Although blood flows through channels immediately after they are made, as demonstrated by the pulsatile spurts of blood that frequently come from epicardial channel openings, a clot soon forms at the epicardial surface. Early claims of prolonged channel patency and resultant direct transmyocardial blood flow[185–188] have mainly been refuted.[189–195] Indeed, more intensive clinical and animal studies, including canine, porcine, and ovine models in both acute and chronic ischemic injury have not demonstrated concomitant long-term patency of the channels.[196–198]

The current hypothesis suggests that TMR stimulates angiogenesis.[181, 182, 199] Myocardial injury arising from thermal, mechanical, and photochemical effects triggers the normal inflammatory responses that result in the formation of new vessels in granulation tissue. Preclinical studies have shown that vascular growth (angiogenesis) after TMR can increase blood reserve by about 30%,[198–200] which may potentially improve symptoms. Additionally, growth of existing vessels is thought to be due to the inflammation occurring in response to the injury around the original laser channels.[201] A third possible mechanism of action of TMR may be denervation of the heart. Myocardial denervation has been seen in laboratory animals.[202] Canine studies using an epicardial transmural laser method resulted in complete denervation by elimination of visceral afferent nerve function,[203] but a percutaneous, nontransmural approach only partially denervates the heart.[204] Less likely mechanisms include a placebo effect of the procedure and the accumulated effect of multiple small myocardial infarcts created by TMR.

Experimental studies in normal and ischemic canine, porcine, and ovine models demonstrate that myocardial laser injury leads to an increase in the density of arterial vessels within and adjacent to channels.[190, 198, 205] In contrast, Whittaker and coworkers found no increase in capillary density 2 months after TMR.[206] The available evidence, therefore, suggests that TMR-induced angiogenesis is likely a nonspecific response of the myocardium to injury and the mechanism of potential clinical importance.[181, 182, 199] Nevertheless, most investigators have not

demonstrated an increase in regional myocardial blood flow after TMR.

Current and future investigation is directed at a clearer elucidation of the mechanism(s) of action of TMR and clinical indications for use. Possible risks include ventricular perforation, pericardial effusion and tamponade, and ventricular septal perforation. The application of angiogenic gene therapy to TMR offers new areas of investigation and possible therapeutic directions.[207] With this proposed mechanism, further stimulation of angiogenesis should be beneficial. Sayeed-Shah and associates recently demonstrated complete reversal of ischemic wall motion abnormalities by combining TMR with the direct injection of an expression plasmid encoding vascular endothelial growth factor (VEGF).[208]

PERIPHERAL VASCULAR REPLACEMENT AND RECONSTRUCTION

Coronary heart disease is the most frequent source of both early and late mortality and morbidity of patients undergoing vascular reconstruction.[48] The mortality rate for elective AAA repair, with or without aortobifemoral reconstruction or infrainguinal arterial reconstruction, is approximately 2 to 5%. MI is the principal cause of early death.

The low early mortality of vascular surgery contrasts with high late death rates; with approximately 50% of patients alive 5 years postoperatively. Almost all late deaths are related to complications of advanced generalized atherosclerosis, chiefly MI.[209] The Framingham Study documented an incidence of coronary artery disease two to five times higher and an increased incidence of cerebrovascular and hypertensive disease in patients with claudication than in those without.[210] Another study demonstrated that approximately 30% of all patients scheduled for aortic aneurysm resection, lower extremity revascularization, or carotid endarterectomy have severe coronary artery disease that warrants myocardial revascularization or is already inoperable.[211] The most significant preoperative risk factor associated with subsequent cardiac mortality and morbidity is a prior history of MI. Some studies suggest that patients operated for peripheral vascular disease have a risk as high as 30% for perioperative reinfarction or cardiac death within 3 months after MI; the risk declines to only 5% 6 months after the infarct. Other studies suggest a protective effect of aortocoronary bypass for patients with obstructive coronary artery disease who undergo elective vascular surgery.

Vascular Graft Pathology

The performance of polyethylene terephthalate (Dacron) grafts in current use is reasonably satisfactory in large-diameter, high-flow, low-resistance locations such as the aorta and the iliac and proximal femoral arteries. In contrast, small-diameter vascular grafts (<6 to 8 mm in diameter) generally perform less well.[48, 212] Expanded polytetrafluorethylene grafts (ePTFE) and autologous saphenous veins are the most widely used small vessel replacements.

Dependence of Patency on Implant Location, Graft Type, and Other Factors

The behavior of prosthetic vascular grafts depends on location, largely related to diameter (and thereby flow rates), with smaller recipient vessels having less favorable short- and long-term patency rates.[48] Aortic interposition grafts rarely occlude. For aortofemoral bypass with fabric grafts, the expected patency is 85% at 5 years, 70% at 10 years, 60% at 15 years, and 55% at 20 years, an attrition rate of 1 to 3% per year.[209] With external velour-knitted Dacron prostheses, the expected 10-year patency rate is 99% at the aortic bifurcation, 79% in the aortofemoral position, and 53% in the above-knee femoropopliteal position.[213] With glutaraldehyde-stabilized human umbilical cord vein grafts, the patency rate at 37 months was 63% in the femoropopliteal position, 54% in the distal tibial position, and 32% in the peroneal site.[214] Thus, in general, the longer the interposed bypass graft and the smaller the recipient vessel, with a corresponding increase in resistance to flow, the less favorable are both short- and long-term patency rates.

In femoropopliteal bypass grafts, five factors significantly influence long-term patency: (1) the nature of the graft, (2) arterio/graphic runoff, (3) indications for operation, (4) site of distal anastomosis, and (5) prior operation in this region. Not only do prosthetic grafts perform less well than grafts of autologous saphenous vein, but also the variables previously discussed have a greater effect on the patency of prosthetic than of vein grafts. Darling and Linton reported that in the femoropopliteal position, the 5-year patency rates were 72% for autogenous saphenous vein and 20% for Dacron prostheses.[215] The patency of femoropopliteal autologous saphenous vein bypass grafts was approximately 50% at 10 years, an attrition of 5% per year.[216]

Graft Healing

Tissue growing into a graft from the host vessel at either its proximal or distal end is called *pannus* and consists primarily of smooth muscle cells and associated extracellular matrix covered by endothelial cells.[48] A varying amount of tissue may be found lining the luminal aspect of a graft continuously or intermittently. Irrespective of its source, its components vary from platelets, fibrin, hematogenous cells, and macrophages to smooth muscle cells, collagen, and endothelial cells (ECs). The interface between this layer and the flowing blood (i.e., the *flow* or the *blood contacting surface*) corresponds to the intimal layer of a natural vessel. It is best termed *neointima* if its surface is lined by endothelial cells and *pseudointima* if the surface is any other biologic material, such as fibrin, platelets, collagen, or smooth muscle cells.

An implanted graft becomes encapsulated in collagen, fibroblasts, blood vessels, and other cellular and extracellular connective tissue elements forming an *outer capsule*. It separates the external surface of the graft from normal surrounding tissue. Initially, graft interstices are filled with edema fluid or fibrin, which are replaced in time by connective tissue. Foreign body giant cells are also found here if the graft has been in situ a long time. A graft enclosed in connective tissue (including an outer capsule, interstices, and lining) is said to be *incorporated*. An incorporated graft lined by neointima is considered to be *healed*.

Three distinct processes could contribute to the formation of a vascular graft's inner lining[48, 213]: (1) host vessel–derived tissue growth across anastomotic sites, (2) transinterstitial tissue migration,[217] and (3) deposition of tissue from blood (Fig. 22-16).[218, 219] ECs could be derived from adjacent vessel, from differentiation of cells growing through graft interstices, or by differentiation of hematogenous cells. In actuality, EC derivation from anastomotic overgrowth occurs to some extent in virtually all cases; transinterstitial growth occurs under special circumstances (see later); and deposition from blood cells capable of generating endothelium may be possible.[218, 219] Intentional pre-implantation seeding of ECs on vascular grafts has yielded mixed results.[220]

For virtually all known vascular replacements, experimental data suggest that ECs and smooth muscle cells derived from the adjacent artery at the anastomosis migrate and proliferate in association with the endothelial growing edge to advance the neointima.[217] This is the

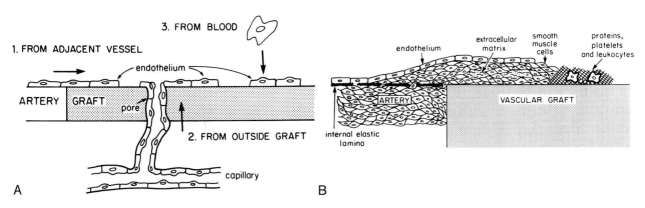

Figure 22-16 • Vascular graft healing. *A*, Possible sources of endothelium on blood-contacting surface of vascular graft: (1) arising from the intima of adjacent artery, (2) by transinterstitial migration of capillaries from the external surface of the graft, and (3) by deposition and differentiation to endothelium of hematogenous cells. *B*, Schematic diagram of pannus formation, the major mode of graft healing with currently available vascular grafts. Smooth muscle cells migrate from the media to the intima of the adjacent artery and extend over and proliferate on the graft surface; this smooth muscle cell layer is covered by a proliferating layer of endothelial cells. (From Schoen FJ: Interventional and Surgical Cardiovascular Pathology: Clinical Correlations and Basic Principles. Philadelphia, WB Saunders, 1989, pp 253, 254)

primary mechanism of graft coverage for solid or low-porosity grafts (comprising most grafts available). Luminal coverage by pannus develops relatively slowly. Furthermore, except in certain experimental species, pannus is generally restricted to a zone near to and contiguous with the viable artery, often despite postoperative intervals of up to many years (see later). Endothelialized neointima that grows over a portion of the luminal surface of vascular prostheses renders the prosthetic surface nonthrombogenic.

Nevertheless, the ability of humans to endothelialize synthetic cardiovascular prostheses is limited.[48] Pathologic examination of Teflon, Dacron, and ePTFE grafts retrieved from patients after months to years of implantation demonstrates that only near an anastomosis does the neointima become well developed; elsewhere the blood-contacting surface generally consists of a compacted platelet-fibrin aggregate (i.e., a pseudointima).[213] A pseudointima composed of nonendothelialized unorganized fibrin or organized fibrous tissue is occasionally noted at large distances from anastomoses in large-bore clinical and experimental fabric grafts. This layer is usually poorly adherent to the underlying graft material. Thus, regardless of the length of time grafts remain in the human host and regardless of the extent of external fibrous tissue incorporation, prostheses remain incompletely healed because of the failure to develop a completely endothelialized flow surface. Typically, ECs ultimately extend 10 to 15 mm across an anastomosis in humans, thereby allowing healing of intracardiac fabric patches and prosthetic valve sewing rings, but not of long vascular grafts. In contrast, after implantation of a cloth vascular prosthesis in some animals (e.g., calf), an extensively endothelialized flow surface (neointima) can form rapidly. Baboons most closely approximate humans with respect to hematologic characteristics and are approximately similar to dogs with respect to the kinetics of healing vascular grafts.

TABLE 22-3 • **Complications of Vascular Grafts**

Thrombosis
Thromboembolism
Infection
Perigraft seroma
Anastomotic pseudoaneurysm
Intimal fibrous hyperplasia
Degradation with fragmentation or dilation

Modified from Schoen FJ: Interventional and Surgical Cardiovascular Pathology: Clinical Correlations and Basic Principles. Philadelphia, WB Saunders, 1989, p 256.

Complications

The major complications of vascular grafts in any site of implantation are thrombosis/thromboembolism, infection, periprosthetic fluid collection, pseudoaneurysm, fibrointimal hyperplasia, and structural degeneration (Table 22-3).[48] With knitted and woven Teflon and Dacron fabric vascular prostheses, the major complications are mural thrombus formation, fragmentation or graft dilation. Failure of small-diameter vascular prostheses is most frequently due to occlusion by thrombus formation or generalized or anastomotic fibrous hyperplasia. Vascular graft biomaterials, like prosthetic materials in general, are less thromboresistant than the normal vascular surface. Thus, blood-contacting surfaces initially have a thin thrombotic covering, and occlusive thrombosis may occur (Fig. 22-17). To a large extent, late thrombosis, periprosthetic fluid collections, anastomotic leaks, infection, and intimal hyperplasia represent defects in healing.

Despite the use of prophylactic systemic antibiotics perioperatively, infection of implanted vascular prostheses occurs in up to 6% of patients (Fig. 22-18). The risk of death after infection of a vascular prosthesis is reported to be 25 to 75%, depending on the infected site and the approach to treatment. Because the anastomotic suture line is almost invariably involved in the septic process, an

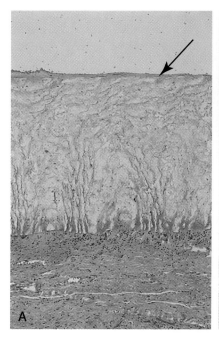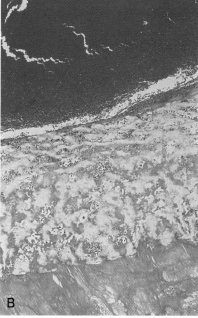

Figure 22-17 • Thrombus associated with vascular grafts. *A,* Thin layer of thrombus lining blood-contacting surface of otherwise patent expanded polytetrafluoroethylene graft (arrow). *B,* Thrombosed expanded polytetrafluoroethylene graft (H&E stain).

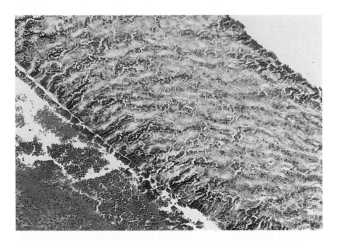

Figure 22-18 • Infection of expanded polytetrafluoroethylene vascular graft, as evidenced by bacteria and dense neutrophilic inflammation surrounding and penetrating graft material (H & E stain).

infected vascular graft is usually a mycotic false aneurysm, and rupture with hemorrhage at the graft site is frequently the presenting sign. Surgical removal of an infected graft is usually necessary to cure the infection.

Prosthetic aortic grafts can have pathologic interactions with the gastrointestinal tract, especially at anastomoses near the third and fourth portions of the duodenum and proximal jejunum. Direct adhesion of the intestine to the aortic graft, most commonly at the proximal anastomosis, can lead to erosion through the bowel wall and subsequent graft infection. In graft-enteric erosion, much less common than graft-enteric fistula, the bowel lumen contacts the external surface of the graft, but the circulatory system is otherwise intact. If the anastomosis is breached, then a direct communication between the lumen of the aortic graft and the lumen of the intestine (graft-enteric fistula) may result. Graft-enteric fistulas occur in 0.4% of patients with abdominal aortic grafts.

A perigraft seroma is a sterile collection of fluid contained within a fibrous capsule around the prosthetic graft. Almost all described cases involve ePTFE or Dacron conduits. The cloudy, pink, viscid fluid often resembles lymph or serum. The etiology is uncertain; postulated pathogenic mechanisms include (1) residual fluid derived from early perigraft hematoma; (2) development of a lymph fistula; (3) locally poor graft incorporation; (4) graft "weeping," either due to inadvertent intraoperative soilage with organic solvents such as alcohol or povidone-iodine or resulting from nonuniform application or uneven resorption of biologic graft sealant or preclot; (5) allergic reactions to the graft material; and (6) graft-induced "fibroblast inhibition."

False aneurysm (pseudoaneurysm) formation occurs in 1 to 4% of grafts, most frequently at the distal anastomoses of aortofemoral grafts. *False aneurysms* can develop at any anastomotic site and commonly lead to hemorrhage. Prosthetic rather than autogenous tissue suture lines are most frequently involved. Although there is a partial separation of the graft from the arterial wall at the anastomosis, allowing blood to escape from the lumen, perianastomotic fibrous tissue may initially prevent immediate gross hemorrhage and permit the formation of a capsule around the hematoma, which gradually expands owing to the pressure transmitted from the arterial lumen. The etiology of anastomotic pseudoaneurysm is multifactorial and includes suture failure; silk and braided Dacron suture materials have been implicated, especially in combination with specific graft types, such as Teflon graft with silk suture. Infection, prosthetic graft defects, systemic hypertension, anastomotic geometry, and native arterial wall degeneration may also contribute.

Late failure of clinical and experimental vascular grafts, especially those less than 8 mm in diameter, is frequently due to diffuse fibrous thickening of the inner capsule (Fig. 22-19). Intimal hyperplasia has been observed in reversed autogenous saphenous veins in the femoropopliteal or aortocoronary position, as well as in endarterectomized arteries and in radial arteries used as aortocoronary bypass grafts, in arteriovenous fistulas constructed for hemodialysis access, and in association with Dacron grafts, bovine heterografts, and ePTFE grafts. In vein grafts, intimal hyperplasia is often diffuse, leading to progressive luminal reduction of the entire graft, but focal lesions can cause isolated stenoses at anastomoses or valve sites. In contrast, synthetic vascular prostheses tend to develop intimal hyperplasia predominantly at or near anastomoses, particularly the distal.

Intimal hyperplasia results primarily from smooth muscle cell migration, proliferation, and extracellular matrix elaboration after and possibly mediated by acute or ongoing EC injury.[221] Contributing factors include (1) surface thrombogenesis, (2) delayed or incomplete endothelialization of the fabric, (3) disturbed flow across the anastomosis, and (4) mechanical factors at the junction of implant and host tissues. Because therapeutic endothelial seeding of vascular grafts has yielded only modest benefit, attempts to seed genetically modified ECs[222] and block smooth muscle cell proliferation[223] are ongoing.

Diffuse or focal graft intimal hyperplasia appears to result from the intimal migration and proliferation of host vessel–derived medial smooth muscle cells with a nonviable (synthetic or chemically cross-linked biologic) vascular graft and from either host vessel or graft itself when the graft has some viable cells (autogenous saphenous vein). Nevertheless, the specific factors that cause this injury are not well understood.

Progressive deterioration of a prosthesis can cause mechanical failure at the anastomotic site or in the body of the prosthesis, leading to aneurysm formation or the formation of false aneurysm due to rupture.[48] The incidence of long-term graft deterioration is unknown. The causes of delayed failure of a synthetic prosthesis include chemical, thermal, or mechanical damage to polymeric yarn materials during manufacture, fabric defects induced during manufacture (e.g., dropped stitches) or during insertion (even "atraumatic" vascular clamps can damage yarn fibers), and postoperative biodegradation of graft material. (Graft complications are also discussed in Chapter 4.)

Endovascular Prosthetic Grafts

The repair of abdominal aortic aneurysms (AAA) by endovascular grafting holds the promise of effective and durable repair, improved morbidity and mortality relative to surgical correction, and reduced hospital costs.[102–104]

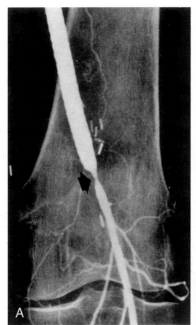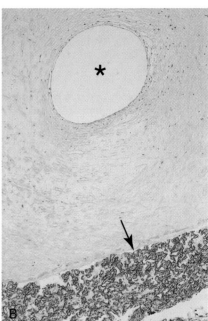

Figure 22-19 • Anastomotic hyperplasia of the distal anastomosis of a synthetic femoropopliteal graft. *A,* Angiogram demonstrating constriction (arrow). *B,* Photomicrograph demonstrating expanded polytetrafluoroethylene graft (arrow) with prominent intimal proliferation and a very small residual lumen designated by an asterisk (*). (*B,* H&E stain). (*A,* Courtesy of Anthony Whittemore, MD, Brigham and Women's Hospital, Boston, MA. From Schoen FJ: Blood vessels. In: Cotran RS, Kumar V, Collins T [eds]: Robbins Pathologic Basis of Disease, 6th ed. Philadelphia, WB Saunders, 1999, p 539)

An endovascular graft consists of a metallic stent covered by a cloth sleeve that resembles a vascular graft (often called a *stent-graft*). Endovascular grafts are either straight with both ends anchored to the infrarenal aorta, or bifurcated with the proximal end attached to the infrarenal aorta and the graft limbs fastened to the iliac arteries. Endovascular grafts are held in place by self-expanding stents or hooks that become embedded in the vessel wall. Clinical success consists of successful deployment of the endovascular device at the intended location without complications.

Reported and potential complications include thrombosis; obstruction owing to device twisting, kinking or oversizing; infection; graft dilation or structural failure with tear or fracture; device migration or change in alignment; erosion of the graft into/through the arterial wall; loss of effective aneurysm exclusion with *endoleak* (persistence of blood flow outside the lumen of the endoluminal graft but within the aneurysm sac) and/or aneurysm expansion, rupture or conversion to open repair.[105, 106] Cardiac deaths, related primarily to coronary artery disease, dominate the early and late mortality rate for both open surgery and endovascular repair of aneurysms. Total morbidity and mortality during the perioperative period is influenced both by comorbid medical conditions and anatomic factors that influence the risk of failed deployment, embolization, and complications related to pelvic ischemia.

In endovascular AAA repair, the aneurysm sac is left intact. Long-term aneurysm exclusion and device stabilization depends on the maintenance of an effective attachment, connection, or seal between the endograft and the host aorta; incomplete exclusion of the aneurysm from the circulation leads to an endoleak. An endoleak may be due to an incomplete "seal" between the endograft and the wall of the blood vessel, inadequate connection between components of a modular prosthesis, fabric defects or porosity, or retrograde blood flow from patent aortic side-branches.[107] The detection, clinical significance, and treatment of endoleaks remain uncertain; however, late explantation of the graft has been necessary in approximately 6% of patients in whom leaks persisted, causing either the AAA to enlarge or the graft to migrate.[108] Since size is the major determinant of the risk of rupture of an AAA, aneurysm growth after endovascular repair suggests that exclusion of the aneurysm wall has been incomplete and risk of rupture remains high.[109] However, an AAA may continue to enlarge after endovascular repair, even in the absence of a detectable endoleak.[110] This phenomenon has been attributed to persistent or recurrent pressurization of an aneurysm sac either due to blood flow that is below the sensitivity limits for detection using current imaging technology or pressure transmission through thrombus or endograft fabric.[111] Moreover, in the study by Blum et al.[104] eight leaks resulted from tears in the polyester fabric covering the stents; this study emphasizes that patients with graft failures and persistent perfusion of the aneurysmal sac have an ongoing risk of rupture. When leaks do not occur and the AAA remains exluded from the circulation, however, remodeling and shrinkage of the aneurysm can occur.

CARDIAC ASSIST AND REPLACEMENT

Mechanical Circulatory Support

Each year in the United States, congestive heart failure is the principal cause of death in 40,000 individuals, a contributing factor in over 200,000 deaths, diagnosed in 400,000 individuals, and the primary diagnosis in over 900,000 hospitalizations. It has been estimated that 60,000 of these persons could benefit from heart transplantation or long-term mechanical support. However, in as much as only 2500 donor hearts are available annually, ventricular-assist devices (VADs) and total artificial hearts

(TAHs) are presently an attractive and the most promising alternative to cardiac allotransplantation.[224, 225]

VADs and TAHs have been used primarily in two settings:

1. Potentially recoverable heart failure, in which cardiac function is likely to recover, should cardiac rest (i.e., ventricular unloading, decreased myocardial work, and increased subendocardial perfusion) be facilitated, while systemic organ perfusion is maintained. Acute cardiac failure after otherwise uncomplicated cardiac surgery (postcardiotomy shock) is the most frequent indication.
2. End-stage cardiac failure not likely to recover and where mechanical support will provide a bridge to transplantation. Indeed some 10 to 30% of patients die while awaiting a transplant, some after an acute deterioration in cardiac function.

Such devices are also being investigated as a long-term/permanent alternative to transplantation for patients with end-stage heart disease who cannot receive transplants and who cannot be removed from cardiac support.

Approximately 62 to 69% of transplant candidates who require some form of mechanical cardiac support eventually undergo transplantation, and their rate of hospital discharge is 65 to 69%.[224] For the subgroup of transplanted patients supported by a mechanical system specifically designed as a bridging device, the hospital discharge rate is approximately 90%. This is comparable to that seen in the general cardiac transplant population not requiring mechanical cardiac support. Indeed, problems due to device complications are balanced by the more complete physical rehabilitation that occurs over the duration of cardiac assist. Of postcardiotomy cardiac shock patients who receive mechanical cardiac assistance, approximately 45% are weaned and 25% survive to discharge.[226] Several thousand such devices have been used, and their use is accelerating.[227]

Ventricular-Assist Devices

In contrast to the widely used intra-aortic ballon pumps, centrifugal pumps, and extracorporeal membrane oxygenation, which provide short-term and incomplete resuscitation, VADs and TAHs can totally replace ventricular function for extended periods. With VADs, the natural heart remains in place and the device is connected via cannulas to the atrium or ventricle (pump inflow) and to the aorta (pump outflow). VADs currently available include univentricular (used as a left or a right ventricular-assist device [LVAD or RVAD, respectively]) and biventricular extracorporeal and implantable pulsatile devices. An assist pump has a single chamber; two must be used to provide bilateral support. In contrast, an artificial heart is composed of two pumping chambers that together replace the heart, analogous to heart transplantation. The pumps have mechanical or bioprosthetic valves to ensure unidirectional flow, fabric and metal conduits, and a blood-containing chamber with an elastomeric moving bladder/membrane in a rigid housing.

Most presently available assist and replacement pumps are energized by pulses of air generated by an external pneumatic unit and transmitted through tubes to the

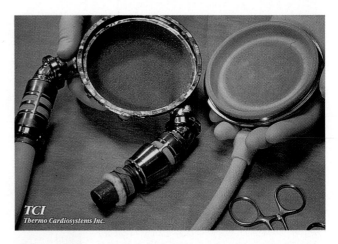

Figure 22-20 • HeartMate left ventricular-assist system with pneumatic actuation. (Courtesy of Thermo CardioSystems, Inc., Woburn, MA.)

pumping unit termed *pneumatic pumps*.[224, 225] Either the air-containing conduits (intrathoracic or intraperitoneal implants) or the blood-carrying lines (extracorporeal devices) necessarily traverse the skin. Two devices are most widely used, the HeartMate device (Thermo Cardio-Systems, Woburn, MA) (Fig. 22-20) and the Novacor (World Heart, Oakland, CA). They are similar with respect to function, implantation techniques, and intended use. Each is pneumatic, involves implantation of the pumping chamber within the abdominal wall, a pump inflow cannula inserted into the left ventricular apex, and an outflow tube anastomosed to the ascending aorta.

The HeartMate device has textured blood-contacting surfaces, which encourage the deposition of circulating cells and coagulation proteins, to form a uniform autologous tissue lining, to yield a stable surface that appears to minimize additional thrombus formation and infection (Fig. 22-21A).[228] The Novacor device uses smooth polyurethane surfaces, requiring that the patient receive long-term anticoagulation therapy with warfarin (see Fig. 22-21B). In each device, inflow and outflow conduits contain bioprosthetic valves (porcine valves in the case of the HeartMate, and pericardial valves in the case of the Novacor) to ensure unidirectional blood flow. Other available mechanical circulatory support systems include (1) the extracorporeal, pneumatically powered Pierce-Donachy device (Thoratec, Thoratec Laboratories, Berkeley, CA), with a seamless polyurethane blood sac with Bjork-Shiley tilting disk valves, (2) the extracorporeal pneumatic Abiomed device (Abiomed, Danvers, MA) with dual-chambered pump having polyurethane trileaflet valves, and (3) the pneumatic but completely implantable Cardiowest TAH (Cardiowest, Tucson, AZ, formerly called the Jarvik or Symbion TAH), with a smooth polyurethane pumping diaphragm and two Medtronic-Hall valves.[224, 225] For patients with these systems, the hospital discharge rate is approximately 90%, comparable with that in the general cardiac transplant population not requiring mechanical support. Recently, technical advances have permitted the development of two electrically (i.e., battery pack) powered, wearable variants of the HeartMate and Novacor LVADs that allow patients to assume some independence outside a hospital.

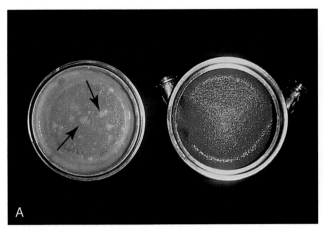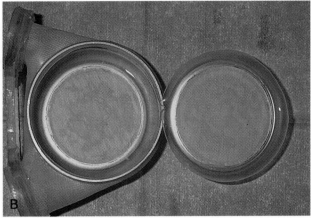

Figure 22-21 • Blood-contacting surfaces after implantation of left ventricular assist systems. *A*, Thermo CardioSystems HeartMate device after 233 days, with a uniform thrombotic coating containing islands of fibrous tissue (arrows). *B*, Novacor left ventricular assist system 90 days after implant. No thrombus is visible.

Three classes of advanced devices under development, include (1) pneumatic devices that are wrapped around the heart and thus do not directly contact blood, (2) compact intracardiac axial-flow pumps, and (3) an electric TAH.[229]

Artificial Heart

The heart can be replaced by two pneumatically powered polyurethane sac-type blood pumps, implanted intrathoracically, that provide both systemic and pulmonary circulations.[224, 230] Tilting-disk–type prosthetic inflow and outflow valves provide unidirectional blood flow in the two ventricles. The Jarvik-7 heart has served as a long-term mechanical cardiac replacement in several individuals since 1982; this and several other types of replacement devices have also been used as a bridge to transplantation. Compact, totally implantable electrical motor–driven ventricular-assist pumps and artificial hearts are being developed for long-term support of the systemic circulation in patients with irreparably damaged ventricles. Among 217 patients in whom a TAH was used clinically, survival was 56%, with average duration of support 26 days (maximum 795 days).[227]

Pneumatic artificial hearts consist of separate right and left ventricles composed of metal and plastic components powered by separate right and left pneumatic power units. Each prosthetic ventricle consists of a rigid outer shell with a flexible polyurethane sac having hydrodynamic flow characteristics. Air pulses from the pneumatic power unit enter the space between the shell and the sac and compress the latter. Inlet and outlet valves, of either a mechanical or a tissue type, ensure unidirectional flow. Each ventricle is attached to the native remnant atrium with an atrial suture cuff, while the outlet port is attached to the aorta or pulmonary artery by a conventional vascular graft. Pneumatic artificial hearts for human use provide a stroke volume of about 70 ml and cardiac output from 4 to 8 L/minute.

Artificial heart implantation is performed in a manner similar to that for heart transplantation. Full cardiopulmonary bypass is employed. The prosthetic atrial cuffs and arterial grafts are sewn into place. Two 6-foot pneumatic lines pass through the chest wall to the pneumatic power unit.

Whereas the pneumatic artificial heart was originally developed as a permanent cardiac substitute, the advent of heart transplantation led to the need for a temporary (days to weeks) cardiac substitute for critically ill patients awaiting heart transplantation. The Jarvik pneumatic heart became commercially available in the mid-1980s and was employed in nearly 200 applications as a bridge to transplantation. Considerable success was reported. However, the best results were obtained when the device was employed for less than 1 week. Infection and thromboembolism were frequent complications and ultimately resulted in withdrawal of the Jarvik heart from the commercial market.[231-234]

Previous clinical studies of artificial heart implantation were of considerable importance. They showed that the available artificial hearts would fit in the chest of an appropriately sized patient, would provide an adequate cardiac output, and could maintain cardiovascular pressures within a physiologic range. In these critically ill individuals, infection and thromboembolism appeared to be more problematic than had been predicted from animal implant studies.

Taking advantage of recent developments in electronics, biomaterials, and other relevant areas, the National Heart, Lung, and Blood Institute, National Institutes of Health are funding several groups to develop an electrically powered artificial heart.

Pathologic Considerations

Complications

The principal complications associated with VADs and TAHs are hemorrhage, infection, and thromboembolism.[229, 231-238] To a lesser extent, device structural failure, right-sided cardiac failure, air embolism, and progressive multisystem organ failure are responsible for morbidity and mortality. Whereas calcification of valves and the pumping bladder is frequent in experimental VAD im-

TABLE 22-4 • **Complications of Circulatory-Assist Devices and Artificial Hearts**

Thrombosis/thromboembolism
Hemorrhage
Endocarditis
Infection external to the pump and cannulas
Hemolysis
Obstruction to flow through conduits
System component mechanical failures
Bladder/valve calcification

Modified from Schoen FJ: Interventional and Surgical Cardiovascular Pathology: Clinical Correlations and Basic Principles. Philadelphia, WB Saunders, 1989, p 222.

plants, this has not been a serious problem noted in removed clinical VADs. These complications are summarized in Table 22-4 and illustrated in Figure 22-22.

Historically, the frequency of thromboembolic events is approximately 20% with either RVADs OR LVADs. Thromboembolism has occurred in most patients having implantation of the Jarvik-7 TAH for temporary or long-term support. Thromboemboli are initiated at the valve rings, at the connection sites to the outflow conduits, and on the diaphragm. In contrast to that with smooth pumping bladders[231, 234-237] the incidence of thromboemboli with textured blood-contacting surfaces has been low, obviating the need for long-term anticoagulation therapy, and allowing only antiplatelet therapy in most recipients.[228, 239]

Infection, either nosocomial or device-related, occurs in 25 to 40% of LVAD and artificial heart recipients (especially after 30 days) and is associated with significant morbidity but does not preclude subsequent successful cardiac transplantation.[233-236, 240-242] The most common infections are those related to the percutaneous drive line; others either occur within the device or are associated with the abdominal wall pocket holding the device.[231, 233] Candida has been noted frequently in infections associated with LVADs.

Bleeding rates are as high as 60% and are related to a coagulopathy induced by hepatic dysfunction, the extensive surgery required to implant the device, and the combined effects on platelet function of cardiopulmonary bypass and the assist pump. Hemolysis is generally not a problem.

Reports of device malfunction have appeared, but failures that compromise the ability of the device to provide adequate blood flow are rare.

Myocardial Changes During Cardiac Assist

During mechanical cardiac support, the pump completely unloads the left ventricle and supports cardiac output. Consequently, patients frequently show improvement in cardiac function during support with assist devices. Indeed, some heart failure patients may ultimately be successfully weaned from cardiac assist. Several factors may modulate the return of cardiac function, including functional recovery of cells in marginally or previously ischemic areas (i.e., myocardial stunning, hibernation), alteration of cardiac geometry by remodeling, and modulation of systemic responses to heart failure and

ongoing myocardial pathology such as hypertrophy, apoptosis, edema, and myocytolysis.[243-248] The propensity for recovery largely reflects the degree of irreversible changes (e.g., primarily myocyte death by necrosis and apoptosis) and myocardial fibrosis that existed before and continue after mechanical cardiac support.

Infection Associated With Cardiac-Assist and Other Prosthetic Devices

Infection occurs in as many as 5 to 10% of patients with implanted prosthetic devices and is a major source of morbidity and mortality.[242, 249-252] Infections associated with medical devices are often resistant to antibiotics and host defenses, frequently persisting until the devices are removed.

Early implant infections (<approximately 1 to 2 months postoperatively) are most likely due to intraoperative contamination from airborne sources or nonsterile surgical technique or to early postoperative complications such as wound infection. In contrast, later infections likely occur by a hematogenous route and are often initiated by bacteremia induced by therapeutic dental or genitourinary procedures. Perioperative prophylactic antibiotics and periodic antibiotic prophylaxis given shortly before diagnostic and therapeutic procedures generally protect against implant infection. Infections associated with implanted medical devices are characterized microbiologically by a high prevalence of *Staphylococcus epidermidis* and other staphylococci, especially *Staphylococcus aureus*. Ordinarily, *S. epidermidis* is an organism with low virulence and thus an infrequent cause of non–prosthesis-associated deep infections. This emphasizes the unique environment in the vicinity of a foreign body.

The presence of a foreign body potentiates infection. The foreign body/biomaterial itself is a critical causal factor in such infections. A seminal experiment reported by Elek and Conen in 1957 indicated that a foreign body (a single silk suture) decreased the threshold infection-producing innoculum of *S. aureus* organisms from 1,000,000 to 100.[253] The factors that predispose a foreign body to infection are poorly understood, but physical form (e.g., roughness, interconnecting porosity), chemical composition (e.g., hydrophobicity), impaired local natural defenses against infection (due to necrotic tissue, loss of vascularity, and interference with phagocytic mechanisms), adherent matrix proteins (e.g., fibronectin), and bacterial biofilms (composed of cellular material, polysaccharides, and debris) probably play a role.

Devices could facilitate infection in several different ways.[242, 249-252] Microorganisms are provided access to the circulation and to deeper tissue by damage to natural barriers against infection during implantation or subsequent function of a prosthetic device. Moreover, an implanted foreign body could (1) limit phagocyte migration into infected tissue or (2) interfere with inflammatory cell phagocytic mechanisms through release of soluble implant components or surface-mediated interactions, thus allowing bacteria to survive adjacent to the implant. Adhesion of bacteria to the prosthetic surface and the formation of microcolonies within an adherent biofilm

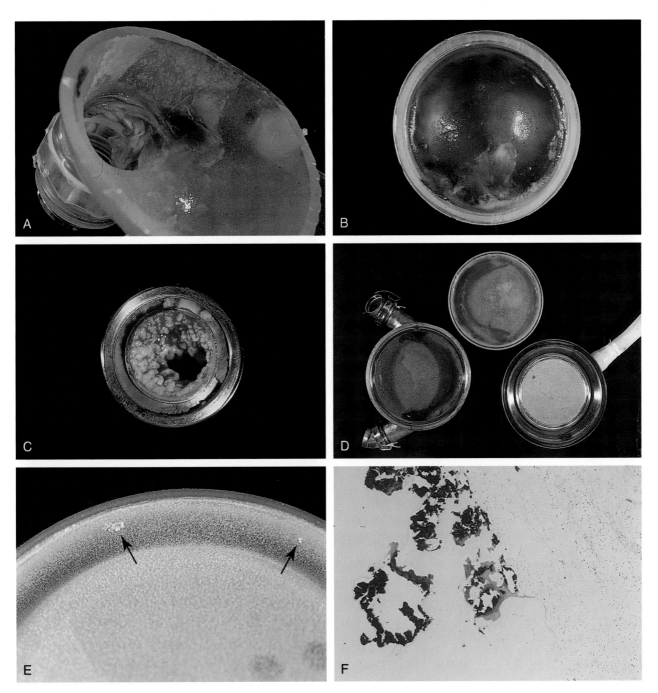

Figure 22-22 • Complications of left ventricular-assist devices (LVADs). *A, B,* Thrombotic deposits at the pump outflow and bladder/housing junction, respectively. *C,* Fungal infection in LVAD outflow graft. *D,* Dehiscence of the bladder of a left ventricular-assist device. *E, F,* Focal calcification of clinical left ventricular-assist device. *E,* A gross photograph with deposits highlighted by arrows. *F,* Histologic section demonstrating calcification (black). (von Kossa stain). (*A, B,* From Fyfe B, Schoen FJ: Pathologic analysis of 34 explanted Symbion ventricular assist devices and 10 explanted Jarvik-7 total artificial hearts. Cardiovasc Pathol 2:187, 1993)

are fundamental steps in the pathogenesis of clinical and experimental infections associated with foreign bodies.

Pathologic Analysis of a Removed Ventricular-Assist Device

Schema have been published to analyze retrieved VADs and TAHs in the context of the entire patient, with emphasis on the local pump-patient interface, remote cardiovascular and end-organ effects, and the impact of circulatory support on the native heart.[254, 255] The specific objectives are to characterize (1) the blood pump, especially blood-contacting surfaces (smooth or textured), valves (mechanical or tissue), conduits, and other components (including energy sources) and (2) other relevant pathology (especially cardiopulmonary and local and distant patient-prosthesis interactions). These goals are best

ANALYSIS OF CARDIAC-ASSIST DEVICE/ARTIFICIAL HEART

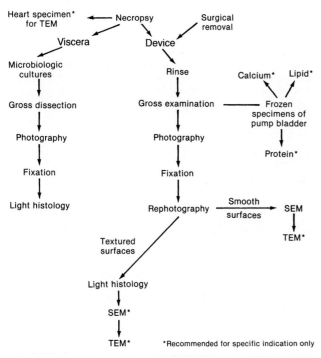

Figure 22-23 • Schema for pathologic analysis of cardiac-assist device/artificial heart. (From Schoen FJ: Interventional and Surgical Cardiovascular Pathology: Clinical Correlations and Basic Principles. Philadelphia: WB Saunders, 1989, p 392)

met by approaching and dissecting the implant (and the recipient if at autopsy) appropriately to ensure adequate retention of information that may be lost when the implant is removed from its anatomic context, photographic documentation, microscopic examination, microbiologic and biochemical assays, and compliance with regulatory and manufacturer requirements.

In brief, a routine autopsy is important in studying deceased patients with these devices, including major viscera, lungs, and brain, and is necessary to document embolic sequelae. The general schema for analysis of a VAD is summarized in Fig. 22-23. The pump should ideally be rinsed with and disassembled while in normal saline solution after removal, and the blood-contacting components should be removed, including pump diaphragm and valves. Consideration should be given to freezing a portion of the pump bladder for later immunohistochemical, biochemical, or mineralization studies. Following careful examination of the pump specimen grossly and under a dissecting microscope and subsequent macroscopic photographic documentation, the pump bladder and valves are radiographed to document calcification. Special attention should be directed toward sampling and culturing fragments of tissue in the implant bed and adjacent to percutaneous electrical and hydraulic lines, all of which are potential sites for infection.

For detailed study of the device, sections for light microscopy and scanning electron microscopy may be selected from the inflow, intermediate, and outflow portions of the pump bladder and valves, as well as any other pertinent areas, and subsequently prepared according to standard procedures. Light microscopy of selected embedded and stained cross sections may be used to map pseudointimal material adherent to the pumping bladder surface and to provide tentative identification of cellular and noncellular components, such as leukocytes, fibroblasts, endothelial cells, fibrin, collagen, and calcium deposits. Scanning electron microscopy can document surface characteristics, such as smoothness, uniformity, and the presence of specific cells and thrombi. Sections of bladder with associated surface deposits should be examined in cross section, preferably after embedding in glycol methacrylate, to facilitate maintaining the tissue-biomaterial interface intact during sectioning. Where the tissue lining a surface is sufficiently thick and fibrous, it may be lifted from the underlying polymer by sharp dissection, with the fragments processed in paraffin or glycol methacrylate. The relation of surface defects in biomaterials to microthrombi or calcification may be assessed by careful dissolution of surface protein layers of mineral deposits, using a dilute solution of proteolytic enzyme (e.g., trypsin) or a decalcification agent, such as RDO Rapid Bone Decalcifier (Dupage Kinetic Labs, Naperville, IL) or 5% formic acid, to expose the underlying surface. However, since proteolytic enzymes may contribute to artifactual polymer degradation under some circumstances, care must be exercised in interpreting such data.

Cardiomyoplasty

Cardiomyoplasty uses a patient's own skeletal muscle to assist the failing heart.[256, 257] This technique wraps a latissimus dorsi muscle around the heart and stimulates it in synchrony with the heart by use of a modified pacemaker. This concept is very attractive because it does not require the use of immunosuppressive drugs or an external power source. However, several factors, such as the need for prolonged conditioning of muscle and the adverse effect of the procedure on ventricular loading in larger hearts, may limit its clinical potential.

Autologous skeletal muscle has been used to provide active cardiac assist in the form of both cardiomyoplasty and skeletal muscle ventricles.[258–260] Chronic low-frequency electrical stimulation of skeletal muscle results in the acquisition by that muscle of fatigue-resistant properties and in accompanying structural and biochemical changes, including increases in capillary density, activity of oxidative enzymes, and mitochondrial volume. Another approach is to use skeletal muscle to power a mechanical VAD. Relevant pathology in these applications has not yet been reported in detail.

Partial Left Ventriculectomy

Batista and coworkers in South America developed an operation for patients with end-stage dilated cardiomyopathy of various etiologies in which the objective is to return the enlarged heart to a normal diameter that will reduce left ventricular wall tension (the mechanism is related to the law of Laplace).[261] Large segments of left ventricular wall are resected (hence, Batista's terminology *partial left ventriculectomy*). The heart is then reconstructed to decrease the left ventricular diameter. Data show that the perioperative mortality is approximately 22% and the 2-year mortality is approximately 45%. Most survivors have an improved clinical condition.

In one study in the United States, although there was a decrease in left ventricular dimensions, a reduction in mitral regurgitation, and an increase in forward ejection fraction after resection, cardiac index did not increase.[262] However, perioperative mortality was low, and at approximately 1 year, survival was 87% and freedom from re-listing for transplantation was 72%. Those investigators concluded that improved selection criteria may avoid early failures and considerable follow-up. Nevertheless, the operation may become a biologic bridge, or even alternative, to transplantation.[262]

ARRHYTHMIA CONTROL

For patients in whom cardiac arrhythmias cannot be controlled by pharmacologic therapy (i.e., antiarrhythmic drugs), two other therapeutic options are available: (1) electrical therapy to control the cardiac rhythm (e.g., direct current cardioversion, implantable electrical devices such as pacemakers and implantable cardioverter-defibrillators) and (2) interventional/surgical therapy to remove the affected tissue (e.g., endocardial resection, cryoablation, and other ablative techniques).

Cardiac Pacemakers

Since about 1960, cardiac pacing has become a well-established therapeutic tool.[263] More than 250,000 new and replacement permanent pacemakers are implanted worldwide each year. Indications for permanent cardiac pacing include sinus node dysfunction, intermittent and incomplete atrioventricular block, and bundle branch block. Most cardiac pacemakers are implanted in patients older than 60 years, but they are also used in children, including infants. Over 100,000 new permanent pacemakers are implanted in the United States each year; pacemaker placement, revision, or removal is a commonly done thoracic and cardiovascular operation.

Cardiac pacing is achieved by a system of interconnected components consisting of (1) a pulse generator that includes a power source (often called the pacemaker) and electric circuitry to initiate the electric stimulus and to sense normal activity, (2) one or more electrically insulated conductors leading from the pulse generator to the heart, with an electrode at the distal end of each; and (3) a tissue, or blood and tissue, interface between electrode and adjacent stimulatable myocardial cells. Pacemaker-related complications are unusual but can be serious.

Cardiac pacing may be either permanent or temporary. Temporary pacing is most frequently done on patients with acute MI complicated by cardiac conduction system disturbances that could progress to complete heart block. Leads for temporary cardiac pacing are generally directed transvenously into the apex of the right ventricle, and the pulse generator is located outside the body. Ultimately, either a temporary pacemaker is replaced by a permanent device or its use is discontinued. Temporary pacing may also be used after cardiac surgery in which the electrodes are usually placed transthoracically onto the anterior surface of the heart to permit easy withdrawal, generally within a few days. Permanent cardiac pacing involves implantation of both pulse generator and leads. The generator is usually placed subcutaneously on the chest; the leads advanced transvenously through a vein, with the electrode terminating at the endocardial surface of the right ventricle (for the most frequently used right ventricular stimulation). Alternatively, the electrodes may be attached to the epicardial surface via the transthoracic route.

With a transvenous insertion, the most commonly used for permanent cardiac pacing, a pulse generator is positioned subcutaneously in the left or right deltopectoral region of the superior thorax. The lead is tunneled through subcutaneous tissue to the subclavian vein and passes along its lumen to the heart. Depending upon the pacing modality, a lead is placed with the electrode at its tip positioned against the endocardium of the right atrium (usually the atrial appendage) for atrial sensing and stimulation and/or near the apex of the right ventricle (Fig. 22-24). If the transthoracic route is used, the pulse gener-

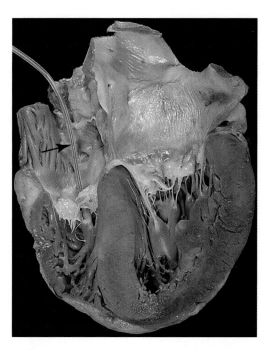

Figure 22-24 • Transvenous pacing lead well-embedded in heart obtained at autopsy. The left ventricle is on the right in this apical four-chamber view of the heart. A pacemaker (arrow) is present with the lead terminating in the right ventricle. This heart also shows hypertensive heart disease with marked concentric thickening of the left ventricular wall causing reduction in lumen size. (From Schoen FJ: The heart. In: Cotran RS, Kumar V, Collins T [eds]: Robbins Pathologic Basis of Disease, 6th ed. Philadelphia: WB Saunders, 1999, p 565)

ator is usually placed in a similar location, and the electrode is inserted directly into the myocardium of the ventricles or atria or attached to their epicardial surfaces. The pacing lead is brought to the heart by an intercostal, subcostal-subxiphoid, or transmediastinal route. In some cases, particularly in infants and young children, in whom the soft tissues of the chest wall are thin, the pulse generator may be placed in an abdominal location.

In *demand* pacing, stimulation is interrupted by any spontaneous cardiac activity. The electrical activity of myocardial depolarization associated with spontaneous contraction of the ventricles is sensed by the same lead used for pacing and inhibits generation of unnecessary stimulation pulses. This is valuable in a patient who has an intermittent conduction disorder or sinus node dysfunction and who may not require pacing much of the time.

The *pacing threshold* is the strength of the pacing stimulus needed to initiate a wave of depolarization through the myocardium, thus allowing the pacemaker to initiate contraction of the chamber being paced. The threshold may be measured as a current (milliamperes) or as an electromotive force (volts), or it may be stated as one of two derived functions: charge (the product of current and time) or energy (the product of voltage, current, and time). Threshold levels (at any given pulse duration) are affected by a variety of factors. Most important, from the pathologist's perspective, are the position of the electrode relative to stimulatable tissue and the nature of the tissue response to the electrode. If an electrode is separated from myocytes by tissue that cannot be stimulated, the stimulus threshold is determined by the distance between the electrode and the excitable tissue through nonexcitable tissue. Note that this explanation does not rely on the misconception that fibrous tissue acts as an electric insulator. In fact, fibrous tissue has about the same conductivity as myocardium. Thus, one may think of the electrode surrounded by nonexcitable tissue as functioning in an equivalent manner, regarding threshold as an imaginary electrode of larger dimensions. A larger electrode has a higher surface area and a lower current density at its boundaries, for the same stimulus current.

Nonstimulatable tissue separating an electrode from myocytes may be fibrosis induced by the electrode itself or myocardial scarring from some other cause, most commonly a healed MI (Fig. 22-25). However, experimental studies show that acute myocardial ischemia causes both an increased stimulation threshold and a decreased threshold for inducing ventricular fibrillation.[264] The threshold several weeks to months after electrode implantation may be two to three times that at implantation, although this is being reduced with improved lead designs, including the use of slow, local release of corticosteroids to reduce fibrosis.[264, 265] The practical point is that, if pulse generator output is not set sufficiently high in the early postoperative phase, loss of pacing with potentially fatal consequences can result. By contrast, maintaining output at such high levels once thresholds have stabilized greatly shortens battery life. Thus, pacemakers with adjustable ("programmable") variations in output have been developed.

From the pathologist's perspective, two additional is-

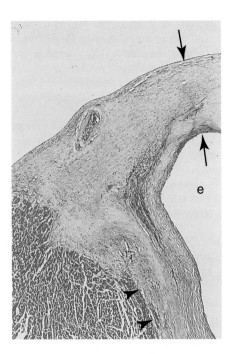

Figure 22-25 • Fibrous capsule surrounding pacemaker electrode at right ventricular apex. Low-power photomicrograph demonstrating space previously occupied by electrode (e), fibrous capsule separating electrode from blood in right ventricular chamber (between arrows) and fibrous capsule separating electrode from surrounding mural myocardium (arrowheads) (Masson trichrome stain).

sues are important with respect to the power source: (1) whether the source has completely discharged, resulting in a failure to pace, and (2) the appropriate means of disposing of a pacemaker at autopsy, particularly of those with nuclear batteries.

Because the success or failure of a pacemaker is largely determined by the tissue response to a lead, and to the electrode in particular, the pathologist is in a key position to describe problems with pacing lead/electrode configurations in clinical use and, in this way, to point to future improvements. Pacing leads may be connected to the heart from either its endocardial or its epicardial aspect. An ideal endocardial pacing lead should provide stable fixation immediately from the time of implantation, achieve and maintain a minimal threshold for stimulation, maximize the amplitude of the cardiac electrogram to facilitate sensing, and function reliably for many years. Electrode fixation may be active or passive. In active fixation, the electrode is designed as a helix or with prongs, to grasp the endocardial surface and achieve immediate fixation at implantation.

A very effective aid to passive fixation is the addition of projecting tines, or fins, in the region of the electrode tip. A quite different approach to improving fixation has been the development of electrodes with porous metal surfaces. An endocardial pacemaker lead may require a special design if it is implanted at a particular site. One example is the J-shaped atrial lead, which is curved to facilitate placing the electrode tip in the right atrial appendage, inherently the most stable site for fixation.

Clinical use of epicardial leads is far less popular because of the entailed need for a thoracotomy. The predominant design is a "corkscrew" electrode in which the helical electrode is insulated over most of its length so that the stimulating surface area at its tip is small. The electrode is screwed into the myocardium; no sutures are needed for attachment. However, the lead is virtually impossible to remove at a later date, except by further surgery.

Complications

Some complications associated with epicardial cardiac pacing are potentially life threatening. Rare intraoperative complications result largely from the route of insertion of a pacing lead. Epicardial pacing involves the risk of complications inherent in a thoracotomy and, in most patients, the associated use of a general anesthetic. In addition, specific complications related to electrode placement are possible. Perforation of the corkscrew type of sutureless epicardial electrode through either the right or the left ventricular wall may occur with a fatal outcome. Transvenous insertion of a pacemaker lead involves different risks such as air embolism, pneumothorax, and perforation of the tricuspid valve[266, 267] or right atrium or the ventricle. Perforation through the right ventricular wall is most common during electrode positioning but may be delayed days or months after insertion. Pacing of the diaphragm or chest wall muscles, chest pain, and/or a pericardial friction rub may result. Such perforation may be asymptomatic[268] but usually causes a loss of pacing. Use of the femoral vein as the site of insertion of temporary pacing leads is associated with several possible acute local complications, including double puncture of the femoral artery and vein[269, 270] and femoral vein thrombosis.[271]

Pulse Generator

Surgical complications relating to implantation of the pulse generator are not unusual. Most common are erosion due to pressure necrosis of the skin overlying the generator, infection of the pacemaker pocket, and either migration or rotation of the pacemaker pack. Under extreme circumstances, the entire pack may extrude from the wound, causing a loss of pacing. Infection of the pacemaker "pocket" by implantation of bacteria at operation represents the most common source of pacemaker-related infection. *S. epidermidis* is most frequently cultured. A local pacemaker pocket infection may lead to the future complication of septicemia[272–274] or endocarditis, the latter caused by propagation of the local infection at the pulse generator site along the pacing lead and into the heart. Complete removal of the pacing system may be necessary.

Loss of Stimulus

Perhaps the most obvious complication related to the pacemaker is loss of the stimulus for pacing attributable either to failure of an electronic component or, more commonly, to battery depletion. Another unusual cause for pulse generator–related loss of pacing is phantom programming, in which the output of the pacemaker is inappropriately reset to a level below the stimulation threshold by electromagnetic interference from a spurious signal, by faulty signals from the programmer circuitry, or by misuse of the device by an uninformed operator.[275, 276] In the past, many reports appeared on interference with pacemaker function by devices ranging from electric razors, toothbrushes, and microwave ovens at home to electrosurgical and diathermy apparatus in hospital. Fortunately, recent generations of cardiac pacemakers have been greatly improved with regard to their resistance to electromagnetic interference.[277, 278]

Rotation may occur spontaneously but usually results when a patient habitually twists the generator within a capacious tissue pocket *(pacemaker twiddler syndrome)*. This can cause dislodgment of the electrode with resulting loss of pacing (1) by the pacing lead being reeled onto the pulse generator like fishing line and (2) by the lead coiling when the pulse generator is rotated on its axis. The interface between a pacing lead and the pulse generator occurs at the connector socket in a pacemaker pack and is a weak link in pacing systems. If the connector seal fails, either fluid or tissue, or both, may enter the socket and cause current leakage with a resultant failure to pace.[279, 280]

Neoplasia in the tissues forming the pacemaker pocket is rare, and given the large numbers of implanted pacemakers and the paucity of case reports of tumors arising from adjacent tissues, there is no reason to consider the association as anything more than coincidental.

Pacing Leads

Complications of endocardial pacing leads include electrode dislodgment, lead fracture, thrombosis and thromboembolism, infection, myocardial penetration or perforation, electrode corrosion and insulation failure, and an unduly high pacing threshold.[281] Complications related to pacing lead(s) may be related to the body of the lead, as distinct from the lead–pacemaker pack interface or the electrode(s). Pacing lead improvements over the years have included helical coil and multifilament designs to decrease electrical resistance and enhance flexibility and durability.

However, some lead fractures continue to occur. Sharp angulation results in increased stress at one point and premature fracture. Because introduction through the subclavian vein is common, the most frequent site of fracture is at the angulation point between the clavicle and the first rib. Lead fracture may cause intermittent or complete pacing failure. Subtle losses of continuity can be discovered at autopsy by measuring the lead resistance. Alternatively, a lead may fail if the insulation layer, usually made of silicone rubber or polyurethane, surrounding the conductor(s) is breached. In this unusual circumstance, a "short circuit" is created, with current leaking into the surrounding blood or tissue fluid instead of exiting from the electrode tip.

Serious and, in some cases, fatal problems were associated with an atrial pacing lead (Telectronics Accufix) owing to fracture from metal fatigue of an electrically inactive J-shaped retention wire.[282] This was caused by repetitive bending induced by cyclic cardiac motion. In approximately 40 patients with these leads, the J retention wire protruded through the polyurethane insulation, causing either laceration of the right atrium with consequent pericardial tamponade or embolization to the pulmonary circulation.

Silicone rubber leads usually fail because of damage at implantation. Some segmented polyether polyurethane leads have failed as a result of biodegradation of the polymer by a process called environmental stress cracking. This requires a sensitive material, reactive chemical media, and tensile stresses. Scanning electron microscopy of suspicious lead surfaces can confirm the characteristic cracking.[283]

An endocardial pacing lead presents a foreign surface to the blood stream. Some thrombus formation is inevitable with conventional silicone rubber lead coatings and even with the newer polyurethane ones. The sheath is well formed within one day and then undergoes organization over several months, forming a fibrous sheath around the lead. This may extend from the site of electrode contact with the endocardium (usually at the right ventricular apex) back across the chordae tendineae and tricuspid valve, to which it may fuse, and into the right atrium.[284, 285] Such lead ensheathment with adhesions to the endocardium and tricuspid valve apparatus usually causes no valve dysfunction and, in this sense, is a "normal" finding (Fig. 22-6). However, if a lead is to be removed, avulsion of part of the tricuspid valve is a possible complication. Most leads can be removed by prolonged gentle traction,[286] but recourse to cardiotomy with cardiopulmonary bypass may be needed if the lead is incarcerated in fibrous tissue.[287–289] Leads that are not removed can later migrate. Increasingly, nonfunctioning pacemaker leads are left in place because they cannot be safely removed; the complication rate of retained leads is low.

In the absence of electrode displacement, an increase in the chronic stimulation threshold exceeding the maximum output of the pulse generator may signify MI, with or without subsequent replacement fibrosis in the region of the electrode; local fibrosis stimulated by electrical injury; corrosion of the electrode; or fragmentation of the electrode lead insulation. Irreparable loss of function of a transvenous electrode catheter, which can be caused by local block of impulse conduction, electrode displacement, lead fracture, or insulation defects, generally requires insertion of a new lead. Removal of the intracardiac lead under these circumstances or when the lead is infected may not be easily done when the defective lead has become encased at one or many points along its transvenous course as described earlier.

Major vein thrombosis and pulmonary thromboembolism may complicate endocardial pacing but are surprisingly infrequent occurrences. Pulmonary thromboemboli arising from a transvenous pacing lead may lead to death.[290] However, asymptomatic pulmonary thromboembolism is more frequent.[291]

Infection is major and not uncommon complication of pacing leads, whether they are endocardial or epicardial.[287–289, 292] The infection may originate in the pacemaker pocket and track along the lead, which acts as a contaminated foreign body; alternatively, it may occur by implantation of bacteria on traumatized endocardium or thrombus contiguous with the lead.[293] Septicemia may develop,[294–296] and septic pulmonary emboli have occurred. The fundamental therapeutic principle in pace-

maker-related endocarditis is removal of at least the lead and, when the pacemaker pocket is involved, the entire pacing system.

An unusual complication peculiar to epicardial leads is migration away from the original site of implantation.[297] When unseated, the tip of the lead most commonly flips into the right ventricular outflow tract or pulmonary artery. An electrode displaced into the inferior vena cava can induce diaphragmatic contractions. An electrode may be malpositioned in the coronary sinus at insertion.[298] The result may be failure to pace due to a high stimulation threshold. It must be appreciated, however, that a transvenous lead may be intentionally implanted in the coronary sinus for atrial pacing.[299, 300]

Once a very common complication of endocardial pacing, electrode dislodgment has been largely obviated by the availability of tined leads for improved passive fixation and various positive fixation designs. Dislodgment generally occurs within the first few days or weeks of electrode insertion. Late displacement is unusual because of fibrous tissue sheath formation around the electrode and body of the lead.

Most pacemaker patients have long-term stimulation threshold stability, but about 20% develop a progressive increase in threshold, which, in some cases, is sufficient to produce exit block. Corticosterioid elution has been incorporated into the design of both endocardial and epicardial electrodes.[265]

Considerations at Autopsy

In examining cardiac pacemakers at autopsy, particularly in a case of sudden death, a pathologist must question whether a malfunction of the implanted hardware or some host reaction to it was responsible for death. This question may be impossible to resolve, but a detailed examination of the pacing system may provide an answer. First, it is essential to document electrical continuity from the pulse generator through the lead(s) to the electrode tip(s). Radiographs (preferably at least two views with one at right angle to another), either taken shortly before death or before commencing the autopsy, can both indicate any lead fractures and locate the position of electrodes.

On opening the body, special care should be exercised to avoid transecting the lead. The pulse generator and lead, including the electrode tip, should be exposed in situ by careful dissection. It is desirable to minimize traction or bending of the lead during this procedure. A search should be made for evidence indicating infection of the pulse generator pouch or of thrombosis along the course of the lead (in the case of transvenous placement), and appropriate photographs taken. Often, a transvenous lead becomes included in a connective tissue sheath along the course of a vein. If thrombi are present along the lead(s), a careful search should be made for pulmonary thromboemboli and any possibility of an infection excluded. The lead(s) and pulse generator can then be separated by removing the lead terminal pin(s) from its (their) socket(s) in the pulse generator. The terminal pin and socket should be carefully examined for evidence of fluid intrusion, which can cause corrosion. Tissue ingrowth into the lead socket is another telltale sign of an electrode seal defect. With the lead and pulse generator separated, the heart can be removed and examined, and photographs taken of the lead(s) in situ.

The lead may be tested after its removal for electrical continuity by measuring the resistance between the electrode tip and the proximal end of the lead. The measured resistance should be in the range of 5 to 50 ohms. If a lead is fractured, resistance should be too high to register on the meter. The lead should be put under tension when measuring resistance, to detect any "make/break" fracture, which is apparent only when the lead is stretched. A more difficult task is to assess whether a pulse generator has failed. This may be attributable to a variety of causes, the most likely of which is battery depletion. Most pathologists do not have at their disposal the electronic equipment necessary for such testing. Therefore, the most practical approach is to turn the pulse generator and lead (preferably without separating them) over to an expert physician who implants pacemakers, a biomedical engineer, or the manufacturer for pulse generator testing. A pathologist should not report battery failure unless battery function is directly tested. It is important to provide relevant clinical and autopsy information when pacing hardware is sent to the manufacturer and to pack it so that there is no danger of disease transmission to those who must transmit or test it but who may not have medical training in handling the explant. It is useful to know that lithium batteries may explode on cremation.

Implanted Cardioverter-Defibrillator

Sudden cardiac death is most often initiated by rapid ventricular tachycardia. The automatic implantable cardioverter-defibrillator has been used to manage patients who have life-threatening ventricular arrhythmias.[276, 301–303] Benefit in overall mortality has been documented.[304, 305]

Complications

Implantable cardioverter-defibrillators are subject to many of the complications and other considerations described previously for implantable pacing systems, but there have been several specific problems. One has been false-positive discharges. Moreover, intrinsic ventricular arrhythmias, both ventricular tachycardia and fibrillation, may go undetected and cause death.

Complications are related to the surgical procedure used for implantation, the number and size of leads, the size of the generator, and the limitations of the system used for arrhythmia detection and termination. Most complications seen perioperatively are related nonspecifically to thoracotomy or subclavian introduction of standard pacing wires. However, the more extensive hardware of the cardioverter-defibrillator system may contribute to an increased frequency of complications (relative to pacemakers), such as infection and late accumulation of serosanguineous pleural fluid. The leads are applied to the epicardium, which involves opening the pericardium and allowing communication between pericardial and pleural spaces. Moreover, the hardware located in the pericardial and pleural spaces may cause local irritation or erosion of the lead into a vital structure such as a coronary artery. Fluid accummulation over the generator box can occur

secondary to the extensive subcutaneous dissection involved with generator placement and subcutaneous tunneling of the leads from the pleural space to the abdominal pocket. The intracardiac leads develop fibrous sheaths similar to those of endocardial pacer leads. As with pacer leads, movement and other factors may alter defibrillation threshold.

The leads and the consequences of repeated defibrillations can cause the following effects: (1) a direct one on the myocardium and vascular structures induced by repeated discharges, (2) possible thrombogenic potential of the indwelling intravascular electrodes, and (3) pericardial changes due to the placement of the apical patch electrodes. One study examined 25 patients at autopsy after implantation of an automatic implantable cardioverter-defibrillator.[306] Pericardial changes were typical of those occurring as a generalized nonspecific response to cardiac surgery, with the addition of localized fibrous adhesions at the sites of apical patch electrodes. Large venous thrombi were present in 20% of patients, and several had asymptomatic pulmonary emboli. Moreover, there was localized contraction band necrosis and myocyte degenerative changes confined to the tissue under the patch electrode but occupying less than 2% of myocardial mass.[306]

Ablation or Excision of Arrhythmogenic Foci

The intentional destruction of arrhythmogenic myocardial tissue, accessory atrioventricular connections, or parts of the specialized conduction system to cure or control cardiac rhythm disturbances is called *ablation.* Ablation is accomplished by either open surgery electrode catheter methods or by delivering pharmacologic substances to the target myocardium. Although the feasibility of treating arrhythmias with ablation was initially demonstrated surgically, catheter ablation of a highly selected region of myocardium has essentially replaced the surgical approach.

The principles of all antiarrhythmic ablation therapy are that (1) the mechanism of the cardiac rhythm can be identified, (2) the site of origin of at least a vulnerable portion of the substrate can be localized, and (3) the site of origin can be ablated.

Electrophysiologic studies are used to (1) provide information on the type of rhythm disturbance, (2) terminate a tachycardia by electrical stimulation, (3) evaluate the effects of therapy, (4) ablate myocardium involved in the tachycardia, and (5) identify patients at risk for sudden cardiac death.[307, 308] Knowledge of the mechanism gives some "dimension" to the substrate. For example, a rhythm that results from abnormal automaticity may well reside in a minute focus of one or only a very few cells and require pinpoint accuracy in ablative methods. By contrast, a large reentrant circuit may be amenable to any method that destroys even a portion of a reentry loop. In an invasive electrophysiologic study, catheter electrodes are introduced into the heart via the venous and/or arterial system to induce and record electrical activity from the atria or ventricles, the His bundle, bundle branches, accessory pathways, and other structures. The risks of undergoing such a study are small but are increased when therapeutic maneuvers (i.e., ablation) are added. In a report of over 10,000 patients who received ablation procedures, complications ranged from 1 to 3%, with procedure-related deaths of approximately 0.2%.[309]

Ablative Techniques

Ablative techniques under investigation or used clinically include excision/incision techniques and a variety of procedures causing thermal injuries employing either cold (cryosurgical freezing) or heat (coagulation, vaporization), or with energy supplied by lasers, radiofrequencies, microwaves, ultrasound, gas expansion, or localized discharge of powerful direct current shocks. The mechanisms whereby injury is achieved vary according to the energy source and include cell rupture from intracellular crystallization and change in permeability (cryosurgery), coagulation (radiofrequency energy, some lasers), physical vaporization (other lasers), and membrane damage due to abrupt local fluxes of ions or pressure transients (direct current shock).

Closed-chest nonsurgical electrode catheter techniques that allow ablation of a site of tachycardia by delivering destructive electrical energy have emerged as an alternative to the direct surgical ablation of resistant arrhythmias. The technique involves delivery of one or more synchronized shocks through an electrode catheter close to the offending tissue, producing a still uncharacterized mixture of electrical, thermal, and barotrauma, which is responsible for both successful ablation and potential complications. Electrical shock fulguration, and laser, radiofrequency, cryoprobe, and other techniques under investigation can be directed either at a tachycardia focus or circuit or at an atrioventricular conduction pathway. Selective fulguration of anomalous conducting tissue, ablation of ventricular tachycardia, and atrial ablation have been done clinically. Catheter-mediated ablation provides an alternative to surgical interruption.

Ablative techniques can be direct or indirect. Direct approaches include division of accessory pathways and removal, interruption, or destruction of areas of reentry or abnormal automaticity. Indirect approaches attempt to modify the substrate of the arrhythmia (e.g., revascularization or sympathectomy) or prevent propagation of the arrhythmia to the adjoining myocardium (e.g., atrial isolation or creation of atrioventricular block in supraventricular tachycardia, ventricular incision for ventricular tachycardia).

Early catheter ablation experiments created atrioventricular block in dogs by placing a pacing catheter at the atrioventricular junction, connecting it to a defibrillator, and delivering a high-voltage shock, which produced a small explosion at the electrode.[310] The heat, barotrauma, and electrical injury produced were effective for ablation. Ablation-induced atrioventricular block has been done in patients suffering from rapid ventricular responses to atrial arrhythmias and in patients with ventricular arrhythmias.[311, 312] The usefulness of electrical ablation was limited by the need for general anesthesia and the concern that the associated trauma could depress ventricular function or cause cardiac perforation.

Radiofrequency catheter ablation uses electrical energy generated from low-power, high-frequency alternating current.[313, 314] The Bovie electrosurgical cutting device uses modulated radiofrequency current.[315] The unmodulated current used in catheter ablation creates tissue desiccation and a focal burn with coagulation necrosis. Radiofrequency current is delivered between an electrode on an endocardial catheter and a large skin electrode. Radiofrequency ablation produces heating without causing propagated depolarizations or ectopic beats and can be performed without general anesthesia.

With the localized injury produced by radiofrequency ablation, it was difficult to achieve a lesion large enough to abolish an arrhythmia, particularly in patients with ventricular tachycardia associated with healed MI. In such cases, the target tissue frequently consists of islands or strips of residual viable myocytes between layers of endocardial fibrosis and dense subendocardial scar.[316] Arrhythmogenic tissue could not be destroyed in 30 to 50% of such cases because when the temperature at the electrode tip reaches 100°C, proteins coagulated on its surface, producing a high-impedance barrier to current flow that prevented further enlargement of ablation lesions.[317, 318] Using a larger electrode surface area reduced the current density at the electrode tip and increased electrode cooling by the circulating blood.[319]

Ventricular tachycardia related to left ventricular scarring is often caused by reentry circuits that are much larger or deeper than typical radiofrequency ablation lesions. Saline-cooled radiofrequency catheter ablation allows creation of larger lesions, presumably increasing the power that can be delivered without coagulum formation.[320–322] Cooling also displaces the region of maximal temperature below the electrode-tissue interface, maintaining lower electrode temperature for a given power application.[323–325] Indeed, in two patients it was shown that ablation lesions could extend to 7 mm deep to the endocardium, and deep to a 4-mm-thick transmural scar. The ablation sites contained coagulation necrosis with hemorrhage, surrounded by a rim of granulation tissue (see Fig. 22-26).[325] This technique may prove useful during ablation of ventricular reentrant circuits in regions of infarction.

The major safety concern regarding cooled radiofrequency ablation is the possibility of achieving a temperature of 100°C below the surface of the tissue, with steam formation and a resultant intramural "explosion" that creates a deep crater and risk of perforation.

Pathologic Considerations

The principal limitation to radiofrequency catheter ablation is the risk of thromboembolism.[326] The incidence is approximately 2% in the left side of the heart, and increases when ventricular tachycardia is present.

Radiofrequency current is an alternating one delivered at cycle lengths of 300 to 750 kHz when used for catheter ablation. It causes resistive heating of the tissue in contact with the electrode.[327] Because the degree of tissue heating is inversely proportional to the radius to the fourth power,[328] the lesions created by radiofrequency energy are small. The primary mechanism of tissue destruction is thermal injury.[329] Irreversible tissue destruction requires a

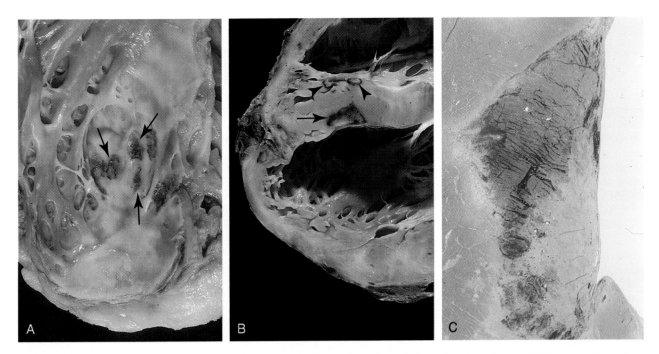

Figure 22-26 • Gross photographs and histologic section of ablation sites of ventricular tachyarrhythmias. *A,* Ablation sites (arrows) on endocardial surface of LV in patient with ischemic heart disease. *B,* Gross cross-sectional slice of heart from patient receiving ablation. Arrow highlights a saline-cooled catheter lesion in the left ventricle while the arrowhead at the right ventricular side of the septum (top) highlights 2 uncooled catheter sites. *C,* Subendocardial myocardial necrosis associated with one of the saline-cooled ablation sites of heart shown in *B* (H & E stain). (From Delacretaz E, Stevenson WG, Winters GL, et al: Ablation of ventricular tachycardia with a saline-cooled radiofrequency catheter: Anatomic and histologic characteristics of the lesions in humans. J Cardiovasc Electrophysiol 10:860, 1999)

tissue temperature of approximately 50°C.[330] In most ablation procedures, the power output of the radiofrequency generator is adjusted manually or automatically to achieve a temperature of 60 to 70°C at the electrode-tissue interface.

The acute lesion created by radiofrequency current consists of a central zone of coagulation necrosis surrounded by a zone of hemorrhage and inflammation. Chronic lesions are characterized by coagulation necrosis and have a discrete border. The arrhythmia may recur if the target tissue is in the zone bordering a lesion instead of in the central area of necrosis.[331] Conversely, the site of origin of an arrhythmia that has not been successfully ablated may later become permanently nonfunctional if it is within the border zone of a lesion and if microvascular injury and inflammation within this zone result in progressive necrosis.[332, 333] Catheter ablation was previously performed with direct-current shocks. Radiofrequency ablation has replaced direct-current ablation because it has several advantages over direct current. These include the absence of skeletal and cardiac muscle stimulation; minimal discomfort during delivery of energy; the possibility of performing the procedure in conscious patients; the absence of barotrauma; the absence of damage to the catheter; the discrete nature of the resulting lesions; and the delivery of energy over a period of 30 to 60 seconds, which allows avoidance of potential complications by terminating the application of energy early.

Histologic studies have been done on the hearts of a few patients whose deaths occurred after, but were not overtly related to, selective transvenous ablation of direct anomalous atrioventricular pathways performed after standard endocardial mapping.[334] Changes ranged from an absence of the target tissue to severe damage and scarring. In a patient who died 5 months after ablation accomplished by a single electrical charge of 280 joules, the atrioventricular node showed intense fibrous scarring that disrupted the outer layer, severing all atrionodal connections, extending to the middle layer, and sparing only part of the innermost layer.[335] The nodal-bundle junction and the beginning of the bundle of His were disrupted by scar. The endocardium over the atrioventricular node and proximal His bundle had marked fibrosis, but the lower part of the His bundle and bundle branches were normal. In another patient in whom death occurred 6 months after ablation by one 275-joule shock, the area immediately anterior to the coronary sinus and adjacent to the insertion of the septal leaflet of the tricuspid valve had no endocardial thickening or scarring, but the atrioventricular nodal tissue was completely replaced by fibrous tissue.[336] An additional patient who died 6 weeks after ablation had marked pathology of the conduction system, including fibroelastosis with chronic inflammatory changes of the atrioventricular node, bundle of His, and bundle branches.[337] Moreover, there were marked inflammatory changes with fibrosis of the atrial septum, adjacent aorta, and summit of the ventricular septum and degenerative changes in the tricuspid and aortic valves.

Catheter modification of posterior accessory atrioventricular pathways has a success rate less than 75%, and there are distinct risks. Complications associated with catheter-mediated ablation include electrical shock–

induced coronary artery injury, whose consequences would be particularly important in a left dominant system or in a right dominant system with a large posterior extension of the right coronary artery. Coronary arteriography done before the ablative procedure may help determine coronary arterial anatomy and thus avoid this complication. Coronary artery spasm has been observed in humans after nearby ablative shocks. Coronary sinus rupture with tamponade occurred in 3 of 19 patients in one study.[338] The patient was salvaged by surgery in all instances, largely because each had been prepared and draped for surgery before the ablative procedure. Electrical discharges delivered close to a direct anomalous pathway can cause permanent and complete block. The pathways most amenable to this technique are those located within the septum or around the left atrial free wall. These areas often can be approached by the coronary sinus, but shocks greater than 100 joules may predispose to rupture. Simultaneous discharges with electrodes on both sides of the interventricular septum may increase effectiveness.[339]

Surgical Treatment of Arrhythmias

Direct surgical treatment of dysrhythmia, whether or not it is due to ischemic heart disease, is accomplished by either isolation or ablation. Ablation stops the dysrhythmia either thermally or by resection or interruption of a reentrant circuit. An open surgical approach can ablate the tissue responsible for atrioventricular junctional reentrant tachycardia, yet preserve normal atrioventricular condition. In the absence of an accessory pathway of conduction, surgical therapy for supraventricular tachycardia must consist of direct ablation of an atrial source of dysrhythmia, exclusion of an atrial focus from propagation through the atria and the atrioventricular junction, or indirect therapy such as ablation or modification of the atrioventricular node–His bundle. Since most patients with recurring symptomatic ventricular tachycardia have a reentry mechanism as a cause, they need only to have the offending tissue interrupted to effect a surgical cure. In contrast, pinpoint accuracy is generally required for the treatment of abnormal automaticity. Isolation limits the exit conduction pathways but does not alter the presence, frequency, or electrophysiologic characteristics of a dysrhythmia.

REPAIRED CONGENITAL HEART DISEASE

Pathologists who evaluate autopsy specimens of operated congenital heart disease must often function as a "medical archeologist," identifying alterations not only associated with the underlying malformations but also related to previous interventional procedures. To provide useful information for one's surgical and clinical colleagues, the following should be evaluated in detail:

1. The underlying congenital cardiac malformations
2. Secondary hypertensive pulmonary vascular disease
3. Extracardiac anomalies, suggestive of a syndrome
4. All interventional procedures, including take-downs
5. Postinterventional enlargement of hypoplastic structures

6. Postinterventional regression of pulmonary vascular disease
7. Postinterventional regression of hypertrophy or dilation
8. Postinterventional complications, including ischemia
9. Late development of valvular regurgitation
10. Evidence of acute or chronic heart failure
11. Evidence of cardiac or extracardiac infections
12. Correlation of the findings with clinical imaging modalities

References are available that describe the pathology of congenital heart disease, the pathology of pulmonary hypertension (see also Chapter 7) the numerous surgical procedures for malformed hearts, nonsurgical interventions (such as balloon valvuloplasty), and postinterventional complications.[340–347] In adults, congenital heart disease can be seen in four settings:

1. No previous diagnosis or treatment of the cardiac anomaly
2. Previous diagnosis and intervention, with no additional intervention needed
3. Previous diagnosis and intervention, with additional intervention needed
4. Previous diagnosis, but no intervention, due to irreversible pulmonary hypertension

Moreover, adults with congenital heart disease may also have coexistent acquired heart disease, such as coronary atherosclerosis, persistent systemic hypertension, and noncongenital valvular disease.

General Approach to Autopsy Specimens

Certain information should be gathered before beginning the dissection, including a history of the underlying malformation, other anomalies, or syndromes and any interventional procedures (both surgical and nonsurgical). One should also ascertain the circumstances surrounding the patient's death (e.g., was it in-hospital or out-of-hospital, witnessed or unwitnessed, postprocedural or not, with attempted resuscitation or not, and expected or sudden and unexpected). If this information cannot be obtained before beginning the dissection, then proceed with caution—like a detective unraveling a complex mystery.

Before evisceration, the position of the heart and the direction of the cardiac apex should be noted. The abdominal cavity should be inspected next for the position and number of spleens, the presence of bowel malrotation, and the "sidedness" of the digestive system. After the thoracic organs have been removed, the cardiac and pulmonary sidedness can also be determined.[348] Initially, the thoracic organs should be kept together as one tissue specimen, such that the heart, lungs, and great vessels, including the entire thoracic aorta and appreciable lengths of the arch vessels, are not separated from one another.

Evaluation of the Heart

If the specimen is to be fixed before dissection, the heart can be distended either by use of a continuous perfusion system or by simple syringe-perfusion of the chambers and vessels. The lungs should be distended to total lung capacity by low-pressure transtracheal perfusion with formalin. The heart and lungs should be kept together in cases either with pulmonary atresia and a ventricular septal defect or with anomalous pulmonary venous connection. Otherwise, the lungs can be removed from the heart by transecting the pulmonary arteries and veins at the hilum.

Dissection of the heart can be achieved by various methods, including the inflow-ouflow, tomographic, base-of-heart, and window techniques.[349, 350] For the inflow-outflow method, one simply opens the heart according to the direction of blood flow, which in complex cases is not necessarily in the direction expected. The tomographic method produces planes of section similar to those achieved by most clinical imaging techniques; the three most popular planes are short-axis, long-axis, and four-chamber. As in living patients, the sequential segmental method is used to evaluate congenital cardiac malformations at autopsy, as described in detail by various authors.[351] A form has been devised to simplify this process (see the Appendix to this chapter).

After the anomalies have been evaluated, the heart and great vessels should be inspected for secondary lesions. These include chamber hypertrophy or dilation, or their regression; valvular or vascular dilation, or their regression; enlargement of a hypoplastic chamber, valve, or vessel; atrophy of a cardiovascular structure; and fibrosis of the myocardium, valves, endocardium, or pericardium. An increase in overall heart weight should be recorded and compared with normal values based on gender and body size.[352, 353]

Evaluation of the Lungs

Pulmonary arteries should be evaluated for thickening and dilation. In some cases, dilated and hypertensive arteries can compress the adjacent tracheobronchial tree and result in recurrent pneumonia. A markedly enlarged heart may also compress adjacent lung tissue and cause partial atelectasis.

In all cases, the upper and lower lobes of each lung should be sampled for a microscopic evaluation of pulmonary vascular and parenchymal disease. Sections are taken such that arteries and airways are cut in cross section, with pleural surfaces included in at least two slides. Sections should be large and the four slides stained with hematoxylin-eosin and elastic–van Gieson.

Patients with congenital cardiac left-to-right shunts can develop progressive plexogenic pulmonary hypertension. In such cases, the pulmonary vasculature should be evaluated for the severity of plexogenic disease, using the modified Heath-Edwards classification (Table 22-5) and for evidence of postoperative regression of disease. Patients with congenital heart disease can also have other types of hypertensive pulmonary vascular disease, for which the Heath-Edwards classification is not applicable. For example, in the setting of chronic heart failure or left-sided obstructive lesions, the changes of pulmonary venous hypertension may be prominent. Also, among patients with tetralogy of Fallot and severely diminished pulmonary blood flow, in situ thrombosis can occur

TABLE 22-5 • **Modified Heath-Edwards Classification for Pulmonary Hypertension Associated With Congenital Cardiac Left-to-Right Shunts**

Grade	Lesion	Reversible
1A	Muscularization of arterioles	Yes
1B	Medial hypertrophy of arteries	Yes
1C	Loss of intra-acinar arteries	Yes*
2	Concentric intimal proliferation	Yes
3	Concentric laminar intimal fibrosis	Borderline†
5	Dilation (angiomatoid) lesions	Borderline†
6	Fibrinoid degeneration	No
6	Necrotizing arteritis	No
4‡	Plexiform lesions	No

* Although arterial loss is irreversible, the percentage of involved vessels is generally small, such that the entire pulmonary vascular bed still exhibits potentially reversible disease.

† If the extent of grade 3 and 5 lesions is mild, pulmonary vascular disease is usually reversible. If moderate, the disease is unpredictable and may regress, remain unchanged, or progress. If severe, the disease tends to be progressive and irreversible.

‡ Because plexiform lesions are now considered to represent the aftermath of necrotizing arteritis and microaneurysm formation, grade 4 lesions follow grade 5 and 6 lesions.

From Edwards WD: Congenital heart disease. In: Damjanov I, Linder J (eds): Anderson's Pathology. 10th ed. St. Louis, Mosby, 1996, p 1339.

within the small pulmonary arteries. In addition, patients with coexistent scoliosis may develop the changes of chronic hypoxic pulmonary hypertension.

General Approach to Surgical Specimens

During operative procedures for congenital cardiac malformations, various cardiac, vascular, or pulmonary specimens may be excised.[354–359] Valves should be evaluated for anomalies, infection, and secondary changes, and the clinical functional state of the valve recorded. Resected endomyocardium, as from the right ventricular outflow tract in a patient with tetralogy of Fallot, generally exhibits myocyte hypertrophy and both interstitial and endocardial fibrosis. Tissue from the ascending aorta, particularly in adults, should be evaluated microscopically for cystic medial degeneration, using an elastic–van Gieson stain. Specimens removed during cardiac transplantation are dissected in a manner similar to that described for hearts removed at autopsy. Lung biopsies are generally performed for the investigation of hypertensive pulmonary vascular disease, and the resected tissues should be processed as described previously for autopsy material.

Surgical and Nonsurgical Interventions

The development of a pump-oxygenator (heart-lung machine) during the early 1950s transformed the vision of open-heart surgery into reality. Since then, creative minds have devised interventional procedures to repair even the most complex cardiac anomalies. Such interventions are now commonplace, are often performed during the first few months of life, and generally have a relatively low mortality rate.

Treatments have become available that have substantially improved the quality of life and increased the longevity of patients with congenitally malformed hearts.

Over 1 million patients with congenital heart disease in North America have survived to adulthood. Nonetheless, all interventions have been associated with various complications, and these need to be identified and assessed during cardiac dissection at autopsy.

From an interventional perspective, congenital heart disease consists of only five types of abnormalities:

1. Extra connections that should not exist (e.g., ventricular septal defect)
2. Absence of connections that should exist (e.g., tricuspid atresia)
3. Obstructed connections (e.g., congenital aortic stenosis)
4. Anomalous connections (e.g., transposition of the great arteries)
5. Regurgitant valves (e.g., Ebstein's anomaly of the tricuspid valve)

Accordingly, interventional procedures include the closure, creation, opening, or repair of the various abnormal connections and the repair or replacement of regurgitant valves.

Because some malformed hearts include combinations of abnormalities, their repair may entail several procedures. For example, the operation for tetralogy of Fallot (with subpulmonary stenosis, a ventricular septal defect, and an overriding aorta) includes relief of the subpulmonary stenosis and closure of the ventricular septal defect so as to direct only left ventricular blood into the ascending aorta. For complex anomalies, several staged operations, performed at different times, may be necessary. Many of the ingenious operations for congenitally malformed hearts carry the name of the surgeon or clinician who devised them (Table 22-6).

Closure of Connections

This category includes the suture or patch closure of an atrial, ventricular, or atrioventricular septal defect *(atrioventricular canal)* and the suture ligation or closure of a patent ductal artery *(patent ductus arteriosus)*. Currently, the surgical mortality for these procedures is very low, and complications are rare. At autopsy, closure sites should be evaluated for incomplete closure (i.e., the presence of a residual shunt), thrombus on a patch, persistent cardiomegaly, and hypertensive pulmonary vascular disease.

Closure of Atrial Septal Defects. For isolated defects, the surgical mortality is less than 1% for all age groups. Postoperative deaths are rare and are generally due to pulmonary hypertension or, in the elderly, to other coexistent cardiac disorders such as mitral regurgitation, ischemic heart disease, or heart failure. Clamshell devices, inserted percutaneously via a transvenous catheter, are also being used to close atrial septal defects nonsurgically.

Closure of Ventricular Septal Defects. Postoperative complications include a residual shunt, conduction disturbances, arrhythmias, and aortic or tricuspid regurgitation. The surgical mortality is less than 1% for infants with

isolated defects and about 10% overall. Early postoperative deaths are usually attributable to acute heart failure, whereas late deaths are often sudden, due to residual pulmonary hypertension or a ventricular arrhythmia.

Repair of Complete Atrioventricular Septal Defect (Complete Atrioventricular Canal). Mitral dysfunction (either regurgitation or stenosis) is the most common postoperative complication, followed by subaortic stenosis, arrhythmias, and progressive pulmonary hypertension. The early postoperative mortality rate is less than 5%, and most deaths are caused by acute heart failure. Coexistent Down syndrome and tetralogy of Fallot increase the surgical risk.

Closure of Patent Ductal Artery. Various potential complications, though rare, include a residual shunt, injury to the phrenic nerve or left recurrent laryngeal nerve, persistent pulmonary hypertension (in adults), and others. The surgical mortality is less than 1% for premature infants, nearly 0% for patients younger than 2 years, and less than 2% for adults.

Creation of Connections

This category includes procedures to create an interatrial shunt, to maintain patency of the ductal artery, and to increase pulmonary blood flow. At autopsy, interventional sites should be assessed for patency and for injury to adjacent structures.

Creation of an Interatrial Shunt. The presence of an unobstructed interatrial communication is needed for the survival of newborns with tricuspid or mitral atresia, total anomalous pulmonary venous connection, or complete transposition of the great arteries with an intact ventricular septum and a closing ductal artery. Nonsurgical balloon atrial septostomy generally results in excellent palliation. Procedural failure is usually due to stretching, rather than tearing, of the valve of the fossa ovalis. Rarely, adjacent structures may be damaged. If the balloon method fails, an interatrial shunt can be created by transcatheter blade septostomy or by a surgical Blalock-Hanlon atrial septectomy.

Maintenance of Ductal Artery Patency. Patency of the ductal artery is necessary if newborns with aortic valve atresia, interrupted aortic arch, pulmonary atresia without collateral arteries, or complete transposition of the great arteries with an intact ventricular septum are to survive. Without intervention, the ductal artery usually closes, despite a fatal outcome. Although prostaglandin E_1 is commonly employed to maintain ductal patency, its prolonged usage causes degenerative changes that weaken the arterial wall. Later surgical closure, during repair of the underlying cardiac malformation, may be complicated by formation of a ductal aneurysm.

Creation of Systemic-to-Pulmonary Arterial Shunts. In patients with decreased pulmonary blood flow (e.g., those with tetralogy of Fallot), a communication may be created between a systemic and a pulmonary artery to increase pulmonary blood flow and to enlarge the pulmonary arteries in preparation for a later reparative operation. Surgical shunts include the Mee, Blalock-Taussig,

TABLE 22-6 • **Eponyms for Surgical Procedures on Congenitally Malformed Hearts**

Eponym	Description of Procedure	Cardiovascular Anomalies
Blalock-Hanlon shunt	Partial atrial septectomy (posterosuperior region)	Complete TGA with intact ventricular septum
Blalock-Taussig shunt	Subclavian-to-pulmonary artery (classic: end-to-side anastomosis; modified: interposed synthetic graft)	Conditions with decreased pulmonary blood flow (tetralogy of Fallot, PA-VSD, and DORV or DILV with PS)
Damus-Kaye-Stansel procedure	Proximal PT to ascending aorta (end-to-side anastomosis); conduit from RV to distal PT; VSD closure	Complete TGA without PS and with or without VSD
Glenn anastomosis	SVC to RPA (end-to-side); ligation of SVC at RA; ligation of proximal RPA (bidirectional Glenn: no ligation of RPA)	Tricuspid atresia, or DILV with PS
Fontan procedure (modified)	Anastomosis of SVC, RA, or RV to RPA or LPA; may include intra-atrial conduit from IVC to SVC	Hearts with single functional ventricle (tricuspid atresia, DILV, etc.)
Jatene procedure	Transection and switching of great arteries and coronary arteries	Complete TGA, and DORV with subpulmonary VSD
Konno procedure	Outlet (infundibular) septostomy, with patch enlargement of LV and RV outflow tracts, and aortic valve replacement	Tunnel subaortic stenosis, and severe hypertrophic cardiomyopathy
Mee procedure	Ascending aorta to MPA (side-to-side anastomosis)	Same as for Blalock-Taussig shunt
Mustard procedure	Resection of atrial septum; intra-atrial baffle directing caval blood to LV, and pulmonary venous blood to RV	Complete TGA
Norwood procedure	Stage 1 (atrial septectomy; PDA ligation; PT transection; aortic incision; reconstruction of aorta with allograft; aorta-PT shunt). Stage 2 (modified Fontan operation)	Aortic atresia (hypoplastic left heart syndrome)
Potts shunt	Descending thoracic aorta to LPA (side-to-side anastomosis)	Same as for Blalock-Taussig shunt
Rastelli procedure	VSD closure directing LV blood to aorta; conduit from RV to distal PT; ligation of proximal PT	PA-VSD, PTA, complete TGA with VSD and PS, and DORV with PS
Ross procedure	Excision of aortic valve; excision of pulmonary valve and insertion into aortic position; insertion of prosthetic pulmonary valve	Severe aortic valve stenosis; tunnel subaortic stenosis
Senning procedure	Use of atrial septum to fashion intra-atrial baffle, similar to Mustard procedure	Complete TGA
Waterston shunt	Ascending aorta to RPA (side-to-side anastomosis)	Same as for Blalock-Taussig shunt

DILV, double inlet left ventricle; DORV, double outlet right ventricle; IVC, inferior vena cava; LPA, left pulmonary artery; LV, left ventricle; PA-VSD, pulmonary atresia with a ventricular septal defect; PDA, patent ductal artery; PS, pulmonary stenosis; PT, pulmonary trunk; PTA, persistent truncal artery; RA, right atrium; RPA, right pulmonary artery; RV, right ventricle; SVC, superior vena cava; TGA, transposition of the great arteries; VSD, ventricular septal defect.

Modified from Edwards WD: Congenital heart disease. In: Damjanov I, Linder J (eds): Anderson's Pathology. 10th ed. St. Louis, Mosby, 1996, p 1339.

Waterston, and Potts procedures (Table 22-6). The Mee and Blalock-Taussig shunts are favored because technically they are the easiest to create and to take down. Shunt failure is the only major complication and is usually the result of thrombosis, kinking of the graft, or progressive anastomotic stricture as the child grows. The surgical mortality is less than 5% overall and is about 1% for classic tetralogy of Fallot.

Relief of Obstructions

Interventions in this category include enlargement of a restrictive ventricular septal defect, reconstruction of the right or left ventricular outflow tract, repair or replacement of stenosed valves, and repair of coarctation of the aorta. At autopsy, surgical sites should be evaluated for intact suture lines, the patency of shunts, conduits, and coarctation sites, and the state of repaired or replaced valves.

Enlargement of a Ventricular Septal Defect. For patients with a restrictive ventricular septal defect and other major cardiac anomalies, surgical repair may include enlarging, rather than closing, the defect. Such procedures include a Rastelli repair for complete transposition or double-outlet right ventricle and a Fontan procedure for transposed great arteries with tricuspid atresia or a double-inlet left ventricle (see Table 22-6). During enlargement of the ventricular septal defect, damage may occur to the adjacent atrioventricular conduction system, ventricular free wall, or epicardial coronary arteries.

Ventricular Outflow Tract Reconstruction. Enlargement or reconstruction of the *right* ventricular outflow tract is employed for patients with classic tetralogy of Fallot and other conotruncal anomalies. For individuals with classic tetralogy, the repair entails the take-down of previous shunts, patch closure of the ventricular septal defect, resection of infundibular myocardium, pulmonary valvotomy, and enlargement of the outflow tract and pulmonary artery with a pericardial or synthetic patch. The most common complications are ventricular tachycardia (in 10%), residual subpulmonary stenosis (10%), and a residual ventricular septal defect (5%). Right ventricular dysfunction and aortic regurgitation are late complications. Early and late postoperative mortality rates are each less than 5%. Late sudden death claims about 2% and is associated with persistent cardiomegaly and postoperative arrhythmias.

For some patients with tetralogy and for other conotruncal anomalies, a Rastelli-type repair (see Table 22-6) is performed using an extracardiac conduit to reestablish communication between the right ventricle and the pulmonary arteries (Fig. 22-27). Conduits include cadaveric aortic or pulmonary homografts and synthetic tube-grafts that contain a bioprosthetic valve. Over time, homograft valves often develop fibrotic retraction, whereas bioprosthetic valves and homograft arteries tend to become calcified (see Chapter 21). Conduit stenosis represents the most common complication and requires reoperation within 5 years in 10% of patients. The most common causes of conduit stenosis are valvular calcification and neointimal hyperplasia (see Fig. 22-27B), accounting for about 90% of the cases. Other postoperative complications include conduit valve regurgitation or infection, residual ventricular septal defect, residual ventricular hypertrophy or dilation, and others. Overall, the early surgical mortality rate is 20% and is usually attributable to acute heart failure, conduit compression, or sepsis. Late postoperative mortality is less than 10% and is often due to chronic heart failure or a sudden fatal arrhythmia.

Reconstruction of the *left* ventricular outflow tract is applicable for the discrete or tunnel forms of subaortic stenosis. Resection of the obstructing tissue may be performed in some (with an early mortality rate of 3%), whereas a Konno procedure, Ross procedure, or use of an extracardiac conduit is necessary in others (see Table 22-6). The mortality rate is 10 to 20%.

Relief of Congenital Aortic and Pulmonary Stenosis. For patients with congenital aortic stenosis, balloon valvuloplasty is successful in 90%. The early postprocedural mortality is 15%, and death generally results from cusp tears with acute aortic regurgitation. Surgical aortic valvuloplasty also carries a 15% early mortality, and most deaths are a result of acute heart failure. Aortic valve replacement is generally well tolerated in children and adults but has an especially poor prognosis in neonates.

Among patients with congenital pulmonary stenosis, transcatheter balloon valvuloplasty is successful in nearly 100%. Complications are rare, and the early mortality rate is nearly 0%. Postprocedural pulmonary regurgitation may occur but is usually well tolerated.

Repair of Coarctation of the Aorta. Coarctation may be repaired by subclavian flap aortoplasty or by segmental resection with end-to-end anastomosis. Complications include postoperative paradoxical hypertension, ischemic abdominal pain, and persistent or recurrent coarctation. Early postoperative mortality rates are 5% for infants and 1% for other age groups. Percutaneous transcatheter balloon aortoplasty can also be used to treat coarctation, either initially or in cases of recurrent coarctation.

Repair of Anomalous Connections

Included in this category are the arterial and atrial switch procedures, conduit operations, and atriopulmonary and cavopulmonary anastomoses. At autopsy, surgical sites should be evaluated for intact suture lines, patent

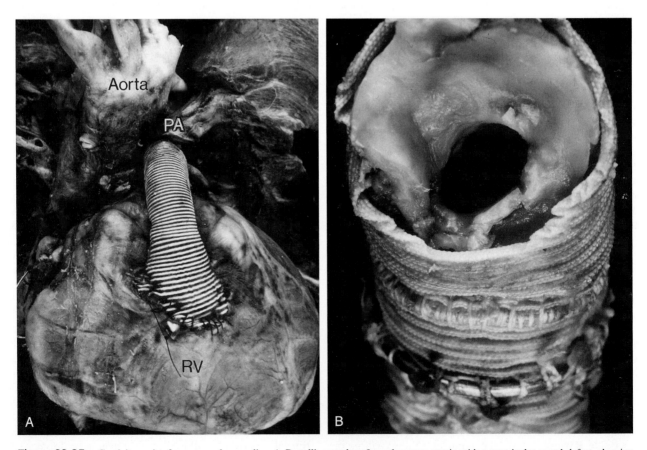

Figure 22-27 • Conduit repair of conotruncal anomalies. *A,* Rastelli procedure for pulmonary atresia with a ventricular septal defect, showing synthetic conduit between right ventricle (RV) and pulmonary arteries (PA) in an anterior view of an autopsy specimen. *B,* Conduit stenosis due to neointimal hyperplasia in a surgical specimen.

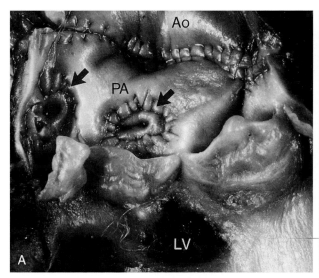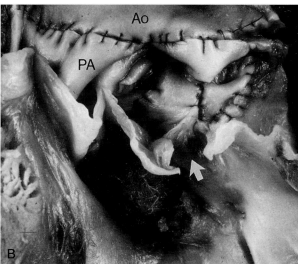

Figure 22-28 • Jatene arterial switch operation for complete transposition of the great arteries. *A,* Intact suture lines between the pulmonary artery (PA) and the ascending aorta (Ao) and at both coronary ostial anastomosis sites (arrows) in an opened left ventricle (LV) from an autopsy specimen. *B,* Acute postoperative aortic regurgitation due to a tear in one "aortic" valve cusp (arrow) adjacent to a coronary ostial anastomosis site in an opened left ventricle from an autopsy specimen.

anastomoses, and injury to coronary ostia or arteries. Hearts should also be assessed for hypertrophy, dilation, and fibrosis. Inspection for acute myocardial injury and myocarditis is important in cases of sudden death.

Complete transposition of the great arteries may exist with or without a ventricular septal defect and with or without pulmonary stenosis. For the resulting four types, numerous ingenious surgical procedures have been devised, including the Jatene, Mustard, Senning, Rastelli, and Damus-Kaye-Stansel operations (see Table 22-6). Only the Jatene arterial switch procedure truly corrects the anomaly both physiologically and anatomically (Fig. 22-28*A*). It usually includes the Lecompte maneuver, in which the pulmonary artery bifurcation is positioned anterior to the aorta. With the Mustard and Senning operations, an intra-atrial baffle reroutes systemic venous blood in the left ventricle and pulmonary artery and redirects pulmonary venous blood into the right ventricle and aorta. Both the Rastelli and the Damus-Kaye-Stansel operations redirect left ventricular blood into the aorta and utilize a valved conduit to reroute right ventricular blood into the pulmonary arteries. The Rastelli procedure requires a ventricular septal defect, which is present in only 30% of the cases. If repair of transposition is performed within the first 6 months of life, progressive pulmonary hypertension rarely develops.

Jatene Arterial Switch Procedure. This operation is generally performed within the first month of life and often during the first week. The two most frequent complications, requiring reoperation in about 15%, are dynamic right ventricular outflow tract obstruction and pulmonary artery stenosis. Coronary artery kinking and coronary ostial stenosis, though uncommon, can cause acute myocardial ischemia or infarction in the immediate postoperative period, with acute heart failure, arrhythmias, or sudden death. Other complications include left ventricular dysfunction, a residual ventricular septal defect, and

"aortic" regurgitation (see Fig. 22-28*B*). The early surgical mortality is less than 5%, due to the complications listed previously, and the late mortality is also less than 5%. Remarkably, the 5-year survival has increased from only 5% in the presurgical era to over 90% in patients currently undergoing an arterial switch operation.

Mustard and Senning Procedures. For the *atrial* switch operations, the morbidity and mortality are somewhat less for the Senning than for the Mustard procedure. Complications include arrhythmias and conduction disturbances, obstruction to systemic or pulmonary blood flow, anastomotic leaks, and tricuspid regurgitation. The two most serious, and potentially fatal, late complications are fibrosis, dilation, and eventual failure of the systemic right ventricle and the development of recurrent ventricular arrhythmias. Early and late postoperative mortality rates are each about 10%, with a 20-year survival rate of 80%.

Rastelli and Damus-Kaye-Stansel Procedures. For both operations, the most frequently encountered postoperative complication is conduit stenosis, which may be assessed in either autopsy or surgical specimens. In patients with a Rastelli repair for complete transposition of the great arteries, the early and late postoperative mortality rates are each about 10%.

Fontan and Glenn Procedures. Atriopulmonary and cavopulmonary anastomoses are applied to hearts with a severely hypoplastic and functionally unusable ventricle. Within this group are two categories of hearts: (1) those with a univentricular atrioventricular connection, including tricuspid atresia, mitral atresia, double-inlet ventricle, and common inlet ventricle, and (2) those with atresia of a semilunar valve and an intact ventricular septum, including aortic atresia (hypoplastic left heart syndrome) and pulmonary atresia. For both operative procedures, the single functional ventricle is used as the systemic pumping chamber, and systemic venous blood is directed to the pulmonary arteries without an intervening ventricle. Forward blood flow through the lungs is maintained by the bellows action of the thorax, the presence of competent left-sided cardiac valves, and the absence of pulmonary hypertension.

Among patients with single functional ventricles, the Fontan procedure has numerous modifications and variations, depending on the complexity of the underlying congenital malformation. It is usually performed when patients are about 2 years old. In general, complications are the result of chronic to-and-fro blood flow in a system lacking a pumping chamber or right-sided valves. Ascites, edema, and chylothorax occur in 15%, and caval and hepatic venous reflux can cause hepatic dysfunction, dilated enteric lymphatics, and protein-losing enteropathy. Right atrial mural thrombus and recurrent ventricular tachycardia can also develop. The early postoperative mortality is 10% for tricuspid atresia and 25% for patients with complex congenital malformations such as the asplenia syndrome. Late postoperative mortality accounts for an additional 15%. Death is usually the result of chronic heart failure, persistent fluid accumulation, reoperation, infection, arrhythmias, or protein-losing enteropathy.

For patients with aortic valve atresia and a hypoplastic left heart syndrome, a Fontan operation represents the second stage of a Norwood procedure (see Table 22-6). The first stage has a 35% early mortality and an additional 15% late mortality, and the second stage a 15% early mortality and an additional 35% late mortality. Death is usually attributable to heart failure. A Glenn cavopulmonary anastomosis (see Table 22-6) is currently recommended for older children in whom a Fontan repair is not feasible and for younger children in whom a Fontan anastomosis will be performed later as a second-stage procedure. Complications are related to nonpulsatile pulmonary blood flow and include the development of pulmonary arteriovenous fistulas. The early postoperative mortality rate is 3%.

Procedures for Valvular Regurgitation

This category includes both valve repair and valve replacement. The functional state of the valve just before death should be recorded, if known. At autopsy, the surgical site should be evaluated for intact suture lines, fibrosis, calcification, infection, and injury to adjacent structures.

Ebstein's Malformation. The most common congenital cause of tricuspid valvular incompetence is Ebstein's anomaly. Surgical intervention includes annular plication, tricuspid valve repair or replacement, reduction right atrioplasty, plication of the atrialized portion of the right ventricle, and closure of any interatrial communication. Potential complications include prosthetic valve dysfunction and infection, persistent right ventricular dysfunction, damage to the atrioventricular conduction system, and kinking of the adjacent right coronary artery. The most common causes of postoperative death are heart failure and fatal arrhythmias.

Late Postoperative Aortic Regurgitation. For certain conotruncal anomalies (tetralogy of Fallot, pulmonary

atresia with a ventricular septal defect, and persistent truncal artery), the ascending aorta or truncal artery is larger than normal. Because patients who underwent Rastelli procedures during childhood are now surviving into adulthood, a significant percentage of those older than 40 years are developing appreciable aortic root dilation and aortic valve regurgitation. In either autopsy or surgical specimens, the aortic valve generally shows stretched cusps with annular dilation, and the ascending aorta may exhibit cystic medial degeneration.

REFERENCES

1. Topol EJ, Serruys PW: Frontiers in interventional cardiology. Circulation 98:1802, 1998
2. www.americanheart.org/statistics/09medicl.html
3. Herrick JB: Clinical features of sudden obstruction of the coronary arteries. JAMA 59:2015, 1912
4. DeWood MA, Spores J, Notske R, et al: Prevalence of total coronary occlusion during the early hours of transmural myocardial infarction. N Engl J Med 303:897, 1980
5. Fuster V: Mechanisms leading to myocardial infarction: Insights from studies of vascular biology. Circulation 90:2126, 1994
6. Theroux P, Willerson JT, Armstrong PW: Progress in the treatment of acute coronary syndromes. A 50-year perspective (1950–2000). Circulation 102:IV-2, 2000
7. Gruppo Italiano Per Lo Studio Della Streptochinasi Nell'Infarct Miocardico (GISSI): Effectiveness of intravenous thrombolytic treatment in acute myocardial infarction. Lancet 1:397, 1986
8. Laffel GL, Braunwald E: Thrombolytic therapy. A new strategy for the treatment of acute myocardial infarction. N Engl J Med 311:710, 770, 1984
9. Lavie CJ, Gersh BJ, Chesebro JH: Reperfusion in acute myocardial infarction. Mayo Clin Proc 65:549, 1990
10. Granger CB, Califf RM, Topol EJ: Thrombolytic therapy for acute myocardial infarction: A review. Drugs 44:293, 1992
11. Cairns JA, Fuster V, Gore J, Kennedy JW: Coronary thrombolysis. Chest 108:401S, 1995
12. Antman EM, Braunwald E: Acute myocardial infarction. In: Braunwald E (ed): Heart Disease: A Textbook of Cardiovascular Medicine. 5th ed. Philadelphia, WB Saunders, 1996, p 1184
13. White HD, Van de Werf JJ: Thrombolysis for acute myocardial infarction. Circulation 97:1632, 1998
14. Topol EJ: Thrombolytic intervention. In: Topol EJ (ed): Textbook of Interventional Cardiology, 3rd ed. Philadelphia, WB Saunders, 1999, p 78
15. Straznicky IT, White HD: Thrombolytic therapy for acute myocardial infarction in the elderly. Coron Artery Dis 11:299, 2000
16. ISIS-2 (Second International Study of Infarct Survival) Collaborative Group: Randomised trial of intravenous streptokinase, oral aspirin, both, or neither among 17,187 cases of suspected acute myocardial infarction: ISIS-2. Lancet 2:349, 1988
17. ISAM (Intravenous Streptokinase in Acute Myocardial Infarction) Study Group: A prospective trial of intravenous streptokinase in acute myocardial infarction (ISAM). N Engl J Med 314:1465, 1988
18. Simes RJ, Topol EJ, Holmes DR Jr, et al, for the GUSTO-I Investigators: Link between the angiographic substudy and mortality outcomes in a large randomized trial of myocardial reperfusion: Importance of early and complete infarct artery reperfusion. Circulation 91:1923, 1995
19. ISIS-3 (Third International Study of Infarct Survival) Collaborative Group: ISIS-3: A randomized trial of streptokinase vs. tissue plasminogen activator vs. anistreplase and of aspirin plus heparin vs. aspirin alone among 41,299 cases of suspected acute myocardial infarction. Lancet 339:753, 1992
20. The GUSTO Angiographic Investigators: The comparative effects of tissue plasminogen activator, streptokinase, or both on coronary artery patency, ventricular function and survival after acute myocardial infarction. N Engl J Med 329:1615, 1993
21. Ohman EM, Califf RM, Topol EJ: Consequences of reocclusion

after successful reperfusion therapy in acute MI. The TAMI Study Group. Circulation 82:781, 1990

22. Reimer KA, Lowe JE, Rasmussen MM, Jennings RB: The wavefront phenomenon of ischemic cell death. I: Myocardial infarct size vs. duration of coronary occlusion in dogs. Circulation 5:786, 1977

23. White HD: Should all occluded infarct-related arteries be opened? Eur Heart J 18:1207, 1997

24. Weaver WD, Simes RJ. Betriu A, et al: Comparison of primary coronary angioplasty and intravenous thrombolytic therapy for acute myocardial infarction: A quantitative view. JAMA 278:2093, 1997

25. The Global Use of Strategies To Open Occluded Coronary Arteries in Acute Coronary Syndromes (GUSTO IIb) Angioplasty Substudy Investigators: A clinical trial comparing primary coronary angioplasty with tissue plasminogen activator for acute myocardial infarction. N Engl J Med 336:1621, 1997

26. Jennings RB, Steenbergen C, Reimer KA: Myocardial ischemia and reperfusion. In: Schoen FJ, Gimbrone MA Jr (eds): Cardiovascular Pathology. Clinicopathologic Correlations and Pathogenetic Mechanisms. Baltimore, Williams & Wilkins, 1995, p 47

27. Buja LM: Modulation of the myocardial response to ischemia. Lab Invest 78:1345, 1998

28. Schoen FJ: The heart. In: Cotran RS, Kumar V, Collins T (eds): Robbins Pathologic Basis of Disease. 6th ed. Philadelphia, WB Saunders, 1999, p 543

29. Piper HM, Garcia-Dorado D: Prime causes of rapid cardiomyocyte death during reperfusion. Ann Thorac Surg 68:1913, 1999

30. Flameng W: Mechanisms underlying myocardial stunning. J Card Surg 8(suppl):275, 1993

31. Appleyard RF, Cohn LH: Myocardial stunning and reperfusion injury in cardiac surgery. J Card Surg 8(suppl):316, 1993

32. Kloner RA, Bolli R, Marban E, et al: Medical and cellular implications of stunning, hibernation, and preconditioning. Circulation 97:1848, 1998

33. Mattfeldt T, Schwarz F, Schuler G, et al: Necropsy evaluation in seven patients with evolving acute myocardial infarction treated with thrombolytic therapy. Am J Cardiol 54:530, 1984

34. Waller BF, Rothbaum DA, Pinkerton CA, et al: Status of the myocardium and infarct-related coronary artery in 19 necropsy patients with acute recanalization using pharmacologic (streptokinase, r-tissue plasminogen activator), mechanical (percutaneous transluminal coronary angioplasty) or combined types of reperfusion therapy. J Am Coll Cardiol 9:785, 1987

35. Cowan MJ, Reichenbach D, Turner P, Thostenson C: Cellular response of the evolving myocardial infarction after therapeutic coronary artery reperfusion. Hum Pathol 22:154, 1991

36. Kloner RA, Ganote CE, Whalen DA Jr, Jennings RB: Effect of a transient period of ischemia on myocardial cells. II. Fine structure during the first few minutes of reflow. Am J Pathol 74:399, 1974

37. Reichenbach D, Cowan MJ: Healing of myocardial infarction with and without reperfusion. Major Probl Pathol 23:86, 1991

38. Maggioni AP, Franzosi MG, Santoro E, et al: The risk of stroke in patients with acute myocardial infarction after thrombolytic and antithrombotic treatment. N Engl J Med 327:1, 1992

39. Landau C, Lange RA, Hillis LD: Percutaneous transluminal coronary angioplasty. N Engl J Med 330:981, 1994

40. Wong JB, Sonnenberg FA, Salem DN, Pauker SG: Myocardial revascularization for chronic stable angina. Analysis of the role of percutaneous transluminal coronary angioplasty based on data available in 1989. Ann Intern Med 113:852, 1990

41. Rosing DR, Cannon RD, Watson RM, et al: Three year anatomic, functional, and clinical follow-up after successful percutaneous transluminal coronary angioplasty. J Am Coll Cardiol 9:1, 1987

42. Kahn JK, Hartzler GO: Frequency and causes of failure with contemporary balloon coronary angioplasty and implications for new technologies. Am J Cardiol 66:858, 1990

43. Myler RK, Shaw RE, Stertzer SH, et al: Lesion morphology and coronary angioplasty: Current experience and analysis. J Am Coll Cardiol 19:1641, 1992

44. Block PC, Bauchman KL, Pasternak RC, Fallon JT: Transluminal angioplasty: Correlation of morphologic and angiographic findings in an experimental model. Circulation 61:778, 1980

45. Baughman KL, Pasternak RC, Fallon JT, Block PC: Transluminal

coronary angioplasty of postmortem human hearts. Am J Cardiol 48:1044, 1981

46. Block PC, Myler RK, Stertzer S, Fallon JT: Morphology after transluminal angioplasty in human beings. N Engl J Med 305:382, 1981

47. Honye J, Mahon DJ, Jain A, et al: Morphological effects of coronary balloon angioplasty in-vivo assessed by intravascular ultrasound imaging. Circulation 85:1012, 1992

48. Schoen FJ: Interventional and Surgical Cardiovascular Pathology: Clinical Correlations and Basic Principles. Philadelphia, WB Saunders, 1989

49. Waller BF: Pathology of new cardiovascular interventional procedures. In: Silver MD (ed): Cardiovascular Pathology. New York, Churchill Livingstone, 1991, p 1683

50. Virmani R, Farb A, Burke AP: Coronary angioplasty from the perspective of atherosclerotic plaque: Morphologic predictors of immediate success and restenosis. Am Heart J 127:163, 1994

51. Lee RT, Loree HM, Cheng GC, et al: Computational structural analysis based on intravascular ultrasound imaging prior to in vitro angioplasty: Prediction of plaque fracture locations. J Am Coll Cardiol 21:777, 1993

52. Ellis SG, Cowley MJ, Whitlow PL, et al: Prospective case-control comparison of percutaneous transluminal coronary revascularization in patients with multivessel disease treated in 1986–1987 versus 1991: Improved in-hospital and 12-month results. Multivessel Angioplasty Prognosis Study (MAPS) Group. J Am Coll Cardiol 25:1137, 1995

53. Bates ER: Ischemic complications after percutaneous transluminal coronary angioplasty. Am J Med 108:309, 2000

54. deFeyter PJ, deJaegere PP, Serruys PW: Incidence, predictors and management of acute coronary occlusion after coronary angioplasty. Am Heart J 127:643, 1994

55. Tan K, Sulke N, Taub N, Sowton E: Clinical and lesion morphologic determinants of coronary angioplasty success and complications: Current experience. J Am Coll Cardiol 24:855, 1995

56. Weyrens FJ, Mooney J, Lesser J, Mooney MR: Intracoronary diltiazem for microvascular spasm after interventional therapy. Am J Cardiol 75:849, 1995

57. The EPIC Investigators: Use of monoclonal antibody directed against the platelet glycoprotein IIb/IIIa receptor in high-risk coronary angioplasty. N Engl J Med 330:956, 1994

58. Aguirre FV, Topol EJ, Ferguson JJ, et al: Bleeding complications with a chimeric antibody to platelet glycoprotein IIb/IIIa integrin in patients undergoing percutaneous coronary intervention. Circulation 91:282, 1995

59. Califf RM, Fortin DF, Frid DJ, et al: Restenosis after coronary angioplasty: An overview. J Am Coll Cardiol 17:2B, 1991

60. Kuntz RE, Baim DS: Defining coronary restenosis. Newer clinical and angiographic paradigms. Circulation 88:1310, 1993

61. Haudenschild CC: Pathobiology of restenosis after angioplasty. Am J Med 94(suppl):40, 1993

62. Epstein SE, Speir E, Unger EF, et al: The basis of molecular strategies for treating coronary restenosis after angioplasty. J Am Coll Cardiol 23:1278, 1994

63. Libby P, Sukhova G, Brogi E, et al: Restenosis as an example of vascular hyperplastic disease: Reassessment of potential mechanisms. Adv Vasc Surg 3:279, 1995

64. Lau KW, Sigwart U: Angioplasty, stenting, atherectomy and laser treatment after coronary artery bypass grafting. Curr Opin Cardiol 8:951, 1993

65. Riessen R, Isner JM: Prospects for site-specific delivery of pharmacologic and molecular therapies. J Am Coll Cardiol 23:1234, 1994

66. Lincoff AM, Topol EJ, Ellis SG: Local drug delivery for the prevention of restenosis. Circulation 90:2070, 1994

67. Casscells W: Growth factor therapies for vascular injury and ischemia. Circulation 91:2699, 1995

68. Bennett MR, Schwartz SM: Antisense therapy for angioplasty restenosis. Circulation 92:1981, 1995

69. Kuntz RE, Hinohara T, Safian RD, et al: Restenosis after directional coronary atherectomy. Effects of luminal diameter and deep wall excision. Circulation 86:1394, 1992

70. Fishman RF, Kuntz RE, Carrozza JP, et al: Long-term results of directional coronary atherectomy: Predictors of restenosis. J Am Coll Cardiol 20:1101, 1992

71. Diethrich EB: Classical and endovascular surgery: Indications and outcomes. Surg Today 24:949, 1994

72. Stertzer SH, Rosenblum J, Shaw RE, et al: Coronary rotational ablation: Initial experience in 302 procedures. J Am Coll Cardiol 21:287, 1993

73. Moscucci M, Mansour KA, Kent KC, et al: Peripheral vascular complications of directional coronary atherectomy and stenting: Predictors, management, and outcome. Am J Cardiol 74:448, 1994

74. Hinohara T, Robertson GC, Selmon MR, et al: Restenosis after directional coronary atherectomy. J Am Coll Cardiol 20:623, 1992

75. Holmes DR Jr, Topol EJ, Adelman AG, et al: Randomized trials of directional coronary atherectomy: Implications for clinical practice and future investigation. J Am Coll Cardiol 24:431, 1994

76. Cesare NB, Popma JJ, Holmes DR, et al: Clinical angiographic and histologic correlates of ectasia after directional coronary atherectomy. Am J Cardiol 69:314, 1992

77. Ruygrok PN, Serruys PW: Intracoronary stenting. From concept to custom. Circulation 94:882, 1996

78. Pepine CJ, Holmes DR: Coronary artery stents. J Am Coll Cardiol 28:782, 1996

79. Holmes DR, Hirshfeld J, Faxon D, et al: ACC expert consensus document on coronary artery stents. J Am Coll Cardiol 32:1471, 1998

80. Phatouros CC, Higashida RT, Malek AM, et al: Carotid artery stent placement for atherosclerotic disease: Rationale, technique, and current status. Radiology 217:26, 2000

81. Topol EJ: Caveats about elective coronary stenting (editorial). N Engl J Med 331:539, 1994

82. Eeckhout E, Kappenberger L, Goy J-J: Stents for intracoronary placement: Current status and future directions. J Am Coll Cardiol 27:757, 1996

83. Al Suwaidi J, Berger PB, Holmes DR Jr: Coronary artery stents. JAMA 284:1828, 2000

84. Serruys PW, Jaegere P, Kiemeneij F, et al: A comparison of balloon expandable stent implantation with balloon angioplasty in patients with coronary artery disease. N Engl J Med 331:489, 1994

85. Fischman DL, Leon MB, Baim DS, et al: A randomised comparison of coronary stent placement and balloon angioplasty in the treatment of coronary artery disease. N Engl J Med 331:496, 1994

86. Savage MP, Douglas JS, Fischman DL, et al: Stent placement compared with balloon angioplasty for obstructed coronary bypass grafts. N Engl J Med 337:740, 1997

87. Laham RJ, Carrozza JP, Berger C, et al: Long-term (4- to 6-year) outcome of Palmaz-Schatz stenting: Paucity of late clinical stent-related problems. J Am Coll Cardiol 28:820, 1996

88. Suryapranata H, van't Hof AW, Hoorntje JC, et al: Randomized comparison of coronary stenting with balloon angioplasty in selected patients with acute myocardial infarction. Circulation 97:2502, 1998

89. Schomig A, Neumann FJ, Kastrati A, et al: A randomised comparison of antiplatelet and anticoagulant therapy after the placement of coronary artery stents. N Engl J Med 334:1084, 1996

90. Teirstein PS, Massullo V, Jani S, et al: Catheter-based radiotherapy to inhibit restenosis after coronary stenting. N Engl J Med 336:1697, 1997

91. Schneider D, Dichek DA: Intravascular stent endothelialisation, a goal worth pursuing? Circulation 95:308, 1997

92. Bailey SR: Local drug delivery: Current applications. Prog Cardiovasc Dis 40:183, 1997

93. Gunn J, Cumberland D: Stent coatings and local drug delivery; state of the art. Eur Heart J 20:1693, 1999

94. Anderson PG, Bajaj RK, Baxley WA, Roubin GS: Vascular pathology of balloon-expandable flexible coil stents in human. J Am Coll Cardiol 19:372, 1992

95. van Beusekom HMM, van der Giessen WJ, van Suylen RJ, et al: Histology after stenting of human saphenous vein bypass grafts: Observations from surgically excised grafts 3 to 320 days after stent implantation. J Am Coll Cardiol 21:45, 1993

96. Kearney M, Pieczek RN, Haley BS, et al: Histopathology of in-stent restenosis in patients with peripheral artery disease. Circulation 95:1998, 1997

97. Kamatsu R, Ueda M, Narukp T, et al: Neointimal tissue response at sites of coronary stenting in humans. Macroscopic, histological and immunohistochemical analyses. Circulation 98:224, 1998

98. Farb A, Sangiorgi G, Carter AJ, et al: Pathology of acute and chronic coronary stenting in humans. Circulation 99:44, 1999

99. Grewe PH, Deneke T, Machraoui A, et al: Acute and chronic tissue response to coronary stent implantation: Pathologic findings in human specimens. J Am Coll Cardiol 35:157, 2000

100. Schwartz RS, Huber KC, Murphy JG, et al: Restenosis and proportional neointimal response to coronary artery injury: Results in a porcine model. J Am Coll Cardiol 19:267, 1992

101. Carter AJ, Laird JR, Kufs WM, et al: Coronary stenting with a novel stainless steel balloon-expandable stent: Determinants of neointimal formation and changes in arterial geometry after placement in an atherosclerotic model. J Am Coll Cardiol 27:1270, 1996

102. Parodi JC: Endovascular repair of abdominal aortic aneurysms and other arterial lesions. J Vasc Surg 21:549, 1995

103. Moore WS, Rutherford RB: Transfemoral endovascular repair of abdominal aortic aneurysm: Results of the North American EVT phase I trial. J Vasc Surg 23:543, 1996

104. Blum U, Voshage G, Lammer J, et al: Endoluminal stent-grafts for infrarenal abdominal aortic aneurysms. N Engl J Med 336:13, 1977

105. Veith FJ, Abbott WM, Tao JST, et al: Guidelines for development and use of transluminally placed endovascular prosthetic grafts in the arterial system. J Vasc Surg 21:670, 1995

106. Dorros G, Parodi J, Schonholz C, et al: Evaluation of endovascular abdominal aortic aneurysm repair: Anatomical classification, procedural success, clinical assessment, and data collection. J Endovasc Surg 4:203, 1997

107. White GH, Yu W, May J, et al: Endoleak as a complication of endoluminal grafting of abdominal aortic aneurysms: Classification, incidence, diagnosis and management. J Endovasc Surg 4:152, 1997

108. Ernst CB: Current therapy for infrarenal aortic aneurysms. N Engl J Med 336:59, 1997

109. Matsumura JS, Moore WS: Clinical consequences of periprosthetic leak after endovascular repair of abdominal aortic aneurysm. J Vasc Surg 27:606, 1998

110. White GH, May J, Waugh RC, et al: Endotension: An explanation for continued AAA growth after successful endoluminal repair. J Endovasc Surg 6:308, 1999

111. Schurink GW, van Baalen JM, Visser MJ, van Bockel JH: Thrombus within an aortic aneurysm does not reduce pressure on the aneurysmal wall. J Vasc Surg 31:501, 2000

112. Eagle KA, Guyton RA, Davidoff R, et al: ACC/AHA guidelines for coronary artery bypass graft surgery: A report of the American College of Cardiology/American Heart Association Task Force on Practice Guidelines (Committee to revise the 1991 guidelines for coronary artery bypass graft surgery). Circulation 100:1464, 1999

113. Yusuf S, Zucker D, Peduzzi P, et al: Effect of coronary artery bypass graft surgery on survival: Overview of 10 year results from randomized trials by the Coronary Artery Bypass Graft Surgery Trialists Collaboration. Lancet 344:563, 1994

114. Cameron AAC, Davis KB, Rogers WJ: Recurrence of angina after coronary bypass surgery. Predictors and prognosis (CASS Registry). J Am Coll Cardiol 26:895, 1995

115. Kirklin JW, Naftel DC, Blackstone EH, Pohost GM: Summary of a consensus concerning death and ischemic events after coronary artery bypass grafting. Circulation 79(suppl I):181, 1989

116. Solomon AJ, Gersh BJ: Management of chronic stable angina: Medical therapy, percutaneous transluminal coronary angioplasty, and coronary artery bypass graft surgery: Lessions from the randomized trials. Ann Intern Med 128:216, 1998

117. Carracciolo EA, Davis KB, Sopko G, et al: Comparison of surgical and medical group survival in patients with left main equivalent coronary artery disease: Long-term CASS experience. Circulation 91:2335, 1995

118. Detre KM, Takaro T, Hultgren H, Peduzzi P: Long-term mortality and morbidity results of the Veterans Administration randomized trial of coronary artery bypass surgery. Circulation 72(suppl V):84, 1985

119. Varnauskas E: Survival, myocardial infarction, and employment

status in a prospective randomized study of coronary bypass surgery. Circulation 72(suppl V):90, 1985

120. Alderman EL, Bourassa MG, Cohen LS, et al: Ten-year follow-up of survival and myocardial infarction in the randomized Coronary Artery Surgery Study (CASS). Circulation 82:1629, 1990

121. Murphy ML, Meadows WR, Thomsen J, et al: The effect of coronary artery bypass surgery on the incidence of myocardial infarction and hospitalization. Prog Cardiovasc Dis 28:309, 1986

122. CASS Principal Investigators and Their Associates: Myocardial infarction and mortality in the Coronary Artery Surgery Study (CASS) randomized trial. N Engl J Med 310:750, 1984

123. Christakis GT, Weisel RD, Fremes SE, et al: Coronary artery bypass grafting in patients with poor ventricular function. J Thorac Cardiovasc Surg 103:1083, 1992

124. Rosengart TK: Risk analysis of primary versus reoperative coronary artery bypass grafting. Ann Thorac Surg 56(suppl):S-74, 1993

125. Kloner RA, Przyklenk K: Hibernation and stunning of the myocardium. N Engl J Med 325:1877, 1991

126. Wijns W, Vatner SF, Camici PG: Hibernating myocardium. N Engl J Med 339:173, 1998

127. Tillisch J, Brunken R, Marshall R, et al: Reversibility of cardiac wall-motion abnormalities predicted by positron tomography. N Engl J Med 314:884, 1986

128. Tamaki N, Kawamoto M, Tadamura E, et al: Prediction of reversible ischemia after revascularization: Perfusion and metabolic studies with positron emission tomography. Circulation 91:1697, 1995

129. Conversano A, Walsh JF, Geltman EM, et al: Delineation of myocardial stunning and hibernation by positron emission tomography in advanced coronary artery disease. Am Heart J 131:440, 1996

130. Kim RJ, Wu E, Rafael A, et al: The use of contrast-enhanced magnetic resonance imaging to identify reversible myocardial dysfunction. N Engl J Med 343:1445, 2000

131. Pocock SJ, Henderson RA, Richards AF, et al: Meta-analysis of randomised trials comparing coronary angioplasty with bypass surgery. Lancet 346:1184, 1995

132. Folland ED, Hartigan PM, Parisi AF: Percutaneous transluminal coronary angioplasty versus medical therapy for stable angina pectoris. J Am Coll Cardiol 29:1505, 1997

133. Anderson WD, King SB 3rd: A review of randomized trials comparing coronary angioplasty and bypass grafting. Curr Opin Cardiol 11:583, 1996

134. Edwards FH, Clark RE, Schwartz M: Coronary artery bypass grafting: The Society of Thoracic Surgeons National Database Experience. Ann Thorac Surg 57:12, 1994

135. Cosgrove DM: Coronary artery surgery in women. In: Proceedings of an N.H.L.B.I. Conference: Cardiovascular Health and Disease in Women. Greenwich, CT, Le Jacq Communications, 1993, p 117

136. Findlay IN: Coronary bypass surgery in women. Curr Opin Cardiol 9:650, 1994

137. Davis KB, Chaitman B, Ryan T, et al: Comparison of 15-year survival for men and women after initial medical or surgical treatment for coronary artery disease: A CASS Registry study. J Am Coll Cardiol 25:1000, 1995

138. Rahimtoola SH, Bennett AJ, Grunkemeier GL, et al: Survival at 15 to 18 years after coronary bypass surgery for angina in women. Circulation 88:II71, 1993

139. Schoen FJ, Fallon JT: Pathologic findings in patients dying early following coronary artery bypass surgery. Lab Invest 52:60A, 1985

140. Vargas SO, Sampson BA, Schoen FJ: Pathologic detection of early myocardial infarction: A critical review of the evolution and usefulness of modern techniques. Mod Pathol 12:635, 1999

141. Chaitman BR, Alderman EL, Sheffield T, et al: Use of survival analysis to determine the clinical significance of new Q waves after coronary bypass surgery. Circulation 67:302, 1983

142. Virmani R, Atkinson JB, Forman MB: Aortocoronary bypass grafts and extracardiac conduits. In: Silver MD (ed): Cardiovascular Pathology. New York, Churchill Livingstone, 1991, p 1607

143. Bourassa MG: Long-term vein graft patency. Curr Opin Cardiol 9:685, 1994

144. Nwasokwa ON: Coronary artery bypass graft disease. Ann Intern Med 123:528, 1995

145. Bulkley BH, Hutchins GM: Myocardial consequences of coronary artery bypass surgery: The paradox of necrosis in areas of revascularization. Circulation 56:906, 1977

146. Vlodaver Z, Edwards JE: Pathologic changes in aortic coronary arterial saphenous vein grafts. Circulation 44:719, 1971

147. FitzGibbon GM, Leach AJ, Kafka HP, Keon WJ: Coronary bypass graft fate: Long-term angiographic study. J Am Coll Cardiol 17:1075, 1991

148. Keon WJ, Heggtveit HA, Leduc J: Perioperative myocardial infarctions caused by atheroembolism. J Thorac Cardiovasc Surg 84:849, 1982

149. Kroncke GM, Kosolcharoen P, Clayman JA, et al: Five-year changes in coronary arteries of medical and surgical patients of the Veterans Administration randomized study of by-pass surgery. Circulation 78(suppl I):144, 1988

150. Hwang MH, Meadows WR, Palac RT, et al: Progression of native coronary artery disease at 10 years: Insights from a randomized study of medical versus surgical therapy for angina. J Am Coll Cardiol 16:1066, 1990

151. Goldman S, Copeland J, Moritz T, et al: Saphenous vein graft patency 1 year after coronary artery bypass surgery and effects of antiplatelet therapy: Results of a Veterans Administration Cooperative Study. Circulation 80:1190, 1989

152. Loop FD, Lytle BW, Cosgrove DM, et al: Influence of the internal-mammary-artery graft on 10-year survival and other cardiac events. N Engl J Med 314:1, 1986

153. Turina M: Coronary artery surgical technique. Curr Opin Cardiol 8:919, 1993

154. Chaikhouni A, Crawford FA, Kochel PJ, et al: Human internal mammary artery produces more prostacyclin than saphenous vein. J Thorac Cardiovasc Surg 92:88, 1986

155. Saber RS, Edwards WD, Holmes DR Jr, et al: Balloon angioplasty of aortocoronary saphenous vein bypass grafts: A histopathologic study of six grafts from five patients, with emphasis on restenosis and embolic complications. J Am Coll Cardiol 12:1501, 1988

156. Wearns JT, Mettier SR, Klempp TG, Zschiesche JL: The nature of the vascular communications between the coronary arteries and the chambers of the heart. Am Heart J 9:143, 1933

157. Jensen D: The hagfish. Sci Am 214:82, 1966

158. Webb GJW: Comparative anatomy of the reptilia. III. The heart of crocodilians and a hypothesis on the completion of the interventricular septum of crocodilians and birds. J Morphol 161:221, 1979

159. Bonnet D, Gautier-Lhermitte I, Bonhoeffer P, Sidi D: Right ventricular myocardial sinusoidal-coronary artery connections in critical pulmonary valve stenosis. Pediatr Cardiol 19:269, 1998

160. Horvath KA, Cohn LH, Cooley DA, et al: Transmyocardial laser revascularization: Results of a multicenter trial with transmyocardial laser revascularization used as sole therapy for end-stage coronary artery disease. J Thorac Cardiovasc Surg 113:645, 1997

161. Burkhoff D, Schmidt S, Schulman SP, et al: Transmyocardial laser revascularisation compared with continued medical therapy for treatment of refractory angina pectoris: A prospective randomised trial. Lancet 354:885, 1999

162. Abramov D, Bhatnagar G, Tamariz M, et al: Current status of transmyocardial laser revascularization: Review of the literature. Can J Cardiol 15:303, 1999

163. Hughes GC, Abdel-Aleem S, Biswas SS, et al: Transmyocardial laser revascularization: Experimental and clinical results. Can J Cardiol 15:797, 1999

164. Lee LY, Rosengart TK: Transmyocardial laser revascularization and angiogenesis: The potential for therapeutic benefit. Semin Thorac Cardiovasc Surg 11:29, 1999

165. Frazier OH, March RJ, Horvath RA: Transmyocardial revascularization with a carbon dioxide laser in patients with end-stage coronary artery disease. N Engl J Med 341:1021, 1999

166. Allen KB, Dowling RD, Fudge TL, et al: Comparison of transmyocardial revascularization with medical therapy in patients with refractory angina. N Engl J Med 341:1029, 1999

167. Schofield PM, Sharples LD, Caine N, et al: Transmyocardial laser revascularization in patients with refractory angina: A randomised controlled trial. Lancet 353:519, 1999

168. Diegeler A, Schneider J, Lauer B, et al: Transmyocardial laser revascularization using the holmium:YAG laser for treatment of end stage coronary artery disease. Eur J Cardiothorac Surg 13:392, 1998

169. Treat MR, Oz MC, Bass LS: New technologies and future applica-

tions of surgical lasers. The right tool for the right job. Surg Clin North Am 72:705, 1992

170. Kornowski R, Bhargava B, Leon MB: Percutaneous transmyocardial laser revascularization: An overview. Cathet Cardiovasc Intervent 47:354, 1999

171. Lauer B, Junghans U, Stahl F, et al: Percutaneous myocardial laser revascularization for patients with end-stage coronary artery disease and refractory angina pectoris. Circulation 98(suppl 1):349, 1998

172. Sanborn TA, Oesterle SN, Heuser RR, el al: Percutaneous laser revascularization (PMR) with a holmium laser: A pilot multicenter feasibility trial. Circulation 98(suppl 1):87, 1998

173. Whitlow PL, Knopf WD, O'Neill WW, et al: Percutaneous transmyocardial revascularization in patients with refractory angina. Circulation 98(suppl 1):87, 1998

174. Kohmoto T, Fisher PE, Gu A, et al: Does blood flow through holmium:YAG transmyocardial laser channels? Ann Thorac Surg 61:861, 1996

175. Hardy RI, Bove KE, James FW, et al: A histologic study of laser induced transmyocardial channels. Lasers Surg Med 6:563, 1987

176. Lutter G, Schwarzkopf J, Lutz C, et al: Histologic findings of transmyocardial laser channels after two hours. Ann Thorac Surg 65:1437, 1998

177. Krabatsch T, Schaper F, Leder C, et al: Histological findings after transmyocardial laser revascularization. J Cardiac Surg 11:326, 1996

178. Gassler N, Wintzer H-O, Stubbe H-M, et al: Transmyocardial laser revascularization. Histological features in human nonresponder myocardium. Circulation 95:371, 1997

179. Sigel JE, Abramovich CM, Ratliff NB: Transmyocardial laser revascularization: Three sequential autopsy cases. J Thorac Cardiovasc Surg 115:1381, 1998

180. Dedic K, Klima T, Cooley DA, et al: Transmyocardial laser revascularization: Histopathological findings. Cardiovasc Pathol 7:63, 1998

181. Whittaker P: Transmyocardial revascularization: The fate of myocardial channels. Ann Thorac Surg 68:2376, 1999

182. Bridges CR: Myocardial laser revascularization: The controversy and the data. Ann Thorac Surg 69:655, 2000

183. Berwing K, Bauer EP, Strasser R, et al: Functional evidence of long-term channel patency after transmyocardial laser revascularization. Circulation 96(suppl 1):564, 1997

184. Horvath KA, Smith WJ, Laurence RG, et al: Recovery and viability of an acute myocardial infarct after transmyocardial laser revascularization. J Am Coll Cardiol 25:258, 1995

185. Cooley DA, Frazier OH, Kadipasaoglu KA, et al: Transmyocardial laser revascularization: Anatomic evidence of long-term channel patency. Tex Heart Inst J 21:220, 1994

186. Horvath KA, Smith WJ, Laurence RG, et al: Recovery and viability of an acute myocardial infarct after transmyocardial laser revascularization. J Am Coll Cardiol 25:258, 1995

187. Mirhoseini M, Shelgikar S, Cayton M: Clinical and histological evaluation of laser myocardial revascularization. J Clin Laser Med Surg 8:73, 1990

188. Yano OJ, Bielefeldl MR, Jeevanandam V, et al: Prevention of acute regional ischemia with endocardial laser channels. Ann Thorac Surg 56:46, 1993

189. Burkhoff D, Fisher PE, Apfelbaum M, et al: Histologic appearance of transmyocardial laser channels after 4½ weeks. Ann Thorac Surg 61:1532, 1996

190. Fisher PE, Kohmoto T, DeRosa CM, et al: Histologic analysis of transmyocardial laser channels: Comparison of CO_2 and holmium:YAG lasers. Ann Thorac Surg 64:466, 1997

191. Kohmoto T, Fisher PE, Gu A, et al: Physiology, histology and 2-week morphology of acute transmyocardial laser channels made with a CO_2 laser. Ann Thorac Surg 63:1275, 1997

192. Krabatsch T, Schaper F, Leder C, et al: Histological findings after transmyocardial laser revascularization. J Card Surg 11:326, 1996

193. Pifarre R, Jasuja ML, Lynch RD, Neville WE: Myocardial revascularization by transmyocardial acupuncture: A physiologic impossibility. J Thorac Cardiovasc Surg 58:424, 1969

194. Kohmoto T, Uzun G, Gu A, et al: Blood flow capacity via direct acute myocardial revascularization. Basic Res Cardiol 92:45, 1997

195. Whittaker P, Kloner RA, Przyklenk K: Laser-mediated transmural

myocardial channels do not salvage acutely ischemic myocardium. J Am Coll Cardiol 22:302, 1993

196. Fleischer K J, Goldschmidt-Clermont PJ, Fonger JD, et al: One-month histologic response of transmyocardial laser channel with molecular intervention. Ann Thorac Surg 62:1051, 1996

197. Kohmoto T, Fisher PE, Gu A, et al: Physiology, histology, and 2-week morphology of acute transmyocardial channels made with a CO_2 laser. Ann Thorac Surg 63:1275, 1997

198. Kohmoto T, DeRosa CM, Yamamoto N, et al: Evidence of vascular growth associated with laser treatment of normal canine myocardium. Ann Thorac Surg 65:1360, 1998

199. Malekan R, Reynolds C, Narula N, et al: Angiogenesis in transmyocardial laser revascularization. A nonspecific response to injury. Circulation 98:I-162, 1998

200. Yamamoto N, Kohmoto T, Gu A, et al: Angiogenesis is enhanced in ischemic canine myocardium by transmyocardial laser revascularization. J Am Coll Cardiol 31:1426, 1998

201. Ware JA, Simons M: Angiogenesis in ischemic heart disease. Nat Med 3:158, 1997

202. Stundt TM 3rd, Kwong KF: Clinical experience with the holmium:YAG laser for transmyocardial laser revascularization and myocardial denervation as a mechanism. J Sem Thorac Cardiovasc Surg 11:19, 1999

203. Kwong KF, Kanellopoulos GK, Nickols JC, et al: Transmyocardial laser treatment denervates canine myocardium. J Thorac Cardiovasc Surg 114:883, 1997

204. Kwong KF, Scheussler RB, Kanellopoulos GK, et al: Nontransmural laser treatment incompletely denervates canine myocardium. Circulation 98 (suppl II):67, 1998

205. Horvath KA, Chiu E, Maun DC, et al: Up-regulation of vascular endothelial growth factor mRNA and angiogenesis after transmyocardial laser revascularization. Ann Thorac Surg 68:825, 1999

206. Whittaker P, Rakusan K, Kloner RA: Transmural channels can protect ischemic tissue. Assessment of long-term myocardial response to laser- and needle-made channels. Circulation 93:143, 1996

207. Sayeed-Shah U, Reul RM, Byrne JG, et al: Combination TMR and gene therapy. Semin Thorac Cardiovasc Surg 11:36, 1999

208. Sayeed-Shah U, Mann MJ, Mastin J, et al: Complete reversal of ischemic wall motion abnormalities by combined use of gene therapy with transmyocardial laser revascularization. J Thorac Cardiovasc Surg 116:763, 1998

209. Crawford ES, Saleh SA, Babb JW, et al: Infrarenal abdominal aortic aneurysm. Factors influencing survival after operation performed over a 25-year period. Ann Surg 193:699, 1981

210. Kannel WB, Skinner JJ, Schwartz MJ, Shurtleff D: Intermittent claudication. Incidence in the Framingham Study. Circulation 41:875, 1970

211. Hertzer NR, Beven EG, Young JR, et al: Coronary artery disease in peripheral vascular patients. A classification of 1000 coronary angiograms and results of surgical management. Ann Surg 199:223, 1984

212. Callow AD: Current status of vascular grafts. Surg Clin North Am 62:501, 1982

213. Davids L, Dower T, Zilla P: The lack of healing in conventional vascular grafts. In: Zilla P, Greisler HP (eds): Tissue Engineering of Vascular Prosthetic Grafts. Texas, RG Landes, 1999, p 3

214. Dardik H, Miller N, Dardik A, et al: A decade of experience with the glutaraldehyde-tanned human umbilical cord vein graft for revascularization of the lower limb. J Vasc Surg 7:336, 1988

215. Darling RC, Linton RR: Durability of femoropopliteal reconstructions. Endocarterectomy versus vein bypass grafts. Am J Surg 123:472, 1972

216. Veith FJ, Gupta SK, Ascer E, et al: Six-year prospective multicenter randomized comparison of autologous saphenous vein and expanded polytetrafluoroethylene grafts in infrainguinal arterial reconstruction. J Vasc Surg 3:104, 1986

217. Clowes AW, Kirkman TR, Reidy MA: Mechanisms of arterial graft healing. Rapid transmural capillary ingrowth provides a source of intimal endothelium and smooth muscle in porous PTFE prostheses. Am J Pathol 123:220, 1986

218. Rafii S, Oz MC, Seldomridge JA, et al: Characterization of hematopoietic cells arising on the textured surface of left ventricular assist devices. Ann Thorac Surg 60:1627, 1995

219. Hammond WP: Surface population with blood-borne cells. In: Zilla P, Greisler P (eds): Tissue Engineering of Vascular Prosthetic Grafts. Texas, RG Landes, 1999, p 379

220. Zilla P: In-vitro endothelialization: Its contribution towards an ideal vascular replacement. In: Zilla P, Greisler HP (eds): Tissue Engineering of Vascular Prosthetic Grafts. Texas, RG Landes, 1999, p 151

221. Libby P, Schoen FJ: Vascular lesion formation. Cardiovasc Pathol 3(suppl):43S, 1993

222. Dunne PF, Newman KD, Jones M, et al: Seeding of vascular grafts with genetically modified endothelial cells. Circulation 93: 1439, 1996

223. Mann MJ, Gibbons GH, Kernoff RS, et al: Genetic engineering of vein grafts resistant to atherosclerosis. Proc Natl Acad Sci U S A 92:4502, 1995

224. Hunt SA, Frazier OH: Mechanical circulatory support and cardiac transplantation. Circulation 97:2079, 1998

225. Goldstein DJ, Oz MC, Rose EA: Implantable left ventricular assist devices. N Engl J Med 339:1522, 1998

226. Mehta SM, Aufiero TX, Pae WE Jr, et al: Results for mechanical ventricular assistance for the treatment of post cardiotomy cardiogenic shock. ASAIO J 42:211, 1996

227. Mehta SM, Aufiero TX, Pae WE Jr, et al: Combined registry for the clinical use of mechanical ventricular assist pumps and the total artificial heart in conjunction with heart transplantation: Sixth official report—1994. J Heart Lung Transplant 14:585, 1995

228. Schoen FJ, Palmer DC, Bernhard WF, et al: Clinical temporary ventricular assist. Pathologic findings and their implications in a multi-institutional study of 41 patients. J Thorac Cardiovasc Surg 92:1071, 1986

229. Clark RE, Zafirelis Z: Future devices and directions. Prog Cardiovasc Dis 43:95, 2000

230. Guy TS: Evolution and current status of the total artificial heart: The search continues. ASAIO J 44:28, 1998

231. Fyfe B, Schoen FJ: Pathologic analysis of 34 explanted Symbion ventricular assist devices and 10 explanted Jarvik-7 total artificial hearts. Cardiovasc Pathol 2:187, 1993

232. Wagner WR, Johnson PC, Kormos RL, Griffith BP: Evaluation of bioprosthetic valve-associated thrombus in ventricular assist device patients. Circulation 88:2023, 1993

233. Kunin CK, Dobbins JJ, Melo JC, et al: Infectious complications in four long-term recipients of the Jarvik-7 artificial heart. JAMA 259:860, 1988

234. DeVries WC: The permanent artificial heart. JAMA 259:849, 1988

235. Pennock JL, Pierce WS, Wisman CB, et al: Survival and complications following ventricular assist pumping for cardiogenic shock. Ann Surg 198:469, 1983

236. Pennington DG, Samuels LD, Williams G, et al: Experience with the Pierce-Donachy ventricular assist device in post-cardiotomy patients with cardiogenic shock. World J Surg 9:37, 1985

237. Eidelman BH, Obrist WD, Wagner WR, et al: Cerebrovascular complications associated with the use of artificial circulatory support. Neurol Clin 11:463, 1993

238. Icenogle TB, Smith RG, Cleavinger M, et al: Thromboembolic complications of the Symbion assist device system. Artif Organs 13:532, 1989

239. Slater JP, Rose EA, Levin HR, et al: Low thromboembolic risk without anticoagulation using advanced-design left ventricular assist devices. Ann Thorac Surg 62:1321, 1996

240. McCarthy PM, Schmitt SK, Vargo RL: Implantable LVAD infections: Implications for permanent use of the device. Ann Thorac Surg 61:359, 1996

241. Holman WL, Murrah CP, Ferguson ER, et al: Infections during extended circulatory support: University of Alabama at Birmingham experience 1989 to 1994. Ann Thorac Surg 61:366, 1996

242. Gristina AG, Dobbins JJ, Giammara B, et al: Biomaterial-centered sepsis and the total artificial heart: Microbial adhesion vs. tissue integration. JAMA 259:870, 1988

243. Levin HR, Oz MC, Chen JM, et al: Reversal of chronic ventricular dilation in patients with end-stage cardiomyopathy by prolonged mechanical unloading. Circulation 91:2717, 1995

244. McCarthy PM, Nakatani S, Vargo R, et al: Structural and left ventricular histologic changes after implantable LVAD insertion. Ann Thorac Surg 59:609, 1995

245. Nakatani S, McCarthy PM, Kotte-Marchant K, et al: Left ventricular echocardiographic and histologic changes: Impact of chronic unloading by an implantable ventricular assist device. J Am Coll Cardiol 27:894, 1996

246. Belland SE, Grunstein R, Jeevanandam V, et al: The effect of sustained mechanical support with ventricular assist devices on myocardial apoptosis in patients with severe dilated cardiomyopathy. J Heart Lung Transplant 17:83, 1998

247. Dipla K, Mattielo JA, Jeevanandam V, et al: Myocyte recovery after mechanical circulatory support in humans with end-stage heart failure. Circulation 97:2316, 1998

248. Mann DL, Willerson JT: Left ventricular assist devices and the failing heart: A bridge to recovery, a permanent assist device, or a bridge too far? Circulation 98:2367, 1998

249. Gristina AG: Biomaterial-centered infection: Microbial adhesion versus tissue integration. Science 237:1588, 1987

250. Schoen FJ: Biomaterial-associated infection, neoplasia, and calcification. Clinicopathologic features and pathophysiologic concepts. Trans Am Soc Intern Organs 33:8, 1987

251. Didisheim P: Current concepts of thrombosis and infection in artificial organs. ASAIO J 40:230, 1994

252. Gristina AG, Naylor PT: Implant-associated infection. In: Ratner BD, Hoffman AS, Schoen FJ, Lemons JE (eds): Biomaterials Science: An Introduction to Materials in Medicine. New York, Academic Press, 1996, p 165

253. Elek SD, Conen PE, et al: The virulence of *Staphylococcus pyogenes* for man: A study of the problems of wound infection. Br J Exp Pathol 38:573, 1957

254. Schoen FJ, Anderson JM, Didisheim P, et al: Ventricular assist device (VAD) pathology analyses: Guidelines for clinical studies. J Appl Biomat 1:49, 1990

255. Borovetz HS, Ramasamy N, Zerbe TR, Portner PM: Evaluation of an implantable ventricular assist system for humans with chronic refractory heart failure. ASAIO J 41:42, 1995

256. Chiu RC-J: Cardiomyoplasty. In: Edmunds LH (ed): Cardiac Surgery in the Adult. New York, McGraw-Hill, 1997, p 1491

257. Furnay AP, Chachques J-C, Moreira LFP, et al: Long-term outcome, survival analysis, and risk stratification of dynamic cardiomyoplasty. J Thorac Cardiovasc Surg 112:1260, 1996

258. Magovern GJ Sr, Simpson KA: Clinical cardiomyoplasty: Review of the ten-year United States experience. Ann Thorac Surg 61:413, 1996

259. el Oakley RM, Jarvis JC: Cardiomyoplasty. A critical review of experimental and clinical results. Circulation 90:2085, 1994

260. Greer KA, Anderson DR, Hammond RL, Stephenson LW: Skeletal muscle as a myocardial substitute. Proc Soc Exp Biol Med 211: 297, 1996

261. Rabbany SY, Kresh JY, Noordergraaf A: Myocardial wall stress: Evaluation and management. Cardiovasc Eng 5:3, 2000

262. McCarthy PM, Starling RC, Wong JW, et al: Early results with partial left ventriculectomy. J Thorac Cardiovasc Surg 114:755, 1997

263. Jeffrey K, Parsonnet V: Cardiac pacing, 1960–1985: A quarter century of medical and industrial innovation. Circulation 97:1978, 1998

264. Chardack WM, Ishikawa H, Fochler FJ, et al: Pacing and ventricular fibrillation. Ann N Y Acad Sci 167:919, 1969

265. Rodovsky AS, Van Vleet JF, Stokes KB, Taker WA Jr: Paired comparisons of steroid-eluting and nonsteroid endocardial pacemaker leads in dogs: Electrical performance and morphologic alterations. Pacing Clin Electrophysiol 11:1085, 1988

266. Gould L, Ramana Reddy CV, Yacob U, et al: Perforation of the tricuspid valve by a transvenous pacemaker. JAMA 230:86, 1974

267. Peterson SR, Small JB, Reeves G, Kocot SL: Tricuspid valve perforation by endocardial pacing electrode. Chest 63:125, 1973

268. Fort ML, Sharp JT: Perforation of the right ventricle by pacing catheter electrode. Am J Cardiol 16:610, 1965

269. Escher DJW, Furman S, Solomon N: Transvenous emergency cardiac pacing. Ann N Y Acad Sci 167:582, 1969

270. Falkoff M, Heinle RA, Ong LS, Baroldi SS: Inapparent double puncture of the femoral artery and vein: An important complication of temporary cardiac pacing by the transfemoral approach. Pacing Clin Electrophysiol 1:49, 1978

271. Cohen SI, Smith CK: Transfemoral cardiac pacing and phlebitis. Circulation 49:1018, 1974

272. Jara FM, Toled-Pereyra MD, Lewis JW Jr, Magilligan DJ Jr: The infected pacemaker pocket. J Thorac Cardiovasc Surg 78:298, 1979

273. Sedaghart A: Permanent transvenous pacemaker infection with septicemia. N Y State J Med 74:868, 1974

274. Siddons H, Nowak K: Surgical complications of implanting pacemakers. Br J Surg 62:929, 1975

275. Fieldman A, Dobrow RJ: Phantom pacemaker programming. Pacing Clin Electrophysiol 1:166, 1978

276. Kelly PA, Cannom DS, Garan H, et al: The automatic implantable cardioverter-defibrillator: Efficacy, complications and survival in patients with malignant ventricular arrhythmias. J Am Coll Cardiol 11:1278, 1988

277. Fetter J, Aram G, Holmes DR, et al: The effects of nuclear magnetic resonance imagers on external and implantable pulse generators. Pacing Clin Electrophysiol 7:720, 1984

278. Irnich W: Interference with pacemakers. Pacing Clin Electrophysiol 7:1021, 1984

279. Cohn JD, Santhanam R, Rosenblood MA, Thorson RF: Delayed pacemaker erosion due to electrode seal defects. Ann Thorac Surg 28:445, 1979

280. Sheridan DJ, Reid DS, Williams DO, Gold RG: Mechanical failure causing current leakage with unipolar pacemakers: Significance and detection. Eur J Cardiol 8:1, 1978

281. De Voogt WG: Pacemaker leads: Performance and progress. Am J Cardiol 83:187D, 1999

282. Kay GN, Binker JA, Kawanishi DT, et al: Risks of spontaneous injury and extraction of an active fixation pacemaker lead: Report of the Accufix Multicenter Clinical Study and Worldwide Registry. Circulation 100:2344, 1999

283. Barbaro V, Bosi C, Caiazza S, et al: Implant effects on polyurethane and silicone cardiac pacing leads in humans: Insulation measurements and SEM observations. Biomaterials 6:28, 1985

284. Huang TY, Baba N: Cardiac pathology of transvenous pacemakers. Am Heart J 83:469, 1972

285. Robboy S, Hawthorne JW, Leinbach RC, et al: Autopsy findings with permanent pervenous pacemakers. Circulation 39:495, 1969

286. Bilgutay AM, Jensen NK, Schmidt WR, et al: Incarceration of transvenous pacemaker electrode. Removal by traction. Am Heart J 77:377, 1969

287. Chavez CM, Conn JH: Septicemia secondary to impacted infected pacemaker wire: Successful treatment by removal with cardiopulmonary bypass. J Thorac Cardiovasc Surg 73:796, 1977

288. Garcia R, Hakimi-Naini M: Bacterial endocarditis and incarceration of a transvenous pacemaker: Removal under cardiopulmonary by-pass after prolonged traction proved ineffective. Henry Ford Hosp Med J 23:135, 1975

289. Yarnoz MD, Attai LA, Furman S: Infection of pacemaker electrode and removal with cardiopulmonary bypass. J Thorac Cardiovasc Surg 68:43, 1974

290. Kinney EL, Allen RP, Weidner WA, et al: Recurrent pulmonary emboli secondary to right atrial thrombus around a permanent pacing catheter: A case report and review of the literature. Pacing Clin Electrophysiol 2:196, 1979

291. Seeger W, Scherer K: Asymptomatic pulmonary embolism following pacemaker implantation. Pacing Clin Electrophysiol 9:196, 1986

292. Firor WB, Lopez JF, Manson EM, Mori M: Clinical management of infected pacemaker. Ann Thorac Surg 6:431, 1968

293. Bryan CS, Sutton JP, Saunders DE, et al: Endocarditis related to transvenous pacemakers: Syndromes and surgical implications. J Thorac Cardiovasc Surg 75:758, 1978

294. Furman S: Complications of pacemaker therapy for heart block. Am J Cardiol 17:439, 1966

295. Schaldach M: New pacemaker electrodes. Trans Am Soc Artif Intern Organs 29:29, 1971

296. Schwartzel EL, Crastnopol P, Hamby RI: Catheter extrusion with infection complicating permanent endocardial pacing. Dis Chest 54:28, 1968

297. Watnick M, Hooshmand I, Spindola-France H: Migration of epicardial pacemaker leads. Clin Radiol 26:483, 1975

298. Meyer JA, Miller K: Malplacement of pacemaker catheters in the coronary sinus. J Thorac Cardiovasc Surg 57:511, 1969

299. Greenberg P, Castellanet M, Messenger J, Ellestad MH: Coronary sinus pacing: Clinical follow-up. Circulation 57:98, 1978

300. Moss AJ, Rivers RJ Jr: Atrial pacing from the coronary vein: Ten-year experience in 50 patients with implanted pervenous pacemakers. Circulation 57:103, 1978

301. Mirowski M, Reid PR, Mower MM, et al: Termination of malignant ventricular arrhythmias with an implanted automatic defibrillator in human beings. N Engl J Med 303:322, 1980

302. Winkle RA, Mead RH, Ruder MA, et al: Long-term outcome with the automatic implantable cardioverter-defibrillator. J Am Coll Cardiol 13:1353, 1989

303. Nisam S, Kaye SA, Mower MM, Hull M: AICD automatic cardioverter defibrillator clinical update: 14 years experience in over 34,000 patients. Pacing Clin Electrophysiol 18:142, 1995

304. The Antiarrhythmics versus Implantable Defibrillators (AVID) Investigators: A comparison of antiarrhythmic-drug therapy with implantable defibrillators in patients resuscitated from near-fatal ventricular arrhythmias. N Engl J Med 337:1576, 1997

305. Moss AJ, Hall WJ, Cannom DS, et al: Improved survival with an implanted defibrillator in patients with coronary artery disease at high risk for ventricular arrhythmia. N Engl J Med 335:1933, 1996

306. Singer I, Hutchins GM, Mirowski M, et al: Pathological findings related to the lead system and repeated defibrillations in patients with automatic implantable cardioverter-defibrillator. J Am Coll Cardiol 10:382, 1987

307. Zipes DP: Genesis of cardiac arrhythmias: Electrophysiological considerations. In: Braunwald E (ed): Heart Disease: A Textbook of Cardiovascular Medicine. Philadelphia, WB Saunders, 1997, p 548

308. Zipes DP, Gillette PC, Myerburg RJ, et al: ACC/AHA Task Force Report: Guidelines for clinical intracardiac electrophysiological and catheter ablation procedures. Circulation 92:673, 1995

309. Scheinman MM: Patterns of catheter ablation practice in the United States: Results of the 1992 NASPE Survey. Pacing Clin Electrophysiol 17:873, 1994

310. Gonzalez R, Scheinman M, Margaretten W, Rubinstein M: Closed-chest electrode-catheter technique for His bundle ablation in dogs. Am J Physiol 241:283, 1981

311. Scheinman MM, Morady F, Hess DS, Gonzales R: Catheter-induced ablation of the atrioventricular junction to control refractory supraventricular arrhythmias. JAMA 248:851, 1982

312. Gallagher JJ, Svenson RH, Kasell JH, et al: Catheter technique for closed-chest ablation of the atrioventricular conduction system. N Engl J Med 306:194, 1982

313. Nath S, Di Marco JP, Haines DE: Basic aspects of radiofrequency catheter ablation. J Cardiovasc Electrophysiol 5:863, 1994

314. Kalbfleisch SJ, Langberg JJ: Catheter ablation with radiofrequency energy: Biophysical aspects and clinical applications. J Cardiovasc Electrophysiol 3:173, 1992

315. McLean A: The Bovie electrosurgical current generator. Arch Surg 18:1863, 1929

316. Bartlett TG, Mitchell R, Friedman PL, Stevenson WG: Histologic evolution of radiofrequency lesions in an old human myocardial infarct causing ventricular tachycardia. J Cardiovasc Electrophysiol 6:625, 1995

317. Morady F, Harvey M, Kalbfleisch SJ, et al: Radiofrequency catheter ablation of ventricular tachycardia in patients with coronary artery disease. Circulation 87:363, 1993

318. Kim YH, Sosa-Suarez G, Trouton TG, et al: Treatment of ventricular tachycardia by transcatheter radiofrequency ablation in patients with ischemic heart disease. Circulation 89:1094, 1994

319. Langberg JJ, Gallagher M, Strickberger SA, Amirana O: Temperature-guided radiofrequency catheter ablation with very large distal electrode. Circulation 88:245, 1993

320. Nakagawa H, Yamanashi WS, Pitha JV, et al: Comparison of in-vivo tissue temperature profile and lesion geometry for radiofrequency ablation with a saline-irrigated electrode versus temperature control in a canine thigh muscle preparation. Circulation 91:2264, 1995

321. Ruffy R, Imran MA, Santel DJ, Wharton JM: Radiofrequency delivery through a cooled catheter tip allows the creation of larger endomyocardial lesions in the ovine heart. J Cardiovasc Electrophysiol 6:1089, 1995

322. Rothman SA, Hsia HH, Chmielewski IL, et al: Standard vs. saline

irrigated-tip radiofrequency ablation: Lesion size in normal vs. scar tissue. J Am Coll Cardiol 29:374A, 1997

323. Nibley C, Sykes CM, Rowan R, et al: Predictors of abrupt impedance rise during chilled-tip radiofrequency catheter ablation. J Am Coll Cardiol 25:293A, 1995

324. Wharton JM, Nibley C, Sykes CM, et al: Establishment of a dose-response relationship for high power chilled-tip radiofrequency current ablation in sheep. J Am Coll Cardiol 25:293A, 1995

325. Delacretaz E, Stevenson WG, Winters GL, et al: Ablation of ventricular tachycardia with a saline cooled radiofrequency catheter: Anatomic and histologic characteristics of the lesions in humans. J Cardiovasc Electrophysiol 10:860, 1999.

326. Zhou L, Keane D, Reed G, Ruskin J: Thromboembolic complications of cardiac radiofrequency catheter ablation: A review of the reported incidence, pathogenesis and current research directions. J Cardiovasc Electrophysiol 10:611, 1999

327. Borggrefe M, Hindricks G, Haverkamp W, Breithardt G: Catheter ablation using radiofrequency energy. Clin Cardiol 13:127, 1990

328. Haines DE, Watson DD: Tissue heating during radiofrequency catheter ablation: A thermodynamic model and observations in isolated perfused and superfused canine right ventricular free wall. Pacing Clin Electrophysiol 12:962, 1989

329. Simmers TA, de Bakker JMT, Wittkampf FHM, Hauer RNW: Effects of heating with radiofrequency power on myocardial impulse conduction: Is radiofrequency ablation exclusively thermally mediated? J Cardiovasc Electrophysiol 7:243, 1996

330. Nath S, Lynch C III, Whayne JG, Haines DE: Cellular electrophysiological effects of hyperthermia on isolated guinea pig papillary muscle: Implications for catheter ablation. Circulation 88:1826, 1993

331. Langberg JJ, Calkins H, Kim YN, et al: Recurrence of conduction in accessory atrioventricular connections after initially successful radiofrequency catheter ablation. J Am Coll Cardiol 19:1588, 1992

332. Langberg JJ, Borganelli SM, Kalbfleisch SJ, et al: Delayed effects of radiofrequency energy on accessory atrioventricular connections. Pacing Clin Electrophysiol 16:1001, 1993

333. Nath S, Whayne JG, Kaul S, et al: Effects of radiofrequency catheter ablation on regional myocardial blood flow: Possible mechanism for late electrophysiological outcome. Circulation 89:2667, 1994

334. Ward DE, Camm AJ: The current status of ablation of cardiac conduction tissue and ectopic myocardial foci by transvenous electrical discharges. Clin Cardiol 9:237, 1986

335. Critelli G, Gallagher JJ, Thiene G, et al: Histologic observations after closed chest ablation of the atrioventricular conduction system. JAMA 252:2604, 1984

336. Ward DE, Davies M: Transvenous high energy shock for ablating atrioventricular conduction in man. Observations on the histological effects. Br Heart J 51:175, 1984

337. Bharati S, Scheinman MM, Morady F, et al: Sudden death after catheter-induced atrioventricular junctional ablation. Chest 88:883, 1985

338. Bardy GH, Ivey TD, Coltoriti F, et al: Developments, complications and limitations of cathether-mediated electrical ablation of posterior accessory atrioventricular pathways. Am J Cardiol 61:309, 1988

339. Davis JC, Finkebeiner W, Ruder MA, et al: Histologic changes and arrhythmogenicity after discharge through transseptal catheter electrode. Circulation 74:637, 1986

340. Edwards WD: Congenital heart disease. In: Damjanov I, Linder J (eds): Anderson's Pathology. 10th ed. St. Louis, Mosby, 1996, p 1339

341. Anderson RH, Becker AE: Pathology of Congenital Heart Disease. London, Butterworth, 1981, p 3

342. Brickner ME, Hillis LD, Lange RA: Congenital heart disease in adults (in two parts). N Engl J Med 342:256, and 334, 2000

343. Kirklin JW, Barratt-Boyes BG: Cardiac Surgery: Morphology, Diagnostic Criteria, Natural History, Techniques, Results, and Indications. 2nd ed. New York, Churchill Livingstone, 1993, p 609

344. Edwards WD: Congenital heart disease. In: Schoen FJ: Interventional and Surgical Cardiovascular Pathology: Clinical Correlations and Basic Principles. Philadelphia, WB Saunders, 1989, p 281

345. Becker AE, Essed CE: The heart after surgery for congenital heart disease. Am J Cardiovasc Pathol 1:301, 1988

346. Van Praagh R, Visner MS: Postoperative pathology of congenital heart disease. Am J Cardiol 38:225, 1976

347. Edwards WD: Pulmonary hypertension and related vascular diseases. In: Stehbens WE, Lie JT (eds): Vascular Pathology. London, Chapman & Hall, 1995, p 585

348. Edwards WD: Classification and terminology of cardiovascular anomalies. In: Emmanouilides GC, Riemenschneider TA, Allen HD, Gutgesell HP (eds): Moss and Adams' Heart Disease in Infants, Children, and Adolescents. 5th ed. Baltimore, Williams & Wilkins, 1995, p 106

349. Edwards WD: Cardiac anatomy and examination of cardiac specimens. In: Emmanouilides GC, Riemenschneider TA, Allen HD, Gutgesell HP (eds): Moss and Adams' Heart Disease in Infants, Children, and Adolescents. 5th ed. Baltimore, Williams & Wilkins, 1995, p 70

350. Ackermann DM, Edwards WD: Anatomic basis for tomographic analysis of the pediatric heart at autopsy. Perspect Pediatr Pathol 2:39, 1988

351. Devine WA, Debich DE, Anderson RH: Dissection of congenitally malformed hearts, with comments on the value of sequential segmental analysis. Pediatr Pathol 11:235, 1991

352. Scholz DG, Kitzman D, Hagen PT, et al: Age-related changes in normal human hearts during the first 10 decades of life. Part I (growth): A quantitative anatomic study of 200 specimens from subjects from birth to 19 years. Mayo Clin Proc 63:126, 1988

353. Kitzman DW, Scholz DG, Hagen PT, et al: Age-related changes in normal human hearts during the first 10 decades of life. Part II (maturity): A quantitative anatomic study of 765 specimens from subjects 20 to 99 years. Mayo Clin Proc 63:137, 1988

354. Dare AJ, Veinot JP, Edwards WD, et al: New observations on the etiology of aortic valve disease: A surgical pathology study of 236 cases from 1990. Hum Pathol 24:1330, 1993

355. Altrichter PM, Olson LJ, Edwards WD, et al: Surgical pathology of the pulmonary valve: A study of 116 cases spanning 15 years. Mayo Clin Proc 64:1352, 1989

356. Hauck AJ, Freeman DP, Ackerman DM, et al: Surgical pathology of the tricuspid valve: A study of 363 cases spanning 25 years. Mayo Clin Proc 63:851, 1988

357. Fugelstad SJ, Puga FJ, Danielson GK, Edwards WD: Surgical pathology of the truncal valve: A study of 12 cases. Am J Cardiovasc Pathol 2:39, 1988

358. Fugelstad SJ, Danielson GK, Puga FJ, Edwards WD: Surgical pathology of the common atrioventricular valve: A study of 11 cases. Am J Cardiovasc Pathol 2:49, 1988

359. Edwards WD, Agarwal KC, Feldt RH, et al: Surgical pathology of obstructed, right-sided, porcine-valved extracardiac conduits. Arch Pathol Lab Med 107:400, 1983

APPENDIX: STANDARDIZED FORM FOR THE AUTOPSY EVALUATION OF CONGENITAL HEART DISEASE*

GENERAL INFORMATION
    Patient name: _____
    Patient I.D. no.: _____

CASE NO.: _____
Age, gender: _____
Date of death: _____

CARDIAC ARRANGEMENT
    Thoracic position: Left-sided   Right-sided   Midline   Unknown   Ectopic _____
    Apical direction: Leftward   Rightward   Inferior   Other: _____
    Displacement: None   Leftward   Rightward   Midline   Unknown
    Morphologic RA: Right-sided   Left-sided   Bilateral   Absent   Indeterminate

PULMONARY ARRANGEMENT
    Morphology of right-sided lung: Right   Left   Indeterminate   Lobes (no.): _____
    Morphology of left-sided lung: Left   Right   Indeterminate   Lobes (no.): _____

ABDOMINAL ARRANGEMENT
    Spleen: Single   Accessory   Polysplenia   Asplenia   Unknown
    Liver: Right-sided   Left-sided   Midline   Unknown   Other: _____
    Bowel: Normal   Malrotation: _____

VISCERAL SIDEDNESS
    Cardiac: Normal   Mirror-image   R. isomerism   L. isomerism   Indeterminate   Unknown
    Pulmonary: Normal   Mirror-image   R. isomerism   L. isomerism   Indeterminate   Unknown
    Abdominal: Normal   Mirror-image   R. isomerism   L. isomerism   Indeterminate   Unknown

ATRIUMS
    Right-sided: RA LA _____
    Left-sided: LA RA _____
    Septum: Intact Patent ASD: _____
    Coronary sinus: Present   Absent _____

ATRIOVENTRICULAR VALVES
    Right-sided: _____ % to RV   _____ % to LV   Morphology: _____
    Left-sided: _____ % to RV   _____ % to LV   Morphology: _____
    Common: _____ % to RV   _____ % to LV   _____

VENTRICLE
    Morphologic RV: Orientation: Normal   Mirror-image   Position: _____
    Morphologic LV: Orientation: Normal   Mirror-image   Position: _____
    Hypoplastic chamber: None   RV   LV _____
    Septal position: Vertical   Oblique   Horizontal   Twisted   Other: _____
    Septum: Intact   VSD: _____

SEMILUNAR VALVES
    Pulmonary: _____ % from RV   _____ % from LV   Morphology: _____
    Aortic: _____ % from RV   _____ % from LV   Morphology: _____
    Truncal: _____ % from RV   _____ % from LV   Morphology: _____

AORTIC VALVE POSITION RELATIVE TO PULMONARY VALVE
    R. post.   Dextroposed   R. lat.   R. ant   Ant.   L. ant.   L. lat.   L. post.   Post.

GREAT ARTERIES
    Pulmonary artery: Present   Hypoplastic   Atretic   Absent   Other: _____
        Systemic collaterals _____
    Thoracic aorta: L. Arch   R. Arch   Double Arch   Coarctation   Other: _____
    Ductal artery: Ligament   Patent   Absent   Other: _____

CORONARY ARTERIES
    Ostia: Normal   Other: _____
    Distribution: Normal   Mirror-image   Other: _____

CONNECTIONS

Venoatrial: Systemic veins: Normal   Other: _____

               Pulmonary veins: Normal   Other: _____

Atrioventricular: Biventricular: Concordance   Discordance   Ambiguous: _____

               Univentricular: Single inlet _____   Double inlet _____   Common inlet _____

Ventriculoarterial: Two arteries: Concordance   Discordance   Double outlet _____

               One artery: Single outlet (Atretic PT)   Common outlet (persistent truncal artery)

CARDIAC MEASUREMENTS

Body size: Height (cm) _____   Weight (kg) _____   BSA (m²) _____

Weights (g):   Heart & lungs _____   R. lung _____   L. lung _____

            Heart _____   Normal mean _____   and range _____

Wall thickness (cm):   LV _____   RV _____   VS _____

Valves (cm):   Aortic _____   Pulmonary _____   Truncal _____

            Mitral _____   Tricuspid _____   Common _____

Shunts (cm):   PFO _____   ASD _____   AVSD _____   VSD _____   PDA _____

SECONDARY CARDIAC EFFECTS

	Hypertrophy	Dilation	Atrophy	Fibrosis	Mural thrombus
LV:					
RV:					
LA:					
RA:					

SECONDARY PULMONARY EFFECTS

Plexogenic pulmonary hypertension: _____

Pulmonary venous hypertension: _____

Other pulmonary hypertension: _____

Pulmonary infection: _____

Other microscopic features: _____

INTERVENTIONAL PROCEDURE

Procedure (date): _____

   Appearance at autopsy: _____

Procedure (date): _____

   Appearance at autopsy: _____

Procedure (date): _____

   Appearance at autopsy: _____

Procedure (date): _____

   Appearance at autopsy: _____

Procedure (date): _____

   Appearance at autopsy: _____

DIAGRAMS

ASD, atrial septal defect; AVSD, atrioventricular septal defect; BSA, body surface area; LA, left atrium; LV, left ventricle; PDA, patent ductus arteriosus; PFA, patent foramen ovale; PT, pulmonary trunk; RA, right atrium; RV, right ventricle; VS, ventricular septum; VSD, ventricular septal defect.

* Modified from Edwards WD: Congenital heart disease. In: Damjanov I, Linder J (eds): Anderson's Pathology. 10th ed. St. Louis, Mosby, 1996, pp. 1390–1391.

Chapter 23

Pathology of Cardiac Transplantation

· · · · ·
Gayle L. Winters • Frederick J. Schoen

GENERAL CLINICOPATHOLOGIC CONSIDERATIONS

Cardiac transplantation is an accepted therapeutic option that provides long-term survival for many patients with end-stage heart failure. More than 45,000 heart transplants at more than 300 centers worldwide were recorded by the International Society for Heart and Lung Transplantation (ISHLT) Registry between 1982 and 1998; approximately 3500 per year are at present done worldwide.[1] The success of heart transplantation over the past decade has been attributed to refinement in candidate selection, use of endomyocardial biopsy to monitor cardiac allograft rejection, and improved immunosuppressive therapies. Actuarial survival is approximately 80% at 1 year and 65% at 5 years.

Recipient and Donor Selection

In the United States, 1 to 2% of the population carries the diagnosis of heart failure, more than one million of these individuals are younger than the age of 70 years, and 40,000 progress to end-stage disease each year.[2–4] The upper age limit beyond which cardiac transplantation was not considered was traditionally set at 55 years. However, since several studies have shown that carefully selected candidates over 55 years of age may successfully undergo the procedure,[5–7] recipient age has been extended into the mid 60s and candidate suitability with respect to age is often more an ethical rather than a medical issue. Comorbid conditions that may be exclusionary include systemic illness with poor prognosis; coexisting neoplasm; irreversible pulmonary, renal, or hepatic disease; pulmonary hypertension with irreversibly high pulmonary vascular resistance; severe peripheral vascular or cerebrovascular obstructive disease or both; insulin-dependent diabetes with end-organ damage; active infection; severe obesity; severe osteoporosis; and either psychosocial instability or substance abuse or both.[1–3, 8, 9]

Donor hearts are procured from individuals with intact circulation and suffering from brain death, usually resulting from blunt injuries sustained in motor vehicle accidents, penetrating head injuries such as gunshot wounds, or from primary central nervous system events. Absolute or relative contraindications for donation include abnormal cardiac structure or function; advanced age; evidence of human immunodeficiency virus (HIV) or hepatitis B or C infection; sepsis; and history of metastatic cancer, carbon monoxide inhalation, or intravenous drug abuse.[10, 11]

Heart donors and recipients are matched for ABO blood group compatibility and body size. Prospective HLA matching is not routinely performed for logistic reasons. A donor-specific lymphocytotoxic cross match is done only if panel-reactive antibody (PRA) analysis has previously demonstrated cytotoxicity when the recipient's serum is mixed with lymphocytes from a panel of randomly chosen individuals.[12, 13] Other considerations in allocation of donor hearts include priority on the United Network for Organ Sharing (UNOS) waiting list and distance between donor and recipient centers.[14] The time from harvesting the donor heart until reestablishment of circulation in the recipient (ischemic time) is limited to 4 to 5 hours maximum, requiring close coordination between donor and recipient operating teams.[11, 15]

The Surgical Procedure

Heart transplantation may be orthotopic, in which the recipient's heart is removed and replaced by a donor organ, or heterotopic, in which a donor heart is added in parallel circuit with the recipient's heart. The orthotopic technique is preferred, is most commonly employed by virtually all transplant centers, and is described in detail below.[16–19] The heterotopic technique has limited indications, primarily for irreversibly high pulmonary vascular resistance in the recipient.[20]

The potential donor heart is carefully examined in situ by the surgeon for evidence of traumatic injury, coronary artery disease, valvular heart disease, or congenital anomaly. The heart is perfused with a cardioplegic solution to achieve electromechanical arrest and is removed by transecting the superior and inferior venae cavae, pulmonary artery, aorta, and pulmonary veins. The organ is further cooled in cold saline and placed in an air-tight sterile container for transport.

Following receipt of the donor heart in the operating room where the recipient has been prepared, including institution of cardiopulmonary bypass, the recipient's diseased heart is removed by incising the right atrium and atrial septum so that the coronary sinus remains with the explanted heart and most of the atrial septum remains behind in the recipient. The aorta and main pulmonary artery are divided closely distal to their respective semilunar valves. The left atrium is then incised, making sure that its atrial appendage is excised and that an adequate cuff of atrial tissue remains anterior to the pulmonary veins for suturing. Anastomoses of the donor to the recipient left atria, right atria, pulmonary arteries, and aortae are completed in that order (Fig. 23-1A). This standard procedure results in bilateral "double" atria, which subsequently produces a double p wave in the recipient's ECG and can lead to stasis, thrombus formation, and suture line complications. A modified procedure, the bicaval technique (Fig. 23-1B) first described in 1991,[21, 22] em-

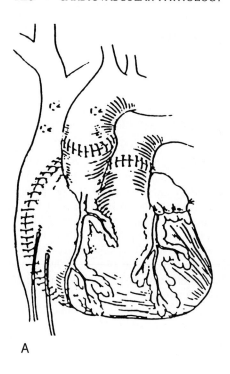

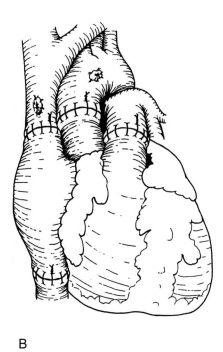

Figure 23-1 • Orthotopic heart transplantation procedures. *A,* Standard technique consists of anastomosing donor and recipient atria, pulmonary arteries, and aortas. *B,* In the bicaval technique, the superior and inferior vena cavae are anastomosed separately along with standard left atrial, pulmonary artery, and aortic anastomoses. (From Winters GL: Transplantation: Explant, biopsy, and autopsy characteristics. In: McManus BM, Braunwald E [eds]: Atlas of Cardiovascular Pathology. Philadelphia, Current Medicine, 2000.)

ploys standard left atrial and separate bicaval anastomoses that maintain intact right atrial anatomy, thereby theoretically reducing complications associated with a double atrium and resulting in improved cardiac function.[23–25]

The Role of Pathology in Heart Transplantation

The contribution of pathology to the success of cardiac transplantation is well established. The most visible role is that of the pathologist who interprets post-transplantation endomyocardial biopsies. The diagnosis and grading of acute rejection and assessment of numerous other biopsy findings are important in guiding the clinical management of recipients. Close collaboration between the pathologist and the transplant clinician is essential for the optimal care of these patients. Pathologists may also make important contributions in examining biopsies of the recipient's native heart as part of the evaluation of the etiology of cardiac failure; in examining explanted recipient hearts; and in evaluating a failed allograft. Moreover, the pathologist has the opportunity and, indeed, is in a rather unique position to add to existing knowledge of the pathobiology of heart failure and transplantation.

PATHOLOGY OF THE EXPLANTED RECIPIENT HEART

In our 15 years of experience with heart transplantation at Brigham and Women's Hospital, more than 90% of more than 400 adult recipients of cardiac allografts have had end-stage heart failure secondary to cardiomyopathy or ischemic heart disease (Fig. 23-2). This experi-

ence parallels that reported by the ISHLT Registry, which collects data annually from nearly 300 transplant centers worldwide.[1] Less common indications for transplantation, in descending order, include valvular heart disease, retransplantation, congenital heart disease, and miscellaneous other conditions. Standardized forms for reporting explanted hearts may be used to provide consistency in format and wording; the form we use appears in Appendix A. Although careful evaluation of an explanted recipient heart confirms clinical diagnoses and adds to the knowledge of the underlying disease, the presence of previously undiagnosed conditions or unexpected findings may affect the prognosis of the recipient.

Eosinophilic Myocarditis

Eosinophilic, or hypersensitivity, myocarditis (see Chapters 9 and 17) has been reported in up to 22% of explanted hearts from patients undergoing cardiac transplantation.[26–28] It is usually considered an incidental finding. Eosinophilic myocarditis differs from cases of usually fatal necrotizing eosinophilic myocarditis in which the terminal event is often an arrhythmia,[29, 30] because the eosinophil-rich inflammatory infiltrate is generally present in a focal or multifocal distribution scattered throughout the myocardium and confined to interstitial and perivascular spaces with little or no associated myocyte necrosis.[31] This disease may occur in association with any form of underlying pathology, including dilated cardiomyopathy, ischemic heart disease, or valvular heart disease. Eosinophilic myocarditis has been related to one or more of the many drugs taken by transplant candidates, including digoxin or furosemide, and an association with dobutamine infusion has recently been reported.[32, 33] Peripheral eosinophilia may be present but is not a consistent finding.

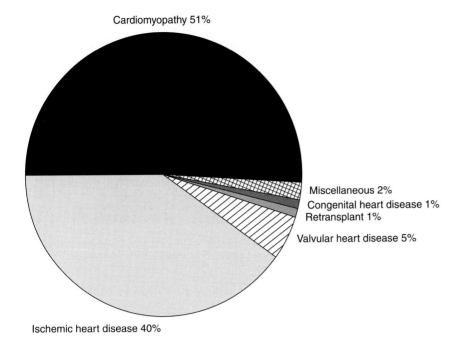

Cardiomyopathy 51%

Miscellaneous 2%
Congenital heart disease 1%
Retransplant 1%
Valvular heart disease 5%

Ischemic heart disease 40%

Figure 23-2 • Indications for heart transplantation at Brigham and Women's Hospital. Cardiomyopathy and ischemic heart disease were the indications in over 90% of more than 400 patients transplanted during a 15-year period. (From Winters GL: Transplantation: Explant, biopsy, and autopsy characteristics. In: McManus BM, Braunwald E [eds]: Atlas of Cardiovascular Pathology. Philadelphia, Current Medicine, 2000.)

Diseases That May Either Recur in the Allograft or Affect Recipient Prognosis

A number of case reports have documented diseases that have recurred in an allograft (Table 23-1).[34, 35] Recurrences have been reported within 6 months or less after transplantation. Endomyocardial biopsy of the recipient's native heart before transplantation may help to document such conditions. Clinicians should be made aware of the presence of any of these findings in the explanted heart, because their recurrence after transplantation, often discovered on routine surveillance endomyocardial biopsy,[35–37] may produce persistent allograft dysfunction. Although patients with sarcoidosis and amyloidosis have undergone successful transplantation, progression of either disease may limit long-term benefits.[38, 39]

Active lymphocytic myocarditis provides the indication for fewer than 1% of heart transplants. However, a retrospective multicenter analysis of 12 patients with active lymphocytic myocarditis in their explanted hearts suggested that such individuals reject their transplanted heart early, at high frequency, and with increased severity compared with heart transplant recipients with other preoperative diagnoses. It is postulated that either a clone of autodirected or crossreactive cytotoxic T cells or autoantibody results in persistent immune-mediated injury to the myocardium. The addition of alloantigens introduced by

heart transplantation could potentiate an already activated immune system, resulting in early, frequent, and severe rejection.[40]

Discordance Between Pretransplant Diagnosis and Pathology of the Explanted Heart

In a small percentage of cases, pathologic evaluation of the explanted recipient heart has yielded findings that did not support the pretransplant clinical diagnosis. One study of more than 200 transplants found a discordance rate of 8% between clinical and pathologic diagnoses.[41] In most cases, the discrepancy involved conditions that mimicked the clinical presentation of dilated cardiomyopathy and included ischemic heart disease and the dilated phase of hypertrophic cardiomyopathy as well as less common entities such as arrhythmogenic right ventricular cardiomyopathy and congenitally corrected transposition of the great arteries.

PATHOLOGY OF THE DONOR HEART

Congenital or Acquired Heart Disease

Gross abnormalities of donor hearts may be detected at their harvesting or during preparation for implantation. Incidental congenital anomalies, such as a bicuspid aortic valve or a patent foramen ovale, do not typically preclude use. A patent foramen ovale is generally sutured at the time of transplantation.

The success of cardiac transplantation has increased the need for an expanded supply of donor hearts. Even in young adults, significant coronary artery disease is not

TABLE 23-1 • **Diseases Reported to Recur in the Allograft**

Amyloidosis
Chagas disease
Fabry disease
Giant cell myocarditis
Melanoma
Sarcoidosis

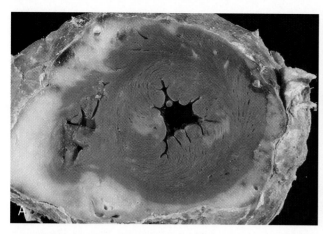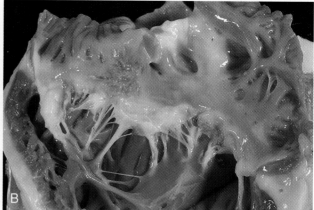

Figure 23-3 • Examples of donor heart disease. *A*, Allograft from a transplant recipient with early graft failure who died 9 days after transplantation. This transverse section through the ventricles stained with triphenyltetrazolium chloride (TTC) demonstrates cardiomegaly (heart weight = 675 g) with concentric left ventricular hypertrophy. The recent subendocardial infarcts (pale areas) of the septal and lateral walls occurred early after transplantation. In addition to hypertrophy, there was also preexisting donor coronary atherosclerosis with 75% stenosis of the left anterior descending and right coronary arteries and 90% stenosis of the left circumflex coronary artery. *B*, Right atrial endocardial donor heart vegetation, likely caused by trauma from a central venous line. It was sterile with no demonstrable organisms. (*A*, From Winters GL: Transplantation: Explant, biopsy, and autopsy characteristics. In: McManus BM, Braunwald E [eds]: Atlas of Cardiovascular Pathology [in press]. *B*, From Schoen FJ: Myocardial, pericardial, and endocardial heart disease. In: Interventional and Surgical Cardiovascular Pathology: Clinical Correlations and Basic Principles. Philadelphia, WB Saunders, 1989, p 188.)

unusual.[42–44] Nineteen percent of 94 male Korean War casualties (mean age 21 years, range 18 to 37 years) had at least one coronary artery narrowing that exceeded 50%; 6% had narrowing in one or more coronary vessel that exceeded 75%.[43] Although routine coronary angiograms of donor hearts are logistically impossible, angiography is often done for male donors who are older than 45 years of age and female donors who are older than 50 years of age or when cardiac risk factors are known.[10, 11] Atherosclerosis in the donor heart may preclude adequate preservation during harvesting and transport, particularly if ventricular hypertrophy is also present (Fig. 23-3*A*). An intravascular ultrasonographic study revealed significant intimal thickening in more than 50% of recipients early after transplantation, suggesting transmission of donor disease.[45] This raised concern that preexistent donor coronary atherosclerosis might accelerate allograft coronary disease. Although one study has shown no acceleration of allograft coronary disease by preexisting donor atherosclerosis within the first few years after transplantation, long-term outcomes of donor transmitted disease will require further evaluation.[46]

Right atrial vegetations in donor hearts are most likely nonbacterial thrombotic endocarditis (NBTE) associated with central venous lines such as Swan-Ganz catheters[47–49] (Fig. 23-3*B*). If infective endocarditis is a consideration, a smear with gram stain and/or frozen section histologic analysis of the vegetation may aid in making the decision about whether a donor heart may be used.

Infections

Transmission of infectious diseases, including cytomegalovirus (CMV) and *Toxoplasma gondii,* from donors to recipients has been well documented.[50] Antibodies to CMV in a donor do not preclude transplantation, but recipients may be at increased risk for reactivation or primary infection, depending on their serologic status before transplantation. CMV-seronegative recipients have a 25 to 40% chance of developing CMV infection.[51] Although most of these infections occur in recipients of CMV-seropositive donors, CMV infection may also occur in 10 to 20% of seronegative recipients of seronegative organs.[52] Primary CMV infections can cause serious complications in the immunosuppressed transplant recipient. In addition, CMV has been implicated as a possible etiologic factor in the development of allograft coronary disease.[53–55]

Despite absence of active infection, a donor may transmit *Toxoplasma gondii* to a recipient through latent myocardial cysts that become reactivated during immunosuppression.[51, 56] Only 5% of *Toxoplasma*-seropositive recipients, regardless of donor serology, develop a clinical infection, and these infections are usually mild. However, *Toxoplasma*-seronegative recipients who receive hearts from *Toxoplasma*-seropositive donors develop a clinical illness in 75% of instances, and these infections carry a high mortality.[57]

Other infectious agents, such as hepatitis B and C and HIV,[58] can potentially be transmitted from donor to recipient.

Ischemic Injury Acquired in the Donor Before Harvesting

Brain death in the donor may induce segmental or global myocardial dysfunction (see Chapter 15). Although the mechanisms are not fully understood, they may be related to (1) high catecholamine levels preceding brain death with norepinephrine release leading to coronary vasospasm or direct myocardial injury; (2) hemodynamic deterioration after brain death leading to stunned myocardium (prolonged postischemic ventricular dysfunction); and (3) reduced circulating triiodothyronine levels, resulting in reduction of oxidative metabolism.[59–62] Moreover, the administration of large doses of vasopressive drugs to support a donor heart before harvesting may cause direct myocyte toxicity or constriction of small intramyocardial vessels with resultant microinfarcts. These lesions, which involve only small clusters of myocytes, may be accompanied by an associated neutrophilic infiltrate similar to that found in perioperative ischemic injury (see later). Lesions resulting from donor or perioperative ischemia may coexist with, and must be differentiated from, acute rejection.

PATHOLOGY OF THE ALLOGRAFT

The major sources of morbidity and mortality after cardiac transplantation are early graft failure (including perioperative ischemic injury), allograft rejection, infection, lymphoproliferative disorders, and allograft coronary disease (Table 23-2). Although particular pathologies are statistically more common at given times after transplantation, considerable overlap exists in their occurrence (Fig. 23-4).

In general, the differential diagnosis of graft failure very early in the post-transplant period includes inappropriate donor selection, anomalous origin of coronary arteries in the donor heart, technical surgical problems, hyperacute rejection, pulmonary hypertension in the recipient, and previous damage to the donor heart from ischemia in the donor or perioperative period. Between 1 month and 1 year after transplantation, acute rejection and infection predominate; however, complications from perioperative ischemic damage may persist, and early manifestations of allograft coronary disease may occur. More than a year after transplantation, allograft coronary disease and malignancy become more common; however, acute rejection and infection remain important considerations at any time.

Hyperacute Rejection

Hyperacute rejection is a rare event with a reported rate of less than 1%. It occurs immediately or within a few hours after heart transplantation.[63, 64] Hyperacute rejection may occur (1) if there are preformed ABO antibodies in the recipient; (2) if preformed antibodies to the HLA system are present in the allograft; (3) if there are preformed antibodies to donor vascular endothelial cell antigens; and (4) after xenotransplantation. Predisposing factors to hyperacute rejection include previous blood transfusions, repeated pregnancies, multiple cardiac surgeries, and previous transplantation.[64]

The pathologic principle underlying hyperacute rejection is that of an antibody-mediated toxicity caused by antibodies present in the recipient at transplantation and directed against antigens in the graft, resulting in its destruction[65–68] (Fig. 23-5). Preformed antibodies (IgG and/or IgM) deposit on donor organ vascular endothelial cells, leading to activation of recipient complement. The combination of antibodies plus complement, as well as other serum factors, leads to endothelial cell activation causing the loss of vascular integrity, enhanced expression of cell surface molecules, cytokine secretion, and activation of clotting and fibrinolytic cascades. The end result is microvascular thrombosis with hemorrhage, myocardial and vascular necrosis, and graft failure.[69, 70]

A diagnosis of hyperacute rejection may be made at endomyocardial biopsy, but this pathology is more often encountered in an explanted heart of a recipient undergoing retransplantation or at autopsy. The heart is typically heavy with diffuse hemorrhagic discoloration of the myocardium (Fig. 23-6A). Histologically, there is diffuse interstitial hemorrhage and edema. Small vessels contain aggregated red cells and fibrin thrombi (Fig. 23-6B). If the patient survives long enough, myocyte and vascular degeneration and eventual necrosis with a neurophilic response ensue.

Right Ventricular Failure

Although right ventricular failure is an important factor in early postoperative cardiac dysfunction after heart surgery in general, acute right ventricular failure and biventricular dysfunction with low output are common causes of death early after cardiac transplantation.[18] Isolated acute right ventricular failure usually results when the normal right ventricle of a donor heart is unable to contract effectively against elevated pulmonary vascular resistance in the recipient. The right ventricle becomes dilated with impaired contractility; inadequate right ventricular output and hypotension result. Endomyocardial biopsy in this setting is frequently not helpful and may show early ischemic injury that may or may not account for the extent of myocardial dysfunction. Left ventricular or biventricular dysfunction is most often caused by myocardial stunning resulting from ischemia or suboptimal myocardial preservation during the operative procedure; this dysfunction usually resolves within 48 to 72 hours.

Both tricuspid and mitral valve regurgitation have been observed in patients after cardiac transplantation, possibly related to altered chamber geometry and size. In most instances, the regurgitation is mild and produces mild or no symptoms. In some cases, however, clinically significant regurgitation may require valvular repair or replacement. Flail tricuspid leaflet as a complication of endomyocardial biopsy (see later) may also result in tricuspid regurgitation.

Perioperative Ischemic Injury

In addition to ischemic injury acquired in the donor, early ischemic injury may occur in the perioperative period during the obligatory ischemic time that accompanies procurement and implantation of a donor heart; such injury may precipitate early graft failure.[34, 49, 63, 71] Three periods of perioperative ischemia occur during donor heart manipulation. They include (1) an interval of warm ischemia from donor cardiectomy to cold storage for transport; (2) an interval of cold ischemia during transport; and (3) the operating ischemia interval from the

TABLE 23-2 • **Differential Diagnosis of Post-Transplant Endomyocardial Biopsy Findings**

	Acute Rejection	Early Ischemic Injury ≤3 mo Post-Transplant	Late Ischemic Injury >3 mo Post-Transplant	Biopsy Site	Quilty Effect	Infection	PTLD
Frequency of finding	10% of bx-ISHLT grade 3A or greater	>80% of pts wk 1–4 post-transplant	Unknown	20–70% of bx	10–20% of bx	<1% of bx	<1% of bx
Pattern of occurrence	Sporadic; common 1st post-transplant yr	Common early	Common in RV and LV in pts with ACD	Common	Often recurrent	Persistent if not treated	Sporadic; rare
Cell population	T-cells, macrophages	Mixed: PMNs, lymphocytes, eosinophils	None; mixed infiltrate, granulation tissue when healing	Mixed; granulation tissue when healing	T and B cells; macrophages; plasma cells	None to mixed	B-cell (most commonly) polyclonal, oligoclonal, multiclonal
Myocyte damage	Grade 2 or >	Coagulation necrosis; contraction bands	SEMV microinfarcts	Localized; myocyte disarray	Focal in Quilty B	Variable	Minimal unless infiltrate is extensive
Other characteristics	Inflammatory infiltrate > myocyte damage	Myocyte damage > inflammatory infiltrate	Positive predictive value for ACD—92%	Overlying fibrin early	Capillary proliferation	Presence of organisms	Cellular atypia; EBV related
Usual clinical response	Consider ↑ immunosuppression	None	Correlate with angiography/ICUS	None	None	Consider ↓ immunosuppression; treat specific agent	Consider ↓ immunosuppression; chemotherapy

PTLD = post-transplant lymphoproliferative disorder; bx = biopsies; pts = patients; RV = right ventricle; LV = left ventricle; PMNs = polymorphonuclear leukocytes; SEMV = subendocardial myocyte vacuolization; EBV = Epstein-Barr virus; ACD = allograft coronary disease; ICUS = intracoronary ultrasound.

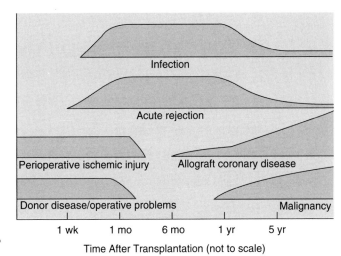

Figure 23-4 • Complications after heart transplantation: relationship to postoperative interval.

Time After Transplantation (not to scale)

time the heart is removed from cold storage to resumption of circulation in the implanted donor heart.

Early ischemic injury is a frequent finding on endomyocardial biopsies obtained during the early post-transplant period and may be diagnosed by conventional histologic criteria. Although the severity and extent of injury may vary, some degree of damage has been noted in up to 89% of biopsies obtained during the first 4 weeks after transplantation.[72]

The morphologic characteristics of early ischemic injury include coagulative myocyte necrosis (Fig. 23-7A, B) and a mixed cellular infiltrate. In very early biopsies (week 1 to 2 after transplantation; Fig. 23-8), coagulative myocyte necrosis, frequently with associated contraction bands and scattered neutrophils, is often the predominant finding. The necrotic cells may be difficult to distinguish in sections stained with hematoxylin and eosin; a Masson trichrome stain may help to make these areas more prominent. The coagulative myocyte necrosis often extends to

the endocardial surface; this is unlike a typical myocardial infarction, which contains an intervening zone of viable myocardium perfused directly by blood in the ventricular cavity.

Subsequent biopsies (week 2 to 4 after transplantation; see Fig. 23-8) may reveal the healing phase of this early ischemic injury. It is characterized by a mixed inflammatory infiltrate consisting of neutrophils, macrophages, lymphocytes, and plasma cells (Fig. 23-7C). At this point, confusion with acute rejection may occur (Fig. 23-7D). The pathologic and clinical features differentiating early ischemic injury from acute rejection are summarized in Table 23-3. The healing inflammatory response following ischemic injury is predominantly in the interstitium or perivascular spaces, not encroaching on, and usually with a clear separation from, adjacent myocytes. Cellular debris is frequently present in the inflammatory foci. Healing fat necrosis and myocyte vacuolization in the adjacent myocardium are often present. The healing response to

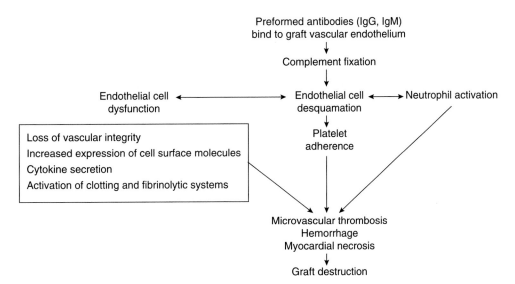

Figure 23-5 • Pathogenesis of hyperacute rejection. (From Winters GL: Transplantation: Explants, biopsy, and autopsy characteristics: In: McManus BM, Braunwald E [eds]: Atlas of Cardiovascular Pathology. Philadelphia, Current Medicine, 2000.)

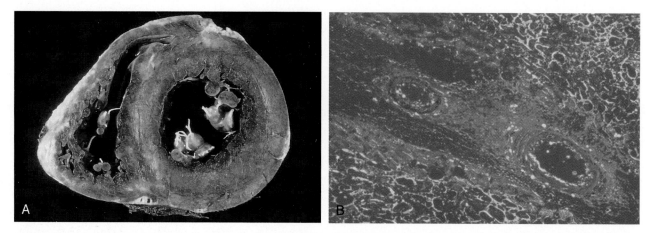

Figure 23-6 • Hyperacute rejection. *A*, Transverse section of allograft weighing 550 g, explanted after 36 hours. There is biventricular dilatation and diffusely hemorrhagic myocardium. *B*, Histologically the myocardium contains extensive interstitial hemorrhage and edema. Fibrin thrombi are present within small vessels. (H&E stain.) (From Winters GL: Transplantation: Explant, biopsy, and autopsy characteristics. In: McManus BM, Braunwald E [eds]: Atlas of Cardiovascular Pathology. Philadelphia, Current Medicine, 2000.)

early ischemic injury may be protracted because of the anti-inflammatory effects of immunosuppression[73] and has been observed more than 6 weeks after transplantation in some patients.

Longer total ischemic time has been associated with increased severity of early ischemic injury.[71, 72] However, distant procurement of donor hearts is a fact of life at most cardiac transplantation centers because it is neces-

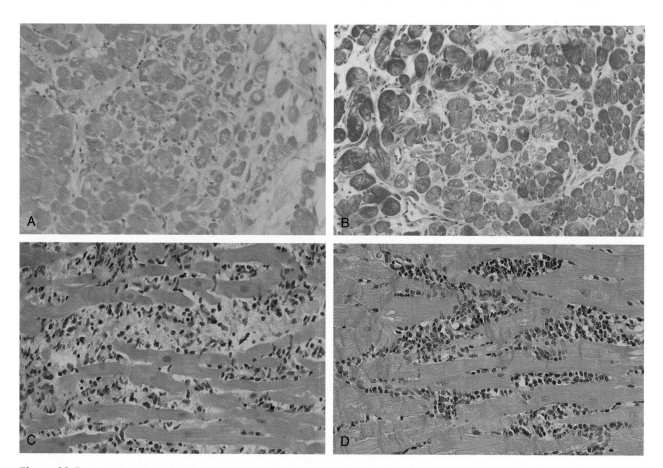

Figure 23-7 • Perioperative ischemic injury. *A*, In early stages, coagulation necrosis is characterized by wavy, eosinophilic myocytes devoid of nuclei. Little or no inflammatory response is present (H&E stain). *B*, Trichrome stain accentuates the necrotic myocytes, which appear purple-gray. *C*, Healing is characterized by a polymorphous inflammatory infiltrate. Necrotic debris is present in the background. *D*, For comparison, acute cellular rejection shows a greater density of lymphocytes with encroachment upon adjacent myocytes and less background debris. (*C* and *D*, H&E stain.)

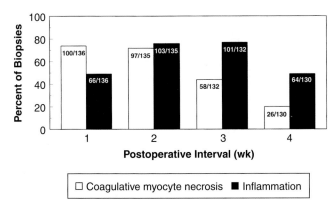

Figure 23-8 • Temporal evolution of coagulative myocyte necrosis and inflammation in perioperative ischemic myocardial injury. Numbers in bars indicate numbers with feature/total biopsies examined at interval. Necrosis was present most frequently in the earliest biopsies (76 and 72% at weeks 1 and 2, respectively); inflammation was maximal at 2 and 3 weeks (76 and 77%, respectively. (From Fyfe B, Loh E, Winters GL, et al: Heart-transplantation-associated perioperative ischemic myocardial injury: Morphological features and clinical significance. Circulation 93:1133, 1996.)

sary to increase the donor pool. An ultrastructural study comparing donor hearts (maximal ischemic times up to 3 hours) with on-site donor hearts consistently revealed capillary endothelial damage in those procured at a distance.[15] These ultrastructural changes were worse after reperfusion. One year after transplantation, ultrastructural changes could not be distinguished in the allografts from the two groups, and no differences in function or survival were detected. However, ISHLT Registry data have consistently shown prolonged ischemic time is a significant risk factor for 1-year and 5-year mortality after heart transplantation.[1]

Although extensive early ischemic injury may have a deleterious effect on short-term survival, the long-term impact, including possible contribution to late allograft dysfunction and/or the development of allograft coronary disease, remains to be established.[15, 74-77] The recognition by pathologists of early ischemic injury in endomyocardial biopsies is important because accurate diagnosis and distinction from rejection decrease unnecessary immunosuppression with its associated sequelae.

Acute Rejection

Pathogenesis[78-80]

Placement of a vascularized allograft induces a complex series of events involving both antigen-specific and nonspecific mechanisms (Fig. 23-9) Graft-derived major histocompatibility complex (MHC) class I and class II antigens in the setting of costimulatory molecules (i.e., CD40, B7-1, B7-2, and others) are recognized by host CD4+ and CD8+ lymphocytes. Antigens may be directly presented by allograft cells or be taken up and presented by host antigen presenting cells. The recognition of allograft class II antigens by host CD4+ T cells results in cytokine production including interleukin-2 (IL-2) and interferon-gamma (IFN-gamma). IL-2 results in further pro-

liferation of CD4+ T cells and can activate CD8+ cytotoxic T cells specific to class I. INF-gamma and other cytokines contribute to macrophage recruitment and activation with secondary cytokine production, all resulting in a delayed type of hypersensitivity response, microvascular injury, and graft destruction. Other cytokines, such as IL-4 and IL-5, may contribute to the effect by driving an antibody response to the allograft.

Morphology[71, 81]

Acute rejection is characterized histologically by infiltrating inflammatory cells and eventual damage to the myocardium and its vasculature. The infiltrate is predominantly lymphocytic but may include macrophages and occasional eosinophils (Fig. 23-10). In the most severe forms of rejection, the infiltrate is polymorphous, consisting of neutrophils and eosinophils as well as lymphocytes. The infiltrating lymphocytes are predominantly T cells comprising a mixture of CD4 and CD8 phenotypes. The proportion of CD4 to CD8 cells, however, has not proved useful in either clinical management of recipients or in predicting clinical outcome.[82] Lymphocyte subtyping, therefore, is not warranted in the routine diagnosis of rejection.

Damage or injury to the myocardium, originally termed "myocyte necrosis," is an important but sometimes difficult feature to identify, and its existence has been questioned.[83] Although readily distinguishable cell necrosis may be a feature of more severe forms of rejection, myocyte damage in milder rejection is often characterized by encroachment of inflammatory cells at the perimeter of myocytes, resulting in irregular myocyte borders, their partial replacement, or in architectural distortion. In severe rejection, vasculitic injury to small vessels results in hemorrhage and edema.

TABLE 23-3 • Differential Pathologic and Clinical Features of Early Ischemic Injury and Acute Rejection

Early Ischemic Injury	Acute Rejection
Pathologic Features	
Coagulative myocyte necrosis, with or without contraction bands	Myocyte fraying and replacement; myocyte damage in advanced grades
Inflammation, a *response* to and usually less than myocyte damage	Inflammmation, *causal* to and usually greater than myocyte damage
PMNs, histiocytes prominent	Lymphocytes prominent; PMNs in grade 4
Vasculitis may be present	Vasculitis may be present in grade 4
Fat necrosis may be present	Fat necrosis is absent
Clinical Features	
Onset early after surgery	Rare within first 2 weeks posttransplant
Usually no clinical symptoms but may cause early graft dysfunction	Usually no clinical symptoms, but higher grades may cause graft dysfunction
No changes in immunosuppressive therapy indicated	Augmented immunosuppression warranted at higher grades

Modified from Fyfe B, Loh E, Winters GL, et al: Heart transplantation-associated perioperative ischemic myocardial injury: Morphological features and clinical significance. Circulation 93:1133, 1996.

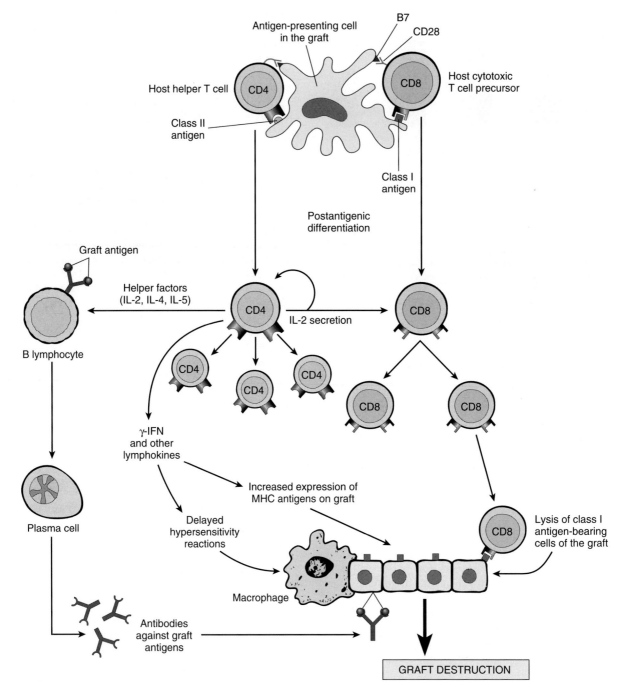

Figure 23-9 • Pathogenesis of acute rejection. (From Kumar V: Disorders of the immune system. In: Kumar V, Cotran RS, Robbins SL [eds]: Basic Pathology. Philadelphia, WB Saunders, 1997, p 97.)

The immunologic mechanism by which infiltrating cells induce myocardial cell injury and the type of injury that occurs in an allograft are not fully understood. Two mechanisms implicated in cell death are necrosis, typically seen after vascular occlusion, and apoptosis, or programmed cell death resulting from direct cytotoxic activity. It was generally assumed that myocyte necrosis was caused by the cytotoxic activity of lymphocytes present in the myocardium during acute rejection. However, CD4+ cells may play an important, and potentially more significant, role via cytokine production with macrophage and/

or endothelial activation. A murine model of cardiac allograft rejection, in which cultured ventricular myocytes were incubated with infiltrating cells, demonstrated that only a small component of myocyte injury could be attributed to direct cytotoxic T lymphocyte killing within the infiltrating cell population.[84]

Apoptosis of cardiac myocytes during acute rejection has been demonstrated and, in one study, correlated with the severity of rejection.[85] In lower grades of rejection, in which myocyte injury is thought to be absent, no apoptotic myocytes were observed. Another study demon-

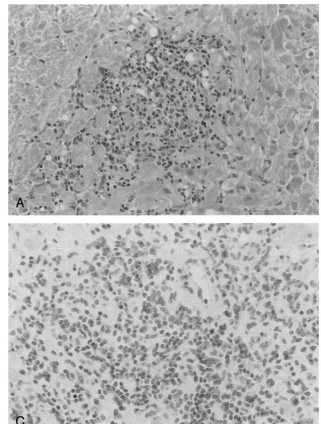

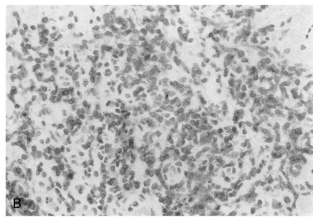

Figure 23-10 • Morphologic features of acute rejection. *A,* Dense cellular infiltrate with associated myocyte damage. *B,* Immunoperoxidase staining (CD3) reveals a predominance of T lymphocytes. *C,* Macrophages make up the other major cellular component of rejection as demonstrated by immunoperoxidase staining with CD68. (*B, C* From Winters GL: Heart transplantation: Explant, biopsy, and autopsy characteristics. In: McManus BM, Braunwald E [eds]: Atlas of Cardiovascular Pathology. Philadelphia, Current Medicine, 2000.)

strated a relationship between apoptosis of cardiac myocytes during acute rejection and the expression of inducible nitric oxide synthase, leading the authors to suggest that apoptosis may be triggered by nitric oxide.[86] Myocyte death by apoptosis may, therefore, contribute to the worsening cardiac function observed during rejection. It should be noted, however, that apoptosis of cardiac myocytes has been observed in diverse cardiac conditions and is not specific for rejection.[87-89] Ischemic injury may also induce nitric oxide synthase and lead to apoptosis.

Numerous indirect or noninvasive approaches to detect or predict allograft rejection have been assessed but none has proved to be as sensitive, specific, or clinically useful in rejection surveillance as the endomyocardial biopsy. Detailed reviews on this topic are available.[90-92] Ancillary diagnostic methods may be divided into two groups: those that monitor myocardial structure and function and those that monitor immunologic events. The former group includes hemodynamic monitoring, electrocardiography, echocardiography, Doppler echocardiography, radionuclide imaging, nuclear magnetic resonance, and positron emission tomography. Immunologic assessment includes monitoring of soluble interleukin 2 receptor levels in serum, monitoring of biochemical byproducts of rejection in urine, and cytoimmunologic monitoring and T-cell analysis of peripheral blood lymphocytes.

Grading Systems for Acute Rejection

Because the clinical therapeutic response to rejection tends to be proportional to the intensity of biopsy pathol-

ogy, the pathologist uses a grading system to maintain consistency in communication of biopsy findings to the transplant physician. In general, increasing grades (representing increasing severity) of rejection are defined by increasing numbers of inflammatory cells and increasing numbers of inflammatory foci associated with increasing amounts of myocyte (and ultimately vascular) damage (Fig. 23-11).

In 1974, Dr. Margaret Billingham of Stanford University established a classification whereby degrees of allograft rejection and related histopathologic features could help guide clinical management of heart allograft recipients.[93] According to her classification, "mild" rejection consisted of a perivascular and/or interstitial infiltrate without evidence of myocyte damage. "Moderate" rejection was characterized by intensification of the inflammatory infiltrate associated with myocyte damage or necrosis. "Severe" rejection consisted of a polymorphous infiltrate, including neutrophils and eosinophils as well as lymphocytes, associated with widespread myocyte necrosis, hemorrhage, edema, and vasculitis.

Dr. Billingham's original classification was used by institutions worldwide. During the next decade and a half, a number of modifications evolved; nevertheless, all grading systems were based on the same premise of increasing inflammatory infiltrates and increasing damage to the myocardium.[49, 71, 94-97] The categories of mild and moderate rejection were often subdivided in an attempt to refine the histologic characteristics that predict progression to higher rejection grades and, therefore, define patients who

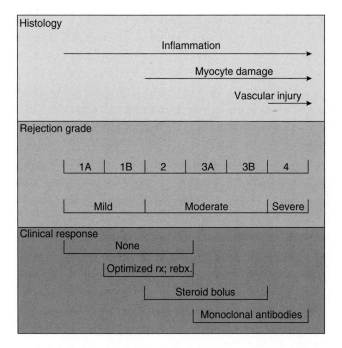

Figure 23-11 • Comparison of histology with rejection grade and clinical response. In general, increasing grades of rejection represent increasing amounts and severity of inflammation and myocyte damage. There is great variation among transplant centers in the clinical response to rejection grades. That response is most uniform at both ends of the spectrum, i.e., grades 0 and 1A are generally not treated; grades 3B and 4 are treated aggressively with augmented immunosuppression. Variation occurs most frequently in response to intermediate grades such as grade 2. rx = therapy; rebx = rebiopsy. (From Winters GL: Heart transplantation: Explant, biopsy, and autopsy characteristics. In: McManus B, Braunwald E [eds]: Atlas of Cardiovascular Pathology. Philadelphia, Current Medicine, 2000.)

should be monitored more closely or receive increased immunosuppression therapy. The proliferation of diverse grading systems, however, impaired effective comparisons of treatment regimens and outcomes from the growing number of transplant centers worldwide.[98, 99]

In 1990, the International Society for Heart and Lung Transplantation grading system for cardiac biopsies[100] (Table 23-4) was established to allow more consistent comparisons of biopsy results between institutions and facilitate multicenter clinical trials. It is as follows:

Grade 0. This represents no evidence of rejection. The myocardial interstitium normally contains a small number of lymphocytes and other interstitial cells that, if cut in cross-section, may resemble lymphocytes. These findings should not be interpreted as rejection. Lymphocytes within adipose tissue or granulation tissue should also not be considered as a sign of rejection.

Grade 1. Figure 23-12*A, B* shows grade 1, "mild" rejection, which consists of perivascular and/or interstitial lymphocytic infiltrates(s) without associated myocyte damage involving one (or more than one) biopsy fragment. Grade 1A (Fig. 23-12*A*), which designates a focal process, and grade 1B (Fig. 23-12*B*), which designates a diffuse process, are considered to be different patterns of the same grade of rejection.

Grade 2. Figure 23-12*C* illustrates grade 2, "focal moderate" rejection, which consists of a single focus of

lymphocytic infiltration with associated myocyte damage. Frequently, the area of infiltration is relatively well circumscribed. Additional foci of inflammatory infiltrates (i.e., grade 1 rejection) may be present elsewhere in the biopsy, but these additional foci should not be associated with myocyte damage.

Grade 3A. Figure 23-12*D* shows grade 3A, "multifocal moderate" rejection, which is characterized by multiple (2 or more) inflammatory foci with associated myocyte damage. The foci may be distributed in one (or more than one) biopsy fragment. Intervening areas of uninvolved myocardium are present between the foci of rejection.

Grade 3B. Figure 23-12*E* depicts grade 3B, "diffuse moderate" rejection, which consists of a diffuse inflammatory process, usually involving several biopsy fragments. Associated myocyte damage is present at multiple locations.

Grade 4. Figure 23-12*F* demonstrates grade 4, "severe" rejection, which is characterized by a diffuse polymorphous infiltrate consisting of lymphocytes, neutrophils, and eosinophils, with multiple areas of associated myocyte damage. Edema and interstitial hemorrhage are usually present and vasculitis is frequently a feature. All, or nearly all, of the biopsy fragments are involved, although the intensity of the infiltrate may vary among fragments. Involvement of the endocardium is common. If a patient has received immunosuppressive therapy before the biopsy, the amount of edema and hemorrhage may be out of proportion to the amount of inflammation.

Improved immunosuppressive regimens in heart transplant recipients have substantially decreased the incidence of serious rejection episodes. Biopsies without evidence of rejection and with grade 1 rejection are the most common, accounting for approximately 80% in large series.

TABLE 23-4 • International Society for Heart and Lung Transplantation Standardized Grading for Cardiac Biopsies

Rejection Grade	Description
0	No evidence of rejection
1 Mild	
A—Focal	Focal perivascular and/or interstitial infiltrate without myocyte damage
B—Diffuse	Diffuse infiltrate without myocyte damage
2 Moderate (focal)	One focus of infiltrate with associated myocyte damage
3 Moderate	
A—Multifocal	Multifocal infiltrate with myocyte damage
B—Diffuse	Diffuse infiltrate with myocyte damage
4 Severe	Diffuse polymorphous infiltrate with extensive myocyte damage, ±edema, ±hemorrhage, ±vasculitis

Nonrejection Biopsy Findings

Quilty effect A and B

Ischemic Injury—Early (≤3 months)
                Late (>3 months)

Infection

Post-transplant lymphoproliferative disorder

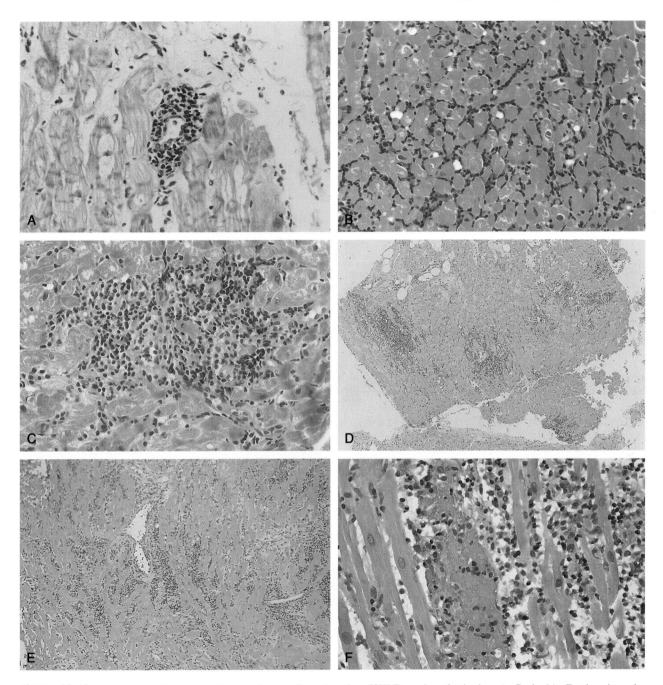

Figure 23-12 • International Society for Heart and Lung Transplantation (ISHLT) grades of rejection. *A*, Grade 1A: Focal perivascular lymphocytic infiltrate without damage to adjacent myocytes. *B*, Grade 1B: Diffuse interstitial lymphocytic infiltrate without damage to adjacent myocytes. *C*, Grade 2: One focus of dense lymphocytic infiltrate with associated myocyte damage. *D*, Grade 3A: Multiple foci of dense lymphocytic infiltrates with associated myocyte damage. There are intervening areas of uninvolved myocardium. *E*, Grade 3B: Diffuse infiltrate with associated myocyte damage. *F*, Grade 4: Polymorphous infiltrate with extensive myocyte damage, edema, and hemorrhage. (H&E stain.)

Grades 2 and 3 rejection each account for approximately 10% of biopsies, and grade 4 rejection is present in fewer than 1% of cases (Fig. 23-13). Most studies agree that the incidence of rejection is highest in the first 3 to 6 months after transplantation and that the incidence falls to 5% or less after 1 year. Although it is reasonable to expect the incidence of rejection would be highest early after transplantation, that incidence may be falsely elevated by the tendency to confuse ischemic injury in early biopsies with

rejection. Because of the low incidence of rejection in later periods after transplantation, the need to perform surveillance biopsies after the first 6 months to 1 year post-transplantation has been questioned.[101-103] However, because rejection can occur years postoperatively, many transplant centers continue to perform late surveillance biopsies at widely spaced intervals or on selected patients.[104]

Several caveats regarding use of the ISHLT grading

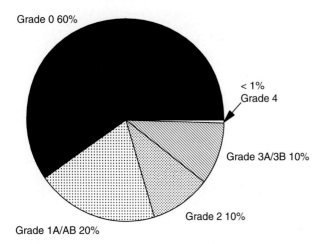

Grade 0 60%

< 1%
Grade 4

Grade 3A/3B 10%

Grade 2 10%

Grade 1A/AB 20%

Figure 23-13 • Incidence of rejection grades. The figure presents the distribution of rejection grade diagnoses, rounded to the nearest 10% as rendered in over 4000 surveillance endomyocardial biopsies obtained at Brigham and Women's Hospital. (From Winters GL: Heart transplantation: Explant, biopsy, and autopsy characteristics. In: McManus BM, Braunwald E [eds]: Atlas of Cardiovascular Pathology. Philadelphia, Current Medicine, 2000.)

system deserve mention.[105] The system is designed to provide a standardized format for conveying histologic biopsy findings. No attempt is made to incorporate clinical parameters or to recommend treatment. A multifocal pattern of rejection consists of discrete foci of rejection with intervening uninvolved myocardium; a diffuse pattern involves nearly the entire tissue fragment and usually the majority of tissue fragments in a biopsy. The rejection grade assigned should reflect the "worst" area of the biopsy. The grading system is based on histologic findings that precede any treatment except for maintenance immunosuppression, which at present includes cyclosporine in virtually all cases. However, biopsies from patients with low cyclosporine levels may contain edema as the predominant histologic finding, reminiscent of biopsies obtained in the precyclosporine era. Biopsies obtained after treatment for rejection may contain residual foci of rejection and/or areas of healing. Whereas the original Stanford grading system allowed for a diagnosis of "resolving" rejection, that terminology is not used in the ISHLT system. Any residual activity should be given a rejection grade. "Resolved" rejection should be designated by grade 0. Immunosuppressive regimens other than the commonly used triple therapy (cyclosporine, azathioprine, and corticosteroids, with or without OKT3 or ATG) may affect the temporal relationship of rejection patterns. The ISHLT system was designed specifically for biopsies and does not apply to autopsy or explanted hearts in which much larger areas of myocardium are available for examination. In these cases, descriptive characterization of rejection (i.e., none, mild, moderate, severe) is preferred. Optimal care of cardiac transplant recipients requires good communication and close collaboration between pathologist and transplant physician. For difficult or borderline biopsy findings, it may not be sufficient to simply report a biopsy grade number. The diagnostic dilemma should be explained to the clinician, and it may be helpful for the clinician to review biopsy slides with the pathologist.

Histologic Indications for Therapeutic Intervention

Clinical response to histologic rejection varies with the rejection grade and depends on particular treatment protocols used at individual transplant centers (see Fig. 23-11). In general, low rejection grades elicit no change in therapy and maximization of maintenance immunosuppression drug levels, with or without repeat biopsy earlier than scheduled. Rejection falling into the middle of the spectrum may be treated with a temporary oral or intravenous increase in corticosteroid dose (pulse). Patients with high grade rejection often receive therapy with monoclonal antibodies, such as OKT3.

However, identifying the exact point in the spectrum of histologic rejection that requires an intensification of immunosuppression remains one of the major unresolved issues in the care of cardiac transplant recipients. The point at which this occurs varies from grade 1B to grade 3A at different heart transplantation centers, with many programs using the presence of any myocyte injury (grade 2) as the threshold for treatment. Low grades of rejection (grades 1A and 1B) in biopsies from asymptomatic patients have been shown to progress to a higher grade of rejection on the next biopsy in approximately 20% of cases.[106–109] The incidence of progression varies inversely with the time after transplantation and drops to as low as 2% of biopsies with grades 1A and 1B rejection obtained more than 1 year after transplantation.[106]

Grade 2 is the most problematic grade of rejection for both clinicians and pathologists.[110, 111] The clinical responses to biopsy findings of asymptomatic grade 2 rejection include no change in therapy, maximization of maintenance therapeutic drug levels, cessation of steroid taper in progress, repeat biopsy earlier than scheduled, or augmentation of immunosuppression. In the Brigham experience over a 9-year period, 85% of biopsies with grade 2 rejection resolved histologically without treatment.[112] However, as with grade 1 rejection mentioned above, the incidence of progression of grade 2 to a higher grade of rejection was greater during the first year after transplantation. Progression of grade 2 in biopsies obtained more than 2 years after transplantation was less than 5% (Fig. 23-14).

For the pathologist, an entire spectrum of grade 2 histologies exists from a minute focus of inflammation with one or two damaged myocytes to a large infiltrate with definite myocyte damage (Fig. 23-15A, B). The difficulty in diagnosing grade 2 often centers around whether myocyte damage is present. As a result, grade 2 proved the least reproducible of the rejection grades. In preparation for a clinical trial of a new immunosuppressive agent, a group of 16 transplant pathologists individually read a series of 23 post-transplant biopsies representing all grades of rejection and other post-transplantation biopsy findings. Whereas the overall concordance was quite high, 81% of major discrepancies and those that would affect treatment in most transplant centers involved the diagnosis of grade 2 rejection.[113] The actual existence of grade 2 rejection has been questioned by Fishbein and colleagues, who demonstrated, using step sectioning and immunohistochemical staining, that 91% of biopsies initially diagnosed as grade 2 rejection were, in fact, Quilty B lesions[114] (see later).

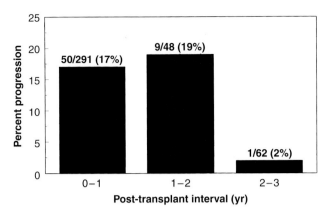

Figure 23-14 • Relationship between post transplant interval and percent progression of International Society for Heart and Lung Transplantation (ISHLT) grade 2 rejection. The probability of progression decreases markedly beyond 2 years after transplantation. (Data from Winters GL, Loh E, Schoen FJ: Natural history of focal moderate cardiac allograft rejection: Is treatment warranted? Circulation 91:1975, 1995.)

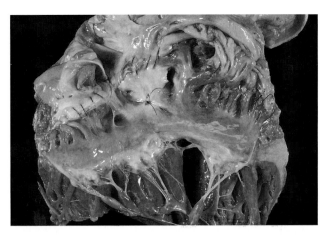

Figure 23-16 • Fatal acute rejection. Gross photograph of allograft right atrium and ventricle showing edematous, mottled, hemorrhagic myocardium that abruptly ends at the atrial suture line. The recipient atrium is tan and pale in comparison. (From Schoen FJ: Myocardial, pericardial, and endocardial heart disease. In: Interventional and Surgical Cardiovascular Pathology: Clinical Correlations and Basic Principles. Philadelphia, WB Saunders, 1989, p 194.)

There is preliminary evidence that some grade 3A rejection also resolves without treatment.[115] At our institution, biopsies with two to three foci of lymphocytic infiltrates and associated myocyte damage are given a separate designation and patients are not routinely treated, allowing the outcome to be followed on subsequent biopsies. Similar to biopsies with grade 2 rejection, 85% resolved without treatment.[112] However, the aforementioned series are small and do not fully explore all parameters required to establish a definite subset of biopsies with grade 3A rejection that do not require treatment. Understandably, there is a reluctance to conduct randomized trials on higher grades of rejection because some patients would not receive standard immunosuppressive therapy.

The decision whether to treat lower grades of acute rejection may have long-ranging implications because the possible contribution of persistent low-grade ("smoldering") rejection to late deterioration of allograft function through immune stimulation or cumulative fibrosis remains an unresolved issue.[112, 116] The possibility that persistent or repetitive untreated low-grade rejection contrib-

utes to allograft coronary disease resulting in graft failure is an important research topic.[117–123]

Fatal Acute Rejection

Despite advances in immunosuppression protocols, acute rejection remains an important cause of death in the first year after heart transplantation. Rejection that was severe enough to cause the death of a recipient is frequently evident grossly and characterized by edematous myocardium with a mottled or hemorrhagic appearance (Fig. 23-16). Histologically, extensive myocyte necrosis with edema and hemorrhage with or without vasculitis is typical. Less severe rejection that is present in a multifocal or focal distribution may be less apparent to gross inspection, and the myocardium should be thoroughly sectioned to ascertain the status of rejection. Fatal acute rejection may occur despite negative biopsies shortly before a patient's death.

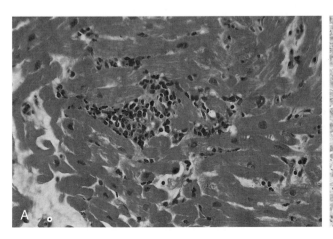

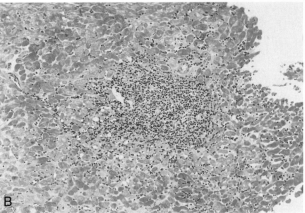

Figure 23-15 • Spectrum of grade 2 histology. *A*, Minute focus of dense lymphocytic infiltrate with focal myocyte damage. *B*, Large area of dense lymphocytic infiltrate with more extensive myocyte damage and replacement. (H&E stain.)

Acute Allograft Dysfunction Without Cellular Infiltrates

Acute changes in allograft function, including decreased contractility, the appearance of new wall motion abnormalities, elevated pulmonary artery wedge pressure, and decreased cardiac index, may occur in the absence of any cellular infiltrates on endomyocardial biopsy. Because rejection may have a patchy distribution, it is always possible that cellular infiltrates may be missed on biopsies obtained from rejecting hearts in a small percentage of cases, even with apparently adequate sampling.

Endomyocardial biopsy findings characterized by interstitial edema or hemorrhage and endothelial cell swelling with or without vasculitis on light microscopy, with vascular deposition of immunoglobulin (IgG or IgM), complement (C3 and/or C1q), and fibrinogen in a vascular pattern on immunofluorescence have been termed "vascular," "humoral," or "microvascular" rejection.[124–127] The role of this process, generally considered to be antibody mediated, in causing allograft dysfunction remains controversial.[128] However, some groups have found that its identification on biopsy, in the absence of cellular infiltrates, correlates with hemodynamic compromise in the allograft. Because most positive immunofluorescence staining occurs on biopsies obtained early after transplantation, routine immunofluorescence studies during this period have been advocated by some groups.[124–127] Immunoglobulin, complement, and fibrinogen deposition on immunofluorescence, however, are nonspecific abnormalities seen in other conditions such as ischemic injury.

The biopsy findings that have been termed vascular rejection may occur independent of, or in conjunction with, acute cellular rejection, and these may be graded independently. Recipients with these biopsy findings have a significantly decreased survival compared with that of recipients with only cellular rejection. However, patients with OKT3 sensitization have a high likelihood of developing these biopsy features, and graft loss may result if OKT3 treatment is not discontinued. This high incidence of graft loss in OKT3-treated recipients may account for at least some of the difference in survival between recipients with cellular rejection and those with the biopsy characteristics described earlier.

The incidence of biopsies with features that may be characterized as vascular rejection varies widely between transplantation centers. It is rare at many centers. In general, patients with these biopsy findings are not treated unless there is concomitant allograft dysfunction, in which case therapeutic options, including corticosteroids, antithymocyte globulin, cyclophosphamide, heparin, and plasmapheresis, have produced variable results.

Depressed myocardial contractile function, which occurs in the absence of cellular infiltrates, may be related to the regulation of endogenous nitric oxide (NO) signaling pathways within the myocardium[129] or to the release of cytokines such as tumor necrosis factor-α (TNF-α).[130] Similarly decreased myocardial contractility in the absence of myocardial inflammatory infiltrates or necrosis has been observed in patients with advanced infection or severe trauma or burns. Cardiac myocytes express consti-

tutive NO synthase (cNOS) and inducible NO synthase (iNOS). Activation of cNOS modulates cardiac myocyte responsiveness to muscarinic cholinergic and β-adrenergic receptor stimulation. Induction of iNOS by soluble inflammatory mediators, including cytokines, depresses myocyte contractile responsiveness to β-adrenergic agonists. Inappropriate activation of cNOS or excessive induction of iNOS in the myocardium may, therefore, contribute to cardiac dysfunction. Clinical and experimental studies[130] strongly support the hypothesis that TNF-α is a mediator of left ventricular systolic and diastolic dysfunction, possibly through secondary mediators or a change in myocardial gene expression.

Endocardial Inflammatory Infiltrates (Quilty Effect)

Endocardial inflammatory infiltrates present on posttransplant endomyocardial biopsies are termed the Quilty effect, or Quilty lesions, after the first patient in whom they were observed. They were first described after the addition of cyclosporine to immunosuppressive regimens. The typical Quilty lesion is a focal flat to nodular densely cellular endocardial nodule (Fig. 23-17A) that may be confined to the endocardium (Quilty A) (Fig. 23-17B) or extend into the underlying myocardium, where associated myocyte damage may be present (Quilty B)[100] (Fig. 23-17C). However, histologic typing of Quilty A or Quilty B lesions does not appear to have any clinical significance.[131] The infiltrates consist predominantly of T lymphocytes with scattered or clustered B lymphocytes and occasional macrophages, plasma cells, and small blood vessels[34, 63, 71, 132, 133] (Fig. 23-17D, E).

Quilty lesions have been reported in approximately 10 to 20% of post-transplant endomyocardial biopsies.[134, 135] They may first appear at any time during the post-transplant course and tend to recur in any given patient. Similar lesions involving the epicardium have been described in autopsy studies of cardiac allografts.[136]

The etiology of Quilty lesions is unknown. Because these lesions were first observed in association with cyclosporine therapy, a relationship was postulated. In a study comparing four immunosuppressive protocols, Quilty lesions were found more commonly in any of three cyclosporine-based protocols compared with azathioprine-corticosteroid immunosuppression.[137] However, other studies demonstrated no relationship between cyclosporine dosage or increased whole blood cyclosporine levels and the presence of Quilty lesions.[138] An autopsy study that examined the hearts of patients who had received cyclosporine but who had not received cardiac allografts failed to reveal any Quilty lesions.[139]

The relationship of the Quilty lesion to acute rejection, if any, remains unknown. Traditionally, this lesion has been considered distinct from rejection, requiring no treatment with intensified immunosuppression. Separate lesions that clearly represent rejection may coexist in the same biopsy. Differentiation of Quilty lesions from acute rejection is not usually a problem when the former are confined to the endocardium. However, when they extend into the underlying myocardium, a tangential cut through

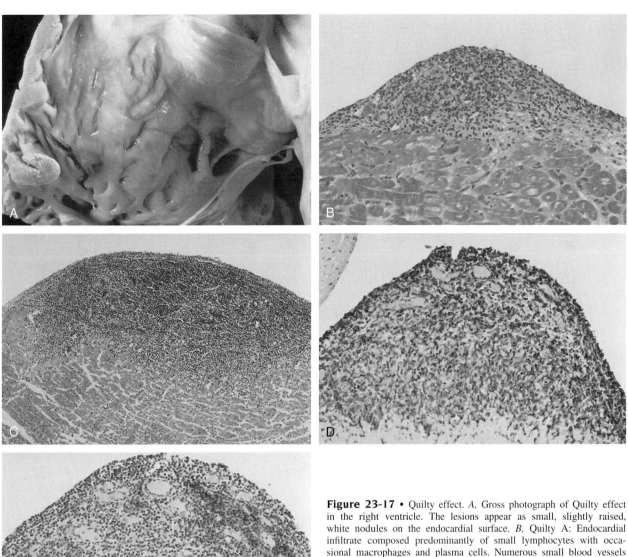

Figure 23-17 • Quilty effect. *A,* Gross photograph of Quilty effect in the right ventricle. The lesions appear as small, slightly raised, white nodules on the endocardial surface. *B,* Quilty A: Endocardial infiltrate composed predominantly of small lymphocytes with occasional macrophages and plasma cells. Numerous small blood vessels are a prominent feature. (*A* and *B*, H&E stain.) *C,* Quilty B: Endocardial infiltrate that extends into the underlying myocardium, where it may be associated with focal myocyte damage (H&E stain). *D,* Immunoperoxidase staining (CD3) reveals a predominance of T lymphocytes. *E,* B lymphocytes are present as scattered individual cells or cluster of cells (immunoperoxidase staining for L26). (From Winters GL: Heart transplantation: Explant, biopsy, and autopsy characteristics. In: McManus BM, Braunwald E [eds]: Atlas of Cardiovascular Pathology. Philadelphia, Current Medicine, 2000.)

the biopsy may not show a connection between the myocardial lesion and the endocardial one, making differentiation from rejection difficult. Cutting additional deeper sections may resolve this dilemma in some cases by demonstrating extension to the endocardium. In the absence of an endocardial extension, the density of the infiltrate, the presence of B cells, and prominent vascularity favor a diagnosis of a Quilty lesion. A study highlighted the difficulty of distinguishing a single focus of rejection from Quilty lesions with no endocardial continuity by demonstrating via step sectioning and immunohistochemical staining that many biopsies originally diagnosed as ISHLT grade 2 rejection were actually Quilty B lesions.[114] Other investigators have suggested that Quilty lesions may be a manifestation of rejection based on the

frequency of association with rejection in the same biopsy or may signal impending rejection in subsequent biopsies.[140, 141] The possibility remains that Quilty lesions are part of the "chronic" rejection process or represent a nonspecific immune response.

An early concern after discovery of Quilty lesions was whether they represented a form of post-transplant lymphoproliferative disorder (PTLD) or were precursors of lymphoma. However, the majority of PTLD have a B-cell phenotype and may be polyclonal, multiclonal, or monoclonal. Quilty lesions consist predominantly of T cells with foci of polyclonal B cells and lack cellular atypia and mitoses. Although an early association between Quilty lesions and Epstein-Barr virus genome was reported[142] using in situ DNA hybridization studies, subse-

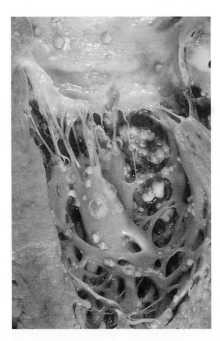

Figure 23-18 • Fatal fungal infection involving an allograft. Gross photograph shows many yellow nodules of *Aspergillus* throughout the left atrium and ventricle from a heart transplant recipient who died of disseminated *Aspergillus* infection. (From Winters GL: Heart transplantation: Explant, biopsy, and autopsy characteristics. In: McManus BM, Braunwald E [eds]: Atlas of Cardiovascular Pathology. Philadelphia, Current Science, 2000.)

quent investigation failed to show a relationship to Epstein-Barr virus or progression to widespread PTLD or monoclonal lymphoma.[143] The characteristics of Quilty lesions compared with those of acute rejection and PTLD are summarized in Table 23-2.

Infection

Like other immunosuppressed individuals, cardiac transplant recipients have an increased risk of infection.

The full spectrum of bacterial, fungal, viral, and protozoal infections either may occur systemically or may involve the heart allograft.[144, 145] In an analysis of 814 patients by the Cardiac Transplant Research Database, CMV was the most commonly reported infection, accounting for 66% of viral and 26% of all infections.[146] Fungal infections, however, were associated with the highest mortality (36%) (Fig. 23-18). The same study found that the most common site of infection was in the lung (28% of all infections), followed by the blood (26%) and the gastrointestinal (17%) or urinary tracts (12%).

During the first month after transplantation, bacterial infections, especially those caused by staphylococcal species, are the most common. Beginning in the second month, opportunistic infections become more common, including those induced by CMV, *Pneumocystis,* and fungal organisms.[51, 146] In recent years, ganciclovir prophylaxis after heart transplantation has reduced both the incidence of CMV disease in CMV-mismatched patients and its morbidity in CMV-positive recipients.

The organisms most commonly diagnosed on endomyocardial biopsy specimens are CVM (Fig. 23-19A) and *Toxoplasma gondii*[34, 63, 147] (Fig. 23-19B). These infections may be either primary or reactivated. The accompanying cellular infiltrate is highly variable, and both CMV and *Toxoplasma* may incite little or no inflammatory reaction. In addition, intensified immunosuppressive therapy used for rejection attenuates the host's response. On histologic examination at low power, an inflammatory infiltrate that accompanies an infection, especially one caused by viral or protozoal organisms, may be reminiscent of acute rejection. A careful search for organisms is, therefore, warranted whenever an unusual infiltrate is encountered or infection is suspected.

CMV infection of the myocardium may produce subtle histologic changes that can be easily missed. In suspected cases, immunohistochemistry to detect viral antigens and in situ hybridization or polymerase chain reaction to detect DNA may be useful adjuncts to histopathology. A

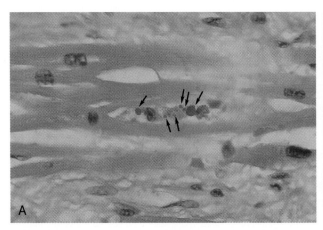
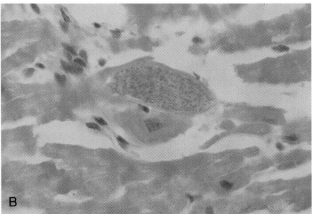

Figure 23-19 • Opportunistic infections detected in heart transplants by endomyocardial biopsy. *A,* Cytomegalovirus (CMV): Multiple inclusions (arrows) are present within a myocyte. There is no associated inflammatory response. *B, Toxoplasma* organisms are present within a myocyte. In some cases (not shown here), there is an associated inflammatory infiltrate that must be differentiated from acute rejection. (H&E stain.) (From Winters GL: Heart transplantation: Explant, biopsy, and autopsy characteristics. In: McManus BM, Braunwald E [eds]: Atlas of Cardiovascular Pathology. Philadelphia, Current Science, 2000.)

Giemsa stain may help to highlight the tachyzoites in *Toxoplasma* cysts.[81]

Infection in patients surviving at least 1 year after heart transplantation is less common than that reported in the early post-transplant period.[148] Community-acquired organisms are responsible for the majority of infections, although the risk for developing opportunistic infections remains. Often a precipitating event requiring augmentation of immunosuppression therapy (i.e., rejection) precedes an infection in this late post-transplant period.[148, 149]

Infection as a cause of death in heart allograft recipients has diminished in frequency since 1990 because of improved diagnostic techniques and therapeutic regimens as well as a more selective use of immunosuppressive agents. Although major infection occurs in less than one third of patients during the first 18 months, it remains a leading cause of post-transplant morbidity and mortality.[146] Because signs and symptoms of infection may be masked before death by immunosuppression, a careful search for infection should be undertaken at autopsy where the heart allograft and other organs may be involved.

Malignancy

Organ transplant recipients who receive long-term immunosuppressive therapy have approximately 100 times greater risk of developing malignant neoplasms relative to an equivalent general population.[150, 151] The overall incidence of cancer in heart transplant recipients is approximately 6%, with an estimated risk of 1 to 2% per year. The predominant tumors are lymphomas (42%) and skin and lip carcinomas, mostly squamous cell carcinomas (28%). Cancers that occur commonly in the nontransplant population (lung, breast, prostate, colon) are not significantly increased in heart transplant recipients.

Marked differences in the incidence of various malignancies have been reported when heart transplant recipients are compared with those having renal allografts.

Heart transplant recipients have a significantly higher incidence of lymphomas compared with kidney recipients (42% vs. 11% of all malignancies). Kidney recipients have a higher incidence of skin cancers and carcinomas of the cervix, vulva, and perineum. Possible explanations for these differences include (1) a higher level of immunosuppression in heart transplantation and the inability to withdraw the therapy; (2) increasing numbers of new immunosuppressive drugs and combinations of these drugs that have emerged during the era of heart transplantation; and (3) longer follow-up of kidney transplant recipients, allowing increased time to develop malignancies that usually appear late after transplantation.[151]

Post-Transplant Lymphoproliferative Disorders

PTLDs are particularly aggressive and not uncommon diseases that occur in approximately 2% of heart transplant recipients.[152] Some reports suggest that the use of specific immunosuppressive agents, such as cyclosporine[153, 154] or OKT3,[155] is associated with a higher incidence and/or earlier onset of PTLDs than when other immunosuppressive agents are employed. However, it is likely that the intensity of immunosuppression is more important than the specific drugs used. A delicate balance exists between providing sufficient immunosuppression to prevent allograft rejection and attempting to limit potentially lethal side effects of immunosuppression such as PTLDs.[152, 156, 157]

PTLDs may (1) develop as localized masses or appear as widely disseminated disease; (2) involve lymph nodes or extranodal sites; and (3) occur early or late in the post-transplant period.[158, 159] Common extranodal sites include the gastrointestinal tract, central nervous system, lungs, and soft tissues. PTLDs involving the allograft (Fig. 23-20*A, B*) may mimic the clinical presentation of acute rejection, in which case endomyocardial biopsy may help differentiate the two processes.[160] However, the distinc-

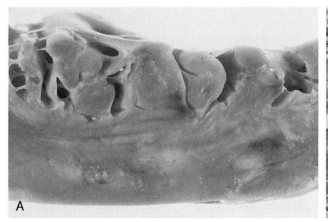
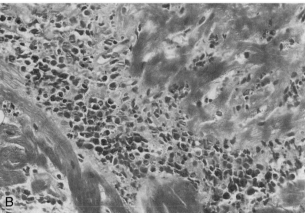

Figure 23-20 • Post-transplantation lymphoproliferative disorder (PTLD). *A,* Transverse section of the left ventricle from a heart transplant recipient who died of PTLD. The white areas within the myocardium represent tumor infiltration. *B,* A diffuse cellular infiltrate composed of large atypical lymphocytes, some with plasmacytoid features, is present within the myocardium. (H&E stain.) Immunoperoxidase staining revealed a predominance of B-cells that were positive for Epstein-Barr virus (EBV). (From Winters GL: Heart transplantation: Explant, biopsy, and autopsy characteristics. In: McManus BM, Braunwald E [eds]; Atlas of Cardiovascular Pathology. Philadelphia, Current Science, 2000.)

tion between PTLD and the reactive lymphocytes of acute rejection can prove extremely difficult, and adjuvant studies, such as immunophenotyping and immunogenetic examination, may be needed for clarification.

Most PTLDs are disorders of B-cell origin, ranging from benign polyclonal B-cell hyperplasias to monoclonal malignant lymphomas with clonal chromosomal abnormalities. Transition from polyclonal to monoclonal B-cell proliferations may occur over a short period in association with the appearance of cytogenetic abnormalities.[161–163] Different clonal immunoglobulin gene rearrangements in lesions obtained from different sites in the same patient indicate multiclonal or oligoclonal B-cell proliferation.[164]

Epstein-Barr virus (EBV), the causative agent for infectious mononucleosis, has been associated with PTLDs.[159, 162, 163] EBV is a herpesvirus that selectively infects EBV-receptor-positive B lymphocytes, resulting in polyclonal activation. The most important factor in controlling EBV-induced B-cell proliferations is the ability to generate EBV-specific cytotoxic T lymphocytes. However, immunosuppressive drugs used to prevent allograft rejection suppress T cell responses, thereby predisposing the transplant recipient to herpesvirus infections, as well as an uncontrolled proliferation of EBV-transformed B lymphocytes.

The mortality of PTLDs exceeds 80%.[162] A high level of suspicion for their development must be maintained, especially in the presence of a viral syndrome, lymphadenopathy, or organ dysfunction. Prompt tissue diagnosis with appropriate studies for clonal analysis, karyotype, and viral analysis are required in planning appropriate therapy. Acyclovir, an antiviral agent that interrupts EBV replication and thus inhibits the continued B-cell proliferation may be effective in some patients during the polyclonal growth phase, but is ineffective once the tumor evolves into a monoclonal lymphoma. Reduction in immunosuppression has resulted in regression of tumors in some patients.[165] Although reduction or cessation of immunosuppression may be possible in renal transplant recipients, acyclovir therapy and only a modest reduction of immunosuppression may be more appropriate in heart transplant recipients in whom allograft rejection can be fatal. Conventional radiation with or without chemotherapy is often used to treat generalized disease.

Allograft Coronary Disease and Late Ischemic Injury

Allograft coronary disease, a diffuse proliferative process that causes obstruction of the coronary vasculature with secondary myocardial ischemic injury, severely limits long-term recipient survival and is the major indication for retransplantation.[1, 166, 167] A number of synonyms are commonly used for this disease, including allograft arteriopathy, accelerated arteriosclerosis, chronic rejection, and transplantation-associated arteriosclerosis. Similar but less extensive changes have been observed in coronary veins; thus, the term graft vasculopathy is also employed. The development of allograft coronary disease has no defini-

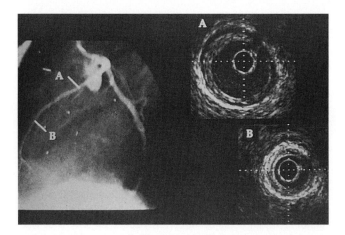

Figure 23-21 • Comparison of coronary angiography (left) and intracoronary ultrasonography (right) from corresponding locations in a transplant recipient with allograft coronary disease. Although no discrete lesions are present angiographically, intracoronary ultrasonography demonstrates intimal thickening at both locations studied (*A* and *B*). (Courtesy of Dr. James Fang, Brigham and Women's Hospital, Boston)

tive relationships with the many usual risk factors for coronary artery disease, commonly affects pediatric recipients, and is unrelated to the etiology of heart failure in the recipient's native heart that prompted transplantation. The incidence of this complication increases progressively after heart transplantation but may become significant at any time during the post-transplant course and progress at variable rates. Clinically significant lesions requiring retransplantation as early as 3 months after the initial transplant have been reported. By 5 years after transplantation, at least 40 to 50% of recipients have angiographically evident disease.[168]

The diffuse nature of allograft coronary disease makes it difficult to detect angiographically, particularly in its early phases when intimal thickening results in expansion of the vessel wall with minimal luminal narrowing. The severity of the disease, therefore, may be significantly underestimated clinically. The development of intracoronary ultrasonography (ICUS) has allowed more sensitive detection of allograft coronary disease. By providing a cross-sectional image, quantitation of intimal thickness, cross-sectional stenosis, and other parameters can be evaluated[169] (Fig. 23-21).

Morphology

Allograft coronary disease has been well described in the coronary arteries of heart allografts and has distinct morphologic features when compared with native artery atherosclerosis[168, 170–174] (Table 23-5). The lesions consist of concentric intimal thickening that diffusely involves the coronary arteries proximally and distally, as well as small intramyocardial branches[175] (Fig. 23-22A, B). The proliferative lesions consist largely of modified smooth muscle cells (Fig. 23-22C) that have most likely migrated from the media, macrophages that contain intracellular and extracellular lipids, collagen, and glycosaminoglycans.[176–182] Whereas necrosis, calcification, and choles-

TABLE 23-5 • **Characteristics of Allograft Coronary Disease vs. Native Vessel Atherosclerosis**

Characteristic	Graft Coronary Disease	Native Vessel Atherosclerosis
Onset	Rapid (mo—yr)	Slow (yr)
Distribution	Diffuse	Focal
Lesions	Concentric	Eccentric
Calcification	Rare	Common
Cellular infiltrates	Common	Variable
Internal elastic lamina	Preserved	Destroyed
Secondary branches and intramural vessels	Affected	Spared

terol clefts are not prominent in typical early proliferative lesions, cholesterol clefts in a band-like distribution and lesions resembling typical atheromatous plaques may arise in the advanced form of the disease, particularly after a long post-transplant interval. The endothelium and internal elastic lamina are nearly completely intact and the media is usually of normal thickness or thinned. Cellular infiltrates, including T-lymphocytes (both CD4+ and CD8+) and macrophages (Fig. 23-22D, E), are frequently present as superficial bands in the subendothelium and deeper within the intima and media.

The importance of allograft coronary disease arises from the consequent distal ischemia it causes, which leads to arrhythmias and myocardial injury. The associated

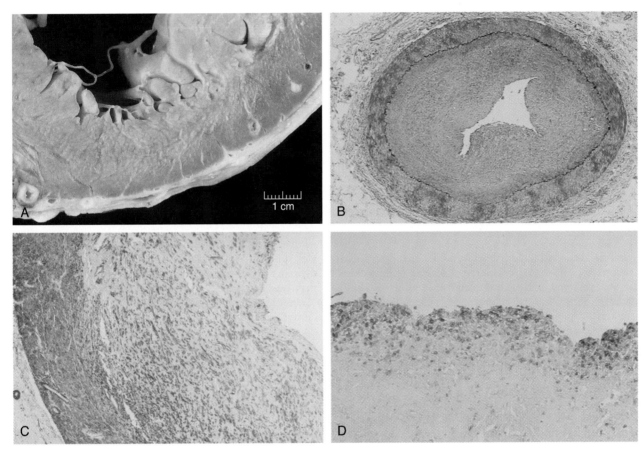

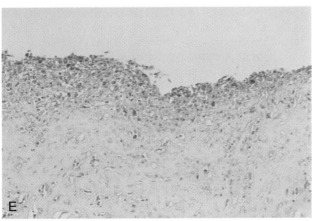

Figure 23-22 • Allograft coronary disease. *A,* Transverse section of the left ventricle from a patient who died of graft coronary disease. There is severe concentric stenosis of epicardial and intramyocardial coronary arteries. *B,* Movat-stained cross-section of an epicardial coronary artery demonstrates concentric intimal proliferation resulting in nearly complete luminal occlusion. The internal elastic lamina is intact. *C,* The intimal lesion consists largely of modified smooth muscle cells that have migrated from the media (immunoperoxidase stained with smooth muscle actin). *D,* The inflammatory component in the thickened intima contains a predominance of T lymphocytes (immunoperoxidase stained with CD3). *E,* Also present are scattered macrophages (immunoperoxidase stained with CD68). (*A,* From Schoen FJ, Libby P: Cardiac transplant graft arteriosclerosis. Trends Cardiovasc Med 1:216, 1991, with permission from Elsevier Science. *B–E,* From Salomon RN, Hughes CCW, Schoen FJ, et al: Human coronary transplantation-associated arteriosclerosis: Evidence for a chronic immune reaction to activated graft endothelial cells. Am J Pathol 138:791, 1991.)

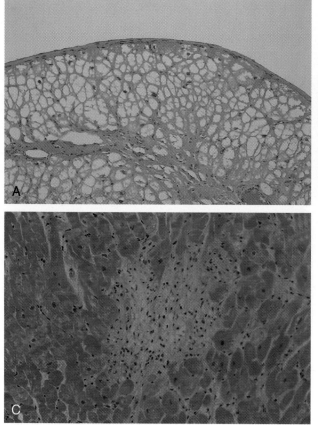

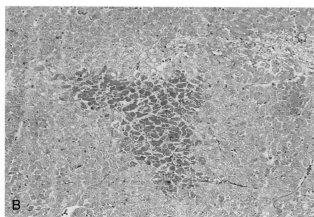

Figure 23-23 • Myocardial lesions in allograft coronary disease. *A,* Subendocardial myocyte vacuolization deep to a thin endocardium and indicating sublethal ischemic injury of viable myocytes. *B,* Microinfarct characterized by small discrete focus of coagulation necrosis suggesting small-vessel obstruction. The lack of inflammatory response suggests depressed healing, possibly resulting from immunosuppressive therapy. *C,* Healing microinfarct consisting of granulation tissue seen in a subendocardial location on endomyocardial biopsy. (H&E stain.)

myocardial lesions include subendocardial myocyte vacuolization (Fig. 23-23*A*), indicating sublethal ischemic injury and regional coagulation necrosis and its healing, indicative of myocardial infarct.[183–186] The microinfarcts characteristic of allograft coronary disease suggest small-vessel involvement (Fig. 23-23*B, C*). Subendocardial and transmural infarcts resemble those that occur secondary to native vessel atherosclerosis; however, healing is frequently delayed because of the immunosuppressive therapy that recipients receive.

Assessing arterial changes of allograft coronary disease in endomyocardial biopsy material is usually precluded by the lack of vessels large enough to permit such an evaluation. However, the ability to detect secondary myocardial changes in endomyocardial biopsy material and the significance of such changes are only beginning to develop. In an autopsy study of failed allografts with graft arteriosclerosis, ischemic myocardial changes were documented in the right as well as the left ventricle; therefore, the assessment of these changes on biopsy is feasible.[183] A review of our experience indicated that late ischemic pathology detected by endomyocardial biopsy has a positive predictive value of 92% in finding significant graft arteriosclerosis at autopsy.[187] However, the absence of ischemic myocardial pathology on endomyocardial biopsy does not indicate an absence of allograft coronary disease.

The difficulty of establishing the clinical diagnosis of graft arteriosclerosis, particularly in its early stages, is well known. A denervated allograft does not allow the recipient to experience angina, and myocardial damage may be far advanced before it becomes clinically evident. Therefore, ischemic myocardial pathology revealed by endomyocardial biopsies may provide clinicians with the opportunity to consider earlier and/or additional assessment of graft arteriosclerosis and possible therapeutic interventions, including timely listing for retransplantation when appropriate.

Pathogenesis

The pathogenetic mechanisms involved in the initiation and progression of allograft coronary disease remain unknown[167, 170, 188, 189] (Fig. 23-24). The limited involvement of the allograft vasculature with sparing of the recipient's native vessels suggests processes that specifically target the allograft and produce endothelial injury and/or derangement in regulation of smooth muscle cell growth. Immunohistochemical studies of allograft coronary disease demonstrate endothelial expression of class I and class II MHC antigens as well as adhesion molecules such as vascular cell adhesion molecule (VCAM-1), intercellular adhesion molecule (ICAM-1), and ELAM (E-selectin), which make the vascular endothelium susceptible to attack by the immune system via a cellular or humoral mechanism.[190–194] The T lymphocytes present in allograft coronary disease express class II MHC antigens such as HLA-DR and are associated with HLA-DR+ macro-

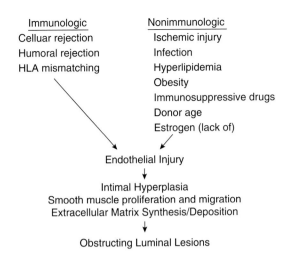

Immunologic
Cellular rejection
Humoral rejection
HLA mismatching

Nonimmunologic
Ischemic injury
Infection
Hyperlipidemia
Obesity
Immunosuppressive drugs
Donor age
Estrogen (lack of)

Endothelial Injury
↓
Intimal Hyperplasia
Smooth muscle proliferation and migration
Extracellular Matrix Synthesis/Deposition
↓
Obstructing Luminal Lesions

Figure 23-24 • Risk factors for the development of allograft coronary disease. (From Winters GL: Heart transplantation: Explant, biopsy and autopsy characteristics. In: McManus BM, Braunwald E [eds]: Atlas of Cardiovascular Pathology. Philadelphia, Current Medicine, 2000.)

phages deep to HLA-DR+ endothelium, leading some authors to suggest that ongoing stimulation of recipient T lymphocytes by HLA-DR+ endothelium of donor coronary arteries contributes to a sustained regional immune response (i.e., a chronic delayed-type hypersensitivity reaction).[170, 177] Although the precise regulatory influences are as yet not completely understood, the progression of lesions most likely depends on a complex interaction among (1) release of cytokines; (2) smooth muscle cell migration to, and proliferation in, the intima; and (3) extracellular matrix synthesis and remodeling.[195–197] Clinicopathologic studies in which acute rejection episodes diagnosed by endomyocardial biopsy were correlated with the development of allograft coronary disease have produced mixed results.[121, 198–200] However, those which showed a correlation between the presence, but not the severity, of acute rejection and allograft coronary disease implied an underlying immune mechanism. Antibody-mediated injury may also have an important role in pathogenesis.[201] Donor-specific circulating antibodies against a family of endothelial cell antigens are a marker of the disease and may be important in its etiology.[202]

Nonimmunologic risk factors including recipient characteristics (age, sex, pretransplant diagnosis, hypertension, cardiac function, obesity, hyperlipidemia, diabetes mellitus, smoking), donor characteristics (age and sex), perioperative ischemic injury, immunosuppressive therapy, and CMV infection have all been implicated as having a causal or contributing role in the development of allograft coronary disease.[203, 204] Of these, ischemic injury[77, 205] and hyperlipidemia[121, 179, 206] are most often implicated. Ischemic damage to the graft during the peritransplant period could injure endothelial cells and thus promote allograft coronary disease by upregulating class I and II antigen expression, activating complement, promoting rejection, increasing susceptibility to infection, and directly damaging the endothelium. Most reports showed that hypercholesterolemia, hypertriglyceridemia, and increased low-den-

sity lipoproteins develop 1 to 2 years after heart transplantation.[207, 208] The pathophysiology of post-transplant hyperlipidemia is complex, and obesity and also steroid and cyclosporine therapy are contributing factors. Most likely, the etiology of graft coronary disease is multifactorial, involving immunologic mechanisms in the setting of nonimmunologic risk factors. Defining the pathogenic mechanism(s) responsible for allograft coronary disease is key to developing effective preventive and treatment strategies, thus reducing both its incidence and progression and routinely allowing a longer survival after heart transplantation.

Animal models of allograft coronary disease are used to study risk factors, pathogenesis, and therapeutic intervention. Models of heterotopic transplantation in rats, rabbits, and dogs require treatment with immunosuppressive drugs to prevent acute rejection. Because the role of immunosuppressive drugs in the pathogenesis of allograft coronary disease remains unknown, animal models that require no immunosuppression hold a distinct advantage. Mouse models using strains that share major MHC antigens but that differ in minor antigens require no immunosuppression.[209, 210] The ability to develop gene-disrupted or "knockout" animal models will allow the study of specific cytokines and adhesion molecules, with or without co-stimulatory molecules, leukocyte subsets, and growth factors. Such models will further the understanding of the molecular pathogenesis of allograft coronary disease.

Other Long-Term Considerations

Myocyte Hypertrophy and Interstitial Fibrosis

Myocyte hypertrophy and interstitial fibrosis are common findings in cardiac allografts and are not necessarily related to the cause of allograft failure.[211, 212] Myocyte hypertrophy is likely a compensatory change in response to reparative or reactive fibrosis and/or systemic hypertension. It is consistently present in allografts more than 1 year after transplantation regardless of ischemic time or use of immunosuppressive therapy. Interstitial and/or replacement fibrosis has been related to both the number of rejection episodes and ischemic time. Although a relationship has been described between increasing amounts of myocardial fibrosis on serial surveillance endomyocardial biopsies and deteriorating cardiac function, fibrosis found in biopsy samples overestimates the degree of deeper fibrosis present in the autopsy hearts from corresponding patients.[213] Fine perimyocyte fibrosis was described in association with cyclosporine therapy; however, this finding has essentially disappeared with reduction of therapeutic cyclosporine levels.

Denervation/Reinnervation

Cardiac transplantation results in immediate afferent and efferent denervation. Interruption of afferent innervation eliminates the ability of the recipient to perceive chest pain during periods of ischemia. The absence of efferent innervation, including vagally mediated parasym-

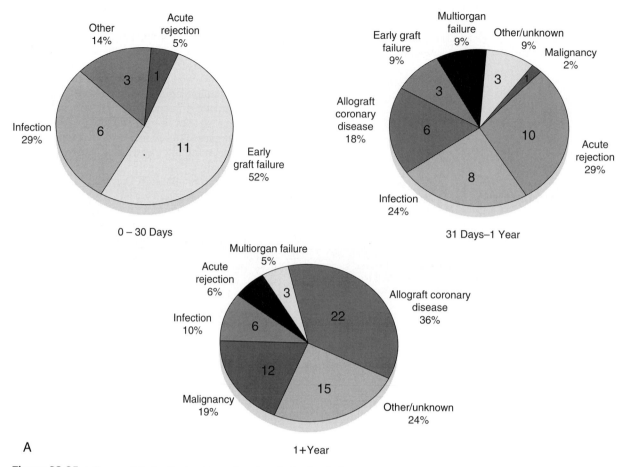

Figure 23-25 • Causes of death after heart transplantation. *A,* One hundred seventeen deaths occurred at Brigham and Women's Hospital, over a 15-year period, divided according to time interval from transplantation and primary etiology.

pathetic influences, causes a higher resting heart rate and loss of vagal signaling from the central nervous system. The absence of autonomic innervation blunts rapid changes in heart rate and contractility in response to exercise.[214]

There is evidence that reinnervation occurs in some patients after transplantation.[215] Nerves can be seen in the transplanted heart but are reduced from the normal number.[216] Angina pectoris has been reported in some heart transplant recipients and suggests that at least partial afferent innervation is present. Tyramine-mediated release of norepinephrine in some recipients implies that limited sympathetic reinnervation may occur.[217] The pattern of reinnervation, however, is extremely variable and its clinical significance is undetermined.[218-220]

Systemic Pathology Secondary to Immunosuppressive Therapy

Systemic pathology secondary to immunosuppressive therapy may be specific to a given drug or result from the cumulative effects of multidrug therapy.[49, 221] Major complications of cyclosporine administration are hypertension and nephrotoxicity.[222] Other adverse effects of this drug include hirsutism, hepatotoxicity, gingival hypertrophy,

and neurotoxicity (especially tremors). Cyclosporine may also affect bile metabolism, leading to cholestasis and gallstone formation. Osteoporosis, a complication of corticosteroid therapy, may result in vertebral compression fractures and avascular necrosis of weight-bearing joints. Corticosteroids also delay wound healing and may obscure major abdominal diseases because of the absence of leukocytosis and abdominal guarding. Hyperlipidemia and obesity are serious problems for recipients who receive triple immunosuppression therapy; these conditions may increase morbidity and mortality and have been implicated in the etiology of allograft coronary disease.

Causes of Death

The predominant causes of death in heart transplant recipients vary with the time interval after transplantation. In the 15 years of heart transplantation at Brigham and Women's Hospital, 117 deaths occurred in over 300 recipients (Fig. 23-25A). Early after transplantation (0 to 30 days), nonspecific graft failure was the most common cause of death, accounting for approximately half of them. In the intermediate period (31 days to 1 year), acute rejection and infection were equally represented.

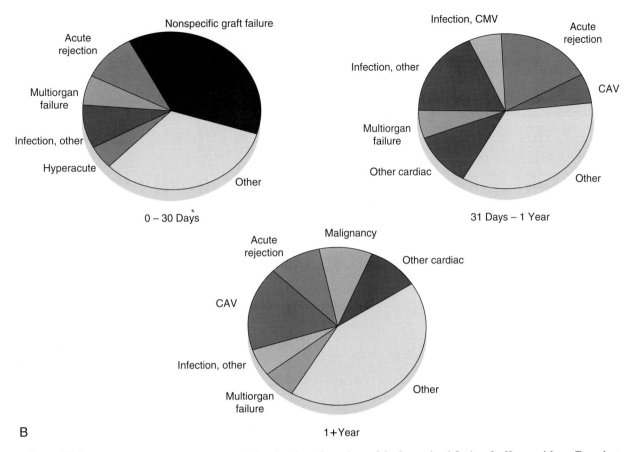

Figure 23-25 • *Continued. B,* For comparison, similar data from the registry of the International Society for Heart and Lung Transplantation, which collects data from nearly 300 heart transplant centers worldwide. (From Hosenpud JD, Bennett LE, Keck BM, et al: The Registry for the International Society for Heart and Lung Transplantation: Fifteenth official report—1998. J: Heart Lung Transplant 17:656, 1998.) CAV = cardiac allograft vasculopathy.

Late after transplantation (more than 1 year), allograft coronary disease and malignancy were the most common causes of death. Our data are similar to those compiled by the ISHLT Registry[1] (Fig. 23-25B). Risk factors that have a statistically significant impact on 1-year mortality include previous transplantation, ventilator dependence before transplantation, long cold ischemic time, and advanced donor and recipient ages.

One large heart transplantation center reviewed the causes of death in their recipients during two eras: an earlier one (1981 to 1986) when recipients were treated predominantly with prednisone/azathioprine or prednisone/cyclosporine immunosuppression; and a later era (1987 to 1994) when recipients received triple-drug immunosuppression.[223] During the first post-transplantation year, recipients in the earlier era were three times as likely to die of acute rejection, reflecting subsequent improvement in diagnosis and treatment. Patients who survived 3 or more years had a similar likelihood of death caused by allograft coronary disease in both eras. In the later era, the risk of dying of malignancy, infection, or other miscellaneous causes was as likely after 3 years as dying of allograft coronary disease. Thus, the long-term consequences of immunosuppression (malignancy and in-

fection) and allograft coronary disease were the major threats to long-term survival.

PATHOLOGY OF THE HEART IN HEART-LUNG TRANSPLANTATION

Combined heart-lung transplantation is a potential therapy for patients with end-stage disease of both heart and lungs and is most frequently performed for primary pulmonary hypertension, congenital heart disease, and Eisenmenger complex. In contrast to heart transplantation, in which male recipients outnumber females, more women than men receive heart-lung transplants because of the higher incidence of conditions such as primary pulmonary hypertension among women.

Heart-lung recipients are typically maintained on higher levels of immunosuppressive therapy and have a much lower incidence of acute cardiac rejection than do heart transplant recipients.[224, 225] Because acute rejection is seen mainly in the transplanted lung, it has been suggested that cardiac biopsies may not be needed for routine surveillance and should be performed only when indicated clinically.[226] The reason for the relative lack of rejection in the heart of heart-lung recipients is not clear. One possibility is that bronchial-associated lymphoid tissue plays an essential role in stimulating the immune response.[227]

Although allograft coronary disease does develop in heart-lung recipients, its incidence is much lower than in heart transplant recipients.[225] An attractive theory is that the low incidence of allograft coronary disease is related to the low incidence of acute cardiac rejection; however, this is speculative because allograft coronary disease is most likely multifactorial. Heart-lung recipients do develop obliterative bronchiolitis in the lung allograft, and that may have immunologic mechanisms in common with allograft coronary disease.

Survival of heart-lung recipients parallels that of lung rather than heart transplant recipients. It is the pulmonary rather than the cardiac pathology that is responsible for most of the morbidity and mortality in these patients. (Lung transplantation is discussed in Chapter 7.)

PATHOLOGIC REVIEW OF AN ENDOMYOCARDIAL BIOPSY

Endomyocardial biopsy is widely used in the diagnosis and management of cardiac diseases, and because histologic findings of rejection frequently precede clinical signs and symptoms, it is particularly valuable for monitoring the status of heart allografts after transplantation. To assess homogeneous myocardial processes, such as cardiac transplant rejection, right ventricular biopsy is preferred because it is technically easier than performing biopsies on the left side of the heart. Recipients undergo regularly scheduled biopsies according to specific protocols set by each transplant center (Fig. 23-26). In general, biopsies are performed more frequently (i.e., weekly) during the early post-transplant period. The interval between biopsies becomes longer with increasing time after transplantation, reaching a frequency of two to four times annually after 1 year. The frequency of endomyocardial biopsies may be increased if there is a change in the clinical status of the recipient or if acute rejection is detected.

The overall complication rate of 3% or less[228–232] associated with an endomyocardial biopsy is not greatly different from that of biopsies of other organs. The most serious complication is right ventricular perforation, with

First post-transplant year	Weekly ×4
	Biweekly ×2
	Monthly ×6
	Every other month ×2
Second post-transplant year	Every 3 months ×2
	Every 6 months
≥Third post-transplant year	Every 6 months

Figure 23-26 • Surveillance endomyocardial biopsy protocol used at Brigham and Women's Hospital. (From Winters GL: Heart transplantation: Explant, biopsy, and autopsy characteristics. In: McManus BM, Braunwald E [eds]: Atlas of Cardiovascular Pathology. Philadelphia, Current Medicine, 2000.)

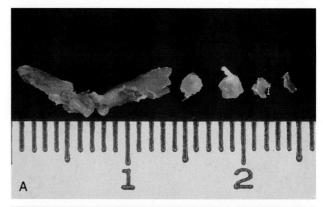

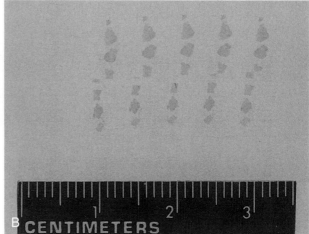

Figure 23-27 • Endomyocardial biopsy samples. *A,* Gross photograph of endomyocardial biopsy; samples are typically 2 to 4 mm. Larger samples (left fragment) are occasionally obtained. *B,* Glass slide showing histologic preparation with multiple levels present.

or without cardiac tamponade, which is reported with a frequency of 0.1 to 0.4%.[231] Arrhythmias, although common during the biopsy procedure, are usually of short duration and resolve spontaneously. Noncardiac complications are related to the method of obtaining vascular access and include pneumothorax, transient nerve injury, thrombosis and embolization, and vessel injury with local thrombus. Rarely, other organs are biopsied.

Specimen Adequacy

Acute rejection and other pathologic processes assessed by endomyocardial biopsy may be focal; therefore, multiple samples of the ventricular endomyocardium are obtained. Biopsy samples should not be divided after they are procured, because this practice results in less representative sampling. It is recommended that four to six samples (depending on the size of the bioptome used) be obtained to produce at least four (minimum three) samples that may be adequately evaluated histologically (Fig. 23-27A). The sensitivity of detecting rejection in right ventricular endomyocardial biopsies ranges from 75 to 98% if three to five samples are obtained.[233, 234] However, once six samples have been examined, obtaining additional tissue does not significantly increase diagnostic yield.[234]

An evaluable endomyocardial biopsy fragment consists of at least 50% myocardium, excluding a previous biopsy site, scar, adipose tissue, or blood clot. Biopsy specimens consisting of less than three pieces of evaluable myocardium should be considered "insufficient for diagnosis," particularly if their purpose is to rule out acute rejection. Although the histologic findings of biopsy tissue obtained are assumed to be representative of the entire allograft, a negative biopsy in the setting of a strong clinical suspicion of rejection must be interpreted cautiously. Additional diagnostic procedures, repeat biopsy, and/or empiric treatment for rejection are sometimes considered.

Specimen Processing

Routine diagnosis and grading of cardiac allograft rejection are performed on formalin-fixed tissue prepared for light microscopy examination. The tissue should be fixed in 10% neutral buffered formalin or other appropriate fixative. All biopsy pieces may be embedded in one paraffin block, which is sectioned at 4μ thickness. Three-step levels with at least three sections at each level should be prepared and stained with hematoxylin and eosin (Fig. 23-27B). A connective tissue stain, such as Masson trichrome, may be helpful in selected cases for assessing myocyte damage as well as myocardial fibrosis. No tissue needs to be routinely fixed for electron microscopy, immunoperoxidase staining, or immunohistochemistry. However, an additional piece of tissue may be frozen in a suitable freezing compound and liquid nitrogen in specific cases or as part of research protocols.

Use of Frozen Sections and Rapid Processing

Acute rejection may be suspected with the onset of new clinical symptoms or alternations in cardiac function, and immediate diagnosis may be obtained by performing a frozen section on endomyocardial biopsy specimens. A review of the Brigham experience with 98 frozen sections over a 9-year period revealed that the frozen sections reflected the pathologic process present on permanent sections in 90% of cases.[235] However, no specific clinical indication (including new onset of arrhythmias, congestive heart failure, echocardiographic abnormalities, hypotension, syncope, etc.) predicted rejection positivity with high sensitivity, either early or late after transplantation. Since the completion of this study, the number of frozen sections requested on endomyocardial biopsies at our institution has fallen dramatically with no apparent clinical consequences.

An alternative to frozen section for immediate biopsy diagnosis is rapid routine processing for paraffin embedding on a shortened processing cycle (i.e., 3 hours). Although rapid processing allows high quality and expeditious preparation of the entire biopsy sample, it requires the availability of specially assigned histology laboratory personnel and equipment.

Specimen Artifacts

The procurement and processing of biopsy samples may result in histologic artifacts, which should not be interpreted as pathologic changes.[236, 237] Biopsy samples must be handled carefully by the clinician who obtains them as well as by the pathologist who processes the tissue. Handling myocardial samples with forceps before fixation may result in *crush artifact,* which distorts tissue and precludes interpretation of any histologic findings in the affected area. A needle is sometimes used to tease the myocardial sample from the bioptome. However, the tissue should not be speared with the needle as it leaves a circular defect in the tissue. Handling and processing of the biopsy specimen may result in separation of the myocardial fibers, simulating *edema* (Figs. 23-28A). Although true edema (Fig. 23-28B) is a component of some pathologic states, such as severe acute rejection, caution should be used in diagnosing edema in the absence of other histologic findings. Similarly, *hemorrhage* may occur secondary to the trauma of the biopsy procedure. *Contraction bands* (Fig. 23-29) are frequently an artifact of the biopsy procedure itself and do not usually indicate myocardial ischemia or catecholamine injury.[238, 239] In contrast

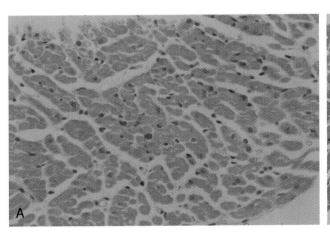
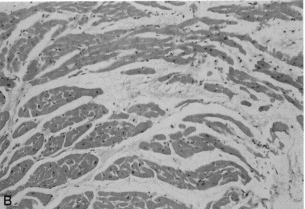

Figure 23-28 • Artifactual and true edema. *A,* Separation of individual myocytes or clusters of myocytes by empty spaces, representing biopsy artifact. *B,* Separation of myocytes with intervening eosinophilic proteinaceous material, representing true edema. (H&E stain.)

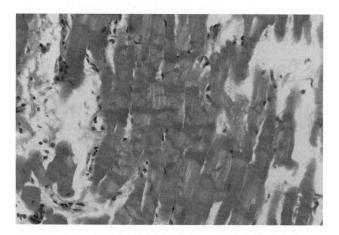

Figure 23-29 • Contraction bands. Contraction bands (dark bands spanning several myocytes) are most often artifactual in biopsy specimens and do not imply myocardial ischemia or necrosis (H&E stain).

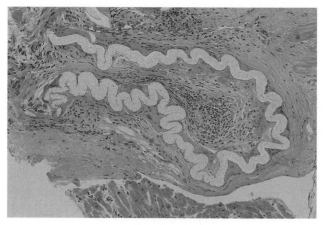

Figure 23-30 • Foreign body giant cell reaction. The foreign material is most likely cotton thread from gauze used to wipe the bioptome (H&E stain). (Courtesy of Dr. Richard N. Mitchell, Brigham and Women's Hospital, Boston.)

to necrosis with contraction bands, artifactual contraction bands often extend across many myocytes that are otherwise normal. (See Chapter 9 also.) Fixing specimens at room temperature, rather than in chilled fixative, reduces this artifact. *Foreign body giant cells containing refractile material*[240] (Fig. 23-30), presumably cotton fibers from gauze used to wipe the bioptome, are sometimes present in endomyocardial biopsies from patients who have undergone previous biopsy procedures.

Sampling artifact and obtaining tissue other than myocardium may pose difficulties in biopsy interpretation. Occasionally, biopsies may contain chordae tendineae, fragments of valvular tissue, or even extracardiac tissue, such as liver. Chordae tendineae that are torn or injured by the bioptome or sheath can sometimes be identified in endomyocardial biopsy specimens[241] (Fig. 23-31) and may result in flail tricuspid leaflet reported in as many as 12% of patients after heart transplantation.[242]

The most common and most problematic entity in this category is a previous *biopsy site* that may be in various stages of healing. The average transplant recipient undergoes as many as 20 biopsies during the first year after transplantation.[71] Because of the rigid structure of the bioptome and the constant configuration of right ventricular trabeculae, the bioptome tends to follow a similar path in any given patient. It is, therefore, not uncommon to rebiopsy a previous biopsy site, a finding observed in as many as 69% of specimens obtained for rejection surveillance.[243] The histology of a biopsy site reflects the degree of healing that has occurred. Immediately after a biopsy procedure, fresh thrombus may overlie areas of acute myocyte injury and hemorrhage (Fig. 23-32A). Although theoretically these thrombi could give rise to minute pulmonary emboli, no clinically significant embolic events have been reported. Progressive healing results in granulation tissue, often containing a leukocytic infiltrate (Fig. 23-32B). It is during this healing phase that a biopsy site may resemble the inflammatory changes present in acute rejection. However, the mixed nature of the healing inflammatory infiltrate and the myocyte disarray frequently

present at the periphery of the biopsy site may aid correct interpretation. In a fully healed biopsy site, granulation tissue is replaced by dense fibrous tissue.

Thrombus in varying stages of organization may be present as part of a pathologic condition that is artificially induced, or it may be the result of a previous biopsy procedure. Thrombus must be distinguished from myocardial tissue, especially necrotic myocardium, which it may sometimes resemble.

Biopsies obtained late in the post-transplant course frequently contain abundant dense *subendocardial fibrous tissue*. The fibrosis may result from organized mural thrombi, healed biopsy sites, or areas of healed rejection. Therefore, attempts to quantify the amount of fibrosis in the underlying myocardium based on biopsy samples result in overestimation.[213]

Intramyocardial *adipose tissue* may be present in many patients, particularly in the right ventricle, where it is within reach of the bioptome. The finding of adipose

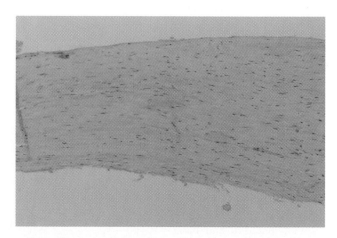

Figure 23-31 • Chorda tendinea in endomyocardial biopsy specimen. A thin chord of dense collagen was obtained from the tricuspid valve during a biopsy procedure (H&E stain).

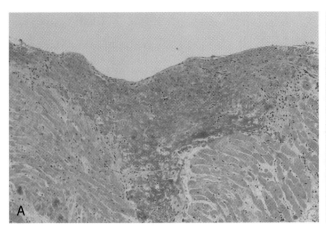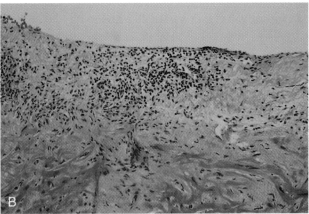

Figure 23-32 • Biopsy site. *A,* At a recent biopsy site, fresh microthrombus overlies the site of the previous biopsy. *B,* Healing biopsy site consisting of granulation tissue with hemosiderin-laden macrophages and a mixed inflammatory infiltrate. The cellular infiltrate at a healing biopsy site must be distinguished from acute rejection. Myocyte disarray is evident deep to the granulation tissue. (H&E stain.)

tissue on endomyocardial biopsy does not necessarily indicate myocardial perforation. Although tissue fragments consisting wholly of hemorrhagic adipose tissue may raise a suspicion of cardiac perforation, only the presence of mesothelial cells provides unequivocal evidence that biopsy-induced perforation has occurred.

Reporting of Endomyocardial Biopsy Results

Endomyocardial biopsy results should be communicated to the transplant clinician in a consistent manner and should contain the following information: (1) time interval from transplantation; (2) number of pieces of evaluable myocardium examined; (3) assessment of rejection, including ISHLT grade; and (4) other (nonrejection) biopsy findings. When more than one pathologist is responsible for reporting biopsy results, a standardized form may be used to provide consistency. This form is easily computerized, which saves transcription time and avoids typing errors. As an example, the form we use at Brigham and Women's Hospital appears in Appendix B. The use of a standardized form, however, should not constrain the pathologist from providing additional narrative interpretation of difficult cases or communicating directly with the clinician.

APPROACH TO THE EXAMINATION OF A FAILED ALLOGRAFT

A failed allograft may become available for examination at the time of retransplantation or at autopsy. We employ the same standardized form (Appendix A) used for explanted native hearts to report explanted failed allografts. The allograft examination should be systematic, yet individualized and based on available clinical information.[71, 244] The approach should include careful study of pericardium, great vessels, chambers, valves, endocardium, myocardium, and coronary arteries. In general, the

major epicardial coronary arteries—left main, left anterior descending, left circumflex, and right—should be sectioned transversely at intervals of 4 to 5 mm, and the overall and maximal luminal narrowing should be assessed. Calcified arteries should be removed from the heart, fixed, and decalcified before sectioning. We do not use postmortem angiography, which is technically difficult in allografts with severe coronary disease and provides little additional information over careful sectioning. The heart may then be sectioned transversely into slices of 1 to 1.5 cm ("bread-loafed") from apex to base, or a four-chamber long axis cut may be used. Transverse sectioning is generally preferable for demonstrating the location and extent of myocardial infarcts. A four-chamber cut is best performed after fixation for evaluation of rejection, chamber dimensions, anastomoses, and intracavitary pathology (fibrosis, thrombus, infection) while keeping the allograft relatively intact.

In long-term survivors, dense pericardial fibrosis may develop and produce constrictive or restrictive hemodynamics. The pulmonary artery should be examined for evidence of atherosclerosis, which may indicate that pulmonary hypertension is responsible for right-sided failure. Regardless of the interval after surgery, anastomoses of left and right atrium, the pulmonary artery, and the aorta should be carefully assessed to ensure that they are intact and without evidence of obstruction. The cardiac chambers should be examined for thrombi. Atria normally have a dilated appearance resulting from the combination of donor and recipient atria. The ventricular cavities are normally mildly to moderately dilated, even in the absence of clinical heart failure. Endocardial and interstitial fibrosis is common. Previous biopsy sites may be present in the right ventricular apical septum. Myocardial hypertrophy is present in virtually all long-term allograft survivors regardless of their clinical course or other pathologic findings.[211]

In addition to ascertaining pathology related specifically to the allograft, efforts should be made to distinguish disorders that originated in the donor, especially preexisting donor atherosclerosis, as well as previously undiagnosed valvular or myocardial disease.

FUTURE CONSIDERATIONS

Despite the success that cardiac transplantation has enjoyed since the mid-1980s many questions remain unanswered. Numerous techniques to assess rejection by noninvasive methods have been explored, but as yet, none has sufficient sensitivity and specificity to supplant the endomyocardial biopsy. Once a diagnosis of rejection is made, when and how to alter immunosuppression remains controversial. Also, the optimal immunosuppressive regimen for control of rejection without increasing side effects remains to be determined. New immunosuppressive drugs with more specific sites of action are under development. The possibility that they or new combinations of drugs will alter classic endomyocardial biopsy findings of rejection must be considered. The ultimate control of rejection would be the ability to induce allograft tolerance by genetic alterations. Understanding the pathogenesis and the developing therapies for allograft coronary disease could prolong the life of many heart transplant recipients. Because heart transplantation will always be limited by donor availability, therapeutic options for patients with end-stage heart failure continue to expand to include aggressive medical therapy, ventriculectomy, cardiomyoplasty, ventricular assist devices, and xenotransplantation. Cardiac transplantation, however, will remain a viable option for carefully selected patients with end-stage heart disease.

REFERENCES

1. Hosenpud JD, Bennett LE, Keck BM, et al: The registry of the International Society for Heart and Lung Transplantation: Fifteenth official report—1998. J Heart Lung Transplant 17:656, 1998
2. Mudge GM, Goldstein S, Addonizio LJ, et al: Twenty-fourth Bethesda conference: Cardiac transplantation: Task force 3: Recipient guidelines/prioritization. J Am Coll Cardiol 22:21, 1993
3. Costanzo MR, Augustine S, Bourge R, et al: Selection and treatment of candidates for heart transplantation: A statement for health professionals from the Committee on Heart Failure and Cardiac Transplantation of the Council on Clinical Cardiology, American Heart Association. Circulation 92:3593, 1995
4. Stevenson LW: Selection and management of candidates for heart transplantation. Curr Opin Cardiol 11:166, 1996
5. Olivari MT, Antolick A, Kaye MP, et al: Heart transplantation in elderly patients. J Heart Transplant 7:258, 1988
6. Blanche C, Takkenberg JJ, Nessim S, et al: Heart transplantation in patients 65 years of age and older: A comparative analysis of 40 patients. Ann Thorac Surg 62:1442, 1996
7. Blanche C, Matloff JM, Denton TA, et al: Heart transplantation in patients 70 years of age and older: Initial experience. Ann Thorac Surg 62:1731, 1996
8. Bourge RC, Naftel DC, Costanzo-Nordin MR, et al: Pretransplantation risk factors for death after heart transplantation: A multiinstitutional study. J Heart Lung Transplant 12:549, 1993
9. Kirsch M, Baufreton C, Naftel DC, et al: Pretransplantation risk factors for death after heart transplantation: The Henri Mondor experience. J Heart Lung Transplant 17:268, 1998
10. Baldwin JC, Anderson JL, Boucek MM, et al: Twenty-fourth Bethesda conference: Cardiac transplantation: Task force 2: Donor guidelines. J Am Coll Cardiol 22:15, 1993
11. Baumgartner WA: Evaluation and management of the heart donor. In: Baumgartner WA, Reitz BA, Achuff SC (eds): Heart and Heart-Lung Transplantation. Philadelphia, WB Saunders, 1990, p 86
12. Norman DJ: Immunogenetics and immunologic mechanisms of rejection. In Hosenpud JD, Cobanoglu A, Norman DJ, Starr A (eds): Cardiac Transplantation: A Manual for Health Care Professionals. New York, Springer-Verlag, 1991, p 15
13. Lavee J, Kormos RL, Duquesnoy RJ, et al: Influence of panel-reactive antibody and lymphocytotoxic crossmatch on survival after heart transplantation. J Heart Lung Transplant 10:921, 1991
14. Hauptman PJ, O'Connor KJ: Procurement and allocation of solid organs for transplantation. N Engl J Med 336:422, 1997
15. Billingham ME, Baumgartner WA, Watson DC, et al: Distant heart procurement for human transplantation: Ultrastructural studies. Circulation 62(suppl):I11, 1980
16. Lower RR, Shumway NE: Studies on orthotopic transplantation of the canine heart. Surg Forum 11:18, 1960
17. Baumgartner WA: Operative techniques utilized in heart transplantation. In: Baumgartner WA, Reitz BA, Achuff SC (eds): Heart and Heart-Lung Transplantation. Philadelphia, WB Saunders, 1990, p 113
18. Cobanoglu A: Operative techniques and early postoperative care in cardiac transplantation. In: Hosenpud JD, Cobanoglu A, Norman DJ, Starr A (eds): Cardiac Transplantation: A Manual for Health Care Professionals. New York, Springer-Verlag, 1991, p 95
19. Emery RW, Arom KV: Techniques in cardiac transplantation. In: Emery RW, Miller LW (eds): Handbook of Cardiac Transplantation. Philadelphia, Hanley & Belfus, 1996, p 61
20. Baumgartner WA: Heterotopic heart transplantation. In: Baumgartner WA, Reitz BA, Achuff SC (eds): Heart and Heart-Lung Transplantation. Philadelphia, WB Saunders, 1990, p 284
21. Sievers H-H, Weyand M, Kraatz EG, Bernhard A: An alternative technique for orthotopic cardiac transplantation, with preservation of the normal anatomy of the right atrium. Thorac Cardiovasc Surg 39:70, 1991
22. Sarsam MAI, Campbell CS, Yonan NA, et al: An alternative surgical technique in orthotopic cardiac transplantation. J Cardiac Surg 8:344, 1993
23. El Gamel A, Yonan NA, Grant S, et al: Orthotopic cardiac transplantation: A comparison of standard and bicaval Wythenshawe techniques. J Thorac Cardiovasc Surg 109:721, 1995
24. Deleuze PH, Benvenuti C, Mazzucotelli JP, et al: Orthotopic cardiac transplantation with direct cavel anastomosis: Is it the optimal procedure? J Thorac Cardiovasc Surg 109:731, 1995
25. Leyh RG, Jahnke AW, Kraatz EG, Sievers H-H: Cardiovascular dynamics and dimensions after bicaval and standard cardiac transplantation. Ann Thorac Surg 59:1495, 1995
26. Gravanis MB, Hertzler GL, Franch RH, et al: Hypersensitivity myocarditis in heart transplant candidates. J Heart Lung Transplant 10:688, 1991
27. Lewin D, d'Amati G, Lewis W: Hypersensitivity myocarditis: Findings in native and transplanted hearts. Cardiovasc Pathol 1:225, 1992
28. de Alava E, Panizo-Santos A, Fernandez-Gonzalez AL, Pardo-Mindan FJ: Eosinophilic myocarditis in patients waiting for heart transplantation. Cardiovasc Pathol 4:43, 1995
29. Herzog CA, Snover DC, Staley NA: Acute necrotising eosinophilic myocarditis. Br Heart J 52:343, 1984
30. Getz MA, Subramanian R, Logemann T, Ballantyne F: Acute necrotizing eosinophilic myocarditis as a manifestation of severe hypersensitivity myocarditis: Antemortem diagnosis and successful treatment. Ann Intern Med 115:201, 1991
31. Burke AP, Saenger J, Mullick F, Virmani R: Hypersensitivity myocarditis. Arch Pathol Lab Med 115:764, 1991
32. Edwards WD, Holmes DR Jr: Transvenous endomyocardial biopsy. In: Brandenburg RO, Fuster V, Giuliani ER, McGoon DC (eds): Cardiology: Fundamentals and Practice. Chicago, Year Book Medical Publishers, 1987, p 506
33. Spear G: Eosinophilic explant carditis with eosinophilia: Hypersensitivity to dobutamine infusion. J Heart Lung Transplant 14:755, 1995
34. Billingham ME: Pathology of human cardiac transplantation. In: Schoen FJ, Gimbrone MA (eds): Cardiovascular Pathology: Clinicopathologic Correlations and Pathogenetic Mechanisms. Baltimore, Williams & Wilkins, 1995, p 108

35. Cantor WJ, Daly P, Iwanochko M, et al: Cardiac transplantation for Fabry's disease. Can J Cardiol 14:81, 1998

36. Gries W, Farkas D, Winters GL, Costanzo-Nordin MR: Giant cell myocarditis: First report of disease recurrence in the transplanted heart. J Heart Lung Transplant 11:370, 1992

37. Oni AA, Hershberger RE, Norman DJ, et al: Recurrence of sarcoidosis in a cardiac allograft: Control with augmented corticosteroids. J Heart Lung Transplant 11:367, 1992

38. Valantine HA, Tazelaar HD, Macoviak J, et al: Cardiac sarcoidosis: Response to steroids and transplantation. J Heart Transplant 6: 244, 1987

39. Hosenpud JD, Uretsky BF, Griffith BP, et al: Successful intermediate-term outcome for patients with cardiac amyloidosis undergoing heart transplantation: Results of multicenter survey. J Heart Transplant 9:346, 1990

40. O'Connell JB, Dec GW, Goldenberg IF, et al: Results of heart transplantation for active lymphocytic myocarditis. J Heart Transplant 9:351, 1990

41. Angelini A, Livi U, Grassi G, et al: Discordance between pre- and post-transplant diagnosis (abstract). J Heart Lung Transplant 13(suppl):S33, 1994

42. Enos WF, Beyer JC, Holmes RH: Pathogenesis of coronary disease in American soldiers killed in Korea. JAMA 158:912, 1955

43. Virmani R, Robinowitz M, Geer JC, et al: Coronary artery atherosclerosis revisited in Korean War combat casualties. Arch Pathol Lab Med 111:972, 1987

44. Wissler RW, Strong JP, and the PDAY Research Group: Risk factors and progression of atherosclerosis in youth. Am J Pathol 153:1023, 1998

45. Tuzcu EM, Hobbs RE, Rincon G, et al: Occult and frequent transmission of atherosclerotic coronary disease with cardiac transplantation: Insights from intravascular ultrasound. Circulation 91: 1706, 1995

46. Botas J, Pinto FJ, Chenzbraun A, et al: Influence of preexistent donor coronary artery disease on the progression of transplant vasculopathy: An intravascular ultrasound study. Circulation 92: 1126, 1995

47. Lange HW, Galliani CA, Edwards JE: Local complications associated with indwelling Swan-Ganz catheters: Autopsy study of 36 cases. Am J Cardiol 52:1108, 1983

48. Rowley KM, Clubb KS, Smith GJW, Cabin HS: Right-sided infective endocarditis as a consequence of flow-directed pulmonary-artery catheterization: A clinicopathological study of 55 autopsied patients. N Engl J Med 311:1152, 1984

49. Schoen FJ: Myocardial, pericardial, and endocardial heart disease. In: Interventional and Surgical Cardiovascular Pathology: Clinical Correlations and Basic Principles. Philadelphia, WB Saunders, 1989, p 173

50. Hakim M, Wreghitt TG, English TAH, et al: Significance of donor transmitted disease in cardiac transplantation. J Heart Transplant 4: 302, 1985

51. Miller LW, Schlant RC, Kobashigawa J, et al: Twenty-fourth Bethesda conference: Cardiac transplantation: Task force 5: Complications. J Am Coll Cardiol 22:41, 1993

52. Przepiorka D, LeParc GF, Werch J, Lichtiger B: Prevention of transfusion-associated cytomegalovirus infection: Practice parameter. Am J Clin Pathol 106:163, 1996

53. Grattan MT, Moreno-Cabral CE, Starnes VA, et al: Cytomegalovirus infection is associated with cardiac allograft rejection and atherosclerosis. JAMA 261:3561, 1989

54. McDonald K, Rector TS, Braunlin EA, et al: Association of coronary artery disease in cardiac transplant recipients with cytomegalovirus. Am J Cardiol 64:359, 1989

55. Kendall TJ, Wilson JE, Radio SJ, et al: Cytomegalovirus and other herpesviruses: Do they have a role in the development of accelerated coronary arterial disease in human heart allografts? J Heart Lung Transplant, 11(suppl):S14, 1992

56. Holliman RE, Johnson JD, Adams S, Pepper JR: Toxoplasmosis and heart transplantation. J Heart Transplant 10:608, 1991

57. Dressler FA, Javier JJ, Salinas-Madrigal, et al: Myocardial toxoplasmosis complicating cardiac transplant. Cardiovasc Pathol 5: 101, 1996

58. Anthuber M, Kemkes BM, Heiss MM, et al: HIV infection after heart transplantation: A case report. J Heart Transplant 10:611, 1991

59. Bolli R: Mechanism of myocardial "stunning." Circulation 82:723, 1990

60. Pilati CF, Bosso FJ, Maron MB: Factors involved in left ventricular dysfunction after massive sympathetic activation. Am J Physiol 263:H784, 1992

61. Mertes PM, Carteaux JP, Jaboin Y, et al: Estimation of myocardial interstitial norepinephrine release after brain death using cardiac microdialysis. Transplantation 57:371, 1994

62. Novitzky D: Selection and management of cardiac allograft donors. Curr Opin Cardiol 11:174, 1996

63. Billingham ME: Cardiac transplantation. In: Waller BF (ed): Contemporary Issues in Cardiovascular Pathology. Philadelphia, FA Davis, 1988, p 185

64. Kemnitz J, Cremer J, Restrepo-Specht I, et al: Hyperacute rejection in heart allografts: Case studies. Path Res Pract 187:23, 1991

65. Forbes RDC, Guttmann RD: Pathogenetic studies of cardiac allograft rejection using inbred rat models. Immunological Rev 77:5, 1984

66. Miyagawa S, Hirose H, Shirakura R, et al: The mechanism of discordant xenograft rejection. Transplantation 46:825, 1988

67. Rose AG, Cooper DKC, Human PA, et al: Histopathology of hyperacute rejection of the heart: Experimental and clinical observations in allografts and xenografts. J Heart Lung Transplant 10: 223, 1991

68. Platt JL, Fischel RJ, Matas AJ, et al: Immunopathology of hyperacute xenograft rejection in a swine-to-primate model. Transplantation 52:214, 1991

69. Forbes RDC, Guttmann RD: Evidence for complement-induced endothelial injury in vivo: A comparative ultrastructural tracer study in a controlled model of hyperacute rat cardiac allograft rejection. Am J Pathol 106:378, 1982

70. Bach FH, Blakely ML, Van der Werf W, et al: Discordant xenografting: A working model of problems and issues. Xeno 1:8, 1993

71. Winters GL: The pathology of heart allograft rejection. Arch Pathol Lab Med 115:266, 1991

72. Fyfe B, Loh E, Winters GL, et al: Heart transplantation-associated perioperative ischemic myocardial injury: Morphological features and clinical significance. Circulation 93:1133, 1996

73. Carrier M, Paplanus SH, Graham AR, Copeland JG: Histopathology of acute myocardial necrosis: Effects of immunosuppression therapy. J Heart Transplant 6:218, 1987

74. Pickering JG, Boughner DR: Fibrosis in the transplanted heart and its relation to donor ischemic time: Assessment with polarized light microscopy and digital image analysis. Circulation 81:949, 1990

75. Wahlers T, Cremer J, Fieguth HG, et al: Donor heart-related variables and early mortality after heart transplantation. J Heart Lung Transplant 10:22, 1991

76. Foerster A, Abdelnoor M, Geiran O, et al: Morbidity risk factors in human cardiac transplantation: Histoincompatibility and protracted graft ischemia entail high risk of rejection and infection. Scand J Thorac Cardiovasc Surg 26:169, 1992

77. Gaudin PB, Rayburn BK, Hutchins GM, et al: Peritransplant injury to the myocardium associated with the development of accelerated arteriosclerosis in heart transplant recipients. Am J Surg Pathol 18: 338, 1994

78. Kumar V: Disorders of the immune system. In: Kumar V, Cotran RS, Robbins SL (eds): Basic Pathology. Philadelpia, WB Saunders, 1997, p 97

79. Hutchinson IV: Effector mechanisms in transplant rejection—an overview. In: Rose ML, Yacoub MH (eds): Immunology of Heart and Lung Transplantation. London, Edward Arnold, 1993, p 3

80. Yowell RL, Araneo BA: Mechanisms of allograft rejection. In: Hammond EH (ed): Solid Organ Transplantation Pathology. Philadelphia, WB Saunders, 1994, p 4

81. McManus BM, Winters GL: Pathology of heart allograft rejection. In: Kolbeck PC, Markin RS, McManus BM (eds): Transplant Pathology. Chicago, ASCP Press, 1994, p 197

82. Weintraub D, Masek M, Billingham ME: The lymphocyte subpopulations in cyclosporine-treated human heart rejection. J Heart Transplant 4:213, 1985

83. Myles JL, Ratliff NB, McMahon JT, et al: Reversibility of myocyte injury in moderate and severe acute rejection in cyclosporin-

treated cardiac transplant patients. Arch Pathol Lab Med 111:947, 1987

84. Wagoner LE, Zhao L, Bishop DK, et al: Lysis of adult ventricular myocytes by cells infiltrating rejecting murine cardiac allografts. Circulation 93:111, 1996

85. Laguens RP, Cabeza Meckert PM, San Martino J, et al: Identification of programmed cell death (apoptosis) in situ by means of specific labeling of nuclear DNA fragments in heart biopsy samples during acute rejection episodes. J Heart Lung Transplant 15: 911, 1996

86. Szabolcs M, Michler RE, Yang X, et al: Apoptosis of cardiac myocytes during cardiac allograft rejection: Relation to induction of nitric oxide synthase. Circulation 94:1665, 1996

87. Narula J, Haider N, Virmani R, et al: Apoptosis in myocytes in end-stage heart failure. N Engl J Med 335:1182, 1996

88. Olivetti G, Abbi R, Quaini F, et al: Apoptosis in the failing human heart. N Engl J Med 336:1131, 1997

89. Yeh ETH: Life and death in the cardiovascular system (editorial). Circulation 95:782, 1997

90. Baughman K: Monitoring of allograft rejection. In: Baumgartner WA, Reitz BA, Achuff SC (eds): Heart and Heart-Lung Transplantation. Philadelphia, WB Saunders, 1990, p 157

91. Valantine HA, Hunt SA: Clinical and non-invasive methods of diagnosing rejection after heart transplantation. In: Rose ML, Yacoub MH (eds): Immunology of Heart and Lung Transplantation. London, Edward Arnold, 1993 p 219

92. Ferraro P, Carrier M: Acute cardiac allograft rejection: Diagnosis and treatment. In: Emery RW, Miller LW (eds): Handbook of Cardiac Transplantation, Philadelphia, Hanley & Belfus, 1996, p 119

93. Caves BC, Billingham ME, Stinson EB, Shumway NE: Serial transvenous biopsy of the transplanted human heart: Improved management of acute rejection episodes. Lancet 1:821, 1974

94. Billingham ME: Diagnosis of cardiac rejection by endomyocardial biopsy. J Heart Transplant 1:25, 1982

95. McAllister HA, Schnee MJ, Radovancevic B, Frazier OH: A system for grading cardiac allograft rejection. Tex Heart Inst J 13:1, 1986

96. Kemnitz J, Cohnert T, Schafers HJ, et al: A classification of cardiac allograft rejection: A modification of the classification by Billingham. Am J Surg Pathol 11:503, 1987

97. Hammond EH, Yowell RL, Nunoda S, et al: Vascular (humoral) rejection in heart transplantation: Pathologic observations and clinical implications. J Heart Transplant 8:430, 1989

98. O'Connell JB, Renlund DG: Variations in the diagnosis, treatment, and prevention of cardiac allograft rejection: The need for standardization? J Heart Transplant 9:269, 1990

99. Billingham ME: Dilemma of variety of histopathologic grading systems for acute cardiac allograft rejection by endomyocardial biopsy. J Heart Transplant 9:272, 1990

100. Billingham ME, Cary NRB, Hammond EH, et al: A working formulation for the standardization of nomenclature in the diagnosis of heart and lung rejection: Heart rejection study group. J Heart Transplant 9:587, 1990

101. Spratt P, Sivathasan C, Macdonald P, et al: Role of routine endomyocardial biopsy to monitor late rejection after heart transplantation. J Heart Lung Transplant 10:912, 1991

102. White JA, Guiraudon C, Pflugfelder PW, Kostuk WJ: Routine surveillance myocardial biopsies are unnecessary beyond one year after heart transplantation. J Heart Lung Transplant 14:1052, 1995

103. Sethi GK, Kosaraju S, Arabia FA, et al: Is it necessary to perform surveillance endomyocardial biopsies in heart transplant recipients? J Heart Lung Transplant 14:1047, 1995

104. Heimansohn DA, Robison RJ, Paris JM: Routine surveillance endomyocardial biopsy: Late rejection after heart transplantation. Ann Thorac Surg 64:1231, 1997

105. Winters GL, Marboe CC, Billingham ME: The ISHLT grading system for cardiac transplant biopsies: Clarification and commentary. J Heart Lung Transplant 17:754, 1998

106. Laufer G, Laczkovics A, Wollenek G, et al: The progression of mild acute cardiac rejection evaluated by risk factor analysis: The impact of maintenance steroids and serum creatinine. Transplantation 51:184, 1991

107. Yeoh TK, Frist WH, Eastburn TE, Atkinson J: Clinical significance of mild rejection of the cardiac allograft. Circulation 86(supp II): 267, 1992

108. Lloveras JJ, Escourrou G, Delisle MB, et al: Evolution of un-

109. Rizeq MN, Masek MA, Billingham ME: Acute rejection: Significance of elapsed time after transplantation. J Heart Lung Transplant 13:862, 1994

110. Winters GL: The challenge of endomyocardial biopsy interpretation in assessing cardiac allograft rejection. Curr Opin Cardiol 12: 146, 1997

111. Winters GL: Grade 2 cardiac rejection: Pathological and clinical controversies. Pathology Case Reviews 3:1, 1998

112. Winters GL, Loh E, Schoen FJ: Natural history of focal moderate cardiac allograft rejection: Is treatment warranted? Circulation 91: 1975, 1995

113. Winters GL, McManus BM, for the Rapamycin Cardiac Rejection Treatment Trial Pathologists: Consistencies and controversies in the application of the ISHLT working formulation for cardiac transplant biopsy specimens. J Heart Lung Transplant 15:728, 1996

114. Fishbein MC, Bell G, Lones MA, et al: Grade 2 cellular heart rejection: Does it exist? J Heart Lung Transplant 13:1051, 1994

115. Janis E, Peng C, Baughman K, et al: Should grade 3A rejection be treated? (abstract). J Heart Lung Transplant 15(suppl): S77, 1996

116. Anguita M, Lopez-Rubio F, Arizon JM, et al: Repetitive non-treated episodes of grade 1B or 2 acute rejection impair long-term cardiac graft function. J Heart Lung Transplant 14:452, 1995

117. Uretsky BF, Murali S, Reddy PS, et al: Development of coronary artery disease in cardiac transplant patients receiving immunosuppressive therapy with cyclosporine and prednisone. Circulation 4: 827, 1987

118. Schutz A, Kemkes BM, Kugler C, et al: The influence of rejection episodes on the development of coronary artery disease after heart transplantation. Eur J Cardiothorac Surg 4:300, 1990

119. Ratkovec RM, Wray RB, Renlund DG, et al: Influence of corticosteroid-free maintenance immunosuppression on allograft coronary artery disease after cardiac transplantation. J Thorac Cardiovasc Surg 100:6, 1990

120. Pucci AM, Forbes RD, Billingham ME: Pathologic features in long-term cardiac allografts. J Heart Transplant 9:339, 1990

121. Winters GL, Kendall TJ, Radio SJ, et al: Post-transplant obesity and hyperlipidemia: Major predictors of severity of coronary arteriopathy in failed human heart allografts. J Heart Transplant 9:364, 1990

122. Stovin PGI, Sharples L, Hutter JA, et al: Some prognostic factors in the development of transplant-related coronary artery disease in human cardiac allografts. J Heart Lung Transplant 10:38, 1990

123. Costanzo-Nordin MR: Cardiac allograft vasculopathy: Relationship with acute cellular rejection and histocompatibility. J Heart Lung Transplant 11(suppl):S90, 1992

124. Hammond EH, Yowell RL, Nunoda S, et al: Vascular (humoral) rejection in heart transplantation: Pathologic observations and clinical implications. J Heart Transplant 8:430, 1989

125. Hammond EH, Hansen JK, Spenser LS, et al: Vascular rejection in cardiac transplantation: Histologic, immunopathologic, and ultrastructural features. Cardiovasc Pathol 2:21, 1993

126. Caple JF, McMahon JT, Myles JL, et al: Acute vascular (humoral) rejection in non-OKT3-treated cardiac transplants. Cardiovasc Pathol 4:13, 1994

127. Lones MA, Czer LS, Trento A, et al: Clinical-pathologic features of humoral rejection in cardiac allografts: A study in 81 consecutive patients. J Heart Lung Transplant 14:151, 1995

128. Bonnaud EN, Lewis NP, Masek MA, Billingham ME: Reliability and usefulness of immunofluorescence in heart transplantation. J Heart Lung Transplant 14:163, 1995

129. Ungureanu-Longrois D, Balligand JL, Kelly RA, Smith TW: Myocardial contractile dysfunction in the systemic inflammatory response syndrome: Role of a cytokine-inducible nitric oxide synthase in cardiac myocytes. J Mol Cell Cardiol 27:155, 1995

130. Pagani FD, Baker LS, Hsi C, et al: Left ventricular systolic and diastolic dysfunction after infusion of tumor necrosis factor-α in conscious dogs. J Clin Invest 90:389, 1992

131. Joshi A, Masek MA, Brown BW, et al: Quilty revisited: A 10-year perspective. Hum Pathol 26:547, 1995

132. Billingham ME: The postsurgical heart: The pathology of cardiac transplantation. Am J Cardiovasc Pathol 1:319, 1988

133. Hunt SA, Tazelaar HD: Use of endomyocardial biopsy in cardiac transplantation. In: Fowles RE (ed): Cardiac Biopsy. Mount Kisco, NY, Futura Publishing Inc., 1992, p 155

134. Kottke-Marchant K, Ratliff NB: Endomyocardial lymphocytic infiltrates in cardiac transplant recipients. Arch Pathol Lab Med 113: 690, 1989

135. Radio SJ, McManus BM, Winters GL, et al: Preferential endocardial residence of B-cells in the "Quilty effect" of human heart allografts: Immunohistochemical distinction from rejection. Mod Pathol 4:654, 1991

136. Luthringer DJ, Yamashita JT, Czer LSC, et al: Nature and significance of epicardial lymphoid infiltrates in cardiac allografts. J Heart Lung Transplant 14:537, 1995

137. Forbes RDC, Rowan RA, Billingham ME: Endocardial infiltrates in human heart transplants: A serial biopsy analysis comparing four immunosuppression protocols. Hum Pathol 21:850, 1990

138. Suit PF, Kotte-Marchant K, Ratliff NB, et al: Comparison of whole-blood cyclosporine levels and the frequency of endomyocardial lymphocytic infiltrates (the Quilty lesion) in cardiac transplantation. Transplantation 48:618, 1989

139. Barone JH, Fishbein MC, Czer LSC, et al: Absence of endocardial lymphoid infiltrates (Quilty lesions) in nonheart transplant recipients treated with cyclosporine. J Heart Lung Transplant 16:600, 1997

140. Pardo-Mindan FJ, Lozano MD: "Quilty effect" in heart transplantation: Is it related to acute rejection? J Heart Lung Transplant 10: 937, 1991

141. Costanzo-Nordin MR, Winters GL, Fisher SG, et al: Endocardial infiltrates in the transplanted heart: Clinical significance emerging from the analysis of 5026 endomyocardial biopsy specimens. J Heart Lung Transplant 12:741, 1993

142. Kemnitz J, Cohnert TR: Lymphoma like lesion in human orthotopic cardiac allografts (abstr). Am J Clin Pathol 89:430, 1988

143. Nakhleh RE, Copenhaver CM, Werdin K, et al: Lack of evidence for involvement of Epstein-Barr virus in the development of the "Quilty" lesion of transplanted hearts: An in situ hybridization study. J Heart Lung Transplant 10:504, 1991

144. Woods G, Linder J: The detection of opportunistic infections in the transplant patient. In: Kolbeck PC, Markin RS, McManus BM (eds): Transplant Pathology. Chicago, ASCP Press, 1994, p 123

145. Fishman JA, Rubin RH: Infection in organ-transplant recipients. N Engl J Med 338:1741, 1998

146. Miller LW, Naftel DC, Bourge RC, et al: Infection after heart transplantation: A multiinstitutional study. J Heart Lung Transplant 13:381, 1994

147. Linder J: Infection as a complication of heart transplantation. J Heart Transplant 7:390, 1988

148. Hosenpud JD, Hershberger RE, Pantely GA, et al: Late infection in cardiac allograft recipients: Profiles, incidence, and outcome. J Heart Lung Transplant 10:380, 1991

149. Winters GL, Costanzo-Nordin MR, O'Sullivan EJ, et al: Predictors of late acute orthotopic heart transplant rejection. Circulation 80 (suppl III): 106, 1989

150. Lanza RP, Cooper DK, Cassidy MJ, Barnard CN: Malignant neoplasms occurring after cardiac transplantation. JAMA 249:1746, 1983

151. Penn I: Incidence and treatment of neoplasia after transplantation. J Heart Lung Transplant 12(suppl):S328, 1993

152. Nalesnik MA, Makowa L, Starzl TE: The diagnosis and treatment of posttransplant lymphoproliferative disorders. Curr Probl Surg 25:367, 1988

153. Bieber CP, Reitz BA, Jamieson SW, et al: Malignant lymphoma in cyclosporine A treated allograft recipients (letter). Lancet 1:43, 1980

154. Calne RY, Rolles K, White DJ, et al: Cyclosporin A initially as the only immunosuppressant in 34 recipients of cadaveric organs: 32 kidneys, 2 pancreases, and 2 livers. Lancet 2:1033, 1979

155. Swinnen LJ, Costanzo-Nordin MR, Fisher SG, et al: Increased incidence of lymphoproliferative disorder after immunosuppression with the monoclonal antibody OKT3 in cardiac transplant recipients. N Engl J Med 323:1723, 1990

156. Penn I: Cancers following cyclosporine therapy. Transplantation 43:32, 1987

157. Penn I: Cancers complicating organ transplantation (editorial). N Engl J Med 323:1767, 1990

158. Craig FE, Gully ML, Banks PM: Posttransplantation lymphoproliferative disorders. Am J Clin Pathol 99:265, 1993

159. Purtilo DT, Harrington D: Malignant neoplasms in organ transplant recipients. In: Kolbeck PR, Markin RS, McManus BM (eds): Transplant Pathology. Chicago, ASCP Press, 1994, p 145

160. Eisen HJ, Hicks D, Kant JA, et al: Diagnosis of posttransplantation lymphoproliferative disorder by endomyocardial biopsy in a cardiac allograft recipient. J Heart Lung Transplant 13:241, 1994

161. Cleary ML, Warnke R, Sklar J: Monoclonality of lymphoproliferative lesions in cardiac transplant recipients: Clonal analysis based on immunoglobulin-gene rearrangements. N Engl J Med 310:477, 1984

162. Hanto DW, Najarian JS: Advances in the diagnosis and treatment of EBV-associated lymphoproliferative diseases in immunocompromised hosts. J Surg Oncol 30:215, 1985

163. Hanto DW, Frizzera G, Gajl-Peczalska KJ, Simmons RL: Epstein-Barr virus, immunodeficiency, and B cell lymphoproliferation. Transplantation 39:461, 1985

164. Cleary ML, Sklar J: Lymphoproliferative disorders in cardiac transplant recipients are multiclonal lymphomas. Lancet 2:489, 1984

165. Armitage JM, Kormos RL, Stuart S, et al: Posttransplant lymphoproliferative disease in thoracic organ transplant patients: Ten years of cyclosporine-based immunosuppression. J Heart Lung Transplant 10:877, 1991

166. Hosenpud JD, Shipley GD, Wagner CR: Cardiac allograft vasculopathy: Current concepts, recent developments, and future directions. J Heart Lung Transplant 11:9, 1992

167. Weis M, von Scheidt W: Cardiac allograft vasculopathy: A review. Circulation 96:2069, 1997

168. Gao SZ, Schroeder JS, Alderman EL, et al: Prevalence of accelerated coronary artery disease in heart transplant survivors: Comparison of cyclosporine and azathioprine regimens. Circulation 80 (suppl III):100, 1989

169. Johnson JA, Kobashigawa JA: Quantitative analysis of transplant coronary artery disease with use of intracoronary ultrasound. J Heart Lung Transplant 14(suppl):S198, 1995

170. Schoen FJ, Libby P: Cardiac transplant graft arteriosclerosis. Trends Cardiovasc Med 1:216, 1991

171. Johnson DE, Alderman EL, Schroeder JS, et al: Transplant coronary artery disease: Histopathologic correlations with angiographic morphology. J Am Coll Cardiol 17:449, 1991

172. Billingham, ME: Histopathology of graft coronary disease. J Heart Lung Transplant 11(suppl):S38, 1992

173. Liu G, Butany J: Morphology of graft arteriosclerosis in cardiac transplant recipients. Hum Pathol 23:768, 1992

174. Rose AG, Viviers L, Odell JA: Pathology of chronic cardiac rejection: An analysis of the epicardial and intramyocardial coronary arteries and myocardial alterations in 43 human allografts. Cardiovasc Pathol 2:7, 1993

175. Lin H, Wilson JE, Kendall TJ, et al: Comparable proximal and distal severity of intimal thickening and size of epicardial coronary arteries in transplant arteriopathy of human cardiac allografts. J Heart Lung Transplant 13:824, 1994

176. Hruban RH, Beschorner WE, Baumgartner WA, et al: Accelerated arteriosclerosis in heart transplant recipients is associated with a T-lymphocyte-mediated endothelialitis. Am J Pathol 137:871, 1990

177. Salomon RN, Hughes CCW, Schoen FJ, et al: Human coronary transplantation-associated arteriosclerosis: Evidence for a chronic immune reaction to activated graft endothelial cells. Am J Pathol 138:791, 1991

178. McManus BM, Malcom G, Kendall TJ, et al: Lipid overload and proteoglycan expression in chronic rejection of the human transplanted heart. Clin Transplant 8:336, 1994

179. McManus BM, Horley KJ, Wilson JE, et al: Prominence of coronary arterial wall lipids in human heart allografts: Implications for pathogenesis of allograft arteriopathy. Am J Path 147:293, 1995

180. Lin H, Wilson JE, Roberts CR, et al: Biglycan, decorin and versican protein expression patterns in coronary arteriopathy of human heart allografts: Distinctness as compared to native atherosclerosis. J Heart Transplant 15:1233, 1996

181. Lin H, Ignatescu M, Wilson JE, et al: Prominence of apolipoproteins B, (a) and E in the intimae of coronary arteries in transplanted human hearts: Geographic relationship to vessel wall proteoglycans. J Heart Lung Transplant 15:1223, 1996

182. Radio S, Wood S, Wilson J, et al: Allograft vascular disease: Comparison of heart and other grafted organs. Transplant Proc 28: 496, 1996

183. Neish AS, Loh E, Schoen FJ: Myocardial changes in cardiac transplant-associated coronary arteriosclerosis: Potential for timely diagnosis. J Am Coll Cardiol 19:586, 1992

184. Edwalds GM, Said JW, Block MI, et al: Myocytolysis (vacuolar

degeneration) of myocardium: Immunohistochemical evidence of viability. Hum Pathol 15:753, 1984

185. Pirolo JS, Hutchins GM, Moore GW: Myocyte vacuolization in infarct border zones is reversible. Am J Pathol 121:444, 1985

186. Clausell N, Butany J, Gladstone P, et al: Myocardial vacuolization, a marker of ischemic injury, in surveillance cardiac biopsies post-transplant: Correlations with morphologic vascular disease and endothelial dysfunction. Cardiovasc Pathol 5:29, 1996

187. Winters GL, Schoen FJ: Graft arteriosclerosis-induced myocardial pathology in heart transplant recipients: Predictive value of endomyocardial biopsy. J Heart Lung Transplant 16:985, 1997

188. Dong C, Redenbach D, Wood S, et al: The pathogenesis of cardiac allograft vasculopathy. Curr Opin Cardiol 11:183, 1996

189. Marboe CC: Cardiac transplant vasculopathy. In: Hammond EH (ed): Solid Organ Transplantation Pathology. Philadelphia, WB Saunders, 1994, p 111

190. Libby P: Do vascular wall cytokines promote atherogenesis? Hosp Prac 27:51, 1992

191. Hosenpud JD, Shipley GD, Wagner CR: Cardiac allograft vasculopathy: Current concepts, recent developments, and future directions. J Heart Lung Transplant 11:9, 1992

192. Allen MD, McDonald TO, Carlos T, et al: Endothelial adhesion molecules in heart transplantation. J Heart Lung Transplantation 11 (suppl):S8, 1992

193. Ardehali A, Laks H, Drinkwater DC, et al: Vascular cell adhesion molecule-1 is induced on vascular endothelia and medial smooth muscle cells in experimental cardiac vasculopathy. Circulation 92:450, 1995

194. Billingham ME: Graft coronary disease: Old and new dimensions. Cardiovasc Pathol 6:95, 1997

195. Molossi S, Elices M, Arrhenius T, et al: Blockade of very late antigen-4 integrin binding to fibronectin with connecting segment-1 peptide reduces accelerated coronary arteriopathy in rabbit cardiac allografts. J Clin Invest 95:2601, 1995

196. Cowan DE, Baron O, Crack J, et al: Elafin, a serine elastase inhibitor, attenuates post-cardiac transplant coronary arteriopathy and reduces myocardial necrosis in rabbits after heterotopic cardiac transplantation. J Clin Invest 97:2452, 1996

197. Libby P: Transplantation-associated arteriosclerosis: Potential mechanisms. In: Tilney NL, Strom TB, Paul LC (eds): Transplantation Biology: Cellular and Molecular Aspects. Philadelphia, Lippincott-Raven, 1996, p 577

198. Costanzo-Nordin MR: Cardiac allograft vasculopathy: Relationship with acute cellular rejection and histocompatibility. J Heart Lung Transplant 11(suppl):S90, 1992

199. Kobashigawa JA, Miller L, Yeung A, et al: Does acute rejection correlate with the development of transplant coronary artery disease? A multicenter study using intravascular ultrasound. J Heart Lung Transplant 14(suppl):S221, 1995

200. Hauptman PJ, Nakagawa T, Tanaka H, Libby P: Acute rejection: Culprit or coincidence in the pathogenesis of cardiac graft vascular disease? J Heart Lung Transplant 14(suppl):S173, 1995

201. Hosenpud JD, Everett JP, Morris TE, et al: Cellular and humoral immunity to vascular endothelium and the development of cardiac allograft vasculopathy. J Heart Lung Transplant 14(suppl):S185, 1995

202. Wheeler CH, Collins A, Dunn MJ: Characterization of endothelial antigens associated with transplant-associated coronary artery disease. J Heart Lung Transplant 14(suppl):S188, 1995

203. Johnson MR: Transplant coronary disease: Nonimmunologic risk factors. J Heart Lung Transplant 11(suppl):S124, 1992

204. Hauptman PJ, Davis SF, Miller L, Yeung AC, on behalf of the Multicenter Intravascular Ultrasound Transplant Study Group: The role of nonimmune risk factors in the development and progression of graft arteriosclerosis: Preliminary insights from a multicenter intravascular ultrasound study. J Heart Lung Transplant 14 (suppl):S238, 1995

205. Day JD, Rayburn BK, Gaudin PB, et al: Cardiac allograft vasculopathy: The central pathogenetic role of ischemia-induced endothelial cell injury. J Heart Lung Transplant 14(suppl):S142, 1995

206. Valantine HA: Role of lipids in allograft vascular disease: A multicenter study of intimal thickening detected by intravascular ultrasound. J Heart Lung Transplant 14(suppl):S142, 1995

207. Keogh A, Simons L, Spratt P, et al: Hyperlipidemia after heart transplantation. J Heart Transplant 7:171, 1988

208. Grady KL, Costanzo-Nordin MR, Herold LS, et al: Obesity and hyperlipidemia after heart transplantation. J Heart Lung Transplant 10:449, 1991

209. Hirozane T, Matsumori A, Furukawa Y, Sasayama S: Experimental graft coronary artery disease in a murine heterotopic cardiac transplant model. Circulation 91:386, 1995

210. Shi C, Russell ME, Bianchi C, et al: Murine model of accelerated transplant arteriosclerosis. Circ Res 75:199, 1995

211. Rowan RA, Billingham ME: Pathologic changes in the long-term transplanted heart: A morphometric study of myocardial hypertrophy, vascularity and fibrosis. Hum Pathol 21:767, 1990

212. Billingham ME: The pathologic changes in long-term heart and lung transplant survivors. J Heart Lung Transplant 11(suppl): S252, 1992

213. Meckel CR, Wilson JE, Sears TD, et al: Myocardial fibrosis in endomyocardial biopsy specimens: Do different bioptomes affect estimation? Am J Cardiovasc Pathol 2:309, 1989

214. Schuler S, Thomas D, Thebken M, et al: Endocrine response to exercise in cardiac transplant patients. Transplant Proc 19:2506, 1987

215. Stark RP, McGinn AL, Wilson RF: Chest pain in cardiac-transplant recipients: Evidence of sensory reinnervation after cardiac transplantation. N Engl J Med 324:1791, 1991

216. Rowan R, Billingham ME: Myocardial innervation in long-term cardiac transplant survivors: A quantitative ultrastructural survey. J Heart Transplant 7:448, 1988

217. Wilson RF, Christensen BV, Olivari MT, et al: Evidence for structural sympathetic reinnervation after orthotopic cardiac transplantation in humans. Circulation 83:1210, 1991

218. Arrowood JA, Goudreau E, Minisi AJ, et al: Evidence against reinnervation of cardiac vagal afferents after human orthotopic cardiac transplantation. Circulation 92:402, 1995

219. Mancini D: Surgically denervated cardiac transplant: Rewired or permanently unplugged? (editorial) Circulation 96:6, 1997

220. Wilson RF: Reinnervation reexamined (editorial) J Heart Lung Transplant 17:137, 1998

221. Cameron DE, Traill TA: Complications of immunosuppressive therapy. In: Baumgartner WA, Reitz BA, Achuff SC (eds): Heart and Heart-Lung Transplantation. Philadelphia, WB Saunders, 1990, p 237

222. Textor SC, Canzanello VJ, Taler SJ, et al: Cyclosporine-induced hypertension after transplantation. Mayo Clin Proc 69:1182, 1994

223. McGiffin DC, Kirklin JK, Naftel DC, Bourge RC: Competing outcomes after heart transplantation: A comparison of eras and outcomes. J Heart Lung Transplant 16:190, 1997

224. Baldwin JC, Oyer PE, Stinson EB, et al: Comparison of cardiac rejection in heart and heart-lung transplantation. J Heart Transplant 6:352, 1987

225. Joshi A, Oyer PE, Berry GJ, Billingham ME: Heart-lung transplantation: Cardiac clinicopathological correlations. Cardiovasc Pathol 5:153, 1996

226. Glanville AR, Imoto E, Baldwin JC, et al: The role of right ventricular endomyocardial biopsy in the long-term management of heart-lung transplant recipients. J Heart Transplant 6:357, 1987

227. Prop J, Kuijpers K, Petersen AH, et al: Why are lung allografts more vigorously rejected than hearts? J Heart Transplant 4:433, 1985

228. Fowles RE, Mason JW: Endomyocardial biopsy. Ann Intern Med 97:885, 1982

229. Fowles RE, Mason JW: Role of cardiac biopsy in the diagnosis and management of cardiac disease. Prog Cardiovasc Dis 27:153, 1984

230. Anastasiou-Nana MI, O'Connell JB, Nanas JN, et al: Relative efficiency and risk of endomyocardial biopsy: Comparisons in heart transplant and nontransplant patients. Cath Cardiovasc Diagn 18:7, 1989

231. Fowles RE, Anderson JL: Instruments and techniques for cardiac biopsy. In: Fowles RE (ed): Cardiac Biopsy. Mount Kisco, NY, Futura Publishing Inc, 1992, p 43

232. Baraldi-Junkins C, Levin HR, Kasper EK, et al: Complications of endomyocardial biopsy in heart transplant patients. J Heart Lung Transplant 12:63, 1993

233. Spiegelhalter DJ, Stovin PGI: An analysis of repeated biopsies following cardiac transplantation. Stat Med 2:33, 1983

234. Zerbe TR, Arena V: Diagnostic reliability of endomyocardial biopsy for assessment of cardiac allograft rejection. Hum Pathol 19:1307, 1988

235. Winters GL, Hauptman PJ, Jarcho JA, Schoen FJ: Immediate eval-

uation of endomyocardial biopsies for clinically suspected rejection after heart transplantation. Circulation 89:2079, 1994

236. Edwards WD: Pathology of endomyocardial biopsy. In: Waller BF (ed): Pathology of the Heart and Great Vessels. New York, Churchill Livingstone, 1988, p 191

237. Hauck AJ, Edwards WD: Histopathologic examination of tissues obtained by endomyocardial biopsy. In: Fowles RE (ed): Cardiac Biopsy. Mount Kisco, NY, Futura Publishing Inc, 1992, p 95

238. Adomian GE, Laks MM, Billingham ME: The incidence and significance of contraction bands in endomyocardial biopsies from normal human hearts. Am Heart J 95:348, 1978

239. Karch SB, Billingham ME: Myocardial contraction bands revisited. Hum Pathol 17:9, 1986

240. Winters GL, Costanzo-Nordin MR: Pathological findings in 2300 consecutive endomyocardial biopsies. Mod Pathol 4:441, 1991

241. Braverman AC, Coplen SE, Mudge GH, Lee RT: Ruptured chor-

dae tendineae of the tricuspid valve as a complication of endomyocardial biopsy in heart transplant patients. Am J Cardiol 66:111, 1990

242. Tucker PA, Jin BS, Gaos CM: Flail tricuspid leaflet after multiple biopsies following orthotopic heart transplantation: Echocardiographic and hemodynamic correlation. J Heart Lung Transplant 13:466, 1994

243. Sibley RK, Olivari MT, Bolman RM, Ring WS: Endomyocardial biopsy in the cardiac allograft recipient: A review of 570 biopsies. Ann Surg 203:177, 1986

244. McManus BM, Markin RS: The role of the autopsy in transplantation. In: Kolbeck PC, Markin RS, McManus BM (eds): Transplant Pathology. Chicago, ASCP Press, 1994, p 309

245. Winters GL: Heart transplantation: Explant, biopsy, and autopsy characteristics. In: McManus BM, Braunwald E (eds): Atlas of Cardiovascular Pathology. Philadelphia, Current Medicine, 2000

· · · · ·

APPENDIX A: EXPLANTED HEARTS

CASE #S_____-_____   RES _____   CARDIAC _____

H1 **HEART (_____ gm):**

H2 **ATHEROSCLEROTIC CORONARY ARTERY AND ISCHEMIC HEART DISEASE**
H3 **IDIOPATHIC DILATED CARDIOMYOPATHY**
H4 **HYPERTROPHIC CARDIOMYOPATHY**
H5 **VALVULAR HEART DISEASE**
H6 **CONGENITAL HEART DISEASE**
H7 **RETRANSPLANT: ACUTE ALLOGRAFT REJECTION** _____
H8 **RETRANSPLANT: GRAFT CORONARY DISEASE**
(−) _____

Configuration
H9 Biventricular hypertrophy and dilatation, mild.
H10 Biventricular hypertrophy and dilatation, moderate.
H11 Biventricular hypertrophy and dilatation, severe.
H12 Left ventricular hypertrophy, mild.
H13 Left ventricular hypertrophy, moderate.
H14 Left ventricular hypertrophy, severe.
H15 Left ventricular dilatation, mild.
H16 Left ventricular dilatation, moderate.
H17 Left ventricular dilatation, severe.
H18 Right ventricular hypertrophy, mild.
H19 Right ventricular hypertrophy, moderate.
H20 Right ventricular hypertrophy, severe.
H21 Right ventricular dilatation, mild.
H22 Right ventricular dilatation, moderate.
H23 Right ventricular dilatation, severe.
H24 Asymmetric septal hypertrophy.
H25 Atrial septal defect, _____ cm, _____
H26 Ventricular septal defect, _____ cm, _____
H27 Patent foramen ovale.
H28 Previous surgical repair, intact, _____
(−) _____

Myocardium
H29 Acute myocardial infarct, transmural, involving _____
H30 Recent myocardial infarct, transmural, involving _____
H31 Remote (healed) myocardial infarct, transmural, involving _____
H32 Acute subendocardial infarct involving _____
H33 Recent subendocardial infarct involving _____
H34 Remote (healed) subendocardial infarct involving _____
H35 Infarct, _____, is approximately _____ old.
H36 Aneurysm (_____ cm) is present involving _____

H37 A mural thrombus is present involving _____

H38 Focal subendocardial myocyte vacuolization suggestive of chronic ischemia.

H39 Diffuse subendocardial myocyte vacuolization suggestive of chronic ischemia.

H40 Focal transmural replacement fibrosis.

H41 Extensive transmural replacement fibrosis.

H42 Microscopic generalized hypertrophy, mild.

H43 Microscopic generalized hypertrophy, moderate.

H44 Microscopic generalized hypertrophy, severe.

H45 Interstitial and/or perivascular fibrosis, mild.

H46 Interstitial and/or perivascular fibrosis, moderate.

H47 Interstitial and/or perivascular fibrosis, severe.

H48 Myofiber disarray, disproportionately involving the interventricular septum.

H49 Active myocarditis, _____

H50 Active myocarditis, eosinophilic, focal (see note).

H51 Active myocarditis, eosinophilic, diffuse (see note).

H52 Acute rejection, _____

H53 No evidence of active myocarditis, acute infarction, or primary valvular disease.

(−) _____

Endocardium

H54 Focal endocardial fibrosis.

H55 Multifocal endocardial fibrosis.

H56 Diffuse endocardial fibrosis.

(−) _____

Valves

H57 Congenitally bicuspid aortic valve.

H58 S/P _____ valve replacement with _____

H59 Valve prosthesis(es) intact; type: _____

(−) _____

Pericardium

H60 Fibrinous pericarditis.

H61 Fibrous pericarditis.

(−) _____

Coronary Arteries

H62 No evidence of coronary atherosclerosis.

H63 Chronic coronary atherosclerosis with luminal narrowing as follows:

H64 Graft coronary disease with luminal narrowing as follows:

H65   LMA _____%

H66   LAD _____%

H67   LCX _____%

H68   RCA _____%

H69 Acute plaque change, _____ , involving _____

H70 S/P saphenous vein bypass graft(s) to _____

H71 S/P internal mammary bypass graft(s) to _____

H72 Bypass graft to _____ with intimal hyperplasia and _____% luminal narrowing.

H73 Bypass graft to _____ with atherosclerosis and _____% luminal narrowing.

H74 Graft coronary disease involves intramural vessels.

(−) _____

Devices

H75 Pacemaker wire present _____

H76 _____ anuloplasty ring present and intact.

H77 S/P placement of defibrillator patches.

H78 S/P placement of ventricular assist device, _____ type.

(−) _____

H79 NOTE: Eosinophilic myocarditis most likely represents a drug-induced hypersensitivity reaction.

. . . . .

APPENDIX B: TRANSPLANT ENDOMYOCARDIAL BIOPSY

CASE #S_____-_____   RES _____   CARDIAC _____

E1 RIGHT VENTRICULAR ENDOMYOCARDIAL BIOPSY
E2 LEFT VENTRICULAR ENDOMYOCARDIAL BIOPSY
(−) _____

Postoperative Interval
E3 _____ days S/P cardiac transplantation.
E4 _____ weeks S/P cardiac transplantation.
E5 _____ months S/P cardiac transplantation.
E6 _____ years S/P cardiac transplantation.

Rejection Grading
E7 No evidence of rejection; ISHLT Grade 0.
E8 Focal perivascular infiltrate without necrosis; ISHLT Grade 1A.
E9 Focal interstitial infiltrate without necrosis; ISHLT Grade 1A.
E10 Diffuse but sparse interstitial infiltrate without necrosis; ISHLT Grade 1B.
E11 Single focus of infiltrate with associated myocyte damage; ISHLT Grade 2.
E12 Two to three foci of infiltrates with associated myocyte damage; ISHLT Grade 2–3A.
E13 Multifocal interstitial infiltrates with associated myocyte damage; ISHLT Grade 3A.
E14 Diffuse inflammatory infiltrates with associated myocyte damage; ISHLT Grade 3B.
E15 Diffuse polymorphous infiltrate with myocyte necrosis, edema, hemorrhage, and/or vasculitis; ISHLT Grade 4.
E16 See note.
(−) _____

Other Biopsy Findings
E17 Tissue insufficient for diagnosis.
     NOTE: The presence of less than four (4) fragments of evaluable myocardium is considered suboptimal to rule
     out rejection with a high degree of certainty.
E18 Focal coagulation necrosis.
E19 Multifocal coagulation necrosis.
E20 Confluent coagulation necrosis.
E21 Focal healing ischemic injury.
E22 Multifocal healing ischemic injury.
E23 Confluent healing ischemic injury.
E24 Focal healing injury.
E25 Multifocal healing injury.
E26 Focal fat necrosis.
E27 Old biopsy site.
E28 Foreign body giant cell reaction.
E29 Dystrophic calcification.
E30 Focal inflammatory infiltrate in fibrous tissue, not considered rejection.
E31 No subendocardial myocyte vacuolization identified.
E32 Mild subendocardial myocyte vacuolization.
E33 Moderate subendocardial myocyte vacuolization.
E34 Severe subendocardial myocyte vacuolization.
E35 Endocardial infiltrate (Quilty A)
E36 Endocardial infiltrate with myocardial extension and encroachment (Quilty B).
     NOTE: Extension of an endocardial infiltrate into the underlying myocardium with or without associated
     myocyte damage is designated as "Quilty effect B" according to the ISHLT Working Formulation. The
     pathobiology of this lesion and relationship to acute rejection and/or other pathologic processes, if any, remains
     undefined.
E37 Mesothelial cells present.

NOTE: The presence of mesothelial cells on endomyocardial biopsy is diagnostic of cardiac perforation; clinical correlation is advised.

E38 See note.

(−) _____

Specimen Adequacy

E39 _____ fragments of diagnostic myocardium.

E40 _____ fragments of fibrous tissue.

E41 _____ fragments of blood clot.

E42 _____ fragments too small to evaluate.

(−) _____

Chapter 24

Genetic Causes of Diseases Affecting the Heart and Great Vessels

Christine Seidman • Barbara Sampson

Genetic studies of human disorders are increasingly defining the molecular basis of disease. Although current success in these endeavors has been limited primarily to studies of monogenic disorders, the future is ripe for expansion to the study of polygenic disease. Elucidation of the role played by genetics in human pathologies has enormous potential for reshaping many aspects of the practice of medicine. Perhaps most immediately, these discoveries will influence how we diagnose disease. Recognition that a gene mutation causes a disorder provides opportunity for diagnosis before clinical signs and symptoms have appeared, during any stage of the pathology, and even after death. The material required for gene-based diagnosis is both small and generic, and DNA from any tissue, viable or preserved, can be used to establish the presence or absence of a disease-causing mutation. For pathologists, the ramifications of gene-based diagnoses are immense. Researchers will have a new foundation for classifying pathologies that should foster better understanding of features that distinguish or link morphologic findings. Practitioners will have both the opportunity to define the causes of clinically quiescent pathology and the responsibility to communicate the import of these data to families and their doctors.

Understanding the clinical importance of discovering molecular causes for human disease requires a familiarity with the basic principles involved in studying inherited human disorders. Although a comprehensive review of this material is beyond the scope of this chapter, definitions of the different modes of inheritance and outlines of linkage studies and mutation detection are provided to enable a fluid description of subsequent studies on the genetic basis of cardiovascular pathologies.

CONCEPTS IN HUMAN MOLECULAR GENETICS

Modes of Inheritance and Penetrance

A wide range of cardiovascular disorders are caused by heritable mutations encoded in DNA sequences in nuclear chromosomes (autosomes 1 through 22, plus sex chromosomes X and Y) or on the single mitochondrial chromosome. The mode of transmission of these mutated genes can be deduced from analyzing pedigrees based on family history and/or clinical evaluation of the first-degree relatives of affected individuals. Definition of the pattern of inheritance of genetic disease is important both for assessing disease risk in family members and for providing critical data to structure research strategies for identifying genetic etiologies. Assignment of the correct pattern of inheritance can be confounded by disease penetrance, which is the likelihood that an individual with a disease-causing mutation exhibits a clinical phenotype. Disease penetrance can depend on the age of an individual as well as on other genetic (gender, modifying genes) or environmental (diet, exercise) factors.

The different modes of inheritance of single-gene (monogenic) cardiovascular disorders are illustrated by the pedigrees in Figure 24–1. Dominant disorders (Fig. 24–1A) are encoded on one of the 22 autosomes and are equally transmitted to men and women within a family. Thus, 50% of the offspring of an affected individual inherit autosomal dominant disease-causing mutations, whereas offspring of a genetically unaffected family have no risk for developing the disorder.

Autosomal recessive disorders occur when an individual inherits one defective copy of the disease gene from each parent. Parents of affected individuals are heterozygous carriers, with one mutated and one normal copy of the disease gene. Their offspring can be homozygous and affected (25% chance), homozygous and unaffected (25% chance), or heterozygous carriers (50% chance), regardless of their sex. Autosomal recessive diseases are more frequent when there is a high prevalence of carriers within the population or with parental consanguinity (Fig. 24–1B), which increases the probability of transmission of a defect inherited by each parent from a common ancestor. The penetrance of autosomal recessive diseases typically approximates 100%, but gene carriers often have no clinical phenotype. Thus, it is frequently impossible to distinguish carriers from genetically unaffected individuals.

X-linked disorders (Fig. 24–1C) are typically quiescent or clinically insignificant in women but fully penetrant in men. Male offspring of female carriers have a 50% chance of inheriting the disease, whereas female siblings of affected males have a 50% risk of being carriers.

Matrilineal transmission (Fig. 24–1D) of a genetic disorder suggests a mitochondrial defect. All offspring of affected women carry the defect and develop disease, but pathology does not occur in the offspring of affected men. The 16,500 nucleotides encoding mitochondrial genes encode proteins involved in the synthesis of adenosine triphosphate (ATP); mutations within these genes produce complex disorders such as Kearns-Sayre syndrome, which involves the central nervous system, kidney, and both skeletal and cardiac muscle. Unlike nuclear

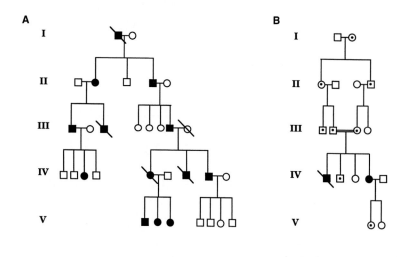

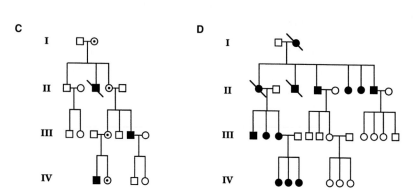

Figure 24-1 • Modes of transmission of inherited cardiovascular pathologies. Squares denote men; circles denote women. Slashes denote deceased individuals. Affection status is shown as follows: filled symbol, affected; clear symbol, unaffected; central dot, carrier. *A*, Note that men and women are equally affected in autosomal dominant disease and that affected individuals are found in each generation. *B*, Autosomal recessive disorders are more common in the offspring of consanguineous marriages (indicated by double bar in generation III). *C*, X-linked disorders can be clinically silent in female carriers, or they can exhibit mild disease. *D*, Mitochondrial traits are recognized by affected status in all offspring of affected women but none of affected men.

genes, hundreds of copies of mitochondrial genes are present in each cell. Mitochondrial genes can exhibit significant heteroplasmy, or normal and abnormal populations within one cell; the degree of heteroplasmy can correlate with the severity of mitochondrial disease.

Identifying Disease Loci, Genes, and Mutations

A key first step in identifying gene mutations that cause heritable cardiovascular disorders is to define the chromosome location of the defect. This is accomplished through linkage or mapping studies in which DNA markers from defined regions of the genome are analyzed to identify those that are coinherited with the disease. For X-linked disorders, analyses are restricted to this chromosome, but for autosomal disorders, analyses are performed for each of the 22 autosomes until linkage is established. This step is unnecessary for mitochondrial disorders, because this small chromosome can be directly screened for mutations by sequence. Successful linkage studies result in the definition of a disease locus or a chromosome region that contains a disease gene.

The efficiency of genetic mapping studies has substantially increased over the past decade, resulting in the identification of many cardiovascular disease loci. However, the rapidity with which the causal disease gene is defined remains quite variable. Two general strategies are usually employed. Genes that have been previously

mapped to the same chromosome region and that are expressed in the heart—called candidate genes—are directly analyzed for potential disease-causing mutations. If sequence analyses do not elucidate causal mutations, other candidate genes are identified and analyzed. At present, demanding molecular technologies are employed to refine the interval of disease loci and to clone novel candidate genes for mutation analyses. With the completion of the Human Genome Project,[1] candidate genes will ultimately be identified through analyses of databases that provide a compilation of sequences within a defined chromosome interval. With this advance, definition of disease genes at disease loci will likely increase quite rapidly.

HERITABLE CARDIOMYOPATHIES

Hypertrophic Cardiomyopathy

Genetic linkage studies in hypertrophic cardiomyopathy (also termed idiopathic subaortic stenosis and asymmetric septal hypertrophy)[2] have demonstrated disease loci on chromosomes 1q31, 3p, 7q3, 11p13-q13, 12q2, 14q1, 15q2, 15q14, and 19p13.2-q13.2.[3-10] Although the disease gene on chromosome 7 remains unknown, analyses of the other loci have led to the identification of mutations in genes encoding contractile proteins: cardiac troponin T, ventricular regulatory light chain, cardiac myosin binding protein C, essential light chain, β cardiac

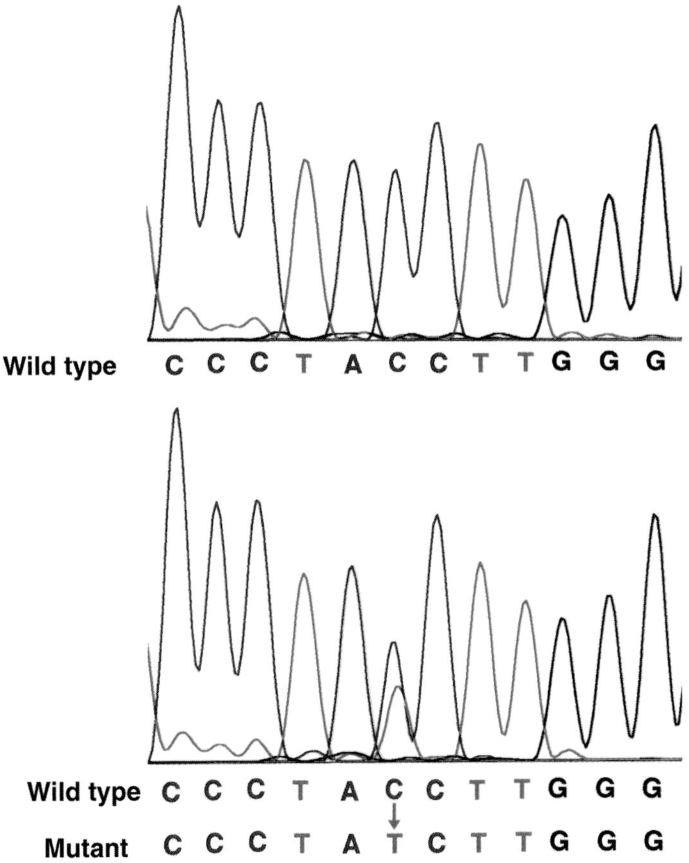

Figure 24–2 • Automated DNA analyses of the β myosin heavy-chain gene comparing wild-type sequences from an unaffected individual and from a patient with hypertrophic cardiomyopathy. Nucleotide residues are identified by color traces (cytosine, blue; thymidine, red; guanine, black; adenine, green) and defined using a single letter code. Note that the affected individual is heterozygous for a mutation (red and blue peaks) that substitutes the conserved glycine residue (position 716) of β cardiac myosin for arginine residue.

myosin heavy chain, α tropomyosin, and α cardiac actin.[11, 12] These genetic data provide a unified basis for hypertrophic cardiomyopathy and define it as a disease of the sarcomere.

Some of the clinical heterogeneity of hypertrophic cardiomyopathy can be accounted for by the substantial diversity of gene defects that cause the condition. Approximately 35% of patients with hypertrophic cardiomyopathy have a β cardiac myosin heavy-chain gene mutation.[13] More than 50 different missense mutations (Fig. 24–2) have been reported to substitute one amino acid within the globular head or head-rod junction of the β cardiac myosin heavy chain.[13–20] These defects are expressed with a high degree of penetrance, and significant myocardial hypertrophy is usually evident by two-dimensional echocardiography early in adulthood; mean maximal left ventricular wall thickness equaled 23.7 ± 7.7 mm in affected individuals from different families.[13] Survival in hypertrophic cardiomyopathy caused by a β cardiac myosin heavy-chain mutation varies considerably and is usually mutation specific.[13, 15, 17] Sudden death and disease-related death from the Arg403Gln and Arg716Trp mutations markedly shorten life expectancy (average age at death is 45 years), whereas survival is near normal for individuals carrying the Val606Met or Leu908Val mutations.[15] Although more data are required to provide a complete profile of the phenotypes associated with each myosin mutation, preliminary data clearly indicate that genotype conveys considerable risk for premature death from this disease.

More than 20 different mutations in the cardiac myosin binding protein C gene, encoded on chromosome 11, have also been identified to cause hypertrophic cardiomyopathy.[21–26] This 137-kD polypeptide is a component of the sarcomere thick filament, with structural and regulatory functions. Phosphorylation of cardiac myosin binding protein C by catecholamine-sensitive pathways[27] provides dynamic regulation of contraction. Several properties of cardiac myosin binding protein C defects distinguish this cause of hypertrophic cardiomyopathy from β cardiac myosin heavy-chain mutations. First, the types of gene defects include missense and splice signal mutations, insertions (Fig. 24–3), and deletions.[21–26] Second, cardiac hypertrophy caused by cardiac myosin binding protein C defects can be absent until late in adult life[23]: only 58% of genetically affected adults fulfilled echocardiographic criteria for disease. Third, with the exception of a Glu451Gln mutation, most cardiac myosin binding protein C defects do not adversely affect life expectancy. Early studies employing linkage analyses estimated that 15% of hypertrophic cardiomyopathy was attributable to cardiac myosin binding protein C mutations.[6] However, recognition of reduced disease penetrance associated with these gene defects, combined with good survival, may have underestimated the incidence of these mutations in hypertrophic cardiomyopathy.

A variety of mutations (missense mutations, small deletions, and mutations in splice signals) in the gene encoding cardiac troponin T cause approximately 15% of all hypertrophic cardiomyopathy.[11, 28–31] There are important

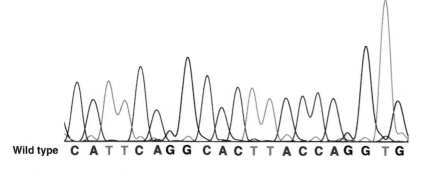

Wild type C A T T C A G G C A C T T A C C A G G T G

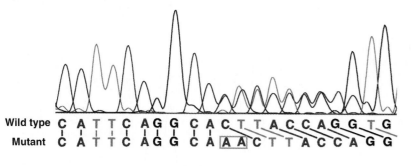

Wild type C A T T C A G G C A C T T A C C A G G T G
Mutant C A T T C A G G C A AA C T T A C C A G G

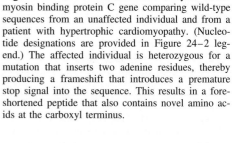

Figure 24–3 • Automated DNA analyses of the myosin binding protein C gene comparing wild-type sequences from an unaffected individual and from a patient with hypertrophic cardiomyopathy. (Nucleotide designations are provided in Figure 24–2 legend.) The affected individual is heterozygous for a mutation that inserts two adenine residues, thereby producing a frameshift that introduces a premature stop signal into the sequence. This results in a foreshortened peptide that also contains novel amino acids at the carboxyl terminus.

differences between the cardiac phenotype produced by defects in this thin filament component and that associated with other hypertrophic cardiomyopathy mutations. These defects generally cause less cardiac hypertrophy (mean maximal left ventricular wall thickness found in six different cardiac troponin T mutations was 16.7 ± 5.5 mm), and some adults with these mutations have normal cardiac wall thickness.[28] Despite incomplete penetrance, cardiac troponin T mutations are usually associated with markedly reduced survival.[28, 30] Genetic diagnosis may therefore be particularly important in identifying individuals at risk for sudden death and for defining hypertrophic cardiomyopathy in sudden death victims with only modest hypertrophy.

Mutations in other thin filament proteins are less common causes of hypertrophic cardiomyopathy, and considerably less is known about their clinical consequences. Six different mutations have been identified in cardiac troponin I, some of which produce a preponderance of apical hypertrophy.[32] Defects in the α tropomyosin gene account for less than 5% of disease,[28, 33–35] and to date, fewer than 10 missense mutations have been identified. The Asp175Asn defect may reflect a mutational hot spot within the gene,[24] as it has arisen independently in many families. Myocardial hypertrophy in response to the α tropomyosin mutation Asp175Asn varies considerably among different families, suggesting that modifying genes or the environment influence this cardiac phenotype. Survival in individuals with this defect is near normal. Fewer than five mutations have been identified in myosin regulatory or essential light chains,[4] and in one kindred a ventricular regulatory myosin defect caused marked midventricular hypertrophy and systolic midcavity obliteration (hourglass morphology). Alpha cardiac actin is the most recently defined hypertrophic cardiomyopathy gene[9]; in one family, a missense mutation (Ala295Ser) caused

highly penetrant disease characterized by a range of morphologic phenotypes.

The disease gene encoded on chromosome 7q3 has not been identified. Individuals with hypertrophic cardiomyopathy caused by this locus typically have morphologic features of disease, and exhibit Wolff-Parkinson-White syndrome.[5, 36] Elucidation of the mechanism for this associated phenotype awaits identification of the causal gene.

Dilated Cardiomyopathy

Dilated cardiomyopathy is increasingly recognized as a heritable disorder. Genetic transmission of disease is recognized in at least 25% of patients.[37–39] Although recessive and X-linked patterns of inheritance are recognized, most pedigrees indicate autosomal dominant transmission. In addition to the pattern of transmission, subgroups of heritable dilated cardiomyopathy vary according to age of onset (pediatric vs. adult) and associated clinical features (e.g., conduction disease or neuromuscular involvement). These features indicate the considerable heterogeneity of dilated cardiomyopathy and, in combination with the substantial impact this disease has on survival and reproductive health, help to explain why few disease genes have been identified.

Six disease genes, on chromosomes 1q32, 2q35, 2q31, 9q13-22, 10q1, and 15q14, cause dilated cardiomyopathy that is inherited as an autosomal dominant trait.[40–45] Although disease onset is variable, affected individuals typically have signs and symptoms of ventricular dilation and systolic dysfunction in late teenage years or early adulthood. Studies of several families with heritable dilated cardiomyopathy identified nonpentrant individuals: gene carriers in whom clinical studies are normal.

Two missense mutations[45] in α cardiac actin (chromosome 15q14)[45] and 1 missense mutation (Ile437Met)[41] in desmin (chromosome 2q35)[41] were identified by direct sequence analyses of these candidate genes in small affected families. As noted earlier, mutations in α cardiac actin are also a rare cause of hypertrophic cardiomyopathy. Based on mutation location, researchers have postulated that the consequences of force generation or force transmission account for an actin defect that causes the hypertrophic or dilated phenotype. Although multiple candidate genes have been identified at other disease loci, disease-causing genes encoded in these regions have not been identified.

Autosomal dominant inheritance of conduction system disease and late-onset dilated cardiomyopathy can be caused by mutations on chromosome 1p-1q21 or 3p25-22.[46, 47] These disorders cause onset of sinoatrial node dysfunction and atrial arrhythmias in the third to fourth decade of life. With age, progressive atrioventricular block occurs (fifth to sixth decade), concurrent with cardiac dilation and failure. Sudden death is common throughout the natural history of disease and appears to reflect unrecognized high-grade atrioventricular block and atrial or ventricular tachyarrhythmias. Pacemaker implantation and antiarrhythmics may delay disease progression, but there is no definitive evidence that these treatments prevent cardiac dilation and heart failure. Pathologic specimens from late affected individuals exhibit typical features of idiopathic dilated cardiomyopathy without inflammation, but they typically show marked fibrosis or fatty infiltration of the conduction system.

The disease gene on chromosome 1p-1q21 has recently been identified to be lamin A/C,[48] which encodes four isoforms of lamin, components of the nuclear envelope.[49] Surprisingly, lamin A/C gene mutations also cause autosomal dominant Emery-Dreifuss syndrome, a muscular dystrophy with childhood onset characterized by contractures of the elbow and Achilles tendons and adult-onset cardiac conduction abnormalities. However, muscular-skeletal abnormalities are not observed in individuals with "isolated" dilated cardiomyopathy and conduction system disease nor are they found in their family members. Determining the mechanisms by which distinct mutations in one gene cause these distinct phenotypes is an area of active research.

An unidentified gene on chromosome 19q13.2-13.3 causes progressive familial heart block (right bundle branch block and complete atrioventricular block), which can evolve into cardiac dilation and heart failure.[50] Interestingly, this genomic region encodes myotonin protein kinase, which is mutated in myotonic dystrophy.[51] Although cardiac conduction defects can occur in myotonic dystrophy, mutations in myotonin have not been demonstrated in individuals with progressive familial heart block.

Mutations in the promoter (5′ regulatory region) of the dystrophin gene cause adult-onset dilated cardiomyopathy that is transmitted as an X-linked trait. Although dystrophin mutations are more typically associated with Duchenne or Becker muscular dystrophy,[52, 53] a cardiac phenotype can predominate in some individuals.[54–56] Immunohistochemical analyses of skeletal muscle biopsies often show classic features of Duchenne or Becker dystrophy despite the absence of symptoms.

A rare disorder characterized by age-dependent sensorineural hearing loss and dilated cardiomyopathy has been mapped to chromosome 6q23-24.[57] Hearing deficits evolve throughout the school-age years and always precede cardiac disease, characterized by progressive chamber dilation and congestive heart failure.

Dilated Cardiomyopathies of Childhood

Pediatric dilated cardiomyopathies often have a genetic cause.[58] Inborn errors of metabolism (amino acid deficiencies), glycogen storage disease, and mucopolysaccharidoses, although rare, are usually recognized through neonatal screening assays or by unique histopathologies. Inherited disorders of fatty acid oxidation occur more commonly, with an incidence of 1 in 15,000 individuals.[59] In the heterozygous state, mutations in the medium-chain acyl-CoA dehydrogenase gene (MCAD, chromosome 1p) or long-chain acyl-CoA dehydrogenase (LCAD, chromosome 7) cause no pathology, but individuals who are homozygous for these defects develop dilated (occasionally hypertrophic) cardiomyopathy in childhood.[60–62] Genetic studies of the MCAD deficiencies indicate that approximately 90% of affected individuals share a common mutation, thereby simplifying DNA analyses of this disorder. Recessive mutations in other carnitine pathways also cause dilated cardiomyopathy of childhood.[63, 64] Carnitine deficiencies result from homozygous mutations in genes encoding transporter proteins that bring substrate into cells or in the translocase, which shuttle carnitine into mitochondria.

Sudden death in dilated cardiomyopathies caused by defects in fatty acid oxidation can be precipitated by periods of fast, when these pathways become important for energy production.[65] Affected patients typically have signs and symptoms of disease throughout the first and second decades of life; subsequently, symptoms abate for unknown reasons. Patient age and history can, therefore, be essential in establishing the diagnosis. Histopathologic findings of cytoplasmic lipid inclusions further support this diagnosis.

Genetic Heterogeneity

At present, one can only speculate whether inherited gene mutations at these or other loci contribute to idiopathic dilated cardiomyopathy. Identification of disease genes at each locus should provide the necessary reagents to address this hypothesis. It is noteworthy that no mutations in the 5′ sequences of dystrophin were found in DNA derived from individuals with idiopathic dilated cardiomyopathy.[66] Given that this is an X-linked cause of dilated cardiomyopathy, this result was not surprising, but it appears to indicate that identification of a considerable fraction of the entire spectrum of human dilated cardiomyopathy genes may be necessary before analyses of nonfamilial cases become worthwhile.

Restrictive Cardiomyopathy

Although familial restrictive cardiomyopathy has been reported, this disorder is exceedingly rare. Its cardiac pathology is not dissimilar from that occurring secondary to systemic disease. Biatrial enlargement is found with normal-sized ventricles; histopathology shows nonspecific features of patchy fibrosis and, notably, an absence of eosinophilia or amyloid.

Two reports[67, 68] indicate that restrictive cardiomyopathies can be transmitted as autosomal dominant traits; however, neither a chromosome location nor disease gene has been identified. The molecular basis for dominant inheritance of restrictive cardiomyopathy accompanied by conduction system disease and skeletal myopathy is mutation of the cytoskeletal protein desmin, encoded on chromosome 2q35.[69] The mechanism by which defects in the rod produce a restrictive cardiomyopathy and skeletal muscle disease whereas mutations in the peptide's carboxyl tail cause isolated dilated cardiomyopathy[41] is unknown.

Arrhythmogenic Cardiomyopathy

Arrythmogenic cardiomyopathy, formerly named arrhythmogenic right ventricular dysplasia, is an unusual disorder with an incidence that approaches 1 in 5000 individuals in certain populations.[70] Pedigree analyses of large kindreds indicate autosomal dominant inheritance with variable penetrance. Genetic linkage studies have defined five disease loci on chromosomes 1q42, 2q32, 3p23, 14q23, and 14q24.[71–75] No disease genes have been identified. Naxos syndrome appears to be a related disorder that has similar cardiac findings, in addition to hyperkeratosis of plantar palmar skin surfaces. Mutations in plakoglobin encoded on chromosome 17q21 cause Naxos syndrome.[76]

As the name of this disorder indicates, right-sided ventricular involvement typically is more substantial than left, although histopathology is usually evident in both chambers. The ventricular myocardium can be "parchment" thin or normal or have increased wall thickness, but it must exhibit localized or widespread fatty or fibrofatty replacement (3% fat and 40% fibrosis). Histologic findings also include myocardial necrosis and lymphocytic infiltration. Ventricular dilation and aneurysm are common.

Clinical symptoms of dyspnea and heart failure are rare in childhood but progress with disease duration.[77] Silent and symptomatic ventricular arrhythmias occur commonly, and sudden death may be the presenting manifestation of disease.[78] In regions of Italy, the disorder appears to be an important cause of sudden death in young adults, accounting for 12.5% of all cases.[70]

HERITABLE CARDIAC ARRHYTHMIAS

Long QT Syndrome

Arrhythmias that occur in the absence of structural cardiac pathology represent a group of clinically challenging disorders. Individuals affected with these disorders manifest syncope, seizures, or sudden death on presentation. Electrocardiographic abnormalities (preexcitation,

long QT interval, ST segment elevation) can be overt, subtle, or absent, but notably, echocardiographic assessment of heart structure and function is normal.[79, 80] Family history is a critical component of diagnosis, in that long QT syndrome,[81] Brugada syndrome,[82] Wolff-Parkinson-White syndrome,[83] atrial fibrillation,[84] and atrioventricular block[85] can each be inherited as autosomal dominant traits. As with cardiomyopathies, the familial nature of these primary arrhythmias has enabled genetic studies that have elucidated the molecular basis for long QT and Brugada syndromes. Disease loci, but not disease genes, have also been identified for familial Wolff-Parkinson-White syndrome with hypertrophic cardiomyopathy (chromosome 7q3)[5, 36] and familial atrial fibrillation (chromosome 10q22-24).[84]

The Romano-Ward syndrome, or autosomal dominant long QT syndrome, causes heightened cardiac excitability and episodic ventricular tachyarrhythmias, such as torsades de pointes and ventricular fibrillation, in otherwise healthy individuals.[79, 80] Diagnosis is made by electrocardiographic demonstration of prolonged QT interval, which may be accompanied by dysmorphic ST-T waves and repolarization abnormalities (aberrant T and U waves). Yet, diagnosis is hindered both by the inconsistency of these findings in affected individuals and by the variation of QT intervals (between 0.38 and 0.47 second) in normal individuals. Pharmacologic agents, including psychoactive and antiarrhythmic medications, also prolong QT intervals.

Mutations in five different genes that encode components of cardiac ion channels cause this disorder. Four genes encode subunits of the slowly and rapidly activating delayed rectifier potassium channels: KVLQT1 (chromosome 11q15.5),[86] HERG (chromosome 7q35-36),[87] and KCNE1 and KCNE2 (chromosome 21q22).[88, 89] Mutations in genes encoding the cardiac sodium channel (SCN5A, chromosome 3p21-24)[90] and an unknown gene on chromosome 4q25-27[91] also cause Romano-Ward syndrome. Although electrocardiographic findings do not discriminate between these distinct genetic etiologies, effective therapies (sodium channel blockage or drugs to open potassium channels) can be predicated on the channel properties perturbed by distinct molecular etiologies. Mutations in potassium channel subunits reduce function and, therefore, prolong action potentials.[92] In contrast, defects in the sodium channel cause a gain of function[93] that destabilizes inactivation of the channel, with resultant repetitive channel opening and prolongation of action potentials.

In addition to autosomal dominant inheritance, long QT syndrome can be transmitted as a recessive trait also called the Jervell and Lange-Nielsen syndrome.[51] This rare variant occurs in fewer than six cases per million individuals and is readily identified by the coinheritance of congenital deafness. Individuals with long QT syndrome and deafness have a high incidence of sudden death and shortened survival. Homozygous mutations of subunits of the cardiac slow delayed rectifier potassium channel encoded by KVLQT1 locus[94, 95] cause the Jervell and Lange-Nielsen syndrome.

As with hypertrophic cardiomyopathy, there is significant complexity in gene-based diagnosis for long QT syndrome, and at present, this remains a research endeavor. Recent genetic analyses of 300 unrelated individuals[96] with known or suspected long QT arrhythmias identified a causal mutation in less than one in three individuals. Missense mutations were most common, and approximately 80% of all reported defects occurred in the KVLQT1 or HERG genes. Continued compilation of the entire spectrum of the clinical consequences of long QT syndrome gene defects should help to delineate appropriate therapeutic options for genetically affected, presymptomatic individuals.

Brugada Syndrome

Inherited arrhythmia in the absence of structural heart disease can also be caused by Brugada syndrome,[82] a rare autosomal dominant disorder diagnosed by electrocardiographic abnormalities, including right bundle branch block with right precordial ST segment elevation (> 0.1 mV in leads V1–V3). Left axis deviation is often present, but the QT interval is not prolonged. Ventricular fibrillation is the most common arrhythmic event, with age of onset usually after the third decade. The electrical manifestations of Brugada syndrome implicate defects in the cardiac sodium channels. Direct sequence analyses of the SCN5A gene in several affected families have identified some disease-causing mutations.[96] The identification of additional mutations and characterization of their clinical consequences can be expected.

HERITABLE CONGENITAL MALFORMATIONS

Congenital heart defects are common human malformations that cause significant morbidity and mortality in addition to substantial social and economic costs. Birth defect registries indicate that congenital heart defects occur in approximately 1% of human live births and 10% of stillbirths.[97, 98] Epidemiologic and pathologic investigations of human congenital heart malformations have identified many teratogens, infectious agents, and factors in the maternal environment as important etiologies for some cardiac defects. However, in most cases, the cause remains unknown. Recent molecular studies indicate that some congenital heart defects are caused by gene mutations that are transmitted as dominant or recessive X-linked or autosomal traits.

Holt-Oram Syndrome

Holt-Oram syndrome is a rare autosomal dominant disorder that occurs in fewer than 1 in 100,000 individuals and causes both upper limb malformations in tissues that evolve from the embryonic radial rays and cardiac septation defects.[99] Skeletal abnormalities range from subtle (radiographically detected) malformations of the carpal bones to more obvious thumb abnormalities (triphalangism or aplasia) and phocomelia. Cardiac abnormalities occur in 85% of individuals with Holt-Oram syndrome and commonly include single or multiple atrial ostium se-

cundum defects or muscular ventricular septal defects. Severely affected individuals may manifest "Swiss cheese" septa, and rare individuals with atrioventricular canal defects have been reported. Conduction disease is a common feature of Holt-Oram syndrome and ranges from sinus bradycardia and first-degree atrioventricular block to atrial fibrillation and high-grade atrioventricular block. Electrical abnormalities are independent of the presence or size of septation defects. Associated cardiac anomalies include anomalous pulmonary venous drainage, abnormal isomerism, mitral valve prolapse, persistent left superior vena cava, and, more rarely, hypoplastic left heart syndrome and tetralogy of Fallot.

Holt-Oram syndrome is genetically homogeneous, and all affected individuals have a mutation in TBX5, encoded on chromosome 12q.[100–102] TBX5 is a member of the T-box transcription gene family, which, like other members, shares a conserved DNA binding motif. In lower species, these genes appear to have critical roles in axial patterning of organs during development. In humans, TBX5 appears to pattern the radial side of the upper limb and, in the heart, may participate in the establishment of axes that ultimately specify the location and development of septal structures.

Congenital Heart Defects and Conduction System Disease

Autosomal dominant transmission of congenital heart defects with a late onset of conduction system disease can be caused by mutations in Nkx2-5, encoded on chromosome 5q.[103] The most common structural malformation is secundum atrial septal defect, but subvalvular aortic stenosis, ventricular septal defects, tetralogy of Fallot, and pulmonary atresia have also been observed. Affected individuals have no evidence of aberrant cardiac electrophysiology at birth, but progressive atrioventricular delay develops late in childhood and beyond. Unrecognized conduction system disease appears to account for the high incidence of sudden death in some affected families.

Situs Abnormalities

Heterotaxy is a primary disorder of left-right axis development during embryogenesis. Heterotaxy disorders can be classified as situs solitus, indicating randomization of left-right orientation, or situs inversus, indicating mirror-image reversal of lateralized structures. Estimates indicate a comparable incidence for situs ambiguus and situs inversus of approximately 1 in 10,000 births.[97] Situs inversus is usually not associated with congenital anomalies, whereas situs ambiguus typically causes complex, often fatal, cardiac defects. Heterotaxy disorders are sporadic or inherited as autosomal recessive, dominant, or X-linked traits.[104] Mutations in the X chromosome gene ZIC-3,[105] a zinc-finger transcription factor, cause situs abnormalities associated with complex heart malformations, and variable combinations of gastrointestinal malrotations with genitourinary and central nervous system defects. Heterozygous women have either no detectable abnormalities or situs inversus.

HERITABLE DISORDERS OF THE GREAT VESSELS

Marfan Syndrome

Marfan syndrome is the most common disorder of connective tissue, with manifestations in three organ systems: skeletal, ocular, and cardiovascular.[106] Affected individuals are usually tall with arachnodactyly and exhibit pectus excavatum and carinatum with kyphoscoliosis, in addition to increased joint laxity, a highly arched palate, and multiple skin striae. Ocular findings include ectopia lentis, myopia, and a predisposition to retinal detachment. Cardiovascular pathology[107] accounts for decreased survival, and individuals typically exhibit myxomatous degeneration of cardiac valves, producing prolapse and insufficiency and enlargement of the aorta. Progressive aortic root dilation at the sinuses of Valsalva contributes to aortic insufficiency and, in conjunction with ascending thoracic aortic aneurysm, accounts for most of the morbidity and mortality of Marfan syndrome. Aneurysm can develop in any aortic segment and affected individuals are at a markedly increased risk for aortic dissection. Contractural arachnodactyly shares skeletal abnormalities with Marfan syndrome but is distinguished by the absence of cardiovascular disease. Mutations in the fibrillin-2 gene on chromosome 5q23 cause congenital contractural arachnodactyly.[108]

Marfan syndrome is transmitted as an autosomal dominant disorder, although approximately 25% of cases reflect de novo mutations.[109] Linkage analysis in affected kindreds indicates that the disease is caused by mutations in fibrillin-1, encoded on chromosome 15q.[110] A second locus has been mapped to chromosome 3p24.2-p25.[111] Fibrillin-1 is a microfilament protein that stabilizes elastic fibers; it is widely expressed in connective tissue. More than 60 unique fibrillin-1 mutations have been identified in unrelated individuals with Marfan syndrome.[110] Most are missense mutations, although small deletions have been noted. In vitro analyses of mutant fibrillin indicate that these defects adversely affect connective tissue integrity.

Familial Aortic Aneurysm

Familial aortic aneurysm developing as an isolated vascular pathology and as a component of a connective tissue syndrome is caused by defects in collagen synthesis or assembly. Most prominent are subtypes of Ehlers-Danlos syndrome.[51] Ehlers-Danlos type IV is an autosomal recessive disorder characterized by hyperextensible joints, thin and fragile skin, and arterial and bowel rupture. The associated cardiovascular phenotypes include mitral valve prolapse, varicose veins, arterial tortuosity, and abdominal aortic aneurysm. Autosomal dominant Ehlers-Danlos type IV exhibits similar skin and skeletal findings with vasculopathy and arterial rupture, but true aneurysm formation is less common. Nonetheless, both forms of Ehlers-Danlos type IV are the result of mutations in the collagen 3A1 gene encoded on chromosome 2q31.[112] Deletions and missense mutations have been noted in this disorder.

Ehlers-Danlos type VI exhibits similar skeletal and dermatologic findings, in addition to ocular and cardiovascular abnormalities (mitral valve prolapse, multiple arterial aneurysms, carotid cavernous fistula, and dissecting aneurysm).[51] Mutations in the lysyl hydroxylase gene encoded on chromosome 1p36.3-p36.2 cause this recessive disorder,[113] presumably by perturbing the formation of hydroxylysine in collagens and collagenous proteins. It is critical for normal cross-linking and assembly into the extracellular matrix.

Supravalvular Aortic Stenosis

Supravalvular aortic stenosis[51, 114, 115] is a rare disorder that occurs in isolation as an autosomal dominant trait or as a component of Williams syndrome (elfin facial features, mental retardation, extroverted personality, and hypercalcemia). In both disorders, stenosis of the peripheral pulmonary vasculature is often evident. Genetic studies[116, 117] of familial supravalvular aortic stenosis have demonstrated that deletion or rearrangements of the elastin gene on chromosome 7q11.2 cause this disorder. Williams syndrome is often associated with complex chromosomal abnormalities[118] that include the elastin gene, possibly indicating an effect on several contiguous genes in addition to elastin. The precise biochemical consequences of elastin mutations remain unknown; however, defects may disrupt elastin assembly into extracellular matrix, as occurs with fibrillin and collagen mutations. Collectively, these studies appear to indicate that vascular malformations reflect perturbations in extracellular matrix synthesis and assembly.

PERSPECTIVES AND FUTURE DIRECTIONS

The first impression of an overview of molecular etiologies of inherited cardiovascular disorders can be daunting in its complexity. A single pathologic entity can result from myriad different mutations in distinct genes. Although at first perplexing, genetic heterogeneity can both help explain clinical diversity and provide insights into pathogenetic mechanisms. For example, patients with familial hypertrophic cardiomyopathy exhibit a wide variation in age of onset, severity of hypertrophy, and survival. Although these factors are certainly influenced in part by lifestyle and environment, correlation of genotype with phenotype has indicated that an individual's genetic basis for disease plays a significant role in gene expression.

Genetic heterogeneity has also provided insights into the mechanism of disease. For example, elucidation of the causes of long QT syndrome, hypertrophic cardiomyopathy, congenital malformations, and heritable vascular disorders led to the discovery that proteins encoded by different mutated genes often have related cellular functions (Table 24–1). Long QT syndrome is a disorder of cardiac ion channels; congenital heart disease is caused by mutations in genes that pattern the human heart. These general

TABLE 24-1 • **Genetic Mutations That Define Pathogenetic Mechanisms of Cardiac Disease**

	Locus	Mutated Gene	Protein Function
Congenital heart defects			
Holt-Oram syndrome	12q2	TBX5	Embryonic transcription factor
ASD, VSD with atrioventricular block	5q35	NKX2-5	Embryonic transcription factor
Heterotaxy	Xq26.2	ZIC3	Embryonic transcription factor
Heritable arrhythmias			
Long QT syndrome	3p21-24	SCN5A	Cardiac ion channel
	4q25-27	?	?
	7q35-36	HERG	Cardiac ion channel
	11p15.5	KVLQT1	Cardiac ion channel
	21q22	KCNE1 and KCNE2	Cardiac ion channel
Brugada syndrome	3p21-24	SCN5A	Cardiac ion channel
Wolff-Parkinson-White syndrome	7q3	?	?
Familial heart block	19q13	?	?
Cardiomyopathy			
Dilated	1q32	?	?
	2q35	Desmin	Cytoskeletal protein
	2q31	?	?
	9q13-22	?	?
	10q1	?	?
	15q14	α Cardiac actin	Cytoskeletal protein
Dilated with conduction system disease	1q21	Lamin A/C	Nuclear cytoskeletal protein
	3p25-22		
Hypertrophic	1q31	Cardiac troponin I	Sarcomere protein
	3p	Regulatory light chain	Sarcomere protein
	7q3	?	?
	11p13-q13	Myosin binding protein C	Sarcomere protein
	12q2	Troponin I	Sarcomere protein
	14q1	β Myosin heavy chain	Sarcomere protein
	15q2	α Tropomyosin	Sarcomere protein
	15q14	Cardiac actin	Sarcomere protein
	19p13.2-q13.2	Essential light chain	Sarcomere protein

classifications have potential importance for understanding related disorders. Recognition of the role of cardiac ion channels in long QT syndrome prompted analyses and led to the identification of the genetic causes for Jervell and Lange-Nielsen syndrome and Brugada syndrome. Knowledge of the molecular etiologies of inherited disorders has also defined gene defects in nonfamilial disease. Approximately 33% of cases of Marfan syndrome and hypertrophic cardiomyopathy occur without recognized family history.[51] Direct sequence analyses of genes involved in the hereditary forms of these pathologies have indicated that de novo mutations in the same genes account for some sporadic cases. Genetic analyses should therefore help in confirming diagnoses and indicating the potential for new onset of familial disease.

Gene-based diagnoses have enormous potential for precisely defining etiology, regardless of confounding variables. The importance of and implicit responsibility associated with this capacity are perhaps most easily recognized when considering the differential diagnosis of sudden death. In the setting of significant coronary disease, active myocardial inflammation, or overt cardiovascular malformation, diagnosis can be straightforward. However, when abnormalities are mild or absent, DNA-based analyses can be invaluable (Fig. 24–4). Extraction of DNA from any tissue or blood generally provides sufficient genetic material to allow multiple analyses. (Preservatives cross-link DNA and reduce the size of fragments obtained; DNA isolation should therefore occur before tissue preservation.) Clearly, the definitive diagnosis of the cause of sudden death has enormous medical, psychological, and ethical import for surviving relatives. As gene-based diagnosis becomes more common, it is imperative that these data be appropriately conveyed to physicians and family members. More immediately, identification of pathologies that are transmitted as heritable traits (see Fig. 24–1) should prompt clinical evaluations of other family members at risk.

Today, gene-based diagnosis is largely a research endeavor. Despite the ever-increasing numbers of disease genes identified and the ease of obtaining genetic material for analysis, multiple issues inflate the time and expense required for DNA analysis. Dominant mutations are often private or family specific, and because affected individuals are heterozygous, analyses must be able to distinguish a single mutant nucleotide in the setting of the normal residues (see Figs. 24–2 and 24–3). Heterogeneous disorders require analyses of multiple, often large genes. For gene-based diagnosis to have clinical usefulness, analyses must, therefore, be sufficiently expeditious and highly accurate. Rapid advances in capillary methodology for automated DNA sequencing and DNA chip technologies indicate a high probability for the evolution of efficient and accurate strategies in genotyping. The educated and ethi-

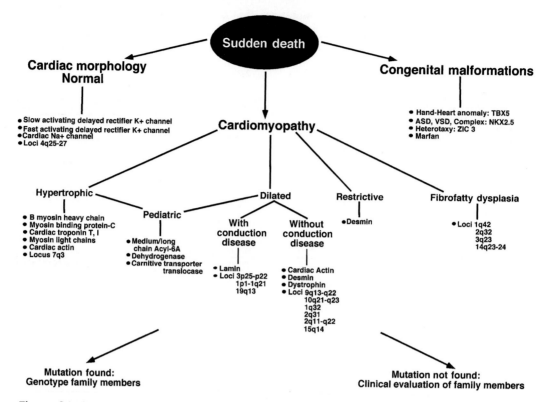

Figure 24–4 • Evaluation of heritable disorders that cause sudden death. Note that pathologic or gene-based diagnosis of a heritable disease should trigger family studies.

cal use of such information toward improved health care delivery remains a critical societal issue.

IMPLICATIONS FOR THE PATHOLOGIST

Many recent developments have defined the genetic causes of abnormalities affecting the heart and great vessels and, in some cases, have permitted an understanding of the mechanism by which they cause disease. From a research perspective, new insights into pathophysiology are particularly well illustrated by studies of Marfan syndrome, hypertrophic cardiomyopathy, and long QT syndrome. In addition, basic mechanisms of development and gene regulation in humans have been elucidated, and definitive links to disease established.

The practical applications of this information for diagnosis, prognosis, and family counseling have enormous potential but remain largely unfulfilled. We believe that after the death of any individual with a suspected family history or morphologic characteristics of any of the known genetic cardiovascular diseases, the heart should receive especially careful examination, including informed and complete dissection and histologic examination. This may require formal consultation with a cardiovascular pathologist. Fresh tissue or tissue in paraffin blocks should be kept indefinitely, because it can be used for DNA analysis, if appropriate. Although routine molecular diagnosis is not widely available at present, it will likely become available in the future. Research laboratories can be consulted on an ad hoc basis.

The importance of genetic diagnosis is particularly well illustrated in sudden cardiac death. As in other cases, the investigation of this type of death must include a complete autopsy with toxicology and appropriate histology, as well as a scene investigation and interviews with family and physicians. However, such a complete workup may reveal only an ostensibly normal heart or one with equivocal gross or microscopic findings. Cases of witnessed, instantaneous death without structurally demonstrable cause at autopsy lead to the compelling conclusion that the decedent had a lethal cardiac arrhythmia, cause unknown. However, pathologists, accustomed to demonstrating a structural basis for all diagnoses, rest uncomfortably with a functionally descriptive cause of death, and molecular biology has taught us that pathologic anatomy at the gross or microscopic level need not be present in some well-defined causes of sudden death.

Indeed, postmortem genetic studies are of special value in instances of sudden cardiac death with equivocal or no anatomic findings. It is likely that the number of deaths due to hypertrophic cardiomyopathy, for example, is vastly underestimated, because the anatomic findings associated with certain mutations (e.g., troponin or myosin binding protein C) are subtle. Correlating sophisticated molecular studies with historical and autopsy data will lead to more precise characterization of this entity and the creation of subgroups. Definition of these subgroups has already revealed important prognostic information. In dilated cardiomyopathy, where the heart is nonspecifically enlarged and dilated and histologically shows myocyte hypertrophy with fibrosis, the underlying cause is usually unknown. However, molecular definition of familial cases has improved diagnostic precision and will likely be of benefit to relatives. The molecular definition of some rhythm disturbances that cannot be demonstrated anatomically (such as the long QT syndrome) has substantial importance.

Family counseling for relatives of those who have died with a defined molecular cardiac defect is also important. Often the forensic pathologist is the sole professional contact for the family, and he or she must recognize the importance of this diagnosis for survivors and suggest consultation with a cardiologist. Screening may identify those in need of therapy and may prevent future deaths. Resources for families include societies dedicated to certain of these diseases and information on the Internet. Finally, the value of providing a precise cause of death for the peace of mind of the decedent's family cannot be overestimated.

Determination of the cause and manner of death in certain instances of apparent sudden cardiac death can have major legal implications. For example, molecular confirmation for classifying the death of an infant or child or of a person in legal detention may exonerate caregivers or custodial personnel. Insurance implications are another consideration, particularly when death occurs at a place of employment.

Numerous problems must be solved before this information can be applied routinely for diagnosis in a hospital or forensic setting. Some of the mutations have incomplete penetrance. Many diseases have a high number of potential mutations in several different genes. These mutations may arise de novo. Opportunity for screening family members at risk must be provided. How should these tests be performed? With the recent advances enabling high throughput analysis of genetic abnormalities (including automated DNA sequencing) facilitated by the Human Genome Project, these problems may be increasingly soluble.

Effective collaboration remains to be established among pathologists, cardiovascular pathologists, and molecular geneticists to identify both the full range of mutations responsible for the diseases discussed in this chapter and those not readily definable with current methods. Eventually, a means for rapid, easy, accurate diagnosis, possibly employing DNA microarray technology, will be established. For example, someday it may be possible to screen for all known mutations related to sudden cardiac death on a single microarray chip. In the meantime, pathologists must acknowledge that there are instances of sudden cardiac death of unknown etiology, classify them as such, and retain tissue for future molecular study.

An additional critical issue is yet unresolved. Contemporary procedures and policies for autopsy permission and other clinical or research use of otherwise discarded tissue do not permit unspecified genetic testing. Additional informed consent is required, because safeguards to preserve patient or source anonymity are not currently in place. Because the generation of genetic data and correlations with pathologic anatomy aid disease diagnosis, enhance understanding of mechanisms of disease, and potentially improve the lives of survivors, it is incumbent on pathologists and other professionals to develop the appropriate legal and ethical framework and the policies and procedures that will permit the full realization of the beneficial potential of genetic testing in this context.

REFERENCES

1. Collins F: Medical and social consequences of the human genome project. N Engl J Med 341:28, 1999
2. Spirito P, Seidman CE, McKenna WJ, et al: The management of hypertrophic cardiomyopathy. N Engl J Med 336:775, 1997
3. Watkins H, MacRae C, Thierfelder L, et al: A disease locus for familial hypertrophic cardiomyopathy maps to chromosome 1q3. Nat Genet 3:333, 1993
4. Poetter K, Jiang H, Hassanzadeh S, et al: Mutations in either the essential or regulatory light chains of myosin are associated with a rare myopathy in human heart and skeletal muscle. Nat Genet 13:63, 1996
5. MacRae CA, Ghaisas N, Kass S, et al: Familial hypertrophic cardiomyopathy with Wolff-Parkinson-White syndrome maps to a locus on chromosome 7q3. J Clin Invest 96:1216, 1995
6. Carrier L, Hengstenberg C, Beckmann JS, et al: Mapping of a novel gene for familial hypertrophic cardiomyopathy to chromosome 11. Nat Genet 4:311, 1993
7. Jarcho JA, McKenna W, Pare JAP, et al: Mapping a gene for familial hypertrophic cardiomyopathy to chromosome 14q1. N Engl J Med 321:1372, 1989
8. Thierfelder L, MacRae C, Watkins H, et al: A familial hypertrophic cardiomyopathy locus maps to chromosome 15q2. Proc Natl Acad Sci U S A 90:6270, 1993
9. Mogensen J, Klausen IC, Pedersen AK, et al: α-Cardiac actin is a novel disease gene in familial hypertrophic cardiomyopathy. J Clin Invest 103:R39, 1999
10. Bhavsar PK, Brand NJ, Yacoub MH, et al: Isolation and characterization of the human cardiac troponin I gene (TNNI3). Genomics 35:11, 1996
11. Thierfelder L, Watkins H, MacRae C, et al: α-Tropomyosin and cardiac troponin T mutations cause familial hypertrophic cardiomyopathy: A disease of the sarcomere. Cell 77:701, 1994
12. Vikstrom KL, Leinwand LA: Contractile protein mutations and heart disease. Curr Opin Cell Biol 8:97, 1996
13. Watkins H, Rosenzweig A, Hwang D-S, et al: Characteristics and prognostic implications of myosin missense mutations in familial hypertrophic cardiomyopathy. N Engl J Med 326:1108, 1992
14. Dausse E, Komajda M, Dubourg O, et al: Familial hypertrophic cardiomyopathy: Microsatellite haplotyping and identification of a hot-spot for mutations in the β-myosin heavy chain gene. J Clin Invest 92:2807, 1993
15. Anan R, Greve G, Thierfelder L, et al: Prognostic implications of novel β-myosin heavy chain gene mutations that cause familial hypertrophic cardiomyopathy. J Clin Invest 93:280, 1994
16. Consevage M, Salada GC, Baylen BG, et al: A new missense mutation, Arg719G1n, in the β-cardiac heavy chain myosin gene of patients with familial hypertrophic cardiomyopathy. Hum Mol Genet 3:1025, 1994
17. Fananapazir L, Dalakas MC, Cyran F, et al: Missense mutations in the β myosin heavy chain gene cause central core disease in hypertrophic cardiomyopathy. Proc Natl Acad Sci U S A 90:3993, 1993
18. Arai S, Matsuoka R, Hirayama K, et al: Missense mutation of the β-cardiac myosin heavy chain gene in hypertrophic cardiomyopathy. Am J Med Genet 58:267, 1995
19. Marian AJ, Yu QT, Mares A, et al: Detection of a new mutation in the β-myosin heavy chain gene in an individual with hypertrophic cardiomyopathy. J Clin Invest 90:2156, 1992
20. Nishi H, Kimura A, Harada H, et al: A myosin missense mutation, not a null allele, causes familial hypertrophic cardiomyopathy. Circulation 91:2911, 1995
21. Watkins H, Conner D, Thierfelder L, et al: Mutations in the cardiac myosin binding protein-C gene on chromosome 11 cause familial hypertrophic cardiomyopathy. Nat Genet 11:434, 1995
22. Bonne G, Carrier L, Bercovici J, et al: Cardiac myosin binding protein-C gene splice acceptor site mutation is associated with familial hypertrophic cardiomyopathy. Nat Genet 11:438, 1995

23. Niimura H, Bachinski LL, Sangwatanaroj S, et al: Mutations in the gene for cardiac myosin-binding protein C and late-onset familial hypertrophic cardiomyopathy. N Engl J Med 338:1248, 1998

24. Rottbauer W, Gautel M, Zehelein J, et al: Novel splice donor site mutation in the cardiac myosin binding protein C gene in familial hypertrophic cardiomyopathy: Characterization of cardiac transcript and protein. J Clin Invest 100:475, 1997

25. Yu B, French JA, Carrier L, et al: Molecular pathology of familial hypertrophic cardiomyopathy caused by mutations in the myosin binding protein C gene. J Med Genet 35:205, 1998

26. Moolman-Smook JC, Mayosi B, Brink P, et al: Identification of a new missense mutation in MyBP-C associated with hypertrophic cardiomyopathy. J Med Genet 35:253, 1998

27. Sata M, Stafford WF, Mabuchi K, et al: The motor domain and the regulatory domain of myosin solely dictate enzymatic activity and phosphorylation-dependent regulation, respectively. Proc Natl Acad Sci U S A 94:91, 1997

28. Watkins H, McKenna WJ, Thierfelder L, et al: Mutations in the genes for cardiac troponin T and α-tropomyosin in hypertrophic cardiomyopathy. N Engl J Med 332:1058, 1995

29. Forissier JF, Carrier L, Farza H, et al: Codon 102 of the cardiac troponin T gene is a putative hot spot for mutations in familial hypertrophic cardiomyopathy. Circulation 94:3069, 1996

30. Moolman JC, Corfield VA, Posen B, et al: Sudden death due to troponin T mutations. J Am Coll Cardiol 29:549, 1997

31. Nakajima-Taniguchi C, Matsui H, Fujio Y, et al: Novel missense mutation in cardiac troponin T gene found in Japanese patient with hypertrophic cardiomyopathy. J Mol Cell Cardiol 29:839, 1997

32. Kimura A, Harada H, Park JE, et al: Mutations in the cardiac troponin I gene associated with hypertrophic cardiomyopathy. Nat Genet 16:379, 1997

33. Watkins H, Anan R, Coviello DA, et al: A de novo mutation in α-tropomyosin that causes hypertrophic cardiomyopathy. Circulation 91:2302, 1995

34. Nakajima-Taniguchi C, Matsui H, Nagata S, et al: Novel missense mutation in α-tropomyosin gene found in Japanese patients with hypertrophic cardiomyopathy. J Mol Cell Cardiol 27:2053, 1995

35. Yamauchi-Takihara K, Nakajima-Taniguchi C, Matsui H, et al: Clinical implications of hypertrophic cardiomyopathy associated with mutations in the α-tropomyosin gene. Heart 76:63, 1996

36. Mehdirad AA, Fatkin D, DiMarco JP, et al: Electrophysiologic characteristics of accessory atrioventricular connections in an inherited form of Wolff-Parkinson-White syndrome. J Cardiovasc Electrophysiol 10:1629, 1999

37. Keeling PJ, Gang G, Smith G, et al: Familial dilated cardiomyopathy in the United Kingdom. Br Heart J 73:417, 1995

38. Grünig E, Tasman JA, Kucherer H, et al: Frequency and phenotypes of familial dilated cardiomyopathy. J Am Coll Cardiol 31:186, 1998

39. Mestroni L, Rocco C, Gregori D, at al: Familial dilated cardiomyopathy: Evidence for genetic and phenotypic heterogeneity. J Am Coll Cardiol 34:181 1999

40. Durand JB, Bachinski LL, Bieling LC, et al: Localization of a gene responsible for familial dilated cardiomyopathy to chromosome 1q32. Circulation 92:3384, 1995

41. Li D, Tapscoft T, Gonzalez O, et al: Desmin mutation responsible for idiopathic dilated cardiomyopathy. Circulation 100:461, 1999

42. Siu BL, Niimura H, Osbourne JA, et al: Familial dilated cardiomyopathy locus maps to chromosome 2q31. Circulation 99:1022, 1999

43. Krajinovic M, Pinamonti B, Sinagra G, et al: Linkage of familial dilated cardiomyopathy to chromosome 9. Am J Hum Genet 57:846, 1995

44. Bowles KR, Gajarski R, Porter P, et al: Gene mapping an autosomal dominant familial dilated cardiomyopathy to chromosome 10q21-23. J Clin Invest 98:1355, 1996

45. Olson TM, Michels VV, Thibodeau SN, et al: Actin mutations in dilated cardiomyopathy, a heritable form of heart failure. Science 280:751, 1998

46. Kass S, MacRae C, Graber HL, et al: A genetic defect that causes conduction system disease and dilated cardiomyopathy maps to 1p1-1q1. Nat Genet 7:546, 1994

47. Olson TM, Keating MT: Mapping a cardiomyopathy locus to chromosome 3p22-p25. J Clin Invest 97:528, 1996

48. Fatkin D, MacRae C, Sasaki T, et al: Missense mutations in the rod domain of the lamin A/C gene as causes of dilated cardiomyopathy and conduction-system disease. N Engl J Med 341:1715, 1999

49. Stuurman N, Heins S, Aebi U: Nuclear lamins: Their structure, assembly and interactions. J Struct Biol 122:42, 1998

50. Brink PA, Ferreira A, Moolman JC, et al: Gene for progressive familial heart block type I maps to chromosome 19q31. Circulation 91:1633, 1995

51. Online Mendelian Inheritance in Man (OMIM). Baltimore, Center for Medical Genetics, Johns Hopkins University, and Bethesda, National Center for Biotechnology Information, National Library of Medicine, 1999. http://www3.ncbi.nlm.nih.gov/omim/

52. Muntoni F, Cau M, Ganau A, et al: Deletion of the dystrophin muscle-promoter region associated with X-linked dilated cardiomyopathy. N Engl J Med 329:921, 1993

53. Milasin J, Muntoni F, Severini GM, et al: A point mutation in the 5′ splice of the dystrophin gene first intron responsible for X-linked dilated cardiomyopathy. Hum Mol Genet 5:73, 1996

54. Muntoni F, Di Lenarda A, Porcu M, et al. Dystrophin gene abnormalities in two patients with idiopathic dilated cardiomyopathy. Heart 78:608, 1997

55. Towbin JA, Hejtmancik F, Brink P, et al: X-linked cardiomyopathy (XLCM): Molecular genetic evidence of linkage to the Duchenne muscular dystrophy (dystrophin) gene at the Xp21 locus. Circulation 87:1854, 1993

56. Mutoni F, Wilson L, Marrosu G, et al: A mutation in the dystrophin gene selectively affecting dystrophin expression in the heart. J Clin Invest 96:693, 1995

57. Schönberger J, Levy H, Grünig E, et al: Dilated cardiomyopathy and sensorineural hearing loss: A heritable syndrome that maps to 6q23-24. Circulation 101:1812, 1999

58. Schwartz ML, Cox GF, Lin AE: Clinical approach to genetic cardiomyopathy in children. Circulation 94:2021, 1996

59. Kelly DP, Strauss AW: Inherited cardiomyopathies. N Engl J Med 330:913, 1994

60. Kelly DP, Whelan AJ, Ogden ML, et al: Molecular characterization of medium-chain acyl-CoA dehydrogenase deficiency. Proc Natl Acad Sci U S A 87:9236, 1990

61. Rocchiccioli F, Wanders RJ, Aubourg P, et al: Deficiency of long-chain 3-hydroxylacyl-CoA dehydrogenase: A cause of lethal myopathy and cardiomyopathy in early childhood. Pediatr Res 28:657, 1990

62. Kelly DP, Hale DE, Rutledge SL, et al: Molecular basis of inherited medium-chain acyl-CoA dehydrogenase deficiency causing sudden child death. J Inherit Metab Dis 15:171, 1992

63. Yokota I, Indo Y, Coates PM, et al: Molecular basis of medium chain acyl-coenzyme A dehydrogenase deficiency: An A to G transition at position 985 that causes a lysine-304 to glutamate substitution in the mature protein is the single prevalent mutation. J Clin Invest 86:1000, 1990

64. Stanley CA, Hale DE, Berry GT, et al: A deficiency of carnitine-acylcarnitine translocase in the inner mitochondrial membrane. N Engl J Med 327:19, 1992

65. Taroni F, Verderio E, Fiorucci S, et al: Molecular characterization of inherited carnitine palmitoyltransferase II deficiency. Proc Natl Acad Sci U S A 89:8429, 1992

66. Michels VV, Pastores GM, Moll PP, et al: Dystrophin analysis in idiopathic dilated cardiomyopathy. J Med Genet 30:955, 1993

67. Aroney C, Bett N, Radford D: Familial restrictive cardiomyopathy. Aust N Z J Med 18:877, 1988

68. Fitzpatrick AP, Shapiro LM, Rickards AF, et al: Familial restrictive cardiomyopathy with atrioventricular block and skeletal myopathy. Br Heart J 63:114, 1990

69. Goldfarb LG, Park K-Y, Cervenakova L, et al: Missense mutations in desmin associated with familial cardiac and skeletal myopathy. Nat Genet 19:402, 1998

70. Thiene G, Basso C, Danieli GA, et al: Arrhythmogenic right ventricular cardiomyopathy. Trends Cardiovasc Med 7:84, 1997

71. Rampazzo A, Nava A, Erne P, et al: A new locus for arrhythmogenic right ventricular cardiomyopathy (ARVD2) maps to chromosome 1q42-q43. Hum Mol Genet 4:2151, 1995

72. Rampazzo A, Nava A, Miorin M, et al: ARVD4, a new locus for arrhythmogenic right ventricular cardiomyopathy, maps to chromosome 2 long arm. Genomics 45:259, 1997

73. Ahmad F, Li D, Karibe A, et al: Localization of a gene responsi-

ble for arrhythmogenic right ventricular dysplasia to chromosome 3p23. Circulation 98:2791, 1998

74. Rampazzo A, Nava A, Danieli GA, et al: The gene for arrhythmogenic right ventricular cardiomyopathy maps to chromosome 14q23-q24. Hum Mol Genet 3:959, 1994

75. Severini GM, Krajiovic M, Pinamonti B, et al: A new locus for arrhythmogenic right ventricular dysplasia on the long arm of chromosome 14. Genomics 31:193, 1996

76. McCoy G, Protonotarios N, Crosby A, et al: Identification of a deletion in plakoglobin in arrhythmogenic right ventricular cardiomyopathy with palmoplantar keratoderma and wooly hair (Naxos disease). Lancet 355:2119, 2000

77. Daliento L, Turrini P, Nava A, et al: Arrhythmogenic right ventricular cardiomyopathy in young versus adult patients: Similarities and differences. J Am Coll Cardiol 25:655, 1995

78. Corrado D, Thiene G, Nava A, et al: Sudden death in young competitive athletes: Clinicopathologic correlation in 22 cases. Am J Med 89:588, 1990

79. Vincent GM, Timothy K, Leppert M, et al: The spectrum of symptoms and QT intervals in carriers of the gene for long QT syndrome. N Engl J Med 327:846, 1992

80. Priori SG, Napolitano C, Schwartz PJ: Low penetrance in the long QT-syndrome: Clinical impact. Circulation 9:529, 1999

81. Moss A, Schwartz PJ, Crampton R, et al: The long QT syndrome: Prospective longitudinal study of 328 families. Circulation 84:1136, 1991

82. Alings M, Wilde A: Brugada syndrome: Clinical data and suggested physiological mechanism. Circulation 99:666, 1999

83. Vidaillet HJ Jr, Pressley JC, Hencke E, et al: Familial occurrence of accessory atrioventricular pathways (preexcitation syndrome). N Engl J Med 317:65, 1987

84. Brugada R, Tapscott T, Czernuszewicz GZ, et al: Identification of a genetic locus for familial atrial fibrillation. N Engl J Med 336:905, 1997

85. Sarachek NS, Leonard JL: Familial heart block and sinus bradycardia: Classification and natural history. Am J Cardiol 29:451, 1972

86. Wnag Q, Curran ME, Splawski I, et al: Positional cloning of a novel potassium channel gene: KVLQT1 mutations cause cardiac arrhythmias. Nat Genet 12:17, 1996

87. Curran ME, Splawski I, Timothy KW, et al: A molecular basis for cardiac arrhythmia: HERG mutations cause long QT syndrome. Cell 80:795, 1995

88. Splawski I, Tristani-Firouzi M, Lehmann MH, et al: Mutations in the hminK gene cause long QT syndrome and suppress IKs function. Nat Genet 17:338, 1997

89. Abbott GW, Sesti F, Splawski I, et al: MiRP1 forms IKr potassium channels with HERG and is associated with cardiac arrhythmia. Cell 97:175, 1999

90. Wang Q, Shen J, Splawski I, et al: SCN5A mutations associated with an inherited cardiac arrhythmia, long QT syndrome. Cell 80:805, 1995

91. Schott J, Charpentier F, Peltier S, et al: Mapping a gene for long QT syndrome to chromosome 4q25-27. Am J Hum Genet 57:1114, 1995

92. Sanguinetti MC, Curran ME, Spector PS, et al: Spectrum of HERG K+ channel dysfunction in an inherited cardiac arrhythmia. Proc Natl Acad Sci U S A 93:2208, 1996

93. Dumaine R, Wang Q, Keating MT, et al: Multiple mechanisms of channel–linked long-QT syndrome. Circ Res 78:916, 1996

94. Splawski I, Timothy KW, Vincent GM, et al: Molecular basis of the long QT syndrome associated with deafness. N Engl J Med 226:1562, 1997

95. Neyroud N, Tesson F, Denjoy I, et al: A novel mutation in the potassium channel gene KVLQT1 causes the Jervell and Lange-Nielsen cardioauditory syndrome. Nat Genet 15:186, 1997

96. Splawski I, Shen J, Timothy KW, et al: Novel mutations in long QT syndrome genes: KVLQT1, HERG, SCN5A, KCNE1, and KCNE2. Circulation 102:1178, 2000

97. Hoffman JIE: Congenital heart disease: Incidence and inheritance. Pediatr Clin North Am 37:25, 1990

98. Roguin N, Du ZD, Barka M: High prevalence of muscular ventricular septal defects in neonates. J Am Coll Cardiol 26:1545, 1995

99. Basson CT, Cowley GS, Solomon SD, et al: The clinical and genetic spectrum of Holt-Oram syndrome (heart-hand syndrome). N Engl J Med 330:885, 1994

100. Basson CT, Bachinsky DR, Lin RC, et al: Mutations in TBX5 cause limb and cardiac malformations in Holt-Oram syndrome. Nat Genet 15:30. 1997

101. Li QY, Newbury-Ecob RA, Terrett JA, et al: Holt-Oram syndrome is caused by mutations in TBX5, a member of the Brachyury (T) gene family. Nat Genet 15: 21, 1997

102. Basson CT, Huang T, Lin RC, et al: Different TBX5 interactions in heart and limb defined by Holt-Oram syndrome mutations. Proc Natl Acad Sci U S A 96:2919, 1999

103. Schott J-J, Benson DW, Basson CT, et al: Congenital heart disease caused by mutations in the transcription factor Nkx2-5. Science 281:108, 1998

104. Alonso S, Pierpont ME, Radtke W, et al: Heterotaxia syndrome and autosomal dominant inheritance. Am J Med Genet 56:12, 1995

105. Gebbia M, Ferrero GB, Pilia G, et al: X-linked situs abnormalities result from mutations in ZIC3. Nat Genet 17:305, 1977

106. Pyeritz RE, McKusick VA: The Marfan syndrome: Diagnosis and management. N Engl J Med 300:772, 1979

107. Marsalese DL, Moodie DS, Vacante M, et al: Marfan's syndrome: Natural history and long-term follow-up of cardiovascular involvement. J Am Coll Cardiol 14:422, 1989

108. Putnam EA, Zhang H, Ramirez F, et al: Fibrillin-2 (FBN2) mutations result in the Marfan-like disorder, congenital contractural arachnodactyly. Nat Genet 11:456, 1995

109. Dietz HC, Cutting GR, Pyeritz, RE, et al: Marfan syndrome caused by a recurrent de novo missense mutation in the fibrillin gene. Nature 352:337, 1991

110. Nijbroek G, Sood S, McIntosh I, et al: Fifteen novel FBN1 mutations causing Marfan syndrome detected by heteroduplex analysis of genomic amplicons. Am J Hum Genet 57:8, 1995

111. Collod G, Babron MC, Jondeau G, et al: A second locus for Marfan syndrome maps to chromosome 3p24.2-p25. Nat Genet 8: 264, 1994

112. Superti-Furga A, Steinmann B, Ramirez F, et al: Molecular defects of type III procollagen in Ehlers-Danlos syndrome type IV. Hum Genet 82:104, 1989

113. Dembure PP, Priest JH, Snboddy SC, Elsas LJ: Genotyping and prenatal assessment of collagen lysyl hydroxylase deficiency in a family with Ehlers-Danlos syndrome type VI. Am J Hum Genet 36:783, 1984

114. Ensing GJ, Schmidt MA, Hagler DJ, et al: Spectrum of findings in a family with nonsyndromic autosomal dominant supravalvular aortic stenosis: A Doppler echocardiographic study. J Am Coll Cardiol 13:413, 1989

115. Chiarella F, Bricarelli FD, Lupi G, et al: Familial supravalvular aortic stenosis: A genetic study. J Med Genet 26:86, 1989

116. Curran ME, Atkinson DL, Ewart AK, et al: The elastin gene is disrupted by a translocation associated with supravalvular aortic stenosis. Cell 73:159, 1993

117. Olson TM, Michels VV, Urban Z, et al: 30 kb Deletion within the elastin gene results in familial supravalvular aortic stenosis. Hum Mol Genet 4:1677, 1995

118. Nickerson E, Greenberg F, Keating MT, et al: Deletions of the elastin gene at 7q11.23 occur in approximately 90% of patients with Williams syndrome. Am J Hum Genet 56:1156, 1995

Acknowledgment

This work was supported by grants from the National Institutes of Health and the Howard Hughes Medical Institutes.

Index

Note: Page numbers in *italics* refer to illustrations; page numbers followed by t refer to tables.

A

A-band(s), in ventricular myocytes, 47, *47*
Abdominal angina, 96
Abetalipoproteinemia (Bassen-Kornzweig disease), 315
Abiomed ventricular-assist device, 698
Abscess, annular, in infective endocarditis, 454–455, *455, 459*
  aortic annular, in infective endocarditis, 454–455, *455–456*
  cerebral, in congenital heart disease, 487
  mitral annular, in infective endocarditis, 455, 457, *457*
  of lung, 190–191
Acquired immunodeficiency syndrome (AIDS), antiviral therapy for, cardiotoxicity of, 550
  cardiac lymphoma associated with, 599
  myocarditis associated with, 273–274, *273*
  opportunistic infections in, myocarditis in, 274, 274t, *275*
  pericarditis in, 391–392, *391*
Acromegaly, cardiovascular effects of, 517
Actin filament(s), in dense peripheral band (DPB), endothelial repair related to, 85
  in endothelial repair, 85
  in smooth muscle cells, modified isotype of, after vascular injury, 85–86
  in ventricular myocytes, 47
  of endothelial cells, in atherosclerotic plaque, 78, *78–79*
    ultrastructure of, 36
  of smooth muscle cells, in atherosclerotic plaque, 79
  rearrangement of, due to shear stress, 85
α Actin gene mutation, in dilated cardiomyopathy, 766–767
  in hypertrophic cardiomyopathy, 766
Acyclovir, for Epstein-Barr virus infection, in heart transplant recipients, 744
Acyl-coenzyme-A dehydrogenase deficiency, cardiovascular effects of, 498–499
Addison's disease, cardiovascular effects of, 493
Adenomatoid tumor, pericardial, 397
Adhesion molecule(s), in allograft coronary disease, 746
Adipose tissue, atrioventricular node replaced by, AV block due to, 615, *616*
  in bundle branches, bundle branch block due to, 616
  in myocardial interstitium, 49
  in sinoatrial node, 615–616
  intramyocardial, in endomyocardial biopsy, of allograft heart, 752–753
  ventricular myocardium replaced by, in arrhythmogenic cardiomyopathy, 307–308, *308–310*, 348, *348*
Adolescent(s), sudden death of, incidence of, 327
Adrenal disorder(s), cardiovascular effects of, 493

β-Adrenergic receptor(s), in catecholamine-induced cardiotoxicity, 545–546
Adrenomedullin, 493
Adria cell(s), in anthracycline-induced cardiomyopathy, 549, *549*
Adriamycin (doxorubicin) toxicity. See *Anthracycline-induced cardiotoxicity.*
Adventitia, aortic, amyloid in, 55
  ultrastructure of, 32
  of large veins, 34–35
  of muscular arteries, 33
  of pulmonary vessels, 35
Aged, autopsy studies of, 54, 55t
  cardiovascular function in, 54
Aging, aortic changes in, 107
  aortic valve and, 56–57, *56*, 620
  conduction system and, 615–616, *616*
  definition of, 54
  degenerative aortic stenosis related to, 421–423, *421–423*, 422t
  endocardial changes in, 56, *56*
  epicardial changes in, 62
  mitral valve and, 57–60, *58–60*
  myocardial changes in, 60–62
  pericardial changes in, 62
  premature disorders of, 64, 64t
  pulmonary circulation and, 167
  pulmonary elastic arteries and, 35
  pulmonary valve and, 60
  pulmonary venules and, 189
  senile cardiovascular amyloid in, 54–56, *55*
  theories on, 54
  tricuspid valve and, 60
  valvular changes in, 406
  vascular changes in, 62–64
AIDS. See *Acquired immunodeficiency syndrome (AIDS).*
Air dissection, of pulmonary artery branches, 187–188, *188*
  air block in, 188
Airway obstruction, sudden death associated with, 328
Alcohol consumption, acute clinical effects of, 556
  "holiday heart" due to, 556
  increased high density lipoprotein levels with, 71
Alcoholic cardiomyopathy, dilated, 556–557
  pathogenesis of, 556–557
  pathology of, 556
Aldosterone excess, cardiovascular effects of, 493
Alkaptonuria, cardiovascular effects of, 493–494, *494*
Allograft heart. See *Heart transplantation.*
Allograft/homograft valve(s), 662–666. See also *Bioprosthetic valve(s).*
  cryopreserved, lack of viable cells in, 665
  mechanisms of deterioration of, 663, *664*, 665–666
  definition of, 632

Allograft/homograft valve(s) *(Continued)*
  mechanisms of deterioration of, 663, 664t
  preservation of, 662
    cryopreservation in, 662–663, *663*
Alveolar capillary(ies), dysplasia of, 181
Alveolus(i), diffuse damage of (DAD), in polyarteritis nodosa, 186
Amebic pericarditis, 390–391
Aminorex, plexogenic pulmonary arteriopathy associated with, 180
  pulmonary hypertension due to, 554
Amniotic fluid embolism, obstructive pulmonary hypertension related to, 175
  of small vessels, 156
Amputated limb(s), specimens from, burial of, by patients, 24
  handling of, 25–26
Amyloid A protein, as marker of myohyperplastic plaque, 245
Amyloidosis, 494–496
  cardiac, autopsy findings in, 496
    clinical features of, 495, *495*
    diagnosis of, 495–496
    gross examination of, 305, *305*
    in restrictive cardiomyopathy, 304–305, *305*
  familial, 305, 496
  hemodialysis-associated, 496
  in bioprosthetic valves, 496
  isolated valvular, 496
  microfibrillar cardiomyopathy due to, 494
  of pulmonary vessels, 181–182
  of small- and medium-caliber vessels, 155
  primary, 304, 494–495
  secondary, 304–305, 495
  senile cardiovascular, 54–56
    aortic amyloid in, 55–56
    in restrictive cardiomyopathy, 305
    isolated atrial amyloid in, 55
    systemic, 55, *55*
  staining technique for, 494
Anabolic steroid(s), cardiovascular effects of, 497, 558
"Anchovy sauce pus," in amebic pericarditis, 390
Andersen disease, 507
Androgen(s), cardiovascular effects of, 496–497
  in anabolic steroids, 497
  polycystic ovaries related to, 497
Anemia, chronic, cardiovascular effects of, 497
  sickle cell, cardiovascular effects of, 522
    small vessel pathology in, 243
Aneurysm(s), aortic. See also *Aorta, aneurysm of.*
  atherosclerotic, of abdominal aorta. See *Aorta, abdominal, atherosclerotic aneurysm of.*
  of thoracic aorta, 95
  berry, mitral valve prolapse associated with, 478